Percutaneous Absorption

Drugs and the Pharmaceutical Sciences: A Series of Textbooks and Monographs

Series Editor Anthony J. Hickey
RTI International, Research Triangle Park, USA

The Drugs and Pharmaceutical Sciences series is designed to enable the pharmaceutical scientist to stay abreast of the changing trends, advances, and innovations associated with therapeutic drugs and that area of expertise and interest that has come to be known as the pharmaceutical sciences. The body of knowledge that those working in the pharmaceutical environment have to work with, and master, has been, and continues, to expand at a rapid pace as new scientific approaches, technologies, instrumentations, clinical advances, economic factors, and social needs arise and influence the discovery, development, manufacture, commercialization, and clinical use of new agents and devices.

Percutaneous Absorption
Drugs, Cosmetics, Mechanisms, Methods, Fifth Edition
Nina Dragićević and Howard I. Maibach

Filtration and Purification in the Biopharmaceutical Industry, Third Edition,
Maik W. Jornitz

Handbook of Drug Metabolism, Third Edition
Paul G. Pearson and Larry Wienkers

The Art and Science of Dermal Formulation Development
Marc Brown and Adrian C. Williams

Pharmaceutical Inhalation Aerosol Technology, Third Edition
Anthony J. Hickey and Sandro R. da Rocha

Good Manufacturing Practices for Pharmaceuticals, Seventh Edition,
Graham P. Bunn

Pharmaceutical Extrusion Technology, Second Edition
Isaac Ghebre-Sellassie, Charles E. Martin, Feng Zhang, and James Dinunzio

Biosimilar Drug Product Development
Laszlo Endrenyi, Paul Declerck, and Shein-Chung Chow

High Throughput Screening in Drug Discovery
Amancio Carnero

For more information about this series, please visit: www.crcpress.com/ Drugs-and-the-Pharmaceutical-Sciences/book-series/IHCDRUPHASCI

Percutaneous Absorption

Drugs, Cosmetics, Mechanisms, Methods

Fifth Edition

Edited by

Nina Dragićević and Howard I. Maibach

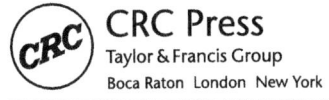

CRC Press
Taylor & Francis Group
Boca Raton London New York

CRC Press is an imprint of the
Taylor & Francis Group, an **informa** business

Fifth edition published 2022
by CRC Press
6000 Broken Sound Parkway NW, Suite 300, Boca Raton, FL 33487-2742
and by CRC Press

2 Park Square, Milton Park, Abingdon, Oxon, OX14 4RN
© 2022 Taylor & Francis Group, LLC

Fourth edition published by CRC Press 2005

Third edition published by CRC Press 1999

CRC Press is an imprint of Taylor & Francis Group, LLC

ISBN: 978-1-138-35123-3 (hbk)
ISBN: 978-1-032-02207-9 (pbk)
ISBN: 978-0-429-20297-1 (ebk)

Typeset in Times LT Std
by KnowledgeWorks Global Ltd.

Contents

Editors

Dr. Nina Dragićević, PhD, is a Professor at the Singidunum University in Belgrade, Serbia. She graduated from the University of Belgrade, Faculty of Pharmacy, in 1999 and subsequently earned a Magister Degree from the University of Belgrade and a PhD (*summa cum laude*, Dr. rer. nat.) in pharmaceutical technology from the Friedrich-Schiller University Jena, Germany. Earlier, Dr. Dragićević worked as an accredited specialist in pharmaceutical technology in the state pharmaceutical chain Apoteka "Beograd" in Belgrade. From 2007 to 2013, she was responsible for the preparation of compounded drugs for different routes of administration in pharmacies of Apoteka "Beograd", and in 2013 was appointed Director of the production department in the same company. She has published in a variety of international journals and was editor of five books.

Prof. Howard I. Maibach, PhD, is currently serving as professor of dermatology at the University of California, San Francisco (UCSF). He earned his MD from Tulane University, New Orleans, Louisiana, in 1955. Later he served in faculty positions in various levels at the UCSF. Dr. Maibach has over 2520 published manuscripts. He has been on the editorial board of more than 30 scientific journals and is a member of 19 professional societies, including the American Academy of Dermatology, San Francisco Dermatological Society, and the Internal Commission on Occupation Health.

Contributors

Marco T.A. Abbate
School of Pharmacy
Queen's University Belfast
Belfast, United Kingdom

Ayse Sermin Filiz Acipayam
Bakirkoy Dr Sadi Konuk Training and
    Research Hospital
Istanbul, Turkey

Yuri G. Anissimov
Queensland Micro-and Nanotechnology Centre
Griffith University
Brisbane, Australia
and
School of Biomolecular and
    Physical Sciences
Griffith University
Gold Coast, Australia

Jacqueline Resende de Azevedo
University of Lyon
Villeurbanne, France

Brian W. Barry
School of Pharmacy
University of Bradford
Bradford, United Kingdom

Nataša Škalko-Basnet
Drug Transport and Delivery
    Research Group
University of Tromsø
The Arctic University of Norway
Tromsø, Norway

Heather A.E. Benson
Curtin Medical School
Curtin Health Innovation Research Institute
Curtin University
Perth, Western Australia

Marie-Alexandrine Bolzinger
University of Lyon
Université Claude
Villeurbanne, France

Michael C. Bonner
School of Pharmacy
University of Bradford
Bradford, United Kingdom

Jordan L. Bormann
University of South Dakota
Sanford School of Medicine
Sioux Falls, South Dakota

Alain Boucaud
Transderma Systems
Rue Giraudeau
Tours, France

Beate Boulgaropoulos
HEALTH – Institute for Biomedicine and
    Health Sciences
Joanneum Research Forschungsgesellschaft
    m.b.H
Graz, Austria

Stéphanie Briançon
University of Lyon
Villeurbanne, France

Thomas Birngruber
HEALTH – Institute for Biomedicine and
    Health Sciences
Joanneum Research Forschungsgesellschaft
    m.b.H
Graz, Austria

Daniel Bucks
Bucks Consulting
Millbrae, California

Joshua J. Calcutt
Queensland Micro-and Nanotechnology Centre
Griffith University
Brisbane, Australia

Myeong Jun Choi
Charmzone Research and Development
    Center, Wonju
Kangwon-do, Korea

Yves Chevalier
University of Lyon
Université Claude
Villeurbanne, France

Rebekka Christmann
Saarland University
Helmholtz-Institute for Pharmaceutical
    Research
Saarland, Saarbrücken, Germany

Julie Christoffel
School of Medicine
University of California
San Francisco, California

Sheree E. Cross
University of Queensland
Princess Alexandra Hospital
    Woolloongabba
Queensland, Australia

Yuri Dancik
Le Studium Loire Valley Institute of Advanced
    Studies, France
Nanomedicines and Nanoprobes, University
    of Tours, Tours, France. Certara UK Ltd,
    Simcyp Division, United Kingdom

Ryan F. Donnelly
School of Pharmacy
Queen's University Belfast
Belfast, United Kingdom

Nina Dragićević
Singidunum University
Danijelova 32
Belgrade, Serbia

Ebtessam A. Essa
Faculty of Pharmacy
Tanta University
Tanta, Egypt

Andrew G.D. Ezersky
University of Southern California
Los Angeles, California

Gøril Eide Flaten
Drug Transport and Delivery Research Group
University of Tromsø
The Arctic University of Norway
Tromsø, Norway

James Forsell
Northern California Transplant Bank
San Rafael, California

Yasmine Gomaa
School of Chemical and Biomolecular Engineering
Georgia Institute of Technology
Atlanta, Georgia
Alexandria University
Alexandria, Egypt

Taís Gratieri
Faculdade de Ciências da Saúde
Universidade de Brasília
Brasília, Brazil

Jeffrey E. Grice
Therapeutics Research Group
The University of Queensland Diamantina
    Institute
University of Queensland
Translational Research Institute
    Woolloongabba
Queensland, Australia

Tracy Hartway
School of Medicine
University of California
San Francisco, California

Sandra Heuschkel
Institute of Applied Dermatopharmacy at
    Martin-Luther-University Halle-Wittenberg
Halle (Saale), Germany

Peter Hoffmann
Biomaterials Engineering and
    Nanomedicine Strand
Future Industries Institute
University of South Australia
Adelaide, South Australia

Aaron. R.J. Hutton
School of Pharmacy
Queen's University Belfast
Belfast, United Kingdom

Xiaoying Hui
School of Medicine
University of California
San Francisco, California

Marjan Koosha Johnson
Western University of Health Sciences
College of Osteopathic
Medicine of the Pacific Pomona
Pomona, California

Yogeshvar N. Kalia
School of Pharmaceutical Sciences
University of Geneva
Institute of Pharmaceutical Sciences of
    Western Switzerland
Geneva, Switzerland

Isadore Kanfer
Rhodes University
Grahamstown, South Africa
and
University of Toronto
Toronto, Canada

Gerald B. Kasting
James L. Winkle College of Pharmacy
The University of Cincinnati
    Medical Center
Cincinnati, Ohio

Nadia Kashetsky
Memorial University of
    Newfoundland
St. John's, Newfoundland, Canada

Victoria Klang
University of Vienna
Vienna, Austria

Melissa Kirkby
School of Pharmacy
Queen's University Belfast
Belfast, United Kingdom

Margaret E.K. Kraeling
Office of Applied Research and Safety
    Assessment Center for Food Safety
    and Applied Nutrition
Food and Drug Administration
Laurel, Maryland

Jürgen Lademann
Humboldt University
Berlin, Germany

Rebecca M. Law
Memorial University of Newfoundland
School of Pharmacy and Faculty of Medicine
St. John's, Newfoundland and Labrador,
    Canada

Jacquelyn Levin
Midwestern University
Arizona College of Osteopathic Medicine
Glendale, Arizona

Dorian Liepmann
University of California
Berkeley, California

Harald Löffler
Philipp University of Marburg
Marburg, Germany

Brigitta Loretz
Helmholtz-Institute for Pharmaceutical
    Research
Saarland, Saarbrücken, Germany

Claire Lotte
Laboratoires de Recherche Fondamentale
L'Oréal
Aulnay sous Bois, France

Laurent Machet
Centre Hospitalier Régional
Universitaire de Tours
INSERM U1253, France

Gamal M. El Maghraby
Tanta University
Tanta, Egypt

Howard I. Maibach
School of Medicine
University of California
San Francisco, California

Ana Melero
University of Valencia
Valencia, Spain

Peter E. McKenna
School of Pharmacy
Queen's University Belfast
Belfast, United Kingdom

Matthew A. Miller
James L. Winkle College of Pharmacy
The University of Cincinnati Medical
    Center
Cincinnati, Ohio

Kurtis J. Moffatt
School of Pharmacy
Queen's University Belfast
Belfast, United Kingdom

Hamid R. Moghimi
School of Pharmacy
Shahid Beheshti University of Medical
    Sciences
Protein Technology Research Center
Tehran, Iran

Yousuf H. Mohammed
Therapeutics Research Group
The University of Queensland
Diamantina Institute
University of Queensland
Translational Research Institute, Woolloongabba
Queensland, Australia

Seyedeh Maryam Mortazavi
School of Pharmacy
Shahid Beheshti University of Medical
    Sciences
Tehran, Iran

S. Narasimha Murthy
The University of Mississippi School of
    Pharmacy
Mississippi
and
Institute for Drug Delivery and Biomedical
    Research
Bengaluru, India

Shivakumar H. Nanjappa
KLE College of Pharmacy
Institute for Drug Delivery and Biomedical
    Research
Bengaluru, India

Reinhard H. H. Neubert
Institute of Applied Dermatopharmacy at
    Martin-Luther-University Halle-Wittenberg
Halle (Saale), Germany

Mai A. Ngo
Memorial University of Newfoundland
School of Pharmacy
St. John's, Newfoundland, Canada
and
California Department of Toxic Substances
    Control
Sacramento, California

Lars Norlén
Karolinska Institutet
Stockholm, Sweden
and
Dermatology Clinic
Karolinska University Hospital
Stockholm, Sweden

Nina Otberg
Humboldt University
Berlin, Germany

Ulrike Blume-Peytavi
Humboldt University
Berlin, Germany

Nicholas Poblete
School of Medicine
University of California
San Francisco, California

Mark R. Prausnitz
School of Chemical and Biomolecular
    Engineering
Georgia Institute of Technology
Atlanta, Georgia

Tarl Prow
Biomaterials Engineering and Nanomedicine
    Strand
Future Industries Institute
University of South Australia
Adelaide, South Australia

Anne S. Raber
Saarland University
Saarbrücken, Germany

Inken K. Ramöeller
School of Pharmacy
Queen's University Belfast
Belfast, United Kingdom

Heike Richter
Humboldt University
Berlin, Germany

Jim E. Riviere
Center for Chemical Toxicology Research and
    Pharmacokinetics
College of Veterinary Medicine
North Carolina State University
Raleigh, North Carolina

Michael S. Roberts
Therapeutics Research Group
The University of Queensland
Diamantina Institute
University of Queensland
Translational Research Institute, Woolloongabba
Queensland, Australia
and
School of Pharmacy and Medical Sciences
University of South Australia
Basil Hetzel Institute for Translational Health
    Research
Adelaide, South Australia

André Rougier
Laboratoire Pharmaceutique
La Roche-Posay
Courbevoie, France

Annick Roul
General Directorate of Civil Security
Ministry of Interior
Paris, France

Hans Schaefer
Humboldt University
Berlin, Germany

Ulrich F. Schaefer
Saarland University
Saarbrücken, Germany

Vinod P. Shah
VPS Consulting
LLC
North Potomac, Maryland

Anuj Shukla
Institute of Applied Dermatopharmacy at
    Martin-Luther-University Halle-Wittenberg
Halle (Saale), Germany

Frank Sinner
HEALTH – Institute for Biomedicine and
    Health Sciences
Joanneum Research Forschungsgesellschaft
    m.b.H
Graz, Austria

Raja K. Sivamani
University of California – Davis
USA Pacific Skin Institute
Sacramento, California

Wolfram Sterry
Humboldt University
Berlin, Germany

Sarah A. Stewart
School of Pharmacy
Queen's University Belfast
Belfast, United Kingdom

Boris Stoeber
University of California
Berkeley, California

Christian Surber
University Hospital Zurich
Zürich, Switzerland

Priya S. Talreja
James L. Winkle College of Pharmacy
The University of Cincinnati Medical Center
Cincinnati, Ohio

Efrem N. Tessema
Institute of Applied Dermatopharmacy
    at Martin-Luther-University
    Halle-Wittenberg
Halle (Saale), Germany

Ethel Tur
Tel Aviv University
Tel Aviv, Israel

Željka Vanic´
University of Zagreb
Zagreb, Croatia

Pranav Vasu
Case Western Reserve University
Cleveland, Ohio

Claudia Vater
University of Vienna
Vienna, Austria

Kenneth A. Walters
An-Ex Analytical Services Ltd
Capital Business Park, Cardiff
Wales, Australia

Boen Wang
Lynbrook High School
San Jose, California

Ronald C. Wester
School of Medicine
University of California
San Francisco, California

Leszek J. Wolfram
Clairol, Inc.
Stamford, Connecticut

Gabriel C. Wu
University of California – Davis
USA Pacific Skin Institute
Sacramento, California

Miko Yamada
Biomaterials Engineering and Nanomedicine
  Strand
Future Industries Institute
University of South Australia
Adelaide, South Australia

Jeffrey J. Yourick
Office of Applied Research and Safety
  Assessment Center for Food Safety and
  Applied Nutrition
Food and Drug Administration
Laurel, Maryland

Hongbo Zhai
School of Medicine
University of California
San Francisco, California

Ying Zou
Shanghai Skin Disease Hospital
Shanghai, P. R. China

1 Molecular Structure and Function of the Skin Barrier

Lars Norlén
Karolinska University Hospital, Stockholm, Sweden

CONTENTS

1.1 INTRODUCTION

Terrestrial life was only made possible through the adaptive evolution of a waterproof barrier in the integument of organisms. This barrier is constituted by a uniquely organized lipid structure situated between the cells of the stratum corneum (Blank, 1952; Breathnach et al., 1973; Elias and Friend, 1975) (Figure 1.1).

The lipid structure's molecular organization has been determined in situ with the aid of a novel experimental approach: high-resolution cryo-electron microscopy of vitreous tissue section (CEMOVIS) defocus series combined with molecular dynamics (MD) simulation and electron microscopy (EM) simulation. It is arranged as stacked bilayers of fully extended ceramides with cholesterol largely associated with the ceramide sphingoid moiety (Iwai et al., 2012; Lundborg et al., 2018a) (Figure 1.2).

Recently, a thermodynamically equilibrated atomistic MD model of the skin's lipid structure has been constructed (Figure 1.2b) and validated against high-resolution CEMOVIS data from near-native skin using EM simulation (Lundborg et al., 2018a) (Figure 1.3). The atomistic MD model of the skin's lipid structure may be used for predicting, and potentially computer screening, percutaneous absorption of drugs and other chemical compounds (Lundborg et al., 2018b).

What follows is a brief account of the structure–function relationships of the human skin's lipid structure.

1.2 SKIN LIPID COMPOSITION AND PHASE STATE

The skin's lipid structure consists of a heterogeneous mixture of saturated, long-chain ceramides (of which about 15% are acyl-ceramides), free fatty acids, and cholesterol in a roughly 1:1:1 molar ratio (Wertz and Norlén, 2003). More than 300 different species have been identified in the ceramide fraction alone (Masukawa et al., 2009).

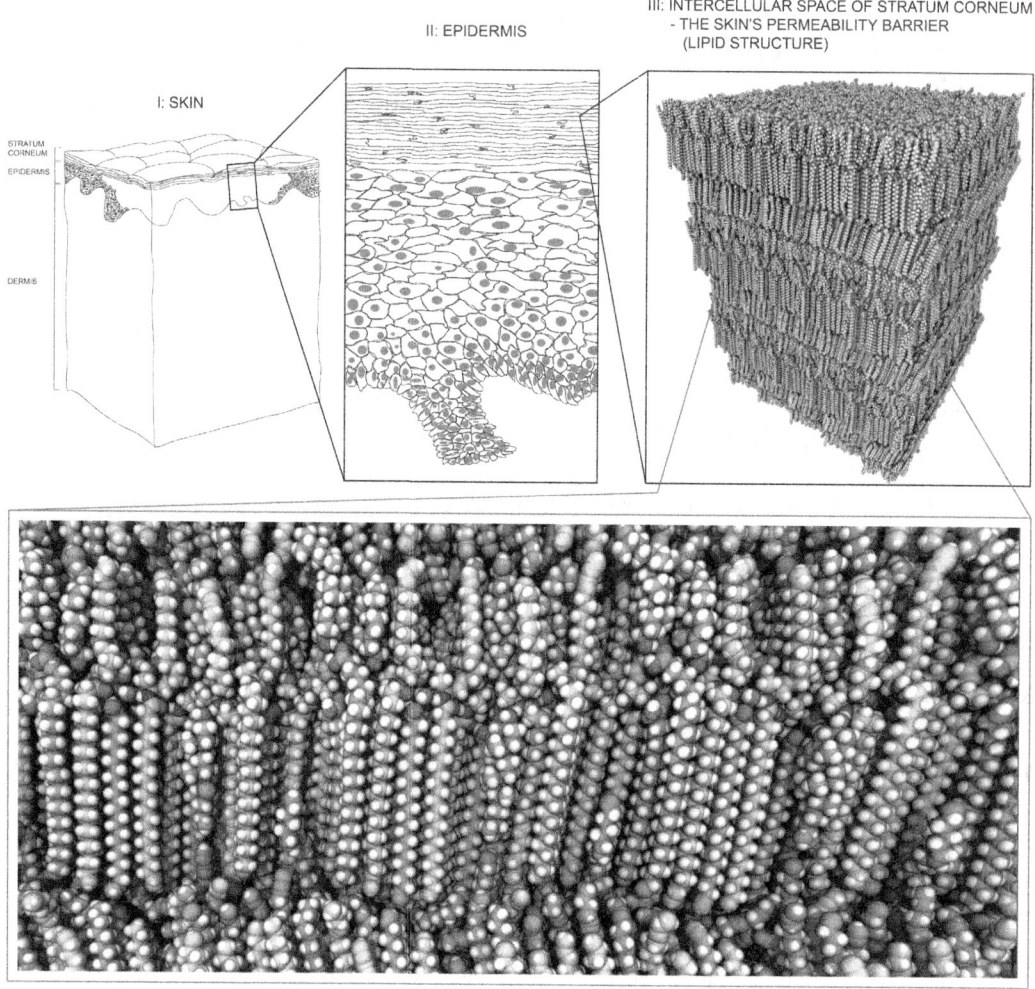

FIGURE 1.1 Schematic drawing of the skin and its lipid structure. Section I: Organ-scale drawing of the skin. Section II: Tissue-scale drawing of the epidermis. Section III: Molecular-scale drawing of the skin's barrier lipid structure.

The characteristic features of the stratum corneum lipid composition (Wertz and Norlén, 2003) are (1) extensive compositional heterogeneity with broad, but invariable, chain length distributions (20 to 32C; peaking at 24C) in the ceramide fatty acid and free fatty acid fractions; (2) almost complete dominance of saturated very long hydrocarbon chains (C20:0 to C32:0); and (3) large relative amounts of cholesterol (about 35 mol%).

These features are the same as those typically stabilizing lipid gel phases. It has therefore been proposed that the skin's lipid structure exists as a single and coherent gel phase (Norlén, 2001b). The viscous gel-like behavior of the lipid structure has been demonstrated in situ by its remarkable malleability (Iwai et al., 2012) and in silico by its gel-like molecular dynamics (Lundborg et al., 2018a).

1.3 SKIN BARRIER STRUCTURE

Using cryo-electron microscopy of near-native skin sections (skin CEMOVIS) combined with MD simulation and EM simulation, it has been shown that the skin's lipid structure is organized as stacked bilayers of fully splayed ceramides with cholesterol largely associated (about 75 mol%) with

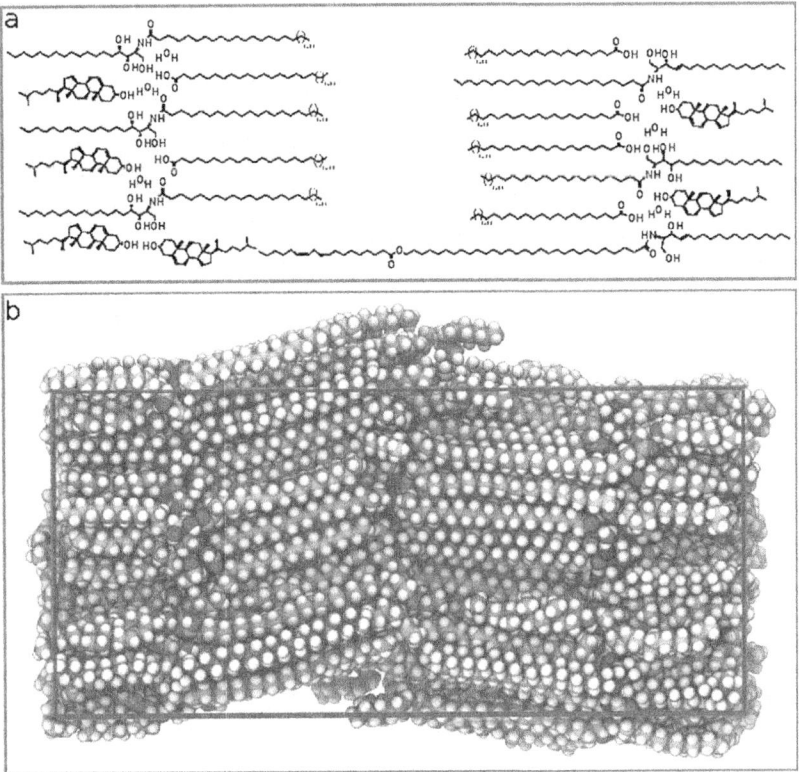

FIGURE 1.2 The molecular organization of the skin's lipid structure. The optimized MD model system for the skin's lipid structure validated against CEMOVIS data from skin. (a) A schematic drawing of the model system, where the ceramide fatty acid and free fatty acid chain lengths are just included as a range. The basic lipid arrangement is that of stacked bilayers of fully extended ceramides with cholesterol largely (about 75%) associated with the ceramide sphingoid moiety. (b) The model system after the MD simulation production phase.

the ceramide sphingoid moiety and all the free fatty acids associated with the ceramide fatty acid moiety. A restricted number of water molecules are associated with the lipid headgroups (about one water per ceramide headgroup), and the lipid structure also contains some acyl-ceramides (about 5 mol%) (Lundborg et al., 2018a) (Figure 1.2a).

Recently, a thermodynamically equilibrated atomistic MD model of the skin's lipid structure has been constructed (Figure 1.2b) and validated against high-resolution CEMOVIS data from near-native skin (Lundborg et al., 2018a) (Figure 1.3). The dynamics of the skin lipid molecules differ along the chains. The mobility is highest at the interface between opposing ceramide fatty acid and free fatty acid chains. Ester-bound linoleic acid chains of the acyl-ceramides accumulate at this interface, contributing, together with the skin lipids' broad ceramide fatty acid and free fatty acid chain length distribution, to the higher lipid chain mobility in this interface region (Lundborg et al., 2018a).

1.4 SKIN BARRIER PERMEABILITY AND THERMOTROPIC BEHAVIOR

The new MD model of the skin's lipid structure has permeability properties, as well as a thermotropic behavior, compatible with that of human skin (Lundborg et al., 2018a,b). Water has a large and complex effect on the skin's permeability depending on the permeant (water or other compound),

Cryo-electron micrograph 1
(defocus -1.3μm)

Cryo-electron micrograph 2
(defocus -2.7μm)

Cryo-electron micrograph 3
(defocus -4.0μm)

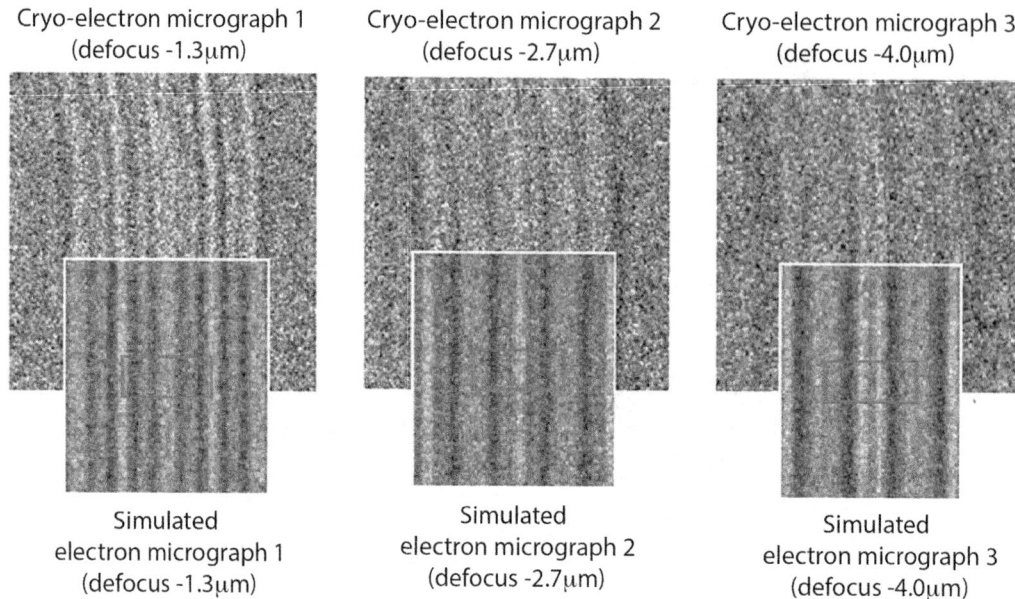

Simulated
electron micrograph 1
(defocus -1.3μm)

Simulated
electron micrograph 2
(defocus -2.7μm)

Simulated
electron micrograph 3
(defocus -4.0μm)

FIGURE 1.3 CEMOVIS micrograph defocus series from human skin (upper/back row) compared with simulated electron micrograph defocus series from the atomistic MD model in Figure 1.2. Upper/back row: Sequential CEMOVIS micrograph defocus series recorded at −1.3 μm, −2.7 μm, and −4.0 μm defocus. Lower/front row: Simulated sequential electron microscopy defocus series recorded at −1.3 μm, −2.7 μm, and −4.0 μm defocus. It is shown that the atomistic MD model in Figure 1.2 accurately accounts not only for the skin's CEMOVIS micrograph intensity patterns at a single defocus but also for the intensity pattern changes observed upon varying the microscope's defocus during image acquisition. Pixel size in the CEMOVIS and in the simulated electron micrographs: 1.88 Å. (Adapted from Iwai et al. 2012 and Lundborg et al. 2018a, respectively, with permission.)

with, e.g., multiple local maxima for the permeation of water as a function of model system water content (Lundborg et al., 2018a,b).

1.5   CEMOVIS

With CEMOVIS, the native tissue is preserved down to the molecular level, and the micrograph pixel intensity is directly related to the local electron density of the specimen (Dubochet et al., 1988; Al-Amoudi et al., 2004; Norlén et al., 2009). As biomolecules are essentially composed of atoms with similar atomic weight (carbon, nitrogen, and oxygen), they generally possess small intermolecular and intramolecular differences in electron density. However, for orderly arranged molecular assemblies, such as lipid headgroups and tails in membranes, even small differences in shape and atomic composition may be amplified due to interference effects that appear in the image phase contrast. During cryo-EM image acquisition, phase contrast is made visible using defocus (cf. e.g., Fanelli and Öktem, 2008).

At very high magnification (pixel sizes of a few Ångström), complex interference patterns can be resolved in CEMOVIS micrographs (Iwai et al., 2012). This can be exploited by recording CEMOVIS micrographs repeatedly at the same position of the tissue sample while increasing step-wise the microscope's defocus, ensuring that differences in the recorded micrographs are exclusively due to the different defocuses used. Thus, the recorded CEMOVIS defocus series images represent a range of unique phase contrast patterns for the underlying biological structure, which can be used for structure determination (Iwai et al., 2012; Lundborg et al., 2018a) (Figure 1.3, upper/back row).

1.6 ANALYSIS OF CRYO-EM (CEMOVIS) DATA USING MD SIMULATION AND EM SIMULATION

Atomistic MD simulation combined with EM simulation may be used to analyze CEMOVIS data. Simulated electron micrographs (cf. Rullgård et al., 2011) are then generated at defocuses corresponding to those of the original cryo-EM defocus series data for different atomistic candidate MD models (Lundborg et al., 2018a) (Figure 1.3, lower/front row).

CEMOVIS image analysis is then based on an iterative process where an MD model is modified in a stepwise fashion until optimal correspondence is achieved between the original CEMOVIS data derived from the biological specimen and the simulated EM data derived from the MD model (Figure 1.4). The major advantages of using CEMOVIS for biological structure determination in situ are the near-native preservation of the analyzed biological structure, the high image resolution and information content of cryo-EM images, and the high sensitivity of the cryo-EM image interference patterns to the microscope defocus levels. An advantage of analyzing CEMOVIS data using MD simulation to generate input for EM simulation is that MD simulation allows for investigation of the thermodynamic and other physicochemical properties of the candidate atomic models. Another advantage is that it ensures a realistic model atomic density irrespectively of model topology. EM simulation errors derived from model artifacts, such as atomic overlapping or void spaces, are thereby avoided.

The procedure for MD-simulation/EM-simulation–based CEMOVIS image analysis is as follows (Figure 1.4): (1) collection of a high-resolution cryo-EM image defocus series, (2) construction of a candidate atomic model using model building software, (3) equilibration of the candidate atomic model using MD simulation, (4) generation of a series of simulated EM images at different microscope defocus levels from the equilibrated atomistic MD model using EM simulation, and finally (5) comparison of the original cryo-EM defocus series images and the simulated defocus series images. The procedure is repeated until optimal correspondence is achieved between simulated and original data (Figure 1.3).

1.7 SKIN LIPID FORMATION

In order to appreciate the structure–function relationships of the skin barrier in vivo, it is important to understand skin lipid formation, as the skin's lipid structure may represent a "frozen-in" or "immobilized" open biological system rather than a primary minimum energy equilibrium system. Skin lipid formation is also central from a dermatological standpoint, since barrier malformation may be an etiological factor in barrier-deficient skin conditions such as eczema, psoriasis, and dry skin.

It has been proposed (Norlén, 2001a) that skin lipid formation proceeds via (1) membrane synthesis in the trans-Golgi of a cubic lipid phase, followed by (2) a nonfusion-dependent secretion of the cubic lipid phase into the intercellular space (den Hollander et al., 2016), a subsequent (3) phase transition from cubic to stacked lamellar membrane morphology (Naragifard et al., 2018) with a concomitant (4) dehydration (Wennberg et al., 2018) and (5) condensation (Wennberg et al., 2018) of the stacked lamellar lipid phase, and with a final internal (6) lipid chain rearrangement from a folded (hairpin) to an extended (splayed) chain conformation (Narangifard et al., 2020).

1.8 SKIN LIPID FUNCTION

Current knowledge suggests that a stacked, fully extended (splayed chain) ceramide bilayer arrangement with a high cholesterol content and a heterogeneous, saturated, long-chain lipid composition (Figure 1.1(III), Figure 1.2) may represent an optimized barrier material for skin. This is because it is largely impermeable to water as well as to both hydrophilic and lipophilic substances (Lundborg et al., 2018a,b) because of its condensed lipid chain packing and its alternating lipophilic (alkyl

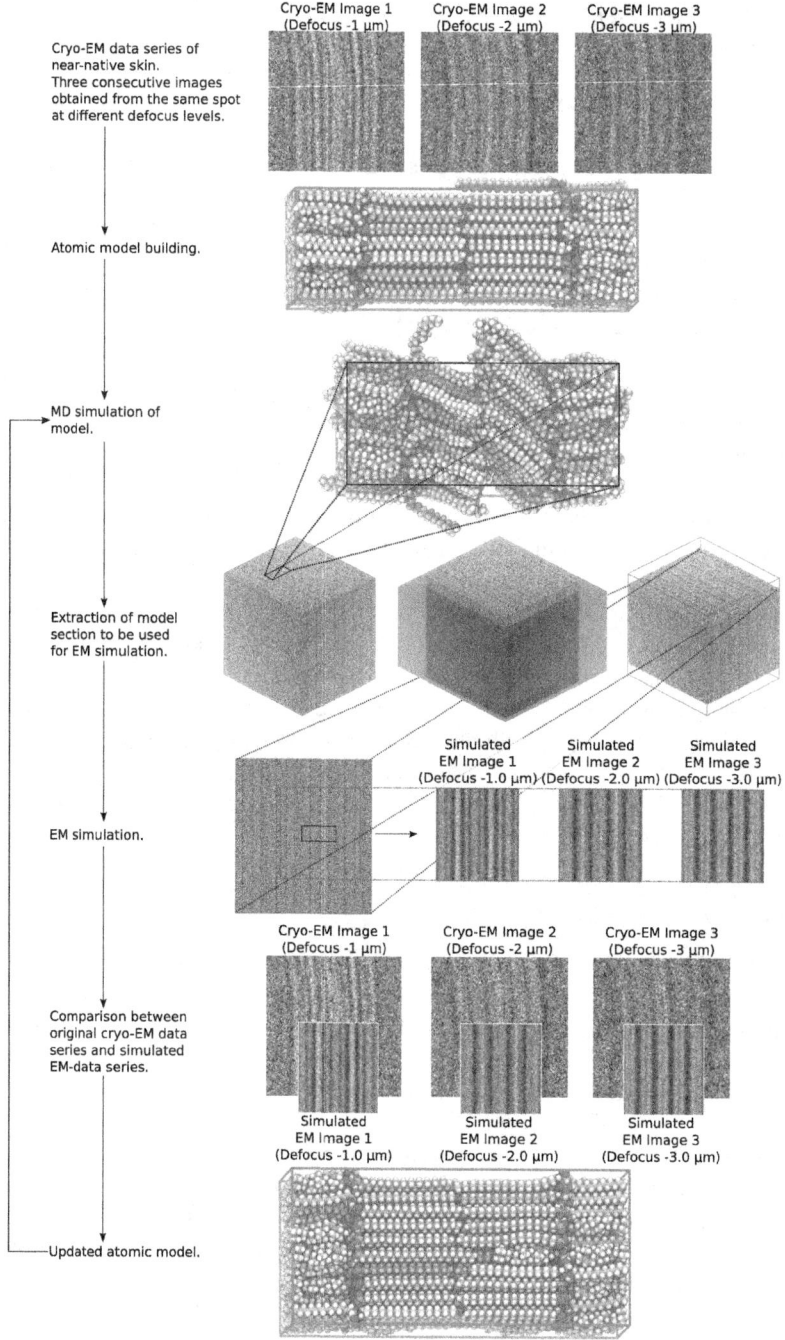

FIGURE 1.4 Experimental procedure for the analysis of cryo-EM (CEMOVIS) data using MD simulation and EM simulation. Outline of the general procedure for analyzing the structure and composition of the system by comparing simulated EM images generated from candidate atomic models after MD simulation with experimental cryo-EM images obtained from near-native human skin, using an iterative approach. The candidate model system is modified (regarding relative ceramide, free fatty acid, and cholesterol concentrations; cholesterol distribution; acyl-ceramide content; and amount of water in the membrane) until good agreement with experimental data is achieved. (Adapted from Lundborg et al., 2018a with permission.)

chain) and hydrophilic (headgroup) layers (Lundborg et al., 2018a). Likewise, it may be resistant to both hydration and dehydration because of its lack of exchangeable water between lipid leaflets. It may also be resistant to temperature and pressure changes because of its heterogeneous lipid composition and high cholesterol content, which stabilize gel-like chain packing (Iwai et al., 2012; Lundborg et al., 2018a) and thereby prevent both lateral domain formation and induction of "pores" or nonlamellar morphologies. Further, this bilayer arrangement may account for stratum corneum cell cohesion without advocating specialized intercellular adhesion structures such as desmosomes. The arrangement may hence allow for sliding of stratum corneum cells to accommodate skin bending. Finally, as the interaction between the individual layers of the lipid structure involves only hydrocarbons, the layers may be relatively free to slide with respect to one another, making the lipid structure pliable. The fully extended ceramide bilayer arrangement with high cholesterol content and heterogeneous saturated long-chain lipid composition may thus meet the barrier needs of skin by being simultaneously impermeable and robust.

1.9 CONCLUSION

Terrestrial life was only made possible through the adaptive evolution of a waterproof barrier in the integument of organisms. This barrier is constituted of a uniquely organized lipid structure situated between the cells of the horny layer of the skin. It was recently shown that this lipid structure is organized in an arrangement not previously described in a biological system—stacked bilayers of fully extended ceramides with cholesterol molecules largely associated with the ceramide sphingoid moiety.

The physical state of the skin's lipid structure is that of a gel phase. Further, the lipid structure is likely formed via a phase transition from cubic-like to stacked lamellar morphology followed by a flip of the constituent lipid components from a folded (hairpin) to an extended (splayed chain) ceramide bilayer conformation.

The skin's lipid structure is responsible for both the skin's low permeability to water and other compounds and for the barrier's robustness to environmental stress, such as hydration and dehydration, temperature and pressure changes, stretching, compression, bending, and shearing.

A validated atomistic MD model of the skin's lipid structure that may be used for predicting, and potentially computer screening, percutaneous absorption of drugs was recently presented.

REFERENCES

Al-Amoudi, A. Chang, J-J. Leforestier, A. McDowall, A. Michel Salamin, L. Norlén, L. Richter, K. Sartori Blanc, N. Studer, D. Dubochet, J. (2004) Cryo-electron microscopy of vitreous sections. EMBO J. 15;23(18):3583–88.

Blank, I.H. (1952) Factors which influence the water content of stratum corneum. J. Invest. Dermatol. 18:433–40.

Breathnach, A.S., Goodman, T., Stolinski, C., Gross, M. (1973) Freeze fracture replication of cells of stratum corneum of human epidermis. J. Anat. 114:65–81.

den Hollander, L. Han, H-M. de Winter, M. Svensson, L. Masich, S. Daneholt, B. Norlén, L (2016) Skin lamellar bodies are not discrete vesicles but part of a tubuloreticular network. *ACTA Dermato-Venereol.* 96(3):303–8

Dubochet, J., Adrian, M., Chang, J.-J., Homo, J.-C., Lepault, J., McDowall, A.W., Schultz, P. (1988) Cryo electron microscopy of vitrified specimens. Q. Rev. Biophys. 21(2):129–228.

Elias, P.M., Friend, D.S. (1975) The permeability barrier in mammalian epidermis. J. Cell. Biol. 65:180–91.

Fanelli, D., Öktem, O. (2008) Electron tomography: a short review with an emphasis on the absorption potential model for the forward problem. Inverse Probl. 24:013001.

Lundborg, M., Narangifard, A., Wennberg, C., Lindahl, E., Norlén, L. (2018a) Human skin barrier molecular structure and function analyzed by cryo-electron microscopy and molecular dynamics simulation. J. Struct. Biol. 203(2):149–61.

Lundborg, M., Wennberg, C., Narangifard, A., Lindahl, E., Norlén, L. (2018b) Predicting drug permeability through skin using molecular dynamics simulation. J. Control Release. 283:269–79.

Iwai, I., Han, H., den Hollander, L., Svensson, S., Öfverstedt, L.-G., Anwar, J., Brewer, J., Bloksgaard Mølgaard, M., Laloeuf, A., Nosek, D., Masich, S., Bagatolli, L., Skoglund, U., Norlén, L. (2012) The human skin barrier is organized as stacked bilayers of fully-extended ceramides with cholesterol molecules associated with the ceramide sphingoid moiety. J. Invest. Dermatol. 132:2215–25.

Masukawa, Y., Narita, H., Sato, H., Naoe, A., Kondo, N., Sugai, Y., Oba, T., Homma, R., Ishikawa, J., Tagaki, Y., Kitahara, T. (2009) Comprehensive quantification of ceramide species in human stratum corneum. J. Lipid Res. 50:1708–19.

Narangifard, A., den Hollander, L., Iwai, I., Han, H., Wennberg, C.L., Lundborg, M., Lindahl, E., Masich, S., Daneholt, B., Norlén, L. (2018) Human skin barrier formation takes place via a cubic to lamellar lipid phase transition. Exp. Cell Res. 366(2):139–51.

Narangifard, A., Wennberg, C., den Hollander, L., Iwai, I., Han, H., Lundborg, M., Masich, S., Lindahl, L., Daneholt, B., Norlén, L. (2020) Molecular reorganization during formation of the human skin barrier studied *in situ*. J. Invest. Dermatol. In press. doi.org/10.1016/j.jid.2020.07.040.

Norlén, L. (2001a) Skin barrier formation: the membrane folding model. J. Invest. Dermatol. 117(4):823–29.

Norlén, L. (2001b) Skin barrier structure and function: the single gel-phase model. J. Invest. Dermatol. 117(4):830–36.

Norlén, L., Al-Amoudi, A., Dubochet, J. (2003) A cryo-transmission electron microscopy study of skin barrier formation. J. Invest. Dermatol. 120:555–60.

Norlén, L., Öktem, O., Skoglund, U. (2009) Molecular cryo-electron tomography of vitreous tissue sections: current challenges. J. Microsc. 235:293–307.

Rullgård, H., Öfverstedt, L.-G., Masich, S., Daneholt, B., Öktem, O. (2011) Simulation of transmission electron microscope images of biological specimens. J. Microsc. 243(3):234–56.

Wennberg, C., Narangifard, A., Lundborg, M., Lindahl, E., Norlén, L. (2018) Structural transitions in ceramide cubic phases during formation of the human skin barrier. Biophys. J. 114(5):1116–27.

Wertz, P., Norlén, L. (2003) "Confidence Intervals" for the "true" lipid compositions of the human skin barrier? In: Skin, Hair, and Nails. Structure and Function. B. Forslind and M. Lindberg, editors. Marcel Dekker. 85–106. Biochim. Biophys. Acta 304:265–75.

2 Mathematical Models in Percutaneous Absorption

Yuri G. Anissimov
Griffith University, Brisbane, Australia
Griffith University, Gold Coast, Australia

Joshua J. Calcutt
Griffith University, Brisbane, Australia

Michael S. Roberts
The University of Queensland, Princess Alexandra
Hospital, Woolloongabba, Australia
University of South Australia, Adelaide, Australia

CONTENTS

A number of mathematical models have been used to describe percutaneous absorption kinetics. In general, most of these models have used either diffusion or compartmental-based equations. The object of any mathematical model is to (1) be able to represent the processes associated with absorption accurately, (2) be able to describe/summarize experimental data with parametric equations or moments, and (3) predict kinetics under varying conditions. However, in describing the processes involved, some developed models often suffer from being too complex to be practically useful. In this chapter, we have attempted to approach the issue of mathematical modeling in percutaneous absorption from four perspectives. These are to (1) describe simple practical models, (2) provide an overview of the more complex models, (3) summarize some of the more important/useful models used to date, and (4) examine some practical applications of the models. This chapter revises an earlier one [1] incorporating some of the more recent findings.

The range of processes involved in percutaneous absorption and considered in developing the mathematical models in this chapter are shown in Figure 2.1. We initially address in vitro skin diffusion models and consider (1) constant donor concentration and receptor conditions, (2) the corresponding flux, donor, skin, and receptor amount–time profiles for solutions, and (3) amount and flux–time profiles when the donor phase is removed. More complex issues such as finite volume donor phase, finite volume receptor phase, the presence of an efflux rate constant at the membrane–receptor interface, and two-layer diffusion are then considered. We then look at specific models and issues concerned with (1) release from topical products; (2) use of compartmental models as alternatives to diffusion models; (3) concentration-dependent absorption; (4) modeling of skin metabolism; (5) role of solute–skin–vehicle interactions; (6) effects of vehicle loss; (7) shunt transport; and (8) in vivo diffusion, compartmental, physiological, and deconvolution models. We conclude by examining topics such as (1) deep tissue penetration, (2) pharmacodynamics, (3) iontophoresis, (4) sonophoresis, and (5) pitfalls in modeling.

Each model is described in diagrammatic and equation form. Given that the analytical solution to most models is in the form of infinite series, often involving solutions to transcendental equations,

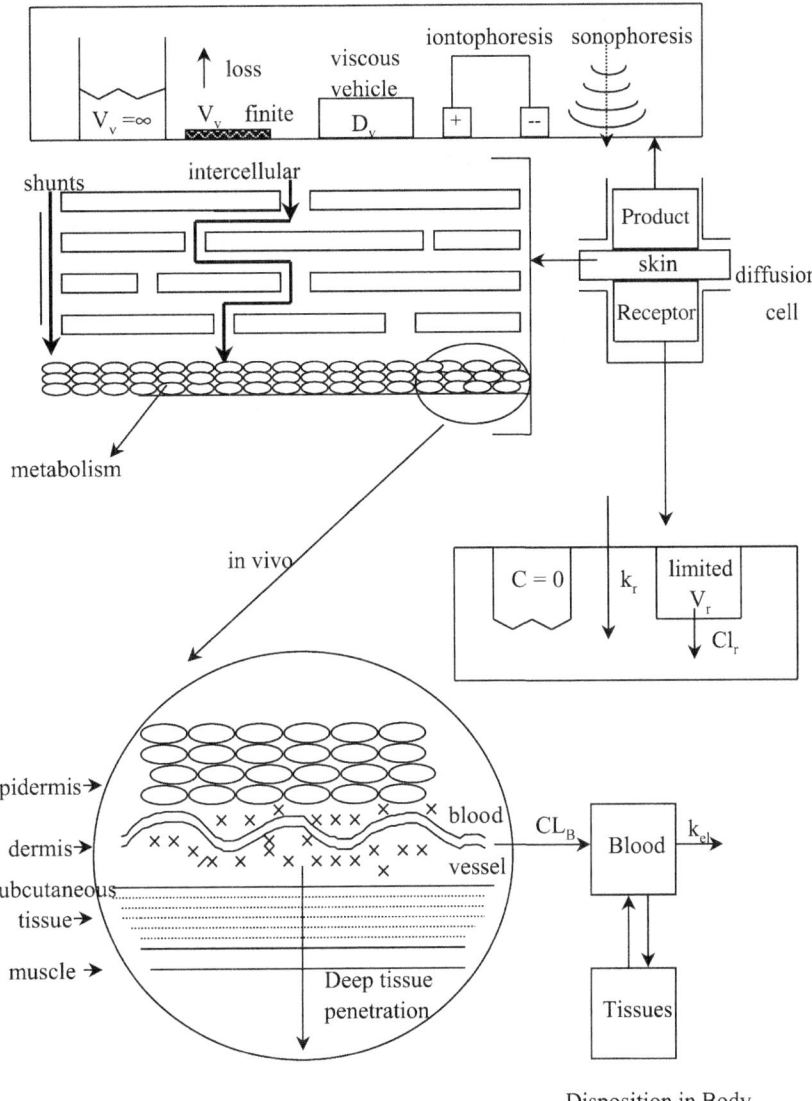

FIGURE 2.1 Diagrammatic overview of percutaneous processes associated with mathematical models.

we have emphasized the Laplace domain and steady-state solutions. Most nonlinear regression programs such as MULTI FILT, MINIM, and SCIENTIST enable analysis of concentration–time data using numerical inversion of Laplace domain solutions. By utilizing this technique, these programs are able to avoid some of the computational difficulties associated with series solutions, especially those involving solving transcendental equations. The steady-state solutions describing the linear portion of a cumulative amount versus time profile for a constant donor concentration are of great practical use. These solutions are described by a linear equation with lag time and steady-state flux as the intercept and the slope, respectively. In order to make equations in this chapter as useable as possible, each equation has been presented in nondimensionless form (all variables have their normal dimensions). Simulations and nonlinear regressions presented in this review were undertaken using either SCIENTIST 2.01 or MINIM 3.09.

2.1   IN VITRO SKIN DIFFUSION MODELS IN PERCUTANEOUS ABSORPTION

We consider first the mathematical models associated with solute penetration through excised skin. The simplest of these models is when a well-stirred vehicle of infinite volume is applied to the stratum corneum (SC) and the solute passes into a receptor sink (Figure 2.2A). The complexity of the model increases when the vehicle volume is finite (Figure 2.2B), when the receptor is no longer a sink (Figure 2.2C), and when the vehicle cannot be considered well-stirred (Figure 2.2D). We examine each of these models in terms of expressions for amount penetrating, flux, and, where possible, summary parameters such as mean absorption time, normalized variance, peak time for flux, and maximum flux.

2.1.1   IN VITRO SKIN PERMEABILITY STUDIES WITH A CONSTANT DONOR CONCENTRATION AND SINK RECEPTOR CONDITIONS

Most in vitro skin permeability studies are carried out assuming that both (1) the concentration of solute in a vehicle applied to the skin and (2) the sink conditions provided by the receptor remain constant

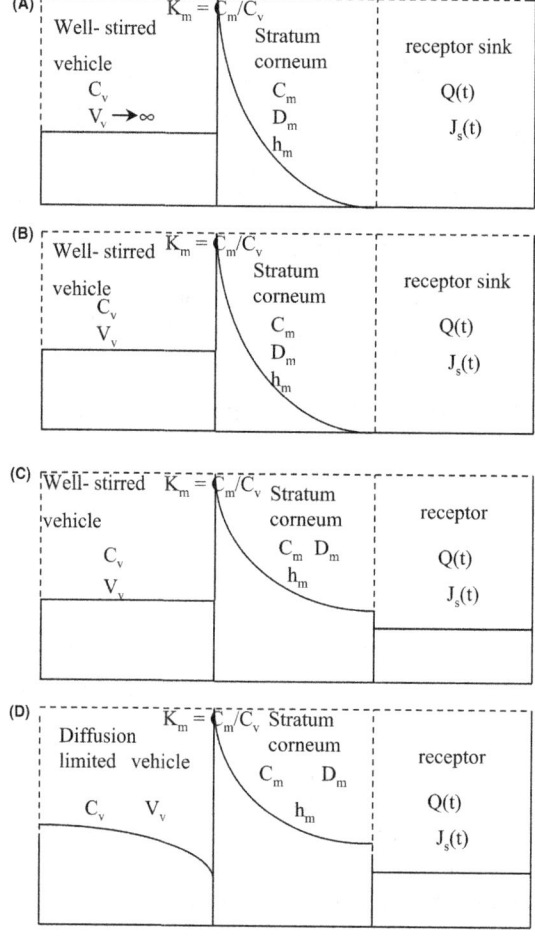

FIGURE 2.2   In vitro skin models of transport. (A) Well-stirred vehicle containing solute concentration C_v in volume V_v (where $V_v = \infty$) adjacent to assumed homogenous SC with solute concentration C_m at distance x from applied vehicle. Solute moves with a diffusion coefficient D_m over an effective path length h_m and penetrates into a receptor sink to give an amount penetrated $Q(t)$ in time t or flux $J(t)$. (B) as for (A), but with V_v finite. (C) as for (B), but the receptor is not a sink. (D) as for (B) but the vehicle is not well-stirred.

over the period of the study. Significant depletion of solute in the donor vehicle or an inadequate receptor sink requires more complex modeling, as discussed later. If transport through the SC is rate limiting, the steady-state approximation of amount of solute absorbed (Q) when concentration Cv is applied to an area of application (A) for an exposure time (T) is given in Equation (2.1) (see Ref. 2):

$$Q = k_p A C_v (T - lag) \qquad (2.1)$$

where k_p is the permeability coefficient (unit: cm/h) of the SC. In reality, absorption does not cease after removal of the vehicle, so that the overall absorption is slightly over $k_p A C_v T$. The permeability coefficient in Equation (2.1) is normally defined in terms of the dimensionless partition coefficient between the SC and vehicle (K_m) and D_m, the diffusivity of a solute in SC over a diffusion path length h_m:

$$k_p = \frac{K_m D_m}{h_m} \qquad (2.2)$$

K_m is defined as the ratio of solute concentrations in the SC (C_m) and vehicle (C_v) under equilibrium i.e., $K_m = C_m/C_v$.

In practice, the permeability coefficient k_p is a composite parameter. When solute transport occurs via both a lipid pathway of permeability coefficient $k_{p.lipid}$ and a polar pathway of permeability coefficient $k_{p.polar}$, an aqueous boundary layer of the epidermis provides a rate-limiting permeability coefficient $k_{p.aqueous}$ and k_p is more properly expressed as:

$$k_p = \left(\frac{1}{k_{p.lipid} + k_{p.polar}} + \frac{1}{k_{p.aqueous}} \right)^{-1} \qquad (2.3)$$

As discussed by Roberts and Walters [2], for most solutes, $k_p \approx k_{p.lipid}$.

Absorption is more commonly expressed in terms of the steady state flux J_{ss} or the absorption rate per unit area:

$$J_{ss} = \frac{Q}{A(T - lag)} = k_p C_v \qquad (2.4)$$

Equations (2.1) and (2.4) are the simplified forms of a more complex expression based on the solution of the diffusion equation for transport of solute in the skin:

$$\frac{\partial C_m}{\partial t} = D_m \frac{\partial^2 C_m}{\partial x^2} \qquad (2.5)$$

the initial condition:

$$C_m(x,0) = 0 \qquad (2.6)$$

and boundary conditions:

$$C_m(0,t) = K_m C_v \qquad (2.7)$$

$$C_m(h_m,t) = 0 \qquad (2.8)$$

Traditionally Equation (2.5) is solved in terms of the amount of solute $Q(t)$ exiting from the membrane in time t and expressed as a series solution [3]:

$$Q(t) = -D_m A \int_0^t \frac{\partial C_m}{\partial x}\bigg|_{x=h_m} dt = K_m A C_v h_m \left(\frac{t}{t_d} - \frac{1}{6} - \frac{2}{\pi^2} \sum_{n=1}^{\infty} \frac{(-1)^n}{n^2} \exp\left(-\frac{t}{t_d} \pi^2 n^2 \right) \right) \qquad (2.9)$$

where the diffusion time is given by:

$$t_d = \frac{h_m^2}{D_m} \tag{2.10}$$

It should be noted that as the exponent of a very large negative number approaches zero, the summation term in Equation (2.9) can be ignored at long times so that Equation (2.9) reduces to the form of Equation (2.1):

$$Q(t) = K_m A C_v h_m \left(\frac{D_m t}{h_m^2} - \frac{1}{6} \right) = k_p A C_v \left(t - \frac{h_m^2}{6 D_m} \right) = k_p A C_v (t - \text{lag}) \tag{2.11}$$

where lag is given by:

$$\text{lag} = \frac{h_m^2}{6 D_m} = \frac{t_d}{6} \tag{2.12}$$

Given the advent of numerical fast inverse Laplace transforms (FILTs) [4–6] with nonlinear regression modeling, we would normally analyze cumulative amount vs. time data numerically, inverting from the Laplace domain using Equation (2.13), where s is the Laplace variable:

$$\hat{Q}(s) = -D_m A \frac{1}{s} \frac{\partial \hat{C}_m}{\partial x} \bigg|_{x=h_m} = \frac{k_p A C_v}{s^2} \frac{\sqrt{s t_d}}{\sinh \sqrt{s t_d}} \tag{2.13}$$

Figure 2.3 shows a plot of the cumulative amount penetrated for the diffusion [Eq. (2.13), curve 2] and steady-state [Eq. (2.11), curve 1] models versus time. Equation (2.9) or (2.13) can be used to analyze in vitro experimental data by nonlinear regression, as shown in Figure 2.4.

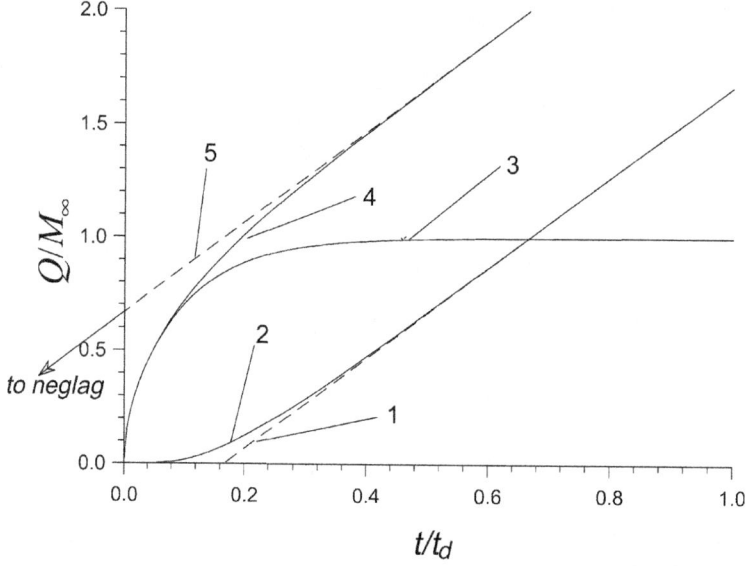

FIGURE 2.3 Normalized cumulative amount of solute penetrating Q/M_∞ [curve 2, Equation (2.13)]; taken up by the SC [curve 3, Equation (2.15)]; and leaving vehicle [curve 4, Equation (2.18)] with normalized time. Curves 1 and 5 represent steady-state approximations of the cumulative amount penetrating the SC [Equation (2.11)] and leaving the vehicle [Equation (2.17)] with normalized time.

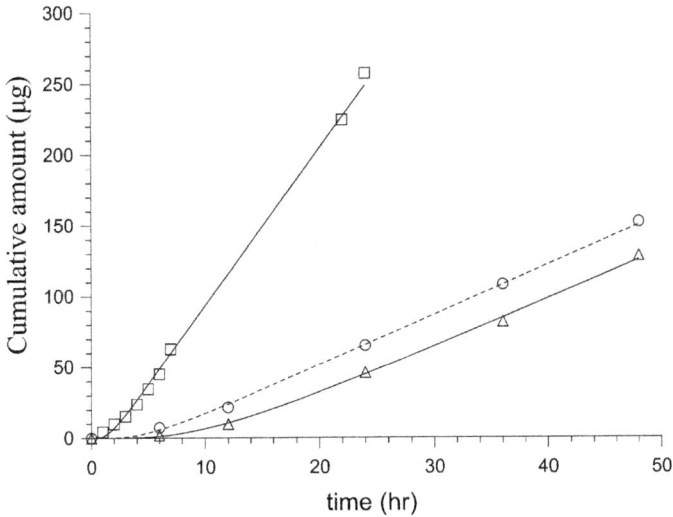

FIGURE 2.4 Nonlinear regressions of cumulative amount penetrating human epidermis with time using Equation (2.13) and a weighting of $1/y_{obs}$. Data correspond to triethanolamine salicylate [□, t_d = 9.8 hr, J_{ss} = 11.1 μg/hr, diclofenac skin 1 (o, t_d = 32.7 hr, J_{ss} = 3.5 μg/hr) and diclofenac skin 2 (Δ, t_d = 68.0 hr, J_{ss} = 3.8 mg/hr)].

Figure 2.3 (curve 3) also shows the amount of solute taken up by the SC with time. These profiles are of interest for those solutes that may be targeted for retention in this tissue, e.g., sunscreens, or that may be sequestered in this tissue, e.g., steroids. The time domain and Laplace domain solutions for the amount of solute $M(t)$ taken up into an assumed homogeneous SC with time are:

$$M(t) = M_\infty \left\{ 1 - \frac{8}{\pi^2} \sum_{n=0}^{\infty} \frac{1}{(2n+1)^2} \exp\left[-\frac{t}{t_d} \pi^2 (2n+1)^2 \right] \right\} \tag{2.14}$$

$$\hat{M}(s) = M_\infty \frac{2}{s} \frac{\cosh\sqrt{st_d} - 1}{\sqrt{st_d}\,\sinh\sqrt{st_d}} \tag{2.15}$$

where M_∞ is the amount of solute in the skin at steady state and is given when a linear concentration gradient is assumed.

The summation of $Q(t)$ and $M(t)$ yields the expression for the amount, which leaves the vehicle $Q_{in}(t)$ (the profile shown in Figure 2.3, curve 4):

$$Q_{in}(t) = K_m AC_v h_m \left[\frac{t}{t_d} + \frac{1}{3} - \frac{2}{\pi^2} \sum_{n=1}^{\infty} \frac{1}{\pi^2} \exp\left(-\frac{t}{t_d} \pi^2 n^2 \right) \right] \tag{2.16}$$

When $t \to \infty$, Equation (2.16) reduces to:

$$Q_{in}(t) = K_m AC_v h_m \left(\frac{t}{t_d} + \frac{1}{3} \right) = k_p AC_v \left(t + \frac{t_d}{3} \right) = k_p AC_v \left(t + \text{neglag} \right) \tag{2.17}$$

Hence, the linear portion of $Q_{in}(t)$ vs. t has a slope of $k_p AC_v$ and intercepts on the negative side of the time axis at a point of neglag = $t_d/3 = h_m^2/3D_m$ (Figure 2.3, curve 5).

The corresponding Laplace domain expression for $Q_{in}(t)$ is:

$$\hat{Q}_{in}(s) = \frac{k_p A C_v}{s^2} \sqrt{s t_d} \coth \sqrt{s t_d} \tag{2.18}$$

The absorption rate or flux of solutes in the period before steady state is important for many agents applied topically for local effects and in the toxicology of agents applied to the skin. The flux of solutes exiting the membrane per unit area, $J_s(t)$, is defined by $J_s(t) = (1/A) \, \partial Q/\partial t$ or $\hat{J}_s(s) = s\hat{Q}(s) / A$ in the Laplace domain. Using Equations (2.9) and (2.13) we find therefore:

$$J_s(t) = -D_m \frac{\partial C_m}{\partial x}\bigg|_{x=h_m} = k_p C_v \left[1 + 2\sum_{n=1}^{\infty} (-1)^n \exp\left(-\frac{t}{t_d} \pi^2 n^2 \right) \right] \tag{2.19}$$

$$\hat{J}_s(s) = \frac{k_p C_v}{s} \frac{\sqrt{s t_d}}{\sinh\left(\sqrt{s t_d} \right)} \tag{2.20}$$

The corresponding equation for the flux of solute from the vehicle into the membrane, $J_{in}(t)$, is:

$$J_{in}(t) = k_p C_v \left[1 + 2\sum_{n=1}^{\infty} \exp\left(-\frac{t}{t_d} \pi^2 n^2 \right) \right] \tag{2.21}$$

$$\hat{J}_{in}(s) = \frac{k_p C_v}{s} \sqrt{s t_d} \coth \sqrt{s t_d} \tag{2.22}$$

Figure 2.5 shows the flux profiles for solutes leaving the membrane and vehicle, respectively.

2.1.2 Amount and Flux–Time Profiles on Removing the Donor Phase After Reaching the Steady State for Conditions Described in Section 2.1.2.A

We now consider the amount and flu–time profiles for the specific case in which the donor phase has been removed after a steady state has been reached. This equates to a number of practical cases of

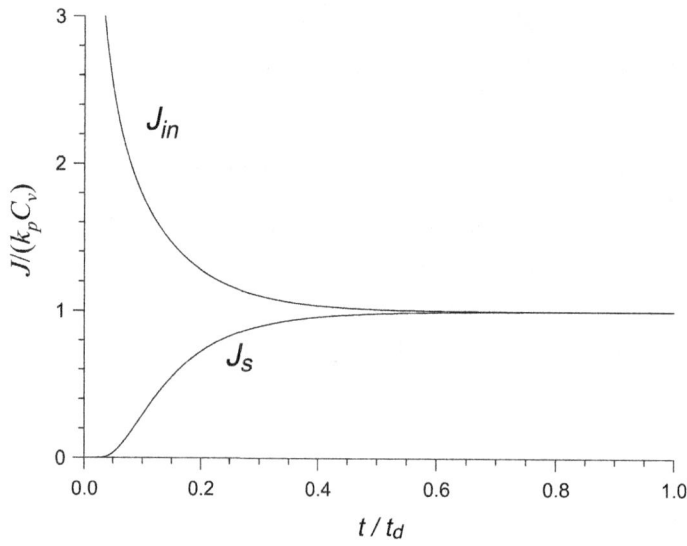

FIGURE 2.5 Normalized flux $(J/k_p C_v)$ against normalized time (t/t_d) for flux of solutes penetrating the SC [J_s, Equation (2.20)] and entering the SC [J_{in}, Equation (2.22)].

interest such as patch removal, sunscreen, and other products and toxins being washed and removed from the skin, when the assumption can be made that there has not been a significant (>10%) depletion in the concentration of solute at the surface. The amount absorbed into a systemic circulation across the skin from the time the dosage form is removed is given by:

$$Q(t) = M_\infty \left\{ 1 - \frac{4}{\pi^3} \sum_{n=0}^{\infty} \frac{(-1)^n}{[n+(1/2)]^3} \exp\left[-\frac{t}{t_d}\pi^2\left(n+\frac{1}{2}\right)^2 \right] \right\} \qquad (2.23)$$

where $M_\infty = K_m C_v A h_m/2 = k_p A C_v t_d/2$ is the amount of solute present in the skin before removal of the vehicle. The Laplace domain equivalent of this expression is:

$$\hat{Q}(s) = \frac{M_\infty}{s^2} \frac{2}{t_d} \left(1 - \frac{1}{\cosh\sqrt{st_d}} \right) \qquad (2.24)$$

The corresponding equations for flux are:

$$J_s(t) = k_p C_v \frac{2}{\pi} \sum_{n=0}^{\infty} \frac{(-1)^n}{n+(1/2)} \exp\left[-\frac{t}{t_d}\pi^2\left(n+\frac{1}{2}\right)^2 \right] \qquad (2.25)$$

$$\hat{J}_s(s) = \frac{k_p C_v}{s} \left(1 - \frac{1}{\cosh\sqrt{st_d}} \right) \qquad (2.26)$$

Figure 2.6 shows the amount and flux–time profiles associated with donor phase removal.

The mean time for absorption of solute from the skin in this case is given by:

$$\text{MAT} = \frac{\displaystyle\int_0^\infty J_s(t)t\,\mathrm{d}t}{\displaystyle\int_0^\infty J_s(t)\,\mathrm{d}t} = -\lim_{s\to 0}\frac{\mathrm{d}}{\mathrm{d}s}\ln(\hat{J}_s) = \frac{5h_m^2}{12D_m} = \frac{5}{12}t_d \qquad (2.27)$$

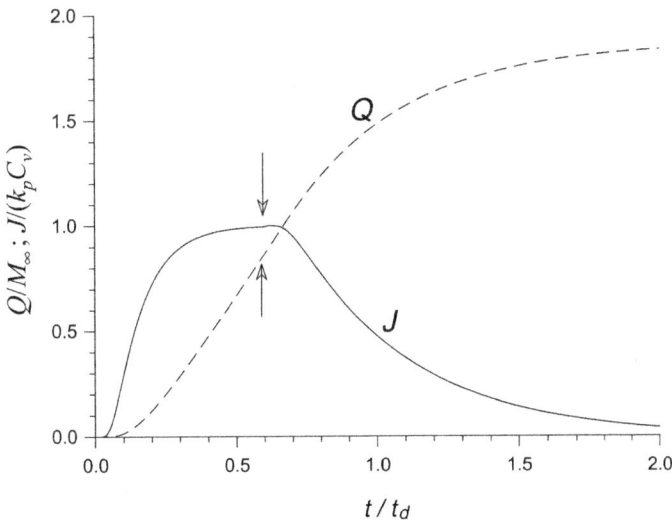

FIGURE 2.6 Changes in normalized cumulative amounts penetrating (Q/M_∞) and flux ($J/k_p C_v$) when the vehicle is removed (as indicated by *arrows*) at a specific normalized time (t/t_d) after application.

The amount absorbed after infinite time is the amount in the skin before the vehicle is removed, which is equal to M_∞.

Given the complexity of solute–distance–time profiles in membranes, the expressions for these profiles are not reproduced here. However, it should be emphasized that these may be important, as illustrated in the use of in vivo attenuated total reflection–Fourier transform infrared spectroscopy (ATR–FTIR) to examine the kinetics of solute uptake into human SC in vivo [7].

2.1.3 IN VITRO PERMEABILITY STUDIES WITH A CONSTANT DONOR CONCENTRATION AND FINITE RECEPTOR VOLUME

In most in vitro studies, it is assumed that sink conditions apply in the receptor phase. However, the receptor phase is a finite volume, and solute accumulation may be possible if there is an inadequate removal rate of the solute penetrating through. Siddiqui et al. [8] related the steady-state flux of steroids through human epidermis to the differences in concentrations between donor C_v and receptor C_{ss} concentrations. In the present notation, this equation is:

$$J_{ss} = k_p \left(C_v - \frac{C_{ss}}{K_r} \right) \tag{2.28}$$

where K_r is the partition coefficient between the membrane and vehicle $K_r = C_r/C_v$ and K_m is the partition coefficient between the membrane and vehicle $K_m = C_m/C_v$. Siddiqui et al. [8] assumed that $K_r = 1$.

Implicit in the underlying boundary conditions for the receptor phase is a constant clearance of solute Cl_r due to repeated sampling or use of a flow-through cell. If such a clearance were absent, C_{ss} would continually increase and approach $C_v K_r$. The value of C_{ss} is defined by the relative magnitudes of the clearance Cl_r and $k_p A/K_r$:

$$C_{ss} = \frac{k_p A C_v}{Cl_r + \left(k_p A / K_r \right)} \tag{2.29}$$

Siddiqui et al. [8] also applied this equation and the dermal clearance of solutes Cl_r to predict the steady-state epidermal concentrations of solutes C_{ss}. Roberts [9] considered the limits of large $k_p A$ as it exists for phenol absorption and low $k_p A$ as it exists for steroid absorption. He suggested that when $k_p A \gg K_r Cl_r$, C_{ss} would eventually approach the donor concentrations used ($C_v K_r$). In contrast, when $k_p A \ll K_r Cl_r$, C_{ss} approaches $k_p A C_v/Cl_r$.

The derivation of the full equation, from which steady-state Equations (2.28) and (2.29) arise, needs to take into account a finite receptor or epidermis volume. The boundary condition at $x = h_m$ in this case is $C_m(h_m, t)/K_m = C_r(t)/K_r$, together with [10]:

$$V_r \frac{dC_r}{dt} = -A D_m \frac{\partial C_m}{\partial x} \bigg|_{x=h_m} - Cl_r C_r \tag{2.30}$$

where Cl_r is the clearance (mL/min) of solution containing solute from the receptor phase, V_r is the volume of the receptor, and C_r is the concentration in the receptor.

Using this boundary condition together with the boundary condition in [7] yields the amount of solute, which penetrated the skin into the receptor (= amount in receptor + amount cleared from receptor), and for the flux of solute into the receptor [9]:

$$\hat{Q}(s) = \frac{k_p A C_v}{s^2} \frac{\sqrt{st_d}}{\sinh\sqrt{st_d} + \left\{ \left[\sqrt{st_d} / (st_d V_{rN} + Cl_{rN}) \right] \cosh\sqrt{st_d} \right\}} \tag{2.31}$$

$$\hat{J}_s(s) = \frac{k_p C_v}{s} \frac{\sqrt{st_d}}{\sinh\sqrt{st_d} + \left\{ \left[\sqrt{st_d} / (st_d V_{rN} + Cl_{rN}) \right] \cosh\sqrt{st_d} \right\}} \tag{2.32}$$

where the dimensionless parameter $Cl_{rN} = Cl_r K_r/(k_p A)$ is a measure of the magnitude of the removal rate from the receptor phase (Cl_r) relative to transport through the membrane $(k_p A)$, and $V_{rN} = V_r K_r/V_m K_m$ is the dimensionless receptor volume defined as the ratio of the amount of drug in the receptor phase and membrane $(C_r V_r/C_m V_m)$, assuming equilibrium exists between phases.

Figure 2.7 shows the effect of receptor volume (as defined by V_{rN}) and clearance of solution from the receptor phase (as defined by Cl_{rN}) on the $J_s(t)$–time profile.

The steady-state approximation of Equation (2.31) is:

$$Q(t) \approx AJ_{ss}\left(t - \text{lag}\right) \tag{2.33}$$

where:

$$J_{ss} = k_p C_v \frac{Cl_r}{Cl_r + \left(k_p A / K_r\right)} = \frac{k_p C_v}{1 + \left(1 / Cl_{rN}\right)} \tag{2.34}$$

and:

$$\text{lag} = \frac{t_d}{6}\left[1 + \frac{2Cl_{rN} - 6V_{rN}}{Cl_{rN}\left(Cl_{rN} + 1\right)}\right] \tag{2.35}$$

We note that if Equation (2.29) is substituted into Equation (2.28), the expression for J_{ss} is identical to Equation (2.34). We also note that when $Cl_r \rightarrow \infty$ (infinite sink), J_{ss} and lag reduce to Equations (2.4) and (2.12), respectively.

The corresponding solution for the receptor/epidermal concentration with the noted boundary conditions is:

$$\hat{C}_r(s) = \frac{k_p A C_v}{s} \frac{\sqrt{st_d}}{\left(V_r s + Cl_r\right)\left\{\sinh\sqrt{st_d} + \left[\sqrt{st_d} / \left(st_d V_{rN} + Cl_{rN}\right)\right]\cosh\sqrt{st_d}\right\}} \tag{2.36}$$

At long times $t \rightarrow \infty$, C_r is defined by Equation (2.29).

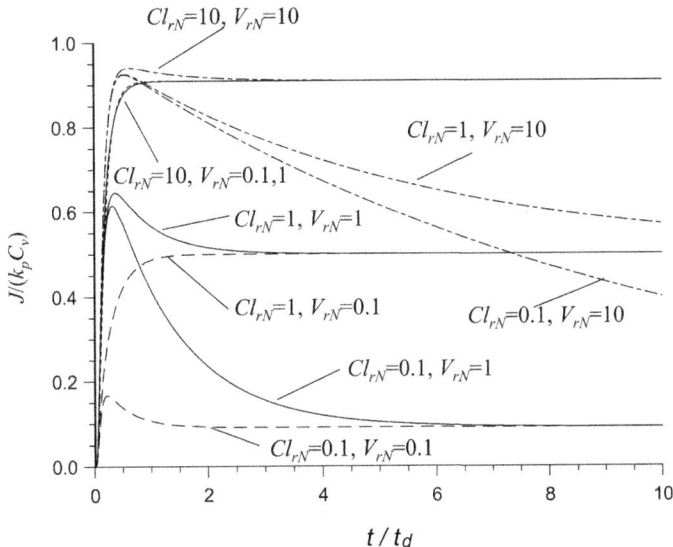

FIGURE 2.7 Normalized flux $(J/k_p C_v)$ versus normalized time (t/t_d) for a finite receptor volume and limited clearance [Equation (2.32)], $Cl_{rN} = Cl_r K_r/k_p A$, $V_{rN} = V_r K_R/V_m K_m$.

Parry et al. [11] has described a percutaneous absorption model in which both the donor and receptor compartments for an in vitro membrane study were well-stirred and finite. Boundary conditions similar in form to that defined by Equations (2.42) and (2.30), but with Clr = 0, were used to describe the disappearance of solute from the donor chamber into the membrane and the efflux of solute from the membrane into the receptor chamber. The resultant expression included a complex function requiring the solution of transcendental equations. It should be emphasized that this model differs from others described in this section in that it does not have a clearance term to account for sampling.

2.1.4 IN VITRO PERMEABILITY STUDIES WITH A CONSTANT DONOR CONCENTRATION OR DEFINED INPUT FLUX AND FINITE CLEARANCE OF SOLUTE FROM THE EPIDERMIS

The importance of receptor conditions on epidermal transport has been the subject of various studies over the last 30 years. Two models are widely used. In the first model, it is assumed that the viable epidermis or aqueous diffusion layer below the SC can exert a significant influence on skin penetration [12, 13]. The second model is one where there is an effectively desorption rate-limited step in partitioning from the membrane to the next phase (e.g., epidermis → receptor solution; SC → epidermis; epidermis → dermis). This rate constant, which we will define as k_c, and the interfacial barrier rate constant are identical if the lag time for the interfacial barrier can be assumed to be negligible. In the specific case of an aqueous diffusion layer being a barrier, $k_c = D_{aq} / l_{aq}^2$ where l_{aq} is the thickness of the layer and D_{aq} is the diffusion coefficient in the layer [13].

Guy and Hadgraft and Guy et al. [14, 15] developed a pharmacokinetic model for skin absorption based on the diffusion model with the boundary conditions defined by (1) the influx into the membrane being related to an assumed exponential decline in vehicle donor concentration and (2) the efflux from the membrane being related to first-order removal at a rate constant k_c. These authors went on to examine short and long time approximations. Kubota and Ishizaki [16] presented a more generalized diffusion model for drug absorption through excised skin by using the boundary conditions of the fluxes (1) into the skin being defined by an arbitrary function $f(t)$ and (2) out of the skin being defined by $ClC(x = h_m)$, where Cl is the clearance from the skin and $C(x = h_m)$ is the concentration of solute at the skin–system interface. They considered a boundary condition at the membrane–vehicle interface defined by an input rate into the membrane $f(t)$ together with a first-order rate constant k_c determining efflux from the membrane. Accordingly, the amount of solute absorbed across the skin $Q(t)$ at various times t is defined in the Laplace domain as:

$$\hat{Q}(s) = \frac{A}{s} \frac{k_c t_d \hat{f}(s)}{\sqrt{st_d} \sinh\left(\sqrt{st_d}\right) + k_c t_d \cosh\left(\sqrt{st_d}\right)} \tag{2.37}$$

Of particular interest in this overview is the case of a constant donor concentration (infinite donor) and sink receptor. $\hat{Q}(s)$ is then defined by:

$$\hat{Q}(s) = \frac{k_p C_v A}{s^2} \frac{k_c t_d \sqrt{st_d}}{\sqrt{st_d} \cosh \sqrt{st_d} + k_c t_d \sinh \sqrt{st_d}} \tag{2.38}$$

Figure 2.8A shows the effect of k_c (as defined by $\alpha = k_c t_d$) on the $Q(t)$ versus time profile.

It is to be noted that at long times, the linear portion of $Q(t)$ [defined by Equation (2.38)] versus t profile describes a steady-state flux J_{ss} and lag time (lag):

$$Q(t) = J_{ss} A(t - \text{lag}) = C_v k_p A \frac{k_c t_d}{1 + k_c t_d} (t - \text{lag}) \tag{2.39}$$

$$\text{lag} = \frac{t_d}{6} \left(1 + \frac{2}{1 + k_c t_d} \right) \tag{2.40}$$

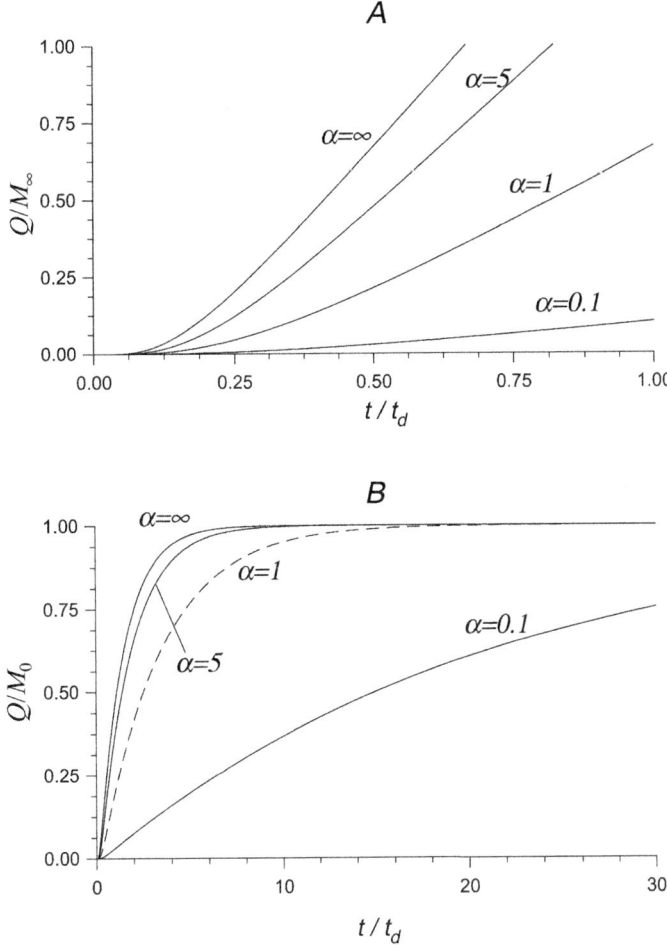

FIGURE 2.8 Effect of interfacial barrier rate constant (expressed as $\alpha = k_c t_d$) on exit from SC on normalized amount penetrating the epidermis with normalized time (t/t_d). (A) constant donor concentration and (B) a finite dose in well-stirred vehicle, where $V_{rN}(= V_r K_R/V_m K_m) = 1$ for time normalized to diffusion time.

Thus, both the slope and lag of the steady-state portion of a $Q(t)$ versus t plot depend on k_c. J_{ss} in Equation (2.39) can be re-expressed as:

$$J_{ss} = C_v k_p \frac{1}{1+(1/k_c t_d)} \tag{2.41}$$

which is identical to Equation (2.34) if $k_c t_d$ is replaced with Cl_{rN}.

Elsewhere we have analyzed a more general case with simultaneous rate limitations due to clearance from the receptor (Cl_r), finite receptor volume (V_r), finite permeability through viable epidermis k_p^{ve}, and finite permeability through the unstirred donor layer k_d^p [10]. Equations (2.31) and (2.38) for $\hat{Q}(s)$ are limiting cases of this more general solution.

2.1.5 In Vitro Skin Permeability Studies with Finite Donor Volume and Receptor Sink Conditions

In practice, the solute concentration applied to the skin does not remain constant but declines due to the finite volumes of vehicles or pure substances applied to the skin. We therefore need to examine solutions for Equation (2.5) in which the boundary condition allows for depletion in solute concentration. We assume initially the simplest boundary conditions applying to the sorption of solutes into a membrane from the well-stirred vehicle at $x = 0$ and from the membrane into a systemic circulation [Equations (2.7) and (2.8)] together with a condition of depletion of concentration in the vehicle at $x = h_v$ [3]:

$$V_v \frac{dC_v}{dt} = AD_m \frac{\partial C_m}{\partial x}\Big|_{x=0} \tag{2.42}$$

where $V_v = Ah_v$ is the volume of the vehicle applied to the skin. The solution of Equation (2.5) with Equations (2.7), (2.8), and (2.42) as boundary conditions gives [17]:

$$Q(t) = M_0 \left\{ 1 - \sum_{n=1}^{\infty} \frac{2\exp\left[-(t/t_d)\gamma_n^2\right]}{\cos\gamma_n\left[1 + V_{vN}\gamma_n^2 + (1/V_{vN})\right]} \right\} \tag{2.43}$$

where $M_0 = C_{v0}V_v = C_{v0}Ah_v$ is the initial amount of solute in the vehicle, C_{v0} is the initial concentration in the vehicle, h_v is the effective thickness of the vehicle, and V_{vN} is a dimensionless parameter defined by:

$$V_{vN} = \frac{V_v}{K_m V_m}$$

and γ_n are positive roots of transcendental equation:

$$\gamma\tan\gamma = \frac{1}{V_{vN}}$$

The Laplace transform of $Q(t)$ is given by [18]:

$$\hat{Q}(s) = \frac{M_0}{s} \frac{1}{V_{vN}\sqrt{st_d}\,\sinh\left(\sqrt{st_d}\right) + \cosh\left(\sqrt{st_d}\right)} \tag{2.44}$$

The corresponding expressions for flux are given by Equations (2.45) and (2.46):

$$J_s(t) = V_{vN}C_{v0}k_p \sum_{n=0}^{\infty} \frac{2\gamma_n^2\exp\left[-(t/t_d)\gamma_n^2\right]}{\cos\gamma_n\left[1 + V_{vN}\gamma_n^2 + (1/V_{vN})\right]} \tag{2.45}$$

$$\hat{J}_s(s) = V_{vN}C_{v0}k_p \frac{t_d}{V_{vN}\sqrt{st_d}\,\sinh\sqrt{st_d} + \cosh\sqrt{st_d}} \tag{2.46}$$

An equation identical to Equation (2.45) was used by Kasting [19] for analysis of the in vitro absorption rates of varying finite doses of vanillylnonanamide applied to excised human skin from propylene glycol.

Figure 2.9 shows the predicted profiles for the flux of solute [Equation (2.46)] with varying $V_{vN} = Vv/(K_m V_m)$. It is apparent that both the peak time and area under the curve decrease with the decreasing V_{vN}. The longer peak time with increasing V_v reflects the movement from a finite to an infinite donor source. The larger area under the curve reflects the higher dose associated with an increase in V_v.

Two summary parameters can be derived from Equation (2.46):

1. Mean absorption time (MAT) measuring from systemic side of the skin is:

$$\text{MAT}_s = \frac{d\left[\ln\hat{J}_v(s)\right]}{ds}\Big|_{s=0} = \frac{1}{2}t_d + V_{vN}t_d \tag{2.47}$$

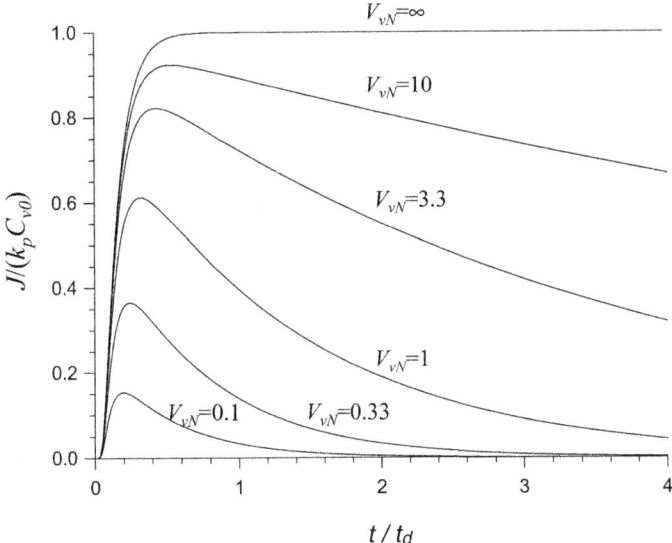

FIGURE 2.9 Normalized flux for penetration of a solute from a finite dose in a well-stirred vehicle $J/k_p C_{vo}$ against normalized time (t/t_d) for diffusion time with varying $V_{rN}(= V_r K_R / V_m K_m)$.

It needs to be emphasized that MATS differs from MTT, which is mean transit time through the SC. MTT can be calculated as:

$$MTT = MAT_s - MAT_v$$

where MAT_v is the mean absorption time from the vehicle:

$$MAT_v = -\frac{d \ln \hat{J}_v(s)}{ds} \bigg|_{s=0}$$

and where $\hat{J}_v(s)$ is the Laplace transform of the flux from the vehicle into the skin. It can be found that:

$$\hat{J}_v(s) = V_{vN} C_{v0} k_p \frac{t_d}{V_{vN} \sqrt{s t_d} \tanh \sqrt{s t_d} + 1}$$

and $MAT_v = V_{vN} t_d$. We therefore have $MTT = t_d/2$.

2. CV^2 for absorption:

$$CV^2 = \frac{d^2/ds^2 \left[\ln \hat{J}_s(s) \right]}{d/ds \left[\ln \hat{J}_s(s) \right]} \bigg|_{s=0} = \frac{2}{3} + \frac{4}{3 \left[2 + 1(1/V_{vN}) \right]^2} \tag{2.48}$$

Another two summary parameters can be derived from Equation (2.46) when $V_{vN} = 1$ ($V_v = V_m K_m$). This applies in a specific case of solvent-deposited solids. Scheuplein and Ross [20] described the application of drugs when 25 µL of acetone is applied to 2.54 cm² and allowed to evaporate, leaving a very thin layer of solid material. When $V_{vN} = 1$ Equation (2.46) reduces to:

$$\hat{J}_s(s) = V_{vN} C_{v0} k_p \frac{t_d}{\cosh \sqrt{s t_d}}$$

and therefore $J(t)$ can be written as:

$$J(t) = V_{vN}C_{v0}k_p f\left(\frac{t}{t_d}\right) = V_{vN}C_{v0}k_p f(\tau)$$

where $\tau = t/t_d$, $f(\tau)$ is a function independent of V_{vN} and whose Laplace transform is $\hat{f}(s) = 1/\cosh\sqrt{s}$. It can be shown by the numerical inversion of $\hat{f}(s)$ that the maximum of the function $f(\tau)$ occurs at $\tau = 1/6$ with the value $f(\tau_{max}) = 1.850$. The maximum flux, J_{max}, and for the time of maximum flux, t_{max}, for finite-dose absorption solvent–deposited solutes are therefore described by the simple equations:

$$J_{max} = 1.85 V_{vN}C_{v0}k_p = \frac{1.85 C_{v0}D_m h_v}{h_m^2}, \quad t_{max} = \frac{t_d}{6} = \frac{h_m^2}{6D_m} \tag{2.49}$$

Hence, the peak time corresponds to the lag time observed after application of a constant donor solution [Equation 2.12]. Scheuplein and Ross [20] provided experimental data to show that (1) J_{max} is proportional to C_{v0} for benzoic acid, (2) t_{max} for different solutes is inversely related to their D_m values, and (3) penetration was facilitated by hydrating the SC.

2.1.6 IN VITRO PERMEABILITY STUDIES WITH A FINITE DONOR VOLUME AND A FINITE CLEARANCE FROM THE EPIDERMIS INTO THE RECEPTOR

Another case of particular practical interest is when the donor phase is assumed to be well-stirred and finite in volume and there is limiting clearance from the epidermis to the receptor phase. Applying the boundary condition defined by Equation (2.42), together with boundary condition for $x = h_m$:

$$D_m \frac{\partial C_m}{\partial x}\bigg|_{x=h_m} = h_m k_c C_m(h_m, t) \tag{2.50}$$

Yields for $\hat{Q}(s)$:

$$\hat{Q}(s) = \frac{M_0}{s} \frac{1}{\sqrt{st_d}\sinh\sqrt{st_d}\left[V_{vN} + (1/t_d k_c)\right] + \cosh\sqrt{st_d}\left[1 + V_{vN}(s/k_c)\right]} \tag{2.51}$$

The profiles for $Q(t)$ versus t defined by Equation (2.51) for different values of k_c ($\alpha = k_c t_d$) and $V_{vN} = 1$ are shown in Figure 2.8B.

A case of finite volume of the vehicle with simultaneous rate limitations due to clearance from receptor (Cl_r), finite receptor volume (V_r), finite permeability through viable epidermis (k_p^{ve}), and finite permeability through unstirred donor layer (k_p^d) were analyzed by Anissimov and Roberts [18]. Equations (2.44) and (2.51) presented here for $\hat{Q}(s)$ are limiting cases of their more general solution.

2.1.7 IN VITRO SKIN PERMEABILITY STUDIES WITH DIFFUSION LIMITED FINITE DONOR AND SINK RECEPTOR CONDITIONS

One of the first attempts at modeling percutaneous absorption with diffusion-limiting uptake from both the vehicle and the skin was made by Kakemi et al. [21]. Their one-dimensional model is shown in Figure 2.2d. Guy and Hadgraft (22) used a similar model with sink receptor conditions, as shown in Figure 2.10.

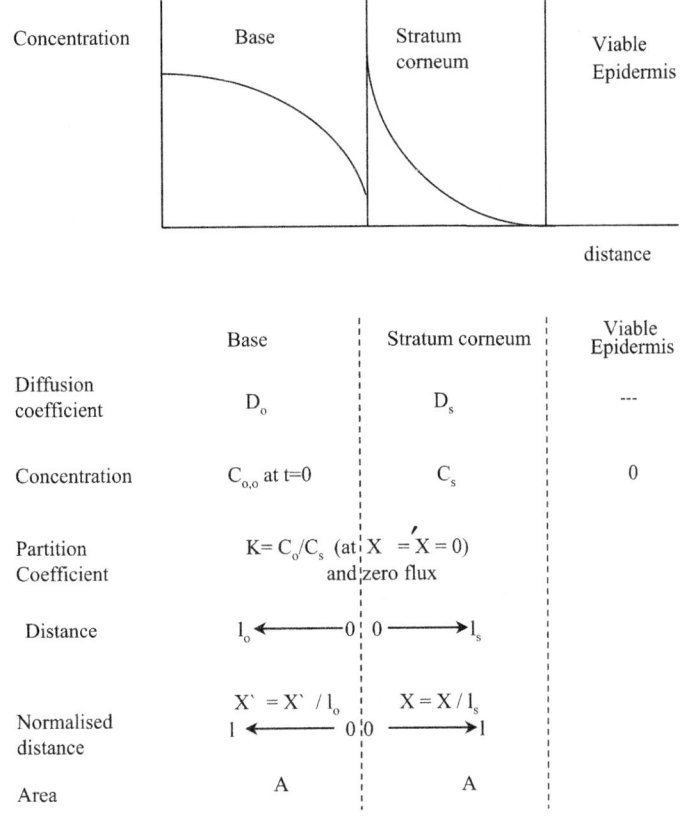

	Base	Stratum corneum	Viable Epidermis
Diffusion coefficient	D_o	D_s	---
Concentration	$C_{o,o}$ at t=0	C_s	0
Partition Coefficient	$K = C_o/C_s$ (at $X' = X = 0$) and zero flux		
Distance	$l_o \longleftarrow 0 \mid 0 \longrightarrow l_s$		
Normalised distance	$X' = X' / l_o$ $1 \longleftarrow 0 \mid 0 \longrightarrow 1$	$X = X / l_s$	
Area	A	A	

FIGURE 2.10 Two-layer diffusion model for *in vitro* percutaneous absorption kinetics as defined by Guy and Hadgraft [22].

In the latter model, the solute has a diffusivity D_v in a finite vehicle of volume V_v, which is in contact with SC in which a solute has a diffusivity D_m down a path length h_m. The Laplace transform for the amount penetrating the epidermis $\hat{Q}(s)$ into an absorbing "sink" is:

$$\hat{Q}(s) = \frac{M_0}{s} \frac{\sinh \sqrt{st_{dv}}}{\sqrt{st_{dv}} \left(V_{vN} \sqrt{t_d / t_{dv}} \sinh \sqrt{st_{dv}} \sinh \sqrt{st_d} + \cosh \sqrt{st_{dv}} \cosh \sqrt{st_d} \right)} \tag{2.52}$$

where, as usual, $M_0 = C_{v0}V_v$ and t_{dv} are the diffusion time in the vehicle, $t_{dv} = h_v^2/D_v$.

When the transport across the epidermis is also dependent on a first-order rate constant k_c for removal from the epidermis, the Laplace transform becomes:

$$\hat{Q}(s) = \frac{M_0}{s} \frac{\sinh \sqrt{st_{dv}}}{\sqrt{st_{dv}}} \left[V_{vN} \sqrt{\frac{t_d}{t_{dv}}} \sinh \sqrt{st_{dv}} \sinh \sqrt{st_d} + \cosh \sqrt{st_{dv}} \cosh \sqrt{st_d} \right.$$
$$\left. + \frac{\sqrt{st_d}}{t_d k_c} \left(V_{vN} \sqrt{\frac{t_d}{t_{dv}}} \cosh \sqrt{st_d} \sinh \sqrt{st_{dv}} + \cosh \sqrt{st_{dv}} \sinh \sqrt{st_d} \right) \right]^{-1} \tag{2.53}$$

Figure 2.11 shows profiles of $Q(t)$ versus t as defined by Equation (2.53) for different vehicle diffusivities ($\gamma = t_{dv}/t_d$) and k_c ($\alpha = k_c t_d$) for $V_{vN} = 1$.

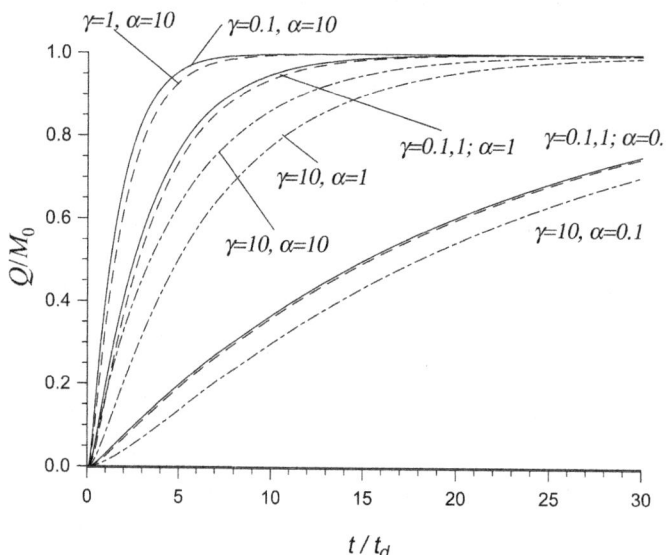

FIGURE 2.11 Cumulative amount penetrated Q normalized for amount applied M versus time normalized for diffusion time t_d for the case of both vehicle and SC limited diffusion. The two parameters varied define the relative diffusion time in vehicle relative to that in SC ($\gamma = t_{dv}/t_d$) and the interfacial barrier rate constant effect on the exit of solutes from the stratum $\alpha = k_c t_d$ [Equation (2.55)].

In the particular cases when $t_{dv} \gg t_d$ and $t_d \gg t_{dv}$ Equation (2.52) reduces to Equations (2.65) and (2.44), respectively.

2.1.8   IN VITRO PERMEABILITY STUDIES WITH TWO-LAYER DIFFUSION LIMITATIONS IN TRANSPORT

The complex cases of diffusion being a limitation in the transport through both the SC and epidermis have been considered by Hadgraft [23, 24]. He considered the case when solute exists as a reservoir in the SC. In his approach, the solute initially present in the SC diffuses from it into and through the epidermis. The case of rate-limiting removal from the epidermis (k_c) was considered.

Cleek and Bunge [25] considered a similar two phases in a series model for the amount of solute entering [Qin(t)] and determined it both as an analytical solution and simulations. This model was then extended to include solute properties as a determinant of uptake [26]. They suggested that steady-state permeability would be underestimated if not corrected for the relative permeabilities of the SC and epidermis. The result of these considerations is a steady-state Equation (2.54) similar to Equations (2.39) and (2.40):

$$Q_{\text{in}}(t) = C_{v0} k_p A \frac{1}{1+B} \left[t + t_{ds} \frac{G(1+3B) + B(1+3BG)}{3G(1+B)} \right] \tag{2.54}$$

where $k_p = K_{sv} D_{sc}/h_{sc}$, $G = t_{ds}/t_{de}$, $B = D_{sc}h_e K_c/D_e h_{sc}$, and K_{sv} is the partition coefficient between SC and the vehicle $K_{sv} = C_{sc}/C_v$.

Seko et al. [27] considered a similar model with the solute metabolism in the second phase (viable epidermis). The resulting equations for the amount exiting the epidermis for drug Q_d and metabolite Q_m are:

$$\frac{A K_{sd} C_v h_s \sqrt{s t_{sd}}}{s^2 t_{sd} \left[\cosh\sqrt{s t_{sd}} \sinh\sqrt{(s+k_m)t_{ed}} + \left(K_{sd} h_s \sqrt{s t_{ed}} / K_{ed} h_e \sqrt{s t_{ed}} \right) \sinh\sqrt{s t_{sd}} \cosh\sqrt{(s+k_m)t_{ed}} \right]} \tag{2.55}$$

$$\hat{Q}_{\mathrm{m}}(s) = \frac{k_{\mathrm{m}}t_{\mathrm{ed}}}{\left(\sqrt{(s+k_{\mathrm{m}})t_{\mathrm{ed}}} - \sqrt{st_{\mathrm{em}}}\right)}\left(\frac{\cosh\sqrt{(s+k_{\mathrm{m}})t_{\mathrm{ed}}}}{\cosh\sqrt{st_{\mathrm{em}}}} - 1\right)\hat{Q}_{\mathrm{d}}(s) \qquad (2.56)$$

where k_{m} is the rate of metabolism in the viable epidermis, $t_{\mathrm{ed}} = h_{\mathrm{e}}^2/D_{\mathrm{ed}}$, $t_{\mathrm{ed}} = h_{\mathrm{s}}^2/D_{\mathrm{sd}}$, $t_{\mathrm{em}} = h_{\mathrm{e}}^2/D_{\mathrm{em}}$, and first subscripts (s and e) denote the SC and the viable epidermis and the second subscripts (d and m) denote the drug and its metabolite, respectively. We note that the boundary conditions used in this work excluded the metabolite from diffusing back into the SC and the donor. This simplifies the solution for the metabolite, but could in some cases slightly overestimate its amount penetrating into the receptor. Two-layer diffusion of the viable epidermis and SC has been described more recently in {Todo, 2013 #1092}. The two-layer model can be described by Fick's second law of diffusion, where there is no impact from metabolism of the drug. Metabolism can occur in the SC layer, the viable epidermis and dermis [121, 122]. The model also compares results to experimental data that was taken in rat skin and within a silicone membrane.

2.1.9 DESORPTION

Although penetration (absorption) experiments are most common in studying percutaneous kinetics, desorption experiments have been used to study SC solute transport [28, 29]. In these desorption experiments, the membrane is initially saturated with the solute so that it is at equilibrium with the donor phase with concentration C_{d}. The membrane is then immersed into the receptor phase with no solute present at time $t = 0$. Assuming sink conditions in the receptor, the initial and boundary conditions for this case are:

$$C_{\mathrm{m}}(x,0) = K_{\mathrm{m}}C_{\mathrm{d}} \qquad (2.57)$$

$$C_{\mathrm{m}}(0,t) = 0 \qquad (2.58)$$

$$C_{\mathrm{m}}(h_{\mathrm{m}},t) = 0 \qquad (2.59)$$

Solving Equation (2.5) with initial and boundary conditions [Equations (2.57 to 2.59)] in the Laplace domain yields for the amount of solute desorbed into the receptor phase:

$$\hat{Q}(s) = \frac{1}{s}\frac{AK_{\mathrm{m}}C_{\mathrm{d}}h_{\mathrm{m}}}{\sqrt{st_{\mathrm{d}}}}2\tan\left(\frac{\sqrt{st_{\mathrm{d}}}}{2}\right) \qquad (2.60)$$

Equation (2.60) could be inverted to the time domain to yield an infinite series solution:

$$Q(t) = M_\infty\left\{1 - \frac{8}{\pi^2}\sum_{n=0}^\infty \frac{\exp\left[-(t/t_{\mathrm{d}})\pi^2(2\pi+1)^2\right]}{(2n+1)^2}\right\} \qquad (2.61)$$

where M_∞ $(= C_{\mathrm{d}}K_{\mathrm{m}}Ah_{\mathrm{m}})$ is the total amount of solute absorbed by the membrane. Equation (2.61) was used by Roberts et al. [29] to fit experimental desorption profiles for some solutes to yield t_{d} and K_{m}. These parameters could then be used to calculate the permeability coefficient:

$$k_{\mathrm{p}} = \frac{K_{\mathrm{m}}h_{\mathrm{m}}}{t_{\mathrm{d}}} \qquad (2.62)$$

The desorption of hydrophilic drugs in the SC has been recently discussed in Miller et al. [1],where two phases of desorption were described. The fast phase happened within a matter of minutes while the slow-phase took a matter of hours. The fast phase was found to be negligible for lipophilic solutes while slow phase desorption was found to be dependent on molecular size, with desorption being slower for solutes that have a larger molecular weight [1].

2.1.10 Modeling the Corneocytes and Lipids Explicitly

Figure 2.12, the brick and mortar approach to SC transport. In this figure, the lipid pathway is shown between the corneocytes and the transcellular pathway is dictated through the corneocytes by D_{cor}.

The development of the brick-and-mortar model was initially discussed within [2] and [3] where two-dimensional microscopic transport of a solute was investigated. The results of implementing this model for four different compounds showed that SC transport may be dependent on both the intercellular and transcellular pathway. This finding contradicts the more commonly expressed doctrine that transdermal drug delivery is predominately through the lipid pathway. For this reason, the brick-and-mortar model was further developed within [7] and [5]. These models incorporated a multi-scale approach where the physical transport properties were determined using quantitative structure-permeability relationships(QSPR) [6].

The brick-and-mortar approach to the SC was applied in [7]. The results of the application of this model was compared to experimental data obtained for nicotine patches. [8] The flux due to diffusion between any neighboring elements that were developed in the matrix could be described by the following mass transfer equation:

$$Q_{ij} = \frac{A}{\dfrac{\delta_i}{D_i} + \dfrac{K_{ij}\delta_j}{D_j}} \left(C_i - K_{ij} C_j \right)$$

The model employs a two-dimensional field which gives important insight into the concentration profile in subcellular areas of the SC. The results exhibit the lipid pathway for diffusion and the "reservoir" effect of the corneocytes. However, the model fails to exhibit the transport mechanics that would be present if the drug permeated through the follicular pathway.

For this reason, the diffusion of a drug through sebum was modeled in silico for caffeine in [6]. The finite difference method was used to develop the governing equations for each grid element the system was split into in the same manner as in [7]. The previous equation was employed to show the mass transfer between each grid element, and the diffusion equation was used to model the diffusive properties within each element. The follicular pathway was shown to be of greater significance to drug transport in the SC. In order to show the impact, [6] compared the disposition of caffeine in the SC when the hair follicles were closed and open. From the results, the hair follicle allowed a greater amount of drug to permeate into deeper layers of the SC. However, the model was only applicable to drugs with a low molecular weight. The diffusion through a two-dimensional representation of the SC when the corneocytes were modelled explicitly was also discussed in [9, 10]. The two-dimensional model was developed within COMSOL and solved numerically by the finite element method. The effect of two different scenarios were investigated; the case when the corneocytes were the main barrier to SC permeability and the case when the lipid pathway was the main barrier. The findings of the model confirmed that the main barrier to SC transport was the lipid layer which corresponded to previous conclusions developed by [9].

A two-dimensional random walk of the transport in the biphasic (lipid and corneocyte) SC has also been employed to model drug transport [11]. Further modelling of the geometry of the SC was performed using a three-dimensional model that used tetrakaidecahedra shapes for the corneocytes. By flattening the tetrakaidecahedra [12], was able to develop a physiological feasible shape for the corneocytes. However, the shape of the corneocytes will be highly volatile from cell to cell. A more asymmetric approach for the corneocyte arrangement should also be considered to investigate the impact of different corneocyte shapes and spacing.

Finally, a multiscale model of diffusion through the SC was considered by [13]. The model expands upon the work of homogenization to find the effective diffusion coefficient, which was discussed in [14] and [15]. In the multiscale model, the microscopic diffusion coefficient in the lipid pathway of the SC was predicted by molecular dynamic simulation. Once simulations are completed, the results are homogenized through the use of a unit cell, and the homogenized results give an effective diffusion coefficient that can be used for finite element analysis [13]. The idea of multiscale modelling is one that has great potential in the future, as molecular simulations may be able to predict pharmacokinetic variables that are hard to come by in in vivo simulations.

2.1.11 Slow Binding in SC

Slow binding in the SC that may occur when molecules diffuse into the corneocytes. Once inside the corneocytes, the molecules may bind and unbind to the keratin fibers that are present before exiting through an arbitrary location on the boundary of the corneocyte. [16]However, the process of slow binding in the corneocytes is highly variable from molecule to molecule and difficult to determine experimentally. By approximating the transport in the SC by not considering the corneocyte diffusion, the following expressions for the unbound and bound concentration can be determined.

$$\frac{\partial C_u}{\partial t} = D\frac{\partial^2 C_u}{\partial x^2} - k_{on}C_u + k_{off}C_b$$

$$\frac{\partial C_b}{\partial t} = k_{on}C_u - k_{off}C_b$$

where C_u is the concentration unbound, C_b is the concentration bound to keratin fibers, k_{on} is the binding rate and k_{off} is the unbinding rate.

By assuming that the donor has a much larger volume than the SC, it could be estimated that the amount of solute at the top of the membrane will be close to the initial amount. Then the unbound concentration at the upper boundary of the SC could be approximated to be:

$$C_u(0,t) = K_{eff}f_uC_o$$

where f_u is the fraction of unbound solute and can be determined by the expression

$$f_u = \left(1 + \frac{k_{on}}{k_{off}}\right)^{-1}$$

Meanwhile at the bottom of the SC, [16] assumed a sink condition so:

$$C_u(h,t) = 0$$

Solving the system in the Laplace domain gives the following expression for the unbound concentration.

$$\hat{C}_u(x,s) = \frac{K_{eff}f_uC_0}{s} \times \left(cos\, h\left(\sqrt{g(s)t_d}\frac{x}{h}\right) - \frac{sinh\left(\sqrt{g(s)t_d}\frac{x}{h}\right)}{tanh\left(\sqrt{g(s)t_d}\right)} \right)$$

When the results of this model were compared to experimental data and water absorption in the SC, it could be seen that the amount of solute desorbed in the skin affected concentration more than slow binding [16, 17]. Another analysis of slow binding was performed in [18] but is instead solved for two layers and not just the one that was used in the previous model.

2.1.12 SC Heterogeneity

A homogeneous membrane model is assumed for the majority of the mathematical analysis of solute transport in SC in this chapter and in most of the literature. In reality the SC consists of at least two phases the stratum disjunctum and stratum compactum and may be seen to be heterogeneous in structure. The applicability of the homogeneity assumption to SC has therefore been questioned [30], and solutions for variable diffusion and partition coefficients in the SC have been presented [31]. In general, penetration flux experiments are relatively insensitive even to extreme values of diffusion and partition coefficient heterogeneity, whereas desorption experiments using Equation (2.62) may lead to a misinterpretation when the SC is heterogeneous. Concentration–distance profiles are the most sensitive to SC heterogeneity. Ignoring partition coefficient heterogeneity in using tape-stripping data to predict penetration flux–time profiles may result in a significant miscalculation of the steady-state flux and lag time values [31].

2.2 RELEASE PROFILES FROM TOPICAL PRODUCTS

A number of transdermal systems are now available for clinical use. Hadgraft [23, 24] considered the solutions for release from patches for a range of boundary conditions. When a drug is contained in both the contact adhesive (priming dose) and patch, the release rate R_s approximates to [32]:

$$R_s = R_0 + H \exp(-at) \tag{2.63}$$

where R_0 is the zeroth-order flux from the patch, assuming no depletion, and H and a are constants defining the release kinetics of the priming dose. Iordanski et al. [33] simulated factors such as matrix diffusion, partition coefficient, and polymer membrane thickness in the modeling of drug delivery kinetics from the adhesive of a transdermal delivery device into skin-imitating membranes.

2.2.1 DIFFUSION-CONTROLLED RELEASE

Of practical interest is a homogenous phase in which the drug is released by diffusion. The expression for the drug release from slabs is well-known to be that of the "burst" effect [3]:

$$Q(t) = M_0 \left\{ 1 - \frac{8}{\pi^2} \sum_{n=1}^{\infty} \frac{1}{(2n+1)^2} \exp\left[-\frac{t}{4t_{dv}} \pi^2 (2n+1)^2 \right] \right\} \tag{2.64}$$

where again $M_0 = C_{v0} V_v$ and $t_{dv} = h_v^2 / D_v$. The Laplace expression for Equation (2.64) is:

$$\hat{Q}(s) = \frac{M_0}{s} \frac{\tanh\sqrt{st_{dv}}}{\sqrt{st_{dv}}} \tag{2.65}$$

At short times when the amount released is less than 30%, Equation (2.64) can be approximated to:

$$Q(t) = 2M_0 \left(\frac{t}{\pi t_{dv}} \right)^{1/2} \tag{2.66}$$

2.2.2 RELEASE OF A SUSPENDED DRUG BY DIFFUSION

Another special case is that for a vehicle or patch containing a suspended drug. In this case, the amount of solute released into a perfect sink is given by [34]:

$$Q(t) = A\sqrt{tD_v (2C_{v0} - C_s)C_s} \tag{2.67}$$

where C_{v0} in this context has the meaning of the total amount of drug (soluble and suspended) in the vehicle per unit volume and C_s is the saturation concentration of the drug in the vehicle.

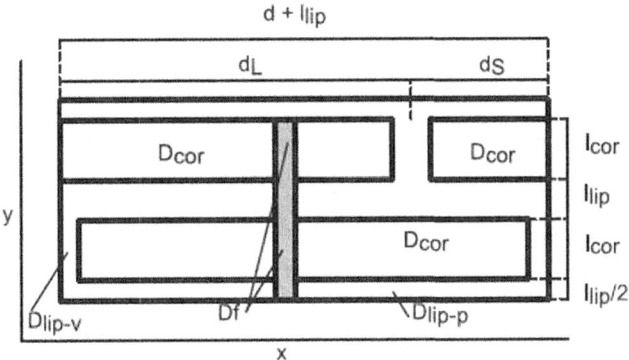

FIGURE 2.12   Examples of compartmental models of skin penetration.

2.3   COMPARTMENTAL MODELS AS AN ALTERNATIVE TO DIFFUSION MODELS IN PERCUTANEOUS ABSORPTION

Riegelman [35] analyzed a range of in vivo skin absorption data using unidirectional absorption and simple compartment-based pharmacokinetic models (Figure 2.12a). A more complex series of models (Figure 2.12b to d) were used by Wallace and Barnett [36] to describe the in vitro methotrexate absorption across the skin. A discussion of the various models and their approximations is given in our earlier version of this chapter [1]. More recently, a comprehensive review of compartmental models has been presented [37].

The key models developed [38] match (1) steady-state SC concentration and penetration rate with an assumption of equilibrium at the two boundaries of the membrane (equilibrium model); (2) steady-state SC concentration, penetration rate, and lag time for all blood and vehicle concentration ratios and for large blood concentrations (general time lag model); (3) as in (2) but for low blood concentrations (simplified time lag model); and (4) the traditional model. The real contribution of this work has been a systematic derivation of equations for coefficients of compartmental models expressed in terms of physicochemical parameters, which are documented in the paper in a readily accessible form.

It could be argued that the model representing SC as five compartments (Figure 2.12e) (39) corresponds best to the diffusion model (Figure 2.13). This model was developed to account for the potential binding of solute to SC proteins for finite vehicle volume.

2.4   OTHER PROCESSES AFFECTING IN VITRO PERCUTANEOUS ABSORPTION

2.4.1   CONCENTRATION-DEPENDENT DIFFUSIVE TRANSPORT PROCESSES

It is well-known that the permeability of solutes through the skin may be affected by their concentration-dependent interaction with the skin, as shown for the alcohols [12] and phenols [40]. At this time, relatively little work has been published on mathematical models for diffusion in a swelling or denaturing skin environment. Wu [41] has attempted to relate water diffusivity $D(C)$ as a function of its water concentration (C) in a keratinous membrane. The expression $D(C) = D_o + AC^B$, where D_o, A, and B are constants, best described the results. Giengler et al. [42] have described the numerical solution of solute concentrations in a system consisting of a polymer film, microporous membrane, adhesive, skin layer, and capillary sink and in which the diffusion coefficients were time dependent.

Higuchi and Higuchi [43] summarized the theory associated with diffusion through heterogeneous membranes and vehicles. They suggested that transport through a two-phase system was a function of the volume fraction and permeability of each phase. They also derived an expression for

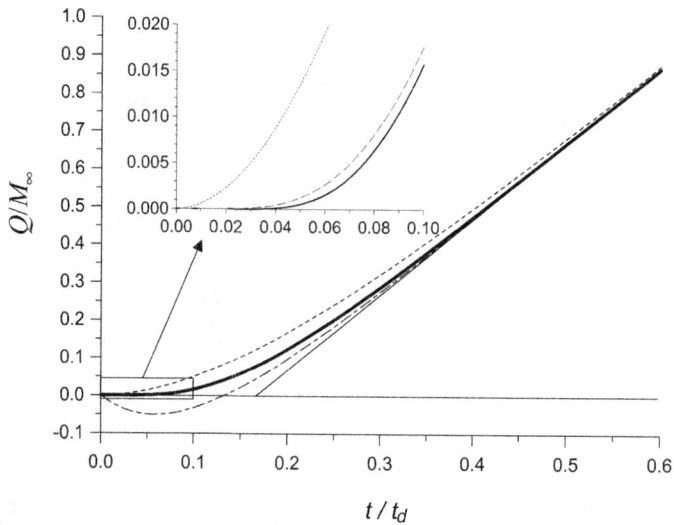

FIGURE 2.13   Normalized cumulative amount penetrated (Q/M_∞) versus normalized time (t/t_d) for diffusion model [*thick solid line*, Equation (2.13)], steady-state approximation of diffusion model [*solid line*, Equation (2.11)], two-compartmental approximations (*short dashed* and *dash dotted lines*, discussed in our earlier version of this chapter; see Ref. 1), and five-compartmental approximation of Zatz [39], assuming no binding in SC (*long dashed*, inset).

lag time across a membrane when simultaneous diffusion and Langmuir adsorption have occurred. The lag time across the membrane is increased by binding of solute to the membrane's binding sites:

$$\text{lag} = \frac{h_m^2}{4D_m} + \frac{h_m^2 A}{2D_m K_1 V_1 C_v} \tag{2.68}$$

where D_m is the effective diffusion constant in heterogeneous membrane, A is the amount of solute taken up by filler per unit volume of membrane material, K_1 is the partition coefficient of the solute in vehicle and phase 1 in the membrane, V_1 is the volume fraction of phase 1, and C_v is the concentration of solute in the vehicle.

When the solute concentration in the vehicle increases, the second term in Equation (2.68) decreases and the overall lag time is shorter.

Chandrasekaran et al. [32, 44] assumed that uptake of solutes by skin was described by a dual-sorption model:

$$Z\frac{dC}{dt} = D\frac{d^2 C}{dx^2} \tag{2.69}$$

where:

$$Z = B\left\{1 + \frac{C_i b / k_D}{\left[1 + (C_D b / kD)\right]^2}\right\}$$

However, these authors then assumed that Z was a constant. This model reduces to the conventional diffusion model in which the effective diffusivity is the diffusion coefficient of free solute modified by the instantaneous partitioning of solute into immobile sites in the diffusion path [45]. Expressions were presented for plasma concentrations and urinary excretion rate profiles after single and multiple patch applications of scopolamine to humans. Kubota et al. [46, 47] applied the dual sorption model to account for the nonlinear percutaneous absorption of timolol. The model accounted for the prolongation in timolol lag time associated with the decrease in applied concentration.

2.4.2   BIOCONVERSION/METABOLISM OF SOLUTES IN THE SKIN

Roberts and Walters [2] related the in vitro (metabolically inactive) skin flux $J_{s,in\ vitro}$ to that in in vivo $J_{s,in\ vivo}$ by a first-pass bioavailability F_s and a fraction released from the product into the skin F_R:

$$J_{s,in\ vivo} = F_s F_R J_{s,in\ vitro} \tag{2.70}$$

The importance of recognizing F_s is illustrated by methylsalicylate where $F_s < 0.05$ [2]. Caution must therefore be applied in extrapolating in vitro data into likely in vivo absorption.

The modeling of percutaneous absorption kinetics in the epidermis when diffusion and metabolic processes occur simultaneously leads to relatively complex solutions. Ando et al. [48] examined the diffusive transport of a solute through a metabolically inactive SC and hence through the epidermis, where it was assumed that there was homogeneous distribution of metabolizing enzymes. Subsequent work developed this model to examine the bioconversion prodrug → drug → metabolite [49, 50]. The work applied the diffusion equation and derived expressions for the steady-state fluxes and cutaneous concentration–distance relationships for each of the species. Yu et al. [51] then solved this model for nonuniform enzyme distribution in the skin. Fox et al. [52] considered Michaelis–Menten kinetics in their examination of prodrug, drug, and metabolite concentrations in the epidermis and dermis. Most recently Seko et al. [27] used a two-layer skin diffusion/metabolism model to describe parabens cutaneous metabolism after topical application [see also Equations (2.55) and (2.56)]. Analysis involved nonlinear regression of numerical inversion of Laplace transform solutions. Approximations to diffusion-based models were applied by Hadgraft [53], Guy and Hadgraft [54], and Kubota et al. [55] to describe the effect of linear and saturable (Michaelis–Menten) epidermal metabolism on percutaneous absorption.

Guy and Hadgraft [56–59] adapted their pharmacokinetic model defined by k_1, k_1, k_2, k_3, and k_4 (Figure 2.14) to include a metabolic step k_5 and removal of metabolite k_6. Linear kinetics was assumed to enable solution in the Laplace domain and inversion to give analytical solutions.

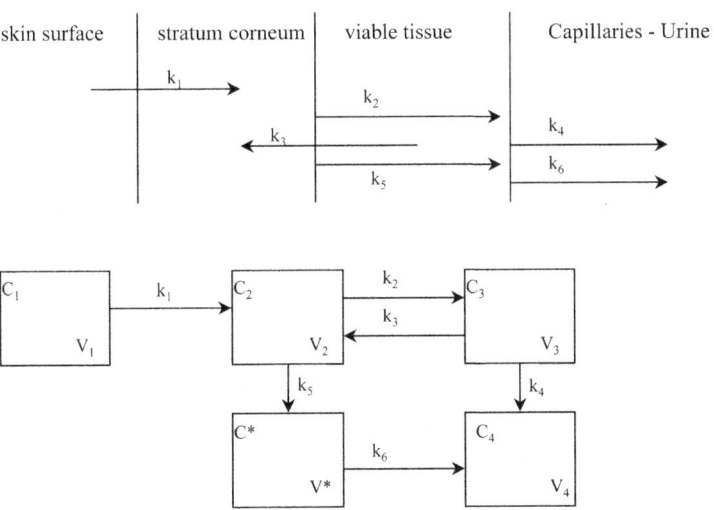

FIGURE 2.14 The compartmental model for skin penetration modified to include epidermal metabolism. (Adapted from reference [57].)

A number of theoretical plasma concentration profiles were then constructed. In reality, Michaelis–Menten kinetics may be operative for a number of solutes.

2.4.3 SOLUTE–VEHICLE, VEHICLE–SKIN, AND SOLUTE–SKIN INTERACTIONS

The practical application of mathematical models in percutaneous absorption to therapeutics or risk assessment is dependent on an understanding of solute–skin, solute–vehicle, and vehicle–skin interactions. Some aspects of each of these areas have been discussed by Roberts and Walters [2], Hadgraft and Wolff [60], Robinson [61], and Roberts et al. [45].

The present analysis has generally been limited to percutaneous absorption kinetics in which the underlying physicochemical parameters are time-independent. In practice, the application of a vehicle to the skin will lead to a time-dependent change in permeability due to either a solute–skin interaction or a vehicle–skin interaction. The solutions of the resultant concentration-dependent diffusion processes also lead to a time- and space-dependent change in solute diffusivity—these are relatively complex and are beyond the scope of this chapter.

Of critical importance in both therapeutics and toxicology is the maximum flux of a solute J_{max}. This flux is normally attained at the solubility of the solute in the given vehicle, S_v, consistent with the solubility of the solute in the SC transport pathway S_m:

$$J_{max} = \frac{D_m K_m S_v}{h_m} = k_p S_v = \frac{D_m S_m}{h_m} \qquad (2.71)$$

The importance of J_{max} as a parameter describing penetration through the skin is in its invariance for a given solute transport from different vehicles, unlike k_p, which is vehicle-dependent. This invariance holds unless the vehicle affects either D_m or S_m [45]. J_{max} (in mol/cm^2 hr) may be expressed in terms of molecular weight (MW), melting point (Mpt), and hydrogen bonding acceptor ability (Ha) [62]:

$$\log J_{max} = -4.35 - 0.0154 MW - 0.293 Mp^* + 0.371 Ha, \quad n = 87, \quad r^2 = 0.937 \qquad (2.72)$$

where J_{max} is in mol/cm^2 hr and the dependence on Mpt is described using the Mpt term: $Mp^* = \Delta S_f$ (Mpt − T) u(Mpt − T)/T, from Yalkowsky's solubility [Equation (2.63)], where T is the temperature, ΔS_f is the entropy of fusion of a solute, and $u(x)$ is the unit step function [i.e., $u(x) = 1$ for $x > 0$ and $u(x) = 0$ for $x < 0$]. Most of the regression variance for J_{max} is defined by MW, showing the dominance of size as a determinant of maximum flux [62]:

$$\log J_{max} = -3.90 - 0.0190 MW, \quad n = 87 \quad r^2 = 0.847 \qquad (2.73)$$

2.4.4 EFFECT OF SURFACE LOSS THROUGH PROCESSES SUCH AS EVAPORATION AND ADSORPTION TO SKIN SURFACE

There is a potential change in solute concentration as a consequence of surface loss during percutaneous absorption. The loss may result in (1) an effective reduction in the volume of the vehicle alone due to evaporation and an increase in solute concentration as a consequence, (2) a reduction in both solute and vehicle due to a removal process, and (3) a loss of solute only due to volatilization or adsorption to the skin surface. For instance, Reifenrath and Robinson [64] have shown that mosquito repellents may be lost due to evaporation at a rate comparable to their percutaneous absorption. The loss of vehicle at a defined rate creates a moving boundary problem and does not appear to have been considered to any great extent in the literature. Guy and Hadgraft [56, 57] examined the first -and zero-order losses of solute from the vehicle surface using diffusion and compartment models, respectively. Recently Saiyasombati and Kasting [65] examined the disposition of benzyl alcohol after topical application to human skin in vitro and showed that evaporation plays a significant role. They found that two-compartment models were adequate to describe the first-order loss of benzyl alcohol from the vehicle surface.

2.4.5 SHUNT TRANSPORT

The importance of shunt transport by appendages has been well-recognized. Scheuplein [66] and Wallace and Barnett [36] assumed a parallel pathway with a minimal lag time relative to transepidermal transport for diffusion and compartmental models, respectively. In our attempted modeling of epidermal and shunt diffusion, we assumed that the overall amount penetrating was the sum of the amounts penetrating through independent epidermal and shunt pathways [8]. The amount penetrating through each pathway was assumed to be defined by Equation (2.9) in which K_m and D_m were defined in terms of the corresponding constants for the two pathways.

More recently, the presence of polar and nonpolar pathways through the intercellular region of the SC has been recognized, as described in Equation (2.3). Mathematical models described include those for steady-state conditions [67, 68] and an infinite dosing condition [69]. Yamashita et al. [70] have presented the Laplace solution for a well-stirred, finite donor phase in contact with SC in which solutes can diffuse through both polar and nonpolar routes. The solute can then diffuse through the epidermis into a sink. Numerical inversion of the Laplace transform with FILT was then undertaken to generate real-time profiles. Edwards and Langer [71] have derived expressions for a range of conditions and suggested their theory confirmed the importance of shunt and intercellular transport for small ions and uncharged solutes, respectively.

More recently, a top down pharmacometrics approach [123], a finite element 2D and 3D simulation approach [124], a multicompartment Simcyp MechDermA PBPK approach [125] and a porous pathway feature in an existing skin diffusion model [126] have been used to analyse the closed and open follicle data for the skin absorption of caffeine [127], with quite disparate results. Each o the models describe parallel SC diffusion and appendageal absorption. These various studies emphasise a move away from conventional analytical diffusion equations into complex and more realistic representations of processes associated with percutaneous absorption by *in silico* driven numerical and quantitative structure -permeability relationships. There are now many papers in this area that are beyond the scope of this overview the on mathematics of skin absorption.

2.4.6 RESERVOIR EFFECT

It is well recognized that significant amounts of solute can accumulate in the SC and be released into lower tissues on rapid skin hydration, the so-called "reservoir" effect [72, 73]. Modeling of this process, including the effects of desquamation, has been undertaken using both diffusion [74] and compartmental models [75]. In the latter model, the kinetics of reservoir depletion was shown to be dependent on solute diffusivity in the SC solute clearance from the underlying tissue and the rate of epidermal turnover. This topic is not discussed here as it is in in some depth in a later chapter in this volume (see chapter 4).

2.5 SIMPLE IN VIVO MODELS IN PERCUTANEOUS ABSORPTION

2.5.1 COMPARTMENTAL PHARMACOKINETIC MODELS

One of the first evaluations of the pharmacokinetics of skin penetration was reported by Riegelman [35]. Absorption of solutes through the skin was generally assumed to follow first-order kinetics with a rate constant k_a (unit: sec^{-1}). Much of the data analyzed appeared to be characterized by "flip-flop" kinetics, where the absorption half-time is much longer than the elimination half-time, as illustrated later in Figure 2.15. This modeling approach has been used by a number of authors, including the

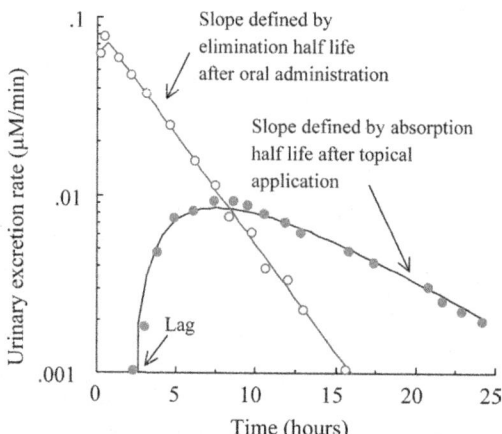

FIGURE 2.15 Simultaneous nonlinear regression of urinary excretion rate–time data for norephedrine hydrochloride administered orally (o) and free base applied topically (•) using a weighting of $1/y_{obs}$ and a common elimination half-life for norephedrine. The regression yielded an absorption half-life of 0.09 hour for oral administration, a lag of 2.2 hours and an absorption half-life of 6.0 hours for topical application, and an elimination half-life of 2.5 hours ($r^2 = 0.999$). (Data from Reference 120.)

recent work of Rohatagi et al. [76]. This work described an integrated pharmacokinetic-metabolic model for selegiline after application of a transdermal system for 24 hours. A series of differential equations and nonlinear regressions were then used to solve drug and metabolite concentrations.

Roberts and Walters [2] have suggested that four processes are commonly used to describe plasma concentrations C_{plasma} with time after topical application, when the body is assumed to be a single compartment, with an elimination rate constant k_{el} and apparent distribution volume V_{B}.

1. Depletion of the applied dose at a first-order rate constant k_a:

$$C_{plasma} = k_a F \quad \text{Dose} \left\{ \exp\left[-k_a \left(t - \text{lag}\right)\right] - \exp\left[-k_{el}\left(t - \text{lag}\right)\right] \right\}, \quad t > lag \quad (2.74)$$

where lag is the lag time for absorption through the skin and F is the fraction that would be absorbed if the product were applied for an infinite time.

Figure 2.15 shows the nonlinear regression of norephedrine urinary excretion rate after topical application using Equation (2.74). Also shown in Figure 2.15 is the profile for an equimolar dose given orally. It is apparent that the topical application is associated with a lag of 2 hours and an absorption half-life (the terminal phase) of 8 hours ($0.693/k_a$). A common elimination half-life ($0.693/k_{el}$) of 3.3 hours is found for both routes of administration.

Cross et al. [77, 78] related the cumulative amount-eluted $Q(t)$–time t profiles after dermal absorption of solutes into a perfused limb preparation to Equation (2.75):

$$Q(t) = M_0 \left[1 + \frac{k_a}{k_{el} - k_a} \exp(-k_{el}t) - \frac{k_{el}}{k_{el} - k_a} \exp(-k_a t) \right] \quad (2.75)$$

where M_0 is the initial amount applied to the dermis, k_a is the absorption rate constant for solute absorption from the dermis defined by the fraction remaining in the dermis with time [$F_{dermins} = \exp(-K_a t)$], and k_{el} is the elimination rate constant from the preparation. It can be shown that after some rearrangement, Equation (2.16) in Williams et al. [79] for the perfused porcine skin flap model (Figure 2.12g) simplifies to Equation (2.75).

Reddy et al. [80] have also described a one-compartment skin pharmacokinetic model to describe in vivo absorption. The model is identical to Model III in Wallace and Barnett

[36] when the shunt transport in the latter is assumed to be negligible. They found that the general time lag model derived by McCarley and Bunge [38], predicted the best diffusion in a membrane for most situations.

Each of these models may lead to erroneous estimates for the absorption rate constant if significant tissue distribution occurs in the body (as represented by the dotted lines in Figure 2.12a). We have recently reported that estimates for k_a based on a single exponential (one compartmental) disposition are often twice those for the more correct biexponential (two compartmental) disposition model [81]. Surprisingly, to date, most analyses of in vivo percutaneous absorption kinetics have assumed monoexponential disposition kinetics and have not considered this potential error.

2. Delivery at a constant rate J_s, for a time period T:

$$C_b = \begin{cases} \dfrac{J_{s,invitro}F}{Cl_{body}}\Big[1-\exp\big(-k_{el}\,[t-lag]\big)\Big], t < lag + T \\[3mm] \dfrac{J_{s,invitro}F}{Cl_{body}}\Big[1-\exp\big(-k_{el}\,[t-lag]\big)\Big]\exp\Big[-k_{el}\,(t-T-lag)\Big], t \ge lag + T \end{cases} \tag{2.76}$$

Singh et al. [82] used Equation (2.76) to describe the in vivo absorption kinetics of a number of solutes iontophoresed transdermally in vivo at a presumed constant flux for a time T. Good fits were obtained in the nonlinear regression of each of the data sets.

Imanidis et al. [83] used a similar approach to describe a constant total flux of acyclovir from a patch $J_T = [C_s/(1/k_{pm} + 1/k_{pp})]$ into the bloodstream when acyclovir disposition is described by a biexponential elimination after intravenous (IV) administration [$C_b = A \exp(-\alpha t) + B \exp(-\beta t)$]. The resulting blood concentration (C_b)–time (t) profile is:

$$C_b = \frac{J_T}{V_c k_{el}}\left[1 + \frac{\beta - k_{el}}{\alpha - \beta}\exp(-\alpha t) + \frac{k_{el} - \alpha}{\alpha - \beta}\exp(-\beta t)\right] \tag{2.77}$$

where C_s is the acyclovir concentration in the patch; k_{pm} is the permeability coefficient of acyclovir in the skin; k_{pp} is the permeability coefficient of acyclovir in the rate-controlling patch of the membrane; V_c is the apparent volume of distribution of the central compartment and A, B, α, and β are constants describing the disposition process. Tegeder et al. [84] described muscle microdialysate after topical application by a first-order absorption process after a lag time (t_{lag}) with a two-compartment disposition model and a fraction of drug unbound to tissue (fu):

$$C_{t,free}(t) = \frac{fuk_{21}Dosek_a}{V_c(\alpha - \beta)}$$
$$\left\{\frac{1}{\beta - k_a}\Big[e^{-k_a(t-t_{lag})} - e^{-\beta(t-t_{lag})}\Big] - \frac{1}{\alpha - k_a}\Big[e^{-k_a(t-t_{lag})} - e^{-\alpha(t-t_{lag})}\Big]\right\} \tag{2.78}$$

Hadgraft and Wolff [60] have recently examined the prediction of in vivo plasma data after topical application. Their modeling appeared to adequately describe the in vivo percutaneous absorption kinetics for a range of drugs.

3. Steady-state conditions:

$$C_{bss} = \frac{FJ_{s,invitro}}{Cl_{body}} = \frac{Fk_pC_vA}{Cl_{body}} \tag{2.79}$$

This equation is a reduced form of Equation (2.76) for $t \rightarrow \infty$ and $t < \text{lag} + T$. Equation (2.79) has been used by Roberts and Walters [2] to define the desired patch release rate for a number of drugs in vivo from a knowledge of the drug's clearance and desired plasma concentration.

4. A time-dependent transdermal flux best analyzed assuming a model deduced from in vitro absorption kinetics (section 2.1.8) or deconvolution analysis (section 2.5.4).
5. Modeling Diffusion Explicitly with Compartmental Models

   Recently, a compartmental model was developed to simulate typical diffusion processes in the SC [19]. The compartments were modeled and compared to a diffusion model. The permeability between each compartment was developed via the resistance of the membrane:

$$k_p^i = (n+1)\frac{D_m}{h_m}$$

Using the permeability of the membrane, [19] was able to develop the following equation for the concentration of the middle compartments.

$$\frac{dC_i}{dt} = \frac{n(n+1)}{t_d}(C_{i-1} + C_{i+1} - 2C_i)$$

When compared to the diffusion model and experimental data, the number of compartments needed to give an adequate representation of the trend was found to be five to ten compartments. The fewer the compartments required to model the trend, the more applicable it is to pharmacists looking for a less numerically challenging form of solution.

2.5.2 Diffusion Pharmacokinetic Models

In vivo absorption models usually represent the body as one or more compartments with input into the body via percutaneous absorption. Cooper [85] derived an expression for the total amount of solute excreted into the urine after topical absorption. Other models of Guy, Hadgraft, Kubota, and Chandrasekaran (described earlier) have adopted a similar approach in describing either plasma concentrations or urinary excretion rates from one- or two- compartment models. Cooper assumed diffusion through the skin according to Equation (2.19) into the body, represented as a single compartment. When his model is modified to include an SC–vehicle partition coefficient K_m, the plasma concentration, $C_p(t)$, and the amount excreted into urine, $M(t)$, are defined by the equations:

$$C_p(t) = \frac{Ak_pC}{V_c}\left\{\frac{1-\exp(-k_{el}t)}{k_a} + 2\sum_{n=1}^{\infty}\frac{(-1)^n}{k_{el}-n^2\pi^2/t_d}\left[\exp\left(-\frac{t}{t_d}n^2\pi^2\right)-\exp(-k_{el}t)\right]\right\} \quad (2.80)$$

$$M(t) = Ak_pC_vk_u\left\{\frac{tk_{el}-1+\exp(-k_at)}{k_{el}^2}\right.$$
$$\left. + 2\sum_{n=1}^{\infty}\frac{(-1)^n}{k_{el}-(n^2\pi^2/td)}\left(\frac{t_d}{n^2\pi^2}\left[1-\exp\left(-\frac{t}{t_d}n^2\pi^2\right)\right]-\frac{1}{k_{el}}\left[1-\exp(-k_{el}t)\right]\right)\right\} \quad (2.81)$$

where k_{el} is the total effective elimination rate constant, k_u is the rate constant for excretion in the urine, and V_c is the total effective volume of the compartment.

The steady-state portion of the $M(t)$ versus t plot from Equation (2.81) yields a slope of $k_uk_pA/k_{el} = f_ek_pA$, where k_p is the permeability coefficient $= K_mD_m/h_m$, A is the area of application, k_{el} is the elimination rate constant of the solute from the body, and f_e is the fraction of the solute excreted in the urine. This plot is associated with a lag time t_L of:

$$t_L = \frac{1}{k_{el}} + \frac{t_d}{6} \tag{2.82}$$

where again $t_d = h^2_m/D$, D is the diffusivity of the solute in an SC and h_m is the distance of the pathway of diffusion. Even for multicompartmental disposition kinetics, the total lag time for elimination of a solute is uncoupled and is the sum of epidermal diffusion and pharmacokinetic lag times [86]. When only a finite dose of solute is applied to the skin, the urinary excretion rate is also a function of the vehicle thickness [17].

In practice, the direct application of Equation (2.19) to in vivo absorption may be limited. Equation (2.32), which takes into account the effectiveness of blood flow in removal of solute from the epidermis and the accumulation of solute in the epidermis in vivo, may be more appropriate. Accordingly, the actual steady-state flux is less than k_pAC_v due to this limitation in blood flow clearance, as defined by Equation (2.34). More recently, Liu et al [128] described the Laplace equivalent solution for 2.81:

$$\hat{M}_{u,sc}(s) = A\hat{J}_{sc}(s)\frac{k_u}{s(s+k_{el})} = A\frac{J_{ss,sc}}{s^2}\frac{\sqrt{st_{d,sc}}}{\sinh\sqrt{st_{d,sc}}}\frac{k_u}{(s+k_{el})} \tag{2.83}$$

Where $\hat{M}_{u,sc}(s)$ is the amount excreted in the urine over time in the Laplace domain for a stratum corneum barrier only, with a diffusion time $t_{d,sc}$ with a steady state flux $\hat{J}_{sc}(s)$ per unit area for an area A, $J_{ss,sc} = k_{p,sc}C$, and where $k_{p,sc}$ is the permeability coefficient of SC barrier only. They then went on to describe the expression for $\hat{M}_{u,epi}(s)$ is the amount excreted in the urine over time in the Laplace domain for when both the stratum corneum and viable epidermis contribute to the skin barrier:

$$\hat{M}_{u,epi}(s) = A\hat{J}_{epi}(s)\frac{k_u}{s(s+k_{el})}$$

$$= A\frac{J_{ss,sc}\sqrt{st_{d,sc}}k_u}{s^2\left(B\frac{\sqrt{st_{d,sc}}}{\sqrt{st_{d,ve}}}\cosh\sqrt{st_{d,sc}}\sinh\sqrt{st_{d,ve}} + \sinh\sqrt{st_{d,sc}}\cosh\sqrt{st_{d,ve}}\right)(s+k_{el})} \tag{2.84}$$

Where Eq. 2.84 is based on the expression for epidermal flux, $\hat{J}_{epi}(s)$ defined by:

$$\hat{J}_{epi}(s) = \frac{J_{ss,sc}\sqrt{st_{d,sc}}}{s\left(B\frac{\sqrt{st_{d,sc}}}{\sqrt{st_{d,ve}}}\cosh\sqrt{st_{d,sc}}\sinh\sqrt{st_{d,ve}} + \sinh\sqrt{st_{d,sc}}\cosh\sqrt{st_{d,ve}}\right)} \tag{2.85}$$

Where the parameter B is that used by Bunge and Cleek [26] used a to define the relative permeability of the SC to the VE, as shown in Eq. 7:

$$B = \frac{D_{sc}h_{ve}K_{ce}}{D_{ve}h_{sc}} = \frac{D_{sc}K_{sc}/h_{sc}}{D_{ve}K_{ve}/h_{ve}} = \frac{k_{p,sc}}{k_{p,ve}} \tag{2.86}$$

where $k_{p,sc}$ and $k_{p,ve}$ are permeability coefficient of SC and VE, respectively

2.5.3 PHYSIOLOGICALLY BASED PHARMACOKINETIC AND PHARMACODYNAMIC (PBPK/PD) MODELS

A number of authors have advocated the use of physiological rather than compartmental representations of the body. McDougal [87] has summarized the modeling in this area. These models utilize the

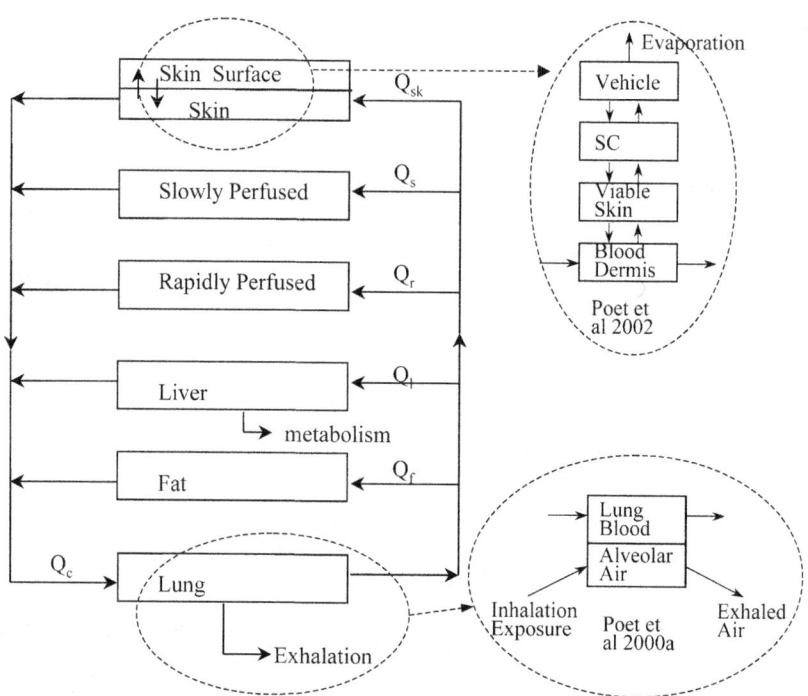

FIGURE 2.16 Physiological pharmacokinetic model for percutaneous absorption. (Adapted from References. 87 and 88.)

numerical integration of a series of differential equations representing each compartment to solve for blood concentration–time profiles after topical application. Individual organs or types of tissues are represented as the compartments with blood flow into and out of the organs defining the transport in the body system. Input into the skin, as a perfused organ, is assumed to follow Fick's first law and may allow for evaporation. Jepson and McDougal (88) have used this model to estimate the permeability constants for halogenated methanes from an aqueous solution after topical application in a whole animal study. Timchalk et al. (89) described an integrated PBPK/PD model for the organophosphate insecticide chlorpyrifos using the McDougal model (Figure 2.16). The percutaneous absorption of perchloroethylene from a soil matrix has been recently described using modification of this model in which solute could evaporate from soil, reversibly partition into SC, and subsequently reversibly partition into dermis [90]. Poet et al. [91, 92] and Thrall et al. [93] used exhaled breath data with the McDougal model to assess the percutaneous absorption of methyl chloroform, trichloroethylene, and toluene. The dermal absorption, evaporation, distribution, metabolism, and excretion of a range of potential toxic solutes has been described using a multicompartment "dermatatoxicokinetic" model based on skin surface, SC dosing device, plasma, tissue, and urine pharmacokinetics after topical and IV administration [94] (Figure 2.17). This modeling has been used to suggest that urinary *p*-nitrophenol may be used as a marker for organophosphate insecticide exposure. The perfuse skin flap enables a simpler model description, as illustrated by its application in the study of jet fuel topical absorption [95].

2.5.4 DECONVOLUTION ANALYSIS IN PHARMACOKINETIC MODELING

Deconvolution analysis is based on the principle that the observed plasma or blood concentration–time profiles, $C_b(t)$, are defined by the percutaneous absorption flux, $J_s(t)$, and the disposition kinetics in the body after a unit IV bolus (impulse) injection, $C_{iv}(t)$:

$$\hat{C}_b(s) = \hat{J}_s(s)\hat{C}_{iv}(s) \tag{2.87}$$

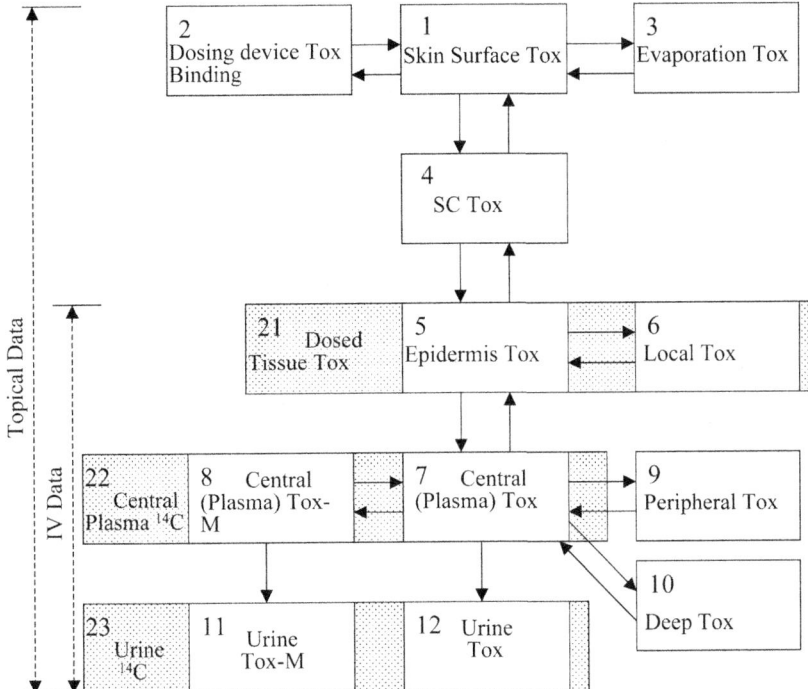

FIGURE 2.17 Dermatotoxicokinetic model for a toxic compound (Tox) and its metabolite (Tox-M). (Adapted from Reference 94.)

Hence from the observed $C_b(t)$ and $C_{iv}(t)$ and inversion of the resulting Laplace domain, expression for $\hat{j}_s(s)$ enables $J_s(t)$ to be defined. This technique is especially useful when the mathematical model for the percutaneous absorption process is not known. A comparison of the observed profile with theoretical profiles may define the underlying model for percutaneous absorption kinetics.

Examples of deconvolution analysis applied in this area include the evaluation of the absorption function from nicotine patches [96], the modeling of subcutaneous absorption kinetics [81], intramuscular absorption kinetics [129] andmodeling of a topically applied local anesthetic agent [97].

2.5.5 Penetration into Tissues Underlying the Topical Application Site

Epidermal concentrations in vivo after topical application, assuming D_e is sufficiently large to approximate a well-stirred state (i.e., compartmental representation), is defined by Equation (2.36) and at long times ($t \rightarrow \infty$) by Equation (2.29) via:

$$C_{ss} = \frac{k_p A C_v}{\mathrm{Cl}_r + \left(k_p A / K_r\right)} \tag{2.88}$$

where Cl_r is the in vivo epidermal clearance.

A similar expression can be defined for subsequent deeper tissues using a compartment in-series model in parallel with removal to the systemic circulation and recirculation (Figure 2.18) after topical application [98]. Transport into deeper tissues could occur by either "convective" blood flow [99] or by diffusion. Nonlinear regressions of experimentally treated and contralateral tissue data with the model used simultaneous numerical integration of a series of differential equations [98, 100, 101]. The analysis showed that, whereas direct deep tissue penetration was apparent at early times, recirculation of drug from the systemic circulation accounted for tissue levels at longer times to

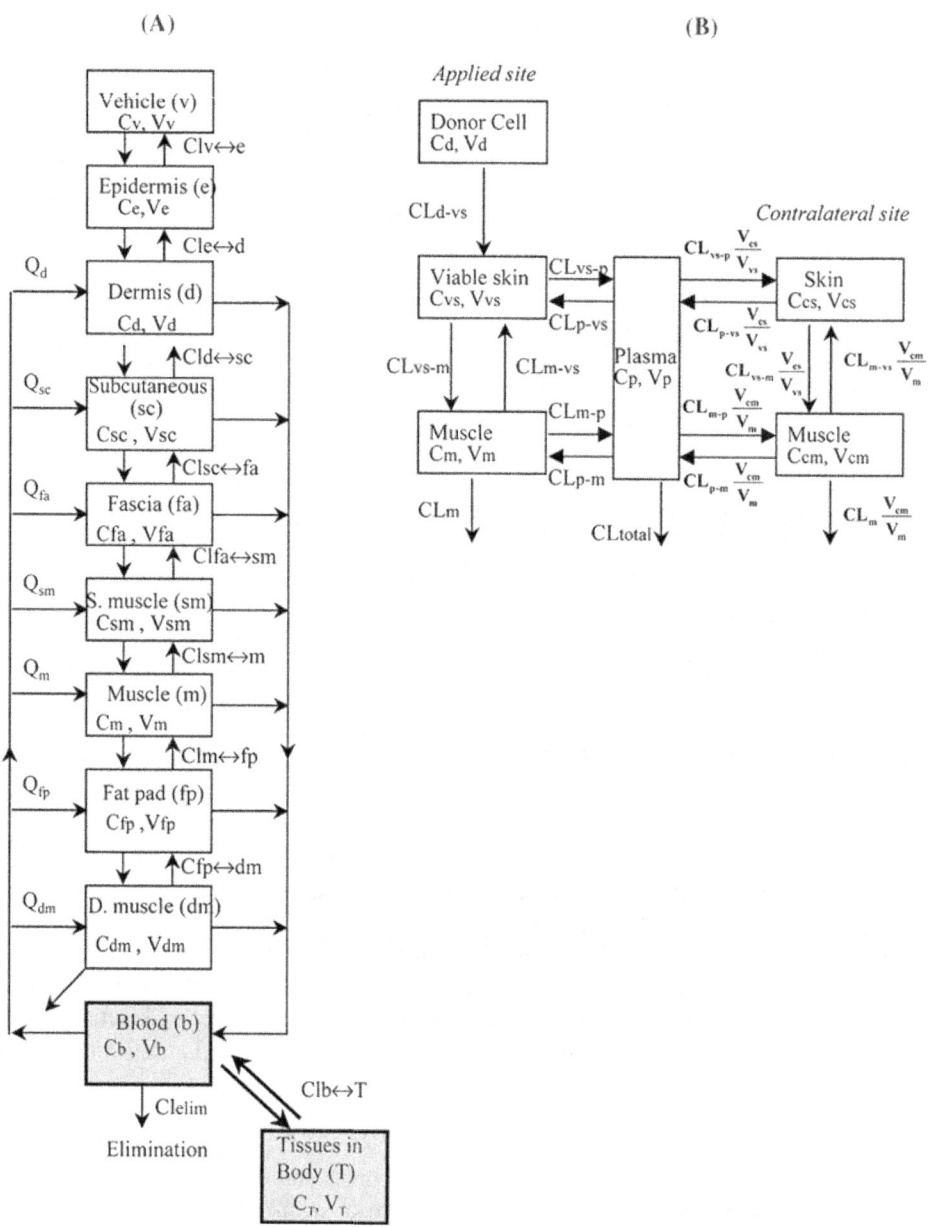

FIGURE 2.18 A pharmacokinetic model for local deep tissue penetration after topical application. The main symbols are Q, blood flow; C, concentration; V, volume; and CL, clearance as they relate to the various tissues and the rest of the body. (Adapted from (A) Reference 98 and (B) Reference 105.)

define deep tissue penetration of dermally applied solutes (Figure 2.18A). Roberts and Cross [102] have suggested that the half-life for elimination of a solute in such tissues is dependent not only on tissue blood flow (Q_p) but also on the fraction unbound of solute in the tissue (fu_T) and blood (fu_B), as well as the apparent unbound volume of distribution (V_T):

$$t_{1/2} \approx \frac{0.693\, fu_B V_T}{fu_T Q_p} \tag{2.89}$$

A further set of studies has been reported using stripped skin and an integrated application site—a contralateral site model (Figure 2.18b) [103, 104]. This work extended earlier work [101, 105–107], which showed significant direct penetration to deeper tissues underlining the topical application site in both rats and in humans. As discussed earlier, Tegeder et al. [84] have described muscle microdialysate pharmacokinetics [Equation (2.78)] after topical application.

More recent work by the authors used a dermal diffusion model in which there is both convective (via the blood supply and lymphatics) and diffusion facilitated transport of solutes in the dermis [130, 131]. This total transport to deeper tissues is described by the dispersion coefficient D_t and is given by the sum of convective and diffusional transport of a solute:

$$D_{\mathrm{disp}} = D_{\mathrm{diff}} + D_{\mathrm{conv}} \tag{2.90}$$

This term is then incorporated in the expressions that describe concentration changes in the dermis and in the blood in pdes:

$$V_d \frac{\partial C_d}{\partial t} = V_d D_t \frac{\partial^2 C_d}{\partial x^2} - ps\left(C_d fu_d - C_b fu_b\right) \tag{2.91}$$

$$V_b \frac{\partial C_b}{\partial t} = -Q_b C_b + ps\left(C_d fu_d - C_b fu_b\right) \tag{2.92}$$

The concentration of solute in the dermis at distance x in the Laplace domain $\hat{C}_d(x,s)$ can be derived from these equations after taking into account the initial and boundary conditions and has been expressed as [132]:

$$\hat{C}_d(x,s) = \frac{J_0}{s\sqrt{\left(s+g(s)\right)D_t}} \exp\left(-x\sqrt{\left(s+g(s)\right)/D_t}\right) \tag{2.93}$$

Where the total diffusivity D_t is the sum of convective and diffusion transport (and, in general, reduces to diffusion only for poorly protein bound drugs), $g(s)$ is defined by

$$g(s) = \frac{fu_d q_b ps + ps fu_d v_b s}{q_b + fu_b ps + v_b s} \tag{2.94}$$

and q_b, ps and v_b are the blood flow rate, the permeability surface area product for blood capillaries and blood capillaries volume per unit volume of dermis, respectively. This modelling allows the half-life described in equation 2.89 to be more fully described in terms of blood flow Q_p and capillary wall permeability surface area product PS [132]:

$$t_{1/2} = \frac{0.693\left(Q_p + fu_B PS\right)V_T}{fu_d Q_p PS}, \; i.e. = \frac{q_b + fu_B ps}{fu_d q_p ps} \tag{2.95}$$

This modelling explains why highly plasma protein bound drugs may be shunted to deeper tissues more so than those which lack this binding – providing targeted drug delivery to inflamed tissues below a topical application site.

More recent modelling has considered the impact of the viable epidermis in series with dermal capillary loops and lymphatic vessels. Capillary loops are responsible for the uptake of low-molecular-weight drugs, while lymphatic vessels redistribute drugs with higher molecular-weight.

One way to model the drug uptake from the capillary loops is through the implementation of a two-layer distributed-elimination model [132]:

$$\frac{\partial C_{ve}}{\partial t} = D_{ve}\frac{\partial^2 C_{ve}}{\partial x^2} \tag{2.96}$$

$$\frac{\partial C_d}{\partial t} = D_d\frac{\partial^2 C_d}{\partial x^2} - k_e C_d \tag{2.97}$$

Where C_{ve} and C_d are solute concnetrations in the viable epidermis and dermis and D_{ve} and D_d is the diffusion coefficient in the epidermis and dermis, k_e is the elimination rate and x is the depth within the dermis.

In previous models, the drug uptake was usually depicted via a sink condition that was placed at an arbitrary depth in the dermis. However, the distributed-elimination model incorporates the capillary network via an elimination rate constant. Solving the two-layer model in the Laplace domain gives the following expressions:

$$C_{ve}^{ss}(x) = \frac{J_{sc}}{\sqrt{D_{ve}k_e}} + \frac{J_{sc}h_{cl}}{D_{ve}}\left(1 - \frac{x}{h_{cl}}\right) \tag{2.98}$$

$$C_d^{ss}(x) = \frac{J_{sc}}{\sqrt{D_d k_e}}\exp\left(\sqrt{\frac{k_e}{D_d}}(h_{cl} - x)\right) \tag{2.99}$$

where J_{sc} is the flux from the SC, h_{cl} is the depth of the capillary loops and ss represents the steady-state.

A three-dimensional capillary loop model that explicitly considers the geometry and spacing of the capillary loops was developed [133]. The capillary loops in this model were presented to give an in silico simulation of typical drug transport in the viable skin. The results of this model were compared to both the distributed elimination model and the sink condition case and showed that the capillary model much more effectively modelled viable skin concentration. This model has now been further developed in a computational form to better understand the impact of elevated skin temperatures on transdermal drug delivery and dermal clearance [63].

2.5.6 Pharmacodynamic Modeling

In principle, established pharmacodynamic models used in whole-body pharmacokinetic modeling can be directly used when solutes are delivered by the skin. Complexities can exist when the site of drug targeting is the skin itself. Imanidis et al. [83] showed that the antiviral efficacy to HSV-1 skin infections of acyclovir was directly related to the logarithm of the flux from transdermal patches—consistent with classical log dose–response relationships. However, an equivalent systemic dose was relatively ineffective.

Beastall et al. [108] examined the onset of erythema (t_E) as a function of solute concentration (C_o). Applying Fick's law of diffusion, they obtained the expression:

$$\log\frac{n_E}{h_m} = \log\left(C_v t_E^{3/2}\right) + \log\left[\frac{K_m}{1 + K_m / p^{1/2}}\right] + \log\left[\frac{8D_{sc}^{3/2}}{\pi^{1/2}h_m^3}\right] - \frac{h_m^2}{9.2D_{sc}t_E} \tag{2.100}$$

where D_{sc} is the diffusion coefficient of nicotinate in the SC, K_m is its partition coefficient between vehicle and skin, h_m is the diffusion path length, p is the ratio of the diffusion coefficients of the nicotinate in the vehicle and the skin, and n_E is the concentration of nicotinate required to trigger erythema. This expression showed a linear relationship should and did exist between $\log C_v t_E^{2/3}$ and $1/t_E$. The gradient of the relationship D_{sc}/h_m^2 was greatly affected by the co-administration of the enhancer urea.

The human skin–blanching assay for evaluating the bioequivalence of topical corticosteroid products should follow standardized guidelines as developed by the U.S. Food and Drug Administration (FDA) in 1995. Demana et al. [109] evaluated the area under the effect curve (AUEC), also called the effect (E), for both visual and chromameter-derived data. The visual data were best described by a sigmoidal E_{max} model [Equation (2.101)] while the chromameter data were described by a simple E_{max}' model [Equation (2.102)]:

$$E = E_0 \pm \frac{E_{max}D}{D + ED_{50}} \tag{2.101}$$

$$E = E_0 \pm \frac{E_{max}D^\gamma}{D^\gamma + ED^\gamma_{50}} \tag{2.102}$$

where E_{max} is the maximal AUEC, D is the dose duration, ED_{50} is the dose duration for half- maximal E, and g is a sigmoidicity factor related to the shape of the curve. The parameter E_0, not explicitly stated in the modeling by Demana et al. [109], should be included in the model fitting to correct for baseline readings [110]. Smith et al. [111] have pointed out that they had corrected for E_0 using unmedicated site values in their earlier work [109]. A key aspect in this mathematical modeling is varying the dose administered by varying the duration of application. Varying dose duration is then used to relate the vasoconstrictor response to a range of corticosteroid amounts. Demana et al. [109] used a weighting of 1/AUEC and a number of goodness-of-fit criteria in their analyses.

More recently, Cordero et al. [112] developed an index to predict topical efficiency of a series of nonsteroidal antiinflammatory drugs. This index took into account both the biopharmaceutical aspect, based on the maximal flux, and the pharmacodynamic aspect, based on the ability to inhibit cyclooxygenase-2 in vitro.

2.6 MODELING WITH FACILITATED TRANSDERMAL DELIVERY

2.6.1 Iontophoresis

A number of mathematical models are used in iontophoresis. As described by Kasting [113], these are generally defined by the Nernst Planck and Poisson equations. Of particular practical usefulness is the iontophoretic flux of a solute through the epidermis. This flux can be incorporated into various pharmacokinetic models for the body to enable the description of plasma concentration and urinary excretion–time data. Singh et al. [82] examined in vivo plasma data after iontophoretic transport with simple pharmacokinetic models. In vivo blood concentrations for most solutes delivered by iontophoresis appear to be able to be described by zero-order input into a one-compartment model [Equations (2.76) and (2.79)] [82].

The iontophoretic flux depends on a number of factors, including solute ionization, interaction of solutes with pore walls, solute size, solute shape, solute charge, Debye layer thickness, solute concentration, and presence of extraneous ions, which are all accounted for. We have recently proposed an integrating expression for the flux of the jth solute [114]:

$$J_{jiont} = C_j \left[\frac{2\mu_j fi_j F z_j I_T \Omega PRT_J}{(k_{s,a} + k_{s,c})\left[1 + fu_i \theta_{ju} + fi_j \theta_{ji}\right]} \pm (1 - \sigma_j) v_m \right] \tag{2.103}$$

where Cj is the concentration of the j-th solute, mj is its mobility, fi_j and fu_i are ionized and unionized fractions of the solute (respectively), z_j is its charge, PRT_j is a partial restriction term, s_j is the reflection coefficient term, v_m is the velocity of water flow across the membrane, IT is the total current across the membrane, O is the permselectivity for cations, $k_{s,a}$ and $k_{s,c}$ are conductivities of the anode and cathode solutions (respectively), y_{ju} and y_{ji} are parameters describing the interaction of unionized and ionized fractions of the solute with the pore, and F is Faraday's constant.

Dermal and subcutaneous concentrations of solutes after in vivo iontophoretic application can also be determined in terms of clearance by blood supply to the tissue, clearance to deeper tissues, and influx by iontophoresis [115].

2.6.2 SONOPHORESIS

The sonophoretic iontophoretic flux can also be included in pharmacokinetic models in a manner analogous to that described under "Iontophoresis." Mitragotri et al. [116] have suggested that sonophoresis induces cavitation. They have suggested that the sonophoretic permeability $k_{p\,sono}$ can be defined in terms of the passive permeability coefficient k_p (unit: cm/hr) and the solute octanol–water partition coefficient Kow as:

$$k_{p\,sono} = k_p + 2.5 \times 10^{-5} K_{ow}^{3/4} \qquad (2.104)$$

Later work examined the threshold frequency dependency [117] and transport at low frequency [118].

2.7 PRACTICAL ISSUES IN APPLYING MATHEMATICAL MODELS TO PERCUTANEOUS ABSORPTION DATA

A major limitation in a number of reported percutaneous absorption studies, including those from our laboratories, has been the assumption of a given mathematical model. Whether that model is strictly the most appropriate one is often difficult to confirm. Most studies appear to have used the simplest model, as defined by Equation (2.1), in which the steady-state flux and lag time are defined by the steady-state portion of the curve. There are a number of limitations in using such a model, as discussed by Robinson [61] and other authors.

Robinson [61] points out that errors can be made if (1) the burst influx and lag containing through flux are represented by a steady-state approximation at early times; (2) an infinite vehicle is assumed when the concentration is actually declining due to the finite volume used; (3) penetration of a solute by passive diffusion also involves modification of the skin barrier properties (solute–skin interactions); (4) vehicle effects on solute concentration, e.g., evaporation or skin permeability (vehicle–skin interactions) exist; (5) skin reservoir effects exist, as illustrated by the extensive uptake of sunscreens into, but not necessarily through, the skin [119]; (6) discrepancies exist between in vitro and in vivo absorption due to the role of capillaries in absorption in vivo; and (7) the resistance barrier of the skin is compromised.

The expressions for a number of the more complex models contain the necessary correction factors to overcome some of the inherent limitations in the simplest model representation of data. For instance, the steady-state flux may be affected by the sampling rate from the receptor compartment, as defined by Equation (2.34). The lag time will be dependent on both this clearance and the volume ratios of the membrane and receptor phases, corrected for partitioning effects, as defined by Equation (2.35). A different set of correction factors apply if an interfacial barrier or desorption rate constant exists [Equations (2.39) and (2.40)]. As Kubota et al. [46, 47] point out, although a simple compartmental model may describe percutaneous penetration kinetics, the parameters obtained may not necessarily represent the membrane diffusion and partition coefficient.

Relating data to a specific model using nonlinear regression techniques also requires an appropriate weighting of the data in accordance with the underlying errors associated with the data. In the absence of known error structures, a weighting of $1/y$obs may be appropriate. This weighting assumes that the coefficient of variation (standard deviation/mean) of the data is relatively constant.

Some of the dilemmas in the mathematical modeling of percutaneous absorption are enunciated in the letters to pharmaceutical research written by Singh et al. [110] and Smith et al. [111], especially in relation to pharmacodynamic modeling of skin blanching after topical application. Issues raised include (1) reliability of visual and chromameter methods; (2) analysis of "naive" pool data by nonlinear regression versus mixed-effect modeling; (3) baseline correction; (4) consistency of parameter values, e.g., sigmoidicity with independent literature estimates; (5) precision of critical small and long dose duration data; and (6) subject (skin) selection. Smith et al. [111] suggest that the current methodology prepared by the FDA requires further evaluation.

Finally, there is probably a greater need for deconvolution techniques to be used with in vivo data. Such techniques do not make any assumption as to the underlying mathematical model of the absorption kinetics. Indeed, such an approach is a powerful way of determining whether assumed models are indeed applicable [81].

2.8   CONCLUSION

This chapter has attempted to review some of the more important mathematical models used in percutaneous absorption. Given the substantive number of reported models and the complexity in many of the models, the overview is limited in its ability to give each of the models the credit they may deserve. However, it is hoped that the emphasis on the more practical models has enabled this fairly complex area to be presented in a manner useful for ready reference.

Our analysis has considered a number of boundary conditions associated with solute transport across a membrane, including clearance from the receptor solution, clearance from the membrane, and diffusion in an underlying layer (e.g., epidermis below the SC). Each situation is defined by a steady-state flux Jss and lag time of the forms:

$$J_{ss} = \frac{k_p C_v}{1 + M} \tag{2.105}$$

$$\text{lag} = \frac{t_d}{6} N$$

where M and N are functions of the transport processes below the membrane. When the clearance of the solute is very high (Cl $\gg k_p$), J_{ss} approaches the usual $k_p C_v$. Approximations for the lag time are less well defined so that the use of lag time as an estimate for td is much less justified. Consequently, there are dangers of parameter misspecification with obvious consequences when extensions such as structure–transport relationships are based on the uncorrected parameters. Ultimately, therefore, mathematical modeling in this area is a balance between simplicity and an accurate representation of the underlying processes.

ACKNOWLEDGMENT

We thank the NH&MRC of Australia, PAH Research Foundation, and the NSW and Qld Lions Medical Research Foundation for the support of this work.

REFERENCES

1. Roberts MS, Anissimov YG, Gonsalvez RA. Mathematical models in percutaneous absorption. In: Bronaugh RL, Maibach HI, eds. Percutaneous Absorption Drugs– Cosmetics–Mechanisms– Methodology. New York: Marcel Dekker, 1999:3–55.
2. Roberts MS, Walters KA. The relationship between structure and barrier function of skin. In: Roberts MS, Walters KA, eds. Dermal Absorption and Toxicity Assessment. New York: Marcel Dekker, 1998.
3. Crank J. The Mathematics of Diffusion. 2nd ed. Oxford: Clarendon Press, 1975.
4. Yano Y, Yamaoka K, Aoyama Y, Tanaka H. Two-compartment dispersion model for analysis of organ perfusion system of drugs by fast inverse Laplace transform (FILT). J Pharmacokinet Biopharm 1989a; 17:179–202.
5. Yano Y, Yamaoka K, Tanaka H. A non-linear least squares program, MULTI(FILT), based on fast inverse Laplace transform (FILT) for microcomputers. Chem Pharm Bull 1989; 37:1535–1538.
6. Purves RD. Accuracy of numerical inversions of Laplace transforms for pharmacokinetic parameter estimation. J Pharm Sci 1995; 84:71–74.

7. Pirot F, Kalia YN, Stinchcomb AL, Keating G, Bunge A, Guy RH. Characterization of the permeability barrier of human skin in vivo. Proc Natl Acad Sci USA 1997; 94(4):1562–1567.

8. Siddiqui O, Roberts MS, Polack AE. Percutaneous absorption of steroids relative contributions of epidermal penetration and dermal clearance. J Pharmacokinet Biopharm 1989; 17(Aug):405–424.

9. Roberts MS. Structure-permeability considerations in percutaneous absorption. In: Scott RC, Guy RH, Hadgraft J, Bodde HE, eds. Prediction of Percutaneous Penetration. 1991. Vol. 2. London: IBC Technical Services:210–228.

10. Anissimov YG, Roberts MS. Diffusion modeling of percutaneous absorption kinetics: Effects of flow rate, receptor sampling rate and viable epidermal resistance for a constant donor concentration. J Pharm Sci 1999; 88(11):1201–1209.

11. Parry GE, Bunge AL, Silcox GD, Pershing LK, Pershing DW. Percutaneous-absorption of benzonic-acid across human skin. 1. In vitro experiments and mathematical modeling. Pharm Res 1990; 7(3):230–236.

12. Scheuplein RJ, Blank IH. Mechanism of percutaneous absorption IV. Penetration of non-electrolytes (alcohols) from aqueous solutions and from pure liquids. J Invest Dermatol 1973; 60:286–296.

13. Roberts MS, Anderson RA, Swarbrick J, Moore DE. The percutaneous absorption of phenolic compounds: the mechanism of diffusion across the stratum corneum. J Pharm Pharmacol 1978; 30(8):486–490.

14. Guy RH, Hadgraft J. Physicochemical interpretation of the pharmacokinetics of percutaneous absorption. J Pharmacokinet Biopharm 1983; 11(2):189–203.

15. Guy RH, Hadgraft J, Maibach HI. Percutaneous absorption: multidose pharmacokinetics. Int J Pharm 1983; 17:23–28.

16. Kubota K, Ishizaki T. A theoretical consideration of percutaneous drug absorption. J Pharmacokinet Biopharm 1985; 13(1):55–72.

17. Cooper ER, Berner B. Finite dose pharmacokinetics of skin penetration. J Pharm Sci 1985; 74(10): 1100–1102.

18. Anissimov YG, Roberts MS. Diffusion modeling of percutaneous absorption kinetics: 2. Finite vehicle volume and solvent deposited solids. J Pharm Sci 2001; 90(4):504–520.

19. Kasting GB. Kinetics of finite dose absorption through skin 1. Vanillylnonanamide. J Pharm Sci 2001; 90(2):202–212.

20. Scheuplein RJ, Ross LW. Mechanism of percutaneous absorption. V. Percutaneous absorption of solvent deposited solids. J Invest Dermatol 1974; 62:353–360.

21. Kakemi K, Kameda H, Kakemi M, Veda M, Koizumi T. Model studies on percutaneous absorption and transport in the ointment. I. Theoretical aspects. Chem Pharm Bull 1975; 23(9):2109–2113.

22. Guy RH, Hadgraft J. Theoretical description relating skin penetration to the thickness of the applied medicament. Int J Pharm 1980; 6:321–332.

23. Hadgraft J. Calculations of drug release rates from controlled release devices. The slab. Int J Pharm 1979; 2:177–194.

24. Hadgraft J. The epidermal reservoir: a theoretical approach. Int J Pharm 1979; 2:265–274.

25. Cleek RL, Bunge AL. A new method for estimating dermal absorption from chemical exposure. 1. General approach. Pharm Res 1993; 10(4):497–506.

26. Bunge AL, Cleek RL. A new method for estimating dermal absorption from chemical exposure: 2. Effect of molecular weight and octanol–water partitioning. Pharm Res 1995; 12(1):88–95.

27. Seko N, Bando H, Lim CW, Yamashita F, Hashida M. Theoretical analysis of the effect of cutaneous metabolism on skin permeation of parabens based on a two-layer skin diffusion/metabolism model. Biol Pharm Bull 1999; 22(3):281–287.

28. Scheuplein RJ, Morgan LJ. "Bound water" in keratin membranes measured by a microbalance technique. Nature 1967; 214(87):456–458.

29. Roberts MS, Triggs EJ, Anderson RA. Permeability of solutes through biological membranes measured by a desorption technique. Nature 1975; 275:225–227.

30. Watkinson AC, Bunge AL, Hadgraft J, Naik A. Computer simulation of penetrant concentration-depth profiles in the stratum corneum. Int J Pharm 1992; 87:175–182.

31. Anissimov YG, Roberts MS. Diffusion modeling of percutaneous absorption kinetics: 3. Variable diffusion and partition coefficients, consequences for stratum corneum depth profiles and desorption kinetics. J Pharm Sci 2004; 93(2):470–487.

32. Chandrasekaran SK, Bayne W, Shaw JE. Pharmacokinetics of drug permeation through human skin. J Pharm Sci 1978; 67(10):1370–1374.

33. Iordanskii AL, Feldstein MM, Markin VS, Hadgraft J, Plate NA. Modeling of the drug delivery from a hydrophilic transdermal therapeutic system across polymer membrane. Eur J Pharm Biopharm 2000; 49(3):287–293.

34. Higuchi WI. Diffusional models useful in biopharmaceutics. Drug release rate process. J Pharm Sci 1967; 56(3):315–324.
35. Riegelman S. Pharmacokinetic factors affecting epidermal penetration and percutaneous adsorption. Clin Pharmacol Ther 1974; 16(5 Part 2):873–883.
36. Wallace SM, Barnett G. Pharmacokinetic analysis of percutaneous absorption: evidence of parallel penetration pathways for methotrexate. J Pharmacokinet Biopharm 1978; 6(4):315–325.
37. McCarley KD, Bunge AL. Physiologically relevant two-compartment pharmacokinetic models for skin. J Pharm Sci 2000; 89(9):1212–1235.
38. McCarley KD, Bunge AL. Physiologically relevant one-compartment pharmacokinetic models for skin. 1. Development of models. J Pharm Sci 1998; 87(4):470–481.
39. Zatz J. Simulation studies of skin permeation. J Soc Cosmet Chem 1992; 43:37–48.
40. Roberts MS, Anderson RA, Swarbrick J. Permeability of human epidermis to phenolic compounds. J Pharm Pharmacol 1977; 29(11):677–683.
41. Wu MS. Determination of concentration-dependent water diffusivity in a keratinous membrane. J Pharm Sci 1983; 72(12):1421–1423.
42. Giengler G, Knoch A, Merkle HP. Modeling and numerical computation of drug transport in laminates: model case evaluation of transdermal delivery system. J Pharm Sci 1986; 75(1):9–15.
43. Higuchi WI, Higuchi T. Theoretical analysis of diffusional movements through heterogeneous barriers. J Am Pharm Assoc Sci Ed 1960; 49(9):598–606.
44. Chandrasekaran SK, Michaels AS, Campbell PS, Shaw JE. Scopolamine permeation through human skin in vitro. AIChE J 1976; 22(5):828–832.
45. Roberts MS, Cross SE, Pellett MA. Skin transport. In: Walters KA, ed. Dermatological and transdermal formulations. New York: Marcel Dekker, 2002:89–195.
46. Kubota K, Sznitowska M, Maibach HI. Percutaneous absorption: a single layer model. J Pharm Sci 1993; 82(5):450–456.
47. Kubota K, Koyama E, Twizell EH. Dual sorption model for the nonlinear percutaneous permeation kinetics of timolol. J Pharm Sci 1993; 82(12):1205–1208.
48. Ando HY, Ho NFH, Higuchi WI. Skin as an active metabolising barrier. 1. Theoretical analysis of topical bioavailability. J Pharm Sci 1977; 66(11):1525–1528.
49. Yu CD, Fox JL, Ho NFH, Higuchi WI. Physical model evaluation of topical prodrug delivery-simultaneous transport and bioconversion of vidarabine 5′-valerate. Part 1. Physical model development. J Pharm Sci 1979; 68(11):1341–1346.
50. Yu CD, Fox JL, Ho NFH, Higuchi WI. Physical model evaluation of topical prodrug delivery-simultaneous transport and bioconversion of vidarabine 5′-valerate. Part 2. Parameter determinations. J Pharm Sci 1979; 68(11):1347–1357.
51. Yu CD, Gordon NA, Fox JL, Higuchi WI, Ho NFH. Physical model evaluation of topical prodrug delivery-simultaneous transport and bioconversion of vidarabine 5′-valerate. Part 5. Mechanistic analysis of influence of non-homogeneous enzyme distributions in hairless mouse skin. J Pharm Sci 1980; 69(7):775–780.
52. Fox JL, Yu CD, Higuchi WI, Ho NFH. General physical model for simultaneous diffusion and metabolism in biological membranes. Computational approach for the steady state case. Int J Pharm 1979; 2:41–57.
53. Hadgraft J. Theoretical aspects of metabolism in the epidermis. Int J Pharm 1980; 4:229–239.
54. Guy RH, Hadgraft J. Percutaneous metabolism with saturable enzyme kinetics. Int J Pharm 1982; 11:187–197.
55. Kubota K, Ademola J, Maibach HI. Simultaneous diffusion and metabolism of betamethasone 17-valerate in the living skin equivalent. J Pharm Sci 1995; 84(12):1478–1481.
56. Guy RH, Hadgraft J. A theoretical description of the effects of volatility and substantivity on percutaneous absorption. Int J Pharm 1984a; 18:139–147.
57. Guy RH, Hadgraft J. Pharmacokinetics of percutaneous absorption with concurrent metabolism. Int J Pharm 1984b; 20:43–51.
58. Guy RH, Hadgraft J. Percutaneous absorption kinetics of topically applied agents liable to surface loss. J Soc Cosmet Chem 1984; 35:103–113.
59. Guy RH, Hadgraft J. Prediction of drug disposition kinetics in skin and plasma following topical administration. J Pharm Sci 1984; 73(7):883–887.
60. Hadgraft J, Wolff HM. In vitro/in vivo correlations in transdermal drug delivery. In: Roberts MS, Walters KA, eds. Dermal Absorption and Toxicity Assessment. New York: Marcel Dekker, 1998.
61. Robinson PJ. Prediction: simple risk models and overview of dermal risk assessment. In: Roberts MS, Walters KA, eds. Dermal Absorption and Toxicity Assessment. New York: Marcel Dekker, 1998.

62. Magnusson BM, Anissimov YG, Cross SE, Roberts MS. Molecular size as the main determinant of solute maximum flux across the skin. J Invest Dermatol 2004;122: 993–999.

63. LaCount TD, Zhang Q, Hao J, Ghosh P, Raney SG, Talattof A, Kasting GB, Li SK. Modeling Temperature-Dependent Dermal Absorption and Clearance for Transdermal and Topical Drug Applications. AAPS J. 2020 May 10;22(3):70.

64. Reifenrath WG, Robinson PB. In vitro skin evaporation and penetration characteristics of mosquito repellents. J Pharm Sci 1982; 71(9):1014–1018.

65. Saiyasombati P, Kasting GB. Disposition of benzyl alcohol after topical application to human skin in vitro. J Pharm Sci 2003; 92(10):2128–2139.

66. Scheuplein RJ. Mechanism of percutaneous absorption. II. Transient diffusion and the relative importance of various routes of skin penetration. J Invest Dermatol 1967; 48(1):79–88.

67. Ghanem AH, Mahmoud H, Higuchi WI, Rohr DD, Borsadia S, Liu P, Fox JL, Good WR. The effects of ethanol on the transport of bestradiol and other permeants in the hairless mouse skin. II. A new quantitative approach. J Control Release 1987; 6:75–83.

68. Hatanaka T, Inuma M, Sugibayashi K, Morimoto Y. Prediction of skin permeability of drugs. II. Development of composite membrane as a skin alternative. Int J Pharm 1992; 79:21–28.

69. Tojo K, Chiang CC, Chien YW. Drug permeation across the skin: effect of penetrant hydrophilicity. J Pharm Sci 1987; 76(2):123–126.

70. Yamashita F, Yoshioka T, Koyama Y, Okamoto H, Sezaki H, Hashida M. Analysis of skin penetration enhancement based on a two layer skin diffusion model with polar and non-polar routes in the stratum corneum: dose-dependent effect of 1-geranylazacyclo- heptan-2-one on drugs with different lipophilicities. Biol Pharm Bull 1993; 16(7):690–697.

71. Edwards DA, Langer R. A linear theory of transdermal transport phenomena. J Pharm Sci 1994; 83(9):1315–1334.

72. Malkinson FD, Ferguson EH. Percutaneous absorption of hydrocortisone-4-C14 in two human subjects. J Invest Dermatol 1955; 25(5):281–283.

73. Vickers CF. Stratum corneum reservoir for drugs. Adv Biol Skin 1972; 12:177–189.

74. Reddy MB, Guy RH, Bunge AL. Does epidermal turnover reduce percutaneous penetration? Pharm Res 2000; 17(11):1414–1419.

75. Roberts MS, Cross SE, Anissimov YG. Factors affecting the formation of a skin reservoir for topically applied solutes. Skin Pharmacol Appl Skin Physiol 2004; 17:3–16.

76. Rohatagi S, Barrett JS, Dewitt KE, Morales RJ. Integrated pharmacokinetics and metabolic modeling of selegiline and metabolites after transdermal administration. Biopharm Drug Dispos 1997; 18(7):567–584.

77. Cross SE, Wu ZY, Roberts MS. Effect of perfusion flow rate on the tissue uptake of solutes after dermal application using the rat isolated perfused hindlimb preparation. J Pharm Pharmacol 1994; 46:844–850.

78. Cross SE, Wu ZY, Roberts MS. The effect of protein binding on the deep tissue penetration and elution of transdermally applied water, salicylic acid, lignocaine and diazepam in the perfused rat. J Pharmacol Exp Ther 1996; 277:366–374.

79. Williams PL, Carver MP, Riviere JE. A physiologically relevant pharmacokinetic model of xenobiotic percutaneous absorption using the isolated perfused porcine skin flap. J Pharm Sci 1990; 79(4):305–311.

80. Reddy MB, McCarley KD, Bunge AL. Physiologically relevant one- compartment pharmacokinetic model for skin. 2. Comparison of models when combined with a systemic pharmacokinetic model. J Pharm Sci 1998; 87(4):482–490.

81. Roberts MS, Lipschitz S, Campbell AJ, Wanwimolruk S, Mcqueen EG, Mcqueen M. Modeling of subcutaneous absorption kinetics of infusion solutions in the elderly using technetium. J Pharmacokinet Biopharm 1997; 25(1):1–19.

82. Singh P, Roberts MS, Maibach HI. Modeling of plasma levels of drugs following transdermal iontophoresis. J Control Release 1995; 33:293–298.

83. Imanidis G, Song W, Lee PH, Su MH, Kern ER, Higuchi WI. Estimation of skin target site acyclovir concentrations following controlled transdermal drug delivery in topical and systemic treatment of cutaneous HSV -1 infections in hairless mice. Pharm Res 1994; 11(7):1035–1041.

84. Tegeder I, Muth-Selbach U, Lotsch J, Rusing G, Oelkers R, Brune K, Meller S, Kelm GR, Sorgel F, Geisslinger G. Application of microdialysis for the determination of muscle and subcutaneous tissue concentrations after oral and topical ibuprofen administration. Clin Pharmacol Ther 1999; 65(4):357–368.

85. Cooper ER. Pharmacokinetics of skin penetration. J Pharm Sci 1976; 65(9):1396–1397.

86. Cooper ER. Effect of diffusional lag time on multicompartmental pharmacokinetics for transepidermal infusion. J Pharm Sci 1979; 68(11):1469–1470.

87. McDougal JN. Prediction-physiological models. In: Roberts MS, Walters KA, eds. Dermal Absorption and Toxicity Assessment. New York: Marcel Dekker, 1998.

88. Jepson GW, McDougal JN. Physiologically based modeling of nonsteady state dermal absorption of halogenated methanes from an aquous solution. Toxicol Appl Pharmacol 1997; 144:315–324.

89. Timchalk C, Nolan RJ, Mendrala AL, Dittenber DA, Brzak KA, Mattsson JL. A physiologically based pharmacokinetic and pharmacodynamic (PBPK/PD) model for the organophosphate insecticide chlorpyrifos in rats and humans. Toxicol Sci 2002; 66(1):34–53.

90. Poet TS, Weitz KK, Gies RA, Edwards JA, Thrall KD, Corley RA, Tanojo H, Hui X, Maibach HI, Wester RC. PBPK modeling of the percutaneous absorption of perchloroethylene from a soil matrix in rats and humans. Toxicol Sci 2002; 67(1):17–31.

91. Poet TS, Thrall KD, Corley RA, Hui X, Edwards JA, Weitz KK, Maibach HI, Wester RC. Utility of real time breath analysis and physiologically based pharmacokinetic modeling to determine the percutaneous absorption of methyl chloroform in rats and humans. Toxicol Sci 2000; 54(1):42–51.

92. Poet TS, Corley RA, Thrall KD, Edwards JA, Tanojo H, Weitz KK, Hui X, Maibach HI, Wester RC. Assessment of the percutaneous absorption of trichloroethylene in rats and humans using MS/MS real-time breath analysis and physiologically based pharmacokinetic modeling. Toxicol Sci 2000; 56(1):61–72.

93. Thrall KD, Weitz KK, Woodstock AD. Use of real-time breath analysis and physiologically based pharmacokinetic modeling to evaluate dermal absorption of aqueous toluene in human volunteers. Toxicol Sci 2002; 68(2):280–287.

94. Qiao GL, Chang SK, Brooks JD, Riviere JE. Dermatoxicokinetic modeling of *p*-nitrophenol and its conjugation metabolite in swine following topical and intravenous administration. Toxicol Sci 2000; 54(2):284–294.

95. Riviere JE, Brooks JD, Monteiro-Riviere NA, Budsaba K, Smith CE. Dermal absorption and distribution of topically dosed jet fuels jet-A, JP-8, and JP-8(100). Toxicol Appl Pharmacol 1999; 160(1):60–75.

96. Benowitz NL, Chan K, Denaro CP, Jacob P. Stable isotope method for studying transdermal drug absorption: nicotine patch. Clin Pharmacol Ther 1991; 50(Sep):286–293.

97. Welin-Berger K, Neelissen JA, Emanuelsson BM, Bjornsson MA, Gjellan K. In vitro–in vivo correlation in man of a topically applied local anesthetic agent using numerical convolution and deconvolution. J Pharm Sci 2003; 92(2):398–406.

98. Singh P, Maibach HI, Roberts MS. Site of effects. In: Roberts MS, Walters KA, eds. Dermal Absorption and Toxicity Assessment. New York: Marcel Dekker, 1998.

99. McNeill SC, Potts RO, Francoeur ML. Local enhanced topical delivery (LETD) of drugs: does it truly exist? Pharm Res 1992; 9:1422–1427.

100. Singh P, Roberts MS. Blood flow measurements in skin and underlying tissues by microsphere method: application to dermal pharmacokinetics of polar non-electrolytes. J Pharm Sci 1993a; 82(9):873–879.

101. Singh P, Roberts MS. Dermal and underlying tissue pharmacokinetics of salicylic acid after topical application. J Pharmacokinet Biopharm 1993; 21(4):337–373.

102. Roberts MS, Cross SE. A physiological pharmacokinetic model for solute disposition in tissues below a topical application site. Pharm Res 1999; 16(9):1392–1398.

103. Nakayama K, Matsuura H, Asai M, Ogawara K, Higaki K, Kimura T. Estimation of intradermal disposition kinetics of drugs: I. Analysis by compartment model with contralateral tissues. Pharm Res 1999; 16(2):302–308.

104. Higaki K, Asai M, Suyama T, Nakayama K, Ogawara K, Kimura T. Estimation of intradermal disposition kinetics of drugs: II. Factors determining penetration of drugs from viable skin to muscular layer. Int J Pharm 2002; 239(1–2):129–141.

105. Singh P, Roberts MS. Effects of vasoconstriction on dermal pharmacokinetics and local tissue distribution of compounds. J Pharm Sci 1994; 83(6):783–791.

106. Cross SE, Anderson C, Thompson MJ, Roberts MS. Is there tissue penetration after application of topical salicylate formulations? Lancet 1997; 350(Aug 30):636.

107. Muller M, Mascher H, Kikuta C, Schafer S, Brunner M, Dorner G, Eichler HG. Diclofenac concentrations in defined tissue layers after topical administration. Clin Pharmacol Ther 1997; 62(3):293–299.

108. Beastall J, Guy RH, Hadgraft J, Wilding I. The influence of urea on percutaneous absorption. Pharm Res 1986; 3(5):294–297.

109. Demana PH, Smith EW, Walker RB, Haigh JM, Kanfer I. Evaluation of the proposed FDA pilot dose-response methodology for topical corticosteroid bioequivalence testing. Pharm Res 1997; 14(3):303–308.

110. Singh GJ, Fleischer N, Lesko L, Williams R. Evaluation of the proposed FDA pilot dose–response methodology for topical corticosteroid bioequivalence testing. Pharm Res 1998; 15(1):4–7.

111. Smith EW, Walker RB, Haigh JM, Kanfer I. Evaluation of the proposed FDA pilot dose–response methodology for topical corticosteroid bioequivalence testing. The authors reply. Pharm Res 1998; 15(1):5–7.
112. Cordero JA, Camacho M, Obach R, Domenech J, Vila L. In vitro based index of topical anti-inflammatory activity to compare a series of NSAIDs. Eur J Pharm Biopharm 2001; 51(2):135–142.
113. Kasting GB. Theoretical models for iontophoretic delivery. Adv Drug Del Rev 1992; 9:177–199.
114. Roberts MS, Lai PM, Anissimov YG. Epidermal iontophoresis: I. Development of the ionic mobility-pore model. Pharm Res 1998; 15(10):1569–1578.
115. Cross SE, Roberts MS. The importance of dermal blood supply and the epidermis on the transdermal iontophoretic delivery of monovalent cations. J Pharm Sci 1995; 84:584–592.
116. Mitragotri S, Blankschtein D, Langer R. An explanation for the variation of the sonophoretic transdermal transport enhancement from drug to drug. J Pharm Sci 1997; 86(10):1190–1192.
117. Tezel A, Sens A, Tuchscherer J, Mitragotri S. Frequency dependence of sonophoresis. Pharm Res 2001; 18(12):1694–1700.
118. Tezel A, Sens A, Mitragotri S. Description of transdermal transport of hydrophilic solutes during low-frequency sonophoresis based on a modified porous pathway model. J Pharm Sci 2003; 92(2):381–393.
119. Jiang R, Roberts MS, Collins DM, Benson HA. Absorption of sunscreens across human skin: an evaluation of commercial products for children and adults. Br J Clin Pharmacol 1999; 48(4):635–637.
120. Beckett AH, Gorrod JW, Taylor DC. Comparison of oral and percutaneous routes in man for systemic administration of ephedrine. J Pharm Pharmacol 1972; 24(Suppl):65–70.
121. Zhang Q, Grice JE, Wang GJ, Roberts MS. Cutaneous metabolism in transdermal drug delivery. Current Drug Metabolism 2009; 10:227–235.
122. Dancik Y, Thörling C, Krishnan G, Roberts MS. Cutaneous Metabolism and Active Transport In Transdermal Drug Delivery. In Toxicology of the skin: Target Organ Toxicity Series. Monteiro-Riviere N (ed.) 2010; 69–82. Boca Raton: Taylor & Francis Group LLC.
123. Liu X, Grice JE, Lademann J, Otberg N, Trauer S, Patzelt A, Roberts MS (2011). Hair follicles contribute significantly to penetration through human skin only at times early after application as a solvent deposited solid in man (ms no. MP-00077-11-AC.R1). Brit J Clin Pharmacol 2011 Nov; 72(5): 768–774.
124. Kattou P, Lian G, Glavin S, Sorrell I, Chen T. Development of a Two-Dimensional Model for Predicting Transdermal Permeation with the Follicular Pathway: Demonstration with a Caffeine Study. Pharm Res. 2017 Oct; 34(10):2036–2048.
125. Martins FS, Patel N, Jamei M, Polak S. Development and Validation of a Dermal PBPK Model for Prediction of the Hair Follicular Absorption of Caffeine: Application of the Simcyp MPML MechDermA model. ISSX 2017. https://www.certara.com/app/uploads/2017/1 Accessed 21 Jan 2021).
126. Kasting GB, Miller MA, LaCount TD, Jaworska J. A Composite Model for the Transport of Hydrophilic and Lipophilic Compounds Across the Skin: Steady-State Behavior. J Pharm Sci. 2019 Jan;108(1):337–349.
127. Otberg N, Patzelt A, Rasulev U, Hagemeister T, Linscheid M, Sinkgraven R, Sterry W, Lademann J. The role of hair follicles in the percutaneous absorption of caffeine. Br J Clin Pharmacol. 2008 Apr;65(4):488–492.
128. Liu X, Yousef S, Anissimov YG, van der Hoek J, Tsakalozou E, Ni Z, Grice JE, Roberts MS. Diffusion modelling of percutaneous absorption kinetics. Predicting urinary excretion from in vitro skin permeation tests (IVPT) for an infinite dose. Eur J Pharm Biopharm.2020 Apr;149:30–44.
129. Mahmood AH, Liu X, Grice J, Medley GA, Roberts MS (2015). Using deconvolution to understand the mechanism for variable plasma concentration-time profiles after intramuscular injection. Int J Pharm 2015; 481(1-2): 71–78.
130. Dancik Y, Anissimov YG, Jepps OG, Roberts MS. Convective transport of highly plasma protein bound drugs facilitates direct penetration into deep tissues after topical application. *Brit J Clin Pharmacol.* 2012;73:564–578.
131. Anissimov YG, Roberts MS. Modelling dermal drug distribution after topical application in man. *Pharm Res* 2011 Sep;28(9): 2119–2129.
132. Anissimov YG, Jepps OG, Dancik Y, Roberts MS (2013). Mathematical and pharmacokinetic modelling of epidermal and dermal transport processes. *Adv Drug Del Rev* 2013;65:169–190.
133. Calcutt JJ, Anissimov YG. Physiologically based mathematical modeling of solute transport in the epidermis and dermis. Int J Pharm. 2019;569:118547.
134. Todo H, Oshizaka T, Kadhum WR, Sugibayashi K. Mathematical model to predict skin concentration after topical application of drugs. Pharmaceutics. 2013 Dec 16;5(4):634–651.

3 In Vivo Percutaneous Absorption

A Key Role for Stratum Corneum/ Vehicle Partitioning

André Rougier

Laboratoire Pharmaceutique, La Roche-Posay, Courbevoie, France

CONTENTS

3.1   INTRODUCTION

Over the past two decades considerable attention has been paid to understanding the mechanisms and routes by which chemical compounds penetrate the skin. Irrespective of the different theories on mechanisms relating to percutaneous absorption, it is well established that the stratum corneum (SC) constitutes the main barrier (1–4). Thus, it is to be expected that the overall kinetic process will depend mainly on the pharmacokinetic parameters governing the penetration of compounds through this membrane.

The interaction between the drug, the vehicle, and the SC as a consequence of their physico-chemical properties is likely to be an important pharmacokinetic parameter in an early step of the absorption process. In studies in rats (5) and humans (6), we have demonstrated a correlation between the amount of the test substance found in the SC at the end of a 30-minute application and the total amount absorbed over four days. The predictive aspect of the so-called "stripping method" was found to take into account the main factors influencing percutaneous absorption (7–10).

It has been suggested that the amount of chemical absorbed within the SC after 30 minutes of application could reflect its SC vehicle partitioning and its rate of entry into the skin (7). Previous studies in hairless rats (8) showed clearly that the amount of various compounds that penetrated in vivo was strictly proportional to the time of application, thus providing indirect evidence that a constant flux of penetration really does exist in vivo.

In light of these results, the present study was carried out to determine whether the stripping method could also be used to predict the in vivo steady-state flux of a test compound.

3.2   MATERIALS AND METHODS

Five radiolabeled compounds (Radiochemical Centre, Amersham, UK) with very different physicochemical properties and belonging to different chemical classes were compared: benzoic acid, caffeine, thiourea, hydrocortisone, and inulin (Table 3.1).

A group of six 12-week-old hairless Sprague-Dawley female rats (IFFA- CREDO, Lyon, France) weighing 200 ± 20 g was used for each compound and each application time.

3.2.1   Percutaneous Absorption Measurements

Each compound (1000 nmol) was applied to a 1-cm^2 area of the back of anesthetized animals (intraperitoneal [IP] injection of gammabutyrolactone, 0.5 mL/kg in 20 μL ethylene glycol/Triton W100 mixtures) (Table 1.1). The treated area was delimited by an open circular cell attached with silicone glue in order to prevent spreading. The application times were from one to five hours.

At the end of the application time, the treated area was washed twice (2×300 μL) with ethanol/water (95/5), rinsed twice with water, and dried with cotton in order to remove excess product. We considered that the compounds had effectively penetrated when they had crossed the SC and reached the viable epidermis. The SC was then stripped 10 times (using adhesive tape 810, 3M USA) in order to exclude any compound that had not penetrated during the time of application (previous histological studies in hairless rats have shown that this procedure almost totally removes the SC). The remaining skin (epidermis plus dermis) was sampled and counted by liquid scintillation (Packard 360, Packard Instruments, Downers Grove, IL, USA) after digestion in Soluene 350 (United Technology, Packard).

The carcasses were then lyophilized and homogenized, and samples were counted by liquid scintillation after combustion (Oxidizer 306, Packard Instruments). In the case of tritiated molecules (caffeine, hydrocortisone, inulin), the water resulting from the lyophilization of the carcasses was sampled and assayed for radioactivity. The radioactivity found was added to that detected in the carcasses, thus obtaining the overall percutaneous absorption values. The urine excreted during the time of application was collected to take into account any product contained therein in the overall absorption. The total amount of each compound penetrating at each application time was determined by summation of the amount found in the epidermis, dermis, and carcass.

3.2.2   Stratum Corneum/Vehicle Partitioning Measurement

Six strippings (using 3M adhesive tape 810) were performed on the treated area of each group of six animals for each compound after a fixed application time of 30 minutes (the reasons for this choice of time are discussed later). The amount of product within the SC was assessed after complete digestion of the keratin material in Soluene 350 by liquid scintillation counting.

TABLE 3.1
Application Conditions

Compound	Specific Activity	Purity (%)	Molecular Weight (Da)	Vehicle
Benzoic acid [7– ^{14}C]	21.3 mCi/mmol	>98	122	Ethylene glycol/Triton × 100 (90/10)
Caffeine [8– ^{3}H]	24 Ci/mmol	>98	194	Ethylene glycol/Triton × 100/water (45/5/50)
Thiourea [^{14}C]	58 mCi/mmol	>98	76	Ethylene glycol/Triton × 100 (90/10)
Hydrocortisone (1.2.6.7)[^{3}H]	98.5 Ci/mmol	>99	362	Ethylene glycol/Triton × 100/isopropanol (72/8/20)
Inulin [^{3}H]	3.2 Ci/mmol	>98	5,200	Ethylene glycol/Triton × 100 (90/10)

Note: Dose applied for all compounds: 1000 nmol/cm^2 in 20-μL vehicle.

3.2.3 Measurement of the Thickness of the Stratum Corneum

The thickness of the SC was measured in biopsies from the backs of six rats according to the technique described by McKenzie (11). Each biopsy was placed on a strip of acetyl cellulose coated with Tekt issue (Miles Scientific, Naperville, IL, USA), then frozen in dry ice. Transverse sections (8 µm) were then cut with the acid of a cryomicrotome (HRLM Slee, London, UK). The sections obtained were fixed for 10 minutes in a 70% alcohol bath, then stained for 30 seconds with a 0.5% aqueous solution of methylene blue. After rinsing with distilled water, the sections were mounted between a slide and a coverslip with the aid of Aqua-Mount (hydrophilic mounting medium). The thickness of the horny layer was measured at 20 different points on each section by means of a semiautomatic image analyzer (Digipet, Reichert, Wien, Austria) connected to a microscope (Polyvar, Reichert, Austria), and hence a mean thickness could be calculated.

3.2.4 Effect of Vehicles Used on the Stratum Corneum Integrity

After anesthesia, 20 µL of each of the vehicles used was applied to a 1-cm² area on the backs of groups of five rats. The area was delimited by an open circular cell as described previously. After five hours of contact, the treated area was washed twice (2 × 300 µL) with water and dried with cotton in order to remove excess vehicle. One hour after completion of the vehicle treatment, transepidermal water loss (TEWL) was measured with an Evaporimeter EP1 (ServoMed, Stockholm, Sweden). The handheld probe was fitted with a 1-cm tail chimney to reduce air turbulence around the hydrosensors and a metallic shield (supplied by ServoMed) to minimize the possibility of sensor contamination. Measurements (G/m²/hr) stabilized within one minute. The effects of total destruction of the SC have also been studied by measuring TEWL from the backs of a group of five animals, five hours after a series of 10 strippings (using 3M adhesive tape 810).

3.2.5 Theory and Data Treatment

The mass transfer of compounds from the surface of the skin to the interior of the body through the SC is generally considered to be due to passive diffusion. A classical but oversimplified description of the transport process is represented in Figure 3.1. The SC is assumed to be a homogeneous membrane (thickness h); D is the diffusion coefficient of the solute through the membrane. The concentration of solute (C) within the outermost layer of the membrane ($x = 0$) depends on the concentration within the vehicle (c_0) and the partition coefficient (K) between the membrane and the vehicle:

$$C = CK_0 \tag{3.1}$$

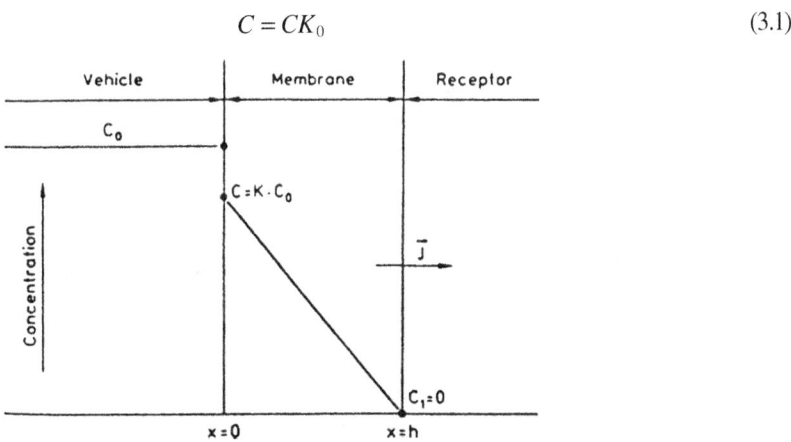

FIGURE 3.1 Concentration profile across homogeneous membrane at steady state (zero-order flux case).

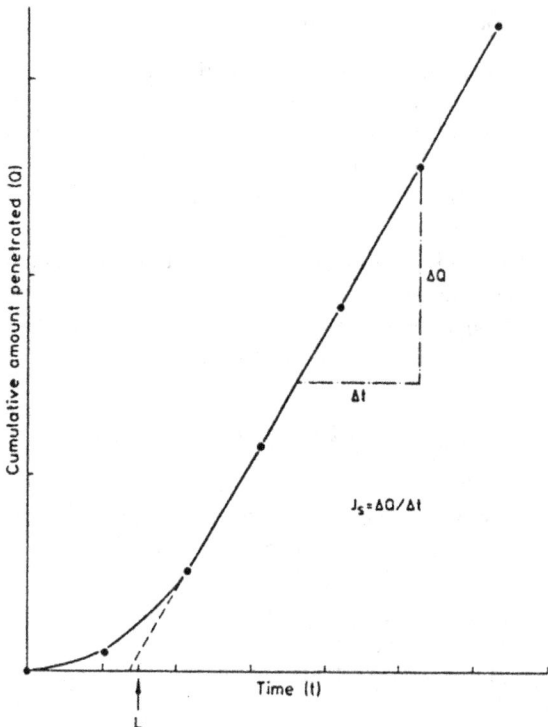

FIGURE 3.2   Typical profile of concentration versus time for diffusion through the stratum corneum.

For all values of time (t), the concentration of solute within the innermost layer of the membrane ($x = h$) is assumed to be negligible (sink condition). The validity of such an assumption is discussed in the "Results" section. The change in the cumulative amount of solute (Q) that passes through the membrane per unit area as a function of time is represented in Figure 3.2. When a steady state is reached, the curve $Q(t)$ is linear and can be described by the equation:

$$Q = J_S(t - L) \tag{3.2}$$

where J_s corresponds to the steady-state flux (the slope of the straight line):

$$J_s = Kc_o d / h \tag{3.3}$$

and L is the lag time (the intercept of the straight line on the time axis):

$$L = \frac{h^2}{6D} \tag{3.4}$$

In practice, J_S and L were calculated for each compound using a linear regression obtained with the aid of a computer (Vax 11/750, Digital Corporation, Bedford, MA, USA) and standard software (RS/Explore BBN Software Product Corporation, Bedford, MA, USA).

3.3   RESULTS

Figure 3.3 shows that, irrespective of the nature of the compound tested, the plot of the cumulative amount of solute that passes through a unit surface area of the SC as a function of the application time appears to be linear ($r = 0.99$, $p < 0.001$). As shown in Figure 3.3 and Table 3.2, the steady-state

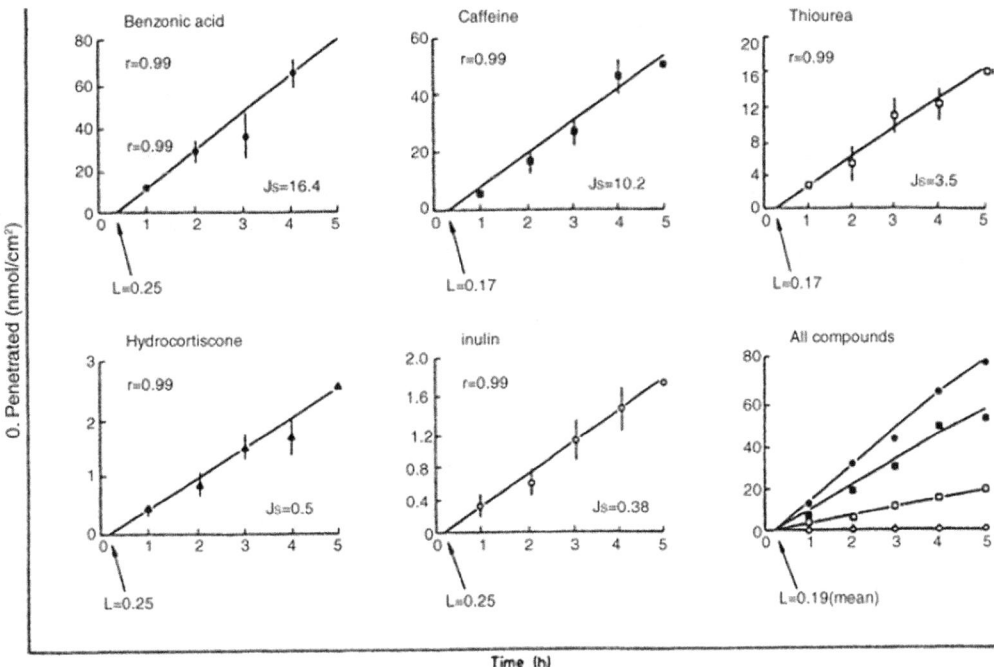

FIGURE 3.3 Cumulative amount of solute penetrating through the stratum corneum as a function of application time. *Abbreviations: J_s*, steady-state flux (nmol/cm²/hr); *L*, lag time (hr).

values (J_S) are strongly molecule dependent. Thus, the values for inulin and benzoic acid differ by a factor of 40. The rank order of the J_S values is inulin < hydrocortisone < thiourea < caffeine < benzoic acid.

In the present case, a constant flux of penetration ought to be attained within a contact time of about 30 minutes (11 × 2.7). According to Zatz (12), the attainment of a constant flux would be expected to coincide with the delivery of a constant amount at the SC. In order to test this hypothesis, we measured the amount present in the horny layer after an application time of 30 minutes (it should be recalled that the time of 30 minutes corresponds to that used in the stripping method).

TABLE 3.2

Amount of Chemical Penetrating Through the Stratum Corneum (nmol/cm²), Measured at the End of the Application Time and the Steady-State Parameters

Compound	Application Time (hr)					Steady-State Flux (J)(nmol/cm²/hr)	Lag Time (hr)
	1	2	3	4	5		
	12.5 (SE 3)	30 (SE 2)	39 (SE 10)	64 (SE 6)	78 (SE 7)	16.4 (SE 0.8)	0.25
Caffeine	7.4 (SE 0.8)	18.6 (SE 2.9)	29.5 (SE 2)	45 (SE 5)	52 (SE 8.5)	10.2 (SE 0.6)	0.17
Thiourea	3 (SE 0.7)	6 (SE 2)	10.7 (SE 2)	13.4 (SE 1.8)	17 (SE 2.2)	3.5 (SE 0.2)	0.17
Hydrocortisone	0.49 (SE 0.05)	0.9 (SE 0.1)	1.5 (SE 0.1)	1.8 (SE 0.3)	2.6 (SE 0.4)	0.5 (SE 0.04)	0.16
Inulin	0.32 (SE 0.04)	0.63 (SE 0.04)	1.1 (SE 0.2)	1.5 (SE 0.2)	1.8 (SE 0.3)	0.38 (SE 0.02)	0.20
						Mean	0.19

Abbreviations: SE, standard error.

TABLE 3.3

Percutaneous Absorption Parameters of the Tested Compounds

Compound	Log p Octanol/ Water[a]	K[b]	Q_{sc}[c] Calculated (nmol/cm²)	Q_{sc} Measured (nmol/cm²)	Steady-State Flux (J_s) (nmol/cm²/hr)	
					Predicted from Equation (3.8)	Measured
Benzoic acid	1.87	0.30	8.77	9.07 (SE 0.66)	15.87 (SE 1.15)	16.4 (SE 0.80)
Caffeine	−0.07	0.14	6.46	5.92 (SE 0.46)	10.36 (SE 0.80)	10.2 (SE 0.60)
Thiourea	−1.02	0.066	3.86	3.34 (SE 0.2)	5.85 (SE 0.35)	3.5 (SE 0.20)
Hydrocortisone	1.61	0.077	0.52	2.36 (SE 0.09)	4.1 (SE 0.16)	0.5 (SE 0.04)
Inulin	−3.58	0.078	0.46	0.85 (SE 0.12)	1.49 (SE 0.20)	0.38 (SE 0.02)

Note: C_0 = solute concentration within the vehicles, taking into account vehicle evaporation (Figure 4): benzoic acid, thiourea, inulin = 4.5×10^4 nmol/cm³; hydrocortisone = 5.2×10^4 nmol/cm³; caffeine = 7.1×10^4 nmol/cm³.

[a] From Reference 12.

[b] Partition coefficient calculated from Equation (3.5) [h = 13 µm; L = 11 minutes; C_0 (see Note)].

[c] Q_{sc} calculated from Equation (3.6) [h = 13 µm, K = calculated from Equation (3.5), C_0 (see Note)].

Abbreviations: SE, standard error.

The results obtained for the five molecules are shown in Table 3.3. The total amounts of solute accumulated in the first six stoppings rank as follows: inulin < hydrocortisone < thiourea < caffeine < benzoic acid.

3.4   DISCUSSION

Our results in vivo, like those in vitro, show that the phenomenon of transport across the SC can be considered a process obeying the general laws governing passive membrane diffusion. Thus, after a time to attain equilibrium, a constant flux of penetration is established. From a theoretical point of view, this can occur only if the solute distribution within the membrane remains constant. This implies that the solute concentration in the outermost layer of the membrane has to remain constant throughout the entire experiment (infinite dose condition) and that the solute concentration in the innermost layer of the membrane has to remain constant and be negligible (sink condition).

As shown in Figure 3.4, the amount of the vehicle applied (20 µL/cm²) changes only during the first hour of administration. Then it remains constant throughout the time of percutaneous absorption measurements of one to five hours. In the case of the most penetrating compound (benzoic acid), the amount that penetrated after five hours of application (78 nmol) was far below the amount applied (1000 nmol). It can therefore be assumed that the solute concentration in the vehicle remained relatively constant between one and five hours. Experimentally, we can consider that the first condition is met.

It can be assumed that the epidermis and the uppermost part of the papillary layer of the dermis constitute a negligible barrier in comparison with the SC (13) and the microvascularization of the dermal papillae prevents solute accumulation in the region of the capillaries. Thus, the solute concentration in the innermost layer of the SC can be considered to be negligible in comparison with the concentration in the outermost layer. Hence, the sink condition is apparently fulfilled.

Although the existence of a steady-state flux of penetration in vivo was predicted about 20 years ago by Tregear (14) and subsequently by others (8, 15, 16), the problem is still the subject of debate (17, 18). Our results clearly demonstrate (Figure 3.3) that a constant flux can be achieved in vivo just as in in vitro experiments. Although this seems to be quite logical in our view, this is the first time that it has been demonstrated experimentally. Our results thus fill a gap in the understanding of the

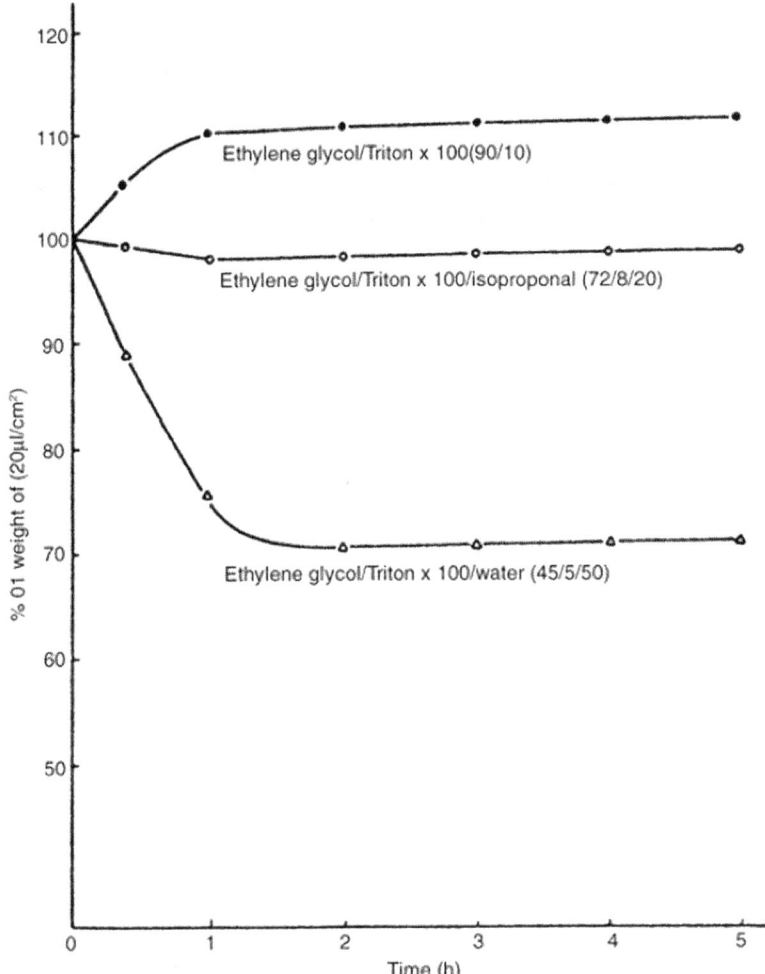

FIGURE 3.4   Modification of the vehicles during their administration (20 μL/cm², room temperature 27°C).

mechanisms governing in vivo percutaneous absorption. It should, however, be emphasized that the existence of such a gap is in no way due to negligence on the part of investigators in the field, but rather to the technical difficulties of measuring a steady-state flux of penetration in vivo.

Our results show (Figure 3.3 and Table 3.2) that lag times for the different molecules tested are very close and extremely short. One explanation is that the vehicles used alter the SC and therefore modify the barrier to penetration. However, Table 3.4 clearly shows that TEWL is not affected by vehicle treatment, whereas removing the SC by 10 successive strippings increases TEWL by a factor of 18.

It is therefore possible to consider that, until the contrary is demonstrated experimentally, such a situation may exist in vivo, even if it upsets some theories that have been built upon in vitro studies. It is important to emphasize that such observations have rarely been made in vitro, perhaps because sink conditions are not necessarily met in vitro. In a dynamic in vitro system, a concentration close to zero in the medium bathing the tissue does not necessarily imply that the concentration in the innermost layer of the membrane is constant with time (13). It is not unusual to observe an increase in the concentration of solute with time in the innermost layers of the epidermis or dermis, depending on the in vitro model adopter (13–20). This increase may be linked either to incomplete resorption by the bathing fluid (21–24) or to a possible affinity of the molecule for these structures (25).

TABLE 3.4

Effect of the Applied Vehicles on the Barrier Function of the Stratum Corneum (Transepidermal Water Loss)

Ethylene Glycol/Triton Xl00 (90/10) (g/m²/hr)	Ethylene Glycol/Triton Xl00/ Water (45/5/50) (g/m²/hr)	Ethylene Glycol/Triton Xl00/ Isopropanol (72/8/20)(g/m²/hr)	Stratum Corneum Removed (10 strippings) (g/m²/hr)
5.8 (SE 0.3)	5.7 (0.4)	5.6 (0.3)	91 (3.0)
Controls:			
5.1 (SE 0.3)	5.3 (0.4)	5.1 (0.3)	5.1 (0.3)

Abbreviations: SE, standard error.

On the basis of knowledge concerning the thickness of the SC ($h = 13 + 2$ μm) and the value for the mean lag time ($L = 11$ minutes), it is possible to deduce a mean value for the apparent diffusion coefficient (D_m) by using Equation (3.4): $D_m = 4.3 \times 10^{-10}$ cm²/sec. This does not mean that the values of the diffusion coefficients for molecules having physicochemical properties as different as those used in this study are identical. It means that it is impossible to control, with the required degree of precision, all the physical, physicochemical, and biological parameters likely to affect diffusion through a membrane as complex as the SC. From a purely practical point of view, it is thus possible, as a first approximation, to consider different molecules as having the same apparent diffusion coefficient in the case of percutaneous absorption in vivo. On the other hand, it is reasonable to ask whether this coefficient may vary as a function of parameters such as animal species, anatomical site, age, etc.

It follows from Equations (3.3) and (3.4) that the flux at equilibrium can be written in the form:

$$J_s = \frac{1}{6} K c_o \frac{h}{L} \tag{3.5}$$

As we have shown earlier, the values of the lag times for the five molecules are similar. This results in the apparent "velocity of diffusion," defined by the ratio h/L, being independent of the nature of the diffusion substance for a given thickness of the horny layer and a given anatomical site. Only the number of molecules in transit (Kc_o) would be characteristic for a given substance and would determine the value of its flux at equilibrium. Since, for a given compound, the value of c_o may be considered to be constant within the time of percutaneous absorption measurements one to five hours, the value of this flux would depend only on the SC/vehicle partition coefficient (K).

Using Equation (3.5) and the values of flux (J_S) determined experimentally (Table 3.3), we have calculated the values of K for each of the five molecules (Table 3.3), taking into account in the C_o values the evaporation of the vehicles (Figure 3.4). The values for the octanol/water partition coefficients (log P) reported in the literature for these five molecules (26) are also shown in Table 3.3. It appears that no relationship exists between these values and the values for flux at equilibrium. Although many examples appear to support the use of log P for predicting the degree of penetration of a molecule (27, 28), there are many others that show the limitations of such a procedure (29–32). The partition coefficient of a given compound between two solvents can be considered a constant physical property of that compound. It is now generally accepted that the percutaneous absorption of a compound can vary considerably as a function of the conditions of administration (vehicle, dose, anatomical site, animal species, etc.). This raises the question: How is it possible to predict the value of a variable parameter only from a constant? Thus, in agreement with Scheuplein (33), we consider that, at present, no solvent system is capable of simulating the extreme complexity of the SC. Only the measurement of the partition coefficient between the SC and the vehicle can be representative of reality.

The amount of substance present in the SC at equilibrium (Q_{sc}) can be measured. According to the model adopted, this quantity is related to the partition coefficient by the equation:

$$Q_{sc} = \frac{1}{2}Kc_o \qquad (3.6)$$

As shown in Table 3.3 and Figure 3.5, very good agreement exists between the values of Q_{sc} measured by stripping the treated area after 30 minutes and the values of Q_{sc} calculated from Equation (3.6) (c_o values take into account vehicle evaporation).

In light of Equations (3.5) and (3.6), the flux at equilibrium can be written:

$$J_s = \frac{Q_{sc}}{3L} \qquad (3.7)$$

Since the lag times of the molecules under study are similar, the fluxes at equilibrium would be expected to depend only on the amount present in the SC.

According to the theoretical model adopted, using Equation (3.7) and a mean lag time of 0.19 hour, the theoretical relationship between J_s and Q_{sc} should be:

$$J_s = 1.75 Q_{sc} \qquad (3.8)$$

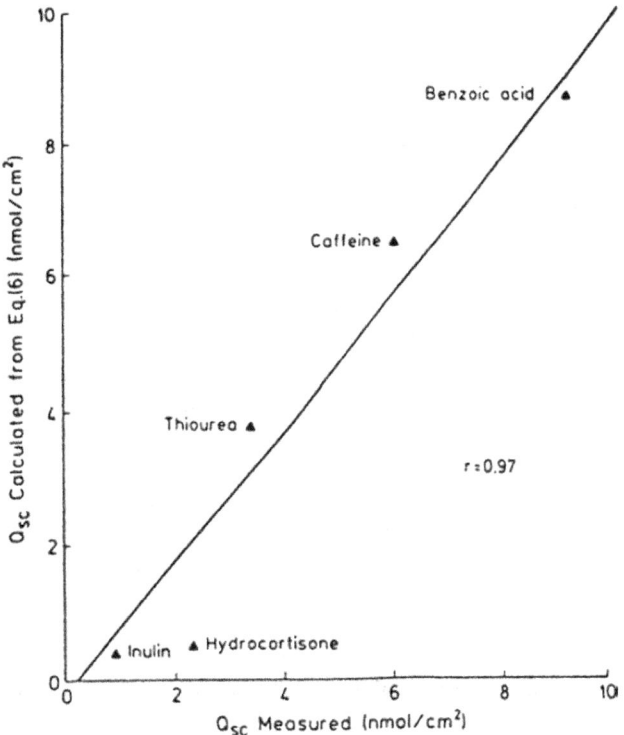

FIGURE 3.5 Relationship between the quantity of chemical within the stratum corneum measured after 30 minutes of contact and predicted using Equation (3.6).

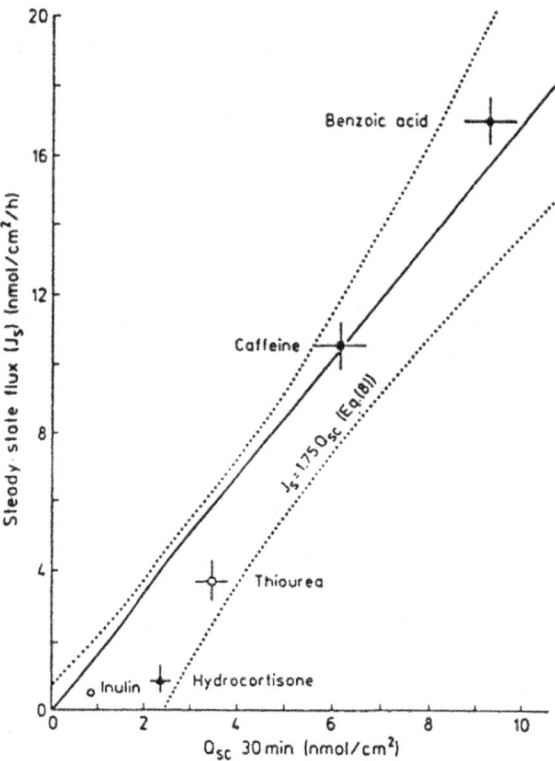

FIGURE 3.6 In vivo relationship between steady-state flux of penetration (J_s) and quantity of solute within the stratum corneum after 30 minutes of contact.

(with J_s being expressed in nmol/cm²/hr). As shown in Figure 3.6, the curve derived from Equation (3.8) is contained within the 5% confidence limits of the experimental values.

In view of the approximations made in the theoretical model and the inevitable errors arising from the inaccuracies of the measurements and biological variation, we can consider that there exists a very satisfactory agreement between experimental values and theory, as in Equation (3.8). Only hydrocortisone does not appear to fit well with the theoretical linear relationship linking steady-state flux of penetration (J_s) and amount in the SC (Q_{sc}). This is not really surprising, since steroids are known to form a depot or reservoir within the SC (34, 35). A fraction of the available molecules may bind to the keratin or other tissue components, while the remainder diffuses slowly downward.

Six years after the development of the stripping method (5–10), the results obtained provide a better understanding of why it is possible to predict the total penetration during four days of a substance administered for 30 minutes with satisfactory precision. As shown in Table 3.3, from a purely practical point of view, the flux of penetration at equilibrium of a substance administered in vivo in a given vehicle can be predicted using Equation (3.8) from the simple measurement of the amount present in the SC (Q_{sc}) after a contact time of 30 minutes. Since the validity of the stripping method has been verified for many molecules administered under different conditions in different species, it is reasonable to think that it would also hold for the predictive assessment of the in vivo steady-state flux of penetration.

Using an original experimental approach, we have obtained data leading to a better understanding of the mechanisms implicated in molecular transport across the SC in vivo. Thus, it appears that the SC/vehicle partitioning plays a determining role in the percutaneous absorption of chemicals in vivo.

We can easily conceive that our results, especially those related to lag times and diffusion coefficients, may not be readily accepted. The strength of the data presented lies in the fact that they are experimental. To reason only in terms of in vitro data would be to admit from the outset that there are no differences between the in vitro and in vivo processes of percutaneous absorption. However, considering the theoretical importance of these results, it would be important to see them verified using other chemicals of widely different physicochemical properties. It would also be interesting to ascertain that the theory we have developed concerning the in vivo mechanism of percutaneous absorption is verified when the same chemical is dissolved in different vehicles.

ACKNOWLEDGMENT

The author thanks Dr. C. Berrebi for her expertise in the histometric measurements and A. M. Cabaillot, C. Patouillet, and M. Zanini for their excellent technical assistance.

REFERENCES

1. Malkinson FD. Studies on percutaneous absorption of ^{14}C labeled steroids by use of the gas-flow cell. J Invest Dermatol 1958; 31:19–28.
2. Marzulli FN. Barrier to skin penetration. J Invest Dermatol 1962; 39:387–393.
3. Stoughton RB. Penetration absorption. Toxicol Appl Pharmacol 1965; 7(Suppl 2):1–6.
4. Vinson LJ, Singer EJ, Koehler WR, Lehmann MD, Masurat T. The nature of the epidermal barrier and some factors influencing skin permeability. Toxicol Appl Pharmacol 1965; 7:7–19.
5. Rougier A, Dupuis D, Lotte C, Roguet R, Schaefer H. Correlation between stratum corneum reservoir function and percutaneous absorption. J Invest Dermatol 1983; 81:275–278.
6. Dupuis D, Rougier A, Roguet R, Lotte C, Kalopissis G. In vivo relationship between horny layer reservoir effect and percutaneous absorption in human and rat. J Invest Dermatol 1984; 82:353–356.
7. Dupuis D, Rougier A, Roguet R, Lotte C. The measurement of the stratum corneum reservoir: a simple method to predict the influence of vehicles on in vivo percutaneous absorption. Br J Dermatol 1986; 115:233–238.
8. Rougier A, Dupuis D, Lotte C. The measurement of the stratum corneum reservoir. A predictive method for in vivo percutaneous absorption studies: influence of the application time. J Invest Dermatol 1985; 84:66–68.
9. Rougier A, Dupuis D, Lotte C, Roguet R, Wester RE, Maibach HI. Regional variation in percutaneous absorption in man: measurement by the stripping method. Arch Dermatol Res 1986; 278:465–469.
10. Rougier A, Lotte C, Maibach HI. In vivo percutaneous absorption of some organic compounds related to anatomic site in man. J Pharmacol Sci 1987; 76:451–454.
11. McKenzie IC. A simple method of orientation and storage of specimens for cryomicrotomy. J Periodont Res 1975; 10:49–50.
12. Zatz JL. Influence of depletion on percutaneous absorption characteristics. J Soc Cosmet Chem 1985; 36:237–249.
13. Schaefer H, Zesch A, Stuttgen G. Skin Permeability. New York: Springer, 1982:607–616.
14. Tregear RT. The permeability of mammalian skin to ions. J Invest Dermatol 1966; 46:16–22.
15. Arita T, Hori R, Anmo T, Washitake M, Akatsu M, Yasima T. Studies on percutaneous absorption of drugs. Chem Pharm Bull 1970; 18:1045–1049.
16. Wepierre J, Corroler M, Didry JR. Distribution and dissociation of benzoyl peroxide in cutaneous tissues after application on skin in the hairless rat. Int J Cosmet Sci 1986; 8: 97–104.
17. Guy R, Hadgraft J. Mathematical models of percutaneous absorption. In: Bronaugh RL, Maibach HI, eds. Percutaneous Absorption. New York: Marcel Dekker, 1985:3–15.
18. Tojo K, Lee AE-RI. A method for predicting steady-state rate of skin penetration in vivo. J Invest Dermatol 1989; 92:105–108.
19. Loden M. The in vivo permeability of human skin to benzene, ethylene glycol, formaldehyde and *n*-hexane. Acta Pharmacol Toxicol 1986; 58:382–389.
20. Zesch A, Schaefer H. Penetration of radioactive hydrocortisone in human skin for various ointment bases. II. In vivo experiments. Arch Dermatol Forsch 1975; 252:245–256.
21. Bronaugh RL. Determination of percutaneous absorption by in vivo techniques. In: Bronaugh RL, Maibach HI, eds. Percutaneous Absorption. New York: Marcel Dekker, 1985:267–279.

22. Bronaugh RL, Stewart RF. Methods for in vitro percutaneous absorption studies. III. Hydrophobic compounds. J Pharm Sci 1984; 73:1255–1258.
23. Bronaugh RL, Stewart RF. Methods for in vitro percutaneous absorption studies. VI. Preparation of the barrier layer. J Pharm Sci 1986; 75:487–491.
24. Scott RC. Percutaneous absorption in vivo-in vitro comparisons. In: Shroot B, Schaefer H, eds. Pharmacology of the Skin. Basel: Karger, 1987:103–110.
25. Miselnicky SR, Lichtin JL, Sakr A, Bronaugh RL. The influence of solubility, protein binding and percutaneous absorption on reservoir formation in skin. J Soc Cosmet Chem 1988; 39:169–177.
26. Hansch C, Leo AJ. Log P Data Base. Pomona, CA: Pomona College Medical Chemistry Project, 1984.
27. Blank HI, Scheuplein RJ. Transport into within the skin. Br J Dermatol 1969; 81(Suppl 4):4–10.
28. Scheuplein RJ, Blank HI. Mechanism of percutaneous absorption. IV. Penetration of non-electrolytes (alcohols) from aqueous solution and from pure liquids. J Invest Dermatol 1973; 60:286–296.
29. Ackerman C, Flynn GL, eds. Ether-water partitioning and permeability through nude mouse skin in vitro. I. Urea, thiourea, glycerol and glucose. Int J Pharmacol 1987; 36:61–66.
30. Blank HI, Scheuplein RJ, McFarlane DJ. Mechanism of percutaneous absorption. II. The effect of temperature on the transport of non-electrolytes across the skin. J Invest Dermatol 1967; 49:582–589.
31. Poulsen BJ, Flynn GL. In vitro methods used to study dermal delivery and percutaneous absorption. In: Bronaugh RL, Maibach HI, eds. Percutaneous Absorption. New York: Marcel Dekker, 1985:431–459.
32. Scheuplein RJ, Blank HI, Branner GJ, McFarlane DJ. Percutaneous absorption of steroids. J Invest Dermatol 1969; 52:63–70.
33. Scheuplein RJ. Mechanism of percutaneous absorption. I. Routes of penetration and the influence of solubility. J Invest Dermatol 1965; 45:334–346.
34. Barry BW. Dermatological formulations: percutaneous absorption. In: Swarbrick J, ed. Drug and Pharmaceutical Sciences. New York: Marcel Dekker, 1983; 18:49–54.
35. Malkinson FD, Ferguson EH. Preliminary and short report. Percutaneous absorption of hydrocortisone 4 C in two human subjects. J Invest Dermatol 1955; 25:281–283.

4 The Skin Reservoir for Topically Applied Solutes

Michael S. Roberts, Sheree E. Cross, and Yuri G. Anissimov
University of Queensland, Queensland, Australia
University of South Australia, Adelaide, South Australia

CONTENTS

4.1 INTRODUCTION

The reservoir function of the skin is an important determinant of the duration of action of a topical solute. The reservoir can exist in the stratum corneum, in the viable avascular tissue (viable epidermis and supracapillary dermis), and in the dermis. There are a number of means by which this reservoir can be formed. A steroid reservoir in the stratum corneum has been demonstrated by the reactivation of a vasoconstrictor effect by occlusion or application of a placebo cream to the skin some time after the original topical application of steroid. Other solutes have also been reported to show a reservoir effect in the skin after topical application. In this work, we develop a simple compartmental model to understand why reactivation of vasoconstriction at some time after a topical steroid application shows dependency on time, topical solute concentration, and product used to cause reactivation. The model is also used to show which solutes are likely to show a reservoir effect and could be potentially affected by desquamation, especially when the turnover of the skin is abnormally rapid. A similar form of the model can be used to understand the promotion of reservoir function in the viable tissue and in the dermis in terms of effective removal by blood perfusing the tissues.

In this overview, we consider published examples consistent with a reservoir effect. In order to understand the effect, we present a simple pharmacokinetic model that we use to explain the reported phenomena. It is recognized that the model used lacks the mathematical rigor and accuracy that would be achieved with the more spatially correct representation of concentration gradients in tissues, as would be defined by diffusion models in series and a convective loss of squamae from the stratum corneum as a result of desquamation. However, the model does provide a simplistic interpretation of events that aids in understanding observed phenomena and in a generalized prediction of likely formation and evidence of a reservoir effect.

4.2 WHAT IS THE SKIN RESERVOIR AND WHY IS ITS UNDERSTANDING IN NATURE IMPORTANT?

Topical applications of medications account for about 5% of all products used for therapeutic purposes and may account for more if their cosmetic and cosmeceutic uses are recognized. Most studies on topical products are concerned with the effective penetration of the agents to cause a local or systemic effect or, from an environmental toxicology perspective, their undesirable penetration. What is less well understood is the sequestration of solutes into components of the skin and their rapid release on appropriate provocation of the skin some time later. In some cases, the amount of solute released is sufficient to yield a pharmacological action that replicates that observed when the solute was first applied. This phenomenon is most widely known as the reservoir effect as a consequence of it being used to show the reactivated steroid vasoconstrictor effect when an occlusive dressing was applied to the original steroid application site several weeks after the original application. The reservoir effect is not, however, limited to steroids or to the stratum corneum.

4.3 HISTORICAL PERSPECTIVE ON THE STRATUM CORNEUM RESERVOIR FOR DRUGS

The existence of a stratum corneum reservoir for drugs has been expressed in two forms. Vickers (1) has suggested a stratum corneum reservoir because a topical agent such as salicylic acid is excreted in the urine more slowly when applied topically than when injected intradermally (2). One could interpret a reservoir in this context as a function of the time lag associated with a drug diffusing through the skin, the time to reach steady state in the presence of a constant application, and the time to desorb after removal of the application. Hence, in this form, the reservoir is most evident for the more slowly diffusing drugs, i.e., those with long lag times. Schaefer et al. (3) also recognized the importance of the stratum corneum barrier as a determinant of reservoir function. They suggested that the reservoir function was the reciprocal function of the multilayer stratum corneum barrier.

The second form of the reservoir is the recognition that the skin may be a depot for drugs. Malkinson and Ferguson (4) first suggested this concept, but as Vickers (1) points out, their data could be explained by a slow diffusion process through the stratum corneum. Potential sites for this depot were suggested to be keratin spaces, follicular openings, and surface folds (5). The first definitive evidence of a stratum corneum depot for topical corticosteroids was presented by Vickers in 1963 (6). He conducted the experiments shown in Figure 4.1. He showed that the initial vasoconstrictor effects of a topical corticosteroid (fluocinolone acetonide or triamcinolone acetonide) occurring after application and occlusion with Saran film first disappeared within 10 to 16 hours, as expected on removal of the film. The vasoconstrictive effect could be reactivated for up to two weeks after topical application by repeated occlusion of the site. If the stratum corneum was stripped prior to the repeated occlusion, no repeat vasoconstriction is evident, providing evidence that the stratum corneum is the main site for the depot (Figure 4.1). Vickers (1) confirmed this site by showing tape strips of stratum corneum and biopsies from nonstripped epidermal sites had high counts after application of radiolabeled steroids, whereas the biopsy from stripped sites had a low count. Interestingly, the number of counts decreased with successive strips (1), as would be anticipated

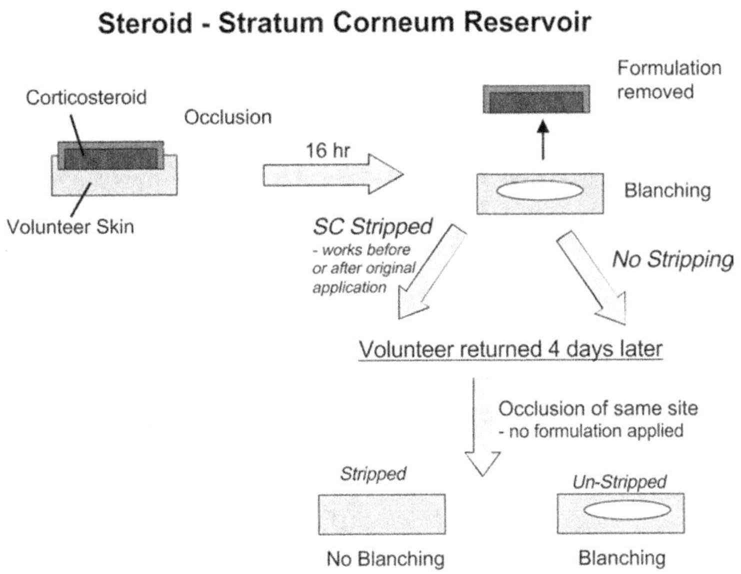

FIGURE 4.1   The reservoir effect as demonstrated by Vickers (6) in 1963.

with concentration distance profiles when a diffusion model is used to characterize the penetration process (7). The presence of a corticosteroid depot has been confirmed in a number of later papers (8, 9). Vickers (1) further observed that the duration of the reservoir depended on the nature of the drug, the vehicle used, the temperature of the skin, and the relative humidity to which the skin is exposed.

4.4   MODELING THE FORMATION AND DURATION OF THE STRATUM CORNEUM CORTICOSTEROID RESERVOIR

We propose that in a simplistic representation, the stratum corneum reservoir is defined by three independent variables: (1) the diffusivity of the drug in the stratum corneum, (2) the amount of drug in the stratum corneum, and (3) clearance of drug from the epidermis.

4.4.1   DIFFUSIVITY

The diffusivity of solutes in the stratum corneum determines the time to reach steady state or to desorb from the stratum corneum. When diffusivity is very slow, sufficient drug will not be taken up into the stratum corneum to be recognized as establishing a reservoir. Vickers (1) recognized that occlusion (via an increased humidity and temperature) was necessary to promote a reservoir effect. Occlusion leads to an increased hydration of the skin and a promotion of diffusivity (10). Further, as shown in Figure 4.2, if the duration of the application is too short relative to the diffusion time of the drug, a reservoir may not be evident. Vickers (1) suggested that, for steroids, ''an occlusion of 8 hr resulted in (if any) a short-lived reservoir that was often not reproducible.'' The increase in the stratum corneum reservoir for sodium fusidate, with increases with both temperature and increase in relative humidity, is consistent with these variables also increasing the percentage of sodium fusidate that had penetrated through the epidermis over 24 hours (1). The duration of the reservoir is also related to the nature of the drug, as shown in Figure 4.3. The duration of the reservoir for aspirin < fusidic acid < fluocinolone acetonide (1). Barry and Woodford (11) have suggested that a corticosteroid reservoir in the skin lasts for 8 to 14 days.

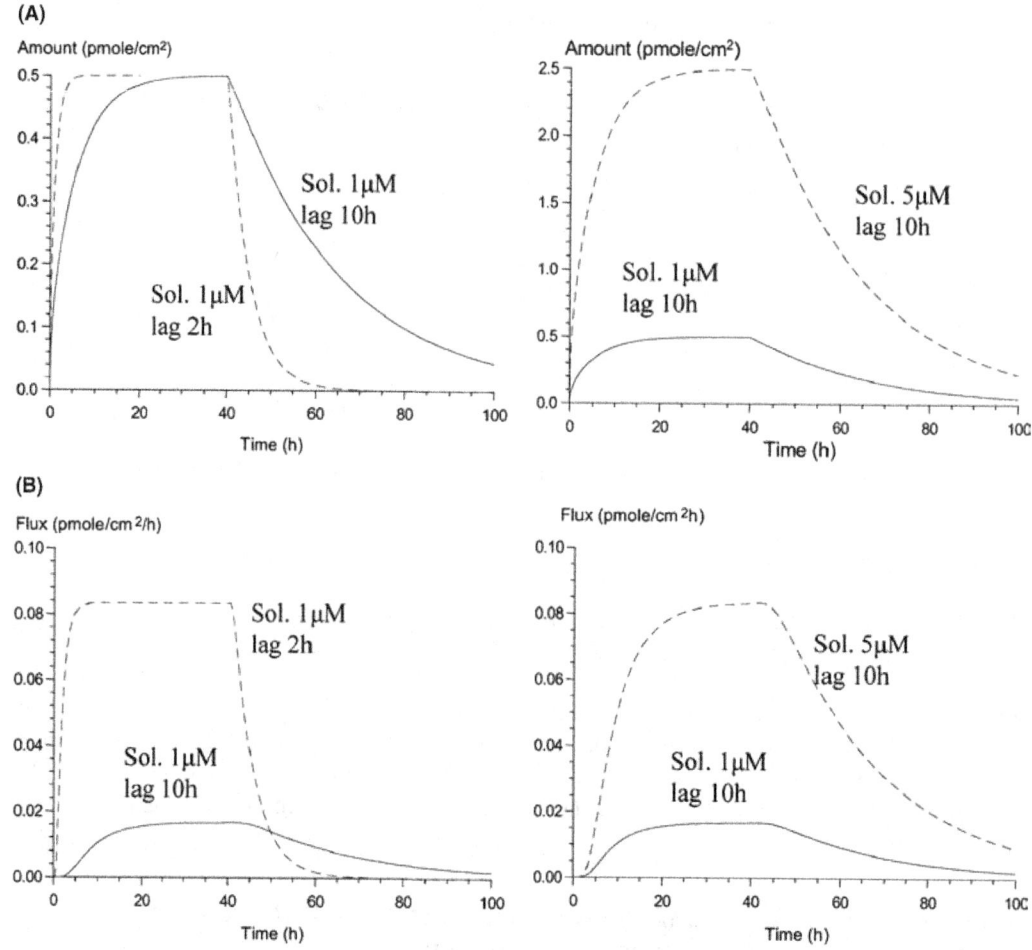

FIGURE 4.2 Amount in the stratum corneum (*a*) and flux through epidermis (*b*) based on a diffusion model for: (A) Two drugs with lag times of 2 and 10 hours and (B) two drugs with stratum corneum solubilities of 1 and 5 μM.

One could, in principle, estimate the duration of the reservoir for a given drug from the time required to reach maximal reservoir concentration (Figure 4.2) or from the epidermal lag times obtained in epidermal penetration studies. Using Equation (49) for lag time and the slowest term in Equation (23) from Roberts et al. (7), the duration time for 10% of the reservoir to remain (i.e., 90% has diffused out) is approximately 5.7 times that of the lag time. The corresponding duration time for 5% to be left remaining in the reservoir is 7.4 times the lag time. Accordingly, using a lag time for aspirin in a hydrated epidermal penetration study of about 0.6 hour (unpublished data) would suggest that 90% of the stratum corneum reservoir would be lost after about 3 to 4 hours. The actual time reported by Vickers (1) is about 240 hours, suggesting that the diffusivity in vivo is about 1/60th that for the hydrated stratum corneum in vitro. An important implication of this difference is that hydration of the stratum corneum by occlusion or other means may substantially increase diffusivity in the stratum corneum. Hydration and various penetration enhancers such as dimethylsulphfoxide have been reported to induce the steroid stratum corneum reservoir effect (1), probably as a result of their increasing drug diffusivity in the stratum corneum.

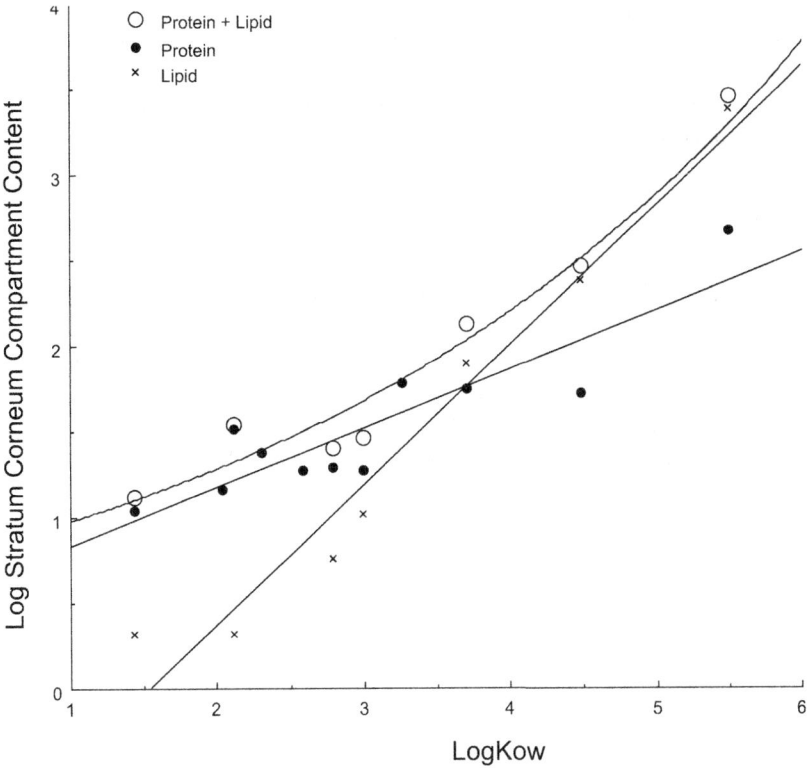

FIGURE 4.3 Plot of log apparent stratum corneum (protein and lipid)–water partition coefficient versus log octanol–water partition coefficient (ratio of 0.85 protein:0.15 lipid). Also shown is the contribution of the stratum corneum protein domain (0.85 protein) and stratum corneum lipid domain (0.15 lipid) to the partition coefficient. (Data abstracted from Reference 12.)

4.4.2 STRATUM CORNEUM PARTITIONING OR CAPACITY

The second determinant of the reservoir effect, the amount of drug in the stratum corneum, is defined by the affinity of the drug for the stratum corneum. In general, "like dissolves like" so that a lipophilic drug dissolved in a polar vehicle such as water will have a high affinity for the stratum corneum, whereas a lipophilic drug dissolved in a nonpolar vehicle such as oil will have a lower affinity. Figure 4.2b shows that increasing the affinity of drug for the stratum corneum results in a greater amount taken up into the stratum corneum but does not affect the time to be taken up or the fractional rate of reservoir depletion. Vickers (1) further suggested that the vehicle in which the steroid was applied was important. He suggested that the average duration of reservoir for 95% alcohol > hydrophilic cream > greasy ointment. If the 95% alcohol effectively left a solvent-deposited solid, the results may arise in part from the partitioning being in the same rank order. However, these vehicles are also likely to affect skin hydration, and stratum corneum diffusivity may be expected to be in the reverse order. Either or a combination of the two effects may explain the reservoir duration results obtained.

The nature of the drug may also affect the amount present in the reservoir. In general, following the principle of "like dissolves like," solutes having the greatest affinity for stratum corneum components would be expected to show the greatest stratum corneum reservoir effect. Figure 4.3 shows that the partitioning of various hydrocortisone-21-esters from water into the stratum corneum increases with lipophilicity, as defined by the octanol–water partition coefficient. These data suggest that partitioning occurs into both the lipid and protein domains of the stratum corneum, showing a higher dependency into the protein domain for the more polar steroids and higher dependency into the lipid domain for the more lipophilic steroids. Other autoradiographic data are consistent with steroids being preferentially located in or close to the intercellular lipids of the stratum corneum, suggesting that the steroid stratum corneum reservoir and lipid transport is in this lipid domain of the stratum corneum (13).

4.4.3 Clearance

In general, removal of solutes from the stratum corneum depends on clearance into the viable epidermis and thence into the dermis. Most of the clearance for steroids from the dermis is due to dermal blood flow (14). Although clearance is normally assumed not to be rate limiting, a sufficiently low clearance may lead to a reduced flux through the stratum corneum and an increased amount retained in the stratum corneum (15). A reduced clearance may arise, for instance, due to vasoconstriction being present or a poor solubility in the viable epidermis or dermis. Figure 4.4 shows that reducing clearance or reducing the partition coefficient between the viable epidermis and stratum corneum increases the duration of the reservoir.

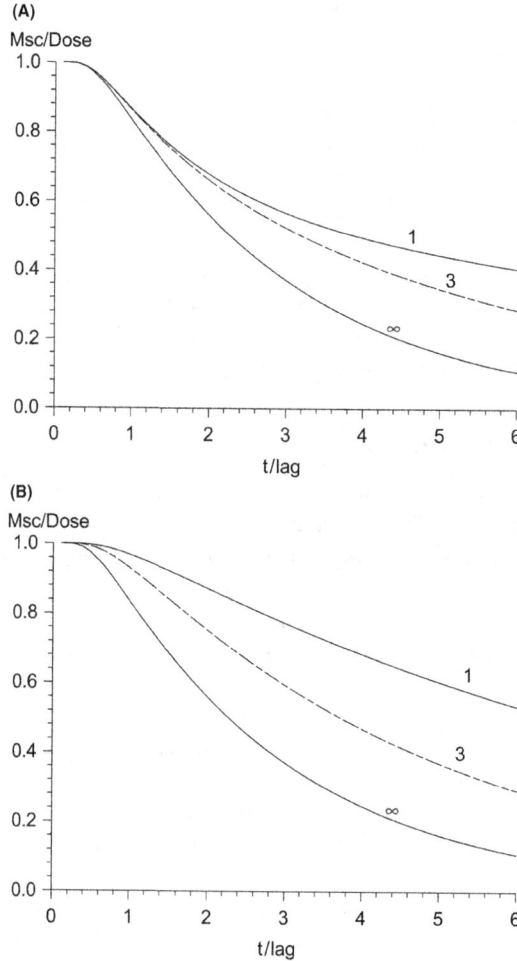

FIGURE 4.4 Effect of (A) blood clearance and (B) viable epidermal resistance relative to that of stratum corneum on the normalized amount remaining in the stratum corneum reservoir (M_{sc}/Dose) with time (t) normalized to lag time (lag time) following application of a solvent-deposited solid and using a diffusion model.

4.5 STRATUM CORNEUM RESERVOIR AND EPIDERMAL FLUX

Epidermal flux (J_{sc}) is defined by the product of the concentration of available drug in the stratum corneum and the diffusivity of a drug in the stratum corneum. Accordingly, percutaneous absorption may be related to the extent of reservoir function. At any given time, the amount of drug in the stratum corneum will be defined by the diffusivity into and affinity for the stratum corneum, as discussed earlier. Dupuis and co-workers (16) in 1984 first showed that the amount of different drugs absorbed in the body of a hairless rat could be correlated with the amounts found in the skin after topical application. This work was then confirmed in man (17) and extended to show that the relationship existed irrespective of anatomical site (18) or type of vehicle used (19).

4.6 STRATUM CORNEUM RESERVOIR AND SUBSTANTIVITY

Substantivity is a measure of the binding of solutes to sites in the stratum corneum, as evident by a resistance to be washed off or removed. Sunscreen substantivity has been defined as resistance to removal by water. The European Cosmetic, Toiletry, and Perfumery Association (COLIPA) has defined a water resistance retention for sunscreens (%WRR) in terms of the sun protection factors prior to (SPF$_{dry}$) and after water immersion (SPF$_{wet}$) (20):

$$\mathrm{WRR}(\%) = \frac{\mathrm{SPF_{wet}} - 1}{\mathrm{SPF_{dry}} - 1} \times 100 \tag{4.1}$$

Stokes and Diffey (20) showed that moisturizing products and sunscreens making no claims about water resistance were readily washed off. Waterproof lotions had the greatest retention of sunscreen (>80% after two applications), followed by water-resistant sunscreens (>60% after two applications). Wester et al. (21) showed that the retention of DDT and benzo[a]pyrene in skin after application in vitro for 25 minutes followed by a soap and water wash was 16.7% and 5.1%, respectively, after acetone application and 0.25% and 0.14%, respectively, after application in soil. Billhimer et al. (22) showed that the amount of 3,4,4'-trichlorocarbanilide remaining on the skin 24 hours after a final soap wash was sufficient to effectively inhibit the growth of *Staphylococcus aureus* added to the skin for 5 hours. A remnant antibacterial effect has been shown for a number of antiseptic products. The substantivity of hair dyes has recently been reviewed (23). Bucks (24) examined the long-term substantivity of hydrocortisone, estradiol, and five phenolic solutes following a one-day and a one-week wash using 10 stratum corneum tape strips after application of radiolabeled solutes to the ventral forearms of healthy male volunteers. He reported retention levels of 0% to 5% of the applied solutes after a week and suggested that the least lipophilic and most poorly penetrating chemicals had the higher substantivity.

4.7 MODELING THE VASOCONSTRICTOR EFFECT ASSOCIATED WITH THE CORTICOSTEROID RESERVOIR

Recently, Clarys et al. (25) carried out a study, which elaborates on the initial work of Vickers. They showed that blanching on reocclusion depended on the time of the reocclusion after the original application, the concentration of steroid, and whether an enhancer was used (Figure 4.5). The extent to which a reservoir is evident after such an application will be dependent on a number of factors (Figure 4.4). First, the reservoir of steroid in the skin achieved after topical application will be depleted (emptied) at a given rate. As Clarys et al. (25) point out, the amount of steroid remaining in the skin after low concentrations of halocinonide (0.005% and 0.05%) is not sufficient to exert a dermal vasoconstrictive effect when the site was reoccluded between 34 and 106 hours after the initial application. However, with 0.2%, a reservoir effect was demonstrated on reocclusion for at least 106 hours. Second, if the enhancement increased more than provided by reocclusion alone,

Steroid - Stratum Corneum Reservoir

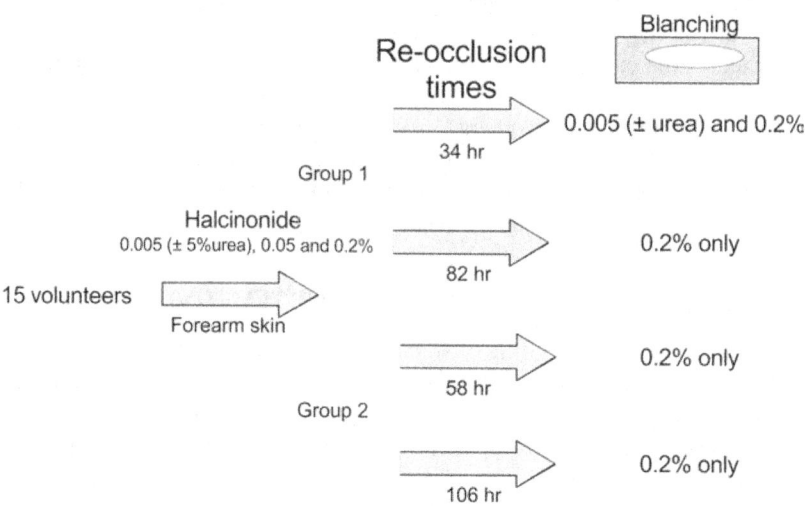

FIGURE 4.5 Time, concentration, and enhancer dependency of the reservoir effect as illustrated for halcinonide. (From Reference 25.)

it is possible that a reservoir effect will be evident with a lower steroid concentration but only for a short time. Clarys et al. (25) showed that when the enhancer urea was included in reocclusion after halcinonide 0.005%, a significant vasoconstriction was achieved when reocclusion was conducted at 34 hours but not at other later times.

Understanding changes in vasoconstriction associated with a stratum corneum reservoir effect through reocclusion or application of an enhancer at a time after the origination application is most easily achieved using an appropriate mathematical model. While a diffusion model may be the most appropriate to describe transport events in the skin and relatively easy to use when expressed in the Laplace domain (7), such a model is difficult to use when model parameters change during the time course of an experiment. Further, precise modeling is further complicated by the known steroid vasoconstrictor nonlinear topical dose–effect relationships (7). Accordingly, for this purpose, we have represented the stratum corneum and viable epidermis as simple, well-stirred compartments (Figure 4.6). We have further limited the model to situations where the reservoir has already been established so as to recognize that this model poorly predicts lag times associated with steady-state epidermal penetration (7, 26). As stated in the introduction, the model has an obvious limitation in that it assumes all of the tissues are well stirred when a diffusional process would better describe the solute transport therein.

The rate constant k_1 is related to the diffusion time, i.e., $k_1 = \pi^2 D_{sc}/4h^2_{sc}$, where D_{sc} is the diffusivity and h_{sc} is the thickness of the stratum corneum. This definition is also equivalent to $\pi^2 k_p A_s/4V_{apsc}$ as $k_p = K_{sc-ve} D_s/h_{sc}$, and $V_{apsc} = K_{sc-ve} V_{sc} = K_{sc-ve} A_s h_{sc}$, where V_{apsc} is the apparent distribution volume of the solute in the stratum corneum and A_s is the area of application. This constant k_1 could be further complicated by also being a function of microconstants defining other transport events in the stratum corneum. The rate constant k_2 is a function of both the diffusion time and stratum corneum–viable epidermis partition coefficient K_{sc-ve}, i.e., k_2 is equivalent to $K_{sc--ve} k_1 V_{sc}/V_{ve}$, where Vve is the volume of distribution of the solute in the viable tissue. It is apparent that when k_2 or K_{sc--ve} is large, a reservoir effect in the stratum corneum is promoted. The rate constant k_3 defines the removal of the solute from the viable tissue and can be derived from the clearance of solute from the tissue as $k_3 = CL_{ve}/V_{ve}$.

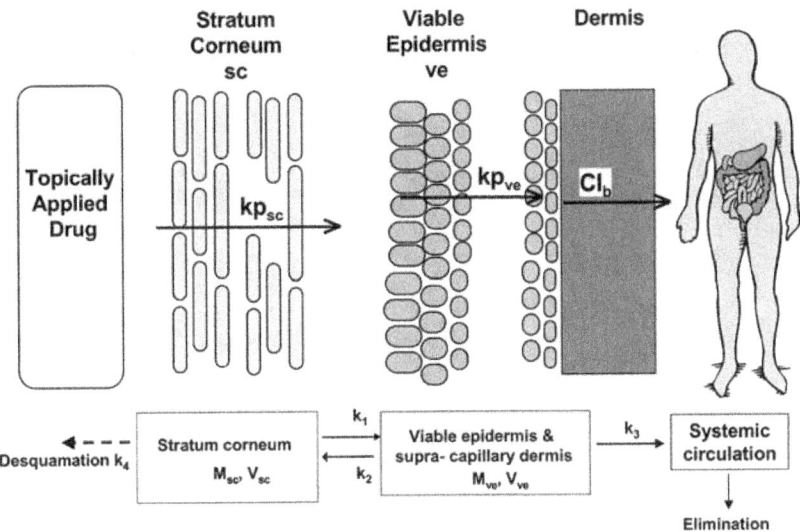

FIGURE 4.6 One-compartmental model representations of stratum corneum and viable avascular tissues used to examine the stratum corneum reservoir effect.

The model differential equations are as follows:

$$\frac{dM_{sc}}{dt} = k_2 M_{ve} - k_1 M_{sc}, \frac{dM_{ve}}{dt} = k_1 M_{sc} - (k_2 + k_3) M_{ve} \qquad (4.2)$$

where M_{ve} is the amount in the viable tissue and M_{sc} is the amount of solute in the stratum corneum. Sink conditions are defined by $k_3 \gg k_2, k_1$; for this special case M_{ve} is relatively small, and we apply an approximation of $M_{ve} \approx 0$ and $dM_{ve}/dt \approx 0$ in Equation (4.2) to give:

$$M_{ve} \approx M_{sc} \frac{k_1}{k_2 + k_3} \qquad (4.3)$$

Equation (4.2) defines the amount of solute in the viable tissue, as well as the concentration C_{ve}, since $C_{ve} = M_{ve}/V_{ve}$. It is evident from Equation (4.3) that an increase in stratum corneum permeability, as evident by an increase in k_1 from, for instance, reocclusion, will increase M_{ve} and therefore, in the case of steroids, the extent of vasoconstriction. The more k_1 is increased, the greater M_{ve} is. It should also be noted that the amount remaining in the stratum corneum is expressed in this case as:

$$M_{sc} \approx M_r \exp(-k_1 t) \qquad (4.4)$$

where M_r is the amount of drug in the stratum corneum reservoir after loading. Hence, an increase in the stratum corneum permeability rate constant k_1 will deplete the amount in the reservoir M_{sc} more rapidly. Also, Equation (4.4) states that the amount in the reservoir M_{sc} is depleting at a rate defined by a rate constant k_1 so that at a sufficient time and in the absence of no further application, the reservoir will be sufficiently depleted so that it no longer exists. Figure 4.7 shows an illustration of these concepts for corticosterone. It is evident that a twentyfold increase in diffusivity as a consequence of occlusion greatly accelerates steroid loss from the stratum corneum reservoir and increases the viable epidermal concentration with the consequential effect of likely vasoconstriction.

In general, the reservoir effect will be observed when a stratum corneum permeability enhancer is applied and causes an increase in the release of the solute from the stratum corneum. In the case of corticosteroids, the most commonly applied enhancer used to demonstrate the reservoir effect is

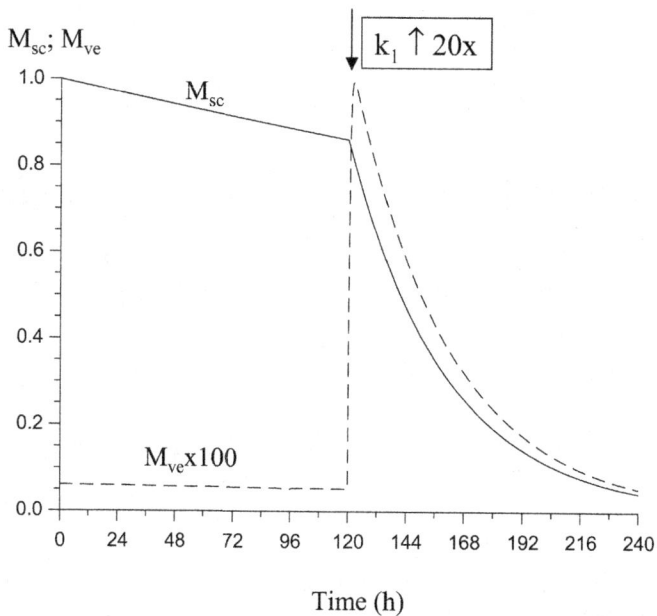

Time (h)

FIGURE 4.7 Amount of corticosterone remaining in the stratum corneum reservoir M_{sc} (—) and in the viable epidermis M_{ve} (x100) (– –) as a function of time based on a simple compartmental model. At 120 hours, it is assumed occlusion has increased stratum corneum diffusivity (k_1 in the compartment model shown in Figure 4.6) 20×. A lag time of 16.5 hours for hydrated epidermis (14), a stratum corneum–viable epidermis partition coefficient of about 0.5 (unpublished data) and k_3 0.3 hr^1 [using dermal clearance (14), and assuming a viable epidermis to stratum corneum thickness ratio of 20].

water (10). Application of an occlusive dressing leads to a reduction of transepidermal water loss and retention of water in the stratum corneum, leading to an increased hydration of various stratum corneum components and an increase in the diffusivity of corticosteroids from the stratum corneum into the viable epidermis and dermis. However, other enhancers such as urea (25) and propylene glycol (27) have also been shown to promote release of steroids from the stratum corneum.

4.8 CHANGES IN PLASMA STEROID LEVELS ASSOCIATED WITH THE CORTICOSTEROID RESERVOIR

Figure 4.8 shows that after topical application of hydrocortisone, a rebound effect in its plasma levels can be achieved when a placebo cream is applied 12 hours after the original product (27). The profiles are consistent with those predicted in Figure 4.7. One possible explanation for the data is a loss of occlusion and decrease in the stratum corneum diffusivity (k_1) between 4 and 12 hours as a result of the cream drying out or subject activity. Application of the placebo cream containing an enhancer leads to an increase in stratum corneum diffusivity and an increase in hydrocortisone release to lower tissues (Figure 4.6) and then into the blood, giving the profile observed in Figure 4.8.

4.9 ROLE OF DESQUAMATION ON STRATUM CORNEUM RESERVOIR EFFECT

In general, it has been asserted that the stratum corneum reservoir is "continuously emptied" by desquamation (28) and that desquamation may have a greater effect on the percutaneous penetration of more lipophilic solutes than would be indicated by the initial partitioning (29). Reddy et al. (30) have recently examined the effects of desquamation on permeation using a theoretical analysis

Steroid - Stratum Corneum Reservoir

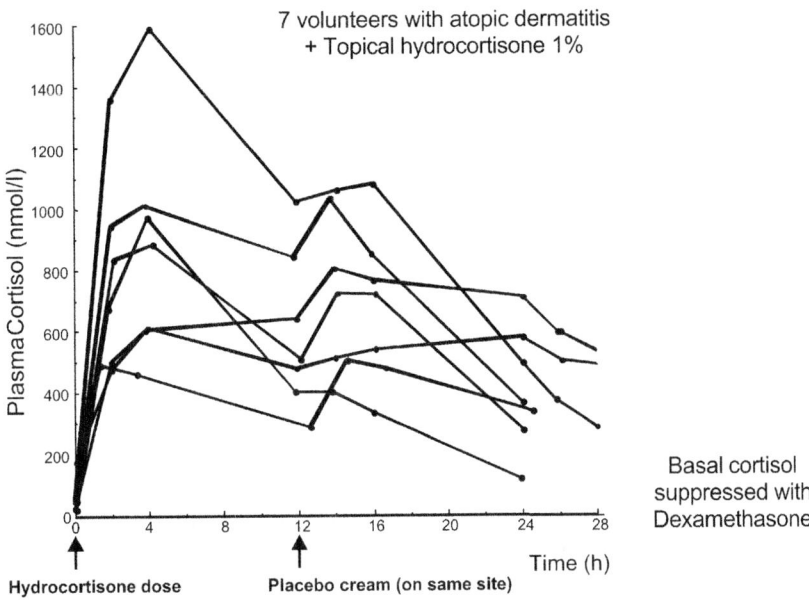

FIGURE 4.8 Evidence of a reservoir effect for hydrocortisone demonstrated by application of a placebo cream 12 hours after the original application of topical hydrocortisone 1%. (Data from Reference 22.)

based on a number of assumptions, including an epidermal turnover time of 14 days, that the viable epidermis turns over at twice the rate of the stratum corneum, and that the viable epidermis is ten-fold the thickness of the stratum corneum. They concluded that significant amounts of drug could be removed if the epidermal turnover was fast relative to the rate of diffusion through the stratum corneum. However, this event was only likely for highly lipophilic or very large solutes.

Desquamation is likely to have a greater effect on the reservoir effect for diseased skin to which corticosteroids are applied. The effect of desquamation can be examined using the simple compartmental model in Figure 4.6 by adding a rate constant k_4 for desquamation. When clearance from the skin is high so that $k_3 \gg k_2$, it is evident that desquamation will only affect the amount of solute remaining in the stratum corneum M_{sc} when the desquamation rate constant k_4 is of a similar order or higher than the diffusion rate constant k_1 through the stratum corneum [Equation (4.5)]:

$$M_{sc} = M_r\left[-\{k_1 + k_4\}t\right] \tag{4.5}$$

It is evident that for the corticosteroid corticosterone, desquamation may increase the rate of depletion of solute from the stratum corneum and that this contribution is likely to be most significant when the epidermis is diseased and has a faster-than-normal turnover rate, as in psoriasis. A flow-on from this analysis is that slowing down the epidermal turnover rate by steroid application is also likely to be associated with an increase in the steroid stratum corneum reservoir at later times (Figure 4.9).

It is to be reemphasized that the model used here is limited by its assumption of a well-mixed compartment for the stratum corneum when the desquamation process is a convective process occurring in the opposite direction to the diffusion-defined chemical concentration–distance gradient in the stratum corneum (Figure 4.10). As Reddy et al. (30) point out, the permeability of

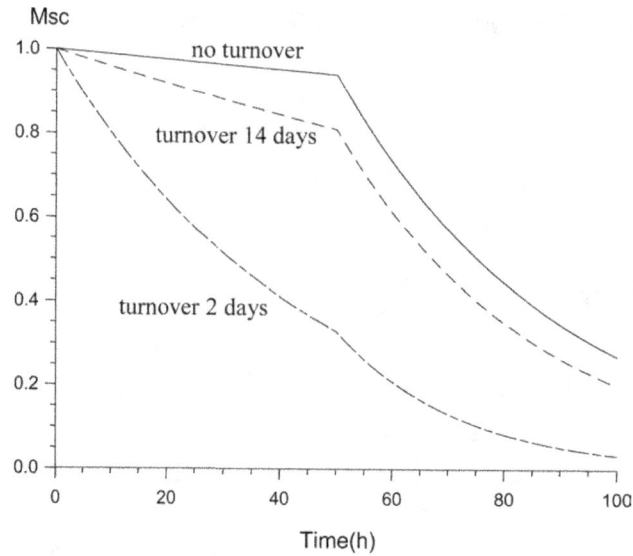

FIGURE 4.9 Amount remaining in stratum corneum reservoir of corticosterone (using hydrated epidermal lag time 16.5 hours and other parameters from Figure 4.7) with no desquamation (—), a normal epidermal turnover of 14 days (– –), and a psoriatic epidermal turnover of 2 days (— –) and the compartmental model described in Figure 4.6.

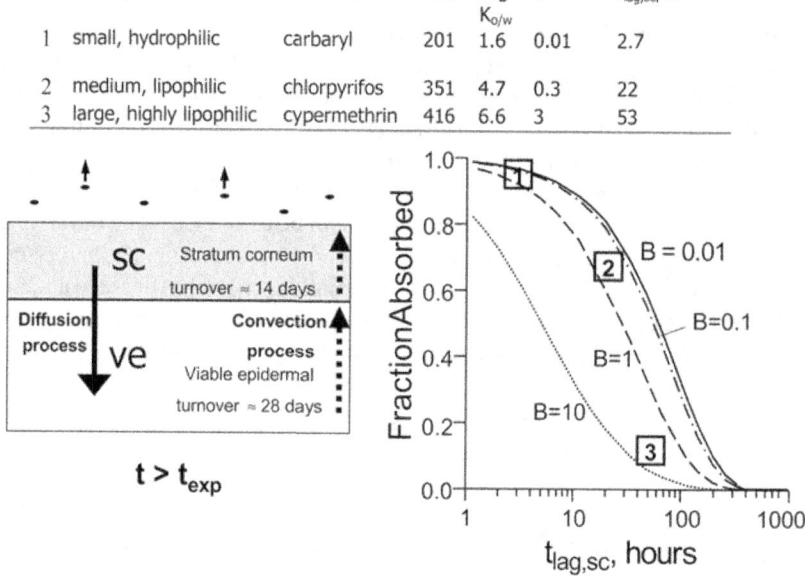

	description	Pesticide	MW	log $K_{o/w}$	B	$t_{lag,sc}$, h
1	small, hydrophilic	carbaryl	201	1.6	0.01	2.7
2	medium, lipophilic	chlorpyrifos	351	4.7	0.3	22
3	large, highly lipophilic	cypermethrin	416	6.6	3	53

FIGURE 4.10 Effect of ratio of stratum corneum to viable epidermis permeabilities (*B*) and diffusional lag time on the fraction absorbed from human stratum corneum with a normal turnover, highlighting differences in absorption for the pesticides carbaryl, chlorpyrifos, and cypermethrin. Based on two convection–diffusion models and a continuity of flux across the stratum corneum–viable epidermal interface. (Adapted from material provided by A. Bunge, personal communication.)

the viable epidermis may also be a determinant of stratum corneum concentrations, leading to a decrease in the loss from the stratum corneum for the more lipophilic solutes. Mimicking an increased resistance from the viable epidermis by reducing in k_3 in the present simple model leads to the amount in stratum corneum being lost at a slower rate [Equations (4.2) and (4.3)]. The use of convection diffusion equations by Reddy et al. (30) provides a more realistic representation of events. Figure 4.10, developed using such a model, shows that when chemicals diffuse slowly (i.e., long lag times—often associated with large molecules), the fraction absorbed from the stratum corneum is likely to be reduced as a result of desquamation. Increasing solute lipophilicity (i.e., increased B) will result in a greater viable epidermal resistance to transport and a reduced fraction of solute likely to be absorbed from the stratum corneum. Figure 4.10 also shows that two of the lipophilic pesticides should have a lower fraction absorbed into the body from the stratum corneum as a consequence of desquamation.

4.10   STRATUM CORNEUM RESERVOIR FOR OTHER SOLUTES

It is to be emphasized that a reservoir effect is not restricted to steroids. Benowitz et al. (31) showed that continued absorption of nicotine from the skin after decontamination is therefore evidence of the stratum corneum acting as a reservoir for nicotine (Figure 4.11). Caffeine has also been shown to have a reservoir in the stratum corneum, and this reservoir is greater for an emulsion than for acetone (32) (Figure 4.12).

Yagi et al. (33) have suggested that cationic beta-blocking drugs may accumulate in stratum corneum intercellular lipids as a consequence of binding to endogenous anionic lipids such as cholesterol-3-sulfate, palmitic acid, stearic acid, and oleic acid. As shown in Figure 4.13, caffeine and a number of sunscreen agents were retained in the stratum corneum and had not penetrated into the epidermis, dermis, or receptor fluid after 16 hours. Other solutes have a high affinity for the stratum corneum, including surfactants testosterone (35). The magnitude of epidermal binding of

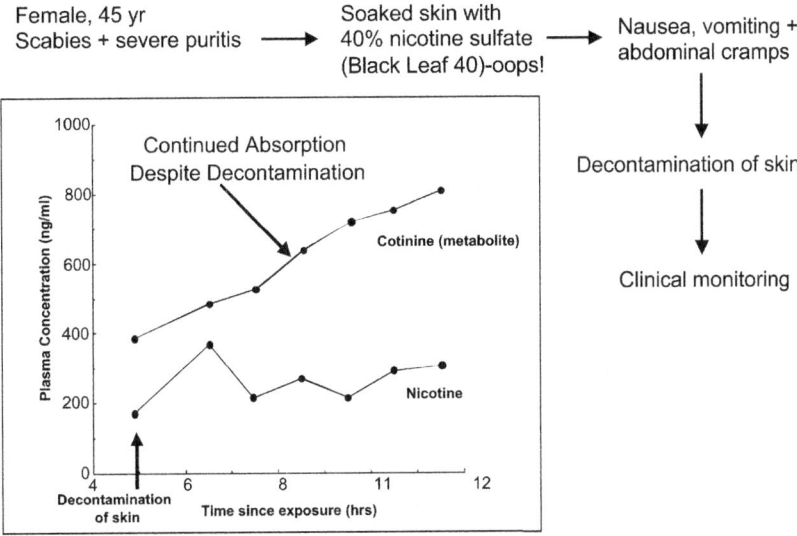

FIGURE 4.11   Evidence of a nicotine reservoir in the skin, as shown by the appearance of nicotine and its metabolite cotinine in plasma after topical decontamination. (From Reference 31.)

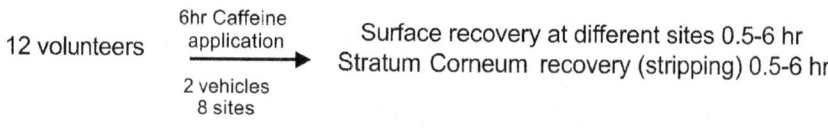

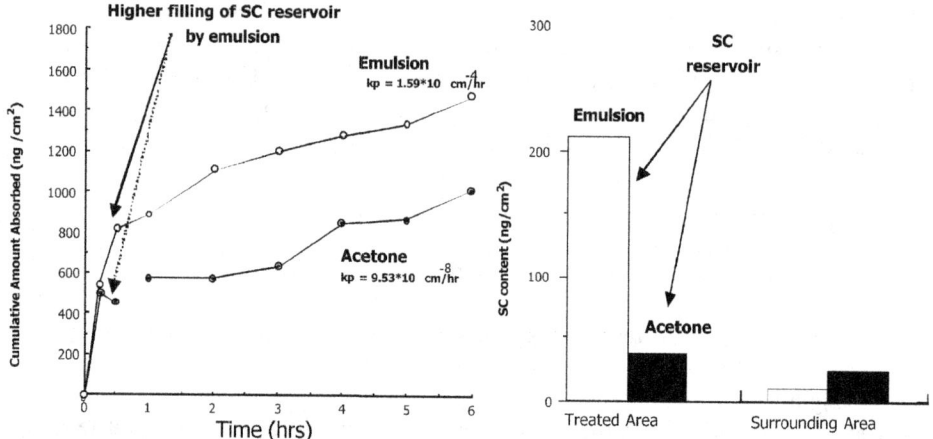

FIGURE 4.12 Effect of formulation on the extent to which a reservoir is formed in the stratum corneum for caffeine. (From Reference 32.)

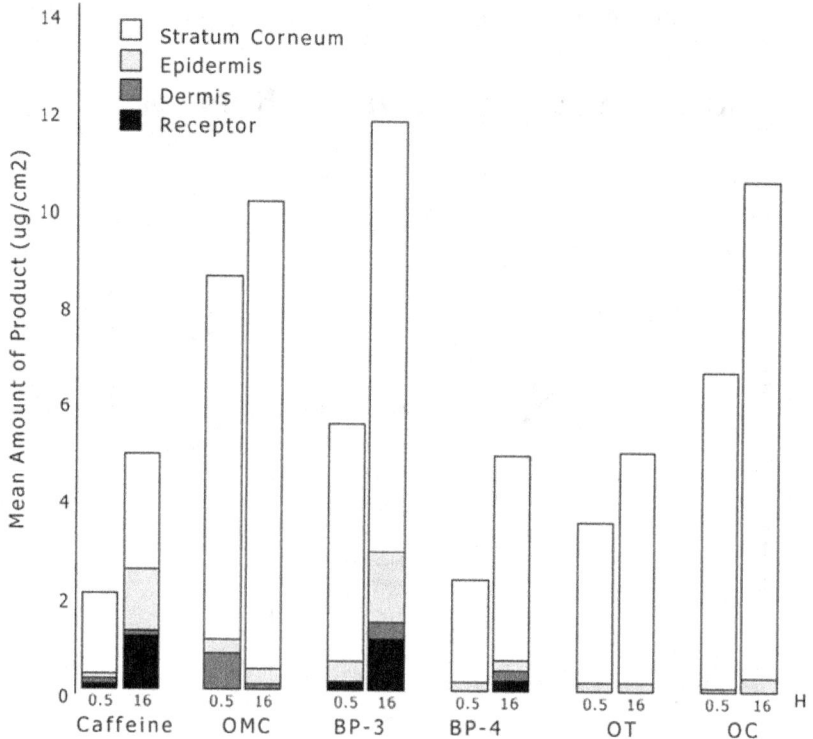

FIGURE 4.13 Differential distributions of caffeine and a number of sunscreens between the stratum corneum, epidermis, dermis, and receptor after in vitro penetration studies. (From Reference 34.)

testosterone exceeds by several-fold that of the dermis, but because of the many-fold thickness of the dermis, far larger amounts are associatively bound from which it is eluted in body fluids. It is plasma protein bound, and therefore its absorption is enhanced. Malathion (36), hair dyes (37), and vitamin E (38) are examples of the many compounds shown to be bound to stratum corneum components.

4.11   VIABLE EPIDERMIS AND DERMAL RESERVOIR

Most studies have emphasized the stratum corneum as a reservoir. However, the viable epidermis, dermis, and underlying tissues may themselves also act as reservoirs. Baker et al. (39) have reported binding of topical steroids to epidermal tissue. The effect of viable epidermal and dermal tissues as reservoirs may be limited by the often-extensive metabolism, which can occur in viable tissue and its location. For beta-estradiol, metabolic activity mainly resided in the basal layer of the viable epidermis (40). Accumulation and the concentration in the basal cell layer of the epidermis are important for many solutes, and it has been suggested that it is the free drug concentration that exerts a pharmacological effect (41). Accumulation in the viable epidermis can be deduced using the model described in Figure 4.6, and this has been used to examine epidermal concentrations of steroids (14). Walter and Kurz (42) have reported that the binding of 10 drugs to both epidermis and dermis was related to the lipophilicity of the drugs. Yagi et al. (33) have commented that binding of beta-blockers to viable epidermis components is an important determinant of the residence time in viable skin. In addition to binding, the rate of removal by the perfusing blood should be a determinant of the extent of reservoir formation in these tissues, as is evident by prolonged anesthesia when a vasoconstrictor is included with a local anesthetic in intradermal injections. Dermal and lower tissue level concentrations are apparent when a drug is applied together with a vasoconstrictor (43).

As an illustration of this principle, the dermal clearance and retention of diclofenac can be shown to depend on both binding to dermal tissues and to blood flow, and this effect is most evident when binding protein is not present in the blood (44).

When dextran rather than albumin is used as the perfusate, diclofenac is retained in the skin after dermal application, and the retention sites are the dermis and subcutaneous tissue (Figure 4.14).

The expression for the retention half-life ($t_{0.5}$) for solutes in the dermis and other tissues can be related to three key parameters: binding to plasma components (fraction unbound [fu_p]), binding to the dermis (fu_T), and the blood flow to the topical site (Q_p), as well as the relative volumes for solute distribution in the plasma (V_p) and in extravascular tissue space (V_{TE}) (44). Drugs such as diclofenac show much greater binding to dermis (and plasma) than some other solutes and therefore are preferentially retained.

4.12   IN VITRO–IN VIVO CORRELATIONS

Recently considerable interest has concerned the skin reservoir associated with in vitro skin penetration studies (45). Conflict presently exists as to whether or not skin levels remaining in the stratum corneum and epidermis/dermis at the end of an in vitro study should be included in the overall estimation of absorbed material. As Yourick et al. (45) point out, guidelines issued by COLIPA and the Scientific Committee on Cosmetic Product and Non-food Products suggest that material remaining in the stratum corneum at the end of a study should not be considered as systemically available, whereas that in the viable epidermis and dermis should. In contrast, the European Centre for Ecotoxicology and Toxicology of Chemicals suggests that percutaneous absorption should be based on receptor fluid concentrations only. The draft Organization for Economic Co-operation and Development guidelines take an intermediate position, namely that the amount of material should include both the skin and receptor fluid unless additional studies can demonstrate that the material in the skin is effectively not available.

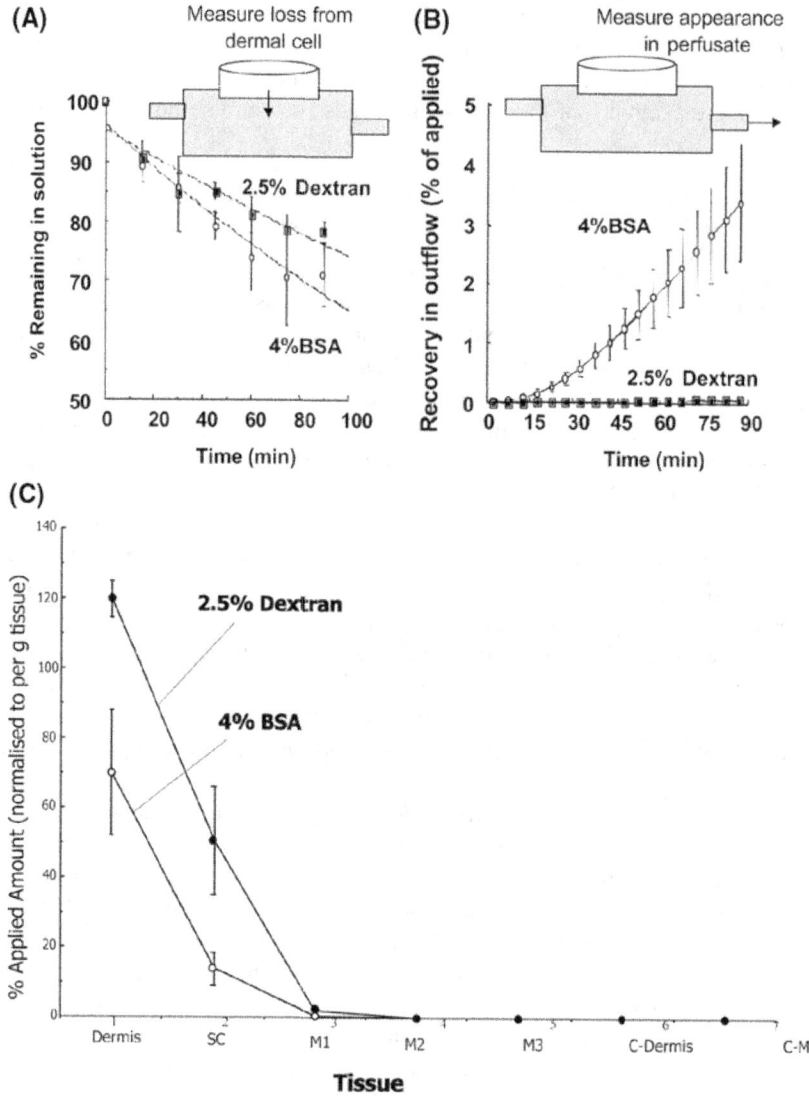

FIGURE 4.14 Amount remaining in (a) dermal absorption cell; (b) eluting in the perfusate; and (c) present in dermis, subcutaneous tissue (SC), muscle (M), and contralateral tissue after dermal application of diclofenac using perfusate, which binds (4% albumin) and does not bind (2.5% dextran) to diclofenac. (From Reference 44.)

As a consequence, any exposure assessment should include an assessment of the likely skin reservoir that exists in terms of whether the chemical in the skin is available for systemic absorption. In principle, the likely extent of the stratum corneum reservoir should be defined at the end of the application together with an estimate of the extent of binding/partitioning to lipid and protein components (Figure 4.3). Prediction of the stratum corneum reservoir is complicated by effects such as binding of solutes to keratin in the stratum corneum and viable epidermis, lipophilicity, and ionization (23, 46, 47); the dependence of the skin reservoir on the nature of formulation used (45, 48); and the use of soaps (49). Further, the stratum corneum and the viable epidermis are not homogenous membranes, but ones in which partitioning may vary with depth from the surface (50, 51) and/or being more evident in specific regions, e.g., around the hair (45).

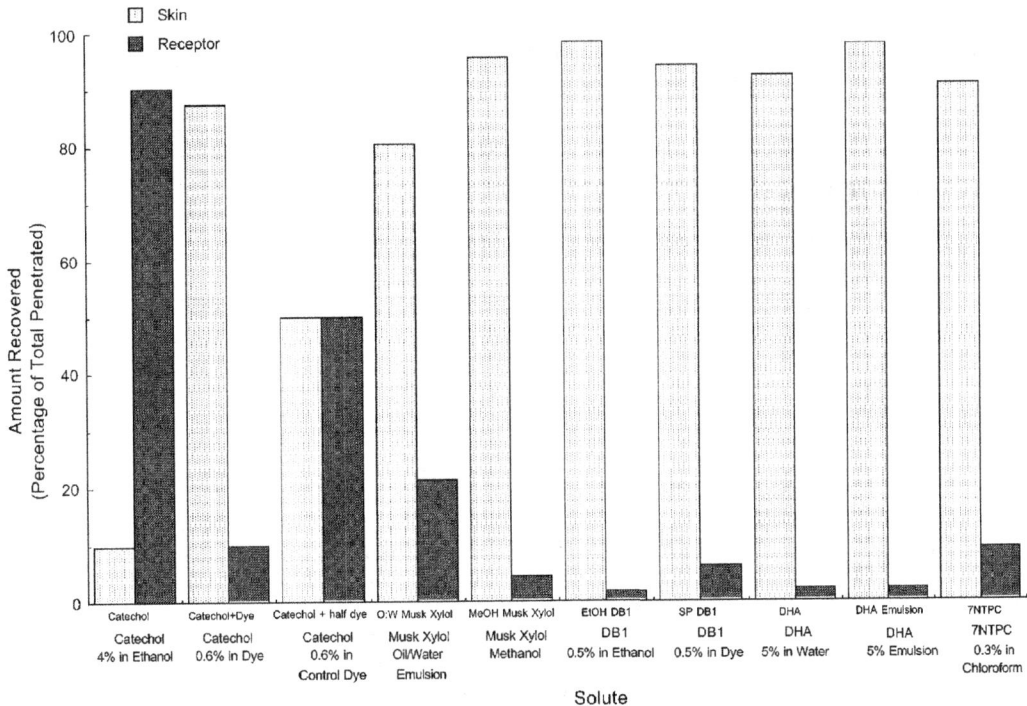

FIGURE 4.15 Comparison of the amount of solute retained in human skin to that penetrating into receptor fluid as a percentage of the total amount penetrated. (Data from References 45, 52, and 53.)

However, a cautious adoption of the present guidelines would suggest that it is the reservoir effect in the viable epidermis and dermis that is of most interest in dermal exposure risk assessment. Of note, it may be that all of the skin will eventually be seen to be important. At this stage there are insufficient data available to be definitive. Yourich et al. (45) point out that when the sun tanning color additive dihydroxyacetone and a fluorescent brightening agent 7-(2H-naphthol[1,2-d]triazole-2-yl)-3-phenylcoumarin are applied to human skin in vitro for 24 hours, the amount remaining in the viable epidermis and dermis constituted 50% or more of the dose calculated to have penetrated. Neither dihydroxyacetone nor 7-(2H-naphthol[1,2- d]triazole-2-yl)-3-phenylcoumarin was metabolized, and only 5% of dihydroxyace- tone was covalently bound to protein. In contrast, the comparable fractions of the amount in the viable epidermis and dermis relative to dose penetrated for the dye agents disperse blue 1 and catechol were small (45, 52). Further, Jung et al. (52) showed that whereas 7% of a catechol dose is absorbed from an ethanol vehicle, less than 0.5% of catechol is absorbed in a consumer permanent hair dye product, with the lower absorption reflecting oxidation of catechol in the latter product. Yurich et al. (45) suggest that it is appropriate to add skin levels to receptor fluids to gain a more realistic measure of dermal absorption when movement of the chemical from the skin to the receptor fluid is known to occur. They further suggest that significant retention in the skin occurs for both polar and nonpolar solutes. Figure 4.15 shows some examples of the relative percentages of solutes penetrating the skin that were recovered in the skin itself and in the receptor fluid. Accordingly, they suggest that further characterization and quantification of the skin reservoir are needed in dermal exposure assessment.

4.13 CONCLUSION

The skin or transdermal reservoir effect is a well-established phenomenon that is both dependent on the amount accumulating in the skin and evident at some time after the original application by application of some type of skin enhancement such as reocclusion or a chemical enhancer.

The time of the follow-up application and the extent of the enhancement will govern the presence of a reservoir effect. Desquamation will only affect the reservoir effect when the penetration rate of the solute is very slow. The reservoir effect is also important in dermal exposure risk assessments.

ACKNOWLEDGMENT

This work was supported by the Australian National Health and Medical Research Council and the Lions Medical Research Foundation. We are grateful to Professor Annette Bunge and Dr. Micaela Reddy for providing us with the material for Figure 4.10. This chapter is an update of our recently published review (54).

REFERENCES

1. Vickers CF. Stratum corneum reservoir for drugs. Adv Biol Skin 1972; 12:177–189.
2. Guillot M. Physiochemical conditions of cutaneous absorption. J Physiol 1954; 46:31–49.
3. Schaefer H, Stuttgen G, Zesch A, Schalla W, Gazith J. Quantitative determination of percutaneous absorption of radiolabeled drugs in vitro and in vivo by human skin. Curr Probl Dermatol 1978; 7:80–94.
4. Malkinson FD, Ferguson EH. Percutaneous absorption of hydrocortisone-4-C14 in two human subjects. J Invest Dermatol 1955; 25:281–283.
5. Sulzberger MB, Hermann F. On some characteristics and biological functions of the skin surface. Dermatologica (Basel) 1961; 123:1–23.
6. Vickers CFH. Existence of reservoir in the stratum corneum—experimental proof. Arch Dermatol 1963; 88:20–33.
7. Roberts MS, Anissimov Y, Gonsalvez R. Mathematical models in percutaneous absorption. In: Bronaugh RL, Maibach HI, eds. Percutaneous Absorption: Drugs Cosmetics Mechanisms Methodology. 3rd ed. New York: Marcel Dekker, 1999:3–55.
8. Carr RD, Wieland RG. Corticosteroid reservoir in the stratum corneum. Arch Dermatol 1966; 94:81–84.
9. Zesch A, Schaefer H, Hoffmann W. Barrier and reservoir function of individual areas of the horny layers of human skin for locally administered drugs. Arch Derm Forsch 1973; 246:103–107.
10. Roberts MS, Walker M. Water—the most natural penetration enhancer. In: Walters KA, Hadgraft J, eds. Skin Penetration Enhancement. New York: Marcel Dekker, 1993: 1–30.
11. Barry BW, Woodford R. Comparative bio-availability and activity of proprietary topical corticosteroid preparations: vasoconstrictor assays on thirty-one ointments. Br J Dermatol 1975; 93:563–571.
12. Anderson BD, Higuchi WI, Raykar PV. Heterogeneity effects on permeability—partition coefficients in human stratum corneum. Pharm Res 1988; 5:566–573.
13. Neelissen JA, Arth C, Wolff M, Schrijvers AH, Junginger HE, Bodde HE. Visualization of percutaneous 3H-estradiol and 3H-norethindrone acetate transport across human epidermis as a function of time. Acta Derm Venereol Suppl (Stockh) 2000; 208:36–43.
14. Siddiqui O, Roberts MS, Polack AE. Percutaneous absorption of steroids: relative contributions of epidermal penetration and dermal clearance. J Pharmacokin Biopharm 1989; 17:405–424.
15. Anissimov Y, Roberts MS. Diffusion modeling of percutaneous absorption kinetics. 1. Effects of flow rate, receptor sampling rate, and viable epidermal resistance for a constant donor concentration. J Pharm Sci 1999; 88:1201–1209.
16. Rougier A, Dupuis D, Lotte C, Roguet R, Schaefer H. In vivo correlation between stratum corneum reservoir function and percutaneous absorption. J Invest Dermatol 1983; 81:275–278.
17. Dupuis D, Rougier A, Roguet R, Lotte C, Kalopissis G. In vivo relationship between horny layer reservoir effect and percutaneous absorption in human and rat. J Invest Dermatol 1984; 82:353–356.
18. Rougier A, Dupuis D, Lotte C, Roguet R, Wester RC, Maibach HI. Regional variation in percutaneous absorption in man: measurement by the stripping method. Arch Dermatol Res 1986; 278:465–469.
19. Dupuis D, Rougier A, Roguet R, Lotte C. The measurement of the stratum corneum reservoir: a simple method to predict the influence of vehicles on in vivo percutaneous absorption. Br J Dermatol 1986; 115:233–238.
20. Stokes RP, Diffey BL. The water resistance of sunscreen and day-care products. Br J Dermatol 1999; 140:259–263.
21. Wester RC, Maibach HI, Bucks DA, Sedik L, Melendres J, Liao C, DiZio S. Percutaneous absorption of [14C]DDT and [14C]benzo[a]pyrene from soil. Fundam Appl Toxicol 1990; 15:510–516.

22. Billhimer WL, Berge CA, Englehart JS, Rains GY, Keswick BH. A modified cup scrub method for assessing the antibacterial substantivity of personal cleansing products. J Cosmet Sci 2001; 52:369–375.
23. Dessler W. Percutaneous absorption of hair dyes. In: Roberts MS, Walters KA, eds. Dermal Absorption and Toxicity Assessment. New York: Marcel Dekker, 1998:489–536.
24. Bucks DAW. Predictive Approaches II. In: Mass-Balance Procedure in Topical Drug Bioavailability, Bioequivalence and Penetration. New York: Plenum Press, 1993:183–195.
25. Clarys P, Gabard B, Barel AO. A qualitative estimate of the influence of halcinonide concentration and urea on the reservoir formation in the stratum corneum. Skin Pharmacol Appl Skin Physiol 1999; 12:85–89.
26. McCarley KD, Bunge AL. Pharmacokinetic models of dermal absorption. J Pharm Sci 2001; 90:1699–1719.
27. Turpeinen M. Absorption of hydrocortisone from the skin reservoir in atopic dermatitis. Br J Dermatol 1991; 124:358–360.
28. Schaefer H, Redelmeier M. Skin Barrier. Basel: Karger, 1996:40–42.
29. Roberts MS, Walters KA. The relationship between structure and barrier function of skin. Dermal Absorp Toxic Assess 1998; 91:1–42.
30. Reddy MB, Guy RH, Bunge AL. Does epidermal turnover reduce percutaneous penetration? Pharm Res 2000; 17:1414–1419.
31. Benowitz NL, Lake T, Keller KH, Lee BL. Prolonged absorption with development of tolerance to toxic effects after cutaneous exposure to nicotine. Clin Pharmacol Ther 1987; 42:119–120.
32. Chambin-Remoussenard O, Treffel P, Bechtel Y, Agache P. Surface recovery and stripping methods to quantify percutaneous absorption of caffeine in humans. J Pharm Sci 1982; 11:1099–1101.
33. Yagi S, Nakayama K, Kurosaki Y, Higaki K, Kimura T. Factors determining drug residence in skin during transdermal absorption: studies on beta-blocking agents. Biol Pharm Bull 1998; 21:1195–1201.
34. Potard G, Laugel C, Schaefer H, Marty J-P. The stripping technique: in vitro absorption and penetration of five UV filters on excised fresh human skin. Skin Pharmacol Appl Skin Physiol 2000; 13:336–344.
35. Menczel E, Maibach HI. Chemical binding to human dermis in vitro testosterone and benzyl alcohol. Acta Derm Venereol 1972; 52:38–42.
36. Menczel E, Bucks D, Maibach H, Wester R. Malathion binding to sections of human skin: skin capacity and isotherm determinations. Arch Dermatol Res 1983; 275:403–406.
37. Bronaugh RL, Congdon ER. Percutaneous absorption of hair dyes: correlation with partition coefficients. J Invest Dermatol 1984; 83:124–127.
38. Lee AR, Tojo K. An experimental approach to study the binding properties of vitamin E (alpha-tocopherol) during hairless mouse skin permeation. Chem Pharm Bull (Tokyo) 2001; 49:659–663.
39. Baker JR, Christian RA, Simpson P, White AM. The binding of topically applied glucocorticoids to rat skin. Br J Dermatol 1977; 96:171–178.
40. Liu P, Higuchi WI, Ghanem AH, Good WR. Transport of beta-estradiol in freshly excised human skin in vitro: diffusion and metabolism in each skin layer. Pharm Res 1994; 11:1777–1784.
41. Borsadia S, Ghanem AH, Seta Y, Higuchi WI, Flynn GL, Behl CR, Shah VP. Factors to be considered in the evaluation of bioavailability and bioequivalence of topical formulations. Skin Pharmacol 1992; 5:129–145.
42. Walter K, Kurz H. Binding of drugs to human skin: influencing factors and the role of tissue lipids. J Pharm Pharmacol 1988; 40:689–693.
43. Singh P, Roberts MS. Effects of vasoconstriction on dermal pharmacokinetics and local tissue distribution of compounds. J Pharm Sci 1994; 83:783–791.
44. Roberts MS, Cross SE. A physiological pharmacokinetic model for solute disposition in tissues below a topical application site. Pharm Res 1999; 16:1394–1400.
45. Yourick JJ, Koenig ML, Yourick DL, Bronaugh RL. Fate of chemicals in skin after dermal application: does the vitro skin reservoir affect the estimate of systemic absorption? Toxical Appl Pharmacol 2004; 195:309–320.
46. Heard CM, Monk BV, Modley AJ. Binding of primaquine to epidermal membranes and keratin. Int J Pharm 2003; 257:237–244.
47. Miselnicky SR, Lichtin JL, Sakr A, Bronaugh RL. The influence of solubility, protein binding, and percutaneous absorption on reservoir formation in skin. J Soc Cosmet Chem 1988; 39(3):169–177.
48. Fang JY, Hwang TL, Leu YL. Effect of enhancers and retarders on percutaneous absorption of flurbiprofen from hydrogels. Int J Pharm 2003; 250:313–325.
49. Loden M, Buraczewska I, Edlund F. The irritation potential and reservoir effect of mild soaps. Contact Dermat 2003; 49:91–96.

50. Mueller B, Anissimov YG, Roberts MS. Unexpected clobetasol propionoate in human stratum corneum after topical application in vitro. Pharm Res 2003; 20:1835–1837.
51. Anissimov YG, Roberts MS. Diffusion modelling of percutaneous absorption kinetics: 3. Variable diffusion and partitioning coefficients. J Pharm Sci 2004; 93:470–487.
52. Hood HL, Wickett RR, Bronaugh RL. In vitro percutaneous absorption of the fragrance ingredient musk oil. Food Chem Toxicol 1996; 34:483–488.
53. Jung CT, Wickett RR, Desai PB, Bronaugh RL. In vitro and in vivo percutaneous absorption of catechol. Food Chem Toxicol 2003; 41:885–895.
54. Roberts MS, Anissimov YG, Cross SE. Factors affecting the formation of a skin reservoir for topically applied solutes. Skin Pharmacol Physiol 2004; 17(1):3–16.

5 Chemical Partitioning into Powdered Human Stratum Corneum

A Useful In Vitro Model for Studying the Interaction of Chemicals and Human Skin

Xiaoying Hui and Howard I. Maibach
University of California, San Francisco, California

CONTENTS

5.1   INTRODUCTION

Chemical delivery/absorption into and through the skin is important in both dermato-pharmacology and dermato-toxicology. The human stratum corneum is the first layer of the skin and constitutes a rate-limiting barrier to the transport of most chemicals across the skin (1). Chemicals must first partition into the stratum corneum before entering the deeper layers of the skin, the epidermis, and the dermis to reach the vascular system. Chemical partitioning proceeds much faster than complete diffusion through the whole stratum corneum, and the process quickly reaches equilibrium. In addition to binding within the stratum corneum, a chemical can be retained within the stratum corneum as a reservoir (2). Thus, understanding the process of chemical partitioning into the stratum corneum becomes important in developing an insight into its barrier properties and transport mechanisms.

Human stratum corneum has been used for decades as an in vitro model to explore both percutaneous absorption and the risks associated with dermal exposure (3–5). The human stratum corneum includes the horny pads of palms and soles (callus) and the membranous stratum corneum covering the remainder of the body (6). The traditional method of preparation is via physical-chemical and enzymological processes to separate the membranous layers of the stratum corneum from whole skin (7, 8). However, it is time consuming and in some cases difficult to control the size and thickness of a sheet of stratum corneum. Moreover, it is often difficult to locate a suitable skin source.

Powdered human stratum corneum (PHSC) prepared from callus (sole) is thus substituted for the intact membranous stratum corneum. Podiatrists routinely remove and discard PHSC from the human foot, so it is easily obtained. The callus can be cut easily and quickly into smaller pieces and ground with dry ice to form a powder. In our laboratory, PHSC particle sizes between 180 and 300 μm were selected with the aid of a suitable sieve. Because a corneocyte is only about 0.5 μm thick and about 30 to 40 μm long, the selected PHSC contains both intact corneocytes and intercellular medium structures and thus retains its original physical-biochemical properties. Moreover, the greater surface area of the PHSC enhances solute penetration. In a typical experimental procedure, a test chemical in a transport vehicle—water—is mixed with the PHSC and the mixture is incubated. After a predetermined period, a solution is separated from the PHSC by centrifugation and samples are measured (9).

This chapter reviews PHSC as an in vitro model for studying chemical interactions with human skin, with reference to studies conducted in our laboratory over the last decades. The results demonstrate that PHSC (callus) offers an experimentally easy in vitro model for the determination of chemical partitioning into the SC and may be useful in many skin research areas.

5.2   PHSC AND PHYSICAL-CHEMICAL PROPERTIES OF THE STRATUM CORNEUM

The callus is derived from human stratum corneum (SC) and thus should retain some of its physical and chemical characteristics (10). SC lipid plays an important role in the determination of skin functions. However, the average lipid content of the SC varies regionally, from 2.0, 4.3, 6.5 to 7.2 wt.% of dry SC from plantar, leg, abdomen, and face, respectively (11). Table 5.1 shows that the average lipid content of the dry PHSC samples derived from various regions were 2.29 and 0.25 wt.% after extraction. This result is consistent with that in human plantar, as determined by Lampe et al. (11).

The water content of the SC is of importance in maintaining SC flexibility. Three possible mechanisms of water absorption and/or retention capacity of the SC have been suggested: (1) Imokawa et al. (12) suggested that SC lipids play a critical role because their removal by the application of

TABLE 5.1
Lipid Content and Water Uptake of Powdered Human Stratum Corneum (PHSC)

Stratum Corneum Source	Lipid Content (% w/w dry PHSC)	Water Uptake (μg/mg dry PHSC)			
		Untreated PHSC	Delipidized PHSC		
			Lipid[a]	Protein[b]	Total
1	2.38	495.85	26.44	452.40	478.84
2	2.21	452.49	39.26	364.96	404.22
3	2.39	585.62	23.09	498.40	521.49
4	2.69	554.27	40.05	492.31	532.36
5	2.08	490.04	49.86	363.30	413.16
6	2.01	381.61	14.82	324.18	339.00
Mean	2.29	493.31	32.26	415.92	448.18
SD	0.25	72.66	12.97	74.50	75.47

[a] Lipid part extracted from the PHSC.
[b] Remaining part of the PHSC after lipid extraction.

acetone/ether decreased absorption/retention capacity. (2) Friberg et al. (13), however, considered that protein might also play an important role in SC water retention. They found that the additional water absorbed after re-aggregation of equilibrated lipids and proteins was equally partitioned between the protein and the natural lipid fraction of the human SC. (3) Middleton (14) considered that water-soluble substances were responsible for water retention and for most of the extensibility of the corneum. He found that powdered SC—but not the intact corneum extracted by water— exhibited lower water retention capacity. He suggested that the powdering procedure ruptures the walls of the corneum cells and allows water to extract the water-soluble substances without a prior solvent extraction. We measured the water retention capacities of untreated PHSC, delipidized PHSC (as the protein fraction), and the lipid content by measuring the amount of [3H]-water (microgram equivalent) per milligram PHSC after equilibration. As shown in Table 5.1, no statistical differences ($p > 0.05$) were observed for untreated PHSC, delipidized PHSC, and the combination of delipidized PHSC and the lipid content. The PHSC can absorb up to 49% by weight of dry untreated PHSC (Table 5.1), which is consistent with literature reports. Middleton (14) found that the amount of water bound to intact, small pieces and powdered guinea-pig footpad stratum corneum was 40%, 40%, and 43% of dry corneum weight. Leveque and Rasseneur (15) demonstrated that the human SC was able to absorb water up to 50% of its dry weight. Our results (Table 5.1) suggest that the protein domain of the PHSC plays an important role in the absorption of water. Depletion of the PHSC lipid content did not affect water retention (16).

5.3 PHSC AND CHEMICAL PARTITIONING

Table 5.2 shows the effect of varying initial chemical concentrations on the partition coefficient (PC) PHSC/w of these compounds (16). Under fixed experimental conditions—two-hour incubation time and 350°C incubation temperature—the concentration required to attain a peak value of the PC varied from chemical to chemical. After reaching the maximum, increases in the chemical concentration in the vehicle did not increase the PC value; rather, it slightly decreased or was maintained at approximately the same level. This is consistent with the results of Surber et al. (3, 4) on whole SC. Chemical partitioning from the vehicle into the SC involves processes in which molecular binding occurs at certain sites of the SC, as well as simple partitioning. Equilibration of partitioning is largely dependent on the saturation of the chemical binding sites of the SC (3, 17). The results also indicate that, under a given experimental condition, the maximum degree of partitioning was compound specific. As the SC contains protein, lipids, and various lower-molecular-weight substances with widely differing properties, the many available binding sites display different selective affinities with each chemical. Thus, the degree of maximum binding or of equilibration varies naturally with molecular structure (17). This result demonstrated that the solubility limit of a compound in the SC was important in determining the degree of partitioning, as suggested by Potts and Guy (5). On the basis of the solubility limit of a chemical, the absorption process of water-soluble or lipid-soluble substances was controlled by the protein domain or the lipid domain, respectively, or a combination of two (18). Since the lipophilicity of the lipid domain in the SC is much higher than that of water, a lipophilic compound would partition into the SC in preference to water. Thus, when water is employed as the vehicle, the PC PHSC/w increases with increasing lipophilicity of solute (19). Conversely, the protein domain of the SC is significantly more polar than octanol and governs the absorption of hydrophilic chemicals (18). For very lipophilic compounds, low solubility in water rather than increased solubility in the SC can be an important factor (19). Moreover, in addition to partitioning into these two domains, some amount of chemicals may be taken into the SC as the result of water hydration. This is the "sponge domain," named by Raykar et al. (18). They assume that this water, having the properties of bulk water, carries an amount of solute into the SC equal to the amount of solute in the same volume of bathing solution. Therefore, for hydrophilic compounds and some lower lipophilic compounds, the partitioning process may include both the protein domain and sponge domain.

TABLE 5.2

Effect of Initial Aqueous Phase Chemical Concentration on Powdered Human Callus/Water Partition Coefficient

Chemical[a] (log $PC_{o/w}$)	Concentration (%, w/v)	Partition (mean)	Coefficient[b] (SD)
Dopamine (−3.40)	0.23	5.42	0.22
	0.46	6.04	0.28
	0.92	5.74	0.28
Glycine (−3.20)	0.05	0.36	0.01
	0.10	0.40	0.02
Urea (−2.11)	0.03	0.26	0.02
	0.06	0.15	0.02
	0.12	0.17	0.02
Glyphosate (−1.70)	0.02	0.79	0.04
	0.04	0.68	0.04
	0.08	0.70	0.01
Theophylline (−0.76)	0.18	0.37	0.02
	0.36	0.43	0.03
	0.54	0.42	0.02
Aminopyrine (0.84)	0.07	0.44	0.09
	0.14	0.46	0.03
Hydrocortisone (1.61)	0.09	0.37	0.01
	0.18	0.34	0.01
	0.36	0.29	0.02
Malathion (2.36)	0.47	0.50	0.09
	0.94	0.40	0.03
	1.88	0.53	0.04
Atrazine (2.75)	0.09	0.53	0.06
	0.14	0.59	0.07
	0.19	0.58	0.03
2,4-D (2.81)	0.27	7.52	0.81
	0.54	7.53	1.01
	0.82	8.39	1.67
Alachlor (3.52)	0.32	1.11	0.05
	0.64	1.08	0.04
	1.28	1.96	0.15
PCB (6.40)	0.04	1237.61	145.52
	0.08	1325.44	167.03
	0.16	1442.72	181.40

[a] PC PHSC/water represents the mean of each test ($n = 5$) ± SD (16).
[b] Log PC (o/w) was cited in Hansch C and Leo A (eds). 1979. (20).
Abbreviations: 2,4-D, 2,4-dichloro-phenoxyacetic acid; *PC*, partition coefficient; *PCB*, polychlorinated biphenyls; *PHSC*, powdered human stratum corneum.

5.4   PHSC AND PERCUTANEOUS ABSORPTION

To evaluate sensitivity of this in the in vitro PHSC model, we examined chemical partitioning into the PHSC as well as that in vitro percutaneous absorption in human skin, and in vivo percutaneous absorption in the rhesus monkey. Table 5.3 shows that the in vivo percutaneous absorption of nitroaniline from surface water following 30-minute exposure was 4.1% and 2.3% of the applied dose. This is comparable with the 5.2% and 1.6% for in vitro absorption with human cadaver skin

TABLE 5.3

In Vivo Percutaneous Absorption of _p_-Nitroaniline in the Rhesus Monkey Following 30 Minutes Exposure to Surface Water: Comparisons to In Vitro Binding and Absorption

Phenomenon	Percent Dose Absorbed/Bound[a]
In vivo percutaneous absorption, rhesus monkey	4.1 ± 2.3
In vitro percutaneous absorption, human skin	5.2 ± 1.6
In vitro binding, powdered human stratum corneum	2.5 ± 1.1

[a] Each number represents the mean $\pm$ SD of four samples.

and the 2.5% and 1.1% bound to PHSC. Wester et al. (10) suggest that this methodology—the systems tested, binding to PHSC, and in vitro and in vivo absorption—can be used to predict the burden on the human body imposed by bathing or swimming.

5.5 PHSC AND THE SKIN BARRIER FUNCTION

The barrier function of the SC is attributed to its multilayered wall-like structure, in which terminally differentiated keratin-rich epidermal cells (corneocytes) are embedded in an intercellular lipid-rich matrix. Any physical factor or chemical reagent that interacts with this two-compartment structure can affect the skin barrier function. Barry (6) described how certain compounds and mechanical trauma can easily dissociate callus cells and readily dissolve their membranes. Thus the amount of protein (keratin) released from the SC after chemical exposure may be a measure of the solvent potential of the chemical. To evaluate this hypothesis, a test chemical in water is mixed with PHSC and incubated. After a predetermined period, a solution is separated from the PHSC by centrifugation. The protein (keratin) content of the solution is then measured. Table 5.4 shows the amount of protein released from the PHSC after incubation with glycolic acid, sodium hydroxide, or water alone at different time points. Sodium hydroxide has a pronounced ability to release protein from PHSC. This ability increases with increasing incubation time. The results suggest that the PHSC model constitutes a vehicle to probe the barrier nature of the stratum corneum and the chemical interactions with the PHSC.

TABLE 5.4

Protein Releasing from PHSC Following Chemical/Water Exposure

Test Chemicals	Protein Content (mg/4mL)[a]		
	10 min	40 min	24 hr
Glycolic acid	0.093	0.175	0.173
	(0.026)	(0.029)	(0.041)
Sodium hydroxide	0.419	0.739	5.148
	(0.054)	(0.301)	(1.692)
Water	0.002	0.135	0.077
	(0.014)	(0.043)	(0.021)

[a] Each number represents the mean (SD) of six samples.

TABLE 5.5

Aqueous Partition Coefficient of Hydrocortisone with Normal and Psoriatic Stratum Corneum

Stratum Corneum Type	Partition Coefficient[a]	
	Mean	SE
Normal sheet (abdominal)	1.04	0.88
Normal powdered (plantar)	1.70	0.47
Psoriatic	1.94	0.42

[a] No statistical significance ($p > 0.05$).

5.6 PHSC AND DISEASED SKIN

The PHSC has potential application in medical treatment. For instance, a set of vehicles can be screened to determine which vehicle most readily releases a given drug into the SC. This information would assist in determining the most effective approaches to drug delivery via the skin. Furthermore, diseases involving the SC can be studied using PHSC. An example is Table 5.5, which is the partitioning of hydrocortisone from normal and psoriatic PHSC. In this case, we have shown that there is no difference in partitioning between normal and psoriatic PHSC. It should be noted that there is no difference between in vivo percutaneous absorption of hydrocortisone in normal volunteers and in psoriatic patients (21).

5.7 PHSC AND ENVIRONMENTALLY HAZARDOUS CHEMICALS

The leaching of environmentally hazardous chemicals from soil and their absorption by the skin of a human body is a major concern. Knowledge of the extent and degree of such absorption will aid in determining the potential health hazards of polluted soil. Our laboratory's interest is in the potential percutaneous absorption of contaminants from soil. Soil can be readily mixed with PHSC, but centrifugation does not separate the two. However, centrifugation readily separates PHSC from any liquid to varying degrees. Thus, the partition coefficients of various liquids may be determined relative to a common third liquid. These relative partitions can then be compared to those of other compounds and to skin absorption values (22–24) to evaluate the degree of hazard. We have determined such coefficients for several environmentally hazardous chemicals partitioning from soil into PHSC (Table 5.6).

TABLE 5.6

Partition Coefficients of Four Environmental Hazardous Chemicals in PHSC/Water and Soil/Water

Test Chemicals	Partition Coefficient	
	PHSC	Soil
Arsenic	1.1×10^4	2.4×10^4
Cadmium chloride	3.6×10^1	1.0×10^5
Arodor 1242	2.6	1.7
Arodor 1254	2.9	2.0

Abbreviation: PHSC, Powdered human stratum corneum.

TABLE 5.7

Decontaminants Selection to Remove Environmental Hazardous Chemical (Alachlor) from Human Skin[a]

	[^{14}C]-Alachlor (%)
PHSC	90.3 ± 1.2
Alachlor in Lasso supernatant	5.1 ± 1.2
Water-only wash of PHSC	4.6 ± 1.3
10% Soap-and-water wash	77.2 ± 5.7
50% Soap-and-water wash	90.0 ± 0.5

[a] [^{14}C]-Alachlor in Lasso EC formulation (1:20 dilution) mixed with powdered human stratum corneum, allowed to set for 30 minutes, then centrifuged. Stratum corneum wash with (1) water only, (2) 10% soap and water, and (3) 50% soap and water.

Abbreviations: PHSC, powdered human stratum corneum.

5.8 PHSC AND CHEMICAL DECONTAMINATION

Our laboratory uses the PHSC model to determine which chemicals might be able to remove (decontaminate) hazardous chemicals from human skin. A contaminant chemical is mixed with PHSC and the decontaminant effects of a series of possible decontaminants are measured. The liquid decontaminant is mixed with contaminated PHSC and, after a predetermined period, a solution is separated from the PHSC by centrifugation. The content of the solution is a measure of the decontaminant's potential. This is shown in Table 5.7, which demonstrates that alachlor readily contaminates PHSC. Water alone removes only a small portion of the alachlor. However, a 10% soap solution removes a larger portion of the alachlor, and a 50% soap solution removes most of it. Perhaps this is an elegant way to show that soapy water is effective in washing one's hands. However, it does illustrate the use of PHSC to determine the effectiveness of skin decontamination (25).

5.9 PHSC AND ENHANCED TOPICAL FORMULATION

Macromolecules have attracted interest as potential drug entities and as modulators to percutaneous delivery systems. Two macromolecular polymers (molecular weight [MW] 2081 and 2565) were developed to hold cosmetics and drugs to the skin surface by altering the initial chemical and skin partitioning. The effect of these polymers on the PC of estradiol with PHSC and water was determined in our laboratory. As shown in Table 5.8, the polymer L had no effect on the estradiol PC between PHSC and water. The polymer H, however, showed a significant increase ($p < 0.01$) in log PC for estradiol concentrations of 2.8 and 0.25 mg/mL. This increase was dependent upon the polymer concentration (26). The results suggest that the PHSC model can help in the development and selection of enhanced transdermal delivery systems.

5.10 PHSC AND QSAR PREDICTIVE MODELING

Many experiments have been conducted to predict chemical partitioning into the SC in vitro. However, most were based on quantitative structure–activity relationships (QSARs) or related chemicals to determine the partitioning process, and few studies focus on structurally unrelated chemicals (15). Since the range of molecular structure and physicochemical properties is very broad, any predictive model must address a broad scope of partitioning behavior.

TABLE 5.8

Effect of Two Polymers (L and H) on the Estradiol PC between PHSC and Water

Test Formulation and Polymer Concentration (%)	Log PC PHSC/Water (mean ± SD, $n = 5$) Estradiol Concentration (µg/mL)		
	2.8	0.028	0.028
Polymer H (hydrophilic polymer)			
10	2.31 ± 0.22[a]	2.36 ± 0.14[a]	2.13 ± 0.07[a]
5	1.93 ± 0.10[b]	2.06 ± 0.21[b]	1.94 ± 0.06[b]
1	1.71 ± 0.10	1.61 ± 0.19	1.59 ± 0.26
Polymer L (lipophilic polymer)			
10	1.74 ± 0.10	1.65 ± 0.07	1.61 ± 0.14
5	1.70 ± 0.20	1.62 ± 0.17	1.65 ± 0.09
1	1.59 ± 0.19	1.57 ± 0.15	1.71 ± 0.07
Control (no polymer)	1.62 ± 0.14	1.68 ± 0.11	1.71 ± 0.13

[a] Statistically significantly different from control ($p < 0.01$).
[b] Statistically significantly different from control ($p < 0.05$).
Abbreviations: PC, partition coefficient; *PHSC*, powdered human stratum corneum.

This study assesses the relationship of a number of chemicals with a broad scope of physicochemical properties in the partitioning mechanism between PHSC and water. Uniqueness and experimental accuracy are added by using PHSC. The experimental approach is designed to determine how the PC PHSC/w is affected by (1) chemical concentration, (2) incubation time, and (3) chemical lipophilicity (or hydrophilicity) and other factors. These parameters are used to develop an in vitro model that will aid in the prediction of chemical dermal exposure to hazardous chemicals.

Figure 5.1 describes a smooth, partially curvilinear relationship between the log PC PHSC/w and the log PC o/w of a number of chemicals. The lipophilicities and hydrophilicities of compounds were defined as log PC o/w larger or smaller than zero, respectively. For lipophilic chemicals, such as aminopyrine, hydrocortisone, malathion, atrazine, 2,4-dichloro phenoxyacetic acid, alachlor, and polychlorinated biphenyls (PCBs), the logarithms of PHSC/water partition coefficients are proportional to the logarithms of the octanol/water partition coefficients:

$$\log \text{PC PHCS/w} = 0.59 \log \text{PC o/w} - 0.72$$

$$\text{Student} - \text{t values } 9.93 \tag{5.1}$$

$$n = 7; \ r^2 = 0.95; \ S = 0.26; \ F = 98.61$$

For hydrophilic chemicals, such as theophylline, glyphosate, urea, glycine, and dopamine, the log PC PHSC/w values are approximately and inversely proportional to log PC o/w:

$$\log \text{PC PHCS/w} = -0.60 \log \text{PC o/w} - 0.27$$

$$\text{Student} - \text{t values}: -4.86 \tag{5.2}$$

$$n = 5; \ r^2 = 0.88; \ S = 0.26; \ F = 23.61$$

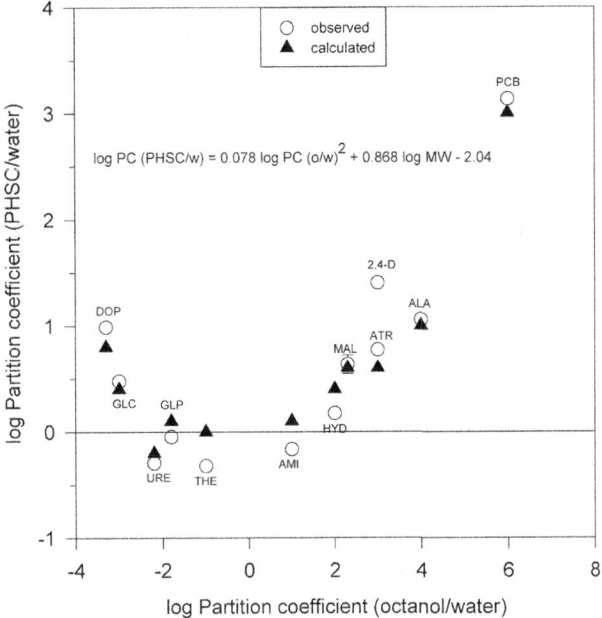

FIGURE 5.1   Correlation of the logarithm of stratum corneum/water partition coefficients (log PC sc/w) and logarithm of octanol/water partition coefficients of the 12 test chemicals. Open symbols express observed values, and each represents the mean of a test chemical ± SD (*n* = 5). Closed symbols express calculated values by Equation (5.3). *Abbreviations: DOP*, dopamine; *GLC*, glycine; *URE*, urea; *GLP*, glyphosate; *THE*, theophylline; *AMI*, aminopyrine; *HYD*, hydrocortisone; *MAL*, malathion; *ATR*, atrazine; *2,4-D*, 2,4-dichlorophenoxyacetic acid; *ALA*, alachlor; *PCB*, polychlorinated biphenyls.

However, the overall relationship of the PC PHSC/w of these chemicals to their PC o/w is nonlinear. This nonlinear relationship is adequately described by the following equation:

$$\log PC\ PHCS/w = 0.078\ \log PC\ o/w^2 + 0.868\ \log MW - 2.04$$

$$\text{Student} - \text{t values}: -8.29\ 2.04 \tag{5.3}$$

$$n = 12;\ r^2 = 0.90;\ S = 0.33;\ F = 42.59$$

The logarithm of MW gave a stronger correlation in this regression than MW (*t* = 1.55) itself. In Figure 5.1, the calculated log PC PHSC/w (Y estimate) values are compared to the corresponding observed values for these chemicals. As shown, the calculated values are acceptably close to the observed values. The correspondence with minimal scatter suggests that this equation would be useful in predicting in vitro partitioning in the PHSC for important environmental chemicals (16).

5.11   CONCLUSION

A new in vitro model employing PHSC (callus) to investigate the interaction between chemicals and human skin has been developed in our laboratory. The PHSC (callus) offers an experimentally easy in vitro model for the determination of chemical partitioning from water into the SC. Due to the heterogeneous nature of the SC, the number and affinity of the SC binding sites may vary from chemical to chemical, depending upon molecular structure. For most lipophilic compounds, the PC PHSC/w was governed by the lipid domain, whereas PCs of the more hydrophilic compounds are determined by the protein domain and, possibly, by the sponge domain (18). These relationships can be expressed by the log PC PHSC/w of these chemicals as a function of the corresponding square of log PC o/w and log MW; see Equation (5.3), which is useful in predicting various chemical partitionings into the SC in vitro. However, a disadvantage in using the human callus is that it may display some differences in water and chemical permeation when compared with membranous SC (6).

This chapter has summarized a variety of potential applications for PHSC, ranging from basic science to applications in medicine and environmental impact studies. The PHSC, imagination, and a balanced study design can add to scientific knowledge.

REFERENCES

1. Blank JH. Cutaneous barriers. J Invest Dermatol 1965; 45:249–256.
2. Zatz JL. Scratching the surface: rationale approaches to skin permeation. In: Zatz JL, ed. Skin Permeation Fundamentals and Application. Wheaten: Allured Publishing Co., 1993;11–32.
3. Surber C, Wilhelm KP, Hori M, Maibach HI, Guy RH. Optimization of topical therapy: partitioning of drugs into stratum corneum. Pharm Res 1990; 7(12):1320–1324.
4. Surber C, Wilhelm KP, Maibach HI, Hall L, Guy RH. Partitioning of chemicals into human stratum corneum: implications for risk assessment following dermal exposure. Fundam Appl Toxicol 1990; 15:99–107.
5. Potts RO, Guy RH. Predicting skin permeability. Pharm Res 1992; 9(5):663–669.
6. Barry BW. Structure, function, diseases, and topical treatment of human skin. In: Barry BW, ed. Dermatological Formulations: Percutaneous Absorption. New York: Marcel Dekker, 1983;1–48.
7. Jublih L and Shelly WB. New Staining techniques for the Langerhans cell. Acta Dermatol (Stockh.) 1977; 57:289–296.
   Knutson K, Potts RO, Guzek DB, Golden DM, McKie JE, Lambert WJ, Higuchi WI. Macro and molecular physical-chemical considerations in understanding drug transport in the stratum corneum. J. contr. Rel. 1985; 2:67–87.
8. Knutson K, Potts RO, Guzek DB, Golden DM, McKie JE, Lambert WJ, Higuchi WI. Macro and molecular physical-chemical considerations in understanding drug transport in the stratum corneum. J. contr. Rel. 1985; 2:67–87.
9. Hui X, Wester RC, Maibach HI, Magee PS. Chemical partitioning into powdered human stratum corneum (callus). In: Maibach HI, ed. Toxicology of Skin. Philadelphia: Taylor & Francis, 2000; 159–178.
10. Wester RC, Mobayen M, Maibach HI. In vivo and in vitro absorption and binding to powdered stratum corneum as methods to evaluate skin absorption of environmental chemical contaminants from ground and surface water. J Toxicol Environ Health 1987; 21:367–374.
11. Lampe MA, Burlingame AL, Whitney J, Williams ML, Brown BE, Roitmen E, Elias PM. Human stratum corneum lipids: characterization and regional variations. J Lipid Res 1983; 24:120–130.
12. Imokawa G, Akasaki S, Hattori M, Yoshizuka N. Selective recovery of deranged waterholding properties by stratum corneum lipids. J Invest Dermatol 1986; 87(6):758–761.
13. Friberg SE, Kayali I, Suhery T, Rhein LD, Simion FA. Water uptake into stratum corneum: partition between lipids and proteins. J Dispersion Sci Technol 1992; 13(3):337–347.
14. Middleton JD. The mechanism of water binding in stratum corneum. Br J Dermatol 1968; 80:437–450.
15. Leveque JL, Rasseneur L. Mechanical properties of stratum corneum: influence of water and lipids. In: Marks RM, Barton SP, Edwards C, eds. The Physical Nature of the Skin. Norwell: MTP Press, 1988; Chapter 17.
16. Hui X, Wester RC, Maibach HI, Magee PS. Chemical partitioning into powdered human stratum corneum: a mechanism study. Pharm Res 1993; 10:S–413.
17. Rieger M. Factors affecting sorption of topically applied substances. In: Zatz JL, ed. Skin Permeation Fundamentals and Application. Wheten: Allured Publishing Co., 1993; 33–72.
18. Raykar PV, Fung MC, Anderson BD. The role of protein and lipid domains in the uptake of solutes of human stratum corneum. Pharm Res 1998; 5(3):140–150.
19. Scheuplein RJ, Bronaugh RL. Percutaneous absorption. In: Goldsmith LA, ed. Biochemistry and Physiology of the Skin. Vol. 1. Oxford: Oxford University Press, 1983; 1255–1294.
20. Hansch C and Leo A (eds). Substituent constants for correlation Analysis in Chemistry and Biology. New York: John Wiley, 1979.

21. Wester RC, Maibach HI. Dermatopharmacokinetics in clinical dermatology. Semin Dermatol 1983; 2(2):81–84.
22. Wester RC, Maibach HI, Sedik L, Melendres J, Di Zio S, Wade M. *In vitro* percutaneous absorption of cadmium from water and soil into human skin. Fundam Appl Toxicol 1992; 19:1–5.
23. Wester RC, Maibach HI, Sedik L, Melendres J, S, Wade M. *In vitro* percutaneous absorption and skin decontamination of arsenic from water and soil. Appl Toxicol 1993; 20:336.
24. Wester RC, Maibach HI, Sedik L, Melendres J. Percutaneous absorption of PCBs from soil: *in vivo* rhesus monkey, *in vitro* human skin, and binding to powdered human stratum corneum. J Toxicol Environ Health 1993; 39:375–382.
25. Scheuplein RJ and Blank JH. Mechanisms of Percutaneous absorption, IV. Penetration of nonelectrolytes (alcohols) from aqueous solutions and from pure liquids. J. Invest. Dermatol. 1973; 60:286.
26. Wester RC, Hui X, Hewitt PG, Hostynet J, Krauser S, Chan T, Maibach HI. Polymers effect on estradiol coefficient between powdered human stratum corneum and water. J Pharm Sci 2002; 91(12):2642–5.

6 Variations of Hair Follicle Size and Distribution in Different Body Sites*

*Nina Otberg, Sora Jung, Heike Richter, Hans Schaefer,
Ulrike Blume-Peytavi and Jürgen Lademann*
Charité - Universitätsmedizin Berlin,
Humboldt-Universität zu Berlin, Berlin, Germany

CONTENTS

6.1 INTRODUCTION

The knowledge of permeation and penetration processes is a prerequisite for the development and optimization of drugs and cosmetics. In the past, percutaneous absorption was described as diffusion through the lipid domains of the stratum corneum. It was presumed that skin appendages, which mean hair follicles and sweat glands, play a subordinate role in absorption processes. Various studies showed that hair follicles play an important role in drug delivery. Blume-Peytavi et al. showed the importance of the follicular pathway for topically applied substances (1). Here, a 5% minoxidil-containing foam was applied in vivo on the skin, while either follicular or percutaneous penetration pathways were blocked by a varnish–wax mixture or both were open. The highest penetration was found when both the follicular and percutaneous pathways were open. The amount of appendages of the total skin surface was estimated to represent up to 0.1% (2). However, previous studies show higher absorption rates in skin areas with higher follicle density (3–7). On the other hand, hair follicle size and density and the amount of the absorbed drug have never been correlated. The variation in the thickness of the stratum corneum in different body areas was considered to be the main reason for the varying absorption rates. Feldman and Maibach (3) and Maibach et al. (4) found regional variations of percutaneous absorption in different skin areas. They assumed that the density and size of hair follicles might be the reason for their findings. More recent studies more strongly suggest that skin appendages play an important role in permeation and penetration processes of topically applied substances. Tenjarla et al. (5) and Hueber et al. (6, 7) found significant differences in percutaneous absorption of appendage-free scarred skin and normal skin. Turner and Guy (8) found a significant iontophoretic drug delivery across the skin via follicular structures. Essa et al. (9) performed an in vitro Franz cell experiment for iontophoretic drug delivery. A new technique

---

* Modified with permission from the *Journal of Investigative Dermatology* (JID).

involving a stratum corneum/epidermis sandwich method was used for blocking the follicular orifice. A five times lower absorption rate was found when the potential shunt routes were blocked.

Moreover Hueber et al. (6, 7) found a follicular reservoir of radiolabeled triamcinolone acetonide in human skin. Lademann et al. (10, 11) found an amount of topically applied titanium dioxide microparticles located in the hair follicles of the forearm. They showed that some follicles were open, whereas others were closed for the penetration process.

It was shown that nanoparticles can penetrate into the hair follicle after topical application (12, 13). Here, the nanoparticles can accumulate, while the hair follicle can serve as a reservoir for nanoparticles, which can be loaded with specific drugs (12).

Patzelt et al. could show that the deepest penetration of nanoparticles could be achieved by nanoparticles sized at around 60 nm in porcine terminal hair follicles (13). By computerized simulation modeling, Radtke et al. showed that this can be explained by a possible ratchet effect by movement of the cuticular hair structure during massaging application of nanoparticle formulations (14).

Another study by Toll et al. in human facial skin found that 7-μm fluorescent polystyrene microbeads showed maximum follicular deposition compared to those of larger or smaller sizes (15). Bigger particles stayed on the surface, while smaller beads showed intercellular penetration into the upper layers of the stratum corneum.

Hair follicle density has mainly been measured for terminal hair follicles on the scalp. Blume et al. (16) determined the vellus hair follicle density on the forehead, cheek, chest, and back by phototrichogram. Seago and Ebling (17) measured hair follicle density on the upper arm and thigh using a classical trichogram. Pagnoni et al. (18) used the cyanoacrylate technique for the measurement of hair follicle density in different regions of the face.

Hair follicles are the most important appendages in terms of surface area and skin depth. An exact knowledge of hair follicle densities, size of follicular orifices, follicular volume, and follicular surface is necessary for the understanding of follicular penetration processes.

Therefore, our aim was to quantify the characteristics of hair follicle sizes. This includes the measurement of the following parameters: density, size of follicular orifice, amount of orifice of the skin surface, hair shaft diameter, volume, and surface of the infundibula in different regions of the body by using noninvasive cyanoacrylate skin surface biopsies and light microscopy. The volume of the follicle infundibula may represent the potential follicular reservoir for topically applied substances.

6.2 MATERIALS AND METHODS

The study was performed on six healthy volunteers (three females and three males) aged 27 to 41 years with normal body mass indices (from 21 to 24). None of the volunteers suffered from any kind of skin disease, hormonal dysregulation, or adiposity.

All volunteers gave written informed consent, and the protocol was approved by the institutional review board. The study was conducted according to the Declaration of Helsinki principles.

Cyanoacrylate surface biopsies were taken from each volunteer from seven different regions of the body (lateral forehead, back, thorax, upper arm, forearm, thigh, and calf region), just below the popliteal space, on the same day under the same conditions, which means the same room temperature and humidity. Figure 6.1 shows the localization of the seven test regions. Hair follicle parameters were measured by light microscopy in combination with digital images. None of the volunteers showed terminal hair growth in the test regions.

Cyanoacrylate is a nontoxic, nonadherent, and optically clear adhesive, which polymerizes and bonds rapidly in the presence of small amounts of water and pressure (19). A drop of cyanoacrylate (UHU GmbH, Brühl, Germany) is placed on the untreated skin and covered with a glass slide under light pressure. After polymerization, which occurs in one minute, the glass slide can be removed. A thin sheet of horny cells, hair shafts, and casts of the follicular infundibula are ripped off with the cyanoacrylate (20–22).

The surface biopsies were investigated using microscopy (Olympus BX60M system-microscope, Tokyo, Japan) in combination with digital image analysis and a special software program (analySIS, Soft Imaging System GmbH SIS, Munster, Germany). The follicular casts were counted in a marked

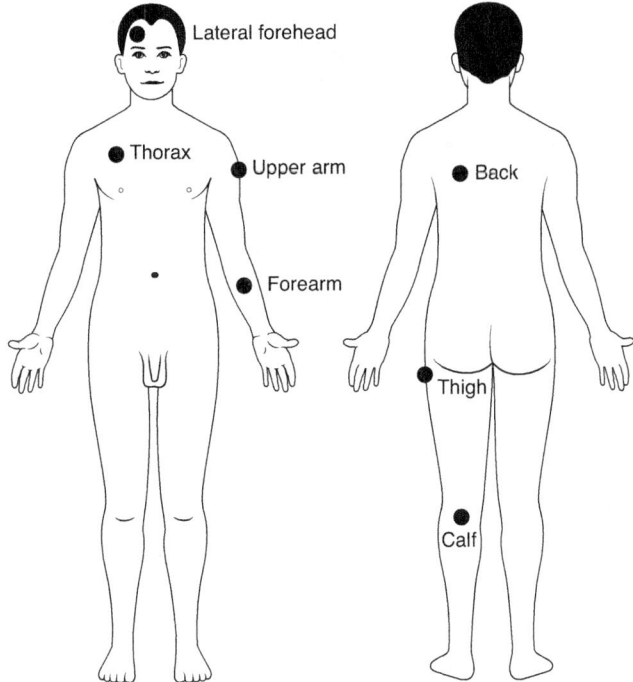

FIGURE 6.1 Localization of the seven test regions.

area of one square centimeter. The diameter of the follicle orifice and of the hair shaft was measured directly. The percentage of orifices of the skin surface can easily be determined by adding all calculated circle areas of the follicular orifices in the labeled biopsy area.

For the measurement of the surface and volume of the infundibula, a special three-dimensional image, extended focal image (EFI), was performed. With the module EFI of the software program, analySIS microscope images can be taken in different focuses and can then be calculated to a three-dimensional picture. With the same software program, length, height, and diameter of the infundibular casts can be measured. Every infundibular cast in the marked square centimeter was divided into truncated cones. Figure 6.2 explains the measurement of the infundibular cast. It shows a cyanoacrylate skin surface biopsy from the lateral forehead.

The volume (V) of each truncated cone was calculated with the following formula:

$$V_n = \pi / 12 h_n \left(d_1^2 + d_1^2 + d_1 d_2 \right) \tag{6.1}$$

where h is the height of the truncated cone and d is the diameter of the covers.

The whole infundibular volume per square centimeter was calculated by adding all single volumes and subtracting the hair shaft volumes. The hair shaft volume (V_{hsn}) was calculated by the following formula:

$$V_{hsn} = \pi / 4 d^2 h_n \tag{6.2}$$

where h is the height of the whole infundibulum and d is the hair shaft diameter.

The surface of the follicular infundibula was measured by calculating the curved surface (A) of the truncated cones by the following formulas:

$$A_n = \pi s \left(d_1 / 2 + d_2 / 2 \right) \tag{6.3}$$

$$s^2 = \left(d_1 / 2 - d_2 / 2 \right)^2 + h_n \tag{6.4}$$

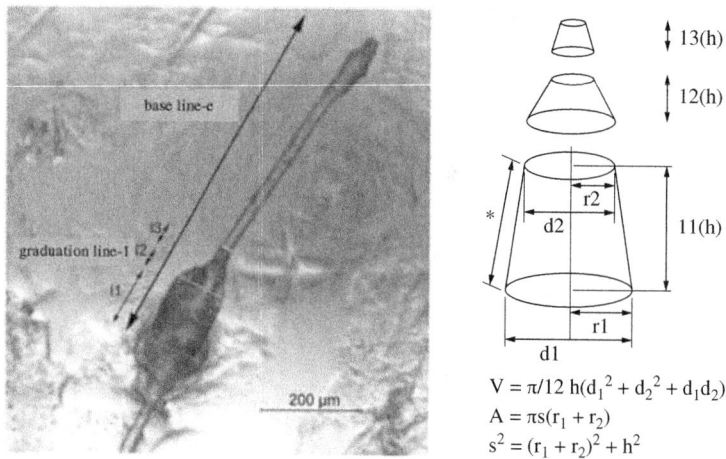

$$V = \pi/12\, h(d_1^2 + d_2^2 + d_1 d_2)$$
$$A = \pi s (r_1 + r_2)$$
$$s^2 = (r_1 + r_2)^2 + h^2$$

FIGURE 6.2 Cyanoacrylate skin surface biopsy with infundibular cast and vellus hair.

where h is the height of the truncated cone and d is the diameter of the covers.

The follicular penetration surface was calculated by adding all curved surfaces within the marked area.

For statistical analysis, we utilized Mann and Whitney's U-test for the comparison of two variables and Kruskal and Wallis's h-test for the comparison of more than two variables and SPSS software (SPSS, Chicago, IL, USA). Data are expressed as mean ± SD, with $p < 0.05$ considered significant, $p < 0.01$ considered very significant, and $p \leq 0.001$ considered highly significant.

6.3 RESULTS

Hair follicle density was measured on seven different body sites in six healthy volunteers. The samples were taken from corresponding areas in the different body areas of the volunteers. Figure 6.3 gives the average density with standard deviation for every test area. The average density was highest on the forehead (292 follicles/cm²), significantly higher than in all other regions ($p \leq 0.001$). The skin regions on the back showed 29, on the thorax 22, on the upper arm 32, on the forearm 18, on the thigh 17, and on the calf region 14 follicles/cm² on average. The back and upper arm showed no significant differences in hair follicle density ($p > 0.05$).

Significant intersite variations of the diameters of the follicular orifices could be found ($p \leq 0.001$). The thigh and calf showed no significant difference in diameters ($p > 0.05$). The diameters

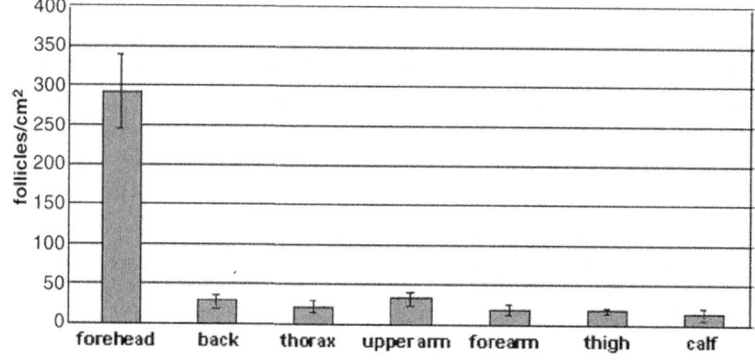

FIGURE 6.3 Hair follicle density on seven body sites.

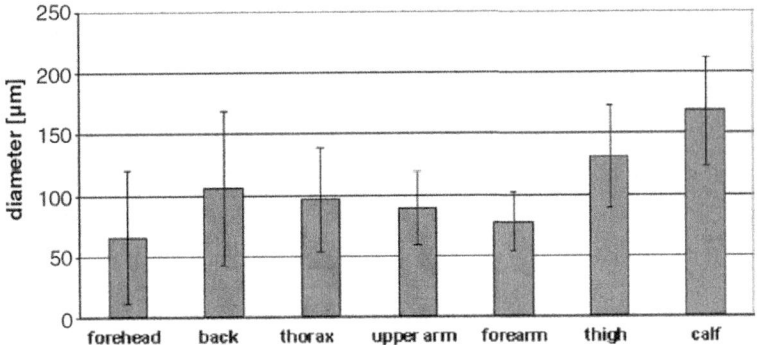

FIGURE 6.4   Diameter of hair follicle orifices on seven body sites.

showed great variations in every body site (Figure 6.4). High standard deviations were found, especially on the forehead and back. These areas belong to the seborrheic regions of the body, where small vellus hair follicles are found together with large sebaceous follicles. Comparing the mean values of diameters of the hair follicle orifices, the smallest diameters were found on the forehead, with 66 μm, and on the forearm, with 78 pm. The calf region showed the largest diameter of the follicular orifices.

The percentage of follicular orifices on the skin surface is given in Table 6.1 for seven different test regions. The amount was calculated by adding all circle areas of the follicle orifices [calculated with the formula for circle areas: $A = \pi(d/2)^2$] in 1 cm^2 of the different test regions.

Although the forehead showed the smallest diameter, it also showed, due to the elevated hair follicle density, the highest percentage of follicular orifices on the skin surface. Significant intersite variations of the percentage of the follicular orifices on the skin surface were found $(p < 0.001)$. The thigh and calf showed no significant difference $(p > 0.05)$.

Additionally, the hair shaft diameter was determined. Figure 6.5 gives the average hair shaft diameters with standard deviation for the seven measured body sites. The hairs on the thigh and calf

TABLE 6.1

Percentage of Follicular Orifices on the Skin Surface in Seven Body Sites

Skin Area	Forehead (%)	Back (%)	Thorax (%)	Upper Arm (%)	Forearm (%)	Thigh (%)	Calf Region (%)
Mean	1.28	0.33	0.19	0.21	0.09	0.23	0.35
(±SD)	(±0.24)	(±0.15)	(±0.08)	(±0.09)	(±0.04)	(±0.12)	(±0.25)

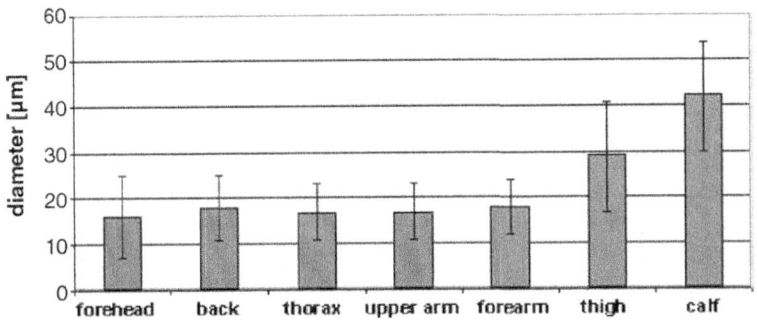

FIGURE 6.5   Hair shaft diameter on seven body sites.

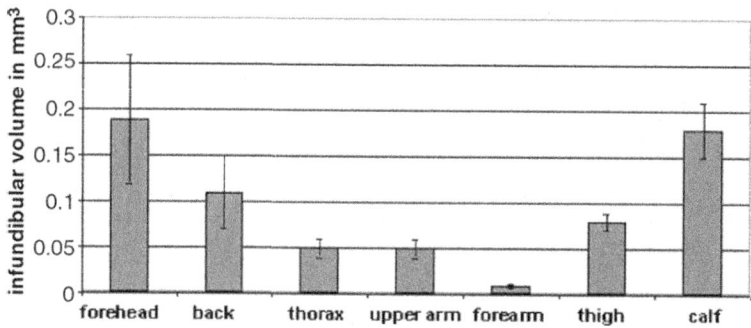

FIGURE 6.6 Volume of the follicular infundibula per square centimeter of skin on seven body sites.

region were significantly thicker compared to the other five regions ($p \leq 0.01$). The lateral forehead, back, thorax, upper arm, and forearm showed no significant differences in hair shaft diameters ($p > 0.05$). The thigh showed hair shaft diameters of 29 μm, the calf region 42 μm.

The volume of the follicular infundibula was measured by dividing the casts on the surface biopsy in truncated cones, calculating each volume, and adding all volumes within 1 cm² and subtracting the hair shaft volumes. The results of these measurements are given in Figure 6.6 related to 1 cm² skin surface. The forehead (0.19 mm³/cm²) and the calf regions (0.18 mm³/cm²) showed the highest volume, with no significant difference ($p > 0.05$), although the hair follicle density is around 20 times higher on the forehead. The forearm shows the lowest volume at 0.01 mm³/cm².

The potential surface for the penetration of topically applied drugs and cosmetics has been estimated as the skin surface, disregarding the fact that substances penetrate into skin appendages (Figure 6.7). The potential penetration surface of the hair follicles was calculated by measuring the curved surface of the follicular casts on the cyanoacrylate biopsy. Significant intersite variations of the surface area were found ($p \geq 0.001$). The largest surface was found on the forehead, with 13.7 mm² on average, or 13.7% of the skin surface. The smallest surface was found on the forearm (0.95 mm²), in accordance with the small follicles and the low follicle density.

6.4   DISCUSSION

The knowledge of hair follicle density and size is important for the understanding and calculation of follicular penetration and permeation processes.

Only a few studies have been performed for determining the vellus hair follicle density on the human body. Blume et al. (16) determined the hair follicle density on the forehead, cheek,

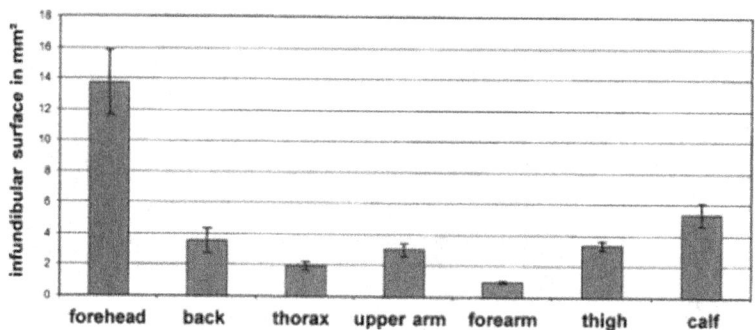

FIGURE 6.7 Surface of the follicular infundibula per square centimeter of skin on seven body sites.

chest, and back. An average density of 423 follicles/cm² was found on the forehead and a mean density of 92 follicles on the back. Pagnoni et al. (18) found a density of 455 hair follicles on the lateral forehead and the highest density on the nasal wing, with 1220 follicles/cm². These results show higher values compared to our findings for the forehead (292 follicles/cm²) and the back (29 follicles/cm²). High standard variations as an expression of intraindividual variations occurred in every study. Even within the forehead region the hair follicle density can differ to a high extent.

Seago and Ebling (17) measured the hair follicle density on the upper arm and thigh using a classical trichogram. They found a mean density of 18 follicles on the upper arm and 17 follicles in the skin area on the thigh, which correspond to our findings.

The mean hair follicle density depends on the skin area because hair follicles are built in the early fetal period. After birth, the body proportions change and the hair follicles move apart according to the growth of body and skin. Because of the relatively lower growth of the head compared to the extremities, hair follicles are much more numerous on the scalp and in the face than on the arms and legs (17, 18). Table 6.2 gives an overview of vellus hair follicle density found in the literature compared to the presented results.

In spite of the fact that the size of hair follicles shows great intraindividual and interindividual differences, hair shaft diameters showed relatively low variations. The thicker hair in the androgen-dependent areas on the thigh and calf, which were thicker than 30 μm, can be regarded as intermediate follicles. This means that these follicles are in a transitional stage between vellus and terminal hair (24).

Our findings show that the assumption of an appendage account of not more than 0.1% of the total skin surface (2) is valid for the forearm. The value of 0.1% corresponds well to our findings on the inner side of the forearm, which is most commonly used as an investigational area for skin penetration experiments. Skin areas with a higher follicle density, such as the forehead, or with larger follicle orifice, such as the calf region, showed much higher values. A higher transfollicular absorption in these areas can be assumed.

TABLE 6.2
Review of Vellus Hair Follicle Density on Different Body Sites

Results (by author)

Body Site	Own Results (cm⁻²)	Pagnoni et al. (18) (cm⁻²)	Blume et al. (16) (cm⁻²)	Seago and Ebling (17) (cm⁻²)	Scott et al. (23) (cm⁻²)
Lateral forehead	292	455	414 ♀ 432 ♂	—	—
Tip of the nose	—	1112	—	—	—
Nasal wing	—	1220	—	—	—
Preauricular region	—	499	—	—	—
Back	29	—	93, 90 <	—	—
Thorax	22	—	—	—	—
Abdomen	—	—	—	—	6
Upper arm	32	—	—	17–19	—
Forearm	18	—	—	—	—
Thigh	17	—	—	14–20	—
Calf	14	—	—	—	—

The measurement of a potential follicular reservoir for topically applied substances showed extreme differences between the investigated body sites. The volume of the infundibula on the forehead was 0.19 mm^3. This is five times less than the volume of the stratum corneum, assuming that the stratum corneum shows a thickness of 10 μm with a volume of 1 mm^3/cm^2 skin surface. The determination of the reservoir function of the stratum corneum is part of recent studies. A study by Jacobi et al. showed that a fluorescent, intravenously applied chemotherapeutic (doxorubicin) can be detected within the sweat glands shortly after the infusion. From here, the chemotherapeutic agent spreads with the sweat on the skin surface as topically applied (25). Huang et al. found that even an orally applied chemotherapeutic drug can be detected on the skin surface (26).

Lademann et al. (10, 27) found that a topically applied substance is found mainly in the upper 20% of the stratum corneum. This means that we have an approximately comparable reservoir volume in the stratum corneum and in the follicles of the forehead, assuming that all follicles are open for the penetration process (11). In contrast to the forehead, the forearm shows a volume of 0.01 mm^3, which is 100 times less than the volume of the stratum corneum. It can be estimated that the hair follicles in this skin area play a minor reservoir function role.

The enlargement of the penetration surface through the follicular epithelium was measured by calculating the surface of the infundibular cast on the cyanoacrylate biopsy. The infundibular surface proved to be 13.7% on the forehead and only 1% on the forearm; thus, only relatively low values for the enlargement of the potential penetration surface could be demonstrated.

A significantly higher amount of drug absorption in skin areas with high follicle densities or large follicles cannot be explained only by an enlargement of the penetration surface through the follicular epithelium. The reason for the better permeation through the hair follicles can likely be found in the ultra structure of the follicular epithelium and in the special environment of the follicular infundibulum. The hair follicle epithelium shows an epidermal differentiation in the infundibulum. The epithelium of the uppermost parts shows no difference to the interfollicular epidermis; in the lower parts of the infundibular epithelium, corneocytes are smaller and appear crumbly. This part of the follicular epithelium can be seen as an incomplete barrier for topically applied substances (28, 29).

Furthermore, using the follicular penetration pathway, a specific drug targeting the sebaceous glands could evolve into new therapeutic options, e.g., for the treatment of acne.

The present study shows body region–dependent hair follicle characteristics concerning follicular size and follicular distribution. Differential evaluation of skin penetration and absorption experiments and the development of new standards for the testing of topically applied drugs and cosmetics on different skin areas are mandatory. By knowing the differences of hair follicle size and density, we suggest performing skin absorption experiments on human skin not only on the inner forearm but also in skin areas with other follicular properties, for example, the forehead or calf.

6.5 CONCLUSION

For the evaluation and quantification of follicular penetration processes, the knowledge of variations of hair follicle parameters in different body sites is basic. Characteristics of follicle sizes and potential follicular reservoir were determined in cyanoacrylate skin surface biopsies taken from seven different skin areas (lateral forehead, back, thorax, upper arm, forearm, thigh, and calf region). The highest hair follicle density, percentage of follicular orifices on the skin surface, and infundibular surface were found on the forehead, while the highest average size of the follicular orifices was measured in the calf region. The highest infundibular volume, and therefore a potential follicular reservoir, was calculated for the forehead and for the calf region, although the calf region showed the lowest hair follicle density. The calculated follicular volume of these two skin areas was as high as the estimated reservoir of the stratum corneum. The lowest values for every other parameter were found on the forearm. The present investigation clearly contradicts the former hypothesis that the amount of appendages of the total skin surface represents not more than 0.1%. Every body region displays its own hair follicle characteristics, which, in the future, should lead us to a differential evaluation of skin penetration processes and a completely different understanding of penetration of topically applied drugs and cosmetics.

ACKNOWLEDGMENTS

The authors are deeply thankful to Prof. Wolfram Sterry, who provided his expertise and assistance for this study.

REFERENCES

1. Blume-Peytavi U, Massoudy L, Patzelt A, Lademann J, Dietz E, Rasulev U, et al. Follicular and percutaneous penetration pathways of topically applied minoxidil foam. Eur J Pharm Biopharm. 2010;76:450–453.
2. Schaefer H, Redelmeier TE. Skin barrier. In: Principles of Percutaneous Absorption. Basel: Karger, 1996:18.
3. Feldmann RJ, Maibach HI. Regional variation in percutaneous penetration of ^{14}C cortisol in man. J Invest Derm. 1967;48(2):181–183.
4. Maibach HI, Feldman RJ, Milby TH, Serat WF. Regional variation in percutaneous penetration in man. Arch Environ Health. 1971;23:208–211.
5. Tenjarla SN, Kasina R, Puranajoti P, Omar MS, Harris WT. Synthesis and evaluzation of N-acetylprolinate esters—Novel skin penetration enhancers. Int J Pharm. 1999;192:147–158.
6. Hueber F, Besnard M, Schaefer H, Wepierre J. Percutaneous absorption of estradiol and progesterone in normal and appendage-free skin of hairless rat: lack of importance of nutritional blood flow. Skin Pharmacol. 1994;7:245–256.
7. Hueber F, Schaefer H, Wepierre J. Role of transepidermal and transfollicular routes in percutaneous absorption of steroids: in vitro studies on human skin. Skin Pharmacol. 1994;7:237–244.
8. Turner NG, Guy RH. Visualization and quantification of iontophoretic pathways using confocal microscopy. J Invest Derm Proc. 1998;3:136–142.
9. Essa EA, Bonner MC, Barry BW. Possible role of shunt route during iontophoretic drug penetration. Perspect Percutan Penetration. 2002;8:54.
10. Lademann J, Weigmann HJ, Rickmeyer C, Bartelmes H, Schaefer H, Muller G, et al. Penetration of titanium dioxide microparticles in a sunscreen formulation into the horny layer and the follicular orifice. Skin Pharmacol Appl Skin Physiol. 1999;12:247–256.
11. Lademann J, Otberg N, Richter H, Weigmann HJ, Lindemann U, Schaefer H, et al. Investigation of follicular penetration of topically applied substances. Skin Pharmacol Appl Skin Physiol. 2001;14(Suppl 1):17–22.
12. Lademann J, Richter H, Schaefer UF, Blume-Peytavi U, Teichmann A, Otberg N, et al. Hair follicles – a long-term reservoir for drug delivery. Skin Pharmacol Physiol. 2006;19:232–236.
13. Patzelt A, Richter H, Knorr F, Schafer U, Lehr CM, Dahne L, et al. Selective follicular targeting by modification of the particle sizes. J Control Release. 2011;150:45–48.
14. Radtke M, Patzelt A, Knorr F, Lademann J, Netz RR. Ratchet effect for nanoparticle transport in hair follicles. Eur J Pharm Biopharm. 2017;116:125–130.
15. Toll R, Jacobi U, Richter H, Lademann J, Schaefer H, Blume-Peytavi U. Penetration profile of microspheres in follicular targeting of terminal hair follicles. J Invest Dermatol. 2004;123:168–176.
16. Blume U, Ferracin J, Verschoore M, Czernielewski JM, Schaefer H. Physiology of the vellus hair follicle: hair growth and sebum excretion. Br J Dermatol. 1991;124:21–28.
17. Seago SV, Ebling FJ. The hair cycle on the human thigh and upper arm. Br J Dermatol. 1995;135:9–16.
18. Pagnoni AP, Kligman AM, Gammal SEL, Stoudemayer T. Determination of density of follicles on various regions of the face by cyanoacrylate biopsy: correlation with sebum output. Br J Dermatol. 1994;131:862–865.
19. Marks R, Dawber RPR. Skin surface biopsy: an improved technique for the examination of the horny layer. Br J Derm. 1971;84:117–123.
20. Plewig G, Kligman M. Sampling of sebaceous follicles by the cyanoacrylate technique. In: ACNE, Morphogenesis and Treatment. Berlin, Heidelberg, New York: SpringerVerlag, 1975:56.

21. Holmes RL, Williams M, Cunliffe WJ. Pilosebaceous duct obstruction and acne. Br J Derm. 1972;87:327.
22. Mills OH, Kligman AM. The follicular biopsy. Dermatologica. 1983;167:57–63.
23. Scott RC, Corrigan MA, Smith F, Mason H. The influence of skin structure on permeability: An intersite and interspecies comparison with hydrophilic penetrants. J Invest Derm. 1991;96(6):921–925.
24. Whiting DA. Histology of normal hair. In: Hordinsky MK, Sawaya ME, Scher RK, eds. Atlas of Hair and Nail. Philadelphia: Churchill Livingstone, 2000:9–18.
25. Jacobi U, Waibler E, Bartoll J, Schulze P, Sterry W, Lademann J. In vivo determination of doxorubicin and its metabolites within the skin using laser scanning microscopy. Laser Phys Lett. 2004;1:100–103.
26. Huang MD, Fuss H, Lademann J, Florek S, Patzelt A, Meinke MC, et al. Detection of capecitabine (Xeloda(R)) on the skin surface after oral administration. J Biomed Opt. 2016;21:47002.
27. Lademann J, Weigmann HJ, Schaefer H, Müller G, Sterry W. Investigation of the stability of coated titanium micropartiles used in sunscreen. Skin Pharmacol Appl Skin Physiol. 2000; 13:258–264.
28. Braun-Falko O, Plewig G, Wolff HH. Dermatologie und Venerologie. Berlin, Heidelberg, New York: Springer-Verlag, 1996.
29. Pinkus H, Mehregan AH. The pilar apparatus. In: A Guide to Dermatopathology. New York: Appleton-Century-Crofts, 1981:S22–S28.

7 In Vivo Relationship between Percutaneous Absorption and Transepidermal Water Loss

André Rougier
Laboratoire Pharmaceutique, La Roche-Posay, Courbevoie, France

Claire Lotte
Laboratoires de Recherche Fondamentale,
L'Oréal, Aulnay sous Bois, France

Howard I. Maibach
University of California,
San Francisco, California

CONTENTS

In its role as a barrier the skin participates in homeostasis by limiting water loss (1, 2) and percutaneous absorption of environmental agents (3, 4).

The stratum corneum's role as a double barrier is intimately linked to its degree of hydration (5, 6), with transport mechanisms being diffusional (3, 7). In humans (8, 9) and in animals (10), an increase in water permeability of the skin corresponds to an increase in permeability to topically applied compounds. However, most of the studies dealing with this topic are only quantitative observations, and the relationship linking these two factors is unknown.

At present, transepidermal water loss (TEWL) can be considered a determinant indicative of the functional state of the cutaneous barrier (11–13). Apart from pathological considerations, the functional state of the cutaneous barrier may vary considerably under physiological conditions (13). Thus, in humans, cutaneous permeability to applied compounds varies from one site to another (14–16). This chapter investigates the influence of anatomical site, age, and sex in humans on both TEWL and percutaneous absorption to establish the precise relationship between these two indicators of the functional state of the cutaneous barrier.

7.1   PERCUTANEOUS ABSORPTION MEASUREMENTS

The penetration of benzoic acid was measured at 10 anatomical sites, the locations of which are shown in Figure 7.1. A group of six to eight informed male volunteers, aged 20 to 30 years, was used for each anatomical site. The influence of aging on skin absorption of benzoic acid was studied on groups of seven to eight male volunteers, aged 45 to 55 years and 65 to 80 years. The anatomical

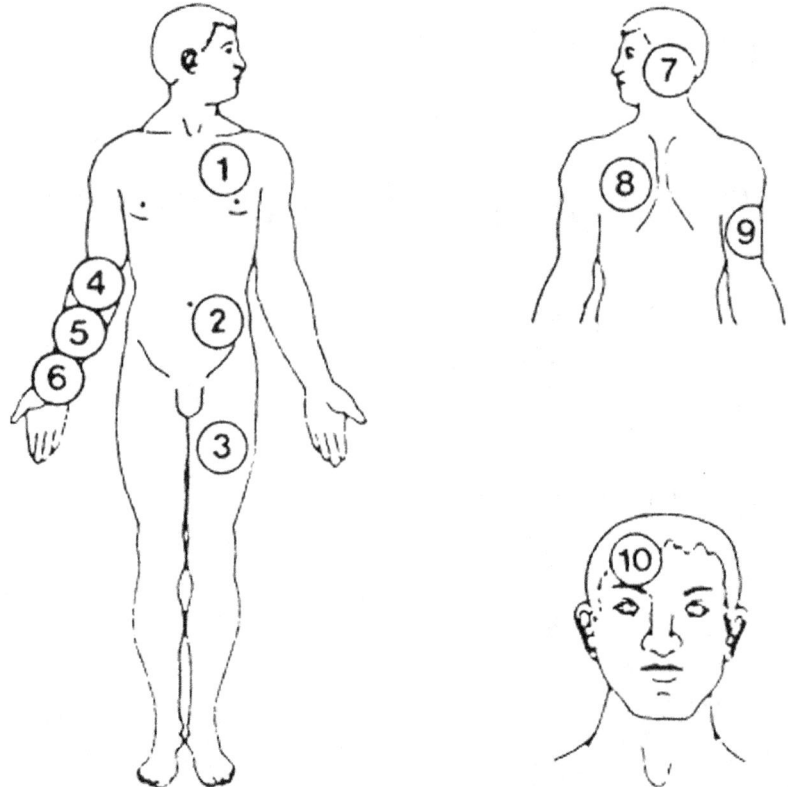

FIGURE 7.1 Anatomical sites tested: 1, chest; 2, abdomen; 3, thigh; 4, forearm (ventral elbow); 5, forearm (ventral mid); 6, forearm (ventral wrist); 7, postauricular; 8, back; 9, arm (upper outer); 10, forehead.

site involved was the upper outer arm. The influence of gender on skin absorption was assessed on the upper outer arms and on the foreheads of groups of seven to eight female volunteers, aged 20 to 30 years.

One thousand nanomoles of benzoic acid (ring-^{14}C) (New England Nuclear) with a specific activity of 10^{-3} μCi/nmol were applied to an area of 1 cm^2 in 20 μL of a vehicle consisting of ethylene glycol to which 10% Triton X-100 had been added as surfactant. The treated area was demarcated by an open circular cell fixed by silicone glue to prevent chemical loss. After 30 minutes, excess chemical was quickly removed by two successive washes (2 × 300 μL) with a 95:5 ethanol/water mixture, followed by two rinses (2 × 300 μL) with distilled water and light drying with a cotton swab.

Benzoic acid was selected because of the rapidity and high level of its urinary excretion. Thus, from literature data on the kinetics of urinary excretion of this compound when administered intravenously and orally (17, 18) or percutaneously (19–21) in different species, the proportion of the total amount of benzoic acid absorbed that would be excreted in the urine within the first 24 hours was 75%. The total quantities absorbed during the four days after application could therefore be calculated, after scintillation counting, from the quantities found in the urine during the first 24 hours.

7.2   TRANSEPIDERMAL WATER LOSS MEASUREMENTS

After completion of the benzoic acid treatment, TEWL was measured with an Evaporimeter EPIC (Servo Med, Sweden) from a contralateral site (same anatomical region) in each subject. The hand-held probe was fitted with a 1-cm tail chimney to reduce air turbulence around the hydrosensors

TABLE 7.1

Influence of Anatomical Site, Age, and Sex on Transepidermal Water Loss (TEWL) and Percutaneous Absorption of Benzoic Acid

Group Number	Volunteers per Group	Anatomical Site	Age (years)	Sex	TEWL[a] (g/m² hr)	Total Penetration of Benzoic Acid within 4 Days[a] (nmol/cm²)
1	8	Arm (upper) outer)	20–30	M	4.24 (0.35)	9.15 (1.01)
2	8	Arm (upper outer)	45–55	M	5.07 (0.23)	10.02 (1.02)
3	7	Arm (upper outer)	65–80	M	4.73 (0.45)	2.53 (0.82)
4	7	Arm (upper outer)	20–30	F	5.12 (0.35)	11.20 (1.20)
5	7	Abdomen	20–30	M	4.40 (0.51)	12.50 (1.64)
6	8	Postauricular	20–30	M	8.35 (0.41)	22.49 (5.14)
7	7	Forehead	20–30	M	10.34 (0.70)	26.80 (3.19)
8	8	Forehead	20–30	F	9.39 (0.73)	28.99 (1.81)
9	7	Forearm (ventral elbow)	20–30	M	2.50 (0.30)	3.48 (0.33)
10	8	Forearm (ventral mid)	20–30	M	4.00 (0.32)	5.51 (1.70)
11	7	Forearm (ventral wrist)	20–30	M	7.19 (0.39)	12.18 (1.62)
12	8	Back	20–30	M	4.51 (0.57)	8.55 (1.32)
13	8	Chest	20–30	M	4.73 (0.26)	11.70 (1.30)
14	7	Thigh	20–30	M	4.39 (0.32)	12.50 (1.43)

[a] Values are means with SD in parentheses.

and a metallic shield (supplied by Servo Med), minimizing the possibility of sensor contamination. Measurements (g/m²hr) stabilized within 30 to 45 seconds. As the room environment was comfortable (room temperature 20°C, relative humidity 70%) and the subjects were physically inactive, the TEWL should closely reflect stratum corneum water flux without significant sweating interference.

Table 7.1 gives the figures for permeability to water (TEWL) and to benzoic acid (percutaneous absorption) according to anatomical site, age, and sex. In male subjects aged from 20 to 30, cutaneous permeability to both water and benzoic acid was as follows: forearm (ventral elbow) < forearm (ventral mid) < back < arm (upper outer) ≤ chest ≤ thigh = abdomen < forearm (ventral wrist) < postauricular < forehead. In the sites studied (upper outer arm, forehead) no differences between sexes were observed.

In relation to age, no alterations in skin permeability appeared to occur before the age of 55. In subjects aged from 65 to 80 (upper outer arm), although there was no change in TEWL, percutaneous absorption of benzoic acid decreased appreciably (factor of 4; $p < 0.001$). Irrespective of anatomical site and sex, a linear relationship exists (Figure 7.2; $r = 0.92$, $p < 0.001$) between total penetration of benzoic acid and TEWL. (Point number 3, corresponding to subjects aged 65 to 80 measured on the upper outer arm, is a special case that will be discussed later and that was not taken into account in the calculation of the correlation coefficient.)

Among factors that might modify skin permeability, both *in vitro* (22) and *in vivo* (14–16, 23, 24), the anatomical location is of great importance, even if the connection between the differences observed, the structure of the skin, and the physicochemical nature of the penetrant remain obscure. As a matter of fact, general reviews often give contradictory explanations of the differences observed from one site to another (22, 25).

The laws describing diffusion through a membrane accord a major role to membrane thickness. These general laws have been applied to several biophysical phenomena, including TEWL and percutaneous absorption. However, examination of the literature shows that it is not unusual that these laws, predicated on pure mathematical logic, are found wanting when applied to a discontinuous

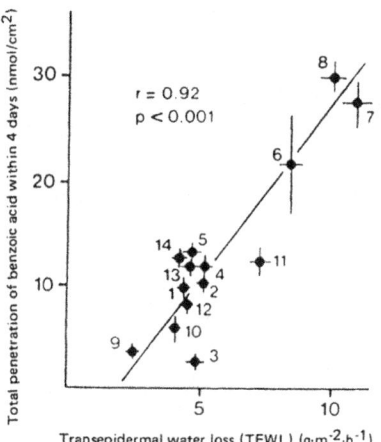

FIGURE 7.2 *In vivo* relationship between transepidermal water loss (TEWL) and percutaneous absorption of benzoic acid according to the anatomical site, age, and sex in humans (Table 7.1).

membrane of great physicochemical complexity such as the stratum corneum. Thus, the skin permeability of the forehead to water and benzoic acid is, respectively, four and eight times higher than on the forearm (ventral elbow), despite the fact that the stratum corneum thicknesses of these two sites are comparable (on average 12 µm and 18 cell layers; see Refs. 26 and 27). This example therefore seems to run counter to the inverse relationship that should exist between permeability and membrane thickness. Hence, simple consideration of the thickness of the stratum corneum cannot, in itself, explain the differences in TEWL and penetration observed between anatomical sites. Other criteria must be considered.

A possible explanation of the higher permeability of the forehead to both benzoic acid and water could partly be because of the great number of sebaceous and sweat glands found in this area. However, even if it is relatively easy to imagine a molecule's penetration by simultaneously adopting the follicular, sweat, and transcorneal routes, it is, unfortunately, difficult to evaluate the relative extent of each route. Because of the density of active sebaceous glands, the forehead is the richest of all the sites tested in terms of sebum. It forms a discontinuous film on the surface of the skin, between 0.4 µm and 4 µm thick (28). It is reasonable to question to what extent the physicochemical nature of benzoic acid interacts with this film and to what extent this initial contact influences its absorption. However, previous studies have shown that the same ratio exists between the permeability levels of areas such as the forehead, which is rich in sebum, and the arm, which has very little sebum, for molecules with totally different lipid/water solubilities (23). Moreover, it has been demonstrated that removing the lipidic film from the skin surface or artificially increasing its thickness has no effect on TEWL (29), which is another indicator of skin permeability.

Regional variations in cell size of the desquaming part of the human stratum corneum have been demonstrated by Plewig and Marples (30) and Marks et al. (31). When taking into account that in all the sites tested, the individual thickness of the corneocytes does not change (32), the relationship between the flat area of corneocytes and barrier function of the horny layer must be addressed.

In permeability phenomena, the current trend is to assign priority to intercellular, rather than transcellular, penetration. Thus, if we consider two anatomical sites with an equal volume of stratum corneum but that contain corneocytes of unequal volume, such as the abdomen and the forehead, it is obvious that the intercorneal space will be greater in the stratum corneum that has smaller corneocytes. In adults (30, 31), the flat surface of the forehead stratum corneum cells is approximately 30% less in area than that of cells from the arm, abdomen, or thigh. Moreover, as a function of the anatomical site, it has been demonstrated that an inverse relationship exists between the area of the horny layer cells and the value of the TEWL (31). What influence the intercorneal volume has on percutaneous absorption presents a question we have undertaken to answer.

As our results show (Table 7.1), there is no difference in benzoic acid absorption and TEWL between the 20 to 30 and 45 to 55 age groups. In subjects aged 65 to 80, on the other hand, absorption of this molecule is greatly reduced (factor of four). These findings agree with those of Malkinson and Fergusson (33), who failed to show any difference in percutaneous absorption of hydrocortisone in adults aged 41 to 58. The reduced absorption of benzoic acid observed in the elderly (65 to 80) was similar to that obtained with testosterone by others (34, 35). It is a reasonable presumption that this change could be partly a consequence of alterations in keratinization and epidermal cell production and itself results in altered structure and function of the stratum corneum. It has been established that corneocyte surface area increases with age (36–38). Moreover, recent studies have shown that, at the same time, a linear decrease occurred in the size of epidermal cells (39).

Although there is no change in total thickness of the stratum corneum with age (40), the question of whether or not there is an increase in surface area of corneocytes concomitant with a decrease in corneocyte thickness has not been finally decided. However, preliminary studies do not suggest that this value alters in aging stratum corneum (31, 41). So, if we assume that this latter factor does not change with advancing age, then the volume of intercellular spaces must decrease as the surface area of the corneocytes increases. The spaces between the corneocytes probably act as the molecular "reservoir" of the stratum corneum (19). For a given molecule, the smaller the capacity of this reservoir, the less it is absorbed (16, 19, 23, 42, 43). As the general morphological organization of the stratum corneum does not appear to be affected by aging (40, 44), it is tempting to conclude that the great differences observed in percutaneous absorption of benzoic acid, according to age, are solely due to the change in corneocyte size. However, this would be too simplistic an approach, and we should take into account other factors that affect the physical and physicochemical properties of the barrier, such as changes in the lipid composition of the intercellular cements; cohesion between corneocytes, which decreases with age (45, 46); or the hydration level of the horny layer (1, 47). Moreover, morphological and functional changes in adjacent structures, in particular the dermis, should also be taken into consideration. Thus, in advancing age, the underside of the epidermis becomes flattened, with this flattening being accompanied by diminution of superficial blood vessels (48, 49). These alterations in the vascular bed and extracellular matrix may lead to decreased clearance of transdermally absorbed materials from the dermis (39, 50).

Although the barrier function of the stratum corneum to the penetration of environmental agents appears to increase with age, we agree with others that TEWL does not statistically vary (45, 46, 51). This is a strange situation because a particular feature of aged skin is the roughness and apparent dryness of its surface. If it is true that the stratum corneum is the differentiated cellular end of the viable epidermis and, as such, must share the general effect of aging that takes place in all cells, the absolute need to maintain homeostasis suggests that to maintain its functional integrity, functional alterations of the horny structure will be subtle and difficult to detect.

In the areas studied (upper outer arm and forehead), no differences have been found between male and female subjects either in percutaneous absorption of benzoic acid or in water loss. There has been no systematic study showing the effects of sex on cutaneous permeability in humans. We cannot therefore compare our results with the literature.

Although most authors recognize the importance of the anatomical site either on the degree of absorption of molecules or on TEWL, the literature does not include any quantitative data on the relationship that may exist in humans between these two functions. Our results show (Figure 7.2) that for the anatomical sites studied, and within the range of TEWL and penetration values determined, a highly significant linear relationship exists ($r = 0.92$, $p < 0.001$) between the permeability of skin to water and the percutaneous absorption of a non-water-soluble compound such as benzoic acid. Only those values obtained for aged subjects (65 to 80 years, upper outer arm, point number 3) do not fit on this correlation curve.

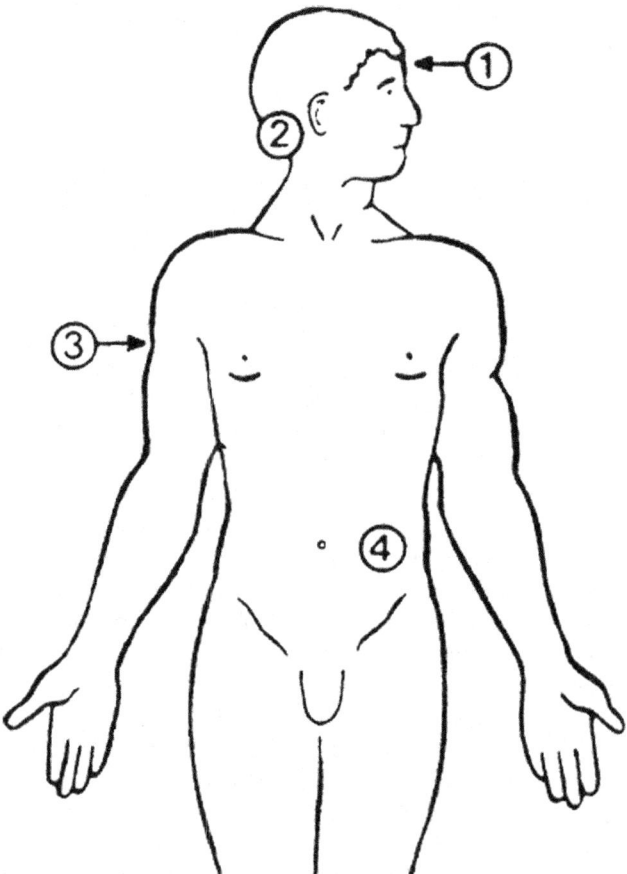

FIGURE 7.3 Anatomical sites tested: 1, forehead; 2, postauricular; 3, arm (upper outer); 4; abdomen.

Although it is generally agreed that either of these factors can be considered a reflection of the functional state and integrity of the cutaneous barrier, our results have demonstrated that they are directly linked. However, before overgeneralizing, we have examined the relationship existing between TEWL and percutaneous absorption of different molecules of varying physicochemical properties. The percutaneous absorption of three radiolabeled compounds (New England Nuclear)—acetylsalicylic acid (carboxyl-^{14}C), caffeine (1-methyl-^{14}C), and benzoic acid sodium salt (ring-^{14}C)—was determined for four anatomical sites, the exact locations of which are shown in Figure 7.3. For each molecule and for each site, six to eight male Caucasian volunteers aged 28 ± 2 years were studied.

One thousand nanomoles of each compound, with a specific activity adjusted to 10^{-3} μCi/nmol, were applied to an area of 1 cm^2 in 20 μL of the appropriate vehicle. The composition of these vehicles, shown in Table 7.2, was selected according to the solubility of each compound. Triton X-100 was added as a surfactant to obtain smooth spreading of the vehicle over the treated area, the boundaries of which were circumscribed by an open circular cell fixed by silicone glue to prevent any chemical loss. After 30 minutes, excess substance was rapidly removed by washing, rinsing, and drying the treated area as previously described.

The molecules tested were selected on the basis of the rapidity and high level of their urinary excretion. In view of the literature concerning urinary excretion kinetics for these substances after administration by various routes in different species (18–21, 43), the total amounts that had penetrated during the four days following application could be calculated, after scintillation counting,

TABLE 7.2
Percutaneous Absorption and Transepidermal Water Loss (TEWL) Values According to Anatomical Site

n and Anatomical Site	Amount in Urine After 24 hr	Total Amount Penetrated Within 4 Days[a]	TEWL	Relative Permeability to Arm	
				Penetration	TEWL[b]
Compound: benzoic acid sodium salt, vehicle A					
6, Arm (upper outer)	3.02 (0.34)	4.02 (0.45)	6.06 (0.36)	1	1
6, Abdomen	5.73 (0.54)	7.65 (0.72)	5.37 (0.46)	1.9	0.9
6, Postauricular	7.54 (0.62)	10.06 (0.82)	7.72 (0.64)	2.5	1.3
8, Forehead	9.31 (1.76)	12.32 (2.30)	12.29 (0.96)	3.1	2
Compound: caffeine, vehicle B					
7, Arm (upper outer)	6.04 (0.92)	12.09 (1.84)	7.04 (0.95)	1	1
6, Abdomen	3.76 (0.67)	7.53 (1.34)	6.05 (0.43)	0.6	0.9
7, Postauricular	5.87 (0.52)	11.72 (1.05)	8.74 (0.62)	1	1.2
6, Forehead	11.17 (1.20)	22.35 (2.39)	12.77 (1.05)	1.9	1.8
Compound: acetylsalicylic acid, vehicle A					
7, Arm	5.27 (0.18)	17.00 (0.37)	5.08 (0.79)	1	1
6, Abdomen	5.34 (1.03)	17.20 (3.35)	5.16 (0.43)	1	1
7, Postauricular	11.04 (2.50)	29.17 (5.37)	9.04 (0.84)	2.1	1.8
6, Forehead	10.89 (1.02)	35.14 (3.29)	11.22 (0.96)	2.1	2.2

Note: Values are expressed in nmol/cm^2 with SD in parentheses. Vehicle A (ethylene glycol/Triton X-100), 90:10; Vehicle B (ethylene glycol/Triton X-100), 90:10/H20;50:50.

[a] Calculated from urinary excretion for benzoic acid sodium salt (amount in urine)/0.75; for caffeine (amount in urine)/0.5; for acetylsalicylic acid (amount in urine)/0.31.

[b] Measured just before the application in g/m^{-2}hr.

from the quantities found in the urine during the first 24 hours. The proportion of the total amounts of benzoic acid sodium salt, caffeine, and acetylsalicylic acid absorbed that were excreted within 24 hours were 75%, 50%, and 31%, respectively.

After topical administration of the tested compound, TEWL was measured from a contralateral site (same anatomical region) in each subject as described earlier. The results (Table 7.2) show that the percutaneous penetration of the test molecules varied with the anatomical location. The area behind the ear and that on the forehead were the most permeable, regardless of the physicochemical properties of the compound tested. In general, the order of cutaneous permeability was as follows: arm ≤ abdomen < postauricular < forehead. Although the literature provides few details about the influence of anatomical site on the absorption of molecules, the rank order obtained here agrees with studies performed with other chemicals (14, 15, 20, 52).

Cutaneous permeability is generally considered a mirror of the integrity of the horny layer. Even in normal skin, the efficacy of this barrier is not constant. Thus, as shown in Table 7.2, for a given anatomical site the permeability varies widely in relation to the nature of the molecule administered because this is related to the physicochemical interactions that may occur between the molecule, the vehicle, and the stratum corneum. For the anatomical sites investigated and for the range of TEWL and penetration observed, there exists a linear relationship between the permeability of the skin to

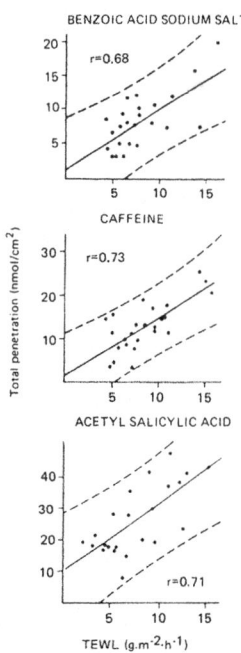

FIGURE 7.4 *In vivo* relationship between transepidermal water loss (TEWL) and percutaneous absorption of some organic compounds according to the anatomical site in humans.

the outward movement of water and the inward uptake of molecules. Table 7.2 shows that this relationship fits with all the compounds tested, with caffeine being an apparent exception (decreased penetration on abdomen and postauricular regions as compared with the arm, whereas TEWL showed a slight decrease on the abdomen and an increase in the postauricular region). It is, however, worth noting that the same relationship, when expressed with individual values (Figure 7.4), shows correlation coefficients between 0.68 and 0.73 ($p < 0.05$), with the latter (and better one) corresponding to caffeine (the confidence limits represent a risk of 5%).

Thus, it appears that the linear relationship linking TEWL and percutaneous absorption is independent of the physicochemical properties of the compound applied. Moreover, with the three molecules investigated, a mean increase of 2.7 in percutaneous absorption corresponded to an increase of 3 in the TEWL value. This fact supports the hypothesis that the efficiency of the barrier is dependent on the physicochemical properties of the molecule administered, but its functional state is independent of these. Consequently, as with determinations of TEWL, percutaneous absorption measurement provides a good marker of the cutaneous barrier integrity.

REFERENCES

1. Blank IH, Moloney J, Emslie AG, Simon I, Apt CH. The diffusion of water across the stratum corneum as a function of its water content. J Invest Dermatol 1984; 82:188–194.
2. Scheuplein RJ, Blank IH. Permeability of the skin. Physiol Rev 1971; 51:702–747.
3. Marzulli FN. Barriers to skin penetration. J Invest Dermatol 1962; 39:387–393.
4. Malkinson FD. Studies on percutaneous absorption of ^{14}C-labelled steroids by use of the Gaz low cell. J Invest Dermatol 1958; 31:19–28.
5. Fritsch WF, Stoughton RB. The effect of temperature and humidity on the penetration of ^{14}C acetylsalicylic acid in excised human skin. J Invest Dermatol 1963; 41:307–311.
6. Wurter DE, Kramer SF. Investigation of some factors influencing percutaneous absorption. J Pharm Sci 1961; 50:288–293.

7. Scheuplein RJ. The skin as a barrier. In: Jarrett A, ed. The Physiology and Pathophysiology of the Skin. Vol. 5. New York: Academic Press, 1978:1669–1692.
8. Guillaume JC, de Rigal J, Leveque JL, Galle P, Touraine R, Dubertret L. Etude comparée de la perée insensible d'eau et de la pénétration cutanïé des corticoides. Dermatologïca 1981; 162:380–390.
9. Smith JG, Fischer RW, Blank IH. The epidermal barrier: a comparison between scrotal and abdominal skin. J Invest Dermatol 1961; 36:337–343.
10. Lamaud E, Lambrey B, Schalla W, Schaefer H. Correlation between transepidermal water loss and penetration of drugs. J Invest Dermatol 1984; 82:556.
11. Maibach HI, Bronaugh R, Guy R, Turr E, Wilson D, Jacques S, Chaing D. Noninvasive techniques for determining skin function. In: Drill VA, Lazar P, eds. Cutaneous Toxicity. New York: Raven Press, 1984:63–97.
12. Surinchak JS, Malinowski JA, Wilson DR, Maibach HI. Skin wound healing determined by water loss. J Surg Res 1985; 38:258–262.
13. Wilson DR, Maibach HI. A review of transepidermal water loss: physical aspects and measurements as related to infants and adults. In: Maibach HI, Boisits EK, eds. Neonatal Skin. New York: Marcel Dekker, 1982:83.
14. Feldman RJ, Maibach HI. Regional variations in percutaneous penetration of ^{14}C cortisol in man. J Invest Dermatol 1967; 48:181–183.
15. Maibach HI, Feldmann RJ, Milby T, Serat W. Regional variation in percutaneous penetration in man. Arch Environ Health 1971; 23:208–211.
16. Rougier A, Dupuis D, Lotte C, Roguet R, Wester R, Maibach HI. Regional variation in percutaneous absorption in man: measurement by the stripping method. Arch Dermatol Res 1986; 278:465–469.
17. Bridges JW, French MR, Smith RL, Williams RT. The fate of benzoic acid in various species. Biochem J 1970; 188:47–51.
18. Bronaugh RL, Stewart RF, Congdon ER, Giles AL. Methods for in vitro percutaneous absorption studies. I. Comparison with in vivo results. Toxicol Appl Pharmacol 1982; 62:474–480.
19. Dupuis D, Rougier A, Roguet R, Lotte C, Kalopissis G. In vivo relationship between horny layer reservoir effect and percutaneous absorption in human and rat. J Invest Dermatol 1984; 82:353–356.
20. Feldmann RJ, Maibach HI. Absorption of some organic compounds through the skin in man. J Invest Dermatol 1970; 54:399–404.
21. Rougier A, Dupuis D, Lotte C, Roguet R, Schaefer H. In vivo correlation between stratum corneum reservoir function and percutaneous absorption. J Invest Dermatol 1983; 81:275–278.
22. Scheuplein RJ. Site variations in diffusion and permeability. In: Jarrett A, ed. The Physiology and Pathology of the Skin. Vol. 5. New York: Academic Press, 1979:1731–1752.
23. Rougier A, Lotte C, Maibach HI. In vivo percutaneous penetration of some organic compounds related to anatomic site in man: Predictive assessment by the stripping method. J Pharm Sci 1987; 76(6):451–454.
24. Wester RC, Maibach HI, Bucks DA, Aufrere MB. In vivo percutaneous absorption of paraquat from hand, leg and forearm of humans. J Toxicol Environ Health 1984; 84:759–761.
25. Idson B. Percutaneous absorption. J Pharm Sci 1975; 64:901–924.
26. Holbrook KA, Odland GF. Regional differences in the thickness (cell layers) of the human stratum corneum: an ultrastructural analysis. J Invest Dermatol 1974; 62:415–422.
27. Pathiak MA, Fitzpatrick TB. The role of natural photoprotective agents in human skin. In: Fitzpatrick TB, ed. Sunlight and Man. Tokyo: University Tokyo Press, 1974:725–750.
28. Kligman AM. The use of sebum. Br J Dermatol 1983; 75:307–319.
29. Kligman AM. A biological brief on percutaneous absorption. Drug Dev Ind Pharm 1983; 9:521–560.
30. Plewig G, Marples RR. Regional differences of cell sizes in human stratum corneum. Part I. J Invest Dermatol 1970; 54:13–18.
31. Marks R, Nicholls S, King CS. Studies on isolated corneocytes. Int J Cosmet Sci 1981; 3:251–258.
32. Plewig G, Scheuber E, Reuter B, Waidelich W. Thickness of corneocytes. In: Marks R, Plewig G, eds. Stratum Corneum. Berlin-Heidelberg, New York: Springer-Verlag, 1983:171–174.
33. Malkinson FD, Ferguson EH. Percutaneous absorption of hydrocortisone-4-^{14}C in two human subjects. J Invest Dermatol 1955; 25:281–283.
34. Christophers E, Kligman AM. Percutaneous absorption in aged skin. In: Montagna W, ed. Advances in Biology of the Skin. New York: Pergamon Press, 1964:163–175.
35. Roskos K, Guy R, Maibach HI. Percutaneous penetration in the aged. Dermatol Clin 1986; 4:455–465.
36. Grove GL. Exfoliative cytological procedures as a nonintrusive method for dermatogerontological studies. J Invest Dermatol 1979; 79:67–69.

37. Plewig G. Regional differences of cell sizes in the human stratum corneum. Part II: Effect of sex and age. J Invest Dermatol 1970; 54:19–23.
38. Grove GL, Lavker RM, Holzle E, Kligman AM. The use of nonintrusive tests to monitor age associated changes in human skin. J Soc Cosmet Chem 1981; 32:15–26.
39. Marks R. Measurement of biological aging in human epidermis. Br J Dermatol 1981; 104:627–633.
40. Lavker RM. Structural alterations in exposed and unexposed aged skin. J Invest Dermatol 1979; 73:59–66.
41. Marks R, Barton SP. The significance of size and shape of corneocytes. In: Marks R, Plewig G, eds. Stratum Corneum. Berlin-Heidelberg, New York: Springer-Verlag, 1983:161–170.
42. Dupuis D, Rougier A, Roguet R, Lotte C. The measurement of the stratum corneum reservoir: a simple method to predict the influence of vehicles on in vivo percutaneous absorption. Br J Dermatol 1986; 115:233–238.
43. Rougier A, Dupuis D, Lotte C, Roguet R. The measurement of the stratum corneum reservoir. A predictive method for in vivo percutaneous absorption studies: influence of application time. J Invest Dermatol 1985; 84:66–68.
44. McKenzye IC, Zimmerman K, Peterson L. The pattern of cellular organization of human epidermis. J Invest Dermatol 1981; 76:459–461.
45. Leveque JL, Corcuff P, de Rigal J, Agache P. In vivo studies of the evolution of physical properties of the human skin with age. Int J Dermatol 1984; 23:322–329.
46. Marks R, Lawson A, Nicholls S. Age-related changes in stratum corneum structure and function. In: Marks R, Plewig G, eds. Stratum Corneum. Berlin-Heidelberg, New York: Springer-Verlag, 1983:175–180.
47. Blank IH. Factors which influence the water content of the stratum corneum. J Invest Dermatol 1952; 18:433–437.
48. Ellis RA. Aging of the human male scalp. In: Montagna W, Ellis RA, eds. The Biology of Hair Growth. New York: Academic Press, 1958:469–485.
49. Montagna W, Carlisle K. Structural changes in aging human skin. J Invest Dermatol 1979; 73:47–53.
50. Küstala G. Dermal epidermal separation: influence of age, sex and body region on suction blister formation in human skin. Ann Clin Res 1972; 4:10–22.
51. Kligman AM. Perspectives and problems in cutaneous gerontology. J Invest Dermatol 1979; 73:39–46.
52. Taskovitch L, Shaw JE. Regional differences in the morphology of human skin: correlation with variations in drug permeability. J Invest Dermatol 1978; 70:217.

8 The Correlation between Transepidermal Water Loss and Percutaneous Absorption

An Updated Overview

Marjan Koosha Johnson
Western University of Health Sciences,
Pomona, California

Jacquelyn Levin
Midwestern University, Glendale, Arizona

Howard I. Maibach
University of California,
San Francisco, California

CONTENTS

8.1 INTRODUCTION

8.1.1 WHAT IS TRANSEPIDERMAL WATER LOSS?

Transepidermal water loss (TEWL) is the outward diffusion of water through the skin (Oestmann et al. 1993). Stated simply, TEWL is a metric of the ability of the skin to retain water (Blattner et al. 2014).

Several methods can be used to measure TEWL. An evaporimeter determines TEWL by measuring the pressure gradient of the boundary layer resulting from the water gradient between the skin surface and ambient air. There are several different evaporimeter devices for TEWL, so baseline TEWL measurements are recorded with results analyzed as a relative change to account for any differences between devices. Generally, as outward water loss across the stratum corneum (SC, Latin for "horny layer") increases, the humidity next to the skin surface rises above ambient humidity, which creates a humidity gradient above the skin surface that is proportional to the SC water loss (Alexander et al. 2018). Raman spectroscopy, an optical imaging technique, is another method to quantify TEWL, but is limited by skin hydration status and must be controlled to minimize error (Blattner et al. 2014). It is also not as commonly employed to determine TEWL as is the evaporimeter method.

Since TEWL measurements can be used to determine the amount of water that crosses the skin epidermis, these values can also be used to estimate the barrier function of the SC. TEWL can therefore reflect the general health of the skin. For example, skin diseases that are associated with impaired barrier function, such as atopic dermatitis (AD), contact dermatitis, psoriasis, and ichthyosis, show increased TEWL (Alexander et al. 2018). TEWL approximations can also assess treatment effectiveness or skin barrier repair by monitoring the change in TEWL over time (Nilsson 1997; Pinnagoda et al. 1990, Zhang et al. 2018). However, TEWL measurements cannot simply be compared across multiple experiments. TEWL measurements are subject to intraindividual variation based on the anatomical site where TEWL was measured. TEWL is high at the palms, soles, axillae, and forehead, and low at the calves and forearms (Alexander et al. 2018). TEWL also depends on interindividual variation based on the extent of skin perspiration and skin surface temperature of the individual tested (Alexander et al. 2018; Pinnagoda et al. 1990). Some works have additionally demonstrated seasonal variation in TEWL and note that TEWL is affected by circadian rhythm and sun exposure (Alexander et al. 2018; Le Fur et al. 2001; Liu et al. 2010). Also, TEWL measurements can be affected by experimental conditions such as air convection, the ambient air temperature and air humidity of the room where the TEWL measurement was taken, and the type of instrument used to gauge TEWL. Although TEWL can be influenced by many variables, experiments show that evaporimeter measurements are generally reproducible *in vitro* and *in vivo* (Alexander et al. 2018; Elkeeb et al. 2010; Fluhr et al. 2006; Pinnagoda et al. 1989, 1990).

8.1.2 What Is Percutaneous Absorption?

Percutaneous absorption refers to the rate of absorption of a topically applied chemical through the skin. The absorption rate is important for determining the effectiveness and/or potential adverse or toxic effects of topically applied compounds. Since many dermally applied formulations are used on diseased skin, where the integrity of the permeability barrier is in doubt, the dose absorbed into the body may vary greatly (Bronaugh 1986). A compound's percutaneous absorption through the skin is rate-limited by the speed of its diffusion through the SC. The rate of absorption through the SC cannot be described by zero- or first-order mathematical rate equations because the SC is a complex system variable in its penetration properties.

Percutaneous absorption and the SC are tightly related. The SC, which serves as the most superficial layer of the epidermis, plays a protective role in skin integrity. While earlier it was thought to serve as the sole skin barrier, it is now known to play a critical (but not solitary) role in the skin's defense system amidst the stratum granulosum and the stratum spinosum and basalis. The SC acts as a resistant barrier against water loss, and along with other dermal layers, functions to regulate temperature and protect against foreign chemicals and bacteria. A substance's ability to penetrate the SC depends on several SC factors, such as the quality of the barrier (including the number of lipids, their chain length, and their organization within the SC), hydration (at the time of substance application), and thickness. Many other factors contribute to the percutaneous absorption of a given chemical. Such examples include methodology, including the effects of application time and method of measurement; physicochemical properties of the topical compound applied; interindividual variation, including the effects of skin condition; age and blood flow of the individual; and intraindividual variation, including the differences between anatomic sites (Noonan and Gonzalez 1990; Wester and Maibach 1993).

It is important to review the relevance of percutaneous absorption as a topic of ongoing research because of its applicability (and benefit) to current practices of pharmaceutical delivery. Percutaneous absorption has gained traction with the surfacing of new research and has the potential to alter the methods of drug delivery in modern medicine (Blattner et al. 2014).

8.1.3 What Is the Significance of a Correlation between TEWL and Percutaneous Absorption?

The extensive procedures required to measure percutaneous absorption versus TEWL enhance our interest to find a correlation between the two measurements to more easily assess skin barrier function and should aid in the understanding and development of penetration enhancers. Recent studies have surmised that heating the skin results in an increased rate of percutaneous absorption of water. In skin diseases like AD and psoriasis, there is increased TEWL as compared to healthy skin. Not all measurements of TEWL are identical in results and should thereby be evaluated further for aspects that may have been overlooked or need further exploration. For example, tape stripping is a widely used method to measure percutaneous penetration of water, limited by its inability to quantify water molecule movement through corneocytes. Barrier function approximations are frequently measured with TEWL quantities and tape stripping by way of gradual corneocyte removal. However, according to a study by van der Molen et al. (1997), histological sections of skin still contained nonstripped skin in the furrows despite 20 replications of tape stripping (van der Molen et al. 1997). All of this becomes important when assessing the relationship between TEWL and percutaneous absorption, which will be further unpacked in this chapter (Blattner et al. 2014).

In an earlier version of this chapter by Levin and Maibach in 2005, nine studies investigating the correlation between TEWL and percutaneous absorption were evaluated. Of the nine studies reviewed, a majority demonstrated a significant quantitative correlation and a few found quantitative correlation. At that time, it was thought that the correlation between TEWL and percutaneous absorption may not hold for in vitro experimentation models, extremely lipophilic compounds, or possibly experiments performed on animal skin. Since then, several other studies have been published that investigated the relationship between TEWL and percutaneous absorption using a lipophilic compound (Hui et al. 2012), in vitro models (Elkeeb et al. 2010; Elmahjoubi et al. 2009; Hui et al. 2012, Guth 2015), and animal skin (Elmahjoubi et al. 2009). All of these studies demonstrated a significant quantitative correlation. In the next section, we review fourteen studies investigating the correlation between TEWL and percutaneous absorption.

8.2 PERTINENT STUDIES INVESTIGATING THE CORRELATION BETWEEN TEWL AND PERCUTANEOUS ABSORPTION

Oestmann et al. (1993) investigated the correlation between TEWL and hexyl nicotinate (HN) penetration parameters in humans. The penetration of HN was indirectly measured using laser-Doppler flowmetry (LDF), which quantifies the increase in cutaneous blood blow (CBF) caused by penetration of HN, a vasodilatory substance. Lipophilic HN was chosen over hydrophilic methyl nicotinate because HN is a slower penetrant (since it is a lipoid compound), hence making it easier to distinguish an intact barrier from an impaired barrier. Again, it is expected that in an impaired barrier, compounds are more rapidly absorbed. The LDF parameters of initial response time (t_o) and time to maximum response (t_{max}) were compared with corresponding TEWL values, and a weak quantitative negative correlation was found ($r = -0.31$, $r = -0.32$). This correlation suggests that when individual initial response time, t_o, was quick, the skin barrier was impaired, whereas in an intact barrier, a slow t_0 would be the expected finding. The weak negative correlation found suggests that LDF is not as reproducible as other methods of measuring percutaneous absorption. Further research should investigate the weak correlation between TEWL and penetration of HN.

Lavrijsen et al. (1993) characterized the SC barrier function in patients with various keratinization disorders using two noninvasive methods: measuring outward transport of water through the skin by evaporimetry, i.e., TEWL, and the vascular response to HN penetration into the skin determined by LDF. Three of the five types of keratinization disorders studied, i.e., autosomal dominant ichthyosis vulgaris, X-linked recessive ichthyosis, and autosomal recessive congenital ichthyosis, have impaired barrier function. On the other hand, for the other two keratinization disorders studied, dyskeratosis follicularis and erythrokeratodermia variabilis, there was no prior information available on barrier impairment. In this experiment, the two methods of barrier function assessment, TEWL and LDF, were correlated for all skin diseases with healthy skin as a control. TEWL measurements and the LDF parameter t_0 showed a strong negative correlation in those with skin disease ($r = -0.64$) and a weaker negative correlation among the healthy skin control group ($r = -0.39$). Since TEWL reflects the steady-state flux of water across the SC and the parameter t_0 is a function of the duration of the lag phase (not a steady-state measurement), this study suggested that these two methods (which measure different variables) should not be considered exchangeable alternatives, but rather complementary tests to assess barrier function. It can thereby be concluded that taken together in sum, measurement of TEWL and of HN penetration are suitable methods to monitor skin barrier function in keratinization disorders.

In a study by Arimoto et al. (2016), seven volunteer subjects (ages 30 to 50, male and female) were compared to determine (1) the absorption into and (2) spreading of moisturizers across the microscopic region of the skin surface using near-infrared (NIR) imaging. Specifically, (1) the time of moisturizer droplet absorption into the skin (of the upper arm) and (2) the area of spreading of the moisturizer droplet across the skin surface were determined. The two measured parameters addressed were skin condition via (1) water content and (2) TEWL. Both the values of (1) and (2) were determined by the use of their own dedicated devices, respectively: Corneometer (CM 825; Courage + Khazaka, Cologne, Germany) and VapoMeter for TEWL (Delfin Technologies Ltd., Kuopio, Finland). Differences between the major constituents (oil and humectants) in the three moisturizer products (M1, M2, and M3) were also considered. Though the major constituents of M1 to M3 were oil and humectants, the number of humectants was the least in M3, and M1 and M2 contained slight amounts of lipophilic humectants. The time-lapse dynamics of the moisturizer droplet on the skin surface was analyzed for evaluating the correlation between water content and TEWL. Not surprisingly, it was found that the skin tissue with high water content and low TEWL tended to absorb the moisturizer more rapidly, while the skin surface spreading of the droplet depended on the constituents of the moisturizers. That is, absorption time was gradual for skin with high water content (and therefore low TEWL) and depended less on the properties of the moisturizer. This can be further extended to suggest that in skin tissue with high water content (and low TEWL), percutaneous absorption will be more rapid, as previously noted. This again exemplifies ways in which TEWL and percutaneous absorption can be related (among elapsed time, droplet area, water content, and TEWL; Arimoto et al. 2016).

Lamaud et al. (1984) investigated whether TEWL correlated to the percutaneous absorption of lipophilic compounds (i.e., hydrocortisone). In part one of the experiment, penetration of 1% hydrocortisone and TEWL rates were recorded for hairless rats in vivo before and after ultraviolet (UV) irradiation (660 J/cm^2). The results demonstrated a correlation between TEWL and the percutaneous absorption of hydrocortisone both before and after UV irradiation for application periods up to one hour. In the second part of the experiment, drug penetration was evaluated by urinary excretion five days after a single 24-hour application of hydrocortisone applied to undisturbed, tape-stripped, or UV-irradiated skin of hairless rats. In this experiment, the quantity of drug eliminated correlated with the level of TEWL for up to two days for all skin conditions. This finding suggests that TEWL can predict the changes in skin permeability to lipophilic drugs in both undisturbed and damaged (tape-stripped or UV-irradiated) skin.

Rougier et al. (1988) attempted to establish a relationship between the barrier properties of the SC using percutaneous absorption and TEWL measurements and discern the surface area of the corneocytes according to the anatomic site, age, and sex in humans. The penetration of benzoic acid (BA) was measured in vivo at seven anatomic sites and compared to the TEWL value measured on the contralateral corresponding sites. The amount of BA penetrated was measured through urinary excretion for up to 24 hours after application. It was discovered that, irrespective of anatomic site and sex, a significant linear relationship ($p < 0.001$, $r = 0.92$) existed between total penetration of BA and TEWL.

Comparing corneocytes within the SC surface area to permeability, Rougier et al. (1988) also found a general correlation of increasing permeability, for both water and BA, with decreasing corneocyte size. The smaller the volume of the corneocyte, the greater the intercellular space between corneocytes available to act as a reservoir for topically applied molecules, ultimately resulting in higher absorption (Dupuis et al. 1984). This thinking is in accord with other studies that have shown that the smaller the capacity of the reservoir, the less the molecule is absorbed (Dupuis et al. 1984; Rougier et al. 1983, 1985, 1987a). Even more recently in a 2016 study by Boer et al., the absorption of substances from the surface of the skin was said to depend to a large degree on the corneocyte size of the SC. Further, absorption was said to be proportional to the capacity of the intercellular space and inversely proportional to the size of the cells (Boer et al. 2016).

To determine the influence of age on corneocyte size, Rougier et al. (1988) investigated corneocyte size in the upper outer arm of three groups of six to eight male volunteers: (1) 20 to 30, (2) 45 to 55, and (3) 65 to 80 years of age. No variation in corneocyte size up to age 55 years was observed. The mean corneocyte size for the 20 to 30 years cohort was 980 ± 34 μm^2 and for the 45 to 55 years cohort, a value of 994 ± 56 μm^2 was recorded. The group aged 65 to 80 years did, however, show significantly larger corneocytes (1141 ± 63 μm^2) relative to the other groups. Comparatively small sample sizes ($n = 6$ to 8) of subjects were used by Rougier et al. (1988), which would likely explain the discrepancies when compared with data from other studies, e.g., Leveque et al. (1984). It is now understood that corneocytes generally increase in size with age (Machado et al. 2010). Similarly, TEWL and percutaneous absorption also increase with age (Roskos and Guy 1989). As such, corneocyte size alone cannot explain the permeability changes in mature skin.

Rougier et al. (1988) used a detergent scrub technique to collect corneocytes at different anatomic sites from a group of six to eight male volunteers, aged 20 to 30 years old. From largest to smallest, the rank order of the corneocyte surface area was elbow (1004 μm^2), ventral-mid forearm (1007 μm^2), upper outer arm (980 μm^2), abdomen (996 μm^2), ventral-wrist (884 μm^2), postauricular (812 μm^2), and forehead (555 μm^2). However, when Rougier et al. (1988) investigated corneocyte size relative to the anatomic site, they found that for certain anatomic sites where corneocyte size was similar (980 to 1000 μm^2), there were differences in permeability. While percutaneous absorption and TEWL are quantitatively correlated, corneocyte size only partially explains the difference in permeability between distinct anatomic sites and different ages of skin.

Lotte et al. (1987) examined the relationship between the percutaneous penetration of four water-soluble chemicals (acetylsalicylic acid, BA, caffeine, and the sodium salt of BA) and TEWL in human skin as a function of the anatomic site. The amount of individual chemical penetration was estimated by urinary excretion for up to 24 hours after dermal application. For a given anatomic site, the permeability varied widely with the nature of the molecule administered due to the physicochemical interactions that occur between the molecule, vehicle of application, and SC. For all anatomic sites investigated, irrespective of the physicochemical properties of the molecules administered, there was a linear relationship between TEWL and percutaneous absorption.

Aalto-Korte and Turpeinen (1993) attempted to find the precise relationship between TEWL and percutaneous absorption of hydrocortisone in patients with active dermatitis. Percutaneous absorption of hydrocortisone and TEWL were studied in three children and six adults with dermatitis.

All the subjects had widespread dermatitis covering at least 60% of their total skin area. Plasma cortisol concentrations were measured by radioimmunoassay before and two and four hours after hydrocortisone application. TEWL was measured in six standard skin areas immediately before the application of the hydrocortisone cream. Each TEWL value was calculated as a mean of these six measurements. The concordance between the post-application increment in plasma cortisol and the mean TEWL was significant, resulting in a correlation coefficient of $r = 0.991$ ($p < 0.001$). In conclusion, this study found a significant correlation between TEWL and percutaneous absorption of hydrocortisone.

Tsai et al. (2001) investigated the relationship between permeability barrier disruption and the percutaneous absorption of various compounds with different lipophilicity. Acetone treatment was used in vivo on hairless mice to disrupt the normal permeability barrier and in vivo TEWL measurements were used to test barrier disruption. The hairless mouse skin was then excised and placed in diffusion cells for obtaining in vitro percutaneous absorption measurements of five model compounds: sucrose, caffeine, hydrocortisone, estradiol, and progesterone. The partition coefficient or lipophilicity of these compounds and compounds used in the subsequent studies are summarized in Table 8.1.

The permeability barrier disruption by acetone treatment and TEWL measurements significantly correlated with the percutaneous absorption of the hydrophilic (sucrose, caffeine) and lipophilic (hydrocortisone) drugs. However, acetone treatment did not alter the percutaneous penetration of the highly lipophilic compounds estradiol and progesterone, suggesting that there is not a correlation between TEWL and the percutaneous absorption of highly lipophilic compounds. The results imply the need to use both TEWL and drug lipophilicity to predict alterations in skin permeability.

Chilcott et al. (2002) investigated the relationship between TEWL and skin permeability to tritiated water (^3H_2O) and the lipophilic sulfur mustard (^{35}SM) in vitro. No correlation was found between basal TEWL rates and the permeability of the human epidermal membrane to ^3H_2O ($p = 0.72$) or sulfur mustard ($p = 0.74$). Similarly, there was no correlation between TEWL rates and the ^3H_2O permeability on full-thickness pig skin ($p = 0.68$). There was also no correlation between

TABLE 8.1

A Summary of the Compounds Used in the Correlation Studies, Their Octanol: Water Partition Coefficient, Solubility Classification, and Whether or Not Their Percutaneous Absorption Correlated with TEWL

Compound	Partition Coefficient ($logP_{octanol/water}$)	Classification	Correlation
Sucrose	−3.7	Hydrophilic	Yes
Caffeine	−0.02	Hydrophilic	Yes
Water	1	Hydrophilic	Yes
ASA	1.13	Hydrophilic	Yes
Hydrocortisone	1.5	Lipophilic	Yes
Benzoic Acid	1.87	Lipophilic	Yes
Estradiol	2.7	Highly Lipophilic	No
Progesterone	3.9	Highly Lipophilic	No
Hexyl Nicotinate	4	Highly Lipophilic	Yes (weak)
Clonidine	5.4	Highly Lipophilic	Yes (weak)

Source: Aalto-Korte and Turpeinen 1987; Atrux-Tallau et al. 2007; Chilcott et al. 2002; Duracher et al. 2015; Elkeeb et al. 2010; Elmahjoubi et al. 2009; Hui et al. 2012; Lamaud et al. 1984; Lavrijsen et al. 1993; Lotte et al. 1987; Nilsson 1997; Oestmann et al. 1993; Rougier et al. 1998; Tsai et al. 2001.

TEWL rates and ^3H_2O permeability following physical damage using up to 15 tape strips ($p = 0.64$) or up to four needle stick punctures ($p = 0.13$). Taken together, these results indicate that under these experimental circumstances (i.e., in vitro human and pig skin), TEWL cannot be used as a measure of the skin's permeability to topically applied lipophilic or hydrophilic compounds. Simply, the authors believe that TEWL rates must not be attributed to alterations in skin barrier function, as other factors may be largely at play for the variation in TEWL rates in vivo. It should also be noted that their p-values were not significant, further weakening that claim.

Elkeeb et al. (2010) compared TEWL to the percutaneous absorption/flux rate of ^3H_2O in in vitro dermatomed, clinically healthy human cadaver skin using three different evaporimeters to measure TEWL. Measurements were taken at baseline (i.e., at the start of the experiment) and then again at several time points over 24 hours. The evaporimeters included an open-chamber evaporimeter A (TEWameter TM 210; Courgae and Khazaka, Cologne, Germany) and two closed-chamber evaporimeters B (VapoMeter; Delfin Technologies, Kuopio, Finland) and C (AquaFlux AF200, Biox Systems, Ltd, London, UK). Open-chamber evaporimeters are open to the ambient air, while closed-chamber evaporimeters are closed systems that are not open to the environment. There has been controversy over the years as to whether open- and closed-chamber evaporimeters are equivalent in providing accurate and precise TEWL measurements. Baseline TEWL measurements with evaporimeters A ($p = 0.04$, $r^2 = 0.34$) and C ($p = 0.00$, $r^2 = 0.50$) correlated with the percutaneous absorption or flux rate of tritiated water (^3H_2O), while evaporimeter B showed no statistically significant correlation ($p = 0.07$, $r^2 = 0.31$). However, the pattern of changing TEWL values over 24 hours was similar to that of the percutaneous absorption or tritiated water flux for all three evaporimeters A, B, and C ($p = 0.04$, $r^2 = 0.34$). The reason that evaporimeter B showed no significant correlation for baseline TEWL measurement remains unknown. Elkeeb et al. (2010) state that the results of this experiment imply the validity of using both open- and closed-chamber evaporimeters in the evaluation of skin barrier function.

Atrux-Tallau et al. (2007) demonstrated a significant correlation between TEWL and the percutaneous absorption of caffeine (a hydrophilic compound) during an ex vivo experiment on heat-separated epidermis and dermatomed human skin ($p < 0.001$, $r^2 = 0.88$). Since caffeine is a hydrophilic compound and has a relatively small molecular weight of 194 Da, it was not surprising to the authors that its permeation behavior resembles that of tritiated water (at a molecular weight of 22 Da).

In a study by Duracher et al. (2015), the dermal absorption of acetyl aspartic acid (A-A-A) was examined using in vitro and in vivo human skin after 6 and 24 hours post-dermal application of a cosmetic formulation containing A-A-A at 1% in a water-in-oil emulsion. Franz-type diffusion cells (effective diffusion area: 3.14 cm^2) containing ex vivo human skin samples were used for the in vitro experiment. For the in vivo experiment, nine (male or female) human volunteers underwent topical application followed by tape stripping after six hours. To control for potential confounding, the volunteers were instructed not to apply any cosmetic or skincare products for up to 12 hours pre-experiment. They were also acclimated for 15 minutes in a room at constant temperature and humidity. Once acclimation was complete, TEWL was measured on the test areas using a closed-chamber device (VapoMeter, Delfin). The goal of both the in vitro and in vivo experiments was to quantify A-A-A in the main skin compartments: skin surface, the SC, and the in vitro skin in the receptor fluid. The results followed that after 24 hours in vitro A-A-A exemplified substantial penetration potential in all of the skin compartments analyzed. That is, 46.2% and 34.9% of applied A-A-A was recovered in the skin surface, 37.7% and 47.5% in the SC, 1.1% and 1.9% in the skin, and 0% and 3.1% A-A-A in the receptor fluid after 6 hours and 24 hours, respectively. According to the Society of Cosmetic Scientists, the amounts retrieved in the skin (without SC) and the receptor fluid are considered dermally absorbed. From 6 to 24 hours, the amount of A-A-A that remained on the surface decreased, which indicates its diffusion from the formulation to the first skin layers relative to time. No statistical difference was observed between the quantities retrieved in the SC after 6 or 24 hours, which might suggest that A-A-A penetrates rapidly and remains in the SC, where it is accumulated over time. Subsequently, the available amount of A-A-A diffused deeper and increasing amounts were retrieved in the skin samples, as well as in the receptor fluid, following 24 hours.

Additionally, after six hours of topical application, the removed tape strips from both the in vitro ($n = 5$) and in vivo ($n = 9$) experiments were analyzed and the profile of A-A-A diffusion was assessed. This aspect of the experiment made it possible to compare in vitro versus in vivo. In vitro, $46.2 \pm 10.5\%$ of A-A-A was retrieved in the first tape strip, with $52.7\% \pm 6.2\%$ in vivo. Although different quantities were attained in the pooled tapes two to three in vitro (29.8%) and in vivo (15.1%), the amounts of A-A-A were alike and declined correspondingly with the SC's depth. The inconsistency seen between both the in vitro and in vivo experiments might be described by interindividual variability and by the origin of skin samples. For the in vitro experiment, skin samples were taken from abdominal tissue, while the in vivo tests were done on the volar forearms of human volunteers. Ultimately it was demonstrated that the diffusion profile observed on the in vitro skin penetration was highly comparable to the in vivo skin in healthy volunteers (Duracher et al. 2015)

Hui et al. (2012) investigated the correlation between TEWL and the percutaneous absorption of clonidine (a lipophilic compound) and ^3H_2O in vitro human cadaver skin. The partition coefficient of clonidine is reported in Table 8.1. TEWL measurements were made with a closed-chamber TEWL meter (AquaFlux AF200). Hui et al. (2012) aimed to discern the potential differences in the correlation between TEWL and lipophilic clonidine, the correlation between TEWL and ^3H_2O percutaneous absorption, and general differences in the percutaneous absorption of clonidine and ^3H_2O. They accomplished this by recording and comparing the flux rate, skin distribution, and total amount of absorption for clonidine and tritiated water. Statistical analysis indicated that the baseline TEWL values weakly correlated with the flux of [^{14}C]-clonidine ($p < 0.03$, $r^2 = 0.36$) and ^3H_2O ($p = 0.04$, $r^2 = 0.34$). The correlation between the fluxes of ^3H_2O and [^{14}C]-clonidine was significant (correlation coefficient = 0.675, $p < 0.001$). In addition, TEWL and permeation data of ^3H_2O expressed as a percent dose of the amount in the receptor fluid correlated throughout the experiment. However, the permeation curve of [^{14}C]-clonidine as a percent dose in the receptor fluid differed from that of ^3H_2O. The variation in the curves is likely secondary to differences between the hydrophilic and lipophilic properties of water versus clonidine. Therefore, as Hui et al. suggest, it may be necessary to combine the TEWL values with factors such as molecular weight and/or hydrophilicity/lipophilicity to gauge percutaneous absorption.

Elmahjoubi et al. (2009) investigated TEWL (using the AquaFlux Evaporimeter) and the percutaneous absorption/flux of ^3H_2O in full-thickness in vitro porcine skin both at baseline and after physical and chemical barrier disruption in multiple different experiments. These experiments aimed to further investigate the relationship between TEWL and ^3H_2O flux using the AquaFlux Evaporimeter (Bio Systems Ltd, USA) and to evaluate the use of porcine skin in vitro as a model to study the human skin barrier.

The first experiment investigated the relationship between baseline TEWL rates and ^3H_2O flux in in vitro healthy, full-thickness porcine skin. The results showed that baseline TEWL values were linearly correlated with baseline ^3H_2O flux values ($r^2 = 0.80$, $n = 63$). The second experiment examined the effect of physical barrier disruption with skin punctures on TEWL measurements. The results did not show a correlation between skin punctures and TEWL measurements. TEWL increased significantly after the first skin puncture and then remained constant for punctures 2, 3, and 4. Another large increase in TEWL was seen with the fifth puncture. However, no changes in TEWL values were seen with the sixth or seventh puncture, suggesting a threshold may have been reached after the fifth puncture. The third and fourth experiments examined TEWL changes after chemical barrier disruption with surfactants. In the third experiment, anionic surfactants of differing alkyl chain lengths were applied to the full-thickness porcine skin in vitro to determine if measuring TEWL values could discern between mild perturbations to the barrier function and severe damage. TEWL was largely unaffected following cutaneous exposure to short and long alkyl chain surfactants; however, it was significantly elevated over control levels following exposure to those with intermediate chain lengths. Exposure to sodium lauryl sulfate (SLS), with an intermediate

12-carbon alkyl chain, produced the greatest increase in TEWL. In the fourth experiment, the effect of varying SLS concentration, volume, and contact time on TEWL in vitro in porcine skin was measured. The results showed a linear trend between TEWL and SLS concentration in the 0% to 1% weight/volume (w/v) concentration range. However, following treatment with 5% w/v SLS, TEWL readings were only slightly higher than those following treatment with 1% w/v surfactant. A linear correlation was also demonstrated between TEWL and surfactant solution volume ($r^2 = 0.87$), which was statistically significant ($p < 0.01$). TEWL also increased as a function of increasing SLS treatment time, when concentration was fixed at 1% w/v and volume fixed at 200 µL. To summarize, Elmahjoubi et al. (2009) found that baseline TEWL values correlated with the percutaneous absorption of ^3H_2O in vitro in healthy porcine skin, and the TEWL measurements linearly correlated with the exposure of porcine skin in vitro to increasing concentrations, time, and volumes of SLS. TEWL measurements did not demonstrate a linear correlation between skin punctures (i.e., skin damage) and TEWL. The authors feel that TEWL measurements in vitro in porcine skin may serve as a model for future studies in this area, in contrast to the previous findings by Chilcott et al. (2002).

8.3 DISCUSSION OF THE ASSUMPTIONS MADE BY THE STUDIES INVESTIGATING THE CORRELATION BETWEEN TEWL AND PERCUTANEOUS ABSORPTION

Many of the experiments investigating TEWL and percutaneous absorption make large assumptions that could affect the results and hence be a source of controversy. For example, Tsai et al. (2001) and Chilcott et al. (2002) assume that in vitro measurements of TEWL and percutaneous absorption are equivalent to in vivo measurements, and Lamaud et al. (1984) assume that animal skin may serve as a permeability model for human skin. Great sources of error and variation can also be induced depending on the measurement device used to record TEWL rates and the choice of the compound and/or method used to measure percutaneous absorption rates. Because we do not completely understand the qualitative relationship between TEWL and percutaneous absorption, it is difficult to establish which assumptions made during the experiment could be affecting the correlation results. The next section investigates various causes that could influence the results of the correlation experiments. Provided in Table 8.2 is a summary of the major assumptions from 12 studies discussed in this chapter.

8.3.1 USING IN VITRO METHODS TO MODEL IN VIVO EXPERIMENTS

Skin permeation can be measured in vivo or in vitro by using excised skin in diffusion cells. In theory, studies using in vitro or ex vivo are feasible models for in vivo experiments because passage through the skin is a passive diffusion process and the SC is nonliving tissue. Many studies comparing in vivo and in vitro TEWL and percutaneous absorption measurements have been conducted, and the results from those experiments support the contention that reliable measurements can be obtained from in vitro studies (Bronaugh et al. 1982a; Duracher et al. 2015; Elkeeb et al. 2010; Elmahjoubi et al. 2009; Hui et al. 2012; Nangia et al. 1993; Noonan et al. 1990). While the consensus is that in vitro experiments are reasonable models for in vivo human experiments, some experiments note significant differences between these methods for measuring skin permeation. The most significant study by Bronaugh and Stewart (1985) found that the effects of UV irradiation could not be duplicated using an in vitro experimentation model, hence suggesting that in vitro experiments examining the TEWL and percutaneous absorption after barrier damage may not be an acceptable model for correlation with in vivo studies. In vitro damage to the SC barrier may not be an accurate model to in vivo SC damage because in vivo exposure to skin irritants result in a cascade of reactions that do not occur in vitro in human cadaver skin (Nangia et al. 1993).

Chilcott et al. (2002) investigated the correlation between TEWL and percutaneous absorption in vitro after inducing different types of barrier damage. This was one of the rare studies that did not

TABLE 8.2

A Summary of the Major Assumptions Made by the Studies Discussed in this Review

Reference	In Vivo versus In Vitro (Percutaneous Absorption)[c]	Skin Type	Percutaneous Absorption Measurement Method	Compound[b]	Healthy Skin versus Damaged Skin	Correlation Results
Duracher et al. 2015	Both	Human	Diffusion Cell	Hydrophilic	Healthy	Yes
Lamaud et al. 1984	in vivo	Animal	Urinary	Lipophilic	Both	Yes
Lavrijsen et al. 1993	in vivo	Human	LDF	Lipophilic	Damaged	Yes
Rougier et al. 1988	in vivo	Human	Urinary	Lipophilic	Healthy	Yes
Lotte et al. 1987	in vivo	Human	Urinary	Hydrophilic and Lipophilic	Healthy	Yes
Aalto-Korte and Turpeinen 1993	in vivo	Human	Plasma Cortisol Level	Lipophilic	Damaged	Yes
Tsai et al. 2001[a]	in vitro	Animal	Diffusion Cell	Hydrophilic and Lipophilic	Damaged	Yes
Tsai et al. 2001[a]	in vitro	Animal	Diffusion Cell	Highly Lipophilic	Damaged	No
Chilcott et al. 2002	in vitro	Both	Diffusion Cell	Hydrophilic and Lipophilic	Both	No
Elkeeb et al. 2010	in vitro	Human	Diffusion Cell	Hydrophilic	Healthy	Yes
Hui et al. 2012	in vitro	Human	Diffusion Cell	Hydrophilic and Lipophilic	Healthy	Yes
Atrux-Tallau et al. 2007	ex vivo	Human	Diffusion Cell	Hydrophilic	Healthy	Yes
Elmahjoubi et al. 2009	in vitro	Animal	Diffusion Cell	Hydrophilic	Both	Yes
Oestmann et al. 1993	in vivo	Human	LDF	Lipophilic	Healthy	Yes

Source: Aalto-Korte et al. 1987; Atrux-Tallau et al. 2007; Chilcott et al. 2002; Elkeeb et al. 2010; Elmahjoubi et al. 2009; Hui et al. 2012; Lamaud et al. 1984; Lavrijsen et al. 1993; Lotte et al. 1987; Nilsson et al. 1997; Oestmann et al. 1993; Rougier et al. 1998; Tsai et al. 2001.

[a] Reference Tsai et al. was divided into two experiments in this table since the study found a correlation between TEWL and percutaneous absorption with some compounds and no correlation with others.

[b] Compounds were classified by their octanol-water partition coefficient, log $K_{octanol/water}$ (Table 8.1). Compounds possessing log $K_{octanol/water}$ values less than 1 are considered hydrophilic, while compounds with log $K_{octanol/water}$ higher than 3 were considered very lipophilic.

[c] TEWL in vivo and in vitro measurements are considered equivalent. We are only concerned with how percutaneous absorption measurements were performed.

observe a correlation between TEWL and percutaneous absorption after barrier damage. It is possible that in vitro methodology in the experimental design may be responsible for the lack of correlation of TEWL to skin damage reported in this study. However, Fluhr et al. (2006) suggest that the conditions used in the study of Chilcott et al. (2002), i.e., the use of heat-split human epidermis and nonpigmented pig skin that had been stored for up to 14 days and penetration studies that extended over 96 hours post-heat separation, likely contributed to their results. Fluhr et al. (2006) state that the extracellular lipid matrix and corneocytes of the SC were potentially compromised from heat separation. In one study, it was found that heating the skin increases the rate of percutaneous absorption of water (Blattner et al. 2014). However, it is this author's opinion that even if the barrier was compromised by heat separation, these changes in barrier function should have been reflected both in the TEWL and percutaneous absorption, and hence should have correlated if both measured variables truly reflect skin barrier function.

In a paper by Günther et al. (2020), the aim was to uncover the degree to which measurements of skin permeation in vitro can be used to predict corresponding permeation in vivo for human pharmacokinetics of dermally applied substances. This was done by using the lipophilic nonsteroidal selective glucocorticoid receptor agonist, BAY1003803, to make the comparison. The neutral drug compound BAY1003803 is almost insoluble in water and has a calculated log P octanol/water of 3.3. [^{14}C]-BAY1003803 was made in several preparations: ointment, hydrophilic cream, lipophilic cream, and milk (thin lotion) for topical application to human skin. For the in vitro skin penetration experiment, full-thickness human skin samples (abdomen, breast, and/or back) were taken from six donors (male and female) aged 30 to 51 years, from St. John's Hospital in the United Kingdom. To measure its permeation in healthy human skin in vitro, static diffusion cells were employed.

Subsequently, percutaneous absorption and dermal delivery were determined for the two selected formulations in vivo in healthy volunteers. It was determined that the absorption in vivo associating ointment and lipophilic cream was correlated with the authors' expectation based on the dermal delivery obtained in vitro. The ointment formulation reached a 2.17-fold higher systemic exposure to BAY1003803. This is in agreement with the 2.74 predicted exposure difference based on in vitro data. It follows, then, that in vitro skin absorption studies using human skin are appropriate for the projection of systemic exposure and preparation effects in vivo. Further, they can be useful to aid in the design of clinical studies of dermatological formulations (Günther et al. 2020).

Since Chilcott and colleagues' original publication in 2002, several studies demonstrating the correlation between TEWL and percutaneous absorption have been conducted in in vitro models (Elkeeb et al. 2010; Elmahjoubi et al. 2009; Hui et al. 2012), and it is more likely that the results of Chilcott et al. (2002) were an exception rather than the rule.

8.3.2 USING ANIMAL SKIN TO MODEL HUMAN SKIN

Comparing the skin morphology and absorption of chemicals through human versus animal skin, it is clear that human skin is unique in both morphology and absorption (Bronaugh and Franz, 1986). An experiment by Bronaugh et al. (1982b) found that depending on the compound and the vehicle used, permeability values obtained using animal skin are well within an order of magnitude of the permeability values for human skin.

Independently, in vitro and animal skin models might not be reliable models to predict percutaneous absorption in human skin in vivo. Rougier et al. (1987b) documented a distinct difference between animal studies performed in vivo versus animal studies performed in vitro when compared to the absorption of compounds through human skin in vivo. This experiment compared the permeability of human skin to hairless rat (Walker et al. 1983) and hairless mouse skin (Bronaugh and Stewart 1986) using molecules of widely different physicochemical properties. The results show that in animal or human skin in vivo, for whatever molecule tested, the permeability ratios remained relatively constant, whereas in vitro, the same does not hold. When application conditions are strictly identical in humans and animals, it may be possible to predict percutaneous absorption in human skin in vivo by measuring in vivo absorption through animal skin, but not using in vitro animal absorption. The inaccurate results obtained when conducting experiments in vitro using animal skin may have affected the results studied by Tsai et al. (2001) and Chilcott et al. (2002), which were the only two studies using in vitro animal skin and showing no correlation between TEWL and percutaneous absorption.

Nevertheless, Lamaud et al. (1984) conducted their study in porcine skin in vivo and Elmahjoubi et al. (2009) conducted their study in porcine skin in vitro, and both found a correlation between TEWL and percutaneous absorption. This suggests that factors other than using the animal in vitro model may have played a role in the lack of correlation found in studies by Tsai et al. (2001) and Chilcott et al. (2002). However, there is no doubt that there are distinct differences between animal skin and human skin when used as a model for human absorption. Whether these differences are large enough to invalidate the use of animal skin as a model for experimentation is less likely. Further research on this topic will be pertinent to clarify this issue.

8.3.3 DIFFERENCES IN TEWL MEASUREMENT METHODS

TEWL meters or evaporimeters can have an open- or closed-chamber system. Open-chamber TEWL meters are open to the environment, and therefore their measurements are influenced by environmental factors such as room temperature and/or humidity. Closed-chamber devices are closed systems that are not dependent on environmental variables. With adequate control of environmental variables, open-chamber TEWL meters can provide reliable and reproducible measurements that are comparable to closed-chamber TEWL meters (Elkeeb et al. 2010; Fluhr et al. 2006; Pinnagoda et al. 1989, 1990). Yet only a limited number of comparisons between different types of TEWL meters have been described in the literature until the last few years, and TEWL meters are known to differ in their measurement range, speed, repeatability, and reproducibility (Hui et al. 2012).

Elkeeb et al. (2010) and Fluhr et al. (2006) performed studies that exemplified the general comparability of TEWL meters but also demonstrated their differences. As mentioned in the previous section, Elkeeb et al. (2010) compared TEWL to the percutaneous absorption/flux rate of ^3H_2O in in vitro human cadaver skin using three different evaporimeters: one open-chamber evaporimeter A (TEWameter TM 210, Courage and Khazaka, Cologne, Germany; Acaderm, Inc., Menlo Park, CA, USA) and two closed-chamber evaporimeters B (VapoMeter, Delfin Technologies, Kuopio, Finland), and C (AquaFlux AF200, Biox Systems, Ltd, London, UK). TEWL values correlated at baseline and over the 24-hour experiment for evaporimeters A and C. However, TEWL values of evaporimeter B only correlated with evaporimeters A and C during the experiment and did not correlate at baseline.

An experiment by Fluhr et al. (2006) compared many different TEWL meters in vivo in human and murine skin and ex vivo in murine skin. TEWL rates obtained with two closed-chamber systems (VapoMeter, Delfin Technologies, Kuopio, Finland) and H4300 (NIKKISO YSI CO., Ltd, Tokyo, Japan) and one closed-loop system (MEECO; MEECO, Warrington, PA, USA) under different experimental in vivo conditions were compared with data from four open-loop instruments, i.e., TEWameter TM 210, TEWameter TM 300, (Courgae and Khazaka, Cologne, Germany), DermaLab (Cortex Technology, Hadsund, Denmark), and EP 1 (ServoMED, Stockholm Sweden). Through these experiments, Fluhr et al. demonstrated the ability of most of the TEWL meters to detect minor, moderate, and severe changes in barrier dysfunction. None of the devices could detect minor improvements in barrier function, and there were differences in the TEWL meters ability to detect differences between severe versus very severe barrier dysfunction. Still, analysis of all the data collected demonstrated a weak correlation between a few TEWL meters but an overall good correlation among all of the TEWL meters.

An additional study by Farahmond et al. (2009) found similar results to Fluhr et al. (2006) when studying the differences between two closed-chamber TEWL measurement instruments. These instruments were designed based on different measurement principles and demonstrated slight differences in their ability to detect changes in skin barrier function despite that the values of all three instruments correlated well with each other ($p < 0.001$).

One more recent paper by Alexander et al. (2018) described the utility in each of several TEWL devices (open chamber, unventilated chamber, condenser chamber). Open-chamber devices have been discussed earlier in this chapter, but the unventilated-chamber and condenser-chamber have not, and will now be briefly mentioned. Unventilated chambers consist of a chamber with a closed upper end to protect from ambient air movement disturbances. The more recently developed condenser chamber has become more often used, as it provides a dynamic reading of TEWL (Alexander et al. 2018; Imhof et al. 2009). A small comparative study of an open-chamber device with an unventilated-chamber and condenser-chamber system found that the condenser-chamber device was the only one to detect the effect of tape stripping on TEWL and the only one able to distinguish between the effects of moisturizers versus petrolatum on skin barrier integrity (Farahmand et al. 2009). This finding thereby suggests that the condenser-chamber method provides greater sensitivity (Alexander et al. 2018).

The studies by Elkeeb et al. (2010), Fluhr et al. (2006), Farahmond et al. (2009), and Alexander et al. (2018) reveal that there are potential limitations to TEWL meters in experimentation and the TEWL meter must be chosen carefully based on the proposed study design. In general, TEWL meters produced comparable and reliable results; however, in the Elkeeb et al. (2010), Fluhr et al. (2006), and Alexander et al. (2018) studies, there were reported TEWL measurements that did not significantly correlate with other measurements. These variations in measurement have the potential to influence experimentation.

8.3.4 INFLUENCES OF PERCUTANEOUS ABSORPTION MEASUREMENT METHODS

The major factor affecting percutaneous absorption measurements is the methodology used (Bronaugh 1989; Wester and Maibach 1992). Methods used for percutaneous absorption measurements are not equal and thus can and do give different results. Table 8.2 (column 3) summarizes the percutaneous absorption measurement methodologies used in these correlation studies.

The most common method for determining percutaneous absorption in vivo is measuring the radioactivity of excreta following the topical application of a labeled compound. Determination of percutaneous absorption from urinary radioactivity does not account for metabolism by skin but has been proven to be a reliable method for absorption measurements and is widely accepted as the "gold standard" when available.

The most commonly used in vitro technique involves placing excised skin in a diffusion chamber, applying the radioactive compound to one side of the skin (the epidermal side), and then assaying the radioactivity in the collection vessel on the other side of the skin (Bronaugh and Maibach 1991). The advantages of using this in vitro technique are that the method is easy to use and that the results are obtained quickly. The disadvantage is that the fluid in the collection bath, which bathes the skin, is saline. This may be appropriate for studying hydrophilic compounds but is not suitable for hydrophobic compounds. If the parent compound is not adequately soluble in water, then determining in vitro permeation into a water receptor fluid will be self-limiting.

When conducting in vitro experiments, animal skin often substitutes human skin. As animal skin has different permeability characteristics than human skin, one should be careful about which type of animal skin is used (see the section on animal vs. human skin). In addition, proper care should be taken in skin preparation of excised skin to not damage the skin barrier integrity. Anatomical site is also important, since skin from different sites shows different permeability, as well as using many different donor skin samples.

The only two experiments that did not find a correlation between TEWL and percutaneous absorption, Tsai et al. (2001) and Chilcott et al. (2002), were experiments that measured percutaneous absorption in vitro. Perhaps using a diffusion cell to measure percutaneous absorption is the reason for not finding a correlation.

Oestmann et al. (1993) and Lavrijsen et al. (1993) used LDF to measure HN penetration. LDF measures the increase in CBF caused by the penetration of HN, a vasoactive substance. One problem with this method is that LDF measurements are not only dependent on the amount of HN absorbed but also on the individual's vasoreactivity, sex, and age. This may be the reason why Oestmann et al. (1993) and Lavrijsen et al. (1993) obtained only a weak correlation between TEWL and percutaneous absorption of HN. Another disadvantage of this method is that LDF measurements have many sources of variation, which make it difficult to compare interlaboratory results.

8.3.5 INFLUENCE OF THE LIPOPHILICITY OR HYDROPHILICITY OF THE COMPOUND STUDIED IN TEWL MEASUREMENT METHODS

The percutaneous absorption rate and/or total absorption of a compound varies greatly depending on the compound and its lipophilicity. Yet many of the papers reviewed did not consider how lipophilicity of the test compound would affect percutaneous absorption and hence affect the correlation between

TEWL and percutaneous absorption. Feldmann and Maibach (1970) measured both the total absorption and maximal absorption rate for 20 diverse compounds of different lipophilicities. The range for total absorption of the 20 compounds tested demonstrated a difference greater than 250 times in total absorption amounts, while the 20 compounds had a difference in maximum absorption rate greater than 1000-fold (Feldmann et al. 1970). Because of the wide range of absorption for topically applied compounds, it seems reasonable to assume that the correlation between TEWL and percutaneous absorption is not independent of the physicochemical properties of the compound applied. TEWL measurements should predict the skin's barrier permeability changes to hydrophilic compounds.

A correlation between TEWL and percutaneous absorption was found in many studies, such as Oestmann et al. (1993), Lamaud et al. (1984), Lavrijsen et al. (1993), Lotte et al. (1987), Aalto-Korte and Turpeinen (1993), Tsai et al. (2001), Elkeeb et al. (2010), Elmahjoubi et al. (2009), Hui (2012), and Atrux-Tallau et al. (2007), which suggests that TEWL can predict the changes in skin permeability to topically applied hydrophilic and lipophilic drugs. However, Tsai et al. (2001) found that the percutaneous absorption of the highly lipophilic progesterone and estradiol did not correlate with TEWL.

Referring back to Table 8.1, the most common lipophilicity scale of molecules is defined by the octanol/water partition coefficient ($K_{oct/w}$= log [$P_{oct/w}$]). Presented in Table 8.1 are the compounds used in the aforementioned studies, their octanol/water partition coefficient, their solubility classification, and whether or not their percutaneous absorption correlated with TEWL. Looking closely at Table 8.1, the highly lipophilic compounds were the compounds that demonstrated a weaker correlation or no evidence of a correlation between percutaneous absorption and TEWL, while the moderately lipophilic compounds such as hydrocortisone and BA and the hydrophilic compounds did show a correlation. This should be further investigated. As stated previously, it may be necessary to use both TEWL and drug lipophilicity to predict alterations in skin permeability.

8.4 CONCLUSION

In an earlier version of this chapter (2005), Levin and Maibach reviewed nine studies investigating the correlation between TEWL and percutaneous absorption of various compounds. At that time, seven of the nine studies demonstrated a quantitative correlation, while two studies did not. The studies that did not confirm a quantitative correlation (Chilcott et al. 2002; Tsai et al. 2001) or observed a weak correlation (Hui et al. 2012; Lavrijsen et al. 1993; Oestmann et al. 1993) used different experimental methods. We conclude that those assumptions and differences in experimental design were likely responsible for the observed lack of correlation. Since then, new studies have been published investigating the use of lipophilic compounds, in vitro models, and animal skin as models for the in vivo human skin barrier (Elkeeb et al. 2010; Elmahjoubi et al. 2009; Hui et al. 2012). In this updated chapter, 12 of the 14 studies discussed here found some degree of correlation between TEWL and percutaneous absorption. Nonetheless, in observation of Table 8.1, it seems probable that TEWL can serve as a correlate for percutaneous absorption in both in vivo and in vitro models in human and animal skin. Also, selection of the type of evaporimeter device used likely does have an even more substantial role in experimental design than was previously assumed.

For this field of research to have more informative and rigorous results in the future, larger sample sizes of comparable tests must be conducted under multiple experimental and control conditions. It is expected that these expanded studies will yield more robust statistical results. Taken together, the weight of evidence suggests a relationship between TEWL and percutaneous penetration of various compounds, yet much remains to be understood.

REFERENCES

Aalto-Korte K, and Turpeinen M. 1993. Transepidermal water loss and absorption of hydrocortisone in widespread dermatitis. Br J Dermatol 128: 663–635.
Alexander H, Brown S, Danby S, and Flohr C. 2018. Research techniques made simple: transepidermal water loss measurement as a research tool. J Invest Dermatol 138:2295–3000.

Arimoto H, Yanai M, and Egawa M. 2016. Analysis of absorption and spreading of moisturizer on the microscopic region of the skin surface with near-infrared imaging. Skin Res Technol 22:505–512.

Atrux-Tallau N, Pirot F, Falson F, Roberts MS, and Maibach HI. 2007. Qualitative and quantitative comparison of heat separated epidermis and dermatomed skin in percutaneous absorption studies. Dermatol Res 299(10):507–511.

Blattner CM, Coman G, Blickenstaff NR, and Maibach HI. 2014. Percutaneous absorption of water in skin: a review. Rev Environ Health. 29:175–180.

Boer M, Duchnik E, Maleszka R, and Marchlewicz M. 2016. Structural and biophysical characteristics of human skin in maintaining proper epidermal barrier function. Postepy Dermatol Alergol 33:1–5.

Bronaugh RL, and Franz RJ. 1986. Vehicle effects on percutaneous absorption: in vivo and in vitro comparisons with human skin. Br J Dermatol 115:1–11.

Bronaugh RL, and Maibach HI. 1989. Percutaneous Absorption, 2nd ed. (New York: Marcel Dekker).

Bronaugh RL, and Maibach HI 1991. In Vitro Percutaneous Absorption. (Boca Raton: CRC Press).

Bronaugh RL, and Stewart RF. 1983. Methods for in vitro percutaneous absorption studies III: hydrophobic compounds. J Pharm Sci 73:1255–1258.

Bronaugh RL, and Stewart RF. 1985. Methods for in vitro percutaneous absorption studies V: Permeation through damaged skin. J Pharm Sci 74:1062–1066.

Bronaugh RL, and Stewart RF. 1986. Methods for in vitro percutaneous absorption studies VI: preparation of the barrier layer. J Pharm Sci 75:487–491.

Bronaugh RL, Stewart RF, and Congdon ER. 1982b. Methods for in vitro percutaneous absorption studies II. Animal models for human skin. Toxicol Applied Pharm 62:481–488.

Bronaugh RL, Stewart RF, Congdon ER, and Giles Jr AL. 1982a. Methods for in vitro percutaneous absorption studies I. Comparison with the in vivo results. Toxicol Applied Pharm 62:474–480.

Chilcott RP, Dalton CH, Emmanuel AJ, Allen CE, and Bradley ST. 2002. Transepidermal water loss does not correlate with skin barrier function in vitro. J Invest Dermatol 118(5):871–875.

Dupuis D, Rougier A, Roguet R, Lotte, C and Kalopissis, G. 1984. In vivo relationship between horny layer reservoir effect and percutaneous absorption in human and rat. J Invest Dermatol 82:353–356.

Duracher L, Visdal-Johnsen L, and Mavon A. 2015. In vitro and in vivo dermal absorption assessment of acetyl aspartic acid: a compartmental study. Int J Cosmet Sci 37(Suppl 1):34–40.

Elkeeb R, Hui X, Chan H, Tian L, and Maibach HI. 2010. Correlation of transepidermal water loss with skin barrier properties in vitro: comparison of three evaporimeters. Skin Res Technol 16(1):9–15.

Elmahjoubi E, Frum Y, Eccleston GM, Wilkinson SC, and Meidan VM. 2009. Transepidermal water loss for probing full-thickness skin barrier function: correlation with tritiated water flux, sensitivity to punctures and diverse surfactant exposures. In Vitro 23(7):1429–1435.

Farahmand S, Tien L, Hui X, and Maibach HI. 2009. Measuring transepidermal water loss: a comparative in vivo study of condenser-chamber, unventilated-chamber and open-chamber systems. Skin Res Technol 15(4):392–398.

Feldmann RJ, and Maibach HI.1970. Absorption of some organic compounds through the skin in man. J Invest Dermatol 54:399–404.

Fluhr JW, Feingold KR, and Elias PM. 2006. Transepidermal water loss reflects permeability barrier status: validation in human and rodent in vivo and ex vivo models. Exp Dermatol 15(7):483–492.

Franz TJ. 1978. The finite dose technique as a valid in vitro model for the study of percutaneous absorption in man. Curr Probl Dermatol 7:58–68.

Günther C, Kowal K, Schmidt T, Jambrecina A, Toner F, and Nave R. 2020. Comparison of in vitro and in vivo percutaneous absorption across human skin using BAY1003803 formulated as ointment and cream. Clin Pharmacol Drug Dev 9:582–592.

Guth K, Schafer-Korting M, Fabian E, Landsiedel R, and van Ravenzwaay B. 2015. Suitability of skin integrity tests for dermal absorption studies in vitro. Toxicol In Vitro, 29: 113–23.

Hui X, Elkeeb R, Chan H, and Maibach HI. 2012. Ability to estimate relative percutaneous penetration via a surrogate maker - trans epidermal water loss? Skin Res Technol 18(1):108–113.

Imhof RE, De Jesus ME, Xiao P, Ciortea LI, and Berg EP. 2009. Closed-chamber Transepidermal Water Loss Measurement: Microclimate, Calibration and Performance. International Journal of Cosmetic Science 31.2: 97–118.

Lamaud E, Lambrey B, Schalla W, and Schaefer H. 1984. Correlation between transepidermal water loss and penetration of drugs. J Invest Dermatol 82:556.

Lavrijsen AP, Oestmann E, Hermans J, Bodde HE, Vermeer BJ, and Ponec M. 1993. Barrier function parameters in various keratinization disorders: transepidermal water loss and vascular response to hexyl nicotinate. Br J Dermatol 129:547–554.

Le Fur I, Reinberg A, Lopez S, Morizot F, Mechkouri M, and Tschachler E. 2001. Analysis of Circadian and Ultradian Rhythms of Skin Surface Properties of Face and Forearm of Healthy Women. J Invest Dermatol 117.3: 718–24.

Leveque JL, Corcuff P, de Rigal J, and Agache P, 1984. In vivo studies of the evolution of physical properties of the human skin with age. Int J Dermatol 23:322–329.

Levin J and Maibach HI. 2005. The correlation between transepidermal water loss and percutaneous absorption: an overview. J Control Release 103(2): 291–299.

Liu Z, Fluhr JW, Song SP, Sun Z, Wang H, Shi YJ, Elias PM, Man MQ. 2010. Sun-induced changes in stratum corneum function are gender and dose dependent in a Chinese population. Skin Pharmacol Physiol. 23(6): 313–319.

Lotte C, Rougier A, Wilson DR, and Maibach HI. 1987. In vivo relationship between transepidermal water loss and percutaneous penetration of some organic compounds in man: effect of anatomic site. Arch Dermatol Res 279: 351–356.

Machado M, Hadgraft H, and Lane ME. 2010. Assessment of the variation of skin barrier function with anatomic site, age, gender and ethnicity. Int J Cosmet Sci 32:397–409.

Van Der Molen, RG, et al. 1997. Tape stripping of human stratum corneum yields cell layers that originate from various depths because of furrows in the skin. Arch Dermatol Res 289(9): 514–518.

Nangia A, Camel E, Berner B, and Maibach HI. 1993. Influence of skin irritants in percutaneous absorption. Pharm Res 10: 1756–1759.

Nilsson GE. 1997. Measurement of water exchange through skin. Med Biol Eng Comput 15: 209–218.

Noonan P and Gonzalez M 1990. Pharmacokinetics and the variability of percutaneous absorption. J Toxicol 9(2):511–516.

Oestmann E, Lavrijsen AP, Hermans J, and Ponec M. 1993. Skin barrier function in healthy volunteers as assessed by transepidermal water loss and vascular response to hexyl nicotinate: intra- and inter- individual variability. Br J Dermatol 128: 130–136.

Pinnagoda J, Tupker RA, Agner T, and Serup J. 1990. Guidelines for transepidermal water loss (TEWL) measurement. Contact Derm 22:164–178.

Pinnagoda J, Tupker R, Coenraads PJ, and Nater JP. 1989. Comparability and reproducibility of the results of water loss measurements: a study of 4 evaporimeters. Contact Derm 20:241–246.

Roskos RV and Guy RH. 1989. Assessment of skin barrier function using transepidermal water loss: effect of age. Pharm Res 6(11):949–953.

Rougier A, Dupuis D, Lotte C, Roguet R, and Schaefer H. 1983. In vivo correlation between stratum corneum reservoir function and percutaneous absorption. J Invest Dermatol 81:275–278.

Rougier A, Dupuis D, Lotte C, and Roguet R. 1985. The measurement of the stratum corneum reservoir. A predictive method for in vivo percutaneous absorption studies: Influence of application time. J Invest Dermatol 84:66–68.

Rougier A, Lotte C, Corcuff P, and Maibach HI. 1988. Relationship between skin permeability and corneocyte size according to anatomic site, age and sex in man. J Soc Cosmet Chem 39:15–26.

Rougier A, Lotte C, and Maibach HI. 1987a. In vivo percutaneous penetration of some organic compounds related to anatomic site in man: Predictive assessment by the stripping method. J Pharm Sci 76:451–454.

Rougier A, Lotte C, Maibach HI. 1987b. The hairless rat: a relevant model to predict in vivo percutaneous absorption in humans? J Invest Dermatol 88:577–581.

Tsai JC, Sheu HM, Hung PL, and Cheng CL. 2001. Effect of barrier disruption by acetone treatment on the permeability of compounds with various lipophilicities: implications for the permeability of compromised skin. J Pharm Sci 90:1242–1254.

Walker M, Dugard PH, and Scott RC. 1983. In vitro percutaneous absorption studies: a comparison of human and laboratory species. Hum Toxicol 2:561–565.

Wester RC and Maibach HI. 1992. Percutaneous absorption in diseased skin. In Maibach and Surber (eds.) Topical Corticosteroids, pp. 128–141 (Basel: Karger).

Wester RC and Maibach HI. 1993. Chair's summary: percutaneous absorption - in vitro and in vivo correlations. In Dermatology: Progress & Perspectives. The Proceedings of the 18th World Congress of Dermatology, pp. 1149–1151 (New York: The Parthenon Publishing Group).

Zhang, Q, Murawsky M, LaCount T, Kasting GB, and Li SK. 2018. Transepidermal water loss and skin conductance as barrier integrity tests. Toxicol In Vitro 51:129–135.

9 Human Percutaneous Absorption and Transepidermal Water Loss (TEWL) Correlation

Howard I. Maibach
University of California, San Francisco, California

CONTENTS

9.1 INTRODUCTION

Percutaneous absorption is defined as the rate and extent that a chemical is absorbed into and through the skin and into the systemic circulation. A major variable in percutaneous absorption is regional variation, where some body sites show extensive skin absorption, while the other sites show less absorption. Also, we are a world of individuals, and percutaneous absorption will vary by individual, as well as anatomic site. Where percutaneous absorption is the passage of chemicals from the outside environment into and through skin, transepidermal water loss (TEWL) is the passage of water in the other direction, from the body through the skin into the outside environment. The question is whether percutaneous absorption and TEWL correlate and are predictable of one another.

9.1.1 PERCUTANEOUS ABSORPTION

The first occupational disease in recorded history was scrotal cancer in chimney sweepers. The historical picture of a male worker holding a sweeper and covered from head to toe with black soot is vivid. But why the scrotum? Percutaneous absorption in man and animals varies depending on the area of the body in contact with a chemical. This is called regional variation. When a certain skin area is exposed, any effect of the chemical will be determined by how much is absorbed through the skin. Where systemic drug delivery is desired, such as transdermal delivery, a high-absorbing area may be desirable to deliver sufficient drug. Scopolamine transdermal systems are supposedly placed in the postauricular area (behind the ear) because at this skin site the percutaneous absorption of scopolamine is sufficiently enhanced to deliver effective quantities of the drug. A different example is with estimating human health hazard effects of environmental contaminants. This could be a chemical warfare agent on exposed parts of the skin (head, face, neck, and hands) and trying to determine the amount of chemical that might be absorbed into the body. The estimate for skin absorption is an integral part of the estimate for potential hazard; thus, accuracy of estimate is very relevant.

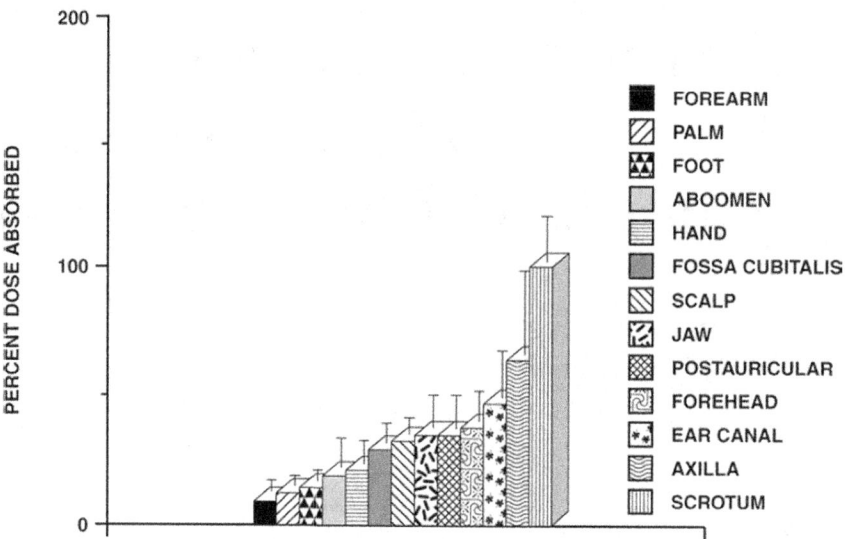

FIGURE 9.1 Anatomical regional variation with parathion percutaneous absorption.

9.1.2 REGIONAL VARIATION IN HUMANS

Feldmann and Maibach (1) were the first to systemically explore the potential for regional variation in percutaneous absorption. The first absorption studies were done with the ventral forearm because this site is convenient to use; however, skin exposure to chemicals exists over the entire body. They first showed regional variation with the absorption of parathion (Figure 9.1). The fact that the scrotum was the highest absorbing skin site (scrotal) cancer in chimney sweeps is the key. Among other body sites, skin absorption was lowest for the foot area and higher around the head and face area.

Data in Table 9.1 illustrate the influence of anatomical region on the percutaneous absorption of two common pesticides, parathion and malathion, in humans (2). There are two major points in this

TABLE 9.1

Effect of Anatomical Region on *In Vivo* Percutaneous Absorption of Hydrocortisone and Two Pesticides, Parathion and Malathion, in Humans *In Vivo*

	Dose Absorbed (%)		
Anatomical Region	Hydrocortisone	Parathion	Malathion
Forearm	1.0	8.6	6.8
Palm	0.8	11.6	5.8
Foot, ball	0.2	13.5	6.8
Abdomen	1.3	18.5	9.4
Hand, dorsum	—	21.0	12.5
Forehead	7.6	36.3	23.2
Axilla	3.1	64.0	28.7
Jaw angle	12.2	33.9	69.9
Fossal cubitalis	—	28.4	
Scalp	4.4	32.1	
Ear canal	—	46.6	
Scrotum	36.2	101.6	

TABLE 9.2
Site Variation and Decontamination Time for Parathion

Skin Residence Time Before Soap and Water Wash[a]	Parathion Dose Absorbed (%)[a]		
	Arm	Forehead	Palm
1 min	2.8	8.4	
5 min			6.2
15 min	6.7	7.1	13.6
30 min		12.2	13.3
1 hr	8.4	10.5	11.7
4 hr	8.0	27.7	7.7
24 hr	8.6	36.3	11.8

[a] Each time is a mean for four volunteers. The fact that there were different volunteers at each time point accounts for some of the variability with time for each skin site.

study. First, regional variation was confirmed with the different chemicals; note that parathion and malathion are chemically related to some chemical warfare agents. Second, those skin areas that would be exposed to the pesticides, the head and face, were of the higher-absorbing sites. The body areas most exposed to environmental contaminants are the areas with the higher skin absorption.

Table 9.2 gives site variability for parathion skin absorption with time. Soap and water wash in the first few minutes after exposure is not a perfect decontaminant. Site variation is apparent early in skin exposure (3).

Van Rooy et al. (4) applied coal tar ointment to various skin areas of volunteers and determined absorption of polycyclic aromatic hydrocarbons (PAH) by surface disappearance of PAH and the excretion of urinary I-OH pyrene. Using PAH disappearance, skin ranking (highest to lowest) was shoulder > forearm > forehead > groin > hand (palmar) > ankle. Using I-OH pyrene excretion, skin ranking (highest to lowest) was neck > calf > forearm > trunk > hand. Table 9.3 compares their results with Guy and Maibach (5).

TABLE 9.3
Absorption Indices of Hydrocortisone and Pesticides (Parathion/Malathion) Calculated by Guy and Maibach (5) Compared with Absorption of Pyrene and Polycyclic Aromatic Hydrocarbons (PAH) for Different Anatomical Sites by Van Rooy et al. (4)

Anatomical Site	Absorption			
	Hydrocortine	Pesticides	Pyrene	PAH
Genitals	40	12	—	—
Arms	1	1	1	1
Hand	1	1	0.8	0.5
Leg/ankle	0.5	1	1.2	0.8/0.5
Trunk/shoulder	2.5	3	1.1	/2.0
Head/neck	5	4	/1.3	1.0

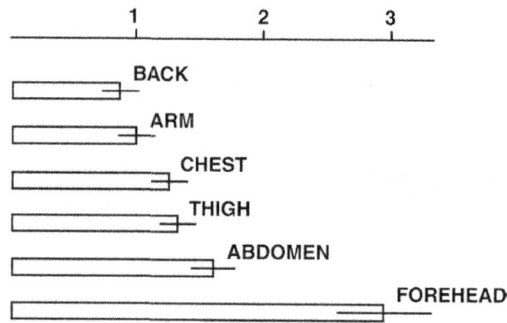

FIGURE 9.2 Relative permeability, ARM = 1.

Rougier et al. (6) examined the influence of anatomical site on the relationship between total penetration of benzoic acid in humans and the quantity present in the stratum corneum (SC) 30 minutes after application. Figure 9.2 shows total penetration of benzoic acid according to anatomical site. Figure 9.3 shows correlation between the level of penetration of benzoic acid within four days and its level in the SC after a 30-minute application relative to anatomical site.

Wertz et al. (7) determined regional variation in permeability through human and pig skin and oral mucosa. In the oral mucosa of both species, permeability ranked floor of mouth > buccal mucosa > palate. Skin remains a greater barrier, with absorption some tenfold less than oral mucosa.

The barrier properties of skin relative to the oral mucosa have been a benefit for longer-term transdermal delivery. Nitroglycerin buccal tablets are effective for about 20 minutes due to rapid buccal absorption. In contrast, transdermal nitroglycerin is prescribed for 24-hour, continuous-dose

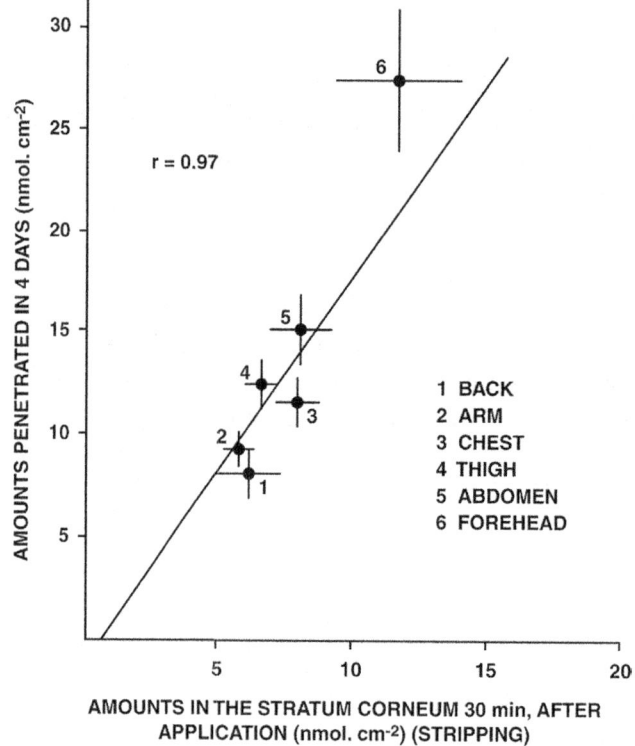

FIGURE 9.3 Human percutaneous absorption and transepidermal water loss.

TABLE 9.4
Site Variation in Transdermal Delivery

Transdermal	Body Site	Reason
Nitroglycerin	Chest	Psychological: the patch is placed over the heart
Scopolamine	Postauricular	Scientific: behind the ear was found to be the best absorbing area
Estradiol	Trunk	Convenience: easy to place and out of view
Testosterone	Scrotum	Scientific: highest skin-absorbing area
Testosterone	Trunk	Scientific/convenience: removal from trunk skin is easier than scrotal skin

delivery. The transdermal nitroglycerin patch is placed on the chest more for psychological reasons than that related to scientific regional variation skin absorption. Some transdermal systems take advantage of regional variations in skin absorption and some do not (Table 9.4).

Shriner and Maibach (8) studied skin contact irritation and showed that areas of significant response were neck > perioral > forehead. The volar forearm was the least sensitive of eight areas tested. This is in contrast to the commonly held belief that the forearm is one of the best locations to test for immediate contact irritation.

9.1.3   INDIVIDUAL VARIATION

It is well understood that chemical trials are designed with multiple volunteers to account for individual subject variation. This extends to *in vivo* percutaneous absorption where individual subject variability has been demonstrated. This subject variation also extends to *in vitro* human skin samples (9). Table 9.5 shows the in vitro percutaneous absorption of vitamin E acetate through human skin *in vitro*. Percent doses absorbed for two formulations, A and B, are shown for 24-hour receptor fluid accumulation and for skin content (skin digested and assayed at 24-hour time point). Assay of skin surface soap and water wash at the end of the 24-hour period gives dose accountability.

TABLE 9.5
***In Vitro* Percutaneous Absorption of Vitamin E Acetate into and through Human Skin**

	Percent Dose Absorbed		
	Receptor Fluid	Skin Content	Surface Wash
Formula A:			
Skin source 1	0.34	0.58	74.9
Skin source 2	0.39	0.66	75.6
Skin source 3	0.47	4.08	89.1
Skin source 4	1.30	0.96	110.0
Mean ± SD	0.63 ± 0.45[a]	1.56 ± 1.69[a]	87.4 ± 16.4
Formula B:			
Skin source 1	0.24	0.38	–
Skin source 2	0.40	0.64	107.1
Skin source 3	0.41	4.80	98.1
Skin source 4	2.09	1.16	106.2
Mean ± SD	0.78 ± 0.87[a]	1.74 ± 2.06[b]	103.8 ± 5.0

[a] $p = 0.53$ (nonsignificant; paired t-test).

The two formulations were the same except for slight variation in pH. Statistically, there was no difference in absorption between the two formulations. However, a careful examination of the individual values in Table 9.5 shows consistency within individuals. Analysis of variance (ANOVA) for individual variation showed statistical significance for receptor fluid ($p = 0.02$) and skin content ($p = 0.000$); therefore, when comparing treatments for *in vitro* percutaneous absorption, it is recommended that each treatment be a part of each skin source.

9.2 TRANSEPIDERMAL WATER LOSS

Water comprises about 60% of adult human body weight. The body obtains water from the intake of foods and fluids and leaves the body visibly via urine, sweat, and feces. Additionally, the body loses water continuously by evaporation from the respiratory passages and skin surface—termed insensible water loss, since we do not feel that we are actually losing water all the time. The amount of water that is leaving the body at rest is about 700 mL/day at an ambient temperature of 20°C (10, 11). The average water loss by diffusion through the skin is 300 to 400 mL/day, even in a person who is born without sweat glands (11) or whose sweat glands are inactivated (12). In other words, the water molecules themselves actually diffuse across the skin (11). This invisible natural process of water diffusion is called TEWL (10).

The TEWL has been related to the skin barrier function by a series of investigations. For instance, studies in the past have established that washing the skin surface with fat solvents did not increase the rate of water loss, but light sandpapering of the skin surface (13) or tape stripping of the whole SC (14, 15) resulted in increased TEWL. As the permeation rate of water across full-thickness skin, epidermis, or SC turned out to be approximately the same, it was realized that SC acts as the principal barrier to TEWL (16). Furthermore, a high rate of TEWL has been detected by patients with SC disorders, like psoriasis or ichthyosis (17). The TEWL is therefore taken as a measure of the skin barrier integrity, which mainly resides in the SC.

Anatomical skin site is an important variable with respect to baseline TEWL, which can be ranked from the highest to the lowest values: palm > sole > forehead = postauricular skin = dorsum of hand > forearm = upper arm = thigh = chest = abdomen = back (18). It can actually be related to the SC thickness of the particular body regions (19). Studies of different areas of the forearms showed the differences between three sites: (1) the site close to the wrist showed the highest values in all cases; (2) the nearest elbow region showed a slightly higher value than the median site; and (3) the median site (20, 21). Statistically, only the wrist region differed significantly from the other sites. The fact that the sweat gland density and activity varied on the forearm increasing towards the wrist could be one, but not the only, explanation for the higher value of the wrist region (22). Another hypothesis is that the wrist region is more exposed to mechanical and atmospheric influences than the others and the SC there could be more easily and regularly irritated, leading to increased TEWL values (22). An emotional influence on the wrist region was also suggested to play a role.

9.2.1 CORRELATION OF PERCUTANEOUS ABSORPTION AND TEWL

Percutaneous absorption can be performed *in vivo* with human volunteers and animals. It can also be done *in vitro* with cadaver skin, human and animal, in a diffusion system. Percutaneous absorption is by passive diffusion only, from a higher concentration progressively to a lower concentration. The TEWL has a passive diffusion component where water from the body (high concentration) passes out through the skin to a lower concentration, the environment. This would be baseline TEWL. The TEWL also has an active component: the release of water through sweat glands for heat dissipation or nervous response. In *vivo* TEWL studies would contain both passive and active water transport; however, cadaver skin in *in vitro* studies would only have the passive transport.

TABLE 9.6

Percutaneous Absorption and Transepidermal Water Loss (TEWL) Values According to Anatomical Site

n	Anatomical Site	Amount in Urine After 24 Hours[a]	Total Amount Penetrated Within 4 Days[b]	TEWL[c]	Relative Permeability to Arm	
					Penetration	TEWL
Compound: benzoic acid sodium salt, vehicle A						
6	Arm (upper, outer)	3.02[d] (0.34)[e]	4.02 (0.45)	6.06 (0.36)	1	1
6	Abdomen	5.73 (0.54)	7.65 (0.72)	5.37 (0.46)	1.9	0.9
6	Postauricular	7.54 (0.62)	10.06 (0.82)	7.72 (0.64)	2.5	1.3
8	Forehead	9.31 (1.76)	12.32 (2.30)	12.29 (0.96)	3.1	2
Compound: caffeine, vehicle B						
7	Arm (upper, outer)	6.04 (0.92)	12.09 (1.84)	7.04 (0.95)	1	1
6	Abdomen	3.76 (0.67)	7.53 (1.34)	6.05 (0.43)	0.6	0.9
7	Postauricular	5.87 (0.52)	11.72 (1.05)	8.74 (0.62)	1	1.2
6	Forehead	11.17 (1.20)	23.35 (2.39)	12.77 (1.05)	1.9	1.8
Compound: benzoic acid, vehicle A						
8	Arm (upper, outer)	6.87 (0.75)	9.15 (1.01)	4.24 (0.35)	1	1
7	Abdomen	10.88 (1.23)	14.52 (1.64)	4.40 (0.51)	1.6	1
8	Postauricular	16.87 (3.85)	22.49 (5.14)	8.35 (0.41)	2.5	1.9
7	Forehead	20.10 (2.39)	26.80 (3.19)	10.34 (0.70)	2.9	2.4
Compound: acetylsalicylic acid, vehicle A						
7	Arm (upper, outer)	5.27 (0.18)	17.00 (0.37)	5.08 (0.79)	1	1
6	Abdomen	5.34 (1.03)	17.20 (3.35)	5.16 (0.43)	1	1
6	Postauricular	11.04 (2.50)	29.17 (5.37)	9.04 (0.84)	2.1	1.8
6	Forehead	10.89 (1.02)	35.14 (3.29)	11.22 (0.96)	2.1	2.2

[a] 24-hour urinary accumulation.

[b] Calculated from urinary excretion: (b) = (a)/0.75.

[c] Measured just before the application, expressed in $g/m^2/hr$.

[d] Expressed in $nmol/cm^2$.

[e] SD.

Abbreviations: vehicle A (ethyleneglycol/triton × 100) (90/10); vehicle B (ethyleneglycol/triton × 100) (90/10)/(H_2O)(50/50).

Lotte et al. (23) studied the relationship between the percutaneous penetration of four chemicals and TEWL *in vivo* in man as a function of anatomical site. The findings showed an appreciable difference in the permeability of the skin from one site to another with regard to both water loss and chemical penetration. In addition, independent of the physicochemical properties of the molecules administered, there was a linear relationship between TEWL and penetration. Table 9.6 gives the results for the four anatomical sites (arm, abdomen, postauricular, and forehead) and the four test chemicals (benzoic acid sodium salt, caffeine, benzoic acid, and acetylsalicylic acid). Figure 9.4 illustrates the correlation between percutaneous absorption and TEWL. Correlations ranged from *r* = 0.62 to 0.73, which are good for an *in vivo* human study. These data confirm both the importance of anatomical site in the degree of permeability of the cutaneous barrier and the utility of determination of TEWL and percutaneous absorption in the evaluation of its functional condition.

Aalto-Karte and Turpeinen (24) studied *in vivo* percutaneous absorption of hydrocortisone in three children and six adults with widespread dermatitis after the application of 1% hydrocortisone cream. Before application of the cream, the TEWL was measured in six skin areas. A highly significant correlation was found between the post-application rise in plasma cortisol level and the

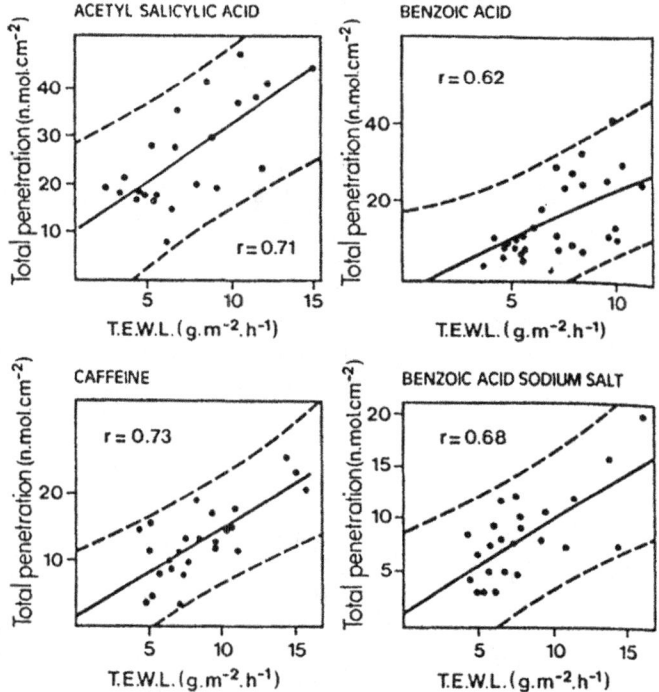

FIGURE 9.4 *In vivo* relationship between transepidermal water loss (TEWL) and percutaneous absorption of different compounds according to the anatomical site in man.

mean TEWL. Figure 9.5 shows the relationship where the correlation coefficient *r* was a significant ($p < 0.001$) 0.991.

The TEWL and percutaneous absorption can also be correlated using *in vitro* diffusion systems. This removes the influence of active water production (sweaty palms), but an *in vitro* system can have its own particular problems. Nangia et al. (25) demonstrated a linear correlation between tritiated water absorbed and TEWL for various sodium lauryl sulfate treatments and for various physical injuries applied to the excised skin (Figure 9.6). Chilcott et al. (26), on the other hand, found no correlation between basal TEWL rates and the permeability of human epidermal membranes to ^3H_2O ($p = 0.72$) or sulfur mustard ($p = 0.74$). Similarly, there was no correlation between TEWL

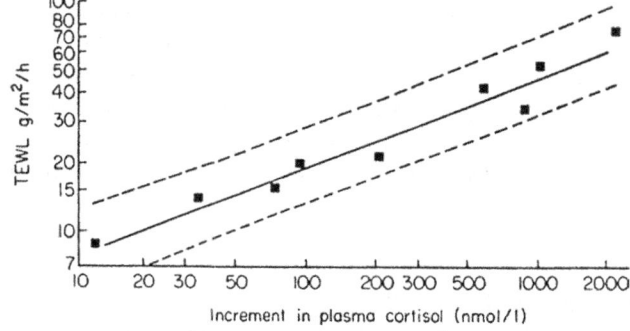

FIGURE 9.5 Relation between TEWL and the increment in plasma cortisol in the percutaneous absorption test, in nine patients with widespread dermatitis. Log_{10} scales have been used to normalize the skewed distributions of the two variables. 95% confidence limits are given. The regression line is log_{10} TEWL= 0.39 log_{10} plasma cortisol + 0.51. Spearman's rank correlation coefficient r_s is 0.991 ($p < 0.001$: 95% confidence limits for r_s 0.955 to 0.998).

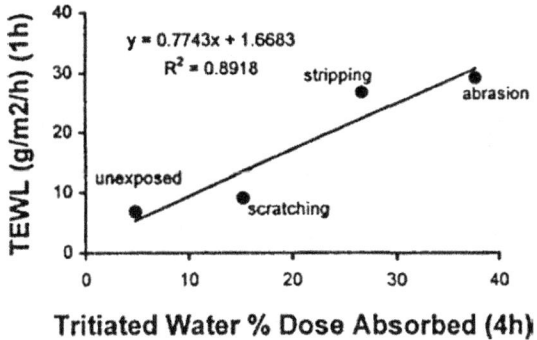

FIGURE 9.6   Linear correlation between TEWL (measured after 1 hour) and the fraction of the dose of tritiated water absorbed (in 4 hours) after various physical injuries applied to excise human skin.

rates and the ^{3}H2O permeability of full-thickness pig skin ($p = 0.68$). There was no correlation between TEWL rate and ^{3}H$_2$O permeability following up to 15 tape strips ($p = 0.64$) or up to four needle stick punctures ($p = 0.13$).

Punnagoda et al. (18) summarized the individual-related variables to TEWL (Table 9.7).

9.3   CONCLUSION

Human skin has barrier properties designed through evolution to protect the inner body from the environment. This barrier property is not absolute, and chemicals on the skin can pass into and through the skin by passive diffusion. These same barrier properties are also leaky to the body's water content, and water escapes, through the skin, also by passive diffusion. This two-way passive travel through the same membrane suggests a correlation between percutaneous absorption and TEWL, especially in the same individual. Science involves seeking a truth among a multitude of variables. Despite the many variables in both percutaneous absorption and TEWL, some statistically positive correlations have been determined between the two. This is not absolute, and negative reports do exist. The TEWL also has the added variable of active water exchange for heat dissipation.

TABLE 9.7
Individual-Related Variables to Transepidermal Water Loss (TEWL)

Age	Baseline TEWL is, for most of the range, independent of age. Premature infants have increased TEWL during their first weeks, and elderly skin may show decreased TEWL.
Sex	Sex as a factor has no apparent effect on baseline TEWL.
Race	There is no apparent difference in baseline TEWL between different human races.
Anatomical sites	Anatomical site is an important variable with respect to baseline TEWL, which can be ranked as follows: palm > sole > forehead = postauricular skin = nail = dorsum of hand > forearm = upper arm = thigh = chest abdomen = back.
Intraindividual and interindividual variation	The intraindividual variation of baseline TEWL values is considerably less than the interindividual variation by sites and by days.
Sweating	Physical, thermal, and emotional sweating are important variables to control for in making accurate TEWL measurements.
Vascular effects	TEWL does not appear to be influenced by simple vasoconstriction and vasodilatation.
Skin surface temperature	Skin temperature is important for TEWL, and preconditioning of the test person is required (see "Sweating"). Skin surface temperature should be measured and reported in publications, particularly if ambient room air temperature deviates from 20 to 22°C.

Source: From Reference 18.

REFERENCES

1. Feldmann RJ, Maibach HI. Regional variation in percutaneous penetration of [14C] cortisol in man. J Invest Dermatol 1967; 48:181–183.
2. Maibach HI, Feldmann RJ, Milby TH, Sert WF. Regional variation in percutaneous penetration in man. Arch Environ Health 1971; 23:208–211.
3. Wester RC, Maibach HI. In vivo percutaneous absorption and decontamination of pesticides in humans. J Toxicol Environ Health 1985; 16:25–37.
4. Van Rooy TGM, De Roos JHC, Bodelier-Bode MD, Jongeneelen FJ. Absorption of polycyclic aromatic hydrocarbons through human skin: differences between anatomic sites and individuals. J Toxicol Environ Health 1993; 38:355–368.
5. Guy RH, Maibach HI. Calculations of body exposure from percutaneous absorption data. In: Bronaugh R, Maibach H, eds. Percutaneous Absorption. New York: Marcel Dekker, 1985:461–466.
6. Rougier A, Dupuis D, Lotte C, Roquet R, Wester RC, Maibach HI. Regional variation in percutaneous absorption in man: measurement by the stripping method. Arch Dermatol Res 1986; 278:465–469.
7. Wertz PW, Swartzendruber DC, Squier CA. Regional variation in the structure and permeability of oral mucosa and skin. Adv Drug Deliv Rev 1993; 12:1–12.
8. Shriner DL, Maibach HI. Regional variation of nonimmunological contact urticaria. Skin Pharmacol 1996; 348:1–11.
9. Wester RC, Maibach HI. Individual and regional variation with in vitro percutaneous absorption. In: Bronaugh R, Maibach H, eds. Vitro Percutaneous Absorption. Boca Raton: CRC Press, 1991:25–30.
10. Rothman S. Insensible water loss. In: Rothman S, ed. Physiology and Biochemistry of the Skin. Chicago: The University of Chicago Press, 1954:233–243.
11. Guyton AC. Textbook of Medical Physiology. Philadelphia: WB Saunders Co, 1991:274–275.
12. Pinson EA. Evaporation from human skin with sweat glands inactivated. Am J Physiol 1942; 137:492–503.
13. Winsor T, Burch GE. Different roles of layers of human epigastric skin on diffusion rate of water. Arch Int Med 1944; 74:428–436.
14. Blank IH. Factors which influence the water content of the stratum corneum. J Invest Dermatol 1952; 18:433–440.
15. Blank IH. Further observations on factors which influence the water content of the stratum corneum. J Invest Dermatol 1953; 21:259–269.
16. Kligman AM. The biology of the stratum corneum. In: Montagna W, Lobitz WCJ, eds. The Epidermis. New York: Academic Press, 1964:387–433.
17. Frost P, Weinstein GD, Bothwell JW, Wildnauer R. Icthyosiform dermatoses III. Studies of transepidermal water loss. Arch Dermatol 98:230–233.
18. Punnagoda J, Tupker RA, Agner T, Serup J. Guidelines for transepidermal water loss (TEWL) measurement. A report from the standardization group of the European Society of Contact Dermatitis. Contact Dermat 1990; 22:64–178.
19. Baker H, Kligman AM. Measurement of transepidermal water loss by electrical hygrometry. Instrumentation and responses to physical and chemical insults. Arch Dermatol 1967; 96:441–452.
20. Martini MC, Cotte J. Influence des produits hygroscopiques et occlusifs sur l'evaporation in vivo de l'eau du stratum corneum. Lab Pharma Probl Technol 1982; 30:547–553.
21. Panisset F, Treffel P, Faivre B, Lecomte PB, Agache P. Transepidermal water loss related to volar forearm sites in humans. Acta Derm Vencreol (Stockh) 1994; 72:4–5.
22. Sam VV, Passet J, Maillois H, Guillot B, Guillot JJ. TEWL measurement standardization: kinetic and topographic aspects. Acta Derm Venereol (Stockh) 1994; 74:168–170.
23. Lotte C, Rougler A, Wilson DR, Maibach HI. In vivo relationship between transepidermal water loss and percutaneous penetration of some organic compounds in man: effect of anatomic site. Arch Dermatol Res 1987; 279:351–356.
24. Aalto-Korte K, Turnpeinen M. Transepidermal water loss and absorption of hydrocortisone in widespread dermatitis. Br J Dermatol 1993; 128:633–635.
25. Nangia A, Berner B, Maibach HI. Transepidermal water loss measurements for assessing skin barrier function during in vitro percutaneous absorption studies. In: Bronaugh R, Maibach H, eds. Percutaneous Absorption, 3rd ed. New York: Marcel Dekker, 1999:587–594.
26. Chilcott RP, Dalton CH, Emmanuel AJ, Allen CE, Bradley ST. Transepidermal water loss does not correlate with skin barrier function in vitro. J Invest Dermatol 2002; 118:871–875.

10 Evaluation of Stratum Corneum Heterogeneity

Gerald B. Kasting, Matthew A. Miller, and Priya S. Talreja
The University of Cincinnati Medical Center, Cincinnati, Ohio

CONTENTS

When confronted with an organ as complex as skin, a biologist tends to want to relate structure to function at the most fundamental level, and indeed an enormous amount of complexity may be found. A physical scientist, on the other hand, looks for simplifying assumptions that allow him to describe the system within a mathematical framework and to make quantifiable predictions about its behavior. There is often a credibility gap between the two approaches, and the appropriate balance point moves as different problems are addressed. There is little doubt that the elegant work of Elias (1, 2), Steinert (3, 4), Wertz (5, 6), and many others in the chemistry and structural biology of the stratum corneum (SC) has enormously increased our understanding of skin barrier function; however, the simplifying framework introduced by Scheuplein and Blank (7) and advanced by others including Flynn (8), Roberts (9, 10), Cooper (11), and Potts and Guy (12) has had a comparable impact on quantifying its properties. The Potts–Guy model for steady-state skin permeability (12) and extensions thereof (13) are arguably the most widely used predictive tools in transdermal drug delivery and dermal risk assessment (14).

Potts and Guy treated skin as a homogeneous lipid membrane, arguing against the need for additional features to explain the steady-state absorption of many organic compounds from aqueous solution (12). The molecular properties determining absorption were molecular weight and octanol–water partition coefficient (K_{oct}). Elaborations on this scheme have included an aqueous barrier in series with the SC (14, 15), a polar pathway in parallel with the lipid pathway (16–18), or both (13, 19), providing reasonable limits to skin permeability for extremely hydrophilic and lipophilic compounds. Other descriptors, notably hydrogen bond donor and acceptor strength (20, 21), have been proposed, as well as quantitative structure-permeability relationships (QSPRs) (22, 23) and neural network approaches (24), yet it is not clear that significant improvements to the basic model have been achieved. Some investigators have considered the tortuosity of the lipid pathway in deriving SC barrier properties (16, 25–27) under the assumption that corneocytes are impermeable. Due to the longer path length, these models yield higher effective diffusivities for permeants in the SC than do homogeneous membrane models. However, Frasch and Barbero's notable analysis (27) shows that diffusion via a tortuous pathway and that through a homogeneous slab cannot be distinguished on the basis of macroscopic observations unless the underlying transport properties are known. Thus, the tortuous pathway formulation of SC permeability leads to predicted permeation profiles similar to those of Potts and Guy (12). More complex behavior is possible if the corneocytes are considered to be permeable (28, 29); however, the full implications of this approach with regard to the time course of permeation have yet to be explored.

10.1   WHAT IS MEANT BY SKIN HETEROGENEITY?

For the purposes of discussion, three levels of heterogeneity in the skin may be distinguished: (1) multiple pathways and barriers for transport through full-thickness skin; (2) the biphasic "brick-and-mortar" structure of the SC; and (3) the variation of SC properties with depth. Much has been learned about the first two levels, as summarized in the preceding paragraph, although complete descriptions of neither are available. Both are considered central to a discussion of barrier function. The impact of the third level, asymmetry of the SC, is less certain. This is an area where effective approximations to the complex structure and composition gradients are essential for predictive transport models because the microscopic transport properties of individual SC layers are not experimentally accessible. Thus, despite the eloquent arguments of Elias (30) and others regarding the biological complexity of the SC barrier, there is still merit to simpler models. This chapter will present a physical chemistry perspective on the factors that must be included in order to make a generally useful description of transport across the SC. The impact of lower skin layers and the cutaneous circulation, although important to a general picture of skin absorption, is not considered here.

10.2   THE ROLE OF APPENDAGES AND THE SKIN'S POLAR PATHWAY

The importance of skin appendages—hair follicles and sweat ducts—to the transport of ions and highly polar molecules across skin is easily established. Examples include the perifollicular wheal and flare response induced by topical application of histamine ($K_{oct} = 0.20$) (31), punctuate patterns of dyes administered to skin via iontophoresis (32, 33), and localized electric fields observed indirectly at the skin surface during passage of mild electric currents (34–36). Peck and coworkers distinguished permeants penetrating via this "polar pathway," which most likely includes microscopic defects in the SC lipid lamellar structure, by their low permeabilities and low activation energies for diffusion relative to lipophilic permeants (17, 18). Appendageal contributions to the transport of lipophilic compounds across the SC are less obvious, but still demonstrable on the basis of transient diffusion analyses (37). Figure 10.1 shows data obtained recently in our laboratory supporting the need for a two-pathway diffusion model to explain transient diffusion profiles for permeants spanning a wide range of lipophilicity. The data were obtained using small doses of radiolabeled compounds applied to split-thickness (250 to 300 μm), cadaveric human skin mounted in Franz diffusion cells and tested according to previously described methods (37, 38). In each case a homogeneous membrane model (37) failed to describe the early stage of the absorption process, which was much more rapid than can be accounted for by diffusion through a slab. In most cases (but not for the flavonoid, kaempferol), permeation after several hours was well described by the single-pathway model. The second pathway having the shorter lag time, but clearly a limited capacity, is most likely related to either skin appendages or to microscopic defects in the SC lipid lamellae. These observations are consistent with the predictions of Scheuplein more than three decades earlier (39) and also with earlier results obtained by one of the authors using aqueous ibuprofen solutions applied to split-thickness skin (40). They may be important for understanding how nicotinate esters cause flushing within minutes of application to skin in vivo (41). It may be concluded that shunt pathways are important for most compounds during the initial transient phase of absorption and at all times for very hydrophilic compounds or for high-molecular-weight species (17) that cannot otherwise penetrate the skin (37, 42).

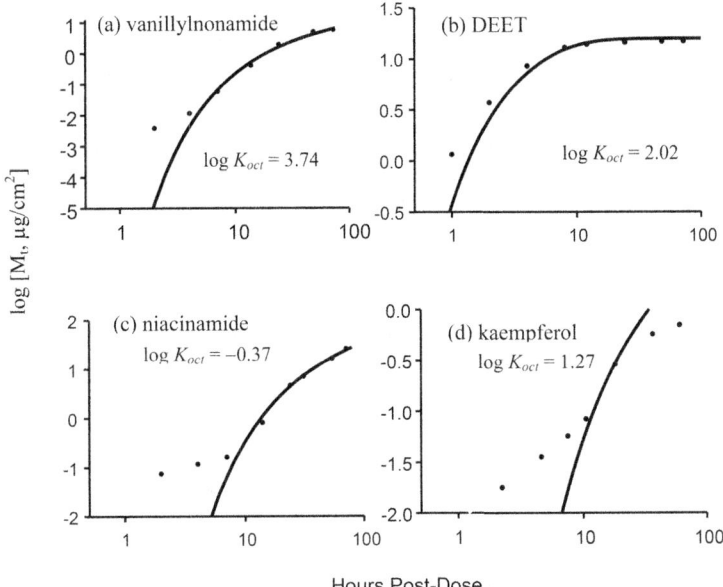

FIGURE 10.1 Permeation time course of four radiolabeled compounds through split-thickness human skin in vitro. The compounds were applied in simple solvent systems (5 μL/0.79 cm² cell) at doses of 10–100 μg/cm². (a) ^{14}C-vanillylnonanamide in propylene glycol (37); (b) ^{14}C-DEET in ethanol; (c) ^{14}C-niacinamide in 1:1 v/v ethanol/water; (d) ^{3}H-kaempferol in propylene glycol. The solid lines are theoretical curves for finite dose permeation through a homogeneous membrane (37) that have been fit to the data. The theory for DEET includes a first-order evaporative loss from the skin surface (42). The positive departures of the data from the theory suggest a second (shunt) pathway through the SC having a very short time lag.

10.3   THE ROLE OF CORNEOCYTES IN THE STRATUM CORNEUM BARRIER

Perhaps the most unfortunate consequence of the "brick-and-mortar" analogy for SC structure is the tendency to think of corneocytes as impermeable obstacles. The body of evidence to the contrary is compelling. First and foremost, immersion in water leads to swelling of the SC to several times its normal thickness in about an hour (43–46). Although a small amount of water may hydrate lipid headgroups in the lipid lamellae (47), the bulk of the water must enter the corneocytes, as the lamellar spacings do not change significantly with hydration (48). Nuclear magnetic resonance (NMR) studies have shown the diffusivity of mobile protons in partially hydrated SC (guinea pig footpad hydrated to ˜43% w/w) to be 2.8×10^{-6} cm²s⁻¹, only tenfold less than the self-diffusivity of water (49, 50). This signal presumably derives largely from water within the corneocytes (50). Water diffusivity in fully hydrated corneocytes is likely to be higher; an estimate from hindered diffusion theory, including keratin–water binding interaction, is 2.2×10^{-7} cm²s⁻¹ (51).

There is a school of thought that it is the cornified cell envelopes (CEs), rather than the keratinized interiors, that leads to corneocyte impermeability. This thinking appears to derive from a consideration of the chemical resistance of the CE, which is indeed formidable. Boiling in alkali is required to degrade these structures. It is supported by microscopic studies of heavy metal distribution in SC that show a higher fraction of metal ions or metal ion precipitates within apical corneocytes following topical administration than in the lower layers (52, 53). The published studies of Hg^{2+} distribution (52, 53) are supported by additional unpublished work with Zn^{2+} and Cu^{2+} (R. R. Warner, personal communication). Investigators have hypothesized that desmosomal degradation in the outer SC leads to breaches in the CEs, allowing ion entry (53). Although there is merit to this idea, an alternative explanation is possible to which we will return momentarily. First, we note that the impermeable CE concept is inconsistent both with spectroscopic studies of water diffusion in SC (49, 50) and with organic solute partitioning and permeability relationships in SC (54, 55), as follows.

Packer and Sellwood studied samples of partially hydrated guinea pig footpad SC by ^{1}H NMR, using both relaxation (49) and pulsed field-gradient spin echo (50) techniques. The latter measurements, which were conducted in oriented SC samples, provided estimates of the diffusivity and the characteristic diffusion length of "mobile protons" within the sample. According to their analysis, the characteristic diffusion length of these protons in the direction perpendicular to the plane of the tissue was 3 to 4 μm, consistent with diffusion within the interior of a partially hydrated corneocyte. Extraction of lipids with 2:1 chloroform:methanol "produced fairly large 'holes' in the cell walls which considerably reduced the degree of restriction in the diffusion of the mobile molecules" (50). If one takes the reasonable position (50, 51) that this signal represents largely water within corneocytes, then it is evident that removal of the noncovalently bound lipid from the SC allowed water to diffuse rapidly between corneocytes. Since the CEs are not disrupted by this extraction, it follows that the primary diffusion barrier for water is the intercellular lipids rather than the CEs.

Evidence for corneocyte permeability to other solutes is provided by Anderson and Raykar's thoughtful analysis of SC/water partition coefficients and their relationship to SC permeability (54, 55). These workers showed that permeability was directly proportional to partition coefficient for the more lipophilic solutes, but not for moderately lipophilic or hydrophilic solutes. These and related data (16, 56) may be understood on the basis of a biphasic SC transport model with transfer of solutes by both lipid-continuous and lipid-corneocyte pathways (28, 29). This is a subject of ongoing research in our laboratory.

We return now to the question of metal ion distribution in skin. The best-known examples are two studies in which Hg^{2+} was driven into the skin (as the chloride) via iontophoresis, then precipitated as the sulfide by exposure to ammonium sulfide vapors and analyzed by transmission electron microscopy (TEM) (52, 53). In both cases the investigators found precipitated HgS within the corneocytes in the outer layers of the SC, but only within the lipid lamellae in the lower SC. It was hypothesized (53) that the corneocytes in the lower SC are impermeable, whereas those in the upper SC are not due to the degradation of the desmosomal linkages between the corneocytes, allowing access to the corneocyte through the degraded areas. These observations led both groups to the conclusion that mercuric chloride penetrates the SC via an intercellular pathway.

We offer the following alternative interpretation. Mercuric chloride is a salt with considerable covalent character and moderate lipophilicity ($K_{oct} = 0.6$ [57]). Mercury is furthermore quite reactive with organic materials and readily forms organometallic compounds that bioaccumulate in the food chain due to their high lipophilicity (K_{oct} for dimethyl mercury, for example, is about 390 [57]). Monteiro-Riviere et al. (53) noted that Hg-containing precipitates found in basal keratinocytes were localized to the mitochondrial membrane; hence, even in a predominately aqueous cellular environment, Hg partitioned into (or absorbed onto) lipid membranes. These observations suggest that the reason that Hg was found in the intercellular lipids of the lower SC is simply equilibrium partitioning rather than corneocyte impermeability. In the upper SC the intercellular lipid content may have been lower due to the desquamation process, leading to more Hg within the corneocytes. According to this reasoning, the pathway for penetration of Hg^{2+} through the tissue cannot be inferred from the distribution of Hg-containing precipitates.

To summarize this section, the partition ratio must always be considered when drawing inferences about transport pathways from steady-state (or pseudo steady-state) tissue distributions. The key property to consider is permeability, P, defined as the product of diffusivity D and partition coefficient K:

$$P = DK \qquad (10.1)$$

As Heisig (28) and others (25) have pointed out, in a structure such as SC with a high "internal" phase volume of corneocytes surrounded by a continuous lipid matrix, the ratio $\sigma = P_{lip}/P_{cor}$ must exceed about 10^4 before the corneocytes may be considered to be effectively impermeable. A detailed analysis allowing for anisotropic transport properties in the lipid phase and in which corneocyte permeability was carefully estimated from partition data (54–56) and hindered diffusion theory (29) suggests that the contribution of corneocytes to transport across the SC is significant for many permeants, although it cannot be estimated from a single parameter ratio, as in Heisig's analysis.

10.4 THE INFLUENCE OF ASYMMETRY ON SC TRANSPORT

The location of the transport barrier in skin was debated until the early 1960s due to the propensity of the tissue to be disrupted (thereby resulting in a "basket-weave" appearance) in routine histological preparations (30). Development of the alkaline swelling technique in Kligman's laboratory (58) was a key step that allowed visualization of the highly organized, compact structure of intact SC. This was complemented by outstanding transport work, much of which was conducted by Scheuplein and Blank (7, 39, 59–63), that established beyond a doubt that the SC was the primary diffusion barrier to water and most other permeants. It was also clear by the mid-1960s that the SC barrier extended across the tissue rather than residing in a thin layer at the base of the SC, as had originally been thought (60). Scheuplein and Blank provide a fascinating summary of these developments in their 1971 review (7).

Scheuplein had several lines of evidence available to support the uniformity of the SC transport barrier. Electron microscopy showed a dense, compact structure (64, 65), although the staining techniques to bring out the intercellular lipids had not yet been developed. Light microscopy using the alkaline swelling technique (58, 66) showed the SC to have a remarkably uniform appearance from top to bottom. An example micrograph from our laboratory is shown in Figure 10.2. Studies in which water transport was measured across sequentially tape-stripped skin suggested a uniform

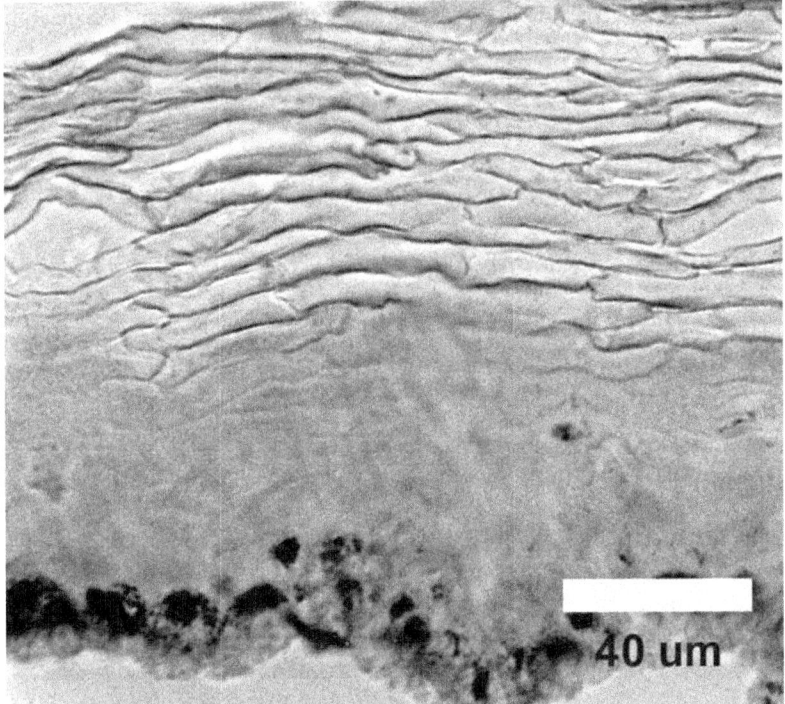

FIGURE 10.2 Brightfield image of alkaline-swollen human SC stained with methylene blue, illustrating partially ordered stacking of corneocytes. (From Reference 26.)

barrier (67). Osmotic shock experiments in which the SC was split into two sections of approximately equal thickness showed both sections to have excellent barrier properties (33). The latter experiments were evidently more qualitative than quantitative in nature, as details of tissue thickness and permeability were not provided. More recently, careful in vivo studies of transepidermal water loss (TEWL) from skin following sequential tape stripping have tended to confirm the picture of a uniform transport barrier, at least for water (68–70).

Detailed examination of SC structure, biochemistry, and transport properties, however, has continued to reveal asymmetric features. The most obvious of these are in the first two categories. It has long been evident that the outer few layers of SC have degraded desmosomes and reduced lamellar lipid content (52, 53, 71). It is likely these layers offer reduced diffusional resistance due to the disruption of the ordered lipid structure. A closely related concept is that of a stratum "conjunctum" and stratum "disjunctum," the former being the compact lower SC, the latter the upper desquamating layers. This distinction was noted in the 1950s and nicely elaborated by Bowser and White (72). Recent examinations of cryopreserved SC obtained from water-exposed skin in vivo have shown that hydration-induced swelling of the SC is also asymmetric (71, 73, 74). According to both reports, the lower three to four layers of the SC do not swell to the same degree as the middle layers. This phenomenon is clearly demonstrated in Figure 10.3. Warner argued that the incomplete breakdown of the filaggrin binding the keratin bundles in the lower SC limits the ability of the keratin to swell; moreover, the osmotic gradient contributing to swelling is not fully established because much of it comes from filaggrin breakdown products, i.e., amino acids derived from proteolytic degradation of filaggrin (71). This observation, combined with the established relationship between SC water content and permeability (44, 51, 75–78), suggests that the lower SC layers may be less permeable than the middle ones, at least for the case of fully hydrated skin. Offsetting this is the fact that the CEs in the lower SC are not fully mature, leading to a distinction between "fragile" (CEf) and "resilient" (CEr) cell envelopes, as identified by mechanical properties and light microscopy (79). The CEr are more prevalent in the apical layers of the SC and the CEf more prevalent in the lower layers (79). If the CEf are, in fact, more permeable than the CEr, then the gradient of SC permeability could be

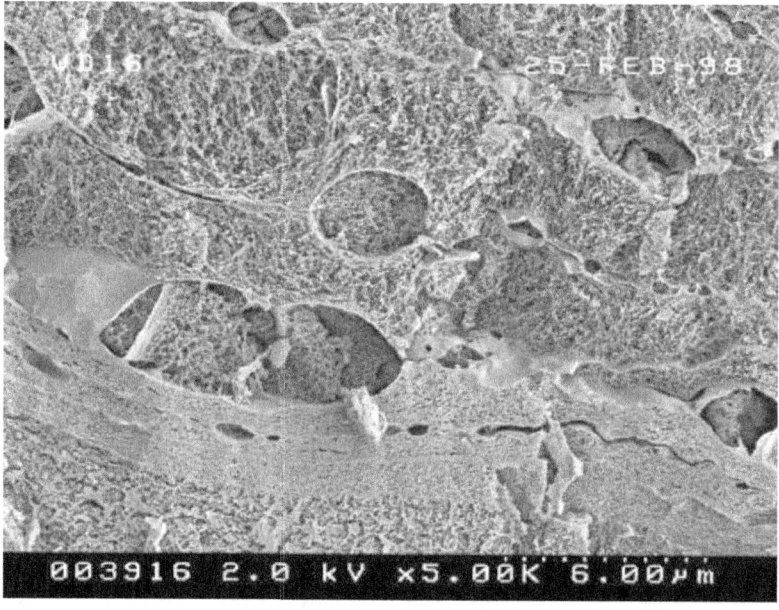

FIGURE 10.3   Cryo-SEM image of human SC following 24-hour exposure to urine *in vivo*. The open arrows mark cisternae in the intercellular regions of the innermost SC layers, which are seen to be much less swollen than the overlying layers. There are three unswollen corneocyte layers in this micrograph. (From Reference 71.)

opposite to that suggested by the swelling behavior. The uncertainty as to which of these features is the more important led us to conduct the studies described next.

Sorption/desorption studies on isolated SC offer a useful complement to permeation studies because different combinations of membrane properties are emphasized. A desorption study readily yields a time constant h^2/D and a partition coefficient K (80–82), whereas permeation studies give direct information on the permeability coefficient DK/h (33). In making these assignments for a heterogeneous membrane, one must recognize that the values of h, D, and K represent, respectively, *effective* thickness, diffusivity, and partition coefficient and are not in most cases equal to the microscopic transport constants (27). Nevertheless, they do characterize the macroscopic transport properties. In principle, permeation studies also yield the time constant from the time lag $h^2/6D$; however, the latter measurement is confounded for a membrane such as SC by the contribution of polar or appendageal pathways to the early time data (Figure 10.1). Sorption or desorption data are less affected by shunt pathways so long as the total shunt surface area is small compared to that of the bulk membrane. This may be seen by considering the effect of a large pinhole on permeation across and desorption from an otherwise homogeneous membrane (Figure 10.4).

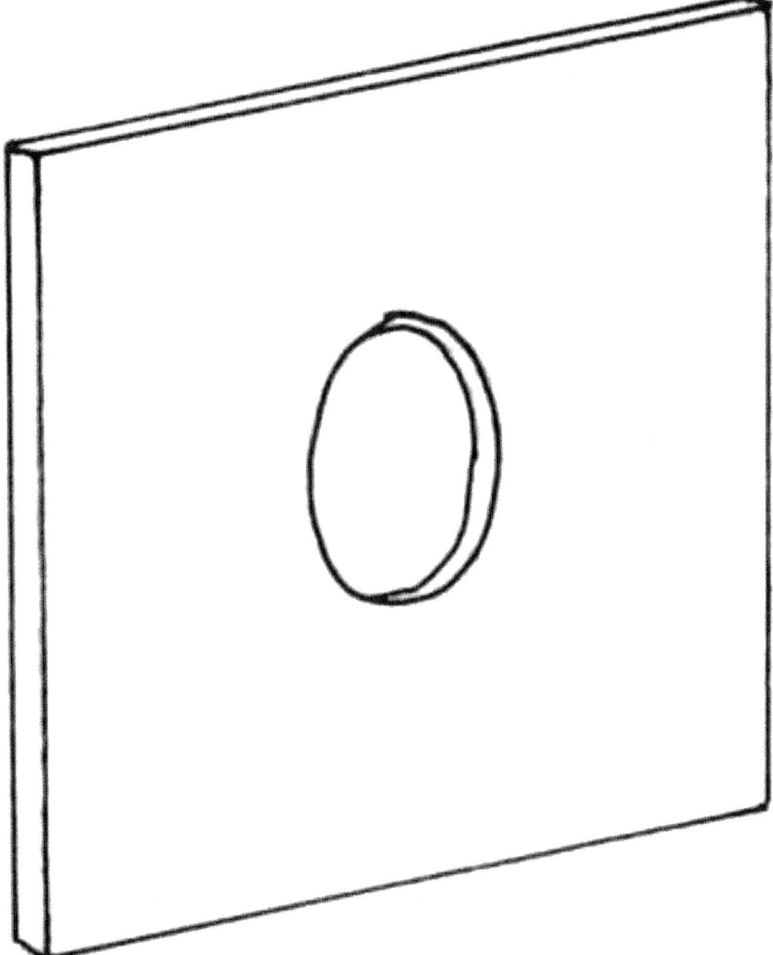

FIGURE 10.4   Illustration depicting a membrane with a large pinhole. The impact of the hole on permeation through the membrane (e.g., left to right) is enormous; however, the impact on desorption of a solute from the membrane is much smaller. For a homogeneous membrane, the contribution of the hole to the initial desorption rate is proportional to the surface area of its perimeter divided by the full surface area of the membrane.

Sorption/desorption studies offer the possibility of studying depth-dependent transport properties of SC because any such dependence destroys the plane of symmetry in the center of the membrane. Anissimov and Roberts (83) have provided an excellent discussion of these effects. They show that permeation and desorption studies are relatively insensitive to variation in D across the membrane but that desorption studies are highly sensitive to variations in K. The latter is of particular significance because experimental work from the same laboratory has shown a profound variation with depth in the SC for the partition coefficient of a lipophilic permeant, clobetasol propionate (84). This result is reproduced in Figure 10.5. Anissimov and Roberts (83) concluded that "partition coefficient heterogeneity can be the reason for higher fluxes predicted using desorption as compared with penetration techniques," citing an earlier experimental study by one of the authors (9) in which this behavior was systematically observed.

We show next without details the results of several experiments from our laboratory supporting the concepts of multiple pathways and moderate asymmetry for the SC barrier. The studies involved a hydrophilic permeant, niacinamide (MW 122, log K_{oct} = −0.37 [85]), and a lipophilic permeant, testosterone (MW 288; log K_{oct} = 3.32 [57]). They were conducted using radiolabeled tracers, ^{14}C-niacinamide and ^{3}H-testosterone, dissolved in pH 7.4 aqueous buffers in the presence of 5 to 10 μg/mL concentrations of unlabeled permeant. All studies were conducted at a skin temperature of 30°C. The first study consisted of permeation measurements across human epidermal membranes (HEM) mounted in Franz diffusion cells and desorption studies conducted with isolated

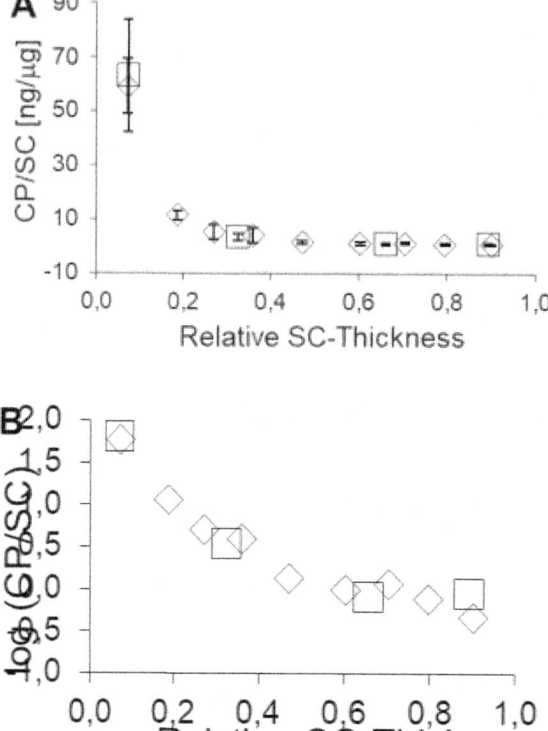

FIGURE 10.5 Variation of clobetasol propionate (CP) concentration with depth in human SC after 48 hours equilibration in a saturated solution of CP in propylene glycol. Since both sides of the membrane were exposed to the donor solution, this is an equilibrium distribution rather than a steady-state transport distribution. The apical (upper) side of the SC corresponds to a relative SC thickness of 0. (A) Linear scale; (B) logarithmic scale. (From Reference 84.)

SC obtained by trypsinization of epidermal membrane samples from the same skin donors (86). The skin samples were prepared by heat separation of freshly excised tissue from breast reduction surgery and were shown to have excellent barrier properties to tritiated water (38). Representative results are shown in Figures 10.6 and 10.7. The average steady-state permeability coefficients of HEM to niacinamide and testosterone, calculated as

$$k_p = J_{ss} / \Delta C_v \qquad (10.2)$$

where J_{ss} is steady-state flux in $\mu g\ cm^{-2}h^{-1}$ and ΔC_v is the concentration difference between the donor and receptor solutions, were 4.9×10^{-5} cm/h and 9.2×10^{-3} cm/h, respectively (Table 10.1). These values are in accord with expectations for high-quality human skin (16). However, for both permeants, skin samples having comparable values of J_{ss} (and, consequently, of k_p) had widely varying time lags to permeation (Figure 10.6). For niacinamide, some samples even showed evidence of a convective burst prior to establishing a steady-state flux (data not shown). Since it is improbable that SC thickness or permeant diffusivities in these skin samples could vary enough to cause large

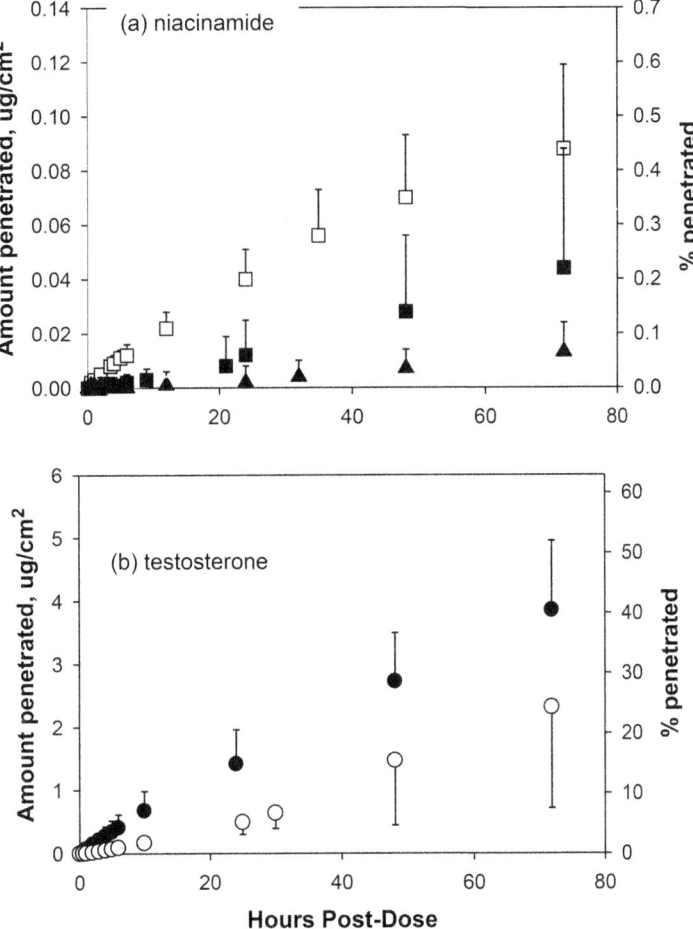

FIGURE 10.6 Permeation of (a) niacinamide and (b) testosterone across freshly excised human epidermal membrane. Each symbol represents the mean ± SE for one donor, $n = 5$–8 samples/donor. The average permeability coefficients calculated from the straight line regions are reported in Table 10.1.

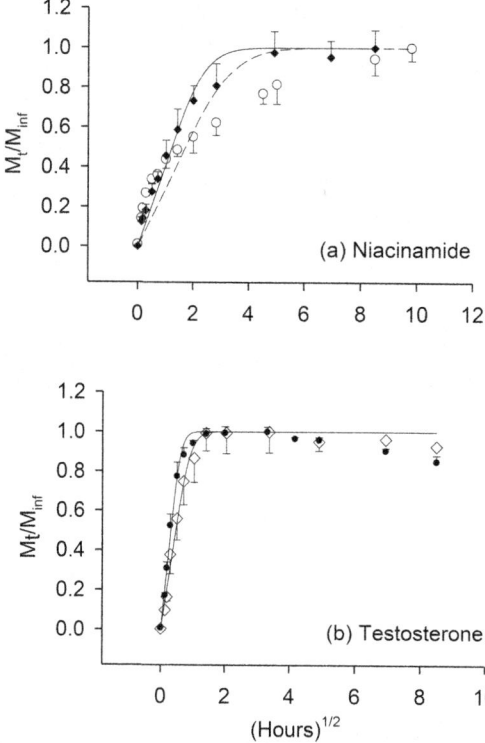

FIGURE 10.7 Desorption of (a) niacinamide and (b) testosterone from isolated human SC *in vitro*. Each symbol represents the mean ± SE for one donor, $n = 3$ samples/donor. (Data from Reference 86 with revised partition coefficient calculation.)

TABLE 10.1

Transport Parameters for Niacinamide and Testosterone in Human SC Obtained From Analysis of Permeation and Desorption Studies According to Homogeneous Membrane Theory

Compound	No. of Donors	$k_p \times 10^5$, cm h^{-1}	h^2/D, h	$D \times 10^{10}$, cm^{2}s^{-1}	K	$P \times 10^{10}$, cm^{2}s^{-1}
Niacinamide						
Permeation	5 (31)	4.9 ± 4.7	50 ± 35[a]	4.4 ± 4.0[a]	0.29 ± 0.13	0.8[b]
Desorption (slow)	5 (14)	-	230 ± 230	0.5 ± 0.5	1.2 ± 0.3	0.6[c]
Desorption (initial)	5 (14)	-	10 ± 5	11 ± 5	1.2 ± 0.3	13[c]
Testosterone						
Permeation	3 (24)	920 ± 470	55 ± 4[a]	3.3 ± 0.1[a]	91 ± 43	160[b]
Desorption	4 (13)	-	3.0 ± 1.4	35 ± 17	7 ± 2	250[c]

Note: The thickness of hydrated SC was taken to be $h = 62.1$ μm as described in (87). Each value represents the mean ± SD
     of 3 to 5 donors with 3 to 10 replicates per donor. The total number of samples is given in parentheses.

[a] Estimated from time lag of selected samples as described in (86).

[b] Calculated as $P = h \times k_p$

[c] Calculated as $P = D \times K$

Source: Data from Reference 86.

changes in h^2/D while maintaining constant k_p, the variable time lags are most likely due to shunt diffusion. Thus, these data support the conclusion stated in a preceding section that shunt pathways contribute significantly to transient diffusion for many compounds.

Desorption of testosterone from isolated SC (Figure 10.7b) was relatively rapid and followed closely the profile expected for a homogeneous membrane (80, 81). The process was essentially complete within 3 hours. A gradual loss of radiolabel at longer times was traced to glass adsorption (86). According to diffusion theory, the initial slope of the plot of amount desorbed from a homogeneous membrane versus the square root of time yields the time constant h^2/D, i.e., (80, 81)

$$M_t / M_\infty = 4\sqrt{\frac{Dt}{\pi h^2}} \tag{10.3}$$

The average time constant so calculated for testosterone was 3.2 ± 1.5 hours (Table 10.1). Desorption of niacinamide was much slower, although many samples had a rapid initial phase in which about 20% of the dose was desorbed (Figure 10.7a). Some samples were still releasing permeant after 100 hours, although others were discharged by 24 hours. Although this behavior was clearly more complex than the homogenous membrane theory, we estimated time constants for the initial phase and the slower phase of desorption according to Equation (10.3). The results varied widely between samples, but averaged about 9 hours for the initial phase and 150 hours for the slow phase (Table 10.1).

Based on the concentrations of radiolabeled permeants in the uptake solutions and the total amounts desorbed, we were able to calculate bulk SC/water partition coefficients from the desorption studies using the relationship

$$K = \frac{\text{DPM} / \text{g wet tissue}}{\text{DPM} / \text{g solution}} \tag{10.4}$$

Note that Equation (10.4) defines K on a wet tissue basis rather than the dry tissue basis used elsewhere (54–56). The results were $K = 1.2 \pm 0.3$ for niacinamide and $K = 7 \pm 2$ for testosterone (Table 10.1). The value of K for niacinamide, combined with its polarity and the fact that the lipid content of hydrated SC is only 3% to 4%, strongly suggests that it partitions into the corneocyte phase. Testosterone, being a highly lipophilic compound, could well achieve its bulk SC/water partition coefficient of 7 by residing primarily in the intercellular lipids. For example, for a 3% lipid content, an SC lipid/water partition coefficient of $7/0.03 = 230$ would be required.

We tested the consistency between permeation and desorption results by further analyzing the data according to homogeneous membrane theory (80). This procedure involved estimating h^2/D for permeation from the permeation time lag $h^2/6D$, followed by calculation of D for both methods using the estimate $h = 62.1$ μm for the thickness of hydrated SC (87). K for permeation was then calculated from the relationship

$$k_p = DK / h \tag{10.5}$$

The details of this analysis are presented elsewhere (86). It can only be viewed as an approximation due to the wide variation in permeation time lags for both compounds and the nonideal shape of the niacinamide desorption curves. The analysis yielded two sets of transport properties, D and K, for testosterone—one from the permeation study and the other from the desorption study—and three for niacinamide. Permeability P was also calculated using $P = h \times k_p$ for permeation and Equation (10.1) for desorption. Considering first the slow phase of niacinamide desorption, it can be seen from Table 10.1 that permeation and desorption studies yielded comparable values for P but different values for its components, D and K. The testosterone results ($D_{\text{desorption}} > D_{\text{permeation}}$) are similar to previous results obtained by Roberts and coworkers for other lipophilic compounds (9) and recently interpreted by the same group on the basis of membrane asymmetry (83, 84). In light of this, we conducted the following experiment to test the symmetry of permeant release from SC.

The test was designed as a desorption study employing the same radiolabeled permeants, ^{14}C-niacinamide and ^{3}H-testosterone, and isolated human SC. In this case, however, the tissue was mounted in side-by-side diffusion cells with attention paid to the orientation of the sample. The study also employed cadaver skin rather than surgical discard skin, which may lead to somewhat higher permeability. Aside from these features, the conditions were the same as those for the experiments in Figure 10.7. The SC was equilibrated with solutions of each compound (2.5 to 5.0 μCi/mL and 5 to 10 μg/mL) in phosphate-buffered saline (PBS), pH 7.4, containing 0.02% sodium azide for two to three days. The SC was then mounted in side-by-side diffusion cells maintained at 32°C, with the apical (upper) side to the left and the proximal (lower) side to the right. Desorption was initiated by simultaneously filling both the left and right compartments with PBS. Sequential samples were then withdrawn from each compartment and replaced with an equal volume of PBS. The results of this study are shown in Figure 10.8. Significant differences (paired t-test, $p < 0.05$) between apical and proximal surfaces were obtained in both the initial desorption rate and the plateau desorption value for both compounds. Similarly to the studies in Figures 10.6 and 10.7, the differences for the hydrophilic and lipophilic permeants were in opposite directions. Niacinamide desorbed more rapidly and extensively from the proximal surface, whereas testosterone did so from the apical surface. Microscopic examination of cross-sectioned, alkaline-expanded sections showed no evidence for residual viable epidermis on the proximal side of the tissue. Thus, the SC samples were clearly asymmetric in a rather interesting manner; however, the magnitude of the asymmetry as measured

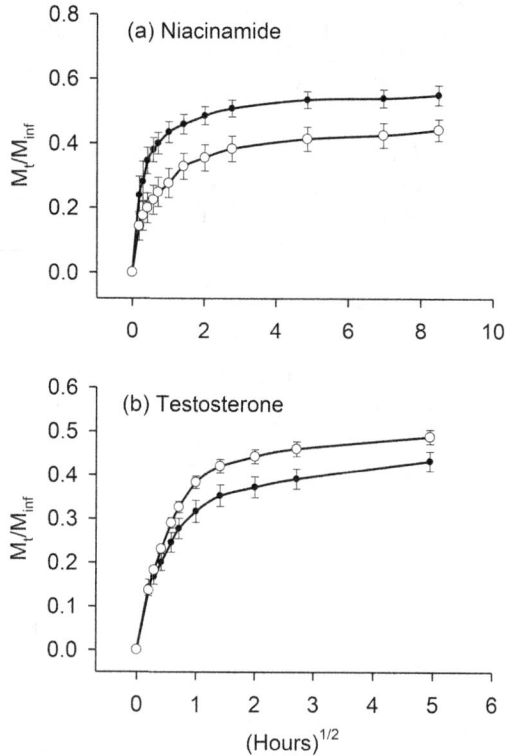

FIGURE 10.8 Desorption of (a) niacinamide and (b) testosterone from isolated human SC mounted in side-by-side diffusion cells. Each point represents the mean ± SE of two donors, $n = 4$–5 samples/donor. The open circles were obtained from the compartment exposed to the apical (upper) surface; the closed circles from the compartment exposed to the proximal (lower) surface.

by this technique was modest. (The reader will note that this method somewhat underestimates differences between apical and proximal surfaces because of the simultaneous transport of permeant through the tissue due to the developing concentration gradient.)

10.5 DISCUSSION

The experiments described in this chapter provide several lines of evidence supporting the premise that SC behaves as a heterogeneous and somewhat asymmetric membrane with respect to transport. The former is not unexpected, based on its brick-and-mortar architecture (Figure 10.2) and numerous transport models based on this structure (16, 25–29). It should be noted that shunt diffusion is a heterogeneous feature of the SC not anticipated by brick-and-mortar models, yet evidently important in the early stages of absorption of many compounds. The results shown in Figures 10.1 and 10.6 establish that shunt diffusion contributes significantly to the transient diffusion of both hydrophilic and lipophilic substances across the SC. Other work has established its importance to the steady-state transport of ions and very polar-neutral molecules across the SC, especially under the influence of an electric field (17, 18, 32, 34–36). We consider the shunts of importance in human skin to be hair follicles, sweat ducts, and microscopic defects in the SC lipid lamellae. These penetration routes may also constitute the skin's "polar pathway"; however, their net contributions to transport appear to extend beyond polar compounds (Figures 10.1a, 10.1b, and 10.6b). Evidence for a fourth potential contributor to the polar pathway—the proteinaceous route consisting of corneocytes and their interconnecting desmosomes—is either weak or nonexistent. Such a pathway would be hard to find experimentally because of the relatively long time lag associated with the filling of the corneocytes.

The symmetry of the SC barrier has been debated for many years, as previously discussed. Recent evidence supporting an asymmetric barrier is presented in this report. The SC swells nonuniformly when exposed to water or urine (Figure 10.3), sorbs and desorbs compounds unevenly with respect to depth or membrane surface (Figures 10.5 and 10.8), and yields different effective transport properties when studied by permeation and sorption methods (Figures 10.6 and 10.7 and Table 10.1). These phenomena inject a note of caution into inference of transport rates from membrane concentration profiles, as in proposed tape-strip bioequivalence methods (88) or inference of transmembrane transport from initial desorption rates (82). The biphasic desorption of niacinamide from SC (Figure 10.7a) and associated high and low diffusivities (Table 10.1) show that considerable error would be incurred by basing transport calculations for this compound on initial desorption rate. A practical take-home from these studies is that traditional permeation studies (rather than desorption studies or tissue concentration profiles) should always be conducted in order to predict flux, as they integrate over asymmetries present in the membrane. From a modeling perspective, some error will be incurred by considering the membrane to be vertically isotropic. However, if the spatial variations are of the order suggested by Figure 10.8, the error is likely to be acceptable. If they are more often like those shown in Figure 10.5 (84), then let the modeler beware! We note that the hydration gradient present in human skin in vivo (89) is a natural factor that is likely to contribute to a permeability gradient across the SC (51). The balance of this feature (which leads to lower permeability of the drier, apical layers) with the desquamation-related loss of lipids from these layers (which leads to higher permeability) may be the reason that the SC presents a remarkably uniform barrier to TEWL (68–70).

For lipophilic permeants, there is a consistency between several sets of observations that should be noted. Desorption studies yielded higher values of diffusivity D than did permeation studies for both testosterone (Table 10.1) and a variety of other compounds (9). This phenomenon is predicted for a membrane with an asymmetric partition coefficient (83). Tissue distribution measurements for another lipophilic solute, clobetasol proprionate, in SC (Figure 10.5) support the premise of an asymmetric partition coefficient, with the higher concentration achieved at the apical (upper) surface. Bidirectional desorption of testosterone from SC (Figure 10.8b) supports that higher equilibrium concentrations of this compound are also attained at the apical surface. A possible reason for the enhanced partitioning of lipophilic compounds into the upper SC layers is the presence of sebaceous lipids in this region. Otherwise, one might expect a lower partition coefficient due to the partial loss of lamellar lipids from the upper SC.

The hydrophilic permeant niacinamide showed behavior qualitatively different from testosterone. It desorbed from SC in a complex manner involving a fast and a slow time constant (Figure 10.7a and Table 10.1). The diffusivity calculated from the slow phase of desorption was smaller than that from permeation, not larger. Niacinamide desorbed more rapidly from the proximal (lower) side of the SC rather than the apical side (Figure 10.8a). These phenomena, combined with the bulk SC/water partition coefficient of 1.2 (Table 10.1), suggest that niacinamide partitions into both protein and lipid regions of the SC and that its diffusion rate between the two regions is restricted. It seems possible that the CEs may play a role in this restriction. If the fragile CEf in the lower SC were more permeable to niacinamide than the rigid CEr in the upper SC, then the desorption pattern in Figure 10.8a is understandable. Thus, detailed comparison of the transport behavior of hydrophilic and lipophilic permeants can provide insights into the permeation mechanism for both.

10.6 CONCLUSION

Careful examination of mass transport processes in the SC, focusing especially on transient diffusion rates determined from permeation and desorption methodologies, reveals the heterogeneous and somewhat asymmetric nature of the SC barrier. Although these features are of interest in elucidating transport mechanisms, the most practical way to deal with them is to conduct experiments (e.g., permeation studies) and develop models that integrate over the entire barrier. The concept of SC as a vertically isotropic diffusion barrier has a solid place in current thinking.

FIFTH EDITION UPDATE

As I review this chapter written some 16 years ago, I find myself in general agreement with the sentiments expressed therein, including those in the conclusion. But a great deal has happened in the intervening period. Some highlights follow.

Experimental developments: A number of experiments have directly or indirectly assessed the matter of corneocyte permeability and the nature of the skin's polar pathway. This work has significantly affected thinking regarding transport pathways in the SC. A highlight is the recent NMR studies of Kodiweera, Bunge, and coworkers (90, 91) in which water and a model lipophilic permeant 2-(trifluoromethyl)benzonitrile (TFMB) were studied in oriented, isolated human SC. Both water and TFMB were found within the corneocytes, the latter at about the proportion expected from its calculated SC/water partition coefficient (90). The diffusivity of water in the corneocyte was found to lie generally within the range of 0.2 to 1.5×10^{-5} cm²/s depending on the orientation and hydration state of the sample (91). These values may be compared to the accepted value of 2.3×10^{-5} cm²/s for the self-diffusivity of water at 25°C.

Our laboratory conducted and analyzed more uptake/desorption studies with human SC of the kind shown in Figure 10.7, focusing on hydrophilic permeants (92, 93). Many of the compounds showed two-phase desorption profiles similar to niacinamide. The magnitude of the calculated SC/water partition coefficients and the slow phase diffusivities were consistent with uniform uptake of the solutes into the corneocyte interior, followed by size-selective desorption from that environment. The slow-phase diffusivities for hydrophilic compounds, excluding water, were in the range of 0.3 to 8.7×10^{-11} cm²/s, whereas those for lipophilic compounds and water (a very small hydrophilic compound) were in the range of 2.2 to 3.5×10^{-9} cm²/s or about 100-fold larger. The results provide a new argument to support the "fourth pathway" for polar permeants described in the first paragraph of the "Discussion" section.

Finally, important progress has been made in characterizing a follicular pathway for penetration of solutes through the SC. The human in vivo study of caffeine absorption by Otberg and coworkers at Charité Hospital in Berlin stands out (94). They used a follicular blocking technique to demonstrate that a substantial fraction of caffeine dermal uptake was due to hair follicles. The difference at short exposure times (<30 min) was remarkable. This research group has published widely in this area for more than a decade, including two recent reviews (94–97). A significant build on the follicular blocking approach was published by Mohd and coworkers in Malaysia and Japan (98). These workers employed a blocking technique on pig ear skin in vitro and obtained evidence to support a strong dependence of follicular delivery on lipophilicity, with the more hydrophilic permeants showing larger follicular contributions.

Theoretical models: There is a wide array of modeling approaches to parameterize SC complexity, ranging from sophisticated QSPR methods (99–103) to highly detailed microstructural models (104–109). Intermediate in complexity but perhaps more accessible to many researchers are pharmacokinetic models (110), analytical (111–115), or finite difference (116–120) approximations to simplified SC structures and finite difference approximations to rectangular brick-and-mortar models (27, 121–128). The various classes of models have been further developed to include tissue binding effects (106, 112, 119, 120, 129, 130), follicular delivery (123, 128, 131), and the impact of multicomponent vehicles (101, 120, 132). Reviews of the field have appeared periodically (133–135).

Of particular interest to our research group is the ongoing discussion regarding transport mechanism(s) for hydrophilic permeants and the impact of SC lipid anisotropy on penetration pathways. The essence of the debate is whether a combination of barely permeable corneocytes plus fairly permeable, isotropic SC lipids, or fairly permeable corneocytes plus strongly anisotropic SC lipids better represents the SC diffusion barrier. A readable discussion from several years back can be found in (136). This debate has sparked a great deal of interest from my colleague Prof. Johannes Nitsche at the University of Buffalo, as well as collaborators Prof. Ludwig Nitsche at the University of Illinois at Chicago and Profs. Arne Naegel and Gabriel Wittum at the University of Frankfurt (104, 105, 107). The recent experimental work from Kodiweera et al. (90, 91) combined with Barbero and Frasch's latest finite element analysis (123) seemed to have tipped the balance in favor of the anisotropic lipid position. Prof. Nitsche (J. M.) has also done his homework in studying the related problem in phospholipid membranes (137–140), for which anisotropy is more easily demonstrated. I am honored to be a part of this research.

I offer my apologies to those whose contributions have been omitted as I try to summarize the last 16 years of research into stratum corneum heterogeneity.

ACKNOWLEDGEMENTS

This work was supported by grant R01 OH007529 from the National Institute for Occupational Safety and Health, a branch of the U.S. Centers for Disease Control. We thank Shreekripa Balasubramanian and Arjun Santhanum for data and analysis associated with Figure 10.1 and Fred Frasch for a helpful discussion of membrane tortuosity. Ron Warner and Randall Wickett contributed significantly to the interpretation of the results.

REFERENCES

1. Lampe, M.A., Williams, M.L. and Elias, P.M. Human epidermal lipids: characterization and modulations during differentiation. J Lipid Res. 24:131–140 (1983).
2. Elias, P.M. Structure and function of the stratum corneum permeability barrier. *Drug Devel Res.* 13:97–105 (1988).
3. Steven, A.C., Bisher, M.E., Roop, D.R. and Steinert, P.M. Biosynthetic pathways of filaggrin and loricrin – two major proteins expressed by terminally differentiated epidermal keratinocytes. J Struc Biol. 104:150–162 (1990).

4. Nemes, Z. and Steinert, P.M. Bricks and mortar of the epidermal barrier. *Exp Molecular Med.* 31:5–19 (1999).

5. Wertz, P.W. Epidermal lipids. *Sem Dermatol.* 11:106–113 (1992).

6. Hill, J.R. and Wertz, P.W. Molecular models of the intercellular lipid lamellae from epidermal stratum corneum. *Biochem Biophys Act.* 1616:121–126 (2003).

7. Scheuplein, R.J. and Blank, I.H. Permeability of the skin. *Physiol Rev.* 51:702–747 (1971).

8. Flynn, G.L. Mechanism of percutaneous absorption from physicochemical evidence. In: Percutaneous Absorption (R.L. Bronaugh, H.I. Maibach, eds), pp. 27–51. Marcel Dekker, New York (1985).

9. Roberts, M.S., Triggs, E.J. and Anderson, R.A. Permeability of solutes through biological membranes measured by a desorption technique. 257:225–227 (1975).

10. Roberts, M.S., Anissimov, Y.G. and Gonsalvez, R.A. Mathematical models in percutaneous absorption. In: Percutaneous Absorption Drugs-Cosmetics-Mechanisms-Methodology (R.L. Bronaugh, H.I. Maibach, eds), pp. 3–56. Marcel Dekker, New York (1999).

11. Kasting, G.B., Smith, R.L. and Cooper, E.R. Effect of lipid solubility and molecular size on percutaneous absorption. *Skin Pharmacol.* 1:138–153 (1987).

12. Potts, R.O. and Guy, R.H. Predicting skin permeability. Pharm Res 9:663–669 (1992).

13. Wilschut, A., ten Berge, W.F., Robinson, P.J. and McKone, T.E. Estimating skin permeation. The validation of five mathematical skin penetration models. Chemosphere 30:1275–1296 (1995).

14. U.S. EPA. Guidelines for Exposure Assessment. Risk Assessment Forum, pp. 22888–938. Federal Register, Washington, DC (1992).

15. Cleek, R.L. and Bunge, A.L. A new method for estimating dermal absorption from chemical exposure. 1. General approach. *Pharm Res.* 10:497–506 (1993).

16. Johnson, M.E., Blankschtein, D. and Langer, R. Evaluation of solute permeation through the stratum corneum: lateral bilayer diffusion as the primary transport mechanism. J Pharm Sci 86:1162–1172 (1997).

17. Peck, K.D., Ghanem, A.-H. and Higuchi, W.I. Hindered diffusion of polar molecules through and effective pore radii estimates of intact and ethanol treated human epidermal membranes. *Pharm Res.* 11:1306–1314 (1994).

18. Peck, K.D., Ghanem, A.-H. and Higuchi, W.I. The effect of temperature upon the permeation of polar and ionic solutes through human epidermal membrane. J Pharm Sci 84:975–982 (1995).

19. Kasting, G.B., Smith, R.L. and Anderson, B.D. Prodrugs for dermal delivery: solubility, molecular size, and functional group effects. In: Prodrugs: Topical and Ocular Drug Delivery (K.B. Sloan, ed), pp. 117–161. Marcel Dekker, New York (1992).

20. Potts, R.O. and Guy, R.H. A predictive algorithm for skin permeability: the effects of molecular size and hydrogen bond activity. *Pharm Res.* 12:1628–1633 (1995).

21. Abraham, M.H., Martins, F. and Mitchell, R.C. Algorithms for skin permeability using hydrogen bond descriptors: The problem of steroids. *J Pharm Pharmacol.* 49:858–865 (1997).

22. Moss, G.P., Dearden, J.C., Patel, H. and Cronin, M.T.D. Quantitative structure-permeability relationships (QSPRs) for percutaneous absorption. *Toxicol in Vitro.* 16:299–317 (2002).

23. Geinoz, S., Guy, R.H., Testa, B. and Carrupt, P.-A. Quantitative structure-permeation relationships (QSPeRs) to predict skin permeation: a critical evaluation. *Pharm Res.* 21:83–92 (2004).

24. Degim, T., Hadgraft, J., Ilbasmis, S. and Ozkan, Y. Prediction of skin penetration using artificial neural networks (ANN) modeling. *J Pharm Sci.* 92:656–664 (2003).

25. Michaels, A.S., Chandrasekaran, S.K. and Shaw, J.E. Drug permeation through human skin: theory and in vitro experimental measurement. *Amer Inst Chem Eng J.* 21:985–996 (1975).

26. Talreja, P.S., Kleene, N.K., Pickens, W., Wang, T.-F. and Kasting, G.B. Visualization of lipid barrier and measurement of lipid path length in human stratum corneum. 3:Article 13 (2001).

27. Frasch, H.F. and Barbaro, A.M. Steady-state flux and lag time in the stratum corneum lipid pathway: results from finite element models. *J Pharm Sci.* 92:2196–2207 (2003).

28. Heisig, M., Lieckfeldt, R., Wittum, G., Mazurkevich, G. and Lee, G. Non steady-state descriptions of drug permeation through stratum corneum. I. The biphasic brick and mortar model. Pharm Res 13:421–426 (1996).

29. Wang, T.-F. Microscopic models for the structure and permeability of the stratum corneum barrier layer of skin. Ph.D. thesis, Department of Chemical Engineering. State University of New York; Buffalo (2003).

30. Elias, P.M. The epidermal permeability barrier: From the early days at Harvard to emerging concepts. J Invest Dermatol. 122:xxxvi–xxxix (2004).

31. Shelley, W.B. and Melton, F.M. Factors accelerating the penetration of histamine through normal intact human skin. *J Invest Dermatol.* 13(2):61–71 (1949).

32. Abramson, H.A. and Gorin, M.H. Skin reactions IX. The electrophoretic demonstration of the patent pores of the living human skin; its relation to the charge of the skin. J Phys Chem. 44:1094–1102 (1940).

33. Scheuplein, R.J. Skin permeation. In: The Physiology and Pathophysiology of the Skin (A. Jarrett, ed.), pp. 1669–1752. Academic Press, New York (1978).

34. Grimnes, S. Pathways of ionic flow through human skin in vivo. Acta Derm Venereol (Stockh) 64:93–98 (1984).

35. Cullander, C. and Guy, R.H. Sites of iontophoretic current flow into the skin: identification and characterization with the vibrating probe electrode. *J Invest Dermatol.* 97:55–64 (1991).

36. Burnette, R.R. and Ongpipattanakul, B. Characterization of the pore transport properties and tissue alteration of excised human skin during iontophoresis. *J Pharm Sci.* 77:132–137 (1988).

37. Kasting, G.B. Kinetics of finite dose absorption 1. Vanillylnonanamide. J Pharm Sci 90:202–212 (2001).

38. Kasting, G.B., Filloon, T.G., Francis, W.R. and Meredith, M.P. Improving the sensitivity of in vitro skin penetration experiments. *Pharm Res.* 11:1747–1754 (1994).

39. Scheuplein, R.J. Mechanism of percutaneous absorption II. Transient diffusion and the relative importance of various routes of skin penetration. *J Invest Dermatol.* 48:79–88 (1967).

40. Keister, J.C. and Kasting, G.B. The use of transient diffusion to investigate transport pathways through skin. 4:111–117 (1986).

41. Tur, E., Maibach, H.I. and Guy, R.H. Percutaneous penetration of methyl nicotinate at three anatomic sites: Evidence for appendageal transport? *Skin Pharmacol.* 4:230–234 (1991).

42. Bhatt, V. and Kasting, G.B. A model for estimating the absorption and evaporation rates of DEET from human skin. American Association of Pharmaceutical Scientists Annual Meeting, Salt Lake City, UT (2003).

43. Anderson, R.L., Cassidy, J.M., Hansen, J.R. and Yellin, W. Hydration of stratum corneum. J Invest Dermatol 12:2789–2802 (1973).

44. Blank, I.H., Moloney, J., Emslie, A.G., Simon, I. and Apt, C. The diffusion of water across the stratum corneum as a function of its water content. *J Invest Dermatol.* 82:183–194 (1984).

45. El-Shimi, A.F., Princen, H.M. and Risi, D.R. Water vapor sorption, desorption, and diffusion in excised skin: Part I. Technique. In: Applied Chemistry at Protein Interfaces (R.E. Baier, ed.), American Chemical Society, Washington (1975).

46. Anderson, R.L., Cassidy, J.M., Hansen, J.R. and Yellin, W. The effect of in vivo occlusion on human stratum corneum hydration-dehydration in vitro. Biopolymers 61:375–379 (1973).

47. Potts, R.O. and Francoeur, M. The influence of stratum corneum morphology on water permeability. J Invest Dermatol 96:495–499 (1991).

48. Bouwstra, J.A., Gooris, G.S., van der Spek, J.A. and Bras, W. Structural investigations of human stratum corneum by small angle X-ray scattering. J Invest Dermatol 97:1005–1012 (1991).

49. Packer, K.J. and Sellwood, T.C. Proton magnetic resonance studies of hydrated stratum corneum. Part 1. Spin-lattice and transverse relaxation. *Chem Soc J Faraday Trans.* 74:1579–1591 (1978).

50. Packer, K.J. and Sellwood, T.C. Proton magnetic resonance studies of hydrated stratum corneum. Part 2. Self-diffusion. *Chem Soc J Faraday Trans.* 74:1592–1606 (1978).

51. Kasting, G.B., Barai, N.D., Wang, T.-F. and Nitsche, J.M. Mobility of water in human stratum corneum. J Pharm Sci. 92:2326–2340 (2003).

52. Bodde, H.E., van den Brink, I., Koerten, H.K. and de Haan, F.H.N. Visualization of in vitro percutaneous penetration of mercuric chloride transport through intercellular space versus cellular uptake through desmosomes. *J Control Rel.* 15:227–236 (1991).

53. Monteiro-Riviere, N.A., Inman, A.O. and Riviere, J.E. Identification of the pathway of iontophoretic drug delivery: light and ultrastructural studies using mercuric chloride in pigs. *Pharmaceut Res.* 11:251–256 (1994).

54. Raykar, P.V., Fung, M.-C. and Anderson, B.D. The role of protein and lipid domains in the uptake of solutes by human stratum corneum. Pharm Res 5:140–150 (1988).

55. Anderson, B.D., Higuchi, W.I. and Raykar, P.V. Heterogeneity effects on permeability—partition coefficient relationships in human stratum corneum. Pharm Res 5:566–573 (1988).

56. Roberts, M.S., Pugh, W.J., Hadgraft, J. and Watkinson, A.C. Epidermal permeability-penetrant structure relationships: 1. An analysis of methods of predicting penetration of monofunctional solutes from aqueous solutions. Int J Pharm. 126:219–233 (1995).

57. Hansch, C. and Leo, A. MEDCHEM database and CLOGP 2.0. BioByte, Inc., (1999).

58. Christophers, E. and Kligman, A.M. Visualization of the cell layers of the stratum corneum. J Invest Dermatol 42:407–409 (1964).

59. Blank, I.H. Factors which influence the water content of the stratum corneum. J Invest Dermatol 18:433–440 (1952).

60. Scheuplein, R.J. Mechanism of percutaneous absorption I. Routes of penetration and the influence of solubility. J Invest Dermatol. 45:334–346 (1965).

61. Blank, I.H., Scheuplein, R.J. and MacFarlane, D.J. Mechanism of percutaneous absorption III. The effect of temperature on the transport of non-electrolytes across the skin. J Invest Dermatol 49:582–589 (1967).

62. Scheuplein, R.J. Molecular structure and diffusional processes across intact epidermis. U.S. Army Edgewood Arsenal (1967).

63. Scheuplein, R.J. and Morgan, L.J. "Bound water" in keratin membranes measured by a microbalance technique. Nature 214:456–458 (1967).

64. Brody, I. The ultrastructure of the horny layer in normal and psoriatic epidermis as revealed by electron microscopy. J Invest Dermatol. 39:519 et seq. (1963).

65. Odland, G.F. The fine structure of the inter-relationship of cells in the human epidermis. J Biophys Biochem Cytol. 4:529 et seq. (1958).

66. Blair, C. Morphology and thickness of the human stratum corneum. Brit J Dermatol 80:430–436 (1968).

67. Monash, S. and Blank, I.H. Location and reformation of the epithelial barrier to water transport. Arch Dermatol (Chicago). 78:710 et seq. (1958).

68. Kalia, Y.N., Pirot, F. and Guy, R.H. Homogeneous transport in a heterogeneous membrane: water diffusion across human stratum corneum in vivo. Biophys J. 71:2692–2700 (1996).

69. Pirot, F., Kalia, Y.N., Stinchcomb, A.L., Keating, G., Bunge, A. and Guy, R.H. Characterization of the permeability barrier of human skin in vivo. *Proc Nat Acad Sci USA*. 94:1562–1567 (1997).

70. Pirot, F., Berardesca, E., Kalia, Y.N., Singh, M., Maibach, H.I. and Guy, R.H. Stratum corneum thickness and apparent water diffusivity: facile and noninvasive quantitation in vivo. Pharm Res. 15:492–494 (1998).

71. Warner, R.R., Stone, K.J. and Boissy, Y.L. Hydration disrupts human stratum corneum ultrastructure. J Invest Dermatol. 120:275–284 (2003).

72. Bowser, P.A. and White, R.J. Isolation, barrier properties and lipid analysis of stratum compactum, a discrete region of the stratum corneum. Brit J Dermatol. 112:1–14 (1985).

73. Warner, R.R., Stone, K.J. and Boissy, Y.L. Hydration disrupts human stratum corneum ultrastructure. J Invest Dermatol 110:675 (1998).

74. Bouwstra, J.A., de Graaff, A., Gooris, G.S., Nijsse, J., Wiechers, J.W. and van Aelst, A.C. Water distribution and related morphology in human stratum corneum at different hydration levels. J Invest Dermatol. 120:750–758 (2003).

75. Stockdale, M. Water diffusion coefficients versus water activity in stratum corneum: a correlation and its implications. J Soc Cosmet Chem 29:625–639 (1978).

76. El-Shimi, A.F. and Princen, H.M. Water vapor sorption and desorption behavior of some keratins. Colloid Polym Sci. 256:105–114 (1978).

77. El-Shimi, A.F. and Princen, H.M. Diffusion characteristics of water vapor in some keratins. Colloid Polym Sci. 256:209–217 (1978).

78. Kasting, G.B. and Barai, N.D. Equilibrium water sorption in human stratum corneum. J Pharm Sci. 92:1624–1631 (2003).

79. Harding, C.R., Long, S., Richardson, J., Rogers, J., Zhang, Z., Bush, A., and Rawlings, A.V. The cornified cell envelope: an important marker of stratum corneum maturation in healthy and dry skin. Int J Cosmet Sci. 25:157–167 (2003).

80. Crank, J. The Mathematics of Diffusion. 2nd ed. Clarendon Press, Oxford (1975).

81. Cooper, E.R. and Berner, B. Skin permeability. In: Methods in Skin Research. (D. Skerrow, C.J. Skerrow, eds), pp. 407–432. John Wiley and Sons, New York (1985).

82. Mitragotri, S. In situ determination of partition and diffusion coefficients in the lipid bilayers of stratum corneum. Pharm Res 17:1026–1029 (2000).

83. Anissimov, Y.G. and Roberts, M.S. Diffusion modeling of percutaneous absorption kinetics: 3. Variable diffusion and partition coefficients, consequences for stratum corneum depth profiles and desorption kinetics. J Pharm Sci. 93:470–487 (2004).

84. Mueller, B., Anissimov, Y.G. and Roberts, M.S. Unexpected clobetasol propionate profile in human stratum corneum after topical application in vitro. Pharm Res. 20:1835–1837 (2003).

85. Charman, W.N., Lai, C.S.C., Finnin, B.C. and Reed, B.L. Self-association of nicotinamide in aqueous solution: mass transport, freezing-point depression, and partition coefficient studies. Pharm Res. 8:1144–1150 (1991).
86. Talreja, P.S. Determination of transport pathways in human stratum corneum: micro and macro measurements. MS thesis. College of Pharmacy, University of Cincinnati, Cincinnati, OH (2000).
87. Barai, N.D. Effect of hydration on skin permeability. MS thesis. College of Pharmacy, University of Cincinnati, Cincinnati, OH (2002).
88. Rougier, A., Lotte, C. and Maibach, H.I. In vivo percutaneous penetration of some organic compounds related to anatomic site in humans: predictive assessment by the stripping method. J Pharm Sci. 76:451–454 (1987).
89. Warner, R.R., Myers, M.C. and Taylor, D.A. Electron probe analysis of human skin: Determination of water concentration profile. J Invest Dermatol 90:218–224 (1988).
90. Kodiweera, C., Romonchuk, W., Yang, Y. and Bunge, A. Characterization of water and a model lipophilic compound in human stratum corneum by NMR spectroscopy and equilibrium sorption. J Pharm Sci 105:3376–3386 (2016).
91. Kodiweera, C., Yang, Y. and Bunge, A.L. Characterization of water self-diffusion in human stratum corneum. J Pharm Sci. 107:1131–1142 (2018).
92. Miller, M.A., Yu, F., Kim, K.-I. and Kasting, G.B. Uptake and desorption of hydrophilic compounds from human stratum corneum. J Control Rel. 261:307–317 (2017).
93. Yu, F. and Kasting, G.B. A geometrical model for transport of hydrophilic compounds in human stratum corneum. Math Biosci. 300:55–63 (2018).
94. Otberg, N., Patzelt, A., Rasulev, U., Hagemeister, T., Linscheid, M., Sinkgraven, R., et al. The role of hair follicles in the percutaneous absorption of caffeine. Brit J Clin Pharmacol. 65 488–492 (2008).
95. Teichmann, A., Otberg, N., Jacobi, U., Sterry, W. and Lademann, J. Follicular penetration: development of a method to block the follicles selectively against the penetration of topically applied substances. Skin Pharmacol Physiol. 19:216–223 (2006).
96. Patzelt, A. and Lademann, J. Drug delivery to hair follicles. Expert Opin Drug Deliv. 10:787–797 (2013).
97. Patzelt, A. and Lademann, J. The increasing importance of the hair follicle route in dermal and transdermal drug delivery. In: Percutaneous Penetration Enhancers Chemical Methods in Penetration Enhancement: Drug Manipulation Strategies and Vehicle Effects (N. Dragicevic, H.I. Maibach, eds), pp. 43–53. Springer-Verlag, Berlin (2015).
98. Mohd, F., Todo, H., Yoshimoto, M., Yusuf, E. and Sugibayashi, K. Contribution of the hair follicular pathway to total skin permeation of topically applied and exposed chemicals. Pharmaceutics 8:32–44 (2016).
99. Muhammad, F., Brooks, J.D. and Riviere, J.E. Comparative mixture effects of JP-8(100) additives on the dermal absorption and disposition of jet fuel hydrocarbons in different membrane model systems. Toxicol Lett. 150:351–365 (2004).
100. Riviere, J.E. and Brooks, J.D. Predicting skin permeability from complex chemical mixtures. Toxicol Appl Pharmacol. 208:99–110 (2005).
101. Karadzovska, D., Brooks, J.D., Monteiro-Riviere, N.A. and Riviere, J.E. Predicting skin permeability from complex vehicles *Adv Drug Del Revs.* 65:265–277 (2013).
102. Baba, H., Ueno, Y., Hashida, M. and Yamashita, F. Quantitative prediction of ionization effect on human skin permeability. Int J Pharm. 522:222–233 (2017).
103. Ashrafi, P., Sun, Y., Davey, N., Wilkinson, S.C. and Moss, G.P. The influence of diffusion cell type and experimental temperature on machine learning models of skin permeability J Pharm Pharmacol. 72:197–208 (2020).
104. Wang, T.-F., Kasting, G.B. and Nitsche, J.M. A multiphase microscopic model for stratum corneum permeability. I. Formulation, solution and illustrative results for representative compounds. J Pharm Sci. 95:620–648 (2006).
105. Wang, T.-F., Kasting, G.B. and Nitsche, J.M. A multiphase microscopic model for stratum corneum permeability. II. Estimation of physicochemical parameters and application to a large permeability database. J Pharm Sci. 96:3024–3051 (2007).
106. Nitsche, J.M. and Frasch, H.F. Dynamics of diffusion with reversible binding in microscopically heterogeneous membranes: general theory and applications to dermal penetration. Chem Eng Sci. 66:2019–2041 (2011).
107. Nitsche, L.C., Kasting, G.B. and Nitsche, J.M. Microscopic models of drug/chemical diffusion through the skin barrier: Effects of diffusional anisotropy of the intercellular lipid. J Pharm Sci. 108:1692–1712 (2019).

108. Naegel, A., Hansen, S., Neumann, D., Lehr, C.-M., Schaefer, U.F., Wittum, G., et al. In-silico model of skin penetration based on experimentally determined input parameters. Part II. Mathematical modelling of in-vitro diffusion experiments. Identification of critical input parameters. Eur J Pharm Biopharm. 68:368–379 (2007).

109. Muha, I., Naegel, A., Stichel, S., Grillo, A., Heisig, M. and Wittum, G. Effective diffusivity in membranes with tetrakaidekahedral cells and implications for the permeability of human stratum corneum. J Membr Sci. 368:18–25 (2011).

110. Van der Merwe, D., Brooks, J.D. and Riviere, J.E. A physiologically based pharmacokinetic model of organophosphate dermal absorption. Toxicol Sci. 89:188–204 (2006).

111. Kasting, G.B. and Miller, M.A. Kinetics of finite dose absorption through skin 2. Volatile compounds. *J Pharm Sci.* 95:268–280 (2006).

112. Anissimov, Y.G. and Roberts, M.S. Diffusion modelling of percutaneous absorption kinetics: 4. Effects of a slow equilibration process within stratum corneum on absorption and desorption kinetics. J Pharm Sci. 98:772–781 (2009).

113. Petlin, D.G., Rybachuk, M. and Anissimov, Y.G. Pathway distribution model for solute transport in stratum corneum. J Pharm Sci. 104:4443–4447 (2015).

114. Frasch, H.F. and Barbero, A.M. The transient dermal exposure: theory and experimental examples using skin and silicone membranes. J Pharm Sci. 97:1578–1592 (2008).

115. Frasch, H.F. and Bunge, A.L. The transient dermal exposure II: post-exposure absorption and evaporation of volatile compounds. J Pharm Sci. 104: 1499–1507 (2015).

116. Kruse, J., Golden, D., Wilkinson, S., Williams, F., Kezic, S. and Corish, J. Analysis, interpretation, and extrapolation of dermal permeation data using diffusion-based mathematical models. J Pharm Sci 96:682–703 (2007).

117. Kasting, G.B., Miller, M.A. and Bhatt, V. A spreadsheet-based method for estimating the skin disposition of volatile compounds: application to N,N-diethyl-m-toluamide (DEET). J Occup Environ Hyg. 10:633–644 (2008).

118. Dancik, Y., Miller, M.A., Jaworska, J. and Kasting, G.B. Design and performance of a spreadsheet-based model for estimating bioavailability of chemicals from dermal exposure Adv Drug Deliv Rev. 65:221–236 (2013).

119. Frasch, H., Barbero, A., Hettick, J. and Nitsche, J. Tissue binding affects the kinetics of theophylline diffusion through the stratum corneum barrier layer of skin. J Pharm Sci. 100:2989–2995 (2011).

120. Chittendon, J.T., Brooks, J.D. and Riviere, J.E. Development of a mixed-effect pharmacokinetic model for vehicle modulated in vitro transdermal flux of topically applied penetrants. J Pharm Sci. 103:1002–1012 (2014).

121. Barbero, A.M. and Frasch, H.F. Transcellular route of diffusion through stratum corneum: Results from finite element models. J Pharm Sci. 95:2186–2194 (2006).

122. Barbaro, A.M. and Frasch, H.F. Modeling of diffusion with partitioning in stratum corneum using a finite element model. Ann Biomed Eng. 33:1281–1292 (2005).

123. Barbero, A.M. and Frasch, H.F. Effect of stratum corneum heterogeneity, anisotropy, asymmetry and follicular pathway on transdermal penetration. J Control Rel. 260:234–246 (2017).

124. Chen, L.J., Lian, G.P. and Han, L.J. Use of "bricks and mortar" model to predict transdermal permeation: Model development and initial validation. Ind Eng Chem Res. 47:6465–6472 (2008).

125. Chen, L., Lian, G. and Han, L. Modeling transdermal permeation. Part I. Predicting skin permeability of both hydrophobic and hydrophilic solutes. AIChE J. 56:1136–1146 (2010).

126. Chen, L., Han, L. and Lian, G. Recent advances in predicting skin permeability of hydrophilic solutes. Adv Drug Deliv Rev. 65:295–305 (2013).

127. Chen, L., Han, L., Saib, O. and Lian, G. In silico prediction of percutaneous absorption and disposition kinetics of chemicals. Pharmaceut Res. 32:1779–1793 (2015).

128. Kattou, P., Lian, G., Glavin, S., Sorrell, I. and Chen, T. Development of a two-dimensional model for predicting transdermal permeation with the follicular pathway: demonstration with a caffeine study. Pharm Res. 34:2036–2048 (2017).

129. Hansen, S., Selzer, D., Schaefer, U.F. and Kasting, G.B. An extended database of keratin binding. J Pharm Sci. 100:1712–1726 (2011).

130. Seif, S. and Hansen, S. Measuring the stratum corneum reservoir: desorption kinetics from keratin. J Pharm Sci. 101:3718–3728 (2012).

131. Kasting, G.B., Miller, M.A., LaCount, T.D. and Jaworska, J. A composite model for the transport of hydrophilic and lipophilic compounds across the skin. J Pharm Sci. 108:337–349 (2019).

132. Miller, M.A. and Kasting, G.B. A spreadsheet-based method for simultaneously estimating the disposition of multiple ingredients applied to skin. J Pharm Sci. 104:2047–2055 (2015).

133. Mitragotri, S., Anissimov, Y.G., Bunge, A.L., Frasch, H.F., Guy, R.H., Hadgraft, J., et al. Mathematical models of skin permeability: An overview. Int J Pharm. 418:115–129 (2011).

134. Frasch, H.F., Bunge, A.L., Chen, C.-P., Cherrie, J.W., Dotson, G.S., Kasting, G.B., et al. Analysis of finite dose dermal absorption data: implications for dermal exposure assessment. J Exposure Sci Environ Epidem. 24:65–73 (2014).

135. Kissel, J.C., Bunge, A.L., Frasch, H.F. and Kasting, G.B. Dermal exposure and absorption of chemicals. In: Comprehensive Toxicology, 3rd ed. Vol. 1, pp. 112–127 Elsevier (2018): Oxford, UK.

136. Kasting, G. and Nitsche, J.M. Mathematical models of skin permeability: microscopic transport models and their predictions In: Computational Biophysics of the Skin (B. Querleux, ed.), pp. 187–215. Pan Stanford Publishing, Singapore (2014).

137. Nitsche, J.M. and Kasting, G.B. Permeability of fluid-phase phospholipid bilayers: assessment and useful correlations for permeability screening and other applications. J Pharm Sci. 102:2005–2032 (2013).

138. Nitsche, J.M. and Kasting, G.B. A correlation for 1,9-decadiene/water partition coefficients. J Pharm Sci. 102 136–144 (2013).

139. Nitsche, J.M. and Kasting, G.B. A critique of Abraham and Acree's correlation for 1,9-decadiene/water partition coefficients. New J Chem. 37:283–285 (2013).

140. Nitsche, J.M. and Kasting, G.B. A universal correlation predicts permeability coefficients of fluid- and gel-phase phospholipid and phospholipid-cholesterol bilayers for arbitrary solutes. J Pharm Sci 105:1762–1771 (2016).

11 Regional Variation in Percutaneous Absorption

Principles and Applications to Human Risk Assessment

Ronald C. Wester and Howard I. Maibach
University of California, San Francisco, California

CONTENTS

11.1 INTRODUCTION

The first occupational disease in recorded history was scrotal cancer in chimney sweepers (1). The historical picture of a male worker holding a sweeper and covered from head to toe with black soot is vivid. But why the scrotum?

Percutaneous absorption in man and animals varies depending on the area of the body on which the chemical resides. This is called regional variation. When a certain skin area is exposed, any effect of the chemical will be determined by how much is absorbed through the skin. Where systemic drug delivery is desired, such as transdermal delivery, a high-absorbing area may be desirable to deliver sufficient drug. Scopolamine transdermal systems are supposedly placed in the postauricular area (behind the ear) because at this skin site the percutaneous absorption of scopolamine is sufficiently enhanced to deliver effective quantities of the drug. A third example is with estimating human health hazard effects of environmental contaminants. This could be pesticide residue on exposed parts of the skin (head, face, neck, and hands) and trying to determine the amount of pesticide that might be absorbed into the body. The estimate for skin absorption is an integral part of the estimate for potential hazard; thus, accuracy of estimate is very relevant.

Therefore, when considering skin absorption in humans, the site of application is important. Principles are reviewed and examples of applications to human risk assessment are given. Human risk assessment assigns a number to skin absorption and multiplies by skin area involved. This should include human anatomy and clothing worn.

11.2 REGIONAL VARIATION IN HUMANS

Feldmann and Maibach (2) were the first to systematically explore the potential for regional variation in percutaneous absorption. The first absorption studies were done with the ventral forearm because this site is convenient to use. However, skin exposure to chemicals exists over the entire body. They first showed regional variation with the absorption of hydrocortisone (Figure 11.1).

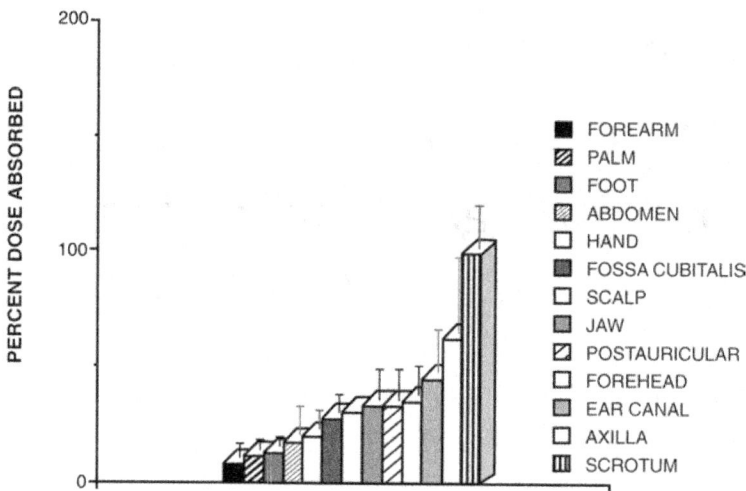

FIGURE 11.1   Anatomic regional variation with parathion percutaneous absorption in humans.

The scrotum was the highest- absorbing skin site (scrotal cancer in chimney sweeps is the key). Skin absorption was lowest for the foot area and highest around the head and face.

Table 11.1 gives the percutaneous absorption of pesticides in humans by anatomical region (3). There are two major points in this study. First, regional variation was confirmed with two different chemicals: parathion and malathion. Second, those skin areas that would be exposed to the pesticides, the head and face, were among the higher-absorbing sites. The body areas most exposed to environmental contaminants are the areas with the higher skin absorption.

Table 11.2 gives site variability for parathion skin absorption with time. Soap and water wash in the first few minutes after exposure is not a perfect decontaminant. Site variation is apparent early in skin exposure (4).

Guy and Maibach (5) took the hydrocortisone and pesticide data and constructed penetration indices for five anatomical sites (Table 11.3). These indices should be used with their total surface areas (Table 11.4) when estimating systemic availability relative to body exposure sites.

TABLE 11.1
Effect of Anatomical Region on In Vivo Percutaneous Absorption of Pesticides in Humans

Anatomical Region	Dose Absorbed (%)		
	Hydrocortisone	Parathion	Malathion
Forearm	1.0	8.6	6.8
Palm	0.8	11.8	5.8
Foot, ball	0.2	13.5	6.8
Abdomen	1.3	18.5	9.4
Hand, dorsum	—	21.0	12.5
Forehead	7.6	36.3	23.2
Axilla	3.1	64.0	28.7
Jaw angle	12.2	33.9	69.9
Fossal cubitalis	—	28.4	—
Scalp	4.4	32.1	—
Ear canal	—	46.6	—
Scrotum	36.2	101.6	—

TABLE 11.2
Site Variation and Decontamination Time for Parathion

Skin Residence Time Before Soap and Water Wash	Parathion Dose Absorbed[a] (%)		
	Arm	Forehead	Palm
1 min	2.8	8.4	—
5 min	—	—	6.2
15 min	6.7	7.1	13.6
30 min	—	12.2	13.3
1 hr	8.4	10.5	11.7
4 hr	8.0	27.7	7.7
24 hr	8.6	36.3	11.8

[a] Each value is a mean for four volunteers. The fact that there were different volunteers at each time point accounts for some of the variability with time for each skin site.

TABLE 11.3
Penetration Indices for Five Anatomical Sites Assessed Using Hydrocortisone Skin Penetration Data and Pesticide (Malathion and Parathion) Absorption Results

Site	Penetration Index Based On	
	Hydrocortisone Data	Pesticide Data
Genitals	40	12
Arms	1	1
Legs	0.5	1
Trunk	2.5	3
Head	5	4

TABLE 11.4
Body Surface Areas Distributed Over Five Anatomical Regions for Adults and Neonates

Anatomical Region	Adult		Neonate	
	Body Area (%)	Area (cm²)	Body Area (%)	Area (cm²)
Genitals	1	190	1	19
Arms	18	3420	19	365
Legs	36	6840	30	576
Trunk	36	6840	31	595
Head	9	1710	19	365
Totals		19,000		1920

TABLE 11.5

Absorption Indices of Hydrocortisone and Pesticides (Parathion/Malathion) Calculated by Guy and Maibach (5) Compared with Absorption Indices of Pyrene and PAH for Different Anatomical Sites by Van Rooy et al. (6)

	Absorption Index			
Anatomical Site	Hydrocortisone[a]	Pesticides[b]	Pyrene[c]	PAH[d]
Genitals	40	12	—	—
Arm	1	1	1	1
Hand	1	1	0.8	0.5
Leg/ankle	0.5	1	1.2	0.8/0.5
Trunk/shoulder	2.5	3	1.1	/2.0
Head/neck	5	4	/1.3	1.0

[a] Based on hydrocortisone penetration data (2).
[b] Based on parathion and malathion absorption data (3).
[c] Based on excreted amount of I–OH–pyrene in urine after coal tar ointment application (6).
[d] Based on the PAH absorption rate constant (K_a) after coal tar ointment application (6).
Abbreviation: PAH, polycyclic aromatic hydrocarbons.

Van Rooy et al. (6) applied coal tar ointment to various skin areas of volunteers and determined absorption of polycyclic aromatic hydrocarbons (PAHs) by surface disappearance of PAH and the excretion of urinary I–OH–pyrene. Using PAH disappearance, skin ranking (highest to lowest) was shoulder > forearm > forehead > groin > hand (palmar) > ankle. Using I–OH–pyrene excretion, skin ranking (highest to lowest) was neck > calf > forearm > trunk > hand. Table 11.5 compares their results with Guy and Maibach (5).

In another study, Wester et al. (7) determined the percutaneous absorption of paraquat in humans. Absorption was the same for the leg ($0.29 \pm 0.02\%$), hand ($0.23 \pm 0.1\%$), and forearm ($0.29 \pm 0.1\%$). Here, the chemical nature of the low- absorbing paraquat overcame any regional variation.

Rougier et al. (8) examined the influence of anatomical site on the relationship between total penetration of benzoic acid in humans and the quantity present in the stratum corneum 30 minutes after application. Total penetration of benzoic acid varied according to anatomical site. There was correlation between the level of penetration of benzoic acid within four days and its level in the stratum corneum after a 30-minute application relative to anatomical site.

Wertz et al. (9) determined regional variation in permeability through human and pig skin and oral mucosa (Table 11.6). In the oral mucosa of both species, permeability ranked floor of mouth > buccal mucosa > palate. Skin remains a greater barrier, absorption of which been some tenfold less than oral mucosa.

TABLE 11.6

Permeability Constants for the Diffusion of ^3H_2O Through Human and Porcine Skin and Oral Mucosa

	K_p (10^{-7} cm/min) (mean ± standard error)	
Site	Human	Pig
Skin	44 ± 4	62 ± 5
Palate	450 ± 27	364 ± 18
Buccal	579 ± 16	634 ± 19
Floor of mouth	973 ± 3	808 ± 23

TABLE 11.7
Site Variation in Transdermal Delivery

Transdermal Drug	Body Site	Reason
Nitroglycerin Scopolamine	Chest Postauricular	Psychological: the patch is placed over the heart Scientific: behind the ear was found to be the best absorbing area
`Estradiol Testosterone	Trunk	Convenience: easy to place, and out of view Scientific: highest
Testosterone	Scrotum	skin absorbing area Scientific/convenience: removal from
	Trunk	trunk skin is easier than scrotal skin

The barrier properties of skin relative to oral mucosa have been a benefit for longer-term transdermal delivery. Nitroglycerine buccal tablets are effective for about 20 minutes due to rapid buccal absorption. In contrast, transdermal nitroglycerin is prescribed for 24 hours of continuous-dose delivery. The transdermal nitroglycerin patch is placed on the chest more for psychological reasons than that related to scientific regional variation skin absorption. Some transdermal systems take advantage of regional variation skin absorption, and some do not (Table 11.7).

Shriner and Maibach (10) studied skin contact irritation and showed that areas of significant response were neck > perioral > forehead. The volar forearm was the least sensitive of eight areas tested. This is in contrast to the commonly held belief that the forearm is one of the best locations to test for immediate contact irritation.

11.3 REGIONAL VARIATION IN ANIMALS

Percutaneous absorption data obtained in man are most relevant for human exposure. However, many estimates for humans are made from animal models. Therefore, regional variation in animals may affect prediction for humans. Also, if regional variation exists in an animal, that variation should be relative to humans.

Bronaugh (11) reported the effect of body site (back vs. abdomen) on male rat skin permeability. Abdominal rat skin was more permeable to water, urea, and cortisone. Skin thickness (stratum corneum, whole epidermis, and whole skin) is less in the abdomen than in the back. With the hairless mouse, Behl et al. (12) showed dorsal skin to be more permeable than abdominal skin (reverse that of the male rat) (Table 11.8). Hairless mouse abdominal skin is thicker than dorsal skin (also reverse that of the male rat) (Table 11.8).

TABLE 11.8
Effect of Body Site on Rat Skin Permeability

Compound	Permeability Constant (cm/hr $\times$ 10^4)
Water	
Back	4.9 ± 0.4
Abdomen	13.1 ± 2.1
Urea	
Back	1.6 ± 0.5
Abdomen	18.8 ± 5.5
Cortisone	
Back	1.7 ± 0.4
Abdomen	12.2 ± 0.6

TABLE 11.9

Percutaneous Absorption of Fenitrothion, Aminocarb, DEET, and Testosterone in the Rhesus Monkey and Rat

Chemical	Species	Applied Dose Absorbed (%) Skin Site		
		Forehead	Forearm	Back
Fenitrothion	Rhesus	49	21	
	Rat			84
Aminocarb	Rhesus	74	37	
	Rat			88
Testosterone	Rhesus	20.4[a]	8.8	
	Rat			47.4
DEET	Rhesus	33	14	
	Rat			36

[a] Scalp.

Skin absorption in the rhesus monkey is considered to be relevant to that of humans. Table 11.9 shows the percutaneous absorption of testosterone (13), fenitrothion, aminocarb, and diethyltoluamide (DEET) (14) (Moody et al., personal communication, 1988) in the rhesus monkey compared with the rat. What is interesting is that for the rhesus monkey there is regional variation between forehead (scalp) and forearm. If one determines the ratio of forehead (scalp/forearm for the rhesus monkey) and compares the results with humans, the similarities are the same (Table 11.10). Therefore, the rhesus monkey probably is a relevant animal model for human skin regional variation.

11.4 APPLICATIONS TO HUMAN RISK ASSESSMENT

Chemical warfare agents (CWAs) are easily and inexpensively produced and are a significant threat to military forces and to the public. The most well-known CWAs are organophosphorus compounds, a number of which are used as pesticides, including parathion. This study determined the in vitro percutaneous absorption of parathion as a CWA stimulant through naked human skin and uniformed skin (dry and sweated). Parathion percentage dose absorbed through naked skin (1.78 ± 0.41) was greater than dry uniformed skin (0.29 ± 0.17; $p = 0.000$) and sweated uniformed

TABLE 11.10

Percutaneous Absorption Ratio for Scalp and Forehead to Forearm in Humans and Rhesus Monkey

Chemical	Species	Percutaneous Absorption Ratio	
		Scalp/Forearm	Forehead/Forearm
Hydrocortisone	Human	3.5	6.0
Benzoic acid	Human		2.9
Parathion	Human	3.7	4.2
Malathion	Human		3.4
Testosterone	Rhesus	2.3	
Fenitrothion	Rhesus		2.3
Aminocarb	Rhesus		2.0
DEET	Rhesus		2.4

TABLE 11.11
VX Systemic Absorption and Toxicity to Uniformed Military Personnel

Exposure time (hr)	Body Exposure	Calculated VX Systemic Dose[a]	
		Compromised[b] (mg)	Protected[c] (mg)
1	Head/neck[d]	4.16	4.16
	Arms and hands[d]	0.52	0.52
	Trunk	4.07	1.35
	Genital-s	0.45	0.15
	Legs	0.68	0.22
	Total	9.87	6.40
8	Head/neck[d]	33.26	33.26
	Arms and hands[d]	4.16	4.16
	Trunk	32.52	10.77
	Genital-s	3.61	1.2
	Legs	5.42	1.8
	Total	78.98	51.18
96	Head/neck[d]	399.16	399.16
	Arms and hands[d]	49.90	49.90
	Trunk	390.29	129.25
	Genital-s	43.37	14.36
	Legs	65.05	21.54
	Total	947.76	614.21

Note: Estimated systemic LD50 of VX is 6.5 mg (human, 70 kg). Systemic concentration is more than 50% lethality dose.

[a] Dose: 4 μg/cm^2 on whole body area (1.8 m^2).
[b] Compromised: uniform with perspiration.
[c] Protected: dry uniform.
[d] Head/neck and arms and hands are unprotected.

skin (0.65 ± 0.16; $p = 0.000$). Sweated and dry uniformed skin absorption was also different ($p = 0.007$) (Table 11.11). These relative dry and sweated uniformed skin absorptions were then applied to VX skin permeability for naked skin (head, neck, arms, and hands) and the remaining uniformed skin over the various regions of the human body. Risk assessment shows VX 50% lethality within the first hour for a soldier wearing a sweated uniform. By eight-hour postexposure to naked skin plus trunk area, lethality was predicted for both dry and sweated uniform, and at 96-hour postexposure, all body regions individually exposed would produce lethality (15).

A second example of human regional variation application is that of permethrin bioavailability and body burden for the uniformed soldier. Permethrin is embedded in military uniform material and is available to the soldier in spray cans for unprotected skin. Permethrin repels insects that could be carrying disease. Permethrin, by design a pesticide, is also toxic. Table 11.12 summarizes predicted permethrin human bioavailability from uniformed and exposed skin at 1.24 mg/kg body burden. The NOEL estimates from animal studies were? at 5 mg/kg, giving a fivefold safety margin.

11.5 CONCLUSION

This chapter outlines 30 years of progress. Careful review of the data shows some general trends; however, most parts of various animal skins have not been explored, and many possible special areas in humans remain unstudied, i.e., finger and toe nails, eyelids, perirectal skin, upper versus lower arm, thigh versus leg, and so on. It is hoped that as more complete maps are available that

TABLE 11.12

Permethrin Bioavailability and Body Burden for Uniformed Soldier

Human Part	Body Surface Area (cm²)	Permethrin Dose[a] (µg/cm²)	Percutaneous Absorption[b]	Body Region Index[c]	Uniform Effect[d]	Total (µg)
Head	1180	4	0.087	×4	1	1642.56
Neck	420	4	0.087	×4	1	584.64
Trunk	5690	125	0.087	×3	0.29	53,834.51
Arms	2280	125	0.087	×1	0.29	7190.55
Hands	840	4	0.087	×1	1	292.32
Genitals	180	125	0.087	×12	0.29	6812.10
Legs	5050	125	0.087	×1	0.29	15,926.44
Feet	1120	4	0.087	×1	1	389.76
Total (µg)						86,672.88
Total (mg)						86.67
Total body burden (mg/70 kg soldier)						1.24 mg/kg

[a] Uniform = 125 µg/cm² (NRC 1994)/spray open skin 4 µg/cm².

[b] 8.7% (0.087) permethrin dose absorbed.

[c] Region body absorption index.

[d] The 0.29 is 29% absorption from cloth relative to open skin (index).

cover a range of chemical moieties, we should be in a position to further refine those aspects of der-matopharmacology and dermatotoxicology that require knowledge of skin penetration. However, the data are sufficient to make reasonable estimates from regional variation percutaneous absorp-tion applied to human risk assessment. Proper risk assessment should also include absorption from clothing, because that is what exists.

REFERENCES

1. Wester RC. Twenty absorbing years. In: Surber C, Elsner P, Bircher AJ, eds. Exogenous Dermatology. Basel: Karger, 1995:112–123.
2. Feldmann RJ, Maibach HI. Regional variation in percutaneous penetration of (14C) cortisol in man. J Invest Dermatol 1967; 48:181–183.
3. Maibach HI, Feldmann RJ, Milby TH, Sert WF. Regional variation in percutaneous penetration in man. Arch Environ Health 1971; 23:208–211.
4. Wester RC, Maibach HI. In vivo percutaneous absorption and decontamination of pesticides in humans. J Toxicol Environ Health 1985; 16:25–37.
5. Guy RH, Maibach HI. Calculations of body exposure from percutaneous absorption data. In: Bronaugh RL, Maibach HI, eds. Percutaneous Absorption. New York: Marcel Dekker, 1985:461–466.
6. Van Rooy TGM, De Roos JHC, Bodelier-Bode MM, Jongeneelen FJ. Absorption of polycyclic aro-matic hydrocarbons through human skin: differences between anatomic sites and individuals. J Toxicol Environ Health 1993; 38:355–368.
7. Wester RC, Maibach HI, Bucks DAW, Aufrere MB. In vivo percutaneous absorption of paraquat from hand, leg and forearm of humans. J Toxicol Environ Health 1984; 14:759–762.
8. Rougier A, Dupuis D, Lotte C, Roquet R, Wester RC, Maibach HI. Regional variation in percutaneous absorption in man: measurement by the stripping method. Arch Dermatol Res 1986; 278:465–469.
9. Wertz PW, Swartzendruber DC, Squier CA. Regional variation in the structure and permeability of oral mucosa and skin. Adv Drug Deliv Rev 1993; 12:1–12.
10. Shriner DL, Maibach HI. Regional variation of nonimmunological contact urticaria. Skin Pharmacol 1996; 348:1–11.
11. Bronaugh RL. Determination of percutaneous absorption by in vitro techniques. In: Bronaugh RL, Maibach HI, eds. Percutaneous Absorption. New York: Marcel Dekker, 1985:267–279.

12. Behl CR, Bellantone NH, Flynn GL. Influence of age on percutaneous absorption of drug substances. In: Bronaugh RL, Maibach HI, eds. Percutaneous Absorption. New York: Marcel Dekker, 1985:183–212.

13. Wester RC, Noonan PK, Maibach HI. Variation on percutaneous absorption of testosterone in the Rhesus monkey due to anatomic site of application and frequency of application. Arch Dermatol Res 1980; 267:229–235.

14. Moody RP, Franklin CA. Percutaneous absorption of the insecticides fenitrothion and aminocarb. J Toxicol Environ Health 1987; 20:209–219.

15. Wester RM, Tanjo H, Maibach HI, Wester RC. Predicted chemical warfare agent VX toxicity to uniformed soldier using parathion in vitro human exposure and absorption. Toxicol Appl Pharmacol 2000; 168:149–152.

12 Effects of Anatomical Location on *In Vivo* Percutaneous Penetration in Man

Jordan L. Bormann
University of South Dakota, Sioux Falls, South Dakota

Howard I. Maibach
University of California, San Francisco, California

CONTENTS

12.1 INTRODUCTION

Percutaneous absorption in vivo in man is a complex process. Percutaneous penetration (absorption) is defined here as the amount of chemical entering into the skin that is likely to be absorbed systemically. As described by Law et al. (1), there are 20+ clinically pertinent factors and observations to consider regarding chemical penetration into and through the cutaneous barrier. One factor explained by Law et al. (1) and previous overviews (2, 3) is regional variability in body application site: differences in stratum corneum thickness, appendage density, blood supply, skin surface conditions, and physico-chemical properties of the chemical being applied can affect chemical absorption at unique body locations. In general, the head and neck are more permeable, while palms and soles remain less permeable (1). In past studies, the ventral forearm was often used as the testing site to quantify percutaneous absorption of chemicals or drugs (4). However, it has been deduced that the absorption at the forearm location may grossly underestimate absorption of the chemical at other anatomical locations (5). The additional experimental quantitative data provided here add some integrity (but also variance) from the 2002 calculations.

The pharmacokinetic differences in absorption caused by regional variation can be disadvantageous. In prior studies, the head and neck region exhibited increased percutaneous absorption compared to other anatomic sites (4). The increased absorption could put occupational workers at increased risk of chemical contamination while not wearing protective head gear. As described by Feldmann and colleagues (4), the scrotum was the most permeable of the tested body regions. For men and children who worked as chimney sweeps, the increased penetrability of scrotal skin led to lesions caused by the permeation of soot through their clothing; this later proved fatal due to the development of scrotal squamous cell carcinoma (6).

Although differences in body region absorption can be hazardous under certain circumstances, the variability can also be advantageous for patients that require drug deliverance via a percutaneous route. There are 19 Food and Drug Administration (FDA)–approved medications offered in the form of transdermal delivery systems (7). These patches and semi-solids have specific guidelines regarding where to place the patch for optimal efficacy. Changes in the location of the patch could potentially increase or decrease drug delivery, leading to differences in drug efficacy/toxicity.

There are limited quantitative data determining in vivo regional variability of percutaneous penetration in man. A prior overview on this topic described two studies utilizing the tape-stripping method and eight studies measuring urinary excretion data (8). Our current study builds on those findings with additional data and incorporation of FDA-approved medication patch regional variability data. Our study is of clinical value because we must acknowledge differences in percutaneous absorption of chemicals and medications in relation to various anatomical sites; recognition and consideration of such data could help risk assessment chemical contamination in occupational roles and maximize efficacy of transdermal medications as they are developed. This research work aims to create an updated, concise overview of the pertinent studies available regarding percutaneous penetration and regional variability.

12.2   MATERIALS AND METHODS

We searched PubMed, Web of Science, Google Scholar, and the FDA's online database for approved transdermal delivery systems from January 1965 to March 2020, with the following search words: percutaneous absorption, regional variation, anatomical location. We further utilized the prior listed search engines to search for published data pertaining to regional differences in percutaneous absorption for each of the FDA-approved medications. If no publication was found, we utilized the Summary Basis of Approval documents for each medication to determine patch application site pharmacokinetics. We utilized both the published paper and Summary Basis of Approval for specific medications if the two sources provided unique data. We reviewed the molecular weights and partition coefficients of the chemicals from each study or Summary Basis of Approval to investigate any associations of those chemical properties with regional variation in percutaneous absorption. Molecular weights and partition coefficients were retrieved from the National Institutes of Health National Library of Medicine PubChem. A flow chart of our methodologies is included (Figure 12.1).

12.3   RESULTS

12.3.1   Urinary Excretion Data

12.3.1.1   Hydrocortisone

In early studies, the ventral forearm served as the reference point for percutaneous absorption of a substance in comparison to other body regions. Feldmann and Maibach (4) tested regional variation in percutaneous absorption of hydrocortisone and suggested that regions with thicker stratum corneum resulted in hindered absorption, while regions with more hair follicles, such as the scalp and forehead, resulted in more absorption. Utilizing urinary excretion data, the body region with the greatest percutaneous absorption was the scrotum, being forty times more permeable than the

Step 1

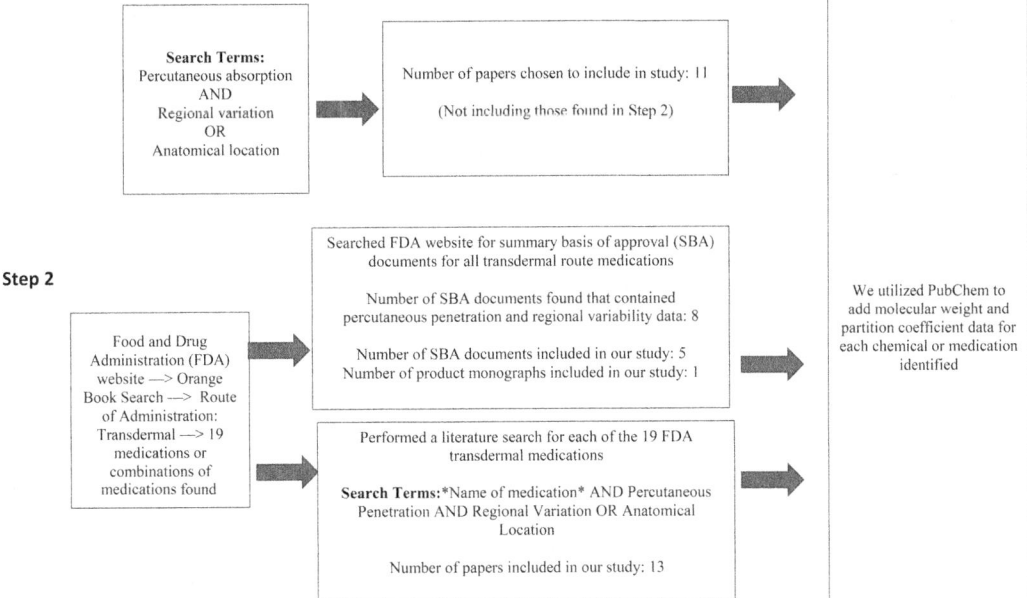

Step 2

FIGURE 12.1   Flow chart of study methods.

ventral forearm (Table 12.1) (Figure 12.2). Britz and colleagues (11) also used urinary excretion measurements to compare hydrocortisone absorption of the ventral forearm and that of the vulva, showing the vulva to be 5.6 times more permeable than the forearm (Table 12.1). Oriba and colleagues (12) reported similar outcomes from urinary excretion data; significantly more absorption of hydrocortisone from vulvar skin occurred compared to the ventral forearm in both premeno-pausal and postmenopausal women (Table 12.1).

12.3.1.2   Testosterone

Oriba and colleagues (12) also compared absorption of testosterone from the vulva and forearm and found that only postmenopausal women exhibited significantly increased absorption of testosterone at the vulvar location compared to the forearm (Table 12.1).

12.3.1.3   Benzoic Acid

Rougier and colleagues (13) utilized urinary excretion data to measure benzoic acid absorption in man. One thousand nmol of benzoic acid ^{14}C was applied for 30 minutes to each of the following locations: upper outer arm, upper back, abdomen, thigh, chest, and forehead. Urinary excretion was measured over the course of four days to calculate total penetration. Penetration was greatest through the forehead, nearly three times more penetrable than the upper outer arm. The following sites are listed in order of decreasing penetrability: forehead, abdomen, thigh, chest, back, and lastly, arm (Table 12.2). The stripping method yielded similar penetration calculated values as when compared to urinary excretion data (13).

Utilizing benzoic acid, Rougier and colleagues (14) suggested that corneocyte size may be a factor in percutaneous absorption. When corneocytes are smaller, there are more spaces between them for chemical to infiltrate. The postauricular area and forehead were most permeable to benzoic acid, and it was acknowledged that both of these regions possess smaller-sized corneocytes compared to other regions. Less permeable regions included the upper outer arm, abdomen, and ventral elbow and ventral wrist (Table 12.1). Interestingly, there were differences in absorption between ventral

TABLE 12.1

Summary of Percutaneous Absorption by Body Region in Reference to Forearm

Chemical/Medication	Hydrocortisone	Hydrocortisone	Hydrocortisone	Testosterone	Benzoic Acid(c)	Parathion	Malathion	Carbaryl	1-OH-pyrene
Reference	(4)	(11)	(12)	(12)	(14)	(16)	(16)	(16)	(17)
Molecular Weight (9)	362.5 g/mol	362.5 g/mol	362.5 g/mol	288.4 g/mol	122.1 g/mol	291.3 g/mol	330.4 g/mol	201.2 g/mol	218.3 g/mol
Partition Coefficient (9)	1.6	1.6	1.6	3.3	1.9	3.8	2.4	2.4	5**
Reference Site	Ventral forearm	Ventral forearm	Ventral forearm	Ventral Forearm	Mid ventral forearm	Forearm	Forearm	Forearm	Forearm
Forearm (no ventral or dorsal designation)									
Forearm (ventral)	1	1	1	1	1(d), 0.6(e), 2.2(f)	1	1	1	1
Forearm (dorsal)	1.1								
Upper Outer Arm					1.7				
Foot arch (plantar)	0.1					1.6	1		
Ankle (lateral or medial)	0.4								
Palm	0.8					1.3	0.9		
Back	1.7								
Scalp	3.5					3.7			
Axilla	3.6					7.4	4.2		
Forehead	6				4.9	4.2	3.4		
Jaw angle	13					3.9		1	
Scrotum	42		2.9(a), 2.8(b)	1.2 (a), 1.7 (b)		11.8			
Vulva		5.6							
Abdomen					2.3	2.1	1.4		1.1
Neck									1.3
Hand dorsum/ventral						2.4	1.8		0.8
Postauricular					4.1	3.9			
Fossa cubitalis						3.3			
Ear canal						5.4			
Calf									1.2

(a) Premenopausal.
(b) Postmenopausal.
(c) Selected for male age group 20–30 years.
(d) Ventral mid-arm.
(e) Ventral forearm at elbow.
(f) Ventral forearm at wrist.
** (10).

Note: Percutaneous absorption was quantified by urinary excretion of chemical or chemical metabolite. Ventral forearm was used as reference site when available. In general, chemical application to the scalp, face, genitalia, and axillae resulted in greater urinary excretion of chemical compared to other body regions.

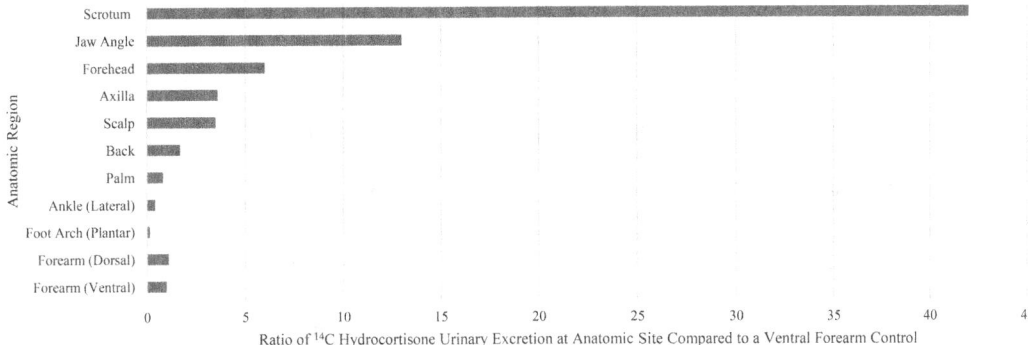

FIGURE 12.2 Percutaneous absorption of ^{14}C hydrocortisone by anatomic region. Percutaneous absorption was measured via urinary excretion at a variety of anatomic sites. This allowed for calculation of a ratio between excretion at each site and a forearm control. (Adapted from 4.)

areas of the forearm; although the mid-ventral forearm is close in proximity to the wrist, the wrist absorbed over two times more chemical (14).

12.3.1.4   Benzoic Acid, Acetylsalicylic Acid, Caffeine, and Benzoic Acid Sodium Salt

Lotte and colleagues (15) utilized benzoic acid, acetylsalicylic acid, caffeine, and benzoic acid sodium salt to determine differences in percutaneous penetration based on anatomic placement of each chemical via urinary excretion results. The postauricular region and forehead were more permeable, while the upper outer arm and abdomen were less so. Of the sites tested, there was a positively associated relationship between transepidermal water loss and the amount of chemical absorbed (Table 12.2) (15).

12.3.1.5   Malathion, Parathion, and Carbaryl

Maibach and colleagues (16) quantified percutaneous penetration of organophosphate chemicals frequently used as pesticides, malathion and parathion. Each pesticide was applied in several anatomic sites and left in place for 24 hours. The radiolabeled pesticide's absorption was then measured via

TABLE 12.2
Summary of Percutaneous Absorption by Body Region in Reference to Upper Outer Arm

Chemical/Medication Tested	Benzoic Acid	Benzoic Acid Sodium Salt	Caffeine	Benzoic Acid	Acetylsalicylic Acid
Reference	(13)	(15)	(15)	(15)	(15)
Molecular Weight (8)	122.1 g/mol	144.1 g/mol	194.2 g/mol	122.1 g/mol	180.2 g/mol
Partition Coefficient (8)	1.9	-2.3	-0.1	1.9	1.2
Upper Outer Arm	1	1	1	1	1
Back	0.9				
Forehead	2.9	3.1	1.8	2.9	2.1
Chest/Shoulder	1.2				
Thigh	1.3				
Abdomen	1.6	1.9	0.6	1.6	1
Postauricular		2.5	1	2.5	1.7

Note: Percutaneous absorption was quantified by urinary excretion of chemical. Data presented here did not include the ventral forearm; therefore, the upper outer arm was used as reference site. Of the body regions tested, the forehead and postauricular region resulted in the most percutaneous absorption and urinary excretion compared to other body sites.

five-day urine analysis. Only parathion was tested on the scrotum; this anatomical location proved most penetrable of all sites tested and was 11 times more penetrable than the forearm. Malathion was placed on the forearm, palm, ball of foot, abdomen, hand dorsum, forehead, and axilla. Of all locations, malathion was most penetrable in the axilla (Table 12.2). Carbaryl was tested on the forearm and jaw angle; however, it was nearly completely absorbed at both sites (Table 12.2) (16).

12.3.1.6   1-OH Pyrene

VanRooij and colleagues (17) determined urinary excretion of 1-OH-pyrene, a metabolite of pyrene (a PAH), from application of PAH to a variety of anatomic locations. There were no significant differences in urinary 1-OH-pyrene metabolite excretion in urine based on body location (Table 12.1); however, there was a significant difference in the duration of time needed to excrete half of the total amount between those anatomic sites (17).

12.3.2   STRIPPING METHODS

12.3.2.1   Estrogen and Testosterone

Oriba and colleagues (12) performed a tape-stripping study on premenopausal and postmenopausal females. Radiolabeled estrogen and testosterone were applied to the mid-labium majus and the ventral forearm, with protective chambers positioned over the application sites for 24 hours. The sites were cleaned at 24 hours, and a covering was placed over the application sites for an additional six days. In premenopausal women, the tape-stripped forearm stratum corneum contained significantly more hydrocortisone than that measured from the vulva. The tape-stripping method retrieved no testosterone from either the vulva or forearm (12). This potentially suggests that testosterone was energetically metabolized by enzymes in the stratum corneum.

12.3.2.2   4-Cyanophenol and Cimetidine

Tsai and colleagues (18) studied 4-cyanophenol (CP) and cimetidine (CM) to determine their permeability through the stratum corneum. CP was applied to the skin for 10 to 15 minutes and CM for three to five hours. At the end of the application periods, patches were removed and skin cleaned, followed by the stripping method and attenuated total reflection–Fourier-transform infrared (ATR-FTIR) spectroscopy of the tape strips. Permeability of both CP and CM was variable among five anatomic sites chosen in the study. CP permeability in descending order was as follows: back, forearm, thigh, leg, and abdomen. Permeability of CM in descending order of anatomic sites was as follows: back, forearm, thigh, leg = abdomen (Table 12.4) (18).

Tsai and colleagues (19) also investigated the effects of sebum production on percutaneous absorption by comparing absorption of CM from the forehead to the forearm and found the forehead absorbed four times more chemical. When they removed sebum from the forehead, there was 22% less absorption from that site. After they supplemented the forearm with sebum, over three times more absorption occurred at that site (Table 12.4) (19).

12.3.3   FIBER-OPTIC LUMINOSCOPE METHODS

12.3.3.1   Polycyclic Aromatic Hydrocarbons

VanRooij and colleagues (17) determined the percutaneous absorption of polycyclic aromatic hydrocarbons (PAH) from coal tar ointment placed on various body regions via fiber-optic luminoscope measurements/fluorescence detection of the chemicals on and within the cutaneous barrier. They found small, yet significant, variations in skin surface absorption of PAH based on body region (Table 12.3). Eleven PAHs were present in the coal tar, determined by fluorescence detection data in combination with high-performance liquid chromatography (17). The regional differences were much less than in other studies involving hydrocortisone or benzoic acid.

TABLE 12.3
Percutaneous Absorption of PAH by Body Region in Reference to Forearm

Chemical	PAH
Reference	(17)
Molecular Weight	Not applicable(a)
Partition Coefficient	Not applicable
Ventral forearm	1
Shoulder	2
Forehead	1
Groin	0.8
Hand (palmar)	0.5
Ankle	0.5

[a] PAH refers to a compound composed of 11 unique PAHs with varying molecular weights and partition coefficients.

Note: VanRooij and colleagues (17) determined skin absorption rate constants of several anatomical locations. The absorption rate constant of the forearm is used as a reference.

12.3.4   PLASMA PHARMACOKINETICS: GELS AND SOLUTIONS

12.3.4.1   Ketoprofen

Shah and colleagues (20) investigated peak plasma concentration of ketoprofen 3% gel when applied to the back, arm, and knee and found no significant differences in absorption when ketoprofen was placed on the back or arm, but there was significantly less absorption at the knee application site, resulting in a decreased peak plasma concentration and Area Under Curve $_{\text{steady state}}$ (AUC_{ss})

TABLE 12.4
ATR-FTIR Spectroscopy Data with Reference to Forearm

Chemical/Medication	Cimetidine	4-cyanophenol	Cimetidine
Reference	(18)	(18)	(19)
Molecular Weight (8)	252.3 g/mol	119.1 g/mol	252.3 g/mol
Partition Coefficient (8)	0.4	1.6	0.4
Forearm	1	1	1
Forearm – sebum supplementation			3.3
Forehead			3.8
Forehead – sebum removed			3
Back	2.2	1.4	
Thigh	0.5	0.7	
Leg	0.4	0.6	
Abdomen	0.5	0.5	

Note: Percutaneous absorption of cimetidine and 4-cyanophenol were measured in several anatomic locations and compared to absorption at the forearm. Additional data comparing sebum removal at the forehead and sebum supplementation at the forearm are shown.

TABLE 12.5

Gel and Solution Percutaneous Absorption: Blood Plasma Pharmacokinetics

Medication	Ketoprofen
Reference	(20)
Molecular Weight (8)	254.3 g/mol
Partition Coefficient (8)	3.1
Reference site	Upper outer arm
Upper outer arm	1(a)
Back	0.9(a), 1.1(b)
Knee	0.7(a)
Measurement Value	$AUC_{(ss)}$(c)

(a) 30 mg 3% gel.

(b) 0.5 m l 60 mg/mL solution.

(c) Area Under the Curve$_{(steady\ state)}$.

Note: Shah et al (1996) utilized plasma pharmacokinetics to determine absorption of two forms of ketoprofen. Area under the curve (AUC) quantified absorption. Data are listed in reference to upper outer arm.

(Table 12.5). In addition to the 3% gel, an equal amount of ketoprofen in a 60 mg/mL solution was applied to the back. There was increased absorption of the solution compared to the gel at that specific anatomic site, as determined by the AUC_{ss} (Table 12.5) (20).

12.3.5 PLASMA PHARMACOKINETICS: PATCHES AND TRANSDERMAL SYSTEMS

New formulations in transdermal delivery systems have been recently developed and serve a role in allowing a means of medication administration in situations where an oral or intravenous route is not optimal. Oftentimes these medications are formulated for application to the buttocks, as this is a discrete, hidden area for such placement. Currently, there are 19 FDA-approved transdermal delivery systems in a variety of formulations (7) (Table 12.6). Here we present the data from Summary Basis of Approval documents, as well as published data, regarding the pharmacokinetics of patch and semi-solid medications. Unless noted otherwise, all data pertain to AUC plasma bioavailability for each anatomic site.

12.3.5.1 Asenapine

Asenapine was similarly absorbed at the upper arm, upper back, upper chest, and hip. The abdomen, however, revealed less absorption when compared to the upper arm (Table 12.7) (28).

12.3.5.2 Buprenorphine

Buprenorphine absorption was similar at the upper outer arm, the upper chest, the midaxillary line, and the upper back (Table 12.7) (29).

12.3.5.3 Clonidine

MacGregor and colleagues (30) applied a clonidine patch to the arm and upper chest. There were no significant differences in mean steady-state plasma concentration at the two sites (Table 12.7). However, Ebihara and colleagues (31) noted the arm showed significantly more absorption than the chest or upper abdomen (Table 12.7).

TABLE 12.6
Summary of FDA-Approved Transdermal Medications (Alone or in Combination)

Medication	Published Research Article (PRA) and/or Summary Basis of Approval (SBA)	Key Mechanism(s) of Action (21)	Clinical Indication(s) (21)
Clonidine	PRA	Centrally acting alpha-adrenergic agonist	Treatment of hypertension
Fentanyl	PRA and SBA	Synthetic phenylpiperidine opioid agonist	Analgesic
Ethinyl estradiol (used alone or in combination with levonorgestrel or norelgestromin)	PRA	Semisynthetic estrogen	Contraceptive
Norelgestromin	PRA	A norgestimate metabolite (22)	Contraceptive
Estradiol (used alone or in combination with levonorgestrel or norethindrone acetate)	PRA	Potent sex hormone that promotes secondary sexual characteristics and supports fertility	Protects against postmenopausal osteoporosis Menopausal symptom therapy Estrogen replacement
Nicotine	PRA	Binds to nicotinic acetylcholine receptors in the central nervous system causing release of dopamine	Prevention of nicotine craving and relief of withdrawal symptoms
Methylphenidate	PRA and SBA	Unknown mechanism in ADHD treatment; may increase release of norepinephrine and dopamine and block their reuptake (23)	Treatment of ADHD
Oxybutynin	PRA	Smooth muscle muscarinic receptor blocker	Relief of overactive bladder contractions
Rivastigmine	PRA	Cholinesterase inhibitor (24)	Treatment of Alzheimer disease
Rotigotine	PRA	Dopamine agonist (25)	Parkinson's disease and restless legs syndrome treatment (25)
Testosterone	PRA	Androgen receptor activator	Treatment of hypogonadism in males
Asenapine	SBA	Unknown; suggested D_2 and 5-HT_{2A} receptor antagonism (26)	Bipolar I disorder (manic or mixed episodes) treatment Schizophrenia treatment
Buprenorphine	SBA	Synthetic opioid that is an antagonist at the kappa-opioid receptor and a practical agonist at the mu-opioid receptor in the central nervous system	Alleviates moderate to severe pain
Selegiline	SBA	Monoamine oxidase (MAO) inhibitor	Major depressive disorder (27)
Levonorgestrel	No Data Found	Progesterone receptor binding resulting in LH suppression and ovulation inhibition	Contraception
Norethindrone acetate	No Data Found	Stimulates nuclear progesterone receptors in the reproductive system and pituitary	Aids in reducing risk of uterine cancer when used in combination with estradiol
Nitroglycerin	No Data Found	A nitrate causing smooth muscle relaxation	Utilized for cardiac conditions (angina)
Granisetron	No Data Found	Antagonizes selective serotonin (5-HT) receptors	Provides antiemetic properties
Scopolamine	No Data Found	Muscarinic acetylcholine antagonist	Antivertigo and antiemetic uses Decreases gut motility Induces cycloplegia and mydriasis Decreases gastric acid and saliva secretion

Note: Nineteen medications were found via the Food and Drug Administration Orange Book Database that are administered transdermally. Summary basis of approval documents and a literature search were utilized for percutaneous penetration data collection. No sources describing percutaneous penetration differences based on regional variability were found for five of the medications, as listed in the table. Key mechanisms of action and clinical indications of each patch are included for clinical relevance; all reference NCIthesaurus (21) unless otherwise listed.

TABLE 12.7
Patch and Semi-solids: Blood Plasma Pharmacokinetics

Medication	Asenapine	Buprenorphine	Clonidine	Clonidine	Fentanyl	Nicotine	Methylphenidate	Methylphenidate	Rivastigmine	Rotigotine
Reference	(28)	(29)	(30)	(31)	(32)	(38)	(39)	(40)	(24)	(25)
Molecular Weight (8)	285.8 g/mol	467.6 g/mol	230.1 g/mol	230.1 g/mol	336.5 g/mol	162.2 g/mol	233.3 g/mol	233.3 g/mol	250.3 g/mol	315.5 g/mol
Partition Coefficient (8)	4.8	5	1.6	1.6	4.1	1.2	0.2	0.2	2.3	4.7
Reference site	Upper arm	Upper outer arm	Arm	Arm	Upper Arm	Upper arm	Hip	Arm	Upper arm	Upper arm
Upper outer arm	1	1			1	1			1	1
Back/Shoulder	1	1			0.9	1	0.8		1.1	1.1
Upper chest/torso	0.9	0.9	1.1	0.8	0.7				1.1	
Arm - unspecified			1	1				1		
Abdomen	0.9			0.7		0.7			0.9	0.9
Midaxillary Line		0.9								
Buccal mucosa								2.9(b)		
Thigh									0.8	0.8
Flank										1
Hip	1						1			0.9
Measurement Value	$AUC_{(0-inf)}$(a)	AUC	% released	$AUC_{(0-120hr)}$	$AUC_{(0hr-inf)}$	$AUC_{(0hr-inf)}$	$AUC_{(0-16hr)}$	Mean % delivered	$AUC_{(0hr-inf)}$	$AUC_{(SSnorm(total))}$

Source: Various Reference Sites.

(a) Area under the Curve.

(b) Buccal measurement after two hours, whereas arm measurement occurred after eight hours.

Note: Medications in patch or semi-solid formulations were placed on several anatomic locations and percutaneous absorption was measured via blood plasma pharmacokinetics. AUC quantified absorption unless otherwise specified. The patches and semi-solids revealed relatively similar absorption values to that of the reference site (e.g., arm, hip).

12.3.5.4   Fentanyl

Fentanyl patches were randomly assigned to subjects for placement on the upper outer arm, back, and chest. When compared to absorption at the upper arm, absorption was 29% lower from the upper chest site and 10% lower for the upper back site (Table 12.7). When the application was repeated at the same sites, there were decreased differences in absorption between all three sites (32).

Solassol and colleagues (33) found no significant differences in estimated percutaneous absorption due to fentanyl patch placement at the arm, shoulder, chest, and back. Absorption was estimated by measuring remaining fentanyl in patches after use.

12.3.5.5   Hormonal Contraceptives

A contraceptive patch containing ethinyl estradiol and gestodene was tested at three location sites: upper outer arm, buttocks, and abdomen. There was no significant difference in percutaneous absorption at any of the sites (Table 12.8) (34). Stanczyk and colleagues (36) found less absorption at the abdomen compared to the back and buttocks of a low-dose ethinyl estradiol patch (Table 12.8). However, therapeutically, all three patch application sites were similar. Abrams and colleagues (22) collected absorption data on a patch containing ethinyl estradiol and norelgestromin also showing decreased absorption of both hormones, yet still within the therapeutic range (Table 12.8). Yet another study regarding 17-B-estradiol absorption showed 88% of the $AUC_{0\text{-last}}$ for an abdominal patch location compared to the buttock (Table 12.8) (37).

12.3.5.6   Nicotine

Nicotine patches were applied to the upper arm, abdomen, and back and percutaneous absorption by Sobue and colleagues (38); they found no significant difference in absorption between the upper arm and back. However, there was significantly less absorption between the upper arm and abdomen (AUC ratio of upper arm to abdomen was 75%) (Table 12.7).

12.3.5.7   Methylphenidate

In two clinical trials, methylphenidate patches were tested for differences in percutaneous absorption (39, 40). The first performed in children showed decreased bioavailability of methylphenidate when applied to the scapula compared to the hip (Table 12.7) (39). The second showed 2.9 times more permeability of methylphenidate when applied to the oral buccal mucosa compared to the arm (Table 12.7) (40).

12.3.5.8   Oxybutynin

Patches were applied for 96 hours in 24 healthy volunteers in a study determining pharmacokinetics of oxybutynin. The abdomen, buttocks, and hip proved bioequivalent (Table 12.8) (41).

12.3.5.9   Rivastigmine

Lefevre and colleagues (24) applied rivastigmine patches to the upper back, chest, upper arm, abdomen, and thigh. Greater adhesive properties of the patch at the thigh and abdomen were found; however, these locations offered less-than-optimal bioavailability compared to the patches placed on the upper back, chest, and upper arm (Table 12.7) (24).

12.3.5.10   Rotigotine

In work performed by Elshoff and colleagues (25), three open-label, randomized, phase 1 multiple-dose studies were pooled and bioavailability of the medication at the shoulder, upper arm, abdomen, flank, hip, and thigh calculated. There were differences in bioavailability; however, there was no significance on outcomes of clinical efficacy (Table 12.7) (25).

TABLE 12.8
Patch and Semi-solids: Blood Plasma Pharmacokinetics

Medication	Ethinyl estradiol	Gestodone	Ethinyl estradiol	Ethinyl Estradiol	Norelgestromin	17-B-estradiol	Oxybutynin	Testosterone
Reference	(34)	(34)	(36)	(22)	(22)	(37)	(41)	(43)
Molecular Weight (8)	296.4 g/mol	310.4 g/mol	296.4 g/mol	296.4 g/mol	327.5 g/mol	272.4	357.5 g/mol	288.42 g/mol
Partition Coefficient (8)	3.7	3.3	3.7	3.7	2.7**	4	4.3	3.3
Buttocks	1	1	1	1	1	1	1	1
Upper Outer Arm	1.2	1.2		1	1			0.9
Back/Shoulder			1					
Upper Chest/Torso				1	1			0.9
Abdomen	0.9	1	0.9	0.8	0.8	0.9	0.9	
Hip							1	
Measurement Value	$AUC_{(0-168hr)}$(a)	$AUC_{(0-168hr)}$	$AUC_{(0-240hr)}$	$AUC_{(0-240hr)}$	$AUC_{(0-240hr)}$	$AUC_{(0-last)}$	$AUC_{(0-inf)}$(b)	$AUC_{(0-27hr)}$

Source: Buttocks

(a) Area under the Curve.

(b) AUC was adjusted for residual oxybutynin from previous treatments.

**(35).

Note: Several transdermal medication delivery systems were tested for their percutaneous absorption capability at several anatomic sites, with the buttocks serving as the reference site. AUC quantified percutaneous absorption. In general, all sites were relatively similar in regard to percutaneous absorption when compared to that of the buttocks.

12.3.5.11 Selegiline

Although no data were found, the Summary Basis of Approval document for selegiline stated that locations at the upper torso or upper thigh provided similar absorption; however, application to the upper buttocks was not bioequivalent and resulted in greater absorption (42).

12.3.5.12 Testosterone

Yu and colleagues (35) determined differences in absorption of testosterone via a transdermal system in hypogonadal men. There were no significant differences in testosterone absorption between application sites of the upper buttocks, back, and upper arms (Table 12.8) (38).

12.4 DISCUSSION

There are many chemical and cutaneous properties to appreciate when suggesting mechanisms for regional variation in percutaneous absorption. As summarized by Law et al. (1), skin is a complex organ with many factors varying by region. There are differences in anatomy from one individual to another, adding yet another layer of complexity (33). Prior studies suggest regional variation in percutaneous absorption by physiological mechanisms such as skin irritation, erythema, and blanching (44). It is beyond the scope of this overview—but of clinical and biological relevance—to relate regional variation in flux to endpoints such as irritant and allergic contact dermatitis (45).

This overview specifically focused on quantifiable data pertaining to percutaneous absorption, such as urinary excretion data, cutaneous disappearance of chemical, and pharmacokinetics of blood plasma. In general, the head, neck, and genital regions appear more absorptive than other body regions. The abdomen, chest, back, and thighs proved less absorptive. Differences at anatomical sites in appendage density, skin anatomy, stratum corneum thickness, sebum production, and proximity of vascular blood supply to the cutaneous surface are factors suggested to affect cutaneous absorption.

There are several ways to calculate percutaneous absorption. It is important to recognize where inaccuracies may arise based on each method used. For example, measuring the amount of chemical that disappears from a solution or a gel without protection on the skin surface over a period of hours or days allows for error (17). Disappearance of the chemicals could be achieved by multiple mechanisms in addition to percutaneous absorption. The studies may have assumed that if the chemical disappeared, its entirety had been percutaneously absorbed. However, the chemical could be rubbed off due to limited or no protective barrier. In addition, the top layers of the stratum corneum slough off over time by physiological mechanisms, so it is possible some of the chemical may have been removed along with the sloughed-off cells in lengthier studies.

The urinary excretion method also allows for error, as chemicals may be excreted via other mechanisms such as exhaled air or feces. In addition, the chemical may build up in other locations in the body and therefore is not excreted in the urine.

Studies quantifying absorption utilizing blood plasma levels are also complex based on where the drug deposits in the body and the effects of renal and fecal excretion, among a myriad of other bodily processes. Although no study method is fully accurate in quantifying percutaneous absorption, the data collected are helpful, as we can create comparisons of the absorption among varying body regions. Guy and Maibach (5) suggested a formula to calculate percutaneous absorption dependent on body region. This can be used as a tool as new transdermal medication patches, gels, and solutions continue to be developed. For example, Wester et al (46) determined percutaneous absorption of piperonyl butoxide and pyrethrin at the forearm and subsequently calculated the percutaneous absorption of those chemicals from the forehead. Such data can be used as an approximate model for future work in the pharmaceutical industry or when determining how to best design protective clothing for the occupation worker.

Interestingly, when using the forearm as a reference, the review data showed similar ratios of absorption for a certain body site for several chemicals regardless of molecular weight or partition coefficient (Table 12.1). This suggests that cutaneous properties are stronger predictors of potential absorption than a chemical's molecular properties. In general, regions with smaller corneocytes, increased appendageal density, thinner stratum corneum, or enclosed protected areas (e.g., axilla, vulva) exhibited increased absorption. However, this observation does not agree with all reported data. For several chemicals, there were virtually no differences in absorption between body locations, suggesting significant complexity of the physiology involved. Standardized experiments investigating chemical percutaneous absorption at a variety of anatomical locations are needed in order to further elucidate these mechanisms.

The prior overview from 2012 by Tev-Lov and colleagues (8) discussed regional variability and percutaneous penetration via both urinary excretion and tape-stripping methods. Our current study highlights these methods, but we also directed our efforts towards the 19 FDA-approved transdermal delivery system medications and their regional variabilities in cutaneous absorption. Most are approved for placement on more than one body region, as multiple locations can achieve the accepted drug efficacy and bioavailability. From limited current data, it appears the upper outer arm provides a delivery site leading to higher drug absorption levels and patient convenience than other locations. Although this increased absorption may not lead to any clinically significant outcomes, it is important to consider this difference when developing drug delivery systems in the future. In addition, some sites may be better able to absorb the medication, but the adhesive ability and the comfort of the patch at such locations must be considered, e.g., scrotum, vulva, and face.

The two main types of experimental data might be examined differently. The Feldmann experiments (4) used finite dosing in which the chemical/drug could exfoliate, rub off, and wash off, while the drug patch data are (almost) an infinite dose in that patches are overloaded and drug continues to be available until the patch is removed.

The basis for marked differences in regional variability remain inadequately studied decades past the Feldmann publication (4). Rougier and colleagues' (13, 14) observations offer some insight, as well as the extensive experimental data on the follicular route (47), yet much remains to be resolved. This area of study holds clinical implications in many different realms, such as occupational contamination and transdermal drug delivery systems. In conclusion, current data permits some extrapolation for all chemicals/drugs, but much remains to be fathomed in terms of mechanisms and predictive formulas. More studies are needed for potential establishment of a regional model of penetrability of human anatomic sites.

12.5 CONCLUSION

1. Consideration of increased percutaneous penetration of the face, neck, and genital regions can aid in counseling patients on occupational work exposure/protection.
2. The practicing clinician should acknowledge and consider the effects of pharmacological patch placement when prescribing such medications to patients.
3. Although quantitative data are minimal, further studies may allow for establishment of a regional model of cutaneous chemical penetrability of human anatomic sites.

REFERENCES

1. Law RM, Ngo MA, Maibach HI. Twenty clinically pertinent factors/observations for percutaneous absorption in humans. Am J Clin Dermatol. 2020;21,85–95.
2. Wester RC, Maibach HI. Cutaneous pharmacokinetics: 10 steps to percutaneous absorption. Drug Metab Rev. 1983;14(2),169–205.
3. Ngo MA, O'Malley M, Maibach HI. Percutaneous absorption and exposure assessment of pesticides. J Appl Toxicol. 2010;30,91–114.
4. Feldmann RJ, Maibach HI. Regional variation in percutaneous penetration of 14C cortisol in man. J Invest Dermatol. 1967;48,181–183.

5. Guy R, Maibach HI. Calculations of body exposure from percutaneous absorption data. In: Bronaugh RL, Maibach HI, editors. Topical Absorption of Dermatological Products. New York, NY: Marcel Dekker; 2002. p. 311–315.

6. Azike JE. A review of the history, epidemiology and treatment of squamous cell carcinoma of the scrotum. Rare Tumors. 2009;1(1),e17.

7. Orange Book: Approved Drug Products with Therapeutic Equivalence Evaluations. Available from: https://www.accessdata.fda.gov/scripts/cder/ob/index.cfm.

8. Lev-Tov H, Maibach HI. Regional variations in percutaneous absorption. J Drug Derm. 2012;11(10),e48–e51.

9. NIH National Medical Library PubChem (Internet). Available from: https://pubchem.ncbi.nlm.nih.gov.

10. Dugheri S, Bonari A, Gentili M, et al. High-throughput analysis of selected urinary hydroxy polycyclic aromatic hydrocarbons by an innovative automated solid-phase microextraction. Molecules. 2018;23980,1869.

11. Britz MB, Maibach HI, Anjo DM. Human percutaneous penetration of hydrocortisone: the vulva. Arch Dermatol Res. 1980;267,313–316.

12. Oriba HA, Bucks DAW, Maibach HI. Percutaneous absorption of hydrocortisone and testosterone on the vulva and forearm: effect of the menopause and site. Br J Dermatol. 1996;134,229–233.

13. Rougier A, Dupuis D, Lotte C, et al. Regional variation in percutaneous absorption in man: Measurement by the stripping method. Arch Dermatol Res. 1986;278,465–469.

14. Rougier A, Lotte C, Corcuff P, et al. Relationship between skin permeability and corneocyte size according to anatomic site, age, and sex in man. J Soc Cosmet Chem. 1988,39:15–26.

15. Lotte C, Rougier A, Wilson DR, et al. In vivo relationship between transepidermal water loss and percutaneous penetration of some organic compounds in man: effect of anatomic site. Arch Derm Res. 1987;279,351–356.

16. Maibach HI, Feldmann RJ, Milby TH, et al. Regional variation in percutaneous penetration in man. Arch Environ Health. 1971;23(3),208–211.

17. VanRooij JGM, De Roos JHC, Bodelier-Bade MM, et al. Absorption of polycyclic aromatic hydrocarbons through human skin: Differences between anatomical sites and individuals. J Toxicol Environ Health. 1993;38,355–368.

18. Tsai JC, Lin CY, Sheu HM, et al. Noninvasive characterization of regional variation in drug transport in human stratum corneum in vivo. Pharm Res. 2003;20(4),632–638.

19. Tsai JC, Lu CC, Lin MK, et al. Effects of sebum on drug transport across the human stratum corneum in vivo. Skin Pharmacol Physiol. 2012;25,124–132.

20. Shah AK, Wei G, Lanman RV, et al. Percutaneous absorption of ketoprofen from different anatomical sites in man. Pharm Res. 1996;13(1),168–172.

21. NCIthesaurus (Internet). National Cancer Institute. Available from: https://ncit.nci.nih.gov/ncitbrowser/pages/home.jsf?version=20.05d

22. Abrams LS, Skee DM, Natarajan J, et al. Pharmacokinetics of a contraceptive patch (Evra™/Ortho Evra™) containing norelgetromin and ethinyloestradiol at four application sites. Br J Clin Pharm. 2002;53,141–146.

23. DAYTRANA® (methylphenidate transdermal system): Highlights of Prescribing Information (Internet) (p. 16). Available from: https://www.accessdata.fda.gov/drugsatfda_docs/label/2010/021514s011lbl.pdf

24. Lefevre G, Sedek G, Huang H-LA, et al. Pharmacokinetics of a rivastigmine transdermal patch formulation in healthy volunteers: relative effects of body site application. J Clin Pharm. 2007;47,471–478.

25. Elshoff J-P, Braun M. Andreas J-O, et al. Steady-state plasma concentration profile of transdermal rotigotine: An integrated analysis of three, open-label, randomized, phase I multiple dose studies. Clin Ther. 2012;34(4),966–978.

26. SECUADO® (asenapine) Transdermal system: Highlights of Prescribing Information (Internet) (p. 22). Available from: https://www.accessdata.fda.gov/drugsatfda_docs/label/2019/212268s000lbl.pdf#page22

27. EMSAM® (Selegiline Transdermal System) (Internet) (p. 2). Available from: https://www.accessdata.fda.gov/drugsatfda_docs/nda/2006/021336s000_021708s000_PRNTLBL.pdf

28. FDA Summary Basis of Approval: Asenapine. FDA study HP-3070-US-03 (Internet) (p. 64–65). Available from: https://www.accessdata.fda.gov/drugsatfda_docs/nda/2019/212268Orig1s000Multidiscipline R.pdf.

29. FDA Summary Basis of Approval: Buprenorphine. FDA Study BP96-0501 (Internet) (p. 94, 121–122). Available from: https://www.accessdata.fda.gov/drugsatfda_docs/nda/2010/021306Orig1s000ClinPharmR.pdf.

30. McGregor TR, Matzek KM, Keirns JJ, et al. Pharmacokinetics of transdermally delivered clonidine. Clin Pharmacol Ther. 1985;38(3):278–284.

31. Ebihara A, Fujimura A, Ohashi K, et al. Influence of application site of a new transdermal clonidine, M-5041T, on its pharmacokinetics and pharmacodynamics in healthy subjects. J Clin Pharm. 1993;33,1188–1191.

32. FDA. Summary Basis of Approval: Fentanyl. FDA study C-2002-047 (Internet) (p. 235–236). Available from: https://www.accessdata.fda.gov/drugsatfda_docs/nda/2009/019813Orig1s044.pdf.

33. Solassol I, Caumette L, Bressolle F, et al. Inter- and intra-individual variability in transdermal fentanyl absorption in cancer pain patients. Oncol Rep. 2005;14,1029–1036.

34. Hochel J, Schuett B, Ludwig M, et al. Implications of different application sites on the bioavailability of a transdermal contraceptive patch containing ethinyl estradiol and gestodene: an open-label, randomized, crossover study. Int J Clin Pharmacol Ther. 2014;52,856–866.

35. PREVRA®. Product Monograph (Internet) (p. 46). Available from: https://s3.pgkb.org/attachment/ Norelgestromin_and_ethinyl_estradiol_HCSC_06_03_15.pdf.

36. Stanczyk FZ, Archer DF, Rubin A, et al. Therapeutically equivalent pharmacokinetic profile across three application sites for AG200-15, a novel low-estrogen dose contraceptive patch. Contraception. 2013;87,744–749.

37. Taggart W, Dandekar K, Ellman H, et al. The effect of site of application on the transcutaneous absorption of 17-beta estradiol from a transdermal delivery system (Climara). Menopause. 2000;7(5),364–369.

38. Sobue S, Sekiguchi K, Kikkawa H, et al. Effect of application sites and multiple doses on nicotine pharmacokinetics in healthy male Japanese smokers following application of the transdermal nicotine patch. J Clin Pharm. 2005;45,1391–1399.

39. Gonzalez MA, Campbell D, Rubin J. Effects of application to two different skin sites on the pharmacokinetics of transdermal methylphenidate in pediatric patients with attention-deficit/hyperactivity disorder. J Child Adolesc Psychopharmacol. 2009;19(3),227–232.

40. FDA Summary Basis of Approval: Methylphenidate. FDA study 17-012. (Internet) (p. 35). Available from: https://www.accessdata.fda.gov/drugsatfda_docs/nda/2006/021514s000_ClinPharmR_P2.pdf.

41. Zobrist RH, Quan D, Thomas HM, et al. Pharmacokinetics and metabolism of transdermal oxybutynin: In vitro and in vivo performance of a novel delivery system. Pharm Res. 2002;20(1),103–109.

42. FDA Summary Basis of Approval: Selegiline. FDA studies 0052, 9806, and 96B. (Internet) (p. 32). Available from: https://www.accessdata.fda.gov/drugsatfda_docs/nda/2006/021336s000_021708s000_ ClinPharmR_Part1.pdf.

43. Yu Z, Gupta SK, Hwang SS, et al. Transdermal testosterone administration in hypogonadal men: comparison of pharmacokinetics at different sites of application and at the first and fifth days of application. J Clin Pharm. 1997;37,1129–1138.

44. Tur E, Maibach HI, Guy RH. Percutaneous penetration of methyl nicotinate at three anatomic sites: Evidence for an appendageal contribution to transport? Skin Pharm. 1991;4,230–234.

45. Leskur D, Bukić J, Petrić A, et al. Anatomical site differences of sodium laurel sulfate-induced irritation: randomized controlled trial. Br J Derm. 2019;181(1),175–185.

46. Wester RC, Buck DAW, Maibach HI. Human in vivo percutaneous absorption of pyrethrin and piperonyl butoxide. Food Chem Toxicol. 1994;32(1),51–53.

47. Elmady A, Hui X, Maibach HI. Role of hair follicle in penetration and decontamination. Forthcoming 2020.

13 Interrelationships in the Dose Response of Percutaneous Absorption

Ronald C. Wester and Howard I. Maibach
University of California, San Francisco, California

CONTENTS

In most medical and toxicological specialties, the administered dose absorbed is defined precisely. This has not always been so in dermatoxicology and dermatopharmacology. The absorbed dose is usually defined as percent applied dose absorbed, flux rate, and/or permeability constant. This may suffice for the person creating the data, but it is incomplete for the person judging the worthiness of the data. Chemical absorbed through skin is usually a low percentage of the applied dose. If 5% is absorbed, it is more than curiosity to question where the other 95% resides. Most critical is whether the remaining dose was in place during the course of the study and whether there is dose accountability. A second critical question is where the clinical or toxicological response lies in relationship to the topically applied dose, the standard safety and efficacy issue that a dose response will provide. The third question is whether absorption is linear to administered dose, i.e., the dose response.

This chapter defines our current, albeit far from perfect, understanding of the relation of applied dose to percutaneous absorption. The dose response is a sound scientific principle, and studies on percutaneous absorption need to apply this principle in some portion of a study.

13.1   DOSE RESPONSE IN REAL TIME

Breath analysis is being used to obtain real-time measurements of volatile organics in expired air following exposure in rats and humans. The exhaled breath data are analyzed using physiologically based pharmacokinetic (PBPK) models to determine the dermal bioavailability of organic solvents. Human volunteers and animals breathe fresh air via a new breath inlet system that allows for continuous real-time analysis of undiluted exhaled air. The air supply system is self-contained and separated from the exposure solvent-laden environment. The system uses a Teledyne 3DQ Discovery ion trap mass spectrometer (MS/MS) equipped with an atmospheric sampling glow discharge ionization source (ASGDI). The MS/MS system provides an appraisal of individual chemical components in the breath stream in the single-digit parts-per-billion (ppb) detectable range for compounds under study, while maintaining linearity of response over a wide dynamic range.

1,1,1-Trichlorethane (methyl chloroform [MC]) was placed in 4 L of water at 1%, 0.1%, and 0.01% concentration (MC is soluble at 0.1% and 0.01% concentrations), and volunteers placed a hand in the bucket of water containing the MC. Figure 13.1 gives the in vivo human dose response. The analytical system measures MC in exhaled breath every four seconds and displays the amount in real time. For investigator "data analysis sanity," 75 four-second data points are averaged each five minutes of elapsed time, as presented in Figure 13.1. At 1% dose MC is immediately and rapidly absorbed through the skin, increasing to over 2500 ppb at two hours when the hand was removed from the solvent/water bucket. Breath MC levels then declined. The 0.1% dose (MC, which is completely soluble in water) peaked at approximately 1200 ppb at 2 hours when the hand was removed from

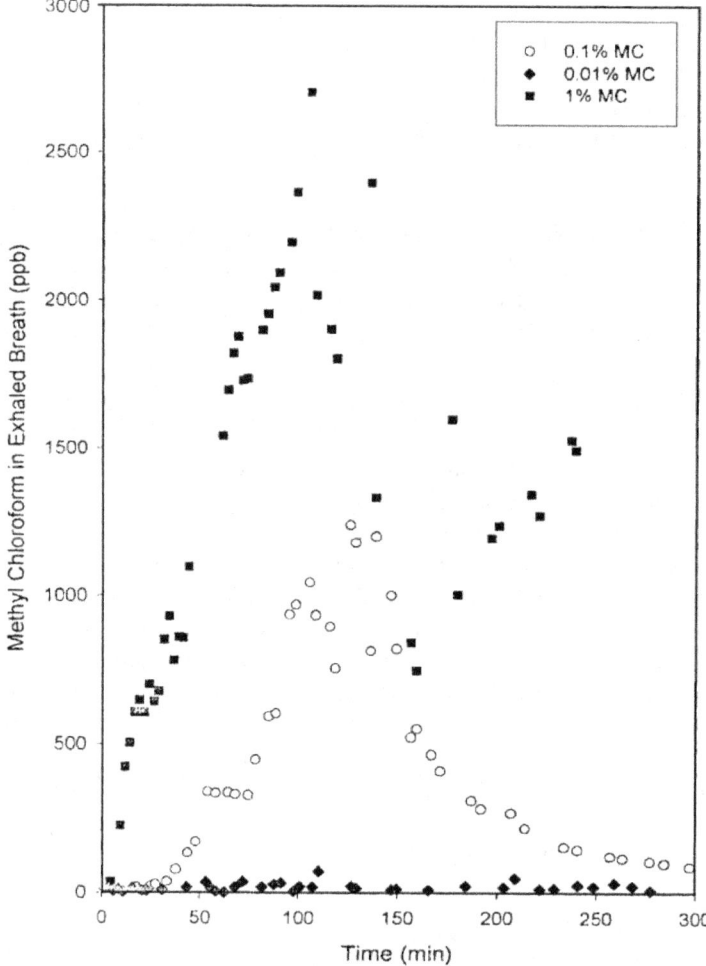

FIGURE 13.1 In vivo real-time absorption of the solvent methyl chloroform (MC) from human volunteers with a hand in 4 L of water containing 1%, 0.1%, or 0.01% solvent. The MC is soluble in water at 0.1% (note lag time) but exceeds solubility at 1% (note no lag time). The hand was removed from the solvent/water at 120 minutes.

the solvent/water exposure. There was an initial delay of 30 to 60 minutes in solvent absorption from the water-soluble dose, which was not seen with the higher dose that exceeded solubility. The lowest dose, 0.01%, was near analytical limitation. These data are then analyzed for human body rate distribution using a PBPK model and appropriate absorption and excretion rates produced (1).

13.2 PHARMACODYNAMIC DOSE RESPONSE

Pharmacodynamics is a biologic response to the presence of a chemical. The chemical needs to be bioavailable for the response to happen, and a dose response within the limits of the biological response can be measured. This can happen with in vivo human skin, and an example is blood flow changes measured by laser Doppler velocimetry (LDV). Minoxidil is a direct-acting peripheral vasodilator originally developed for hypertension, but is now available to promote hair growth. In a double-blind study, balding volunteers were dosed with 0%, 1%, 3%, and 5% minoxidil solutions once each day on two consecutive days and blood flow was measured by LDV (Figure 13.2).

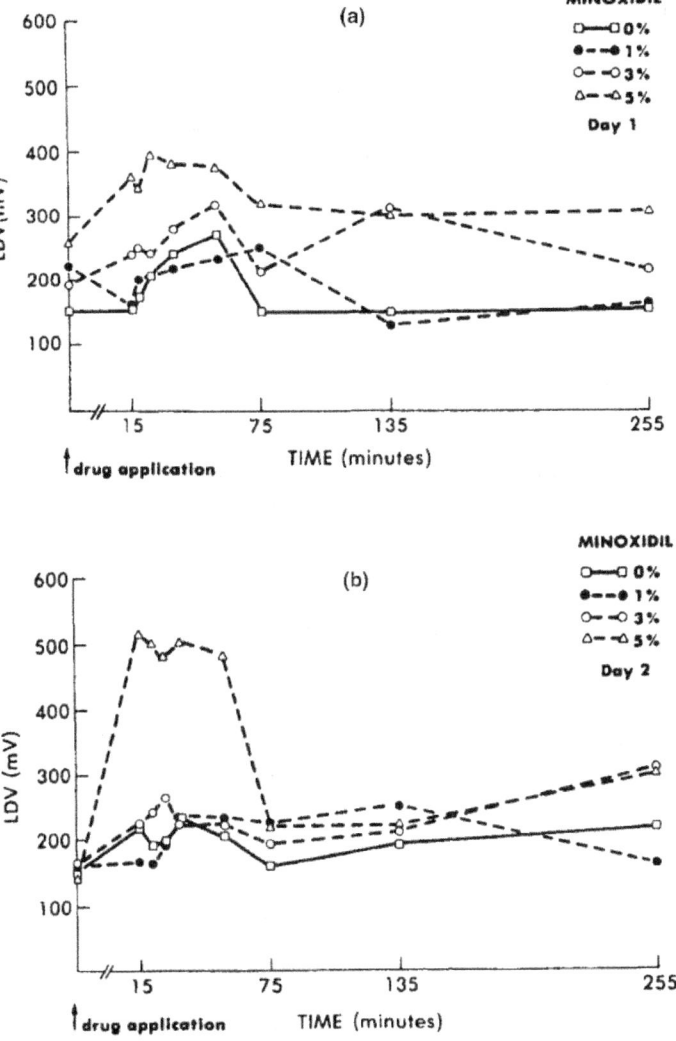

FIGURE 13.2 Pharmacodynamic laser Doppler velocimetry dose response of minoxidil stimulating skin blood flow in the balding scalp of male volunteers. (a) Day 1 and (b) Day 2.

On day 1 an LDV dose response showed the highest blood flow from the 5% dose, followed by the 3% dose, with the 1% dose giving no response above control. Day 2 results clearly showed a pharmacodynamic response for the 5% solutions ($p < 0.0001$), but the other doses were near that of control (2).

This effect of concentration on percutaneous absorption also extends to the penetration of corticoids as measured by the pharmacodynamic vasoconstrictor assay. In this type of assay Maibach and Stoughton (3) showed that, in general, there is a dose-response relationship, with increasing efficacy closely following increased dose. A several-fold difference in dose can override differences in potency between the halogenated analogues. If this applies to corticoids, it could also apply for other chemicals.

Biological response differs from straight chemical analyses (only limited by analytical sensitivity) in that a threshold is probably needed to initiate the response and there are probably limits to the extent that the biology can respond. However, within these parameters some dose response should exist.

13.3   DOSE-RESPONSE INTERRELATIONSHIPS

The interrelationships of dose response in dermal absorption are defined in terms of accountability, concentration, surface area, frequency of application, and time of exposure. Accountability is an accounting of the mass balance for each dose applied to the skin. Concentration is the amount of applied chemical per unit skin surface area. Surface area is usually defined in square centimeter of skin application or exposure. Frequency is either intermittent or chronic exposure. Intermittent can be one, two, and so on exposures per day. Chronic application is usually repetitive and on a continuing daily basis. Time of exposure is the duration of the period during which the skin is in contact with the chemical before washing. Such factors define skin exposure to a chemical and subsequent percutaneous absorption.

13.4   ACCOUNTABILITY (MASS BALANCE)

Table 13.1 gives the in vivo percutaneous absorption of dinoseb in the rhesus monkey and rat. The absorption in the rat over a dose range of 52 to 644 µg/cm² is approximately 90% for all of the doses (4). Conversely, absorption in the rhesus monkey for the dinoseb dose range of 44 to 3620 µg/cm² is approximately only 5%. There is an obvious difference because of species (rat and rhesus monkey). The question then becomes one of mass balance to determine dose accountability. (If dinoseb was not absorbed through the skin, then what happened to the chemical?) Table 13.1 shows that at least

TABLE 13.1
In Vivo Percutaneous Absorption of Dinoseb in Rhesus Monkey and Rat[a]

Applied Dose (µg/cm²)	Skin Penetration (%)	Dose Accountability (%)
Rat		
51.5	86.4 ± 1.1	87.9 ± 1.8
128.8	90.5 ± 1.1	91.5 ± 0.6
643.5	93.2 ± 0.6	90.4 ± 0.7
Rhesus monkey		
43.6	5.4 ± 2.9	86.0 ± 4.0
200.0	7.2 ± 6.4	81.2 ± 18.1
3620.0	4.9 ± 3.4	80.3 ± 5.2

[a] Rat = acetone vehicle; 72-hour application; Monkey—Premerge-3 vehicle; 24-hour application.

TABLE 13.2

Percutaneous Absorption and Accountability of Dinoseb In Vivo Study in the Rhesus Monkey

	Applied Dose ($\mu g/cm^2$)		
Disposition Parameter	43.6	200.00 Applied Dose Accountability (%)	3620.0
Urine	3.3 ± 1.8	4.4 ± 23.9	3.0 ± 2.1
Feces	0.8 ± 0.5	1.0 ± 0.6	3.0 ± 1.7
Contaminated solids	0.03 ± 0.02	0.02 ± 0.02	0.07 ± 0.08
Pan wash	0.04 ± 0.03	0.8 ± 1.1	0.4 ± 0.3
Skin wash	81.1 ± 4.0	75.0 ± 22.9	73.8 ± 6.8
Total Accountability	**86.0 ± 4.0**	**81.2 ± 18.1**	**80.3 ± 5.2**

80% of the applied doses can be accounted for (rat and rhesus monkey) and Table 13.2 that in the rhesus monkey the dinoseb remained on the skin (skin wash recovery 73.8 ± 6.8) and was not absorbed over the 24-hour application period.

13.5 EFFECTS OF CONCENTRATION ON PERCUTANEOUS ABSORPTION

Maibach and Feldmann (5) applied increased concentrations of testosterone, hydrocortisone, and benzoic acid from 4 $\mu g/cm^2$ in three steps to 2000 $\mu g/cm^2$ (4 $\mu g/cm^2$ is approximately equivalent to the amount applied in a 0.25% topical application; 2000 $\mu g/cm^2$ leaves a grossly visible deposit of chemical). Increasing the concentration of the chemical always increased total absorption. These data suggest that as much as gram amounts of some compounds can be absorbed through normal skin under therapeutic and environmental conditions.

Wester and Maibach (6) further defined the relationship of topical dosing. Increasing concentration of testosterone, hydrocortisone, and benzoic acid decreased the efficiency of percutaneous absorption (percent dose absorbed) in both the rhesus monkey and man (Table 13.3), but the total amount of material absorbed through the skin always increased with increased concentration. Schuplein and Ross (7) also showed in vitro that the mass of material absorbed across skin increased when the applied dose was increased. The same relationship between dose applied and dose absorbed is also seen with the pesticides parathion and lindane in Table 13.4.

Wedig et al. (9) compared the percutaneous penetration of different anatomical sites. A single dose of a ^{14}C-labeled magnesium sulfate adduct of dipyrithione at concentrations of 4, 12, or 40 $\mu g/cm^2$ per site was applied for an eight-hour contact time to the forearm, forehead, and scalp of human volunteers. The results again indicated that as the concentration increased, more was absorbed. Skin permeability for equivalent doses on different sites assumed the following order: forehead was equal to scalp, which was greater than forearm. The total amounts absorbed increased even when the percentage of dose excreted at two doses remained approximately the same. On the forehead, proportionately more penetrated from the 40 $\mu g/cm^2$ than from the 4 and 12 $\mu g/cm^2$ doses. On the scalp the difference was even more striking, with almost twice as much proportionately penetrating from 40 $\mu g/cm^2$ than from 4 and 12 $\mu g/cm^2$. Thus, as the concentration of applied dose increased, the total amount of chemical penetrating the skin (and thus becoming systemically available) also increased for all the anatomical sites studied. Therefore, for exposure of many parts of the body, absorption can take place from all of the sites. As the concentration of applied chemical and the total body exposure increase, the subsequent systemic availability will also increase.

TABLE 13.3

Percutaneous Absorption of Increased Topical Dose of Several Compounds in Rhesus Monkey and Man

Compound (µg/cm²)	Totals for Rhesus		Totals for Man	
	%	Micrograms	%	Micrograms
Testosterone				
34	18.4	0.7	11.8	0.4
30	—	—	0.88.	2.6
40	6.7	2.7	—	—
250	2.9	7.2	—	—
400	2.2	8.8	2.8	11.2
1600	2.9	46.4	—	—
4000	1.4	56.0	—	—
Hydrocortisone				
4	2.9	0.1	1.6	0.1
40	2.1	0.8	0.6	0.2
Benzoic acid				
3	—	—	37.0	1.1
4	59.2	2.4	—	—
40	33.6	134.4	25.7	102.8
2000	17.4	348.0	14.4	288.0

Source: From References 5 and 6.

Although the penetration at these doses varied between anatomical sites, the percentage of the dose penetrating was similar at the three doses on the forearm and the forehead. However, on the occiput of the scalp, there was an increasing percentage of penetration with increasing dosage. In other words, at the highest dose, the efficiency of penetration was the greatest.

Reifenrath et at. (10) determined the percutaneous penetration of mosquito repellents in hairless dogs. As the topical dose increased in concentration, the penetration in terms of percentage

TABLE 13.4

Effect of Applied Topical Concentration on Human Percutaneous Absorption

Compound (µg/cm²)	Total	
	%	(mg)
Parathion		
4	8.6	0.3
40	9.5	3.8
400	4.8	19.2
2000	9.0	18.0
Lindane		
4	9.3	0.4
40	8.3	3.3
400	5.7	22.8
1000	3.4	34.0
2000	4.4	88.0

Source: From Reference 8.

TABLE 13.5

Percutaneous Penetration and Total Absorption of Repellents in Relation to Dose of Chemical Applied to Hairless Dog

Compound	Topical Dose ($\mu g/cm^2$)	Penetration (% of Applied Dose)	Mean Total Absorbed ($\mu g/cm^2$)
Ethyl hexanediol	4	8.8	0.35
	320	10.3	33.0
N,N-diethyl-m-toluamide	4	12.8	0.51
	320	9.4	30.1
Sulfonamide[a]	100	9.1	9.1
	320	7.5	24.0
	1000	5.4	54.0

Source: From Reference 10.

[a] *n*-Butane sulfonamide cyclohexamethylene.

of applied dose was about the same (Table 13.5). However, the mean total amount of material absorbed increased dramatically. An application of 4 $\mu g/cm^2$ of N,N-diethyl-m-toluamide gave a 12.8% absorption, resulting in a total absorption of 0.5 $\mu g/cm^2$. An increase in the dose to 320 $\mu g/cm^2$ decreased the percentage absorbed to 9.4; however, the total amount of material absorbed was now up to 30.1 $\mu g/cm^2$, an increase of 60 times!

Roberts and Horlock (11) examined the effects of concentration and repeated skin application of percutaneous absorption. Following single-treatment application with 1%, 5%, and 10% ointments, the penetration fluxes for salicylic acid in hydrophilic ointment increased as the concentration increased (Table 13.6). With extended application on a daily basis, a change in flux was also observed, the skin underwent a change, and subsequently the penetration flux changed.

Wester (unpublished observations) looked at percutaneous absorption of nitroglycerin. The topical concentration of nitroglycerin was increased stepwise from 0.01 to 10 mg/cm². The percentage dose absorbed remained basically the same between 0.01 and 1 mg/cm² (Table 13.7). But as this dose increased 10 times, the amount of material becoming systemically available increased 10 times. At 10 mg/cm² the percentage dose absorbed had markedly decreased. This suggests that the percentage of absorption could become saturated at a high concentration.

TABLE 13.6

Mean Penetration Fluxes of Salicylic Acid in Hydrophilic Ointment Base Through Excised Rat Skin after Single Treatment

Salicylic Acid Concentration (w/w)	Penetration Flux of Salicylic Acid (mg/cm² hr, ± SE)
1	0.014 ± 0.002
5	0.061 + 0.003
10	0.078 ± 0.003

Source: From Reference 11.

TABLE 13.7

Percutaneous Absorption of Nitroglycerin: Topical Concentration versus Absorption for Neat Liquid Application

Topical Nitroglycerin concentration (mg/cm²)	Absorption	
	%	Total (µg)
0.01	41.8	0.004
0.1	43.5	0.04
1.0	36.6	0.4
7.0	26.6	1.9
10.0	7.8	0.8

Source: From Reference 27 (unpublished observations).

Howes and Black (12) determined the comparative percutaneous absorption of sodium and zinc pyrithione in shampoo through rat skin. As the concentrations of material in shampoo increased from 0.1% to 2%, the penetration also increased from 0.7 to 1 µg/cm² (Table 13.8).

13.6   CONCENTRATION AND NEWBORNS

Wester et al. (13) compared the percutaneous absorption in newborn versus adult rhesus monkeys. The total amount absorbed per square centimeter of skin again increased with increased applied dose and was further increased when the site of application was occluded. In the newborn the question of concentration may have special significance because surface area/body mass ratio is greater than in the adult. Therefore, the systemic availability per kilogram of body weight can be increased by as much as threefold.

13.7   CONCENTRATION AND WATER TEMPERATURE

Cummings (14) determined the effect of temperature on rate of penetration on *n*-octylamine through human skin. Increasing the temperature increased the rate of penetration, as evidenced by octylamine-induced wheal formation and erythema. The increase in cutaneous blood flow mainly involved areas of the wheal. The increase in cutaneous blood flow mainly involved areas of the epidermal factors. Therefore, increased temperature along with increased concentration will increase the percutaneous absorption.

TABLE 13.8

The Effect of Concentration of Sodium Pyrithione in Shampoo on Absorption through Rat Skin

Concentration in Shampoo (% w/v)	Total Absorption (%)
0.1	0.07
0.5	0.27
1.0	0.62
2.0	1.02

Source: From Reference 12.

TABLE 13.9
Effect of Duration of Occlusion on Percutaneous
Absorption of Malathion in Man

Duration (hr)	Absorption (%)
0[a]	9.6
0.5	7.3
1	12.7
2	16.6
4	24.2
8	38.8
24	62.8

[a] Immediate wash with soap and water.
Source: From Reference 8.

13.8 CONCENTRATION AND DURATION OF CONTACT

Howes and Black (15) studied percutaneous absorption of triclocarban in rats and humans. As the duration of contact increased, penetration increased.

Nakaue and Buhler (16) examined the percutaneous absorption of hexachlorophene in adult and weanling male rats at exposure times from 1.5 to 24 hours and determined the plasma concentrations of hexachlorophene. The plasma concentrations of hexachlorophene increased with time from a low of just a few ng/mL of plasma up to 80+ ng/mL.

Duration of occlusion enhances percutaneous absorption. The significance of time in occlusion was shown by Feldmann and Maibach (8), who concluded that the longer clothing occludes a pesticide, the greater the contamination potential becomes (Table 13.9).

13.9 CONCENTRATION, DURATION OF CONTACT, AND MULTIPLE-DOSE APPLICATION

Black and Howes (17) studied the skin penetration of chemically related detergents (anionic surfactants) through rat skin and determined the absorption for multiple variables, mainly concentration of applied dose, duration of contact, and the effect of multiple-dose applications. With alcohol sulfate and alcohol ether sulfate, as the concentration of applied dose increased and the duration of contact increased, penetration increased. With multiple applications there was also an increase in penetration (Table 13.10). Therefore, again the systemic availability and potential toxicity of a chemical depend on many variables. One of these, the concentration, was discussed in the preceding paragraphs. Other variables, such as duration of contact and multiple application, are also important.

13.10 CONCENTRATION AND SURFACE AREA

Sved et al. (18) determined the role of surface area on percutaneous absorption of nitroglycerin. As the surface area of applied dose increased, the total amount of material absorbed and systemic availability of nitroglycerin increased. This was confirmed by the percutaneous absorption studies of Noonan and Wester (19), but there was no linear relationship between the size of the surface area and increase in absorption. However, the same information held. The surface area of applied dose determined systemic availability of the chemical.

TABLE 13.10

Concentration, Duration of Contact, and Multiple Application as Variables in Penetration of Anionic Surfactant through Rat Skin

Variable	Penetration ($\mu g/cm^2$)
Concentration (% w/v)	
0.2	0.02
0.5	0.11
1.0	0.23
2.0	0.84
Duration of contact (min)	
1	0.25
5	0.47
10	0.69
20	0.97
Multiple application ($\times$ 5 min)	
1	0.14
2	0.25
4	0.36

Source: From Reference 17.

13.11 EFFECT OF APPLICATION FREQUENCY

Wester et al. (20, 21) studied the effect of application frequency on the percutaneous absorption of hydrocortisone. Material applied once or three times a day showed a statistical difference ($p < 0.05$) in the percutaneous absorption. One application each 24 hours of exposure gave a higher absorption than material applied at a lower concentration but more frequently, namely, three times a day. This study also showed that washing (effect of hydration) enhanced the percutaneous absorption of hydrocortisone. This relationship between frequency of application and percutaneous absorption is also seen with testosterone.

The aforenoted studies used intermittent application per single day of application. Another consideration is extended versus short-term administration and the subsequent effect on percutaneous absorption. Wester et al. (22) examined the percutaneous absorption of hydrocortisone with long-term administration. The work suggests that extended exposure had some effect on the permeability characteristics of skin and markedly increased percutaneous absorption.

With malathion, which apparently has no pharmacological effect on skin, the dermal absorption from day 1 was equivalent to day 8 application (23).

Therefore, for malathion, the single-dose application data are relevant for predicting the toxic potential for longer-term exposure.

13.12 APPLICATION FREQUENCY AND TOXICITY

There is a correlation between frequency of application, percutaneous absorption, and toxicity of applied chemical. Wilson and Holland (24) determined the effect of application frequency in epidermal carcinogenic assays. Application of a single large dose of a highly complex mixture of petroleum or synthetic fuels to a skin site increased the carcinogenic potential of the chemical compared with smaller or more frequent applications (Table 13.11). This carcinogenic toxicity correlated well with the results of Wester et al. (20, 21), in which a single applied dose increased the percutaneous absorption of the material compared with smaller or intermittent applications.

TABLE 13.11
Incidence of Tumors after Application of Shale Oils

Shale Oil	Dose and Frequency	Total Dose Per Week (mg)	Number of Animals with Tumors
OCSO No. 6	10 mg, 4 times	40	2
	20 mg, 2 times	40	4
	40 mg, once	40	13
PCSO II	10 mg, 4 times	40	11
	20 mg, 2 times	40	17
	40 mg, once	40	19

Source: From Reference 24.

13.13   CONCLUSION

Many variables affect percutaneous absorption and subsequent dermal toxicity. Increased concentration of an applied chemical on skin increases the body burden, as does increasing the surface area and the time of exposure. The opposite also holds true, namely, dilution of a chemical will decrease the effects of the applied concentration, provided other factors do not change (such as diluting the chemical but spreading the same total dose over a larger surface area). The body burden is also dependent on the frequency of daily application and on possible effects resulting from long-term topical exposure. Dose accountability (mass balance) completes a dose-response study.

The current data provide a skeleton of knowledge to use in the design and interpretation of toxicological and pharmacological studies to increase their relevance to the most typical exposures for man. In essence, we have just begun to define the complexity of the interrelationships between percutaneous absorption and dermatoxicology (Table 13.12) (25, 26). Until an appropriate theoretical

TABLE 13.12
Factors in the Dose-Response Interrelationships of Percutaneous Absorption

Concentration of applied dose ($\mu g/cm^2$)
Surface area of applied dose (cm^2)
Total dose
Application frequency
Duration of contact
Site of application
Temperature
Vehicle
Substantivity (nonpenetrating surface adsorption)
Wash-and-rub resistance
Volatility
Binding
Individual and species variations
Skin condition
Occlusion

Source: From Reference 25.

basis that has been experimentally verified becomes available, quantitating the various variables listed herein will greatly improve the usefulness of biologically oriented procedures such as LDV, transepidermal water loss, and real-time solvent assay in pulmonary breath exhalation and will expand our knowledge of not only skin dose-response but the use of skin absorption and dynamics to better the human race.

REFERENCES

1. Wester RC, Hui X, Maibach HI, Thrall KD, Poet TS, Corley RA, Edwards JA, Weitz KK. Utility of real time breath analysis and physiologically based pharmacokinetic modeling to determine the percutaneous absorption of methyl chloroform in rats and humans. Toxicol Sci 2000; 54: 42–51.
2. Wester RC, Maibach HI, Guy RH, Novak E. Minoxidil stimulates cutaneous blood flow in human balding scalps: pharmacodynamics measured by laser Doppler velocimetry and photopulse plethysmography. Invest Dermatol 1984; 82: 515–517.
3. Maibach HI, Stoughton RB. Topical corticosteroids. Med Clin N Am 1973; 57: 1253–1264.
4. Shah PV, Fisher HL, Sumler MR, Monroe RJ, Chernoff N, Hall LL. A comparison of the penetration of fourteen pesticides through the skin of young and adult rats. J Toxicol Enviorn Health 1987; 21: 353–366.
5. Maibach HI, Feldmann RJ. Effect of applied concentration on percutaneous absorption in man. Invest Dermatol 1969; 52: 382.
6. Wester RC, Maibach HI. Relationship of topical dose and percutaneous absorption on Rhesus monkey and man. Invest Dermatol 1976; 67: 518–520.
7. Scheuplein RJ, Ross LW. Mechanism of percutaneous absorption V. Percutaneous absorption of solvent-deposited solids. J Invest Dermatol 1974; 62: 353–360.
8. Feldmann RJ, and Maibach HI. Systemic absorption of pesticides through the skin of man. In occupational exposure to pesticides: Report to the Federal Working Group on Pest Management from the task group on occupation exposure to pesticides. Appendix B 1979; 120–127.
9. Wedig JH, Feldmann RJ, Maibach HI. Percutaneous penetration of the magnesium sulfate adduct of dipyrithione in man. Toxicol Appl Pharmacol 1977; 41: 1–6.
10. Reifenrath WG, Robinson PB, Bolton VD, Aliff RE. Percutaneous penetration of mosquito repellents in the hairless dog: effect of dose on percentage penetration. Food Cosmet Toxicol 1981; 19: 195–199.
11. Roberts MS, Horlock E. Effect of repeated skin application on percutaneous absorption of salicylic acid. J Pharm Sci 1978; 67: 1685–1687.
12. Howes D, Black JG. Comparative percutaneous absorption of pyrithiones. Toxicology 1975; 5: 209–220.
13. Wester RC, Noonan PK, Cole MP, Maibach HI. Percutaneous absorption of testosterone in the newborn Rhesus monkey: comparison to the adult. Pediatr Res 1977; 11: 737–739.
14. Cummings EG. Temperature and concentration effects on penetration of N-octylamine through human skin in situ. J Invest Dermatol 1969; 53: 64–79.
15. Howes D, Black JG. Percutaneous absorption of triclocarban in rat and man. Toxicology 1976; 6: 67–76.
16. Nakaue HS, Buhler DR. Percutaneous absorption of hexachlorophene in the rat. Toxicol Appl Pharmacol 1976; 35: 381–391.
17. Black JG, Howes D. Skin penetration of chemically related detergents. Soc Cosmet Chem 1979; 30: 157–165.
18. Sved S, McLean WM, McGilveray IJ. Influence of the method of application on pharmacokinetics of nitroglycerin from ointment in humans. Pharm Sci 1981; 70: 1368–1369.
19. Noonan PK, Wester RC. Percutaneous absorption of nitroglycerin. Pharm Sci 1980; 69: 385.
20. Wester RC, Noonan PK, Maibach HI. Frequency of application on percutaneous absorption of hydrocortisone. Arch Dermatol Res 1977; 113: 620–622.
21. Wester RC, Noonan PK, Maibach HI. Variations in percutaneous absorption of testosterone in the Rhesus monkey due to anatomic site of application and frequency of application. Arch Dermatol Res 1980; 267: 299–335.
22. Wester RC, Noonan PK, Maibach HI. Percutaneous absorption of hydrocortisone increases with long-term administration. Arch Dermatol Res 1980; 116: 186–188.

23. Wester RC, Maibach HI, Bucks DAW, Guy RH. Malathion percutaneous absorption following repeated administration to man. Toxicol Appl Pharmacol 1983; 68: 116–119.
24. Wilson JS, Holland LM. The effect of application frequency on epidermal carcinogenesis assays. Toxicology 1982; 24: 45–54.
25. Wester RC, Maibach HI. Cutaneous pharmacokinetics: 10 steps to percutaneous absorption. Drug Metab Rev 1983; 14: 169–205.
26. Wester RC, and Maibach HI. In vivo percutaneous absorption. In: Marzuui F, Maibach HI, eds. Dermatotoxicology, 2d ed. Washington, DC: Hemisphere, 1982: 131–146.
27. Wester RC, Maibach HI, Guy RH, and Novak E. Pharmacodynamics and percutaneous absorption. In: Bronaugh R, Maibach H, eds. Percutaneous Absorption, New York: Marcel Dekker, Inc., 1985:547–560.

14 Effects of Occlusion
Percutaneous Absorption

Nina Dragićević
Singidunum University, Danijelova 32, Belgrade, Serbia

Howard I. Maibach
University of California, San Francisco, California

CONTENTS

14.1 INTRODUCTION

Occlusion means the skin covered by tape, gloves, impermeable dressings, or transdermal devices. In healthy skin, the stratum corneum typically has a water content of 10% to 20% and provides a relatively efficient barrier against percutaneous absorption of exogenous substances (1). Skin occlusion can increase stratum corneum hydration, and hence influence percutaneous absorption by altering partitioning between the surface chemical and the skin due to the increasing presence of water, swelling corneocytes, and possibly altering the intercellular lipid-phase organization, also by increasing the skin surface temperature and increasing blood flow (2–4). Occlusion may enhance drug efficacy (5–10). Actually, skin occlusion is a complex event producing profound changes and influencing skin biology as well as wound healing processing (11–27). In general, occlusion can, with exceptions (2, 4, 28, 29), increase percutaneous absorption of topically applied compounds (30–42); even a short time (30 minutes) of occlusion can result in significantly increased penetration and horny layer water content (43). However, the effects of occlusion on absorption may also depend on the anatomic site as well as vehicle and penetrant (32, 37, 44, 45).

As to the nature of the vehicle, i.e., drug delivery system (DDS), the effectiveness of some DDSs, such as deformable liposomes, was attributed, besides to the physicochemical properties of vesicles, to application conditions, i.e., to their open application (nonocclusive application to the skin), as explained by the inventors of ultra-deformable vesicles named Transfersomes (46–48). Certain topical vehicles may also act as "occlusive dressings" if they contain fats or some polymer oils, reducing water loss to the atmosphere. Some nanocarriers may act as occlusive vehicles, such as lipid nanoparticles (solid lipid nanoparticles [SLNs] and nanostructured lipid carriers [NLCs]) (49, 50). These nanocarriers occlude the skin by forming a continuous thin film when the water from the formulation evaporates due to their adhesive properties (49). This occlusion reduces water evaporation from the skin, which increases the hydration of the stratum corneum, and the corneocytes become less compact while the inter-corneocyte gaps become wider. These changes increase the stratum corneum permeability, which can promote drug penetration (51). SLNs and NLCs differ in the extent of occlusion which they provide, i.e., SLNs have a higher occlusion property at similar lipid concentrations (49, 52).

Dermal and transdermal drug delivery systems have a high level of interest; in practice, skin is not readily breached in the therapeutic level because of barrier resistance. Various approaches have been employed to enhance absorption. Occlusion, perhaps due to its simplicity and convenience, has been extensively adopted to increase absorption. This chapter focuses on the effect of occlusion on percutaneous absorption and summarizes related details. Table 14.1 summarizes the brief data of the effect of occlusion on percutaneous absorption.

14.2   PERCUTANEOUS ABSORPTION IN VITRO

Gummer and Maibach (30) examined the penetration of methanol and ethanol through excised, full-thickness, guinea pig skin in vitro at varying volumes and under a variety of occlusive conditions over a period of 19 hours. Neither compound showed an increase in penetration with increasing dose volume. But occlusion significantly enhanced ($p < 0.01$) penetration of both when compared to non-occluded skin. The nature of the occlusive material significantly influenced the penetrated amounts of both compounds, as well as the profiles of the amount penetrating per hour.

Hotchkiss et al. (31) evaluated absorption of model compounds nicotinic acid, phenol, and benzoic acid and the herbicide triclopyr butoxyethyl ester (triclopyr BEE) with in vitro flow-through diffusion cells using rat and human skin. After application, the skin surface was either nonoccluded or covered with Teflon caps as an occlusion device. The absorption of each compound across the skin and into the receptor fluid at 72 hours was calculated. Occlusion significantly ($p < 0.05$) enhanced absorption of the model compounds, but varied with the compound and the skin (rat or human) used. They observed the effect of vehicle and occlusion on the in vitro percutaneous absorption of [methylene-^{14}C]-benzyl acetate (1.7 to 16.6 mg/cm^2) in diffusion cells using full-thickness skin from male Fischer 344 rats (32). When benzyl acetate in ethanol was applied to the skin and occluded with Parafilm, the extent of absorption at 48 hours was not significantly different from nonoccluded skin, but at 6 hours, as the ethanol content of the application mixture was increased, the absorption of benzyl acetate through occluded skin was enhanced proportionally ($r = 0.99$). With phenylethanol as a vehicle, the extent of the benzyl acetate absorption through occluded skin at 48 hours was significantly ($p < 0.05$) enhanced compared with nonoccluded skin, but this did not correlate with the proportion of phenylethanol in the application mixture. With dimethyl sulfoxide as a vehicle, the extent of benzyl acetate absorption through occluded skin at 48 hours was enhanced ($p < 0.05$) compared with nonoccluded skin; when dimethyl sulfoxide content of the application mixture was increased, the absorption of benzyl acetate was enhanced proportionally. The researchers concluded that occlusion often significantly enhanced absorption, but the effect varied with time and vehicle.

Cross and Roberts (53) confirmed that the occlusion effect on drug penetration through the skin strongly depends on the vehicle used. They evaluated in vitro human epidermal penetration of a mixture of paraben ester preservatives from a commercially available test ointment and two commonly employed solvent vehicles (acetone and ethanol), together with the effect of occlusion. Parabens were applied in finite doses and occlusion was achieved by the placement of a piece of high-density polyethylene over the application site immediately after dosing (53). There was a significant difference in the epidermal flux of paraben esters from each of the vehicles following occlusion. Increases of drug flux were observed for acetone and ethanol vehicles, while a decrease was seen following occlusive application of the ointment formulation. This decrease in flux appeared to be a result of a significant decrease in the epidermal partitioning of the esters following occlusion of the ointment, while the increased flux of parabens from solvents resulted from an increase in the epidermal diffusivity of parabens following occlusion of the solvent vehicles (53).

TABLE 14.1
Summary of the Effect of Occlusion on Percutaneous Absorption

Models				
In Vitro	In Vivo		Compounds	Results and References
	Animals	Humans		
Guinea pig skin			Methanol and ethanol	Enhanced the penetration of both chemicals. The nature of the occlusive material influenced the occlusion effect (30).
Human skin			Citropten and caffeine	Increased the permeation of citropten (lipophilic compound) but not of caffeine (amphiphilic compound). They found that occlusion does not increase the percutaneous absorption of all chemicals (28).
Human skin			Salicylic acid and formaldehyde	Occlusion affected the percutaneous penetration of the lipophilic salicylic acid more than of the hydrophilic formaldehyde. Thus, occlusion did not have a significant enhancing effect on both chemicals, i.e., a strong correlation was seen between occlusion and their partition coefficients (44).
Rat and human skin			Nicotinic acid, phenol, benzoic acid, and triclopyr butoxyethyl ester	Significantly enhanced the percutaneous absorption of the compounds but varied with the compound under study and the skin (rat or human) used (31).
Rat skin Human epidermis			Benzyl acetate in different vehicles (in ethanol, phenylethanol, and dimethyl sulfoxide) Parabens in different vehicles (in acetone, ethanol, and ointment formulation)	Significantly enhanced absorption, but the effect varied with time and vehicle (32). Increased flux from acetone and ethanol and a decreased flux upon the occlusive application of the ointment formulation. The effect depended on the vehicle used (53).
Isolated perfused porcine skin flap			Phenol and PNP in two different vehicles (acetone and ethanol)	Increased the penetration of both compounds, but affected by used vehicles. The penetration was vehicle, occlusion, and penetrant dependent (45).
Rabbit ear skin			Progesterone in microemulsions with different ethanol content, saturated drug solution, and propylene glycol–water mixture	Occlusion enhanced drug flux from all formulations. The highest drug flux was obtained from microemulsions, i.e., the flux increase was vehicle dependent. Besides occlusion, supersaturation also played an important role (54).
Human skin			Estradiol in ultra-deformable vesicles	Occlusion resulted in a significant reduction of the transdermal flux of the drug from deformable vesicles compared to their nonocclusive application. Thus, the occlusion effect was vehicle dependent (58).
Rat and human skin			2-Phenoxyethanol applied in methanol	Reduced evaporation and increased total absorption (33).
Human skin	Rhesus monkeys		Safrole, cinnamyl anthranilate, cinnamic alcohol, and cinnamic acid	Resulted in greater permeation of all compounds. No correlation was found between skin penetration of compounds and their partition coefficients (34).

(Continued)

TABLE 14.1 *(Continued)*
Summary of the Effect of Occlusion on Percutaneous Absorption

	Models			
	In Vivo			
In Vitro	**Animals**	**Humans**	**Compounds**	**Results and References**
	Weanling pigs		Parathion and its major metabolites	Increased the absorption and shortened the mean residence time; the effect of occlusion on percutaneous absorption was affected by anatomical site (35–37).
	Weanling pigs		Pentachlorophenol	Absorption on occluded dosed site was significantly enhanced (by more than three times) when compared to nonoccluded site (38).
	Rhesus monkeys	Humans	Benzyl acetate and five other benzyl derivatives	Increased the penetration with variability between compounds (39).
	Rats		2',3'-Dideoxyinosine	Gave a more uniform plasma profile but did not increase the bioavailability (40).
		Humans	Hydrocortisone	Significantly increased (tenfold) the cumulative absorption (41).
		Humans	Pesticide malathion	Significantly increased malathion penetration. Duration of occlusion affected the penetration, i.e., increasing duration increased penetration (76).
		Humans	Hexyl nicotinate	Significantly increased the peak height and AUC, and the onset of action and time to peak were significantly shortened; also showed a significant correlation between stratum corneum water content and area under the LDV response–time curve (42, 43).
		Humans	Hydrocortisone, estradiol, testosterone, and progesterone	Significantly increased percutaneous absorption of the lipophilic steroids estradiol, testosterone, and progesterone but did not affect the penetration of the most water-soluble steroid hydrocortisone (29).
		Humans	Elastic surfactant-based vesicles	Fast penetration of intact elastic vesicles into the stratum corneum after nonocclusive treatment. Occlusive treatment provided very few intact vesicles in the deeper layers of the stratum corneum (75).
	Pigs		Ketoprofen in deformable vesicles Transfersomes	Occlusion disables penetration-enhancing effect of ultra-deformable, hydrophilic carriers by eliminating transcutaneous hydration gradient that normally drives carriers across the skin. These vesicles enhance drug penetration under nonocclusive application in vivo (65).

Abbreviations: AUC, area under the curve; *LDV*, laser Doppler velocimetry; *PNP*, *p*-nitrophenol.

Roper et al. (33) tested the absorption of 2-phenoxyethanol applied in methanol through nonoccluded rat and human skin in vitro in two diffusion cell systems over 24 hours. 2-Phenoxyethanol was lost by evaporation with both nonoccluded cells, but occlusion of the static cell reduced evaporation and increased total absorption to $98.8 \pm 7.0\%$.

El Maghraby et al. (54) investigated the transdermal delivery of progesterone from microemulsions (MEs) under occlusive and open application. This study tested an ME formulation containing oleic acid, Tween 80, propylene glycol, and water. The ME system was used neat or with ethanol (20% or 40%) as a volatile co-surfactant. Results of this study indicated that ME formulations enhanced progesterone transdermal flux compared to the saturated drug solution in 14% aqueous propylene glycol (control). Ethanol-containing ME (EME) was more effective than the ethanol-free system (EFME), with the flux increasing upon increasing the ethanol concentration in the ME (54). Occlusive application of 20% EME increased the transdermal flux by 5.7-fold compared to the control and by 2.3-fold compared to the EFM. Occlusive application of 40% EME further increased the transdermal progesterone flux, with the values being 9-fold compared to the control and 3.7-fold compared to EFME. Open application of EFME produced a minor decrease in drug flux compared to occlusive application. For EME, open application significantly reduced the flux by 26% to 28% compared to occlusive application of the same formulation, indicating the importance of occlusion on increasing the drug flux. However, the flux of EME when using open application remained significantly higher than that obtained with EFME regardless if occlusive or open application of EFME was used. This proposed the importance of supersaturation with the contribution of ethanol in the achieved skin penetration enhancement. To confirm this, the authors evaluated the transdermal delivery of progesterone from 40% ethanol in water (ETW) under occlusive and open application. The sum of fluxes obtained from ETW and EFME was lower than that obtained from EME under both application conditions. It was concluded that supersaturation played an important role in enhanced transdermal drug delivery and also occlusion. The authors introduced ME formulations containing volatile components as candidates for the formulation of sprays for dermal application (54).

Treffel et al. (28) compared permeation profiles of two molecules with different physicochemical properties under occluded vs. nonoccluded conditions in vitro over a period of 24 hours. Absorption was determined using human abdominal skin in diffusion cells under occluded and nonoccluded conditions. Occlusion increased the permeation of citropten (a lipophilic compound; partition coefficient = 2.17) 1.6 times ($p < 0.05$) greater than the nonoccluded permeation. However, the permeation of caffeine (an amphiphilic compound; partition coefficient = 0.02) did not show significant differences ($p = 0.18$) between occlusive and nonocclusive conditions. They confirmed the view, i.e., occlusion does not necessarily increase the percutaneous absorption of all chemicals (2, 4, 29).

Hafeez et al. (44) investigated the skin penetration of [14C]-formaldehyde and [14C]-salicylic acid in vitro in human skin under nonocclusion as well as under various occlusive time periods (one, four, and eight hours). The radioactivity recovery as percentage of applied dose of [14C]-salicylic acid was significantly higher under occlusion versus nonocclusion in the epidermis, dermis, and receptor fluid after 24 hours. For [14C]-formaldehyde, no significant statistical difference was observed under occlusion versus nonocclusion. The occlusion duration affected the percutaneous penetration of the lipophilic salicylic acid more than the hydrophilic formaldehyde. Further, a strong correlation between occlusion-enhanced penetration and partition coefficients of salicylic acid and formaldehyde was observed (44).

Brooks and Riviere (45) utilized an isolated perfused porcine skin flap (IPPSF) to determine the percutaneous absorption of [14C]-labeled phenol versus p-nitrophenol (PNP) at two concentrations (4 µg/cm^2 versus 40 µg/cm^2) in two vehicles (acetone versus ethanol) under occluded versus nonoccluded dosing conditions over eight hours Occlusion increased the absorption, penetration into tissues, and total recoveries of phenol when compared to nonoccluded conditions. Absorption and penetration of phenol into tissues were greater with ethanol than with acetone under nonoccluded conditions, but the opposite was observed under occluded conditions. Phenol in acetone had a greater percentage of applied dose penetration into tissues with low doses than high doses, suggesting a fixed absorption rate. This was also seen for PNP, but only under occluded conditions. Neither phenol dose, vehicle, nor occlusion had a significant effect on the labeled phenol seen in the stratum corneum or on time of peak flux, a finding that limits the usefulness of noninvasive stratum corneum sampling to assess topical penetration. Neither PNP dose, vehicle, nor occlusion had a significant effect on total recovery of labeled PNP. The researchers suggested that comparative absorption of phenol and PNP are vehicle, occlusion, and penetrant dependent.

In contrast to most penetration studies, which use mainly occlusive application of drug formulations onto the skin, Cevc and Blume (46) highlighted the importance of the nonocclusive application of drug-loaded deformable vesicles, Transfersomes, onto the skin to preserve the "hydrational driving force" across the epidermis, which should, according to the authors, "push" the deformable vesicles across the epidermis. According to Cevc and Blume (45), the osmotic gradient, which is created by the difference in the total water concentrations between the skin surface and the skin interior, provides one possible source of such driving force. This force would be, according to the authors, sufficiently strong to "push" at least 0.5 mg of lipids per hour and cm^2 through the skin permeability barrier into the region of the stratum corneum (45). Thus, the ability of deformable vesicles to penetrate the intact skin, carrying their encapsulated drugs, is attributed to their xerophobia (tendency to avoid dry surroundings and hence move along with the hydration gradient) and to their deformation ability to "pull" through the skin under nonocclusion (46–48, 55, 56). It has also been shown in murine stratum corneum ex vivo and in vivo that Transfersomes, after nonocclusive application, penetrate into the stratum corneum through preexisting channels, i.e., through the "intercluster" pathway (mostly) between groups of corneocytes that only partly overlap (low-resistance route) with a barrier maximum at around 10 μm and the "intercorneocyte" pathway between individual corneocytes (high-resistance route) with a barrier maximum at around 4 to 7 μm (57). Occlusion would therefore be detrimental for vesicle penetration into intact skin and their penetration-enhancing effect.

El Maghraby et al. (58) investigated in vitro in human skin the transdermal delivery of estradiol from ultra-deformable liposomes after their occlusive and nonocclusive application (using an "open stratum corneum protocol," thus preserving the transepidermal hydration gradient). Occlusion resulted in a significant reduction of the transdermal flux of the drug, which confirms the importance of the "open-application protocol" for the transdermal drug delivery from ultra-deformable vesicles. Therefore, as occlusion is believed to abolish the driving force for the penetration of deformable vesicles into the skin, these vesicles (e.g., Transfersomes, invasomes, ethosomes, etc.) are applied in skin penetration studies, as well as for the evaluation of their therapeutic effectiveness, always under nonocclusive condition (58–67). Thus, when applied onto the skin only under nonocclusion, drug-loaded ultra-deformable vesicles achieve their therapeutic effectiveness, as shown in many studies, such as for the antiacne effect of retinoic acid (66), antiinflammatory effect of ammonium glycyrrhizinate (67), antiinflammatory effect of ketoprofen (56, 65, 68), hypoglycemic effect of insulin (69), etc. For more information on the application conditions for different deformable vesicles and their mechanism of action, one should refer to Refs. (48, 63, 70–75).

14.3   PERCUTANEOUS ABSORPTION IN VIVO

14.3.1   ANIMALS

Bronaugh et al. (34) measured the percutaneous absorption of cosmetic fragrance materials safrole and cinnamyl anthranilate, as well as of cinnamic alcohol and cinnamic acid, at occluded and nonoccluded application sites over a 24-hour period. They determined the absorption in the rhesus monkey in vivo and also measured the absorption value through excised human skin in diffusion cells. Each radiolabeled compound was applied in an acetone vehicle at a concentration of 4 μg/cm^2. Occlusion was accomplished by taping plastic wrap to the skin application site for in vivo experiments and by sealing the tops of the diffusion cells with Parafilm. Occlusion of the application sites resulted in large increases in absorption, an effect consistent with the volatility of permeating molecules. When evaporation of the compounds was prevented, 75% of the applied cinnamic alcohol and 84% of the cinnamic acid were absorbed compared to 25% and 39%, respectively, without occlusion. In vitro experiments showed that the percutaneous absorption of these compounds was increased under occlusion in comparison to nonocclusion conditions (open to the air). The greatest difference between in vivo and in vitro absorption values occurred with safrole, which was the least well absorbed and the most volatile compound. Subsequently, they determined the percutaneous absorption of the fragrance benzyl acetate (octanol–water partition coefficient = 1.96) and five other benzyl derivatives (benzyl alcohol, octanol–water partition coefficient = 0.87; benzyl benzoate, octanol–water partition coefficient = 3.97; benzamide, octanol–water partition coefficient = 0.64; benzoin, octanol–water partition coefficient = 1.35; and benzophenone, octanol–water partition coefficient = 3.18) in vivo in rhesus monkeys and human models (39). Two occlusion methods (plastic wrap and glass chamber) were employed for 24 hours. In general, absorption through occluded skin was high. Differences in absorption were observed between the methods. The low percentage absorbed for benzyl acetate was noted with plastic wrap compared to the nonoccluded site, where glass chamber occlusion resulted in the greatest bioavailability. This discrepancy might be due to compound sequestration by the plastic. No correlations were found between skin penetration of these compounds and their octanol–water partition coefficients. Under nonoccluded conditions skin penetration was reduced; there was great variability between compounds, possibly because of variations in the rates of evaporation from the application site.

Qiao et al. (35) described an in vivo female weanling pigs model to quantify disposition of parathion (PA) and its major metabolites for human dermal risk assessment following ^{14}C PA topical (occluded and nonoccluded dose of 300 µg, 40 µg/cm[2] on the abdomen and back) and intravenous (300 µg) application. Total ^{14}C PA and its major metabolites in plasma, urine, blood, stratum corneum, dosed tissues, dosing device, and evaporative loss were determined. Occlusion enhanced the partition of both PA and PNP into the stratum corneum from the dosed skin surface and slowed down the distribution of PA and PNP in the local dosed tissues. Occlusion also altered the first-pass biotransformation of PA in the epidermis. They further analyzed these data, focusing on a quantitation of the effects of application site (back vs. abdomen) and dosing method (occluded vs. nonoccluded) on in vivo disposition of both the parent PA and its sequential metabolites (36). They concluded that occlusion not only increased ^{14}C absorption and shortened the mean residence time in most compartments but also altered the systemic versus cutaneous biotransformation pattern. They investigated the effects of anatomical site and occlusion on the percutaneous absorption and residue pattern of total ^{14}C following topical application of PA onto four skin sites (300 µg/10 µCi; 40 µg/cm[2]) in weanling swine using occluded and nonoccluded dosing systems (37). Total excretion (% dose) of urinary and fecal was determined after 168-hour dosing onto the abdomen, buttocks, back, and shoulder ($N = 4$/site), and the % dose of excretion was 44%, 49%, 49%, and 29% in the occluded system and 7%, 16%, 25%, and 17% in the nonoccluded system, respectively. The percutaneous absorption from the shoulder was much lower than that from the other three sites under occluded conditions. However, in the nonoccluded system, absorption from the abdomen was the lowest, with shoulder and buttocks being similar, and the back the highest. The researchers suggested that anatomic site may influence the effect of occlusion. They utilized the same model to determine the pentachlorophenol (PCP) dermal absorption and disposition from soil under occluded and nonoccluded conditions for 408 hours (38). The absorption on the occluded dosed site (100.7%) was significantly enhanced (by more than three times, $p < 0.0005$) when compared to the nonoccluded site (29.1%).

Mukherji et al. (40) evaluated the topical application of 2',3'-dideoxyinosine (ddI), a nucleoside analog used for treating patients with acquired immunodeficiency syndrome. A dose of ddI (approximately 80 mg/kg) dispersed in approximately 1 g ointment base was applied to the back of high follicular density (HFD) and low follicular density (LFD) rats with or without occlusion. At 24 hours the experiment was terminated and skin sections at the application site removed. After

24 hours topical application, average plateau plasma levels of about 0.6 μg/mL were achieved within
1 to 2 hours and maintained for 24 hours. Occlusion gave a more uniform plasma profile but did not
increase bioavailability. The researchers thought that the transfollicular absorption route for ddI did
not act as an important role due to the similar bioavailability in the HFD and LFD rats.

14.3.2 MAN

Feldmann and Maibach (41) correlated the increased pharmacological effect of hydrocortisone
(HC) by occlusive conditions with the pharmacokinetics of absorption. [^{14}C]-HC in acetone was
applied to the ventral forearm. The application site was either nonoccluded or occluded with plastic
wrap. After 24 hours application, the nonoccluded site was washed. At the occluded site, the wrap
remained for 96 hours post-application before washing the site. The percentage of the applied dose
excreted into the urine, corrected for incomplete renal elimination, was 0.46 ± 0.2 (mean ± SD)
and 5.9 ± 3.5 under nonoccluded and occluded conditions, respectively. The occlusive condition
significantly increased (tenfold) the cumulative absorption of HC (total excretion was occluded =
4.48% vs. nonoccluded = 0.46%). They noted that the difference of application duration (24 hours
exposure on nonoccluded site vs. 96 hours exposure on occluded site) could influence the absorption as determined by the cumulative measurement of drug excreted into urine, but the significant
difference in percent dose at 12 and 24 hours between nonoccluded and occluded was not expected
to be dependent upon differences in washing times.

Malathion, a pesticide, was intensively studied to determine the effect of duration of occlusion
(76). In as little as one hour (13% of absorption), there was a significant increase in penetration, and
in two hours 17%; in four hours this was 24%, and in eight hours 39%.

Ryatt et al. (42) developed a human pharmacodynamic model to measure the enhanced skin penetration of hexyl nicotinate (HN) using laser Doppler velocimetry (LDV). Before applying HN, the
application site was either untreated (control) or subjected to one of four 30-minute pretreatments:
(1) occlusion with a polypropylene chamber; (2) occlusion [as in (1)] in the presence of 0.3 mL of the
vehicle; (3) occlusion [as in (1)] in the presence of 0.3 mL of the vehicle containing 25% 2-pyrrol-
idone; (4) occlusion [as in (1)] in the presence of 0.3 mL of the vehicle containing 25% laurocapram
(1-dodecylhexahydro-2H-azepin-2-one). The onset of action, time to peak, peak height, area under
the curve (AUC), time course, and magnitude of the LDV response were calculated. The onset of
action and time to peak were significantly shortened, and the peak height and AUC significantly
increased with pretreatments (1) to (4) (i.e., under occlusion conditions). Ryatt et al. (43) explored
the relationship between increased stratum corneum hydration by occlusion and enhanced percutaneous absorption in vivo in man. Percutaneous absorption of HN was monitored noninvasively
by LDV following each of three randomly assigned pretreatments: untreated control, 30-minute
occlusion with a polypropylene chamber, and 30-minute occlusion followed by exposure to ambient conditions for one hour. Stratum corneum water content after the same pretreatments was
measured with the dielectric probe technique. The local vasodilatory effect of the nicotinic acid
ester was quantified using LDV by the onset of increased blood flow, time of maximal increase
in response, magnitude of the peak response, and the area under the response–time curve. A
30-minute period of occlusion significantly shortened ($p < 0.05$) both the time of onset of the LDV-
detected response to HN and the time to peak response when compared to the untreated controls.
The stratum corneum water content values showed the same pattern, where the horny layer water
content after 30-minute occlusion was significantly elevated ($p < 0.001$). There was a significant
correlation between stratum corneum water content and area under the LDV response–time curve
after 30-minute occlusion ($r = 0.8$; $p < 0.05$).

Bucks et al. (29) measured the percutaneous absorption of steroids (hydrocortisone, estradiol,
testosterone, and progesterone) in vivo in man under occluded and "protected" (i.e., covered but
nonocclusive) conditions. The ^{14}C-labeled chemicals were applied in acetone to the ventral forearm of volunteers. After vehicle evaporation, the site was covered with a semirigid, polypropylene

chamber for 24 hours. The intact chambers were employed as the occlusion condition and by boring several small holes through the chamber as the "protected" conditions (i.e., the roof of chamber was covered with a piece of water-permeable membrane). Urine was collected for seven days post-application. Steroid absorption increased with increasing lipophilicity up to a point, but the penetration of progesterone (the most hydrophobic analog studied) did not continue the trend and was presumably at least partly rate-limited by slow interfacial transport at the stratum corneum. Twenty-four-hour occlusion significantly increased ($p < 0.01$) percutaneous absorption of estradiol, testosterone, and progesterone but did not affect the penetration of hydrocortisone. The penetration of the more lipophilic steroids was enhanced by occlusion but not the penetration of the most water-soluble steroid (i.e., hydrocortisone).

Honeywell-Nguyen et al. (75) investigated surfactant-based elastic vesicles, which could be used as drug carrier systems, in vivo in human skin under occlusive vs. nonocclusive application and performed afterwards a series of tape strippings, which were visualized by freeze fracture electron microscopy. The results have shown a fast penetration of intact elastic vesicles into the stratum corneum after nonocclusive treatment, frequently via channel-like regions. Intact vesicles could reach the ninth tape strip after the one-hour nonocclusive treatment. After the four-hour treatment, vesicle material could be found in the fifteenth tape strip. However, micrographs of the four-hour treatment showed extensive vesicle fusion both at the skin surface and in the deeper layers of the stratum corneum. A higher volume of application resulted in an increase in the presence of vesicle material found in the deeper layers of the stratum corneum (76). In contrast, micrographs after occlusive treatment revealed very few intact vesicles in the deeper layers of the stratum corneum, but the presence of lipid plaques was frequently observed. Thus, it has been shown in vivo in man that nonocclusive application is preferred for the use of elastic vesicles as potential drug carrier systems, since they provide deeper drug carrier penetration into the skin.

14.4   DISCUSSION

Skin, particularly the stratum corneum, serves as a barrier that prevents or limits the entrance of substances from the environment and also modulates the balance of water loss from body fluids. Occlusion has the immediate effect of completely blocking diffusional water loss (22). The consequence is the increase of stratum corneum hydration, and thus the swelling of the corneocytes and promoting the uptake of water into intercellular lipid domains (2, 4). Occlusion can increase stratum corneum water content from a normal range of 10% to 20% up to 50% and can increase the skin temperature from 32°C to 37°C (2, 4). Occlusion also prevents the accidental wiping or evaporation (volatile compound) of the applied compound, in essence maintaining a higher applied dose (77). Therefore, skin absorption of volatile substances is enhanced under their occlusive application and, thus, volatility is crucial for determining safety and efficacy of cutaneous exposures and therapies (78). However, in some cases in order to enhance drug penetration into the skin, open application of the drug formulation containing volatile and nonvolatile solvents onto the skin surface is required. This is the case when the drug has higher solubility in the volatile solvent than in the nonvolatile components of the formulation. In this case, evaporation of the volatile component after open application will be associated with a linear reduction in the solubility, creating a transient supersaturation state. The challenge here is to maintain the supersaturation for a long time, which is the driving force for the drug penetration into the skin. Further, in infinite-dose studies performed under occlusion, drug permeation into the skin increased linearly with increasing the degree of drug saturation (79). In addition, occlusion has a reservoir effect of the drug in penetration rates as a result of hydration (80). Initially, a drug enters the stratum corneum under occlusion. After the occlusive dressing is removed and the stratum corneum dehydrates, the movement of drug is slower and the stratum corneum becomes a reservoir (77, 80). Hydration increased the penetration of lipid-soluble, nonpolar molecules but had less effect on polar molecules (28, 29). The absorption of more lipophilic steroids was enhanced by occlusion but not the absorption of the most water-soluble steroid (i.e., HC) (29). It is implied that the rate-determining role of the sequential steps involved in percutaneous absorption can be revealed by experiments of the type described using a related series of homologous or analogous chemicals. However, in these studies a trend of occlusion-induced absorption enhancement with increasing penetrant lipophilicity was apparent (28, 29). An earlier report by Feldmann and Maibach (41) observed an increase in percutaneous absorption of HC under occlusion conditions. Bucks et al. (2) and Bucks and Maibach (4) explained these contrary data and suggested that they may be due to an acetone solvent effect. Topical application of acetone can disrupt barrier function by extracting stratum corneum lipids (81, 82). It is conceivable that 1 mL of acetone over an area of 13 cm^2 skin might compromise stratum corneum barrier function and hence increase the penetration of HC under occlusion conditions. Experimental data are required to clarify this issue.

In practice, to increase skin penetration rates of applied drugs is far from simple. The skin barrier function can be ascribed to the macroscopic structure of the stratum corneum, which consists of alternating lipoidal and hydrophilic regions. For this reason, the physicochemical characteristics of the drug, such as partition coefficient, structure, and molecular weight, play an important role in determining the facility of percutaneous absorption (83, 84). It has been shown in some studies that occlusion-enhanced hydration of the stratum corneum increases the percutaneous absorption of lipophilic molecules more than of hydrophilic molecules. However, extensive research of published studies showed that this effect was not consistent, i.e., many studies did not find that the penetrant's lipophilicity/hydrophilicity reliably predicted occlusion's effect on penetration. In these studies, lipophilic compounds did not demonstrate increased percutaneous absorption under occlusion (85). Another factor to consider in dermal/transdermal drug delivery is the vehicle in which the drug is formulated as it acts on drug release from the formulation (32, 45). The use of drug carriers (nanocarriers), such as vesicles or nanoparticles, also affects the drug delivery to the skin under occlusion (49, 58, 70–75, 87). Moreover, vehicles may also interact with human stratum corneum, thereby affecting its barrier function. Vehicles may contain surfactants and other penetration enhancers influencing the drug penetration from the vehicle into and through the skin. Subsequently, dosing conditions, such as humidity, temperature, and occlusion, also have their impact on the actual input (rate) of drug through human skin.

14.5   CONCLUSION

In conclusion, from the described studies in this chapter and from reviews analyzing research studies on occlusion and its effect on drug penetration (85, 86), one can conclude the following: (1) occlusion enhances the percutaneous absorption of many, but not all, compounds; (2) penetration can increase as the amount of time of occlusion increases; and (3) in some studies occlusion enhanced the penetration of very lipophilic compounds more than that of very hydrophilic compounds, but it has been shown that (4) partition coefficients cannot reliably predict the effect of occlusion on percutaneous penetration in vitro. This suggests skin occlusion may be more complex than previously thought.

The effect of occlusion on percutaneous absorption may be affected by the physicochemical properties of the drug (such as volatility, partition coefficient, and aqueous solubility), vehicle properties, use of drug-loaded nanocarriers, and the anatomical site where the drug is applied. In addition, when ultra-deformable vesicles are applied, occlusive application may be detrimental to their penetration-enhancing effect.

REFERENCES

1. Baker H. The skin as a barrier. In: Rook A, Wilkinson DS, Ebling FJG, eds. Textbook of Dermatology, 2d ed. Oxford: Blackwell Scientific Publications, 1972:249–255.
2. Bucks D, Guy R, Maibach HI. Effects of occlusion. In: Bronaugh RL, Maibach HI, eds. In Vitro Percutaneous Absorption: Principles, Fundamentals, and Applications. Boca Raton: CRC Press, 1991:85–114.

3. Haftek M, Teillon MH, Schmitt D. Stratum corneum, corneodesmosomes and ex vivo percutaneous penetration. Microsc Res Tech, 1998;43:242–249.

4. Bucks D, Maibach HI. Occlusion does not uniformly enhance penetration in vivo. In: Bronaugh RL, Maibach HI, eds. Percutaneous Absorption: Drug-Cosmetics-Mechanisms-Methodology. 3d ed. New York: Marcel Dekker, 1999:81–105.

5. Garb J. Nevus verrucosus unilateralis cured with podophyllin ointment. Arch Dermatol, 1960; 81:606–609.

6. Scholtz JR. Topical therapy of psoriasis with fluocinolone acetonide. Arch Dermatol, 1961;84:1029–1030.

7. Sulzberger MB, Witten VH. Thin pliable plastic films in topical dermatological therapy. Arch Dermatol, 1961;84:1027–1028.

8. McKenzie AW. Percutaneous absorption of steroids. Arch Dermatol, 1962;86:91–94.

9. McKenzie AW, Stoughton RB. Method for comparing percutaneous absorption of steroids. Arch Dermatol, 1962;86:88–90.

10. Kaidbey KH, Petrozzi JW, Kligman AM. Topical colchicine therapy for recalcitrant psoriasis. Arch Dermatol, 1975; 111:33–36.

11. Aly R, Shirley C, Cunico B, Maibach HI. Effect of prolonged occlusion on the microbial flora, pH, carbon dioxide and transepidermal water loss on human skin. J Invest Dermatol, 1978;71:378–381.

12. Rajka G, Aly R, Bayles C, Tang Y, Maibach HI. The effect of short-term occlusion on the cutaneous flora in atopic dermatitis and psoriasis. Acta Dermatol Venereol, 1981;61:150–153.

13. Faergemann J, Aly R, Wilson DR, Maibach HI. Skin occlusion: effect on pityrosporum orbiculare, skin P CO_2, pH, transepidermal water loss, and water content. Arch Dermatol Res, 1983;275:383–387.

14. Alvarez OM, Mertz PM, Eaglstein WH. The effect of occlusive dressings on collagen synthesis and re-epithelialization in superficial wounds. J Surg Res, 1983;35:142–148.

15. Eaglstein WH. Effect of occlusive dressings on wound healing. Clin Dermatol, 1984;2:107–111.

16. Mertz PM, Eaglstein WH. The effect of a semiocclusive dressing on the microbial population in superficial wounds. Arch Surg, 1984;119:287–289.

17. Berardesca E, Maibach HI. Skin occlusion: treatment or drug-like device? Skin Pharmacol, 1988;1:207–215.

18. Silverman RA, Lender J, Elmets CA. Effects of occlusive and semiocclusive dressings on the return of barrier function to transepidermal water loss in standardized human wounds. J Am Acad Dermatol, 1989;20:755–760.

19. Zhai H, Maibach HI. Effect of Occlusion and Semi-occlusion on Experimental Skin Wound Healing: A Reevaluation. Wounds, 2007;19(10):270–276.

20. Matsumura H, Oka K, Umekage K, Akita H, Kawai J, Kitazawa Y, Suda S, Tsubota K, Ninomiya Y, Hirai, H, Miyata K, Morikubo K, Nakagawa M, Okada T, Kawai K. Effect of occlusion on human skin. Contact Dermatitis, 1995;33:231–235.

21. Berardesca E, Maibach HI. The plastic occlusion stress test (POST) as a model to investigate skin barrier function. In: Maibach HI, ed. Dermatologic Research Techniques. Boca Raton: CRC Press, 1996:179–186.

22. Kligman AM. Hydration injury to human skin. In: Van der Valk PGM, Maibach HI, eds. The Irritant Contact Dermatitis Syndrome. Boca Raton: CRC Press, 1996:187–194.

23. Leow YH, Maibach HI. Effect of occlusion on skin. J Dermatol Treat, 1997;8:139–142.

24. Denda M, Sato J, Tsuchiya T, Elias PM, Feingold KR. Low humidity stimulates epidermal DNA synthesis and amplifies the hyperproliferative response to barrier disruption: implication for seasonal exacerbations of inflammatory dermatoses. J Invest Dermatol, 1998;111:873–878.

25. Kömüves LG, Hanley K, Jiang Y, Katagiri C, Elias PM, Williams ML, Feingold KR. Induction of selected lipid metabolic enzymes and differentiation-linked structural proteins by air exposure in fetal rat skin explants. J Invest Dermatol, 1999;112:303–309.

26. Fluhr JW, Lazzerini S, Distante F, Gloor M, Berardesca E. Effects of prolonged occlusion on stratum corneum barrier function and water holding capacity. Skin Pharmacol Appl Skin Physiol, 1999;12:193–198.

27. Warner RR, Boissy YL, Lilly NA, Spears MJ, McKillop K, Marshall JL, Stone KJ. Water disrupts stratum corneum lipid lamellae: damage is similar to surfactants. J Invest Dermatol, 1999;113:960–966.

28. Treffel P, Muret P, Muret-D'Aniello P, Coumes-Marquet S, Agache P. Effect of occlusion on in vitro percutaneous absorption of two compounds with different physicochemical properties. Skin Pharmacol, 1992;5:108–113.

29. Bucks DA, McMaster JR, Maibach HI, Guy RH. Bioavailability of topically administered steroids: a "mass balance" technique. J Invest Dermatol, 1988;91:29–33.

30. Gummer CL, Maibach HI. The penetration of [¹⁴C] ethanol and [¹⁴C] methanol through excised guinea-pig skin in vitro. Food Chem Toxicol, 1986;24:305–309.

31. Hotchkiss SA, Hewitt P, Caldwell J, Chen WL, Rowe RR. Percutaneous absorption of nicotinic acid, phenol, benzoic acid and triclopyr butoxyethyl ester through rat and human skin in vitro: further validation of an in vitro model by comparison with in vivo data. Food Chem Toxicol, 1992;30:891–899.

32. Hotchkiss SA, Miller JM, Caldwell J. Percutaneous absorption of benzyl acetate through rat skin in vitro. 2. Effect of vehicle and occlusion. Food Chem Toxicol, 1992;30:145–153.

33. Roper CS, Howes D, Blain PG, Williams FM. Percutaneous penetration of 2-phenox-yethanol through rat and human skin. Food Chem Toxicol, 1997;35:1009–1016.

34. Bronaugh RL, Stewart RF, Wester RC, Bucks D, Mailbach HI, Anderson J. Comparison of percutaneous absorption of fragrances by humans and monkeys. Food Chem Toxicol, 1985;23:111–114.

35. Qiao GL, Williams PL, Riviere JE. Percutaneous absorption, biotransformation, and systemic disposition of parathion in vivo in swine. I. Comprehensive pharmacokinetic model. Drug Metab Dispos, 1994;22:459–471.

36. Qiao GL, Riviere JE. Significant effects of application site and occlusion on the pharmacokinetics of cutaneous penetration and biotransformation of parathion in vivo in swine. J Pharm Sci, 1995;84:425–432.

37. Qiao GL, Chang SK, Riviere JE. Effects of anatomical site and occlusion on the percutaneous absorption and residue pattern of 2,6-[ring-¹⁴C] parathion in vivo in pigs. Toxicol Appl Pharmacol, 1993;122:131–138.

38. Qiao GL, Brooks JD, Riviere JE. Pentachlorophenol dermal absorption and disposition from soil in swine: effects of occlusion and skin microorganism inhibition. Toxicol App Pharmacol, 1997;147:234–246.

39. Bronaugh RL, Wester RC, Bucks D, Maibach HI, Sarason R. In vivo percutaneous absorption of fragrance ingredients in rhesus monkeys and humans. Food Chem Toxicol, 1990;28:369–373.

40. Mukherji E, Millenbaugh NJ, Au JL. Percutaneous absorption of 2',3'-dideoxyinosine in rats. Pharm Res, 1994;11:809–815.

41. Feldmann RJ, Maibach HI. Penetration of ¹⁴C hydrocortisone through normal skin: the effect of stripping and occlusion. Arch Dermatol, 1965;91:661–666.

42. Ryatt KS, Stevenson JM, Maibach HI, Guy RH. Pharmacodynamic measurement of percutaneous penetration enhancement in vivo. J Pharma Sci, 1986;75:374–377.

43. Ryatt KS, Mobayen M, Stevenson JM, Maibach HI, Guy RH. Methodology to measure the transient effect of occlusion on skin penetration and stratum corneum hydration in vivo. Br J Dermatol, 1988;119:307–312.

44. Hafeez F, Chiang A, Hui X, Maibach H. Role of partition coefficients in determining the percutaneous penetration of salicylic acid and formaldehyde under varying occlusion durations. Drug Dev Ind Pharm, 2014;40(10):1395–1401.

45. Brooks JD, Riviere JE. Quantitative percutaneous absorption and cutaneous distribution of binary mixtures of phenol and para-nitrophenol in isolated perfused porcine skin. Fundam Appl Toxicol, 1996;32:233–243.

46. Cevc G, Blume G. Lipid vesicles penetrate into intact skin owing to the transdermal osmotic gradients and hydration force. Biochim Biophys Acta, 1992;1104(1):226–232.

47. Cevc G, Gebauer D. Hydration driven transport of deformable lipid vesicles through fine pores and the skin barrier. Biophys J, 2003;84:1010–24.

48. Cevc G, Chopra A. Deformable (Transfersome®) vesicles for improved drug delivery into and through the skin. In: Dragicevic N, Maibach H, eds, Percutaneous Penetration Enhancers Chemical Methods in Penetration Enhancement: Nanocarriers. New York, Dordrecht, London: Springer Berlin Heidelberg, 2016: 39–60.

49. Müller RH, Alexiev U, Sinambela P, Keck C. Nanostructured Lipid Carriers (NLC) – the second generation of solid lipid nanoparticles. In: Dragicevic N, Maibach H, eds, Percutaneous Penetration Enhancers Chemical Methods in Penetration Enhancement: Nanocarriers. New York, Dordrecht, London: Springer Berlin Heidelberg, 2016: 161–186.

50. Pardeike J, Schwabe K, Müller RH. Influence of nanostructured lipid carriers (NLC) on the physical properties of the Cutanova Nanorepair Q10 cream and the in vivo skin hydration effect. Int J Pharm, 2010;396(1–2):166–173.

51. Schäfer-Korting M, Mehnert W, Korting H-C. Lipid nanoparticles for improved topical application of drugs for skin diseases. Adv Drug Deliv Rev, 2007;59(6):427–443.

52. Souto EB, Wissing SA, Barbosa CM, Müller RH. Development of a controlled release formulation based on SLN and NLC for topical clotrimazole delivery. Int J Pharm, 2004;278(1):71–77.

53. Cross SE, Roberts MS. The effect of occlusion on epidermal penetration of parabens from a commercial allergy test ointment, acetone and ethanol vehicles. J Invest Dermatol, 2000;115, 914–918.

54. El Maghraby GM. Occlusive and non-occlusive application of microemulsion for transdermal delivery of progesterone: mechanistic studies. Sci Pharm, 2012;80(3):765–778.

55. Cevc G, Vierl U, Mazgareanu S. Functional characterisation of novel analgesic product based on self-regulating drug carriers. Int J Pharm, 2008;360(1-2):18–28.

56. Cevc G, Mazgareanu S, Rother M. Preclinical characterisation of NSAIDs in ultradeformable carriers or conventional topical gels. Int J Pharm, 2008;360(1-2):29–39.

57. Schätzlein A, Cevc G. Non-uniform cellular packing of the stratum corneum and permeability barrier function of intact skin: a high-resolution confocal laser scanning microscopy study using highly deformable vesicles (Transfersomes). Br J Dermatol, 1998;138(4):583–592.

58. El Maghraby GM, Williams AC, Barry BW. Skin hydration and possible shunt route penetration in controlled skin delivery of estradiol from ultradeformable and standard liposomes in vitro. J Pharm Pharmacol, 2001;53:1311–1322.

59. El Maghraby GM. Occlusive versus non-occlusive application in transdermal drug delivery. In Dragicevic N, Maibach Hi, eds, Percutaneous Penetration Enhancers – Drug Penetration into/through the Skin: Methodology and General Considerations. New York, Dordrecht, London: Springer Berlin Heidelberg:27–44.

60. Ascenso A, Raposo S, Batista C, Cardoso P, Mendes T, Garcia Praça F, Vitória Lopes Badra Bentley M, Simões S. Development, characterization, and skin delivery studies of related ultradeformable vesicles: transfersomes, ethosomes, and transethosomes. Int J Nanomed, 2015;10:5837–5851.

61. Dragicevic-Curic N, Scheglmann D, Albrecht V, Fahr A. Temoporfin-loaded invasomes: development, characterization and in vitro skin penetration studies. J Control Release, 2008;127(1):59–69.

62. Dragicevic-Curic N, Scheglmann D, Albrecht V, Fahr A. Development of different temoporfin-loaded invasomes-novel nanocarriers of temoporfin: characterization, stability and in vitro skin penetration studies. Colloids Surf B Biointerfaces, 2009;70(2):198–206.

63. Dragicevic N, Verma DD, Fahr A. Invasomes–vesicles for enhanced skin delivery of drugs. In: Dragicevic N, Maibach HI, eds, Percutaneous Penetration Enhancers – Chemical Methods in Penetration Enhancement: Nanocarriers. New York, Dordrecht, London: Springer Berlin Heidelberg, 2016:77–92.

64. Dragicevic-Curic N, Gräfe S, Albrecht V, Fahr A. Topical application of temoporfin-loaded invasomes for photodynamic therapy of subcutaneously implanted tumours in mice: a pilot study. J Photochem Photobiol B, 2008,91(1):41–50.

65. Cevc G, Mazgareanu S, Rother M, Vierl U. Occlusion effect on transcutaneous NSAID delivery from conventional and carrier-based formulations. Int J Pharm, 2008;359(1–2):190–197.

66. Shamma RN, Sayed S, Sabry NA, El-Samanoudy SI. Enhanced skin targeting of retinoic acid spanlastics: in vitro characterization and clinical evaluation in acne patients. J Liposome Res, 2019;29(3):283–290.

67. Barone A, Cristiano MC, Cilurzo F, Locatelli M, Iannotta D, Di Marzio L, Celia C, Paolino D. Ammonium glycyrrhizate skin delivery from ultradeformable liposomes: a novel use as an anti-inflammatory agent in topical drug delivery. Colloids Surf B Biointerfaces, 2020;193:111152.

68. Sardana V, Burzynski J, Zalzal P. Safety and efficacy of topical ketoprofen in transfersome gel in knee osteoarthritis: a systematic review. Musculoskeletal Care, 2017;15(2):114–121.

69. Cevc G. Transdermal drug delivery of insulin with ultradeformable carriers. Clin Pharmacokinet. 2003;42(5):461–474..

70. Touti R, Noun M, Guimberteau F, Lecomte S, Faure C. What is the fate of multi-lamellar liposomes of controlled size, charge and elasticity in artificial and animal skin?. Eur J Pharm Biopharm, 2020;151:18–31.

71. Abd El-Alim SH, Kassem AA, Basha M, Salama A. Comparative study of liposomes, ethosomes and transfersomes as carriers for enhancing the transdermal delivery of diflunisal: In vitro and in vivo evaluation. Int J Pharm, 2019;563:293–303.

72. Ainbinder D, Godin B, Touitou E. Ethosomes: enhanced delivery of drugs to and across the skin. In: Dragicevic N, Maibach Hi, eds, Percutaneous Penetration Enhancers – Chemical Methods in Penetration Enhancement: Nanocarriers. New York, Dordrecht, London: Springer Berlin Heidelberg, 2016:61–75.

73. Khan MA, Pandit J, Sultana Y, Sultana S, Ali A, Aqil M, Chauhan M. Novel carbopol-based transfersomal gel of 5-fluorouracil for skin cancer treatment: in vitro characterization and in vivo study. Drug Deliv, 2015;22(6):795–802.

74. El Maghraby GM, Ultradeformable vesicles as skin drug delivery systems: mechanism of action. In: Dragicevic N, Maibach Hi, eds, Percutaneous Penetration Enhancers – Chemical Methods in Penetration Enhancement: Nanocarriers. New York, Dordrecht, London: Springer Berlin Heidelberg, 2016:137–145.

75. Honeywell-Nguyen PL, Wouter Groenink HW, de Graaff AM, Bouwstra JA. The in vivo transport of elastic vesicles into human skin: effects of occlusion, volume and duration of application. J Control Release, 2003;90(2):243–255.

76. Task Group on Occupational Exposure to Pesticides: Occupational Exposure to Pesticides. Washington, DC: Federal Working Group on Pest Management, 1974.

77. Wester RC, Maibach HI. Cutaneous pharmacokinetics: 10 steps to percutaneous absorption. Drug Metab Rev, 1983;14:169–205.

78. Rouse NC, Maibach HI. The effect of volatility on percutaneous absorption. J Dermatolog Treat, 2016;27(1):5–10.

79. Santos P, Watkinson AC, Hadgraft J, Lane ME. Formulation issues associated with transdermal fentanyl delivery. Int J Pharm, 2011;416(1):155–9. doi: 10.1016/j.ijpharm.2011.06.024.

80. Ezzedeen FW, Stohs SJ, Kilzer KL, Makoid MC, Ezzedeen NW. Percutaneous absorption and disposition of iodochlorhydroxyquin in dogs. J Pharm Sci,1984;73:1369–1372.

81. Elias PM. Epidermal lipids, barrier function, and desquamation. J Invest Dermatol, 1983;80:44–49.

82. Grubauer G, Feingold KR, Harris RM, Elias PM. Lipid content and lipid type as determinants of the epidermal permeability barrier. J Lipid Res, 1989;30:89–96.

83. Hostýnek JJ, Magee PS, Maibach HI. QSAR predictive of contact allergy: scope and limitations. Curr Probl Dermatol. 1996;25:18–27.

84. Wiechers JW. The barrier function of the skin in relation to percutaneous absorption of drugs. Pharma Week Sci Edit, 1989;11:185–198.

85. Hafeez F, Maibach H. Do partition coefficients (liphophilicity/hydrophilicity) predict effects of occlusion on percutaneous penetration in vitro: a retrospective review. Cutan Ocul Toxicol, 2013;32(4):299–303.

86. Hafeez F, Maibach H. Occlusion effect on in vivo percutaneous penetration of chemicals in man and monkey: partition coefficient effects. Skin Pharmacol Physiol, 2013;26(2):85–91.

87. Dragicevic-Curic, N., Gräfe, S., Gitter, B., Winter, S., Fahr, A. Surface charged temoporfin-loaded flexible vesicles: in vitro skin penetration studies and stability. Int. J. Pharm, 2010;384 (1–2):100–108.

15 Occlusion Does Not Uniformly Enhance Penetration *In Vivo*

Daniel Bucks
Bucks Consulting, Millbrae, California

Howard I. Maibach
University of California, San Francisco, California

CONTENTS

15.1 INTRODUCTION

Mammalian skin provides a relatively efficient barrier to the ingress of exogenous materials and the egress of endogenous compounds, particularly water. Loss of this vital function results in death from dehydration. Compromised function is associated with complications seen in several dermatological disorders. Stratum corneum intercellular lipid domains form a major transport pathway for penetration (1–4). Perturbation of these lamellar lipids causes skin permeation resistance to fall and has implicated their crucial role in barrier function. Indeed, epidermal sterolo-genesis appears to be modulated by the skin's barrier requirements (5). Despite the fact that the skin is perhaps the most impermeable mammalian membrane, it is permeable to a degree, that is, it is semipermeable; as such, the topical application of pharmaceutical agents has been shown to be a viable route of entry into the systemic circulation, as well as an obvious choice in the treatment of dermatological ailments. Of the various approaches employed to enhance the percutaneous absorption of drugs, occlusion (defined as the complete impairment of passive transepidermal water loss at the application site) is the simplest and perhaps one of the most common methods in use. In this chapter we have summarized the literature to evaluate the effect of occlusion on the percutaneous absorption of topically applied compounds and to look at how certain compound physicochemical properties (such as volatility, partition coefficient, and aqueous solubility) may predict what effect occlusion may have.

The increased clinical efficacy of topical drugs caused by covering the site of application was first documented by Garb (6). Subsequently, Scholtz (7), using fluocinolone acetonide, and Sulzberger and Witten (8), using hydrocortisone, reported enhanced corticoid activity with occlusion in the treatment of psoriasis. The enhanced pharmacological effect of topical corticosteroids under occlusion was further demonstrated by the vasoconstriction studies of McKenzie (9) and McKenzie and

Stoughton (10). Occlusion has also been reported to increase the percutaneous absorption of various other topically applied compounds (11–17). However, as shown later, short-term occlusion does not necessarily increase the percutaneous absorption of all chemicals.

15.2 PERCUTANEOUS ABSORPTION OF PHENYLENEDIAMINE (PPDA) IN GUINEA PIGS

The *in vivo* percutaneous absorption of *p*-phenylenediamine (PPDA) from six occlusive patch test systems was investigated by Kim et al. (18). The extent of absorption was determined using ^{14}C radiotracer methodology. The ^{14}C-PPDA was formulated as 1% PPDA in petrolatum (U.S. Pharmacopeia [USP]) and applied from each test system at a skin surface dose of 2 mg/cm^2. Thus, the amount of PPDA was normalized with respect to the surface area of each patch test system (and, hence, to the surface area of treated skin). A sixfold difference in the level of skin absorption ($p < 0.02$) was found between the patches (Table 15.1). It should be noted that a nonocclusive control was not included in this study.

The rate of ^{14}C excretion following topical application of the radiolabeled PPDA in the various patch test systems is shown in Figure 15.1. Clearly, the rate and extent of PPDA absorption were dependent upon the patch test system employed. The mechanism responsible for differences in PPDA percutaneous absorption from these patch test systems is unknown. However, the magnitude of occlusiveness of each dressing is hypothesized to correspond to enhanced absorption.

15.3 PERCUTANEOUS ABSORPTION OF VOLATILE COMPOUNDS

The effect of occlusion on the *in vivo* percutaneous absorption of two fragrances (safrole and cinnamyl anthranilate) and two chemical analogs (cinnamic alcohol and cinnamic acid) in rhesus monkeys was evaluated by Bronaugh et al. (19). Each compound was applied at a topical dose of 4 µg/cm^2 from a small volume of acetone. Occlusion was achieved by covering the site of application with plastic wrap (Saran Wrap, a chlorinated hydrocarbon polymer) after the acetone had

TABLE 15.1
Percutaneous Absorption of PPDA from Patch Test Systems

Patch Test System	Mean % Dose Absorbed (SD)
Hill Top chamber	53 (21)
Teflon (control)	49 (9)
Small Finn chamber	30 (9)
Large Finn chamber	23 (7)
AL-Test chamber	8 (1)
Small Finn chamber with paper disc insert	34 (20)

Source: Data from Reference 18.

Note: The rate of ^{14}C excretion following topical application of the radiolabeled PPDA in the various patch test systems is shown in Figure 15.1. The extent of PPDA absorption was dependent upon the occlusive patch test system employed. It should be noted that a nonocclusive control study was not conducted. The test system used 2 mg/mm^2 PPDA for 48 hours on the dorsal mid-lumbar region of the guinea pig.

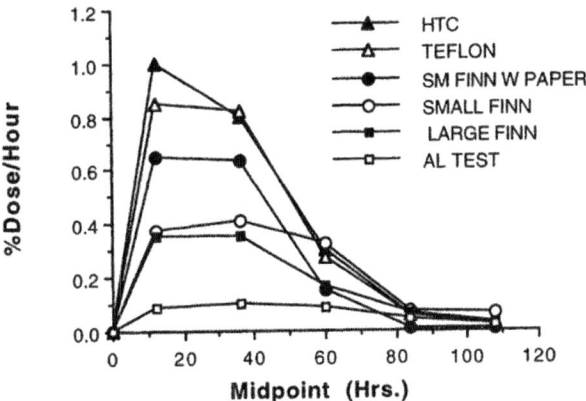

FIGURE 15.1   *In vivo* percutaneous absorption of PPDA (2 mg/mm^2) following a 48-hour exposure on the dorsal lumbar region of guinea pigs. *Abbreviations*: *HTC*, Hill Top chamber; *Teflon*, sheet of Teflon; *sm Finn w paper*, small Finn chamber with paper insert included; *small Finn*, small Finn chamber with paper insert removed; *large Finn*, large Finn chamber with paper insert removed. (Redrawn from Reference 18.)

evaporated from the skin surface. The extent of absorption following single-dose administration was determined using ^{14}C radiotracer methodology. The fragrance materials were well absorbed through monkey skin. Plastic wrap occlusion of the application site resulted in large increases in absorption (Table 15.2). The authors also presented *in vitro* data documenting the significant increase in percutaneous absorption of these chemicals under occluded compared to nonprotected conditions, that is, left open to the air.

Investigation of the effect of occlusion on the percutaneous absorption of six additional volatile compounds (benzyl acetate, benzamide, benzoin, benzophenone, benzyl benzoate, and benzyl alcohol) was conducted using the same *in vivo* methodology. These studies included occlusion of the site of application with a glass cylinder secured to the skin by silicone glue and capped with Parafilm, occlusion with plastic wrap, and nonprotected conditions (20). As shown in Table 15.3, occlusion in general enhances the percutaneous absorption of these compounds. However, differences in percutaneous absorption were observed between plastic wrap and "glass chamber" occlusive conditions. The absorption of benzoin and that of benzyl acetate were lower under plastic wrap compared to the

TABLE 15.2
In Vivo Percutaneous Absorption of Fragrances in Monkeys

	Percent Dose Absorbed[a]	
	Nonprotected	Plastic Wrap Occlusion
Cinnamyl anthranilate	26.1 (4.6)	39.0 (5.6)
Safrole	4.1 (1.6)	13.3 (4.6)
Cinnamic alcohol	25.4 (4.4)	74.6 (14.4)
Cinnamic acid	38.6 (16.6)	83.9 (5.4)

Source: Data from Reference 19.

Note: Values were corrected for incomplete renal elimination. Mean ± SD ($N = 4$).

[a] Single 4-µg/cm^2 dose with a 24-hour exposure prior to soap and water washing.

TABLE 15.3

In Vivo **Percutaneous Absorption of Benzyl Derivatives in Monkeys**

| | | % Dose Absorbed[a] | | |
	Nonprotected	Plastic-Wrap Occlusion	Glass Chamber Occlusion	Log $K_{o/w}$
Benzamide	47 (14)	85 (8)	73 (20)	0.64
Benzyl alcohol	32 (9)	56 (29)	80 (15)	0.87
Benzoin	49 (6)	43 (12)	77 (4)	1.35
Benzyl acetate	35 (19)	17 (5)	79 (15)	1.96
Benzophenone	44 (15)	69 (12)	69 (10)	3.18
Benzyl benzoate	57 (21)	71 (9)	65 (20)	3.97

Source: Data from Reference 20.

[a] Single 4-μg/cm^2 dose with a 24-hours exposure prior to soap and water washing.

Note: Values corrected for incomplete renal elimination. Mean ± SD ($N = 4$).

nonprotected condition. This discrepancy might be due to compound sequestration by the plastic wrap. Glass chamber occlusion resulted in greater bioavailability than nonprotected or plastic wrap occlusion except for benzyl benzoate, where plastic wrap conditions resulted in greater absorption, and for benzophenone, where glass chamber and plastic wrap conditions resulted in the same magnitude increase over nonprotected test conditions.

An attempt was made to correlate occlusion-enhanced bioavailability with each compound's octanol/water partition coefficient. Unexpectedly, no apparent trends were noted for these volatile fragrance compounds. Absence of a trend is in contradiction to results obtained with steroids and phenol derivatives discussed later, given the range of log $K_{O/W}$ evaluated with these fragrances.

Gummer and Maibach (16) studied the penetration of methanol and ethanol through excised, full-thickness guinea pig skin. Occlusion significantly enhanced the cumulative amount penetrating, as well as the profiles of the amount penetrating per hour for both methanol and ethanol. Consistent with results from other investigators reported already, occlusion-induced penetration enhancement was dependent upon the nature of the occlusive material, with the greatest enhancement observed with a plastic Hill Top chamber (21). Intuitively, occlusion-induced enhancement in the penetration of volatile compounds should be one of the items related to the degree to which the occlusive device inhibits evaporative loss of compound from the skin surface.

15.4 PERCUTANEOUS ABSORPTION OF STEROIDS IN HUMANS

The earliest attempt to correlate the increased pharmacological effect of hydrocortisone under occlusive conditions with the pharmacokinetics of absorption was reported by Feldmann and Maibach (12). In this study, the rate and extent of ^{14}C-labeled excretion into the urine following topical application of [^{14}C] hydrocortisone to the ventral forearm of normal human volunteers were measured. Radiolabeled hydrocortisone (75 μg) was applied in acetone solution (1000 μL) as a surface deposit over 13 cm^2 of skin. The authors estimated that this was equivalent to a sparing application of a 0.5% hydrocortisone topical preparation (5.8 μg/cm^2). The site of application was either nonprotected or occluded with plastic wrap (Saran Wrap). When the skin was

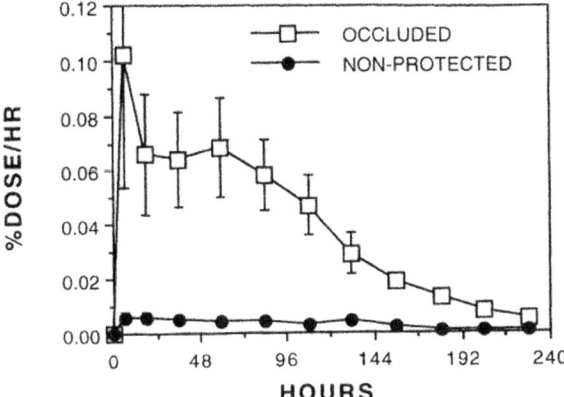

FIGURE 15.2 Percutaneous absorption of hydrocortisone in humans. Human 96-hour occluded versus 24 hours nonprotected exposure of hydrocortisone at 4 $\mu g/cm^2$ prior to soap and water washing. Occlusion was with plastic wrap. (Data from Reference 12.)

nonprotected, the dosing site was washed 24 hours post-application. On the other hand, when the skin was occluded, the plastic wrap remained in place for 96 hours (four days) post-application before the application site was washed. The percentage of the applied dose excreted into the urine, corrected for incomplete renal elimination, was (mean ± SD) 0.46 ± 0.20 and 5.9 ± 3.5 under nonprotected and occluded conditions, respectively (Figure 15.2). A paired *t*-test of the results indicates a significant difference ($p = 0.01$) in cumulative absorption of hydrocortisone between the two exposure conditions. Quantitatively, the occlusive conditions employed increased the cumulative absorption of hydrocortisone (HC) by about an order of magnitude. However, note that the occlusive system retained the drug in contact with the skin for 96 hours compared to the 24-hour exposure period under nonprotected conditions, and this could affect absorption as measured by the cumulative measurement of drug excreted into the urine, but the dramatic difference in percent dose absorbed per hour between occluded and nonprotected at 12 and 24 hours is not expected to be dependent upon differences in times of washing. This enhancement in HC absorption afforded by occlusion is not consistent with the additional studies reported next and may be associated with the large volume of acetone applied per square centimeter of skin (76.9 $\mu L/cm^2$) disrupting stratum corneum barrier function.

Guy et al. (13) investigated the effect of occlusion on the percutaneous absorption of steroids *in vivo* following single and multiple applications. The extent of absorption of four steroids (progesterone, testosterone, estradiol, and hydrocortisone), using radiotracer elimination into the urine following topical application to the ventral forearm of male volunteers, was reported. The chemical dose was 4 $\mu g/cm^2$ over an application area of 2.5 cm^2. The ^{14}C-labeled chemicals were applied in 20 μL acetone (8 $\mu L/cm^2$). In the occlusive studies, after evaporation of the vehicle, the site of application was covered with a plastic (polyethylene–vinyl acetate copolymer, Hill Top) chamber. In all cases, after 24 hours, the site of application was washed with soap and water using a standardized procedure (22). In the occlusive studies, the administration site was then covered again with a new chamber. An essentially identical protocol was also performed following a multiple dosing regimen (23). Daily topical doses of three of the steroids (testosterone, estradiol, and hydrocortisone) were administered over a 14-day period. The first and eighth doses were ^{14}C-labeled, and urinary excretion of radiolabeling was followed. As described earlier, the 24-hour washing procedure was performed daily and a new chamber was applied. Occlusive chambers and washes were collected and assayed for residual surface chemical. The results of

TABLE 15.4

Percutaneous Absorption of Steroids in Humans

	Mean % Applied Dose Absorbed ($\pm$ SD)	
	Nonprotected	Occluded
Hydrocortisone		
Single application	2 ± 2[a]	4 ± 2
Multiple application		
First dose	3 ± 1	4 ± 1
Eighth dose	3 ± 1	3 ± 1
Estradiol		
Single application	11 ± 5[a]	27 ± 6
Multiple application		
First dose	10 ± 2	38 ± 8
Eighth dose	11 ± 5	22 ± 7
Testosterone		
Single application	13 ± 3[a]	46 ± 15
Multiple application		
First dose	21 ± 6	51 ± 10
Eighth dose	20 ± 7	50 ± 9
Progesterone		
Single application	11 ± 6[a]	33 ± 9

[a]*Source:* Data from References 11, 23, and 42.

this study are summarized in Table 15.4. Steroid percutaneous absorption as a function of penetrant octanol/water partition coefficient ($K_{O/W}$) is shown in Figure 15.3. The studies indicate that:

1. The single-dose measurements of the percutaneous absorption of hydrocortisone, estradiol, and testosterone are predictive of percutaneous absorption following a comparable multiple-dose regimen under both occluded and nonoccluded conditions.
2. Occlusion significantly ($p < 0.05$) increased the percutaneous absorption of estradiol, testosterone, and progesterone but not that of hydrocortisone (the compound with the lowest $K_{o/w}$ value in this series of steroids).

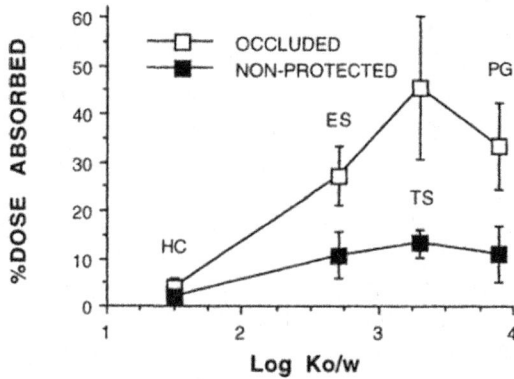

FIGURE 15.3   Percutaneous absorption of four steroids in humans as a function of penetrant octanol/water partition coefficient. Exposure period 24 hours at 4 µg/cm² prior to soap and water washing. *Abbreviations*: *HC*, hydrocortisone; *ES*, estradiol; *TS*, testosterone; *PG*, progesterone. (From Reference 13.)

TABLE 15.5
Accountability of Applied Dose[a] in Occluded Studies

	Absorbed (%)	Removed from Skin (%)	Total % Dose
Hydrocortisone			
Single dose[b]	4 ± 2	64 ± 5	68 ± 4
First MD[c]	4 ± 1	82 ± 5	85 ± 4
Eighth MD[d]	3 ± 1	78 ± 2	81 ± 3
Estradiol			
Single dose[b]	27 ± 6	60 ± 12	87 ± 13
First MD[c]	38 ± 8	62 ± 6	100 ± 4
Eighth MD[d]	22 ± 7	59 ± 8	81 ± 6
Testosterone			
Single dose[b]	46 ± 15	44 ± 7	90 ± 8
First MD[b]	51 ± 10	48 ± 9	99 ± 4
Eighth MD[d]	50 ± 9	42 ± 9	92 ± 17
Progesterone			
Single dose[b]	33 ± 9	47 ± 10	80 ± 6

Source: Adapted from Reference 43.

Note: Values corrected for incomplete renal elimination, mean ± SD. Occluded with a plastic (Hill Top) chamber.

[a] Single 4-μg/cm^2 dose with a 24-hour exposure prior to soap and water washing.

[b] Single-dose study.

[c] First dose of a 14-day multiple-dose study.

[d] Eighth dose of a 14-day multiple-dose study.

3. Percutaneous absorption increases with increasing $K_{o/w}$ up to testosterone but declines for progesterone under occluded and nonoccluded conditions.
4. The occlusive procedure generally permits excellent dose accountability (Table 15.5).

The percutaneous absorption of these same four steroids under "protected" (i.e., covered but nonocclusive) conditions has also been measured *in vivo* (11, 24) using the same methodology. The data obtained from these later experiments permitted the effect of occlusion to be rigorously assessed (since complete mass balance of the applied dose was possible). With the exception of hydrocortisone (Table 15.6), occlusion significantly increased the percutaneous absorption

TABLE 15.6
Percutaneous Absorption of Steroids in Humans:
Single-Dose Application for 24 Hours at 4 μg/cm^2

	Mean % Dose Absorbed (± SD; $N > 5$)	
	Protected[a]	Occluded[b]
Hydrocortisone	4 ± 2	4 ± 2
Estradiol	3 ± 1	27 ± 6
Testosterone	18 ± 9	46 ± 15
Progesterone	13 ± 6	33 ± 9

Source: Data from References 11, 13, and 43.

[a] Dose site covered with a ventilated plastic chamber.

[b] Dose site covered with an occlusive plastic chamber.

TABLE 15.7

Accountability of Applied Dose[a] in Protected Studies Using Ventilated Plastic Chambers

	Absorbed	Removed from Skin (%)	Total % Accounted For
Hydrocortisone	4 ± 2	85 ± 6	89 ± 6
Estradiol	3 ± 1	96 ± 1	100 ± 1
Testosterone	18 ± 9	77 ± 8	96 ± 2
Progesterone	13 ± 6	82 ± 7	96 ± 3

Source: Data from References 11 and 24.

[a] Single 4-μg/cm^2 dose with a 24-hour exposure prior to soap and water washing; penetration corrected for incomplete renal elimination.

($p < 0.01$) of the steroids. These results were in excellent agreement with the comparable nonprotected studies described earlier. As stated before, excellent dose accountability was reported (Table 15.7).

To investigate the apparent discrepancy between the effect of plastic wrap occlusion (12) and that of the plastic chamber on hydrocortisone absorption (13), we repeated the measurements of penetration using plastic wrap (Saran Wrap) with the experimental protocol of Guy et al. (13). Under these circumstances, we found no difference between plastic wrap and plastic chamber occlusion on the percutaneous absorption of hydrocortisone (Table 15.8).

15.5   PERCUTANEOUS ABSORPTION OF PHENOLS IN HUMANS

We subsequently investigated the effect of occlusion on the *in vivo* percutaneous absorption of phenols following single-dose application. The occlusive and protective chamber methodology described by Bucks et al. (24, 25) was utilized. Nine ^{14}C-ring–labeled *para*-substituted phenols (4-aminophenol, 4-acetamidophenol, 4-propionylamidophenol, phenol, 4-cyanophenol, 4-nitrophenol, 4-iodophenol, 4-heptyloxyphenol, and 4-pentyloxyphenol) were used. As in the earlier steroid studies, the site of application was the ventral forearm of male volunteers and the area of application was 2.5 cm^2. Penetrants were applied in 20 μL ethanol (95%). The chemical dose was 2 to 4 μg/cm^2. After vehicle evaporation, the application site was covered with either an occlusive or protective device. After 24 hours, the patch was removed and the site washed with a standardized procedure (22). The application site was then recovered with a new chamber of the same type. Urine was collected for seven days. On the seventh day, (1) the second chamber was removed, (2) the dosing site was washed with the same procedure, and (3) the upper layers of stratum corneum from the

TABLE 15.8

Percutaneous Absorption of Hydrocortisone in Humans

	Plastic Dose Absorbed[a]
Plastic wrap occlusion	4.7 ± 2.1
Plastic chamber occlusion	4.0 ± 2.4
"Protected" condition	4.4 ± 1.7

Source: Adapted from Reference 43.

[a] Single 4-μg/cm^2 dose with a 24-hour exposure prior to soap and water washing; penetration corrected for incomplete renal elimination.

application site were removed by cellophane tape stripping. Urine, chambers, washes, and skin tape strips were collected and assayed for the radiolabel. Percutaneous absorption of each compound under protected and occluded conditions is presented in Figures 15.4 to 15.12. Phenol percutaneous

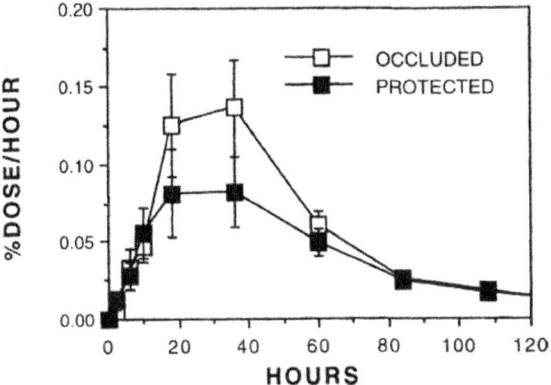

FIGURE 15.4 Percutaneous absorption of acetaminophen in man under occluded and protected conditions (mean ± SEM, $N = 6$). Exposure 24 hours prior to soap and water washing. (Redrawn from References 34 and 35.)

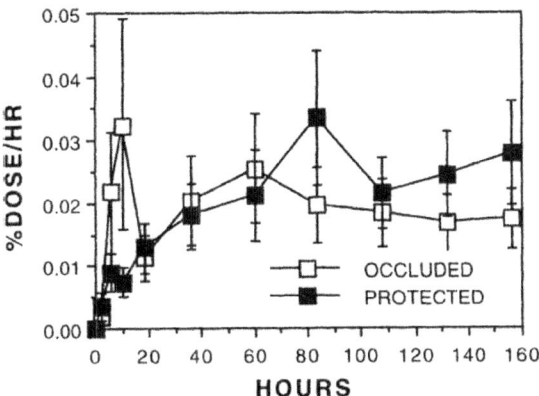

FIGURE 15.5 Percutaneous absorption of acetaminophen in man under occluded and protected conditions (mean ± SEM, $N = 6$). Exposure 24 hours prior to soap and water washing. (Redrawn from References 34 and 35.)

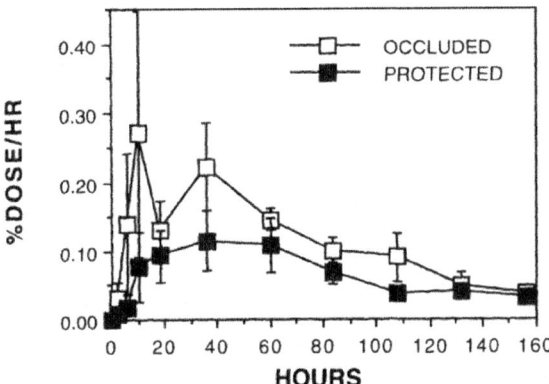

FIGURE 15.6 Percutaneous absorption of phenol in humans under occluded and protected conditions (mean ± SEM, $N = 6$). Exposure 24 hours prior to soap and water washing. (Redrawn from References 34 and 35.)

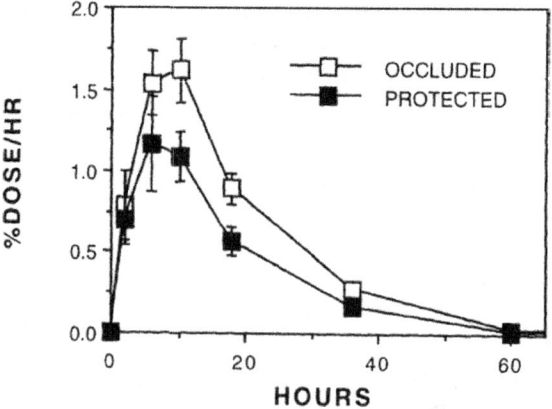

FIGURE 15.7   Percutaneous absorption of phenol in humans under occluded and protected conditions (mean ± SEM, $N = 6$). Exposure 24 hours prior to soap and water washing. (Redrawn from References 34 and 35.)

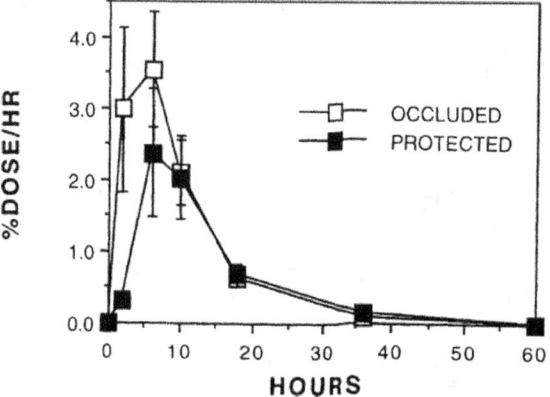

FIGURE 15.8   Percutaneous absorption of nitrophenol in humans under occluded and protected conditions (mean ± SEM, $N = 6$). Exposure 24 hours prior to soap and water washing. (Redrawn from References 34 and 35.)

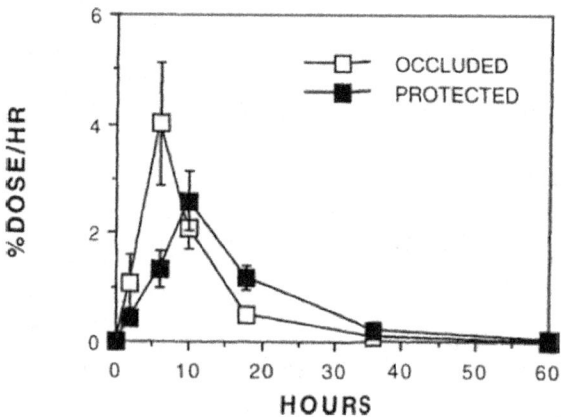

FIGURE 15.9   Percutaneous absorption of nitrophenol in humans under occluded and protected conditions (mean ± SEM, $N = 6$). Exposure 24 hours prior to soap and water washing. (Redrawn from References 34 and 35.)

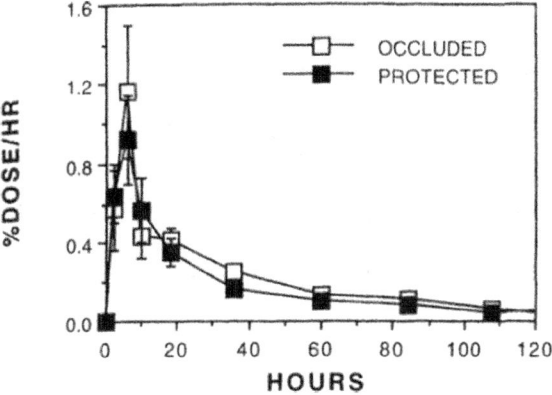

FIGURE 15.10 Percutaneous absorption of iodophenol in humans under occluded and protected conditions (mean ± SEM, $N = 6$). Exposure 24 hours prior to soap and water washing. (Redrawn from References 34 and 35.)

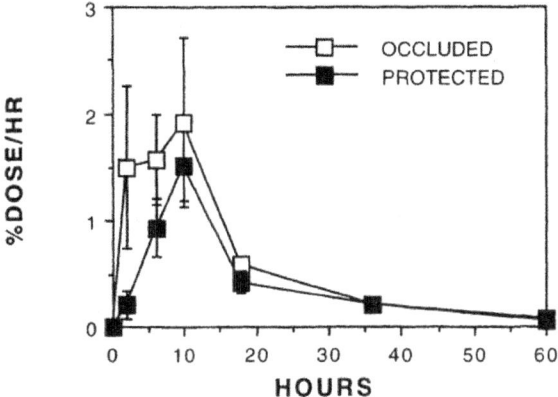

FIGURE 15.11 Percutaneous absorption of heptyloxyphenol in humans under occluded and protected conditions (mean ± SEM, $N = 6$). Exposure 24 hours prior to soap and water washing. (Redrawn from References 34 and 35.)

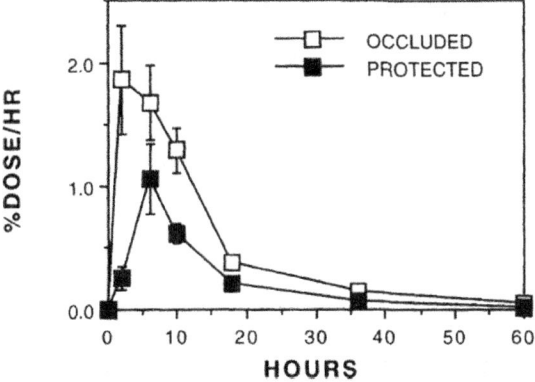

FIGURE 15.12 Percutaneous absorption of phenols in humans under occluded and protected conditions as a function of penetrant octanol/water partition coefficient ($K_{o/w}$). (Redrawn from References 34 and 35.)

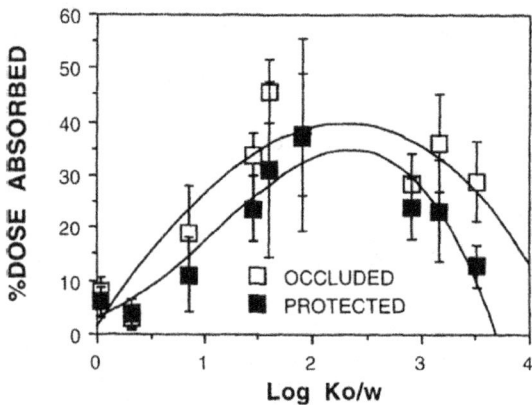

FIGURE 15.13 Percutaneous absorption of phenols in humans under occluded and protected conditions as a function of penetrant octanol/water partition coefficient ($K_{o/w}$). (Redrawn from References 34 and 35.)

absorption as a function of the penetrant $K_{O/W}$ is shown in Figure 15.13. Phenol percutaneous absorption is summarized in Table 15.9. The methodology permitted excellent dose accountability (Tables 15.10 and 15.11). The studies indicate that:

1. Occlusion significantly increased (unpaired t-test, $p < 0.05$) the absorption of phenol, heptyloxyphenol, and pentyloxyphenol.
2. Occlusion did not statistically enhance the absorption of aminophenol, acetaminophen, propionylamidophenol, cyanophefiol, nitrophenol, and iodophenol.
3. The methodology employed again permitted excellent dose accountability.
4. In general, the two compounds with the lowest $K_{o/w}$ values of this series of compounds showed the least enhancement in absorption afforded by occlusion.

TABLE 15.9
Percutaneous Absorption of Phenols[a] in Humans

Compound	Log $K_{o/w}$	Mean % Dose Absorbed (SD)	
		Occluded	Protected
Aminophenol	0.04	8(3)	6(3)
Acetaminophen	0.32	3(2)	4(3)
Propionylamidophenol	0.86	19(9)	11 (7)
Phenol[b]	1.46	34(4)	24 (6)[c]
Cyanophenol	1.60	46 (6)	31 (16) 38 (11)
Nitrophenol	1.91	37 (18)	
Iodophenol	2.91	28 (6)	24 (6)
Heptyloxyphenol	3.16	36 (9)	23 (10)[d]
Pentyloxyphenol	3.51	29 (8)	13 (4)[c]

Source: Data from References 34 and 35.

[a] Single-dose application from 95% ETOH ($N = 6$) at 2–4 µg/cm² to the ventral forearm; 24 hours exposure prior to soap and water washing.

[b] Data analysis accounts for 27.2% of applied dose evaporating off the skin surface during application.

[c] Significant difference at $p < 0.01$.

[d] Significant difference at $p < 0.05$.

TABLE 15.10
Accountability of Applied Dose[a] in Occluded Studies: Mean Percent Dose Absorbed (SD)

Compound	Absorbed (%)	Removed from Skin (%)	Total % Dose
Aminophenol	8(3)	55 (18)	63 (17)
Acetaminophen	3(2)	61 (24)	64 (24)
Propionylamido-phenol	19(9)	77 (9)	96 (2)
Phenol[b]	34(4)	61 (13)	95 (10)
Cyanophenol	46 (6)	41 (9)	87 (7)
Nitrophenol	37 (18)	50 (11)	87 (13)
Iodophenol	28 (6)	63 (4)	91 (3)
Heptyloxyphenol	36 (9)	59 (7)	95 (3)
Pentyloxyphenol	29 (8)	71 (8)	100 (2)

Source: Data from References. 34 and 35.

[a] Single-dose application from 95% ETOH ($N = 6$) at 2–4 µg/cm^2 to the ventral forearm; 24 hours exposure prior to soap and water washing.

[b] Data analysis accounts for 27.2% of applied dose evaporating off the skin surface during application.

15.6 DISCUSSION

A predominant effect of occlusion is to increase hydration of the stratum corneum, thereby swelling the corneocytes and promoting the uptake of water into intercellular lipid domains. The magnitude of increased stratum corneum hydration is related to the degree of occlusion exerted and is dependent upon the physicochemical nature of the dressing (26). The normal water content of stratum corneum is 5% to 15%, a value that can be increased up to 50% by occlusion (27, 28). Upon removal of a plastic occlusive dressing after 24 hours of contact, transepidermal water loss values are increased by an order of magnitude (24); the elevated rate then returns rapidly (~15 min) to normal with extraneous water dissipation from the stratum corneum. With occlusion, skin temperature generally increases from 32°C to as much as 37°C (29). Faergemann et al. (30) showed that occlusion (1) increases the transepidermal flux of chloride and carbon dioxide, (2) increases microbial counts on skin, and (3) increases the surface pH of skin from a preoccluded value of 5.6 to 6.7. Anhidrosis

TABLE 15.11
Accountability of Applied Dose[a] in Protected Studies: Mean Percent Dose Absorbed (SD)

Compound	Absorbed (%)	Removed from Skin (%)	Total % Dose
Aminophenol	6(3)	85 (4)	91 (2)
Acetaminophen	4 (3)	93 (5)	97 (4)
Propionylamido-phenol	11 (7)	84 (7)	95 (2)
Phenol[b]	24 (6)	68 (15)	92 (18)
Cyanophenol	31 (16)	70 (12)	101 (5)
Nitrophenol	38 (11)	65 (12)	103 (4)
Iodophenol	24 (6)	73 (7)	97 (2)
Heptyloxyphenol	23 (10)	71 (10)	95 (4)
Pentyloxyphenol	13(4)	85 (3)	98 (2)

Source: Data from References 34 and 35.

[a] Single-dose application from 95% ETOH ($N = 6$) at 2–4 µg/cm^2 to the ventral forearm; 24 hours exposure prior to soap and water washing.

[b] Data analysis accounts for 27.2% of applied dose evaporating off the skin surface during application.

results from occlusion (31, 32). Plastic chamber occlusion can also cause skin irritation (personal observation). Occlusion-induced increases in the mitotic rate of skin and epidermal thickening have been documented by Fisher and Maibach (33).

With respect to percutaneous absorption, occlusion or a protective cover may prevent loss of the surface-deposited chemical by evaporation, friction, and/or exfoliation; bioavailability may thereby be increased. However, comparison of the data in Tables 15.6 and 15.8 for the percutaneous absorption of steroids under nonprotected and protected conditions shows clearly that the potential increase in bioavailability from protection of the site of application does not explain the increase in steroid absorption under occluded conditions.

Occlusion does not necessarily increase percutaneous absorption through normal healthy skin. HC absorption under occluded conditions was not enhanced in single-dose or multiple-dose application studies (Table 15.12). This lack of penetration enhancement under occluded conditions has also been observed with certain para-substituted phenols (34, 35), as well as with ddI (2',3'-dideoxyinosine, aqueous solubility of 27.3 mg/mL at pH ~6) (36). However, a trend of occlusion-induced absorption enhancement with increasing penetrant lipophilicity is apparent. This trend is also supported by the results of Treffel et al. (37), who have shown that the *in vitro* permeation of citropten (a lipophilic compound) increased 1.6 times under occlusion, whereas that of caffeine (an amphiphilic compound) remained unchanged. However, the degree of lipophilicity (such as measured by $K_{O/W}$)

TABLE 15.12
Percutaneous Absorption of Hydrocortisone in Humans Following Application from Acetone Solution

	Percent Dose Absorbed[a]	Applied Dose µg/cm²)
Plastic wrap occlusion; single dose[b]	9(6)	5.8
Plastic wrap occlusion; single dose[c]	5(2)	4.0
Plastic chamber occlusion[d]	4(2)	4.0
Plastic chamber occlusion[e]	4(1)	4.0
Plastic chamber occlusion[f]	3(1)	4.0
"Protected" condition; single dose[g]	4(2)	4.0
Nonprotected; single dose[h]	1(0.3)	5.8
Nonprotected; single dose[i]	2(2)	4.0
Nonprotected; multiple dose[j]	3(1)	4.0
Nonprotected; multiple dose[k]	3(1)	4.0

[a] Absorption values, mean (SD), corrected for incomplete renal elimination.

[b] Occluded for four days, washed 96 hours post-application with soap and water (12).

[c] Occluded for one day, washed 24 hours post-application with soap and water (35).

[d] Single dose occluded for seven days, washed 24 hours post-application with soap and water (13).

[e] Percentage of first dose absorbed following daily doses. Occluded for 14 days, washed 24 hours post-application with soap and water (13).

[f] Percentage of eighth dose absorbed following daily doses. Occluded for 14 days, washed 24 hours post-application with soap and water (13).

[g] Site covered for seven days with a ventilated plastic chamber, washed 24 hours post-application with soap and water (11, 24).

[h] Site washed 24 hours post-application with soap and water (12).

[i] Site washed 24 hours post-application with soap and water (42).

[j] Percentage of first dose absorbed following daily doses or 14-day site washed 24 hours post-application with soap and water (23).

[k] Percentage of eighth dose following daily doses or 14-day site washed 24 hours post-application with soap and water (23).

exhibited by a penetrant in order for occlusion-induced enhanced skin permeation to be manifested is not clear and may be chemical class dependent.

The increase in percutaneous absorption of HC under occlusive conditions observed by Feldmann and Maibach (12) may be due to an acetone solvent effect. In this early work, the chemical was applied in 1.0 mL acetone over an area of 13 cm. Might the pretreatment of the skin with a large volume of acetone compromise stratum corneum barrier function? It has been reported that acetone can damage the stratum corneum (38, 39). It is conceivable that the large volume of acetone used ($76.9\ \mu L/cm^2$) may be responsible for the observed increase in HC penetration under plastic wrap occlusion. In addition, it is reasonable to suggest that the increased duration of exposure (96 hours compared to 24 hours) may contribute to the increase in observed HC percutaneous absorption. This enhancement in absorption was not observed in the experiments with HC under occlusion (24) when the acetone surface concentration was only $8.0\ \mu L/cm^2$ ($20\ \mu L$ over $2.5/cm^{-2}$) and skin surface exposure was limited to 24 hours.

The occlusion-induced enhancement of lipophilic compounds may be understood by considering the steps involved in the percutaneous absorption process. Minimally, after application in a volatile solvent, the penetrant must (1) dissolve/partition into the surface lipids of the stratum corneum, (2) diffuse through the lamellar lipid domains of the stratum corneum, (3) partition from the stratum corneum into the more hydrophilic viable epidermis, (4) diffuse through the epidermis and upper dermis, and (5) encounter a capillary of the cutaneous microvasculature and gain access to the systemic circulation (Figure 15.14).

As stated earlier, occlusion hydrates the stratum corneum, and if the effect of hydration were simply to decrease the viscosity of the stratum corneum intercellular domain, then the penetration of all chemicals should be equally enhanced by occlusion. In other words, the relative increase in the effective diffusion coefficient of the penetrant across the stratum corneum would be independent of the nature of the penetrant. But this is not the situation observed; the degree of enhancement is compound specific. To account for this effect, we postulate that stratum corneum hydration alters the stratum corneum–viable epidermis partitioning step. Occlusion hydrates the keratin in corneocytes and increases the water content between adjacent intercellular lipid lamellae. A penetrant diffusing through the intercellular lipid domains will distribute between the hydrophobic bilayer interiors and the aqueous regions separating the head groups of adjacent bilayers. Stratum corneum hydration magnifies the latter environment and increases the "hydrophilic" character of the stratum corneum somewhat. It follows that this leads, in turn, to a reduction in the stratum corneum–viable epidermis partition coefficient of the penetrant (because the two tissue phases now appear more similar). The decrease should facilitate the kinetics of transfer of penetrant through the stratum

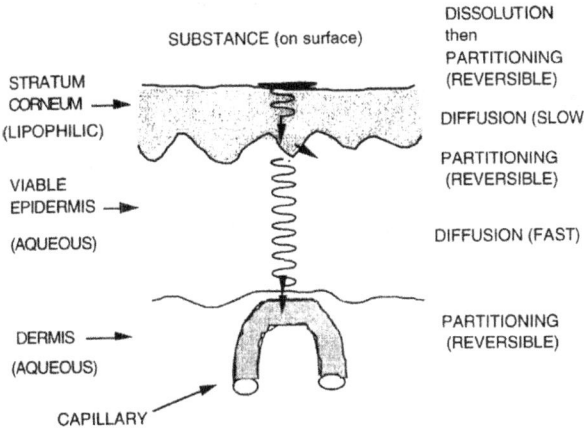

FIGURE 15.14 Schematic depiction of percutaneous absorption.

corneum and from the stratum corneum to the viable epidermis, and the relative effect on this rate should become greater as the lipophilicity of the absorbing molecule increases (40). The limit of this mechanism of enhancement would occur when penetrant is either (1) completely insoluble in the aqueous phases of the stratum corneum or (2) sterically hindered from penetrating the skin at a measurable rate due to, for example, large molecular size.

The importance of the partitioning step is implied by the dependence of percutaneous absorption with compound lipophilicity, as would be predicted if the skin behaved as a simple lipid membrane. Attenuation in absorption may be explained by a shift in the rate-limiting step from diffusion through the stratum corneum to the transfer across the stratum corneum–viable epidermis interface with increasing compound lipophilicity. The effect should be most apparent when the penetrant's aqueous solubility is extremely low; thus, it follows that this transfer process, or partitioning into the viable epidermis, should become slower as penetrant lipophilicity increases. This suggested mechanism is further supported by results obtained with the para-substituted phenols described earlier (25, 41) (Fig. 15.13).

Restricting evaporative loss of volatile compounds using plastic wrap occlusion enhances percutaneous absorption (38). Clearly, this effect may increase the extent of absorption of these lipophilic volatile compounds in addition to the possible enhancement afforded by occlusion-induced hydration of the stratum corneum.

As noted earlier, occlusion does not always increase the percutaneous absorption of topically applied agents. Furthermore, the extent of penetration may depend upon the method of occlusion. This finding has important implications in the design of a transdermal drug delivery system (TDS) for which the duration of application exceeds 24 hours. We have found that about a third of normal, healthy, male volunteers experience plastic chamber occlusion–induced irritation following contact periods greater than 24 hours; however, we have not observed any irritation of the skin using the nonocclusive patch system (made from these occlusive chambers) on the same volunteers following identical contact periods with the same penetrant. In those situations for which occlusion does not significantly increase the percutaneous absorption of a topically applied drug or an occlusion-induced enhancement in percutaneous absorption is not required, a nonocclusive TDS is an approach worthy of consideration.

15.7 CONCLUSION

Conclusions drawn from the preceding discussion are as follows:

1. Studies from multiple investigators indicate that the extent of percutaneous absorption may depend upon the occlusive system used (16, 18–20).
2. Occlusion does not necessarily increase percutaneous absorption. Penetration of hydrophilic compounds (e.g., compounds with low $K_{o/w}$ values), in particular, may not be enhanced by occlusion.
3. Mass balance (dose accountability) has been demonstrated using occlusive and nonocclusive patch systems *in vivo* in humans. Dose accountability rigorously quantifies percutaneous absorption measured using radiotracer methodology and allows objective comparison between different treatment modalities.
4. Occlusion, per se, can cause local skin irritation: which may enhance penetration and has implications in the design of transdermal delivery systems.

REFERENCES

1. Elias PM, Brown BE. The mammalian cutaneous permeability barrier. Lab Invest 1978; 39:574–583.
2. Elias PM, Cooper ER, Korc A, Brown B. Percutaneous transport in relation to stratum corneum structure and lipid composition. J Invest Dermatol 1981; 76:297–301.
3. Elias P. Epidermal lipids, barrier function, and desquamation. J Invest Dermatol 1983; 80:44s–49s.

4. Golden GM, Guzek DB, McKie JE, Potts RO. Role of stratum corneum lipid fluidity in transdermal drug flux. J Pharm Sci 1987; 76:25–31.

5. Menon GK, Feingold KR, Moser AH, Brown BE, Elias PM. De novo sterologenesis in the skin. II. Regulation by cutaneous barrier requirements. J Lipid Res 1985; 26:418–427.

6. Garb J. Nevus verrucosus unilateralis cured with podophyllin ointment. Arch Dermatol 1960; 81:606–609.

7. Scholtz JR. Topical therapy of psoriasis with fluocinolone acetonide. Arch Dermatol 1961; 84:1029–1030.

8. Sulzberger MB, Witten VH. Thin pliable plastic films in topical dermatological therapy. Arch Dermatol 1961; 84:1027–1028.

9. McKenzie AW. Percutaneous absorption of steroids. Arch Dermatol 1962; 86:91–94.

10. McKenzie AW, Stoughton RB. Method for comparing percutaneous absorption of steroids. Arch Dermatol 1962; 86:88–90.

11. Bucks DAW, McMaster JR, Maibach HI, Guy RH. Bioavailability of topically administered steroids: a "mass balance" technique. J Invest Dermatol 1988; 90:29–33.

12. Feldmann RJ, Maibach HI. Penetration of ^{14}C hydrocortisone through normal skin. Arch Dermatol 1965; 91:661–666.

13. Guy RH, Bucks DAW, McMaster JR, Villaflor DA, Roskos KV, Hinz RS, Maibach HI. Kinetics of drug absorption across human skin *in vivo*. In: Shroot B, Schaefer H, eds. Skin Pharmacokinetics. Basel: Karger, 1987:70–76.

14. Wiechers JW. The barrier functions of the skin in relation to percutaneous absorption of drugs. Pharm Weekbl [Sci] 1989; 11:185–198.

15. Qiao GL, Riviere. Significant effects of application site and occlusion on the pharmacokinetics of cutaneous penetration and biotransformation of parathion *in vivo* in swine. J Pharm Sci 1995; 84:425–432.

16. Gummer CL, Maibach HI. The penetration of [^{14}C]ethanol and [^{14}C]methanol through excised guinea-pig skin *in vitro*. Food Chem Toxicol 1986; 24:305–306.

17. Riley RT, Kemppainen BW, Norred WP. Penetration of aflatoxins through isolated human epidermis. J Toxicol Environ Health 1985; 15:769–777.

18. Kim HO, Wester RC, McMaster JR, Bucks DAW, Maibach HI. Skin absorption from patch test systems. Contact Dermatitis 1987; 17:178–180.

19. Bronaugh RL, Stewart RF, Wester RC, Bucks DAW, Maibach HI. Comparison of percutaneous absorption of fragrances by humans and monkeys. Food Chem Toxicol 1985; 23: 111–114.

20. Bronaugh RL, Wester RC, Bucks DAW, Maibach HI, Sarason R. *In vivo* percutaneous absorption of fragrance ingredients in rhesus monkeys and humans. Food Chem Toxicol 1990; 28:369–373.

21. Quisno RA, Doyle RL. A new occlusive patch test system with a plastic chamber. J Soc Cosmet Chem 1983; 34:13–19.

22. Bucks DAW, Marty J-PL, Maibach HI. Percutaneous absorption of malathion in the guinea pig: effect of repeated skin application. Food Chem Toxicol 1985; 23:919–922.

23. Bucks DAW, Maibach HI, Guy RH. Percutaneous absorption of steroids: effect of repeated application. J Pharm Sci 1985; 74:1337–1339.

24. Bucks DAW, Maibach HI, Guy RH. Mass balance and dose accountability in percutaneous absorption studies: development of non-occlusive application system. Pharm Res 1988; 5:313–315.

25. Bucks DAW, McMaster JR, Maibach HI, Guy RH. Percutaneous absorption of phenols *in vivo* [abstr]. Clin Res 1987; 35:672A.

26. Berardesca E, Vignoli GP, Fideli D, Maibach H. Effect of occlusive dressings on the stratum corneum water holding capacity. Am J Med Sci 1992; 304:25–28.

27. Blank IH, Scheuplein RJ. The epidermal barrier. In: Rook AJ, Champion RH, eds. Progress in the Biological Sciences in Relation to Dermatology. Vol 2. Cambridge: Cambridge University Press, 1964:245–261.

28. Potts RO. Stratum corneum hydration: experimental techniques and interpretation of results. J Soc Cosmet Chem 1986; 37:9–33.

29. Kligman AM. A biological brief on percutaneous absorption. Drug Dev Ind Pharm 1983; 9:521–560.

30. Faergemann J, Aly R, Wilson DR, Maibach HI. Skin occlusion: effect on Pityrosporum orbiculate, skin permeability of carbon dioxide, pH, transepidermal water loss, and water content. Arch Dermatol Res 1983; 275:383–387.

31. Gordon B, Maibach HI. Studies on the mechanism of aluminum anhidrosis. J Invest Dermatol 1968; 50:411–413.

32. Orentreich N, Berger RA, Auerbach R. Anhidrotic effects of adhesive tapes and occlusive film. Arch Dermatol Res 1966; 94:709–711.

33. Fisher LB, Maibach HI. The effect of occlusive and semipermeable dressings on the mitotic activity of normal and wounded human epidermis. Br J Dermatol 1972; 86:593–600.
34. Bucks DAW. Prediction of Percutaneous Absorption. Ph.D. dissertation, University of California, San Francisco, 1989.
35. Bucks D, Guy R, Maibach H. Effect of occlusion. In: Bronaugh RL, Maibach HI, eds. *In vitro* Percutaneous Absorption: Principles, Fundamentals, and Applications. Boston: CRC Press, 1991:85–114.
36. Mukherji E, Millenbaugh HJ, Au JL. Percutaneous absorption of 2′,3′-dideoxyinosine in rats. Pharm Res 1994; 11:809–815.
37. Treffel P, Muret P, Muret-D'Aniello P, Coumes-Marquet S, Agache P. Effect of occlusion on *in vitro* percutaneous absorption of two compounds with different physicochemical properties. Skin Pharmacol 1992; 5:108–113.
38. Bond JR, Barry BW. Damaging effect of acetone on the permeability barrier of hairless mouse skin compared with that of human skin. Int J Pharmaceut 1988; 41:91–93.
39. Schaefer H, Zesch A, Stuttgen G. Skin Permeability. Berlin: Springer-Verlag, 1982: 541–896.
40. Guy RH, Hadgraft J, Bucks DAW. Transdermal drug delivery and cutaneous metabolism. Xenobiotica 1987; 17:325–343.
41. Bucks DAW, McMaster JR, Maibach HI, Guy RH. Prolonged residence of topically applied chemicals in the stratum corneum: effect of lipophilicity [abstr]. Clin Res 1987; 35:672A.
42. Feldmann R, Maibach HI. Percutaneous absorption of steroids in man. J Invest Dermatol 1969; 52:89–94.
43. Bucks DAW, Maibach HI, Guy RH. Occlusion does not uniformly enhance penetration *in vivo*. In: Bronaugh R, Maibach H, eds. Percutaneous Absorption. Vol. 2. New York: Marcel Dekker, 1989:77–94.

16 Effect of Single versus Multiple Dosing in Percutaneous Absorption

Howard I. Maibach
University of California, San Francisco, California

CONTENTS

16.1 INTRODUCTION

Standard pharmacokinetic practice is to first do a single-dose application to determine bioavailability. This standard application is no different for percutaneous absorption, and most absorption values are for single doses. But think of topical application (or any drug dosing), and the procedure is repeated, whether once per day for several days (or longer) or multiple times during the day, which also can go on for several days (or longer). There are few one-dose magic bullets in pharmaceutics. Therefore, it becomes important to view multiple topical dosing, especially if that is the standard procedure with which a topical drug is used or if such exposure occurs for a hazardous environmental chemical.

16.1.1 SINGLE DAILY DOSE APPLICATION OVER MANY DAYS: HUMAN

Figure 16.1 illustrates the method used in this type of study (1, 2). [^{14}C]malathion was applied to the skin of human volunteers on day 1. For days 2 to 7, nonradioactive malathion was applied once per day to the same skin site. The radioactivity excretion curve for days 1 to 7 represents the single first daily dose. On day 8, the [^{14}C] malathion was applied again (note that malathion had been applied the previous seven days). The radioactivity–excretion curve for days 8 to 14 represents the multiple daily dose. Figure 16.1 shows no difference in the percutaneous absorption of malathion in man for single daily dose (exposure) over several days. This same method was used by Bucks et al. (3) to study several steroids in humans. Table 16.1 shows no difference in the absorption of a single daily topical steroid dose over several days. The results are exactly like that with malathion (Figure 16.2).

There is an exception to the clear results presented earlier. Azone (l-dodecylazacycloheptan-2-one) is an agent that has been shown to enhance the percutaneous absorption of drugs. It is believed to act on the stratum corneum (SC) by increasing the fluidity of the lipid bilayers. Because

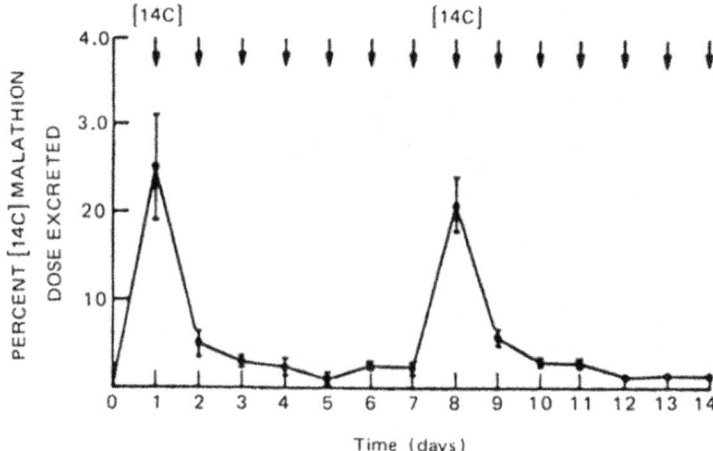

FIGURE 16.1 Percutaneous absorption of [^{14}C]malathion after single and repeated topical application (5 mg/cm^2) to the ventral forearm of a human. Arrow represents application of malathion, and ^{14}C represents when [^{14}C]malathion was applied.

Azone is nonpolar, it is thought to act by partitioning into the lipid bilayers, thereby disrupting the structure and potentially allowing drug penetration to increase. Previous clinical studies with single-dose administration show neat Azone percutaneous absorption to be <1%. A short-term, four-day dosing sequence gave absorption of 3.5 ± 0.3%. However, the effect of long-term multiple dosing on the percutaneous absorption of Azone has never been assessed. A study such as this is important because the mechanism of Azone—disruption of the lipid bilayer structure—suggests a potential for enhanced percutaneous absorption with chronic administration.

Excretion from days 1 to 7 topical application gave a single-dose percutaneous absorption of 1.84 ± 1.56% dose. Percutaneous absorption from days 8 to 15 skin application was 2.76 ± 1.91%, and

TABLE 16.1
Percutaneous Absorption of Steroids in Humans

	Mean % Applied Dose Absorbed (±SD)	
	Nonprotected	Occlusion
Hydrocortisone		
Single application	2 ± 2	4 ± 2
Multiple application		
First dose	3 ± 1	4 ± 1
Eighth dose	3 ± 1	3 ± 1
Estradiol		
Single application	11 ± 5	27 ± 6
Multiple application		
First dose	10 ± 2	38 ± 8
Eighth dose	11 ± 5	22 ± 7
Testosterone		
Single application	13 ± 3	46 ± 15
Multiple application		
First dose	21 ± 6	51 ± 10
Eighth dose	20 ± 7	50 ± 9

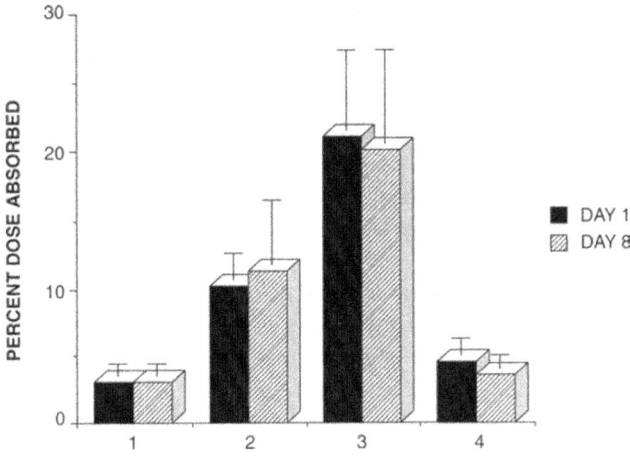

FIGURE 16.2 Skin absorption single (day 1) and multiple (day 8) dose in humans.

the absorption from days 15 to 21 skin application was $2.72 \pm 1.21\%$. Statistical analysis showed a significant difference for day 1 dosing versus day 8 dosing ($p < 0.001$) and for day 1 dosing versus day 15 dosing ($p < 0.008$). No difference was observed in percutaneous absorption for day 8 versus day 15 dosing (Figure 16.3). The daily excretion patterns show that peak excretion occurred at 24 or 48 hours following topical application. The results show that an increase occurs in the absorption of Azone with long-term multiple application, but that this enhanced self-absorption occurs early in use, and a steady-state absorption amount is established after the initial enhancement (4).

16.1.2 TRIPLE DAILY DOSE APPLICATION: HYDROCORTISONE

16.1.2.1 Study Design

The study was specifically designed to compare a single low dose ($13.33\ \mu g/cm^2$) to a single larger dose ($40.0\ \mu g/cm^2$; three times the amount) and to three multiple-application therapy ($13.33\ \mu g/cm^2 \times 3 = 40.0\ \mu g/cm^2$) treatments. Student two-tailed, paired t-tests were employed to

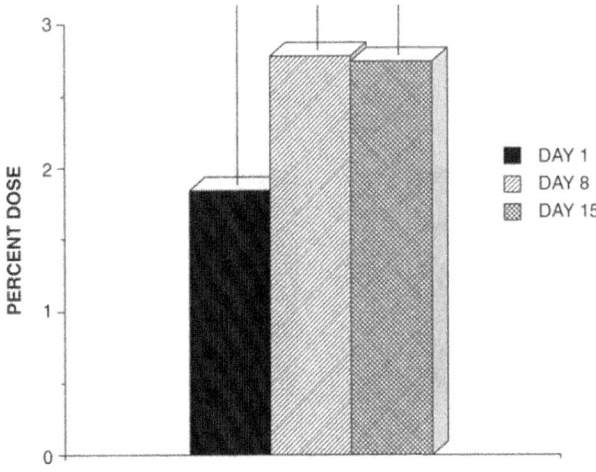

FIGURE 16.3 Azone multiple dosing in human volunteers.

compare the percentage of the applied dose absorbed and observed mass absorbed per square centimeter between each of the treatments:

- Treatment 1 — one bolus application of 1.0 μCi/13.33 μg/cm^2 on the right arm, 3 in. from the antecubital fossa. The dose was exposed to the skin for 24 hours, followed with removal by washing.
- Treatment 2 — one bolus application of 1.0 μCi/40.0 μg/cm^2 on the left arm, 3 in. from the antecubital fossa. The dose was exposed to the skin for 24 hours, followed with removal by washing.
- Treatment 3 — Three repeat applications of 1.0 μCi/13.33 μg/cm^2 on the left ventral forearm, 1 in. from the antecubital fossa. One dose was applied, followed by identical doses 5 and 12 hours after the initial dose. The site was washed 24 hours after the initial dose was applied.

Treatment	Dose per Application (μgc/cm^2)	Cumulative Dose (μgc/cm^2)	Total Vehicle volume (μL)	
			Acetone	Cream
1[a]	13.33	13.33	20	100
2[b]	40.00	40.00	20	100
3[c]	13.33	40.00	60	100

[a] Single dose of 13.33 μg/cm^2 administered in 20 μL of vehicle.
[b] Single dose of 40.00 μg/cm^2 administered in 20 μL of vehicle.
[c] Three serial 13.33 μg/cm^2 doses, each administered in 20 μL of vehicle (total 60 μL).

16.1.3 HYDROCORTISONE DOSING SEQUENCE

Figures 16.4 and 16.5 show the predicted and observed hydrocortisone in vivo percutaneous absorption in acetone or cream vehicles dosed at 13.3 μg/cm^2 × 1 (single low dose), 40.0 μg/cm^2 × 1 (single high dose and an amount three times that of the low dose), and 13.3 μg/cm^2 × 3 (multiple dose, which is three times the single low dose and equal in total amount to the 40 μg/cm^2 in the single high dose). The predicted amounts are multiples (three times) of that of the observed single-dose value.

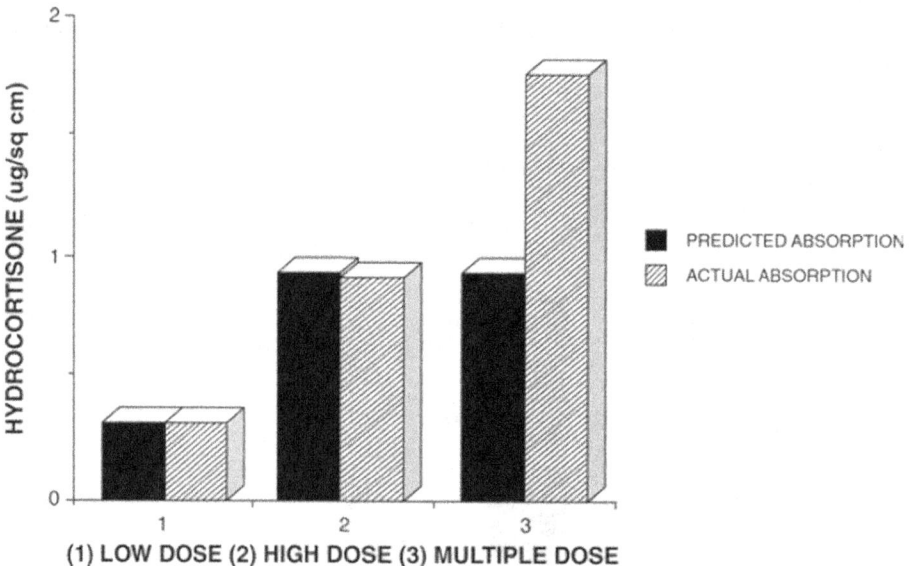

FIGURE 16.4 Hydrocortisone in vivo human skin absorption in cream vehicle.

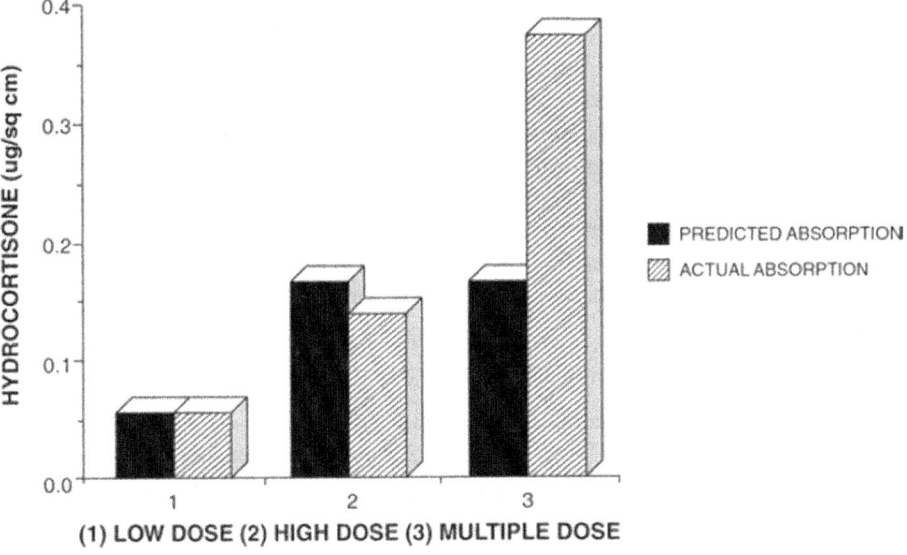

FIGURE 16.5   Hydrocortisone in vivo human skin absorption in acetone vehicle.

With the acetone vehicle, 0.056 ± 0.073 µg/cm² hydrocortisone was absorbed for the low dose. The single high-dose absorption was 0.140 ± 0.136 µg/cm²—a value near its predicted linear amount of 0.168. The multiple-dose absorption should have been the same predicted 0.168; however, the absorption was 0.372 ± 0.304 µg/cm², a value statistically ($p < 0.05$) greater than that of the single high dose (Figure 16.4).

With the cream vehicle, the same pattern emerged. The single high dose absorbed [0.91 ± 1.66 µg/cm²] was three times that of the low dose absorbed 0.31 ± 0.43 µg/cm²). The multiple dose absorbed (1.74 ± 0.93 µg/cm²) exceeded the predicted amount and was statistically ($p < 0.006$) greater than that of the single high dose.

Table 16.2 gives the predicted and observed in vitro hydrocortisone percutaneous absorption. The receptor fluid accumulations (absorbed amounts) show the same trend as that seen *in vivo*. In

TABLE 16.2

Predicted and Observed Hydrocortisone Absorption: In Vitro

		Hydrocortisone (µg/cm²)			
		Receptor Fluid		Skin	
Vehicle	Dosing Sequence	Predict	Observe	Predict	Observe
Acetone[a]	13.3 µg/cm² × 1	—	0.13 ± 0.05	—	0.87 ± 0.23
	40.0 µg/cm² × 1	0.39[b]	0.35 ± 0.22	2.61[b]	2.21 ± 2.05
	13.3 µg/cm² × 3	0.39	0.55 ± 0.75	2.61	2.84 ± 2.05
Cream[a]	13.3 µg/cm² × 1	—	$0.053 + 0.029$	—	0.30 ± 0.24
	40.0 µg/cm² × 1	0.16[b]	0.23 ± 0.03	0.90[b]	0.86 ± 0.53
	13.3 µg/cm² × 3	0.16	0.27 ± 0.21	0.90	1.19 ± 0.43

[a] $n = 3$; mean ± SD.

[b]   0.39 µg/cm² is three times the measured value of 0.13 µg/cm²; 2.61 µg/cm² is three times the measured value of 0.87 µg/cm²; 0.16 µg/cm² is three times the measured value of 0.053 µg/cm²; 0.90 µg/cm² is three times the measured value of 0.30 µg/cm².

vitro studies also allowed the human skin to be assayed for hydrocortisone content following the 24-hour dosing interval. The skin content values markedly reflect those seen with the receptor fluid values. Only three observations were made per dosing sequence, so statistically no differences exist. The same human skin sources were used for both acetone and cream vehicles, so these absorption amounts can be compared. Hydrocortisone absorption is greater with the acetone vehicle (5, 6).

Little information is available on the most effective topical corticosteroid or other topical formulation dosing regimen regarding the number of skin applications in one day. Multiple applications for an ambulatory patient with a readily accessible skin site are common practice. However, for hospitalized patients or patients where multiple dosing would be difficult, a single effective dose of hydrocortisone will eventually do the task.

16.1.4 TRIPLE DAILY DOSE APPLICATION: DICLOFENAC

Diclofenac, a nonsteroidal antiinflammatory drug, has been widely used in the treatment of rheumatoid arthritis and osteoarthritis. However, oral delivery of this drug poses certain disadvantages, such as fast first-pass metabolism and adverse side effects (including gastrointestinal reactions and idiosyncratic drug reactions). Therefore, alternative routes of administration have been sought. The skin has become increasingly important to this effect, and many drugs have been formulated in transdermal delivery systems, including diclofenac itself. However, diclofenac sodium is not easily absorbed through the skin due to its hydrophilic nature. Much work has concentrated on using percutaneous absorption enhancers or cosolvents to increase penetration. A new diclofenac sodium lotion named Pennsaid has been developed for topical application. Pennsaid includes the absorption enhancer dimethylsulfoxide (DMSO). It is expected that the addition of DMSO may increase the in vivo permeation rate of diclofenac through the skin into the deeper target tissues beneath the skin.

Tables 16.3 and 16.4 show that multiple doses of Pennsaid lotion (2 μg/cm^2 and 5/d/cm^2 3×/day) delivered a total of 40.1 ± 17.6 μg and 85.6 ± 41.4 μg diclofenac, respectively, at 48 hours, compared to only 9.4 ± 2.9 μg and 35.7 ± 19.0 μg absorbed after topical application of diclofenac as an aqueous solution ($P < 0.05$). A single-dose study showed no statistical difference between diclofenac delivered in Pennsaid lotion or in aqueous solution. Over 48 hours the total absorption for Pennsaid lotion was 10.2 ± 6.7 and 26.2 ± 17.6 μg (2 and 5 μL/cm^2, respectively) compared to 8.3 ± 1.5 and 12.5 ± 5.7 μg from an aqueous solution. Both single doses of Pennsaid lotion and aqueous diclofenac showed decreased diclofenac absorption into the receptor fluid between 12 and 24 hours. However,

TABLE 16.3
In Vitro Percutaneous Absorption of Diclofenac from Pennsaid Lotion and Aqueous Solution in Viable Human Skin

	Dosing Regimen	Diclofenac Absorbed (μg/cm^2)[a]
A	30 μg/cm^2 single-dose Pennsaid	10.2 ± 6.7
B	75 μg/cm^2 single-dose Pennsaid	26.2 ± 17.6
C	30 μg/cm^2 single-dose aqueous	8.3 ±1.5
D	75 μg/cm^2 single-dose aqueous	12.3 ± 5.6
E	240 μg/cm^2 multidose Pennsaid	40.1 ± 17.6
F	600 μg/cm^2 multidose Pennsaid	85.6 ± 41.4
G	240 μg/cm^2 multidose aqueous	9.4 ± 2.9
H	600 μg/cm^2 multidose aqueous	35.7 ± 19.0

Note: Absorbed cumulative amount in receptor fluid plus skin.

[a] Mean ± SD (n = 4 or 5).

TABLE 16.4
**Statistical Summary: Diclofenac Absorption
in Viable Human Skin**

Treatment	Statistic[a] ($p =$)
Pennsaid lotion	
A vs. B—single dose	0.09[b]
E vs. F—multiple doses	0.05[c]
A vs. E—single vs. multiple	0.007[c]
B vs. F—single vs. multiple	0.02[c]
Aqueous solution	
C vs. D—single dose	0.16[b]
G vs. H—multiple doses	0.02[c]
C vs. G—single vs. multiple	0.42[b]
D vs. H—single vs. multiple	0.03[c]
Pennsaid lotion vs. aqueous solution	
A vs. C—single dose	0.57[b]
B vs. D—single dose	0.13[b]
E vs. G—multiple doses	0.005[b]
F vs. H—multiple doses	0.04[c]

[a] Student's *t*-test.
[b] Nonsignificant.
[c] Statistically significant.

when applied multiple times, absorption from Pennsaid lotion was continually increasing up to 48 hours (7). Clinically, Pennsaid lotion has been shown to be effective in a multidose regimen.

These studies with hydrocortisone and diclofenac show enhanced human skin absorption from a multidose (defined as three times per day application) regimen. The key for diclofenac is the Pennsaid formulation and, probably, the inclusion of the penetration enhancer DMSO. For hydrocortisone, it may simply be the continuing application of vehicle that "washes" the drug through the skin.

16.1.5 ANIMAL MODELS

There are several multidose studies in the literature using animals (8–12), which give mixed results when compared to subsequent human studies. A key animal study is that by Bucks et al. (13), where percutaneous absorption of malathion multidose in the guinea pig is similar to multidose in humans. except where skin washing is introduced into the study design. Skin washing enhances multidose malathion percutaneous absorption. In human studies, skin washing is not a consideration because bathing is an everyday event. In animal experiments, treatment of skin may compromise skin integrity (application of keratolytic agents or soap and water washing), and this can result in altered percutaneous absorption.

16.2 CONCLUSION

Percutaneous absorption with single-dose regimens is generally the only type of study done to determine typical bioavailability. Tradition and regulatory requirements are probably the driving forces. In actual clinical use, the multidose regimen is probably the more widely practiced treatment. Two types of experimental designs have been tested. The one of a single daily dose over the course of a few weeks probably does not affect percutaneous absorption unless the skin is compromised by disease (14) or if some key ingredient in the formulation is an absorption enhancer, such as Azone, and Azone seems to have only influenced the early part of the dosing period. The more intriguing multidose regimen is the multiple-dose application during a single day. Both formulation (as seen with hydrocortisone) and formulation ingredients (DMSO in Pennsaid lotion) can enhance skin absorption. The combined (and relevant) study of multidoses within each day over several days dosing has not been done. Neither have longer-term studies using multidose daily regimens been done to assess percutaneous absorption and diseased skin and the potential compromise of keratolytic agents such as salicylic acid and hydrocortisone.

REFERENCES

1. Wester RC, Maibach HI, Bucks DAW, Guy RH. Malathion percutaneous absorption after. repeated administration to man. J Pharm Sci 1983; 65:116–119.
2. Wester RC, Maibach HI, Bucks DAW, Guy RH. Malathion percutaneous absorption after repeated administration to man. Toxicol Appl Pharmacol 1983; 68:116–119.
3. Bucks DAW, Maibach HI, Guy RH. In vivo percutaneous absorption: effect of repeated application versus single dose. In: Bronaugh R, Maibach H, eds. Percutaneous Absorption. 2nd ed. New York: Marcel Dekker, 1989:633–651.
4. Wester RC, Melendres J, Sedik L, Maibach HI. Percutaneous absorption of Azone following single and multiple doses to human volunteers. J Pharm Sci 1994; 83:124–125.
5. Melendres J, Bucks DAW, Camel E, Wester RC, Maibach HI. In vivo percutaneous absorption of hydrocortisone: multiple-application dosing in man. Pharm Res 1992; 9:1164–1167.
6. Wester RC, Melendres J, Logan F, Maibach HI. Triple therapy: multiple dosing enhances hydrocortisone percutaneous absorption in vivo in humans. In: Smith E, Maibach H, eds. Percutaneous Penetration Enhancers. Boca Raton: CRC Press, 1995:343–349.
7. Hewitt PG, Poblete N, Wester RC, Maibach HI, Shainhouse JZ. In vitro cutaneous disposition of a topical diclofenac lotion in human skin: effect of a multi-dose regimen. Pharm Res 1998; 15(7):988–992.
8. Roberts MS, Horlock E. Effect of repeated skin application on percutaneous absorption of salicylic acid. J Pharm Sci 1978; 67:1685–1687.
9. Wester RC, Noonan PK, Maibach HI. Frequency of application on percutaneous absorption of hydrocortisone. Arch Dermatol 1997; 113:620–622.
10. Wester RC, Noonan PK, Maibach HI. Variations in percutaneous absorption of testosterone in the Rhesus monkey due to anatomic site of application and frequency of application. Arch Dermatol Res 1980; 267:229–235.
11. Wester RC, Noonan PK, Maibach HI. Variations in percutaneous absorption of hydrocortisone increases with long-term administration: in vivo studies in the Rhesus monkey. Arch Dermatol Res 1980; 116:186–188.
12. Courtheoux S, Pechnenot D, Bucks DA, Marty JPL, Maibach H, Wepierre J. Effect of repeated skin administration on in vivo percutaneous absorption of drugs. Br J Dermatol 1986; 115:49–52.
13. Bucks DAW, Marty JPL, Maibach HI. Percutaneous absorption of malathion in the guinea pig: effect of repeated skin application. Food Chem Toxic 1958; 23:919–922.
14. Wester RC, Maibach HI. Percutaneous absorption in diseased skin. In: Maibach H, Surber C, eds. Topical Corticosteroids. Basel: Karger, 1992:128–141.

17 Influence of Formulation on Topical and Transdermal Drug Delivery

Heather A.E. Benson
Curtin University, Perth, Western Australia

Hamid R. Moghimi
Shahid Beheshti University of Medical Sciences,
Tehran, Iran

Jeffrey E. Grice
University of Queensland, Woolloongabba,
Queensland, Australia

Michael S. Roberts
University of Queensland, Woolloongabba,
Queensland, Australia
University of South Australia, Adelaide,
South Australia

CONTENTS

17.1   INTRODUCTION

Topically applied products may target sites in one or more different skin layers (i.e., epidermis, dermis, and hypodermis), the skin appendages (e.g., hair follicles with associated sebaceous glands, sweat glands, and nails), and underlying tissues. Identifying the specific target region and formulating to deliver the therapeutic compound to that target is a key objective in topical product design. The skin surface is the target for cosmetics, sunscreens, and insect repellents, so the aim is to target actives to the skin surface with minimal absorption to deeper skin layers. The key target region for the majority of topically applied products is the viable epidermis and dermis, and sites targeted here include nerves, keratinocytes, melanocytes, Langerhans cells, and hair follicles. Deeper tissues associated with muscles and joints may also be targeted, such as topical products for musculoskeletal pain and inflammation. Transdermal products target the systemic circulation.

The barrier function of the skin limits and controls the dose that is absorbed into or through the skin. Thus, the primary aim of a topical or transdermal formulation is generally to present the applied drug in a form that can be absorbed and possibly enhance its permeation or target delivery to a site within the skin, to deeper tissues beneath the skin, or to the cutaneous circulation for localized or systemic outcome, respectively. Emulsions are the most widely used topical formulations for dermatological, cosmetic, or personal care products because they provide excellent solubilizing capacities for both lipophilic and hydrophilic active ingredients and good skin feel and consumer acceptability. The type of emulsion (oil in water [o/w] or water in oil [w/o]), droplet size, properties of the emollient/oil and emulsifier(s), and surfactant organization (micelles, lyotropic liquid crystals) in the emulsion may affect the skin delivery [1, 2]. A range of pharmaceutical formulation approaches are deployed to increase topical and transdermal delivery. These include permeation enhancers that modulate the skin barrier or by manipulating the thermodynamic activity and hence driving force for drug delivery within the skin. The rationale, mechanism, and application of these formulation approaches to topical and transdermal delivery is the focus of this chapter.

17.2   DRUG TRANSPORT THROUGH THE SKIN

The transdermal permeation process and pathways through the stratum corneum have been considered in detail in Chapter 1. In brief, percutaneous absorption can occur via the appendages (pilosebaceous units, eccrine and apocrine ducts; collectively described as the "shunt" route), through the intercellular lipid domains, or by a transcellular route. Although these three routes can all contribute to percutaneous absorption, the proportional contribution of each route varies depending on the permeant physicochemical characteristics and can be influenced by the formulation vehicle in which it is applied to the skin. It should be noted that the intercellular route is not exclusively lipoidal, as there are desmosomes, proteins, and a thin layer of water associated with the polar head groups in the lipid domains, all contributing to more polar areas within the lipid regions that can facilitate passage of a hydrophilic permeant. Roberts proposed the "mixed permeation model" to describe how most drugs permeate via the intercellular route, but could access microroutes of lipid and polar regions within the lipid bilayers, depending on the partition coefficient of the permeant [3].

Drug permeation through the skin can be described by Fick's laws of diffusion, which in their simplest form state that steady-state flux (J) through the skin into an infinite sink (skin tissues, cutaneous circulation, or the receptor compartment in an *in vitro* experimental diffusion cell) can be calculated by:

$$J = Kp \times C \qquad (17.1)$$

where Kp is the permeability coefficient of the permeant in the skin and C is the concentration of the permeant in the applied formulation vehicle. The permeability coefficient is a composite parameter:

$$Kp = P.D/h \tag{17.2}$$

where P is the partition coefficient of the permeant between the skin and the applied formulation vehicle, D, is the diffusion coefficient of the permeant in the skin, and h is the skin thickness (or, more accurately, the length of the diffusional pathway through the stratum corneum intercellular route).

Although the mathematical modeling of skin diffusion can be considered in far more complex ways (Chapter 2), this simple form of Fick's law is useful to illustrate that percutaneous permeation through the stratum corneum can be enhanced by increasing partitioning or diffusivity, and forms the basis of the range of formulation approaches to skin drug delivery. For example, chemical permeation enhancers that disrupt the stratum corneum intercellular lipid packing will increase diffusivity, whereas solvents present in a formulation vehicle may permeate with the permeant into the stratum corneum to promote partitioning from the vehicle to the skin.

17.3 SKIN PERMEANT PROPERTIES

The ideal physicochemical properties for passive skin delivery are low molecular weight (<500 daltons), moderate lipophilicity (log $P_{o/w}$ 1–4), melting point <200°C, and good potency (daily systemic dose ≤20 mg). Quantitative structure permeation relationships (QSPR) studies [4, 5] have shown that small solute size is important for facilitating the diffusion process, while adequate lipophilicity is required to provide sufficient solubility in the stratum corneum. Drug potency is an important consideration, as demonstrated for a series of antiinflammatory drugs [6]. Although the maximum flux of diclofenac (with a log P > 4) was lower than other antiinflammatory drugs, with log P in the range of 2.7 to 3.1, it had the highest efficacy coefficient ratio (the ratio of maximum flux and drug potency dose), since the antiinflammatory effect of a drug also depends on lipophilicity, thus providing higher potency. Permeant solubility is an important consideration in flux and in formulation design. Although lipophilicity is required for uptake into the stratum corneum and diffusion within the intercellular lipid domains, there is a need to ensure sufficient aqueous solubility to minimize donor depletion from an aqueous-based formulation over the period of application to the skin.

Permeants that are weak acids or bases can dissociate depending on the pH of the topical formulation and the stratum corneum, resulting in poor skin delivery. There is the potential to mitigate this through ion pairs [7–9] and pH adjustment in the formulation [10, 11]. Ion pairing involves addition of an oppositely charged counter-ion to form a neutral pair, with increased lipophilicity and improved stratum corneum diffusivity. The ion pair can dissociate in the viable epidermis or deeper tissue to release the parent compound. The pH of the formulation can be used to alter the degree of ionization, as has been shown with a 50-times difference in the permeability coefficient of lidocaine with pH adjustment [11]. Again, one factor cannot be considered in isolation, as was illustrated by the increase in flux of diclofenac (pKa of 4.7) from pH 3 to 7 in the vehicle [12]. As the diclofenac ionization increased with pH, the permeability coefficient decreased, but was offset by the increased solubility of the ionized species in the vehicle.

17.3.1 HANSEN SOLUBILITY PARAMETERS (HSP) AS A TOOL FOR PREDICTING VEHICLE/DRUG UPTAKE AND ENHANCEMENT

The polarity of the permeant in relation to those of the formulation and membrane is an important parameter in drug permeation through biological barriers, including skin. Polarity is a relative property (not absolute), and different scales are used to express this property, including partition coefficient (PC), solubility parameter (δ), dielectric constant (ε), surface tension (γ), and hydrophilic-lipophilic balance (HLB) [13, 14], each with special applications. Partition coefficient is generally used to express the relative affinity of a permeant to the formulation and the membrane in a passive permeation process, as is seen in Fick's law (Equation 17.2). In applying this concept, it is usually assumed that the formulation stays unchanged on the skin surface and the permeant leaves it toward the skin (static condition). However, we know that there are many situations in which the whole or a part of the formulation/solvent enters the skin and carries the drug into the skin (dynamic conditions). Both dynamic and static conditions might be addressed by different polarity scales. Here, HSP are introduced as a tool that can predict the possible affinity of a drug and formulation to the skin, and even the possibility of its retention within the skin.

The solubility parameter, defined as the square root of cohesive energy density, was first introduced by Hildebrand and Scott [15] and then was optimized by Hansen [16]. The HSP are based on the cohesive energy that arises from (atomic) dispersion forces (δD), bipolar molecular forces (δP), and hydrogen bonding (δH) [17]. Comparison of the HSP values of two systems shows the extent of their affinity to each other. The closeness of the HSP of two systems is evaluated by calculating the HSP distance (R_a, Equation 17.3) [16, 17]. Two systems with similar or close HSP values show smaller R_a and are expected to be compatible or dissolve in each other; this is what is usually expressed as "like likes like" or "like dissolves like."

$$R_a^2 = 4(\delta D_2 - \delta D_1)^2 + (\delta P_2 - \delta P_1)^2 + (\delta H_2 - \delta H_1)^2 \qquad (17.3)$$

This concept can be used to predict the affinity of materials to each other and is used in a range of areas, including drug design and delivery. For example, HSP values have been used to predict nail interactions for the design of nail medicines [18], drug distribution in microspheres [19], and in transdermal drug delivery [20].

To evaluate the affinity of drugs, excipients, and formulations to the skin, we need HSP values of the skin barrier and the interacting material. HSP of different materials are available. For example δD, δP, and δH of dimethyl sulfoxide (DMSO), a known permeation enhancer, are reported to be 18.4, 16.4, and 10.2 (all in MPa$^{1/2}$), respectively, and those of ethanol, a common solvent with permeation enhancement properties, are 15.8, 8.8, and 19.4, respectively [17]. Data are also available for the skin barrier, based on a range of sources. Hansen evaluated HSP values of human skin to be 17.6, 12.5, and 11.0 (MPa$^{1/2}$) for δD, δP, and δH, respectively [17], based on permeation data from Ursin et al. [21]. Two other sets of data are from human psoriatic scales measured through swelling studies [22] and an estimated system for human skin by Abbott [23], as shown in Table 17.1. The main barrier against permeation of drugs through the skin is the stratum corneum. The only available HSP values for human stratum corneum are from Ezati et al. [24], measured at 32°C through uptake studies using 18 different solvents (Figure 17.1 and Table 17.1). HSP values of fingernails and toenails have also been measured by Hossin et al. [18], using a swelling method (Table 17.1).

The enhancement action of permeation enhancers is mostly related to their uptake by the stratum corneum. Ezati et al. [24] used relative energy difference (RED) to investigate the correlation between the enhancement ratios and HSP values. RED (Equation. 17.4) is the ratio of R_a (HSP distance, Equation 17.3) and R_0 (the radius of the interaction sphere). The HSP sphere, or interaction sphere, is a spherical space in the three-dimensional graph of δD, δP, and δH (Figure 17.1 for an example), where the good solvents are inside the sphere and bad solvents are outside of it. The center of this sphere is the HSP, and its radius is R_0 [17]. Equation 17.4 shows the affinity of the materials

TABLE 17.1

HSP Values of Dispersion Forces (δD), Bipolar Molecular Forces (δP), and Hydrogen Bonding (δH) Reported for Human Skin, the Stratum Corneum (SC), and Nails.

Sample	HSPs (MPa$^{1/2}$)			References
	δD	δP	δH	
Human stratum corneum	16.5	12	7.7	[24]
Human skin	17.6	12.5	11	[17]
Human skin	17	8	8	[23]
Psoriatic scales	24.6	11.9	12.9	[22]
Fingernail	17.7	20.9	18.6	[18]

Source: Table is Reproduced after Ezati et al. [24] with permission from the Copyright Owner.

to each other in a way that RED values of close to or lower than 1 indicate high affinity and RED values of markedly greater than 1 indicate low affinity [17].

$$RED = R_a / R_0 \tag{17.4}$$

Using published enhancement data from Lee et al. [25] and stratum corneum HSP values from their own work [24], Ezati et al. calculated RED values and showed that a good correlation exists between flux and reduction of RED for the effects of ethanol and tricaprylin on the skin permeation of tegafur [24]. They applied the same analysis to the published data for the enhancement effects of isopropyl myristate and N-methyl pyrrolidone on lidocaine flux across human skin [26] and again observed a good correlation between the RED reduction and enhancement ratio [24].

HSP can also be used for formulation design. Using HSP values of 17, 8, 8 (δD, δP, δH, respectively) for human skin and HSP distance (R$_a$), Roberts group [27] showed that solubilities of caffeine (a hydrophilic drug) and naproxen (a lipophilic drug) in various solvents and enhancer-containing nanoemulsions increase by decreasing HSP distance (R$_a$) and are at their highest values when the

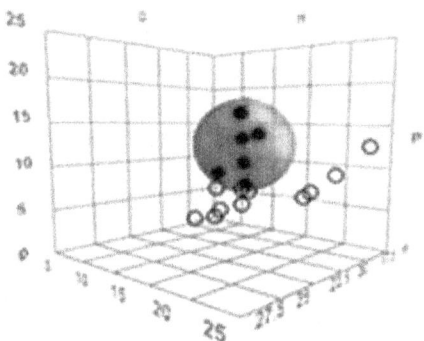

FIGURE 17.1 HSP plot of human stratum corneum at 32°C and the position of interaction sphere (or HSP sphere) showing good solvents (inside) and bad solvents (outside) of the sphere. The center of the spheres shows the HSP values for the SC: δD = 16.5, δP = 12, δH = 7.7 (all in MPa$^{1/2}$), and the radius of the interaction sphere is 6.3. (From Ezati et al. [24] with permission from the copyright owner.)

drugs and vehicles are most similar in their various solubility parameters (HSP). They also showed that solvent uptake into the stratum corneum obeys the same rule. The uptake of formulations into the stratum corneum increases as R_a decreases, and the uptake is highest for formulations that are most similar to the stratum corneum in terms of solubility parameters [27]. Ezati [24] also showed that when the HSP of nanoemulsions are very close to that of human stratum corneum, the formulation will be taken up very well by the stratum corneum, but is then entrapped in this membrane due to high affinity (similarity in HSP values), resulting in decreased permeation.

To conclude, it is clear that solubility parameters can be used as an effective tool in formulation design for optimized dermal/transdermal drug delivery and enhancement. However, we are in the early stages of using this concept for skin drug delivery and formulation design, and further investigation is required to enable us to find truly predictive equations.

17.4 PERCUTANEOUS PERMEATION ENHANCEMENT APPROACHES

The stratum corneum is an effective barrier that limits skin permeation and consequently the extent to which the skin can be effectively used to deliver compounds for therapeutic outcomes in the skin, underlying tissues, or systemically. Many compounds do not possess the ideal physicochemical criteria to passively permeate the skin in therapeutic quantities, thus limiting the potential for topical and transdermal delivery. Many different approaches to enhance delivery into the skin have been investigated. "Passive" technologies involve the use of formulation design and excipients, chemical permeation enhancers, and various types of microtechnology- and nanotechnology-based delivery systems. Technologies using an external driving force ("active" or "physical" enhancement methods) have employed electrical (iontophoresis and electroporation), thermal (laser and radio-frequency thermal ablation), ultrasound, magnetic, heat, mechanical (microneedles), and velocity (jet injector) based energies. In this chapter the focus is on formulation-based approaches to enhance skin delivery. Other permeation enhancement methods have been reviewed elsewhere.

17.5 FORMULATION APPROACHES TO ENHANCE AND/OR TARGET SKIN DELIVERY

Formulation encompasses multiple processes that lead eventually to a successful product in the market. There are many considerations in the selection of a suitable topical formulation, including the physicochemical properties of the permeant, the stability and compatibility of the permeant and excipients, and the cosmetic acceptability of the product. Dosage form design, composition design, packaging design, and industrial scaleup are also essential parts of the formulation development process, but the focus of this chapter is on the use of the formulation to optimize skin delivery.

Based on the theoretical requirements described in previous sections, improved skin delivery of a solute can be achieved by increasing its concentration in the stratum corneum and its rate of transport in this barrier. Table 17.2 summarizes formulation-based approaches for percutaneous absorption enhancement and their possible effect on the amount of permeant retained in the stratum corneum (R_m) and/or the rate constant of permeant transfer in the stratum corneum (T_r) [28]. Formulation-based approaches to enhance percutaneous permeation are discussed in the following sections, including manipulation of permeant thermodynamic activity, chemical permeation enhancers, advanced formulations based on nanosystems and microsystems, and briefly transdermal patch design.

17.5.1 PERMEANT CONCENTRATION AND THERMODYNAMIC ACTIVITY

Fick's law illustrates that the flux through skin is dependent on the concentration, or more accurately, the thermodynamic activity of the permeant in the applied formulation vehicle. Maximal flux is achieved when a saturated solution is applied to the skin surface because at saturation

TABLE 17.2

Formulation-Based Enhancement Strategies and Their Possible Effects on Solute Diffusivity (D) and Retention in Stratum Corneum (R_m) [28]

Approaches	Mechanisms	Potential Effects
Thermodynamic activity	Supersaturation	Increase partitioning, may increase R_m
	Formulating for efficacy	Increase partitioning and/or R_m; (potentially) increase D
Chemical permeation enhancer	Stratum corneum lipid alteration, e.g., fluidized lipid bilayer, lipid Extraction, polar head group alteration, hydrophobic lipid	Increase D
	Stratum corneum desmosomes and protein alterations	Increase D
	Corneocytes alteration	Increase D
	Shift stratum corneum solubility closer to that of permeant	Increase R_m and or partitioning
	Increase solute solubility in the stratum corneum because of solvent-drag mechanism	Increase partitioning and or R_m
Ion pairs and complex coacervates	Increase lipophilicity	Increase partitioning
Eutectic mixture	Decrease melting point	Increase R_m

(the dissolved permeant molecules are in equilibrium with its pure solid), the thermodynamic activity is 1 and the permeant has the highest tendency to "escape" from the donor solution and partition into the stratum corneum [29]. Indeed, in the absence of solute–skin and/or vehicle–skin interactions, the percutaneous absorption is directly related to the thermodynamic activity [30]. One of the considerations in topical formulation design is to maximize permeant thermodynamic activity in the vehicle by controlling the extent of permeant solubility in the formulation vehicle. This was clearly demonstrated by Barry's group, who examined the vapor and liquid diffusion of the volatile model permeant benzyl alcohol across human skin when applied in a range of binary solvent mixtures and correlated this with their thermodynamic activity [31, 32]. In the case of benzyl alcohol, the vapor flux was linearly correlated to the activity, suggesting that percutaneous absorption is controlled by thermodynamic activity when the vehicle has no effect on the stratum corneum barrier [31]. This showed that the thermodynamic activity of benzyl alcohol was directly related to the vapor flux across human skin

17.5.1.1 Supersaturation

Supersaturation can occur when the concentration of the permeant in the formulation vehicle is greater than the equilibrium solubility value and results in a thermodynamic activity greater than 1 for the permeant in that vehicle. This can occur when a topical formulation is applied to the skin. A cream or hydro-alcoholic gel rubbed into the skin will break down, with the potential for volatile solvents, such as alcohols, to evaporate, leaving the permeant in the residual nonvolatile components of the vehicle. If the permeant is poorly water soluble, this can increase its thermodynamic activity in the residual formulation and thereby enhance its partitioning into the skin.

The application of this supersaturation approach to enhanced percutaneous absorption is challenging because generating a supersaturated state through evaporation of volatile solvents leads to poor stability and therefore difficulty in predicting and controlling delivery to the skin.

However, supersaturated states can be achieved for more prolonged periods with suitable mixed solvent systems, leading to increased membrane flux, as has been demonstrated with poorly water soluble drugs such as estradiol [33], ibuprofen [34], and piroxicam [35, 36]. Approximate linear relationships between the degree of saturation (and consequent increase in permeant thermodynamic activity) and skin flux have been reported [33, 35]. In addition, these systems can be stabilized by the addition of antinucleating polymers, such as hydroxypropylmethyl cellulose, hydroxypropyl cellulose, polyvinylpyrrolidone, and polyvinyl alcohol, which act to prevent nucleation and subsequent crystallization of the permeant. Pellet et al. [35] suggested that human skin may also provide antinucleant properties based on their determination of piroxicam in stratum corneum tape strips and viable skin layers following administration of solutions with up to four degrees of saturation. Despite the antinucleating polymers' inability to enter the skin, a linear relationship existed between the degree of saturation and the amount of piroxicam in the stratum corneum and the viable layers of the skin. This may occur as a result of the antinucleating ability of the intercellular lipids of the stratum corneum [35].

Alternative formulations apply the same principles but offer more stable systems. For example, a water-free microemulsion base saturated with bupranolol applied to rabbits with an occlusive patch was converted *in situ* to a microemulsion from the transepidermal water accumulated under the occlusive patch [37]. The decreasing bupranolol solubility with increasing water content resulted in supersaturation, with the pharmacodynamic effect of the bupranolol monitored over a 10-hour period. The effect vs. time curves were inversely correlated with the solubility vs. water content curves.

Marc Brown's group have further applied this principle to a quick drying spray that can be applied to the skin as a metered dose aerosol [38–40]. Buprenorphine dipropionate was formulated in hydrofluoroalkane propellant 134a, ethanol, and polyvinyl pyrrolidone. The drug was supersaturated on the skin surface as the ethanol evaporated. With a similar approach, the skin delivery of betamethasone valerate was increased by six times compared to a conventional cream.

17.5.1.2 Formulating for Efficacy (FFE)

Johann Wiechers introduced the concept of "formulating for efficacy" [41, 42], which was aimed at aiding the rational design of topical formulations for skin delivery, and cosmetic applications in particular. He developed FFE to combine two contradictory properties that are required by a formulation, namely, (1) the formulation has maximum solubility for the permeant in order to accommodate the required therapeutic dose and (2) the formulation should have the minimum solubility for the permeant so as to promote its release from the formulation and partitioning into the stratum corneum. A Relative Polarity Index (RPI) provides a measure of the polarity difference between the permeant and the vehicle. To achieve the first property, the composition of the formulation vehicle (solvent or emollient) is chosen that will provide a low RPI. However, as this has a similar polarity to the permeant, they are mutually soluble, and the escaping tendency of the permeant is low. Therefore, a second solvent or emollient is added to the formulation to adjust the formulation vehicle to the required solubility to solubilize the permeant only to the amount of the required therapeutic dose; then a second vehicle component (solvent or emollient with a large RPI) is added that will reduce the permeant solubility. In 2012, Wiechers published a practical application of the principles of FFE based on his investigation of the *in vitro* human epidermal permeation of four model permeants (testosterone, hydrocortisone, 5-fluorouracil, and ketoconazole) applied in five different formulations (a hydro-alcoholic gel, an o/w emulsion, a w/o emulsion, a microemulsion, and an oil) [43]. He showed that the maximum flux of each permeant was related to its size and polarity and that enhanced permeation fluxes can be achieved by appropriate choice of emollients/solvents in the formulation.

17.5.2 Barrier Modulation by Chemical Permeation Enhancers

The ability of formulation components to alter permeant flux has long been recognized, with extensive research devoted to understanding their mechanism of action and how they can be applied to enhance skin and target delivery. Barry's papers in the early 1990s [44, 45] brought together the large body of research in the area and efficiently described the mechanisms of chemical permeation enhancement, and, together with Williams, their excellent 2004 review [46] remains one of the most highly cited. Dragicevic and Maibach provided a book series devoted to percutaneous permeation enhancers, with their 2015 volume focused entirely on chemical methods [47].

Chemical permeation enhancers can act by a number of mechanisms. The primary mechanisms are those that act by altering stratum corneum lipids and/or proteins and/or affect permeant partitioning behavior, described as the lipid–protein-partitioning theory of skin permeation enhancement [44].

Interaction (disordering/fluidizing) the stratum corneum intercellular lipids: Chemical permeation enhancers disrupt the highly ordered packing arrangements of the intercellular lipids to facilitate permeant diffusion through the primary skin permeation route. The intercellular lipid lamellae are organized into (1) highly ordered, densely packed orthorhombic phase (crystalline; low permeability); (2) ordered, less densely packed hexagonal phase (gel-like; more permeable); and (3) a disordered, liquid phase (highly permeable) [48], as described in Chapter 1. In healthy skin, the orthorhombic phase predominates, and clearly any disruption of this ordered structure will alter percutaneous absorption. Chemical permeation enhancers with lipid chains (e.g., oleic acid, lauric acid, stearic acid, Azone) can insert into the intercellular lipids, with the enhancement efficiency related to the lipid chain length and number of *cis*-double bonds, reflecting the ability to disorder the intercellular lipid structure. Other permeation enhancers that interact with the lipid domains, such as DMSO and terpenes, distort the ordered intercellular lipid packing by associating with the polar head groups of the lipids. Water and surfactants have the potential to cause phase separation within the lipid domains, and solvents such as acetone can cause lipid extraction.

Interaction with the corneocytes: Keratolytic agents, such as urea, act on the corneocytes, possibly reducing the diffusional pathway, or by an indirect influence on the intercellular lipids, or by splitting the desmosomes that act as molecular rivets between the corneocytes. Urea is also a humectant, increasing hydration within the stratum corneum Other agents that have a direct action on keratin within the corneocytes (e.g., DMSO and surfactants) also act on the lipid bilayers, demonstrating the mixed mechanisms that exist.

Altering partitioning between the formulation vehicle and the stratum corneum: Increasing partitioning from the applied formulation vehicle to the skin can be achieved by altering the permeant (e.g., prodrug) or the vehicle to increase the thermodynamic activity of the permeant (e.g., solubility, supersaturation). Administration of a solvent that permeates into the skin can increase the permeant solubility within the stratum corneum, creating a "sink" for partitioning and a reservoir of permeant in the stratum corneum. Ethanol, pyrrolidone, and propylene glycol act in this way, potentially also enhancing the permeation of other enhancers in the formulation to further increase permeant flux. Many semisolid topical formulations contain vegetable oils that are composed of enhancers such as oleic acid, lauric acid, and stearic acid (e.g., olive oil, arachis oil, coconut oil) that when used in conjunction with water, propylene glycol, or Transcutol, can provide synergistic enhancement that leads to high loading of a permeant within the stratum corneum and the potential for sustained or prolonged skin delivery.

17.5.3 HYDRATION

Stratum corneum hydration was first demonstrated to be a major determinant in percutaneous absorption in the 1950s and 1960s by some of the pioneer scientists in percutaneous absorption (including Irvin Blank, Howard Maibach and Robert Scheuplein) [49–52]. Under normal conditions, water makes up 15% to 20% of the dry weight of stratum corneum, but when exposed to occlusion, soaking, or very high humidity, the water content can increase up to 400% of its dry weight [53]. Indeed, water is the safest and most widely chemical permeation enhancer in topical formulations and is likely to be a primary contributor to the effectiveness of highly occlusive products such as ointments and patches through increased drug diffusivity in the stratum corneum.

The exact mechanism of action of water has not been established, but it is likely to alter permeant solubility in the stratum corneum, thereby altering partitioning (release) from the vehicle to the skin. The skin permeation of lipophilic permeants, such as steroids, also benefits from occlusion and increased hydration, suggesting that another mechanism may contribute. It has been proposed that water may influence the tightly packed intercellular lipids, reducing their rigid structure and resulting in an increased rate of skin delivery [54]. The stratum corneum lipid bilayers are known to exist as both rigid (crystalline, orthorhombic) structures and more mobile (gel-like, hexagonal) lipid structures. The increase in the ratio of mobile lipids with hydration [55] suggests that both fluidization of the intercellular lipid bilayers and partitioning modification contribute to the effect of hydration on percutaneous absorption [56].

Hydration can be influenced by several means, including formulation excipients such as humectants (e.g., urea, glycerol, glycols) and those that contribute occlusive properties. Urea, applied as a 10% cream, can increase the water-holding capacity of the stratum corneum by 100% [55, 57] and has been shown to significantly enhance the skin permeability of both lipophilic and hydrophilic permeants [58–60]. Occlusive systems that can increase skin hydration include occlusive dressings (e.g., Tegaderm patches used with the local anesthetic cream EMLA), transdermal patches, ointments, and w/o emulsions [61, 62]. In their review of the literature on the effect of hydration on skin permeation, Roberts et al. [63] found that although hydration was generally positive for skin permeation, there were some cases where there is no apparent relationship between hydration and permeation.

17.5.4 PERMEATION RETARDANTS

Skin is exposed to environmental hazards, different irritants, or toxicants in daily life, some of which can permeate the stratum corneum barrier in toxic amounts to cause a range of problems such as allergies, dermatitis, systemic toxicity, and even death. Physical damage to the skin barrier, such as burns, cuts, etc., and certain skin conditions that weaken the stratum corneum barrier can worsen and complicate the problem. There are many examples of significant toxic consequences following skin exposure of chemicals such as carbon tetrachloride (liver injury) [64]; pesticides such as malathion and related organophosphorus compounds (nerve damage); and warfare agents including Soman, VX and Sarin, which can cause severe toxicity and death following skin contact [65]. Detailed discussion of the range of skin hazards is beyond the scope of this chapter, and the reader is referred to Grandjean's 1990 report for the Commission of the European Communities that considers the many chemicals that are identified skin hazards in different countries [66]. Clearly there is a need for personnel in many industries that utilize these hazardous chemicals to prevent skin absorption and protect against their toxic consequences. A range of strategies are employed to protect the skin from environmental hazards, including protective clothing, gloves, barrier creams, personal and environmental hygiene [67], and the application of percutaneous absorption retardants, the subject of the present section.

In addition, some topical products, such as sunscreens, insect repellents, and skin cleansers, are intended for local effects at or near the skin surface, and their percutaneous absorption is not favorable. Formulations that decrease permeation to deeper regions are therefore desirable. There are also examples where it is desirable to target a specific region, such as the cutaneous nerves in the case of local anesthetics, and limit uptake to the cutaneous blood vessels to enhance and prolong efficacy.

The considerable body of knowledge on skin permeation and the influence of permeant and vehicle characteristics is mostly focused on enhancing skin delivery, but can also be used to limit and retard percutaneous absorption. The ideal physicochemical properties for passive skin delivery (outlined in Section 17.3) can inform how to choose or manipulate a chemical to limit permeation. For example, the molecular weight can be increased by complexation with large molecules such as polymers and dendrimers. Moghimi and Shakerinejad [68] showed significantly decreased permeation flux and lag time of nitroglycerin through rat skin (by two to four times and four times, respectively) when applied with the high-molecular-weight compounds β-cyclodextrin and polyethylene glycol 1540. They attributed the retardation effects of the polymers to reduction of both the diffusion coefficient of nitroglycerin through the skin (possibly due to H-bonding) and its thermodynamic activity in the systems. A similar effect on the flux and lag time of nicotine was shown for different polyethylene glycols and β-cyclodextrin, attributed to either film formation on the skin or complexation with this alkaloid [69]. Other polymers that retard skin permeation include the very hydrophilic and reactive polyanhydride that decreased rat skin permeation of nitrofurazone (by about five times) and nitroglycerin (by about two times), and completely stopped nicotine permeation [70]. The effect on permeation was shown to be affected by the polymer concentration, polymer molecular weight, and type of permeant. Moghimi et al. [71] demonstrated the potential of dendrimers to retard permeation. Generation 5 (G5) polyamidoamine (PAMAM) dendrimer (MW 28800 Da), when applied as either a co-treatment or pretreatment on rat skin, reduced the permeation of furfural (2-furanaldehyde, known to cause contact dermatitis) in a concentration-dependent manner (Figure 17.2). The reduction was attributed to both the chemical interaction between the nucleophilic groups of PAMAM (–NH) and electrophilic group of furfural (COH–) and the physical entrapment of furfural within the dendrimer network.

Another approach is to include chemicals within the formulation that will increase the integrity or reduce the fluidity of the stratum corneum. It has been shown that a chemical that acts as an enhancer can become a retardant, or vice versa, depending upon the vehicle in which it is applied to the skin. For example, Kaushik et al. [72] studied the permeation of the insect repellent diethyl-m-toluamide (DEET) in the presence of laurocapram and iminosulfurane analogues from different

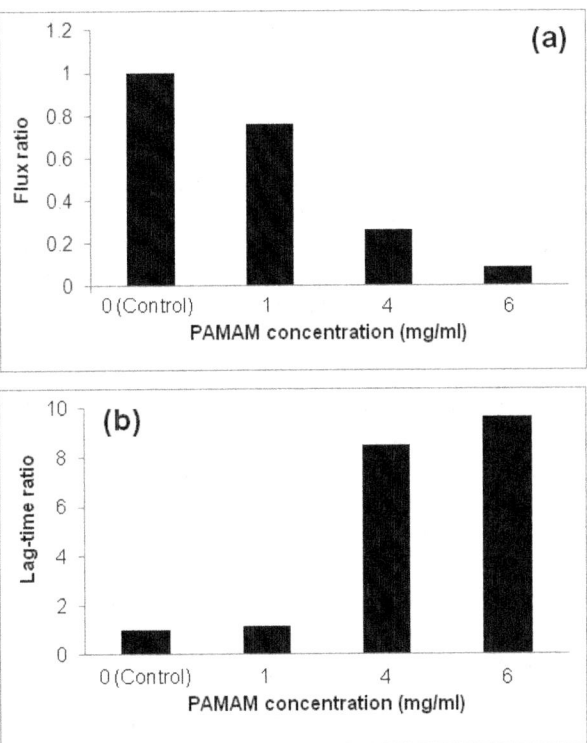

FIGURE 17.2 Retardation effects of PAMAM dendrimer toward permeation of furfural through rat skin, resulting in reduction of flux (a) and elongation of lag time (b). Ratios are PAMAM-treated over untreated values. (Graphs are drawn from raw data published by Moghimi et al. 71.)

solvents. Laurocapram enhanced and retarded DEET permeation in propylene glycol and poly-ethylene glycol 400 (PEG 400), respectively. Dimethyl-N-(2-methoxycarbonyl benzene sulfonyl) iminosulfurane retarded permeation of DEET with ethanol and PEG 400, but not with water or propylene glycol. Mechanistic studies by differential scanning calorimetry and infrared spectros-copy techniques showed that the permeation modifiers that enhanced permeation acted mainly by disruption and fluidization of the lipid bilayers, whereas permeation retardation was mainly through strengthening of the lipid–protein complex and improved organization of the stratum corneum lipids through H-bonding [73].

17.6   FORMULATION COMPOSITION

A typical topical formulation is composed of a number of ingredients that provide a physically stable product with good efficacy, skin feel, and patient acceptance. Common ingredients are:

- Dispersing and/or solubilizing agent (e.g., water, propylene glycol, ethanol)
- Emollient (oil, humectant)
- Emulsifier (most commonly a combination of nonionic surfactants)
- Viscosity modifier (e.g., carbomer, carrageenan, alginates, cellulose derivative)
- Preservatives
- Coloring, fragrance (volatile oils, terpenes)

17.6.1   SOLVENTS AND COSOLVENTS

One of the primary ingredients in a topical formulation is a solubilizing agent, chosen based on the hydrophilic or hydrophobic nature of the permeant. It is common practice to apply the cosolvent method, where two miscible solvents are mixed, to increase solubility in a formulation [10, 74]. For example, the solubility of the lipophilic, active compounds ibuprofen and estradiol in ethanol:water cosolvent mixtures can be increased by 5500-fold and 30-fold relative to their aqueous solubility, respectively, as the amount of ethanol is increased from 0% to 100% [75].

As discussed earlier, many of the solvents and cosolvents used in topical formulations are known to influence the barrier properties of the skin. Ethanol and other small alcohols, such as isopropyl alcohol, are commonly used in topical and personal care formulations (e.g., hydroalcoholic gels) and transdermal patches. They permeate rapidly into the stratum corneum and can enhance the flux of both hydrophilic and lipophilic permeants [76–78]. They are miscible with water and form opti-mal cosolvent mixtures at particular compositions (e.g., around 60% ethanol:water), above which permeation enhancement declines, most likely due to dehydration of the stratum corneum at high alcohol content. At high concentrations, ethanol may extract intercellular lipids.

The fatty alcohol propylene glycol is a colorless and viscous liquid that is commonly used as a cosolvent in topical formulations at 1% to 10% [79, 80]. It acts in a similar way to ethanol but is a milder solvent that is less likely to extract lipids. A binary mixture of propylene glycol:water was shown to provide a linear enhancement in ibuprofen flux across excised skin with increasing pro-pylene glycol content, with the effect attributed primarily to increased solubility and partitioning of ibuprofen [10]. Propylene glycol has also been shown to act synergistically with other enhancers, including Azone, oleic acid, and terpenes.

Grice and colleagues [81] investigated the influence of ternary combinations of ethanol:propylene glycol:water on minoxidil uptake into appendages, stratum corneum, and through human skin *in vitro*, reporting a change in the transport mechanism of minoxidil over time. At early time points (up to 12 hours), formulations containing the highest ethanol:propylene glycol ratio provided higher minoxidil uptake, which was attributed to the evaporation of volatile ethanol leading to increased minoxidil concentrations in the skin. After 12 hours the maximal flux was obtained from the formulation with the lowest ethanol:propylene glycol ratio, which the authors suggested was due to the action of the propylene glycol within the stratum corneum that provided enhanced minoxidil flux.

Vehicle uptake into the membrane can strongly influence skin permeation. We have shown that the maximum flux across human epidermis for a series of 10 similarly sized phenols with a range of lipophilicities was determined by solute solubility in the stratum corneum [82], which was dependent on the amount of vehicle penetrating into the stratum corneum [83]. The maximum flux and stratum corneum solubilities generally increased with the percentage of propylene glycol in the binary propylene glycol:water solvent system (60%, 40%, or 0%) but that the estimated phenol diffusivities appeared to be vehicle independent. The maximum fluxes were related to vehicle-dependent stratum corneum solubilities, which depended on the amount of vehicle absorbed into the stratum corneum and the amount of phenolic compound dissolved in that absorbed vehicle. In a subsequent study, this was extended to include other polar and lipophilic vehicles (mineral oil, isopropyl myristate) [84]. In this case maximum fluxes for the phenols were similar for mineral oil and water. However, for the isopropyl myristate and propylene glycol:water vehicles, the fluxes were higher for the more polar phenols due to a higher diffusivity and higher solubility in the stratum corneum, respectively. Whereas the maximum flux for the phenols was directly related to solubility in the stratum corneum independent of vehicle, increasing phenol lipophilicity increased and decreased the permeability coefficient for aqueous and lipophilic solvents, respectively. The authors also noted that although the maximum fluxes for phenols with a similar molecular size and varying lipophilicity were comparable between water and mineral oil vehicles, they were higher for the isopropyl myristate and propylene:glycol water vehicles.

Attempts have been made to relate vehicle physicochemical properties and flux across the skin, most importantly by the use of solubility parameters (δ), as described earlier in this chapter. Given the importance of formulation vehicle solvents to skin delivery via both diffusivity and membrane partitioning effects, a means of predicting their effect based on the properties of the permeant and vehicle would be very useful.

17.6.2 EMULSIFIERS

Surfactants are included in many topical products to solubilize lipophilic ingredients and stabilize emulsion-based formulations. They are generally composed of a lipophilic fatty chain and a hydrophilic head group, a structure that allows them to lower interfacial tension between oil and water, thus stabilizing one phase as dispersed droplets within the other. Surfactants are categorized according to the ionic nature of their head group: anionic (negative charge), cationic (positive charge), nonionic, or zwitterionic (amphoteric: carry both cationic and anionic moieties). As surfactants are common ingredients in topical formulations, their effect on percutaneous absorption has been extensively studied. Anionic (e.g., sodium lauryl sulphate) and cationic surfactants tend to be an irritant, causing transepidermal water loss and damage to the stratum corneum. They can modify the binding of water, possibly through extraction of natural moisturizing factor and/or stratum corneum lipids, leaving the skin dry and brittle. Nonionic surfactants (e.g., poloxamers [Pluronics, Kolliphor], sorbitan esters [Spans], polysorbates Tweens]) are less irritating and are more widely used, but have low direct permeation enhancement activity, though their presence in a formulation may facilitate solubility and permeation.

17.6.3 VISCOSITY MODIFICATION

Topical products are required to spread easily and smoothly on the skin, with good skin retention. This is achieved through modification of the viscosity, with a wide range of polymers available for the purpose, including carbomers (Carbopol), celluloses, and carrageenan. Incorporating viscosity modifiers in a formulation may hinder drug diffusion from the formulation into the skin, but the evidence is controversial. Although the permeability coefficient of estradiol was significantly reduced when 4% Carbopol 940 was added to thicken the microemulsion [85], addition of the same polymer to thicken a microemulsion containing triptolide did not alter its steady-state flux [86]. It has been suggested that the better contact between thickened microemulsions and the skin surface could aid drug permeation [86, 87]. In examining the skin permeation of the sunscreen oxybenzone, Cross et al. [88] reported that the viscosity of the formulation had different effects depending on the dose applied. Thickening agents retarded skin permeation in a manner consistent with diffusional resistance in the formulation when applied as an infinite dose. However, when applied as a thick, *"in use"* type dose, thickening agents promote permeation. They suggested that the thickened formulation enhanced hydration, which increased the oxybenzone diffusivity in the stratum corneum. Clearly the viscosity of the applied formulation can affect percutaneous absorption by a number of different, and often conflicting, mechanisms.

17.7   ADVANCED FORMULATIONS: VESICLES AND NANOSYSTEMS

Advanced formulation systems used in skin delivery are typically lipid-based and include nanoemulsions (NEs), liposomes or flexible vesicles, nanostructured lipid carriers (NLCs), and solid lipid nanoparticles (SLNs) (Figure 17.3). These nanosystems offer the potential to improve percutaneous absorption, bioavailability, and efficacy; target delivery to specific skin regions and follicles; increase the stability of the permeant in the topical product; and facilitate the formulation of poorly water-soluble compounds.

NEs and microemulsions (MEs) are transparent, monophasic, optically isotropic colloidal dispersions composed of oil, water, surfactant, and cosurfactant with droplet sizes less than 1000 nm and low polydispersity [90]. MEs are thermodynamically stable, whereas NEs are kinetically stable. There is considerable flexibility in their formulation, with a wide choice of components, including the potential to include components with chemical permeation enhancement properties such as terpenes. There is a substantial body of research literature examining these systems and their ability to enhance skin delivery [90]. They have been shown to enhance permeation into the skin because of

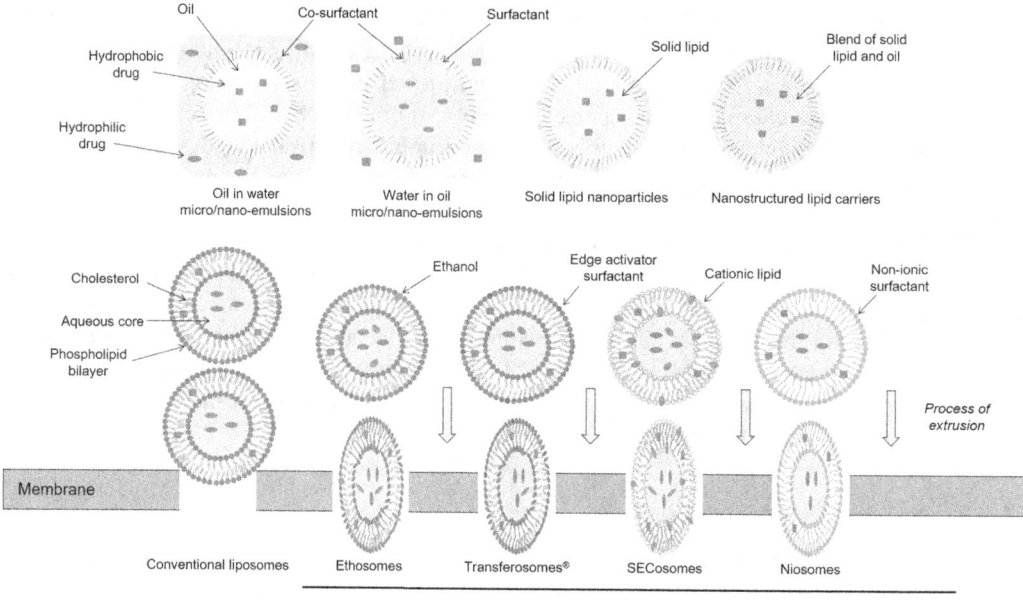

FIGURE 17.3   Nanodelivery systems for topical and transdermal drug delivery. (Adapted with permission from Roberts et al. 89.)

the following: (1) their high solubilization capacity for both lipophilic and hydrophilic compounds provides increased loading capacity and dose application on the skin; (2) their large surface area and good skin contact, coupled with their occlusive nature, ensure surface contact with the stratum corneum; and (3) their oil and surfactant components may have a direct permeation enhancement effect on the stratum corneum lipid structure. We have shown significantly enhanced skin deposition and flux of the lipophilic antioxidant resveratrol with NEs containing terpenes, with the increase in resveratrol flux correlated with increasing lipophilicity of the terpene [91]. The NE containing limonene had the highest resveratrol flux through the skin, whereas the NE containing eugenol showed the highest resveratrol deposition in the stratum corneum and epidermis–dermis–follicle region. We have also examined the increased flux of hydrophilic caffeine and lipophilic naproxen across human epidermis *in vitro* when applied as a NE containing the skin permeation enhancers oleic acid or eucalyptol [27]. There was a modest increase in caffeine solubility within the stratum corneum, showing that the increase in flux was due primarily to the direct effect of the NE excipients on caffeine diffusivity within the stratum corneum. In contrast, increased flux of the lipophilic naproxen was primarily due to NE increased solubility of naproxen in the stratum corneum, with only a modest increase in diffusivity.

Liposomes and vesicles are composed of materials that will aggregate into bilayer structures to form spherical vesicles, with many different compositions explored for skin delivery. Liposomes are generally composed of phospholipid, with or without cholesterol that increases rigidity in the bilayer structure. The first marketed topical liposome product was Pevaryl Lipogel (Cilag AG Switzerland, 1988) containing 1% econazole in a liposomal gel, though the main focus of formulation development since has been on vesicle compositions that provide more flexibility in the vesicle structure to better facilitate skin permeation. Many of these compositions include materials with established permeation enhancement properties, including niosomes (nonionic surfactants) [92, 93], ethosomes (phospholipids with a high proportion of ethanol) [94–96], Transfersomes (phospholipids with the surfactant sodium cholate) [97–100], invasomes (phosphatidylcholine, ethanol, and a mixture of terpene permeation enhancers) [101, 102], SECosomes (surfactant, ethanol, and cholesterol) [103, 104], and a "catch-all" group called permeation enhancer–containing vesicles (PEVs) [105–107]. Multiple mechanisms have been suggested for flexible vesicle enhanced skin permeation: (1) the vesicles disintegrate on the skin surface and their components permeate into the stratum corneum, mixing with and modifying the lipid bilayers to enhance permeation [108, 109]; and (2) Cevc and Gebauer [110] suggested that intact Transfersomes permeate into and through the stratum corneum due to the hydration gradient ($\approx$20% at the skin surface to $\approx$100% at the epidermal–dermal junction), deforming to fit through "pores" within the lipid bilayers to reach the deeper hydrated tissues. The evidence of intact Transfersomes in deep tissues remains controversial, with high-resolution technologies such as multiphoton excitation fluorescence microscopy imaging and cross correlation-raster image correlation spectroscopy (CC-RICS) [111], as well as stimulated emission depletion microscopy (STED) and CC-RICS [108], failing to show evidence of intact vesicles within the skin. These powerful technologies (STED provide image resolution to 20 nm, and CC-RICS allows tracking of two fluorescent probes so that intact vesicles can be resolved) showed that when vesicles and flexible vesicles incorporating sodium cholate (mean diameter 96 nm) were applied to freshly excised human skin for four to eight hours, a large number of vesicles remained at the skin surface, particularly in the skin furrows, with very few intact vesicles in the stratum corneum. Although a smaller proportion of the flexible vesicles remained intact on the skin surface and there was significantly more fluorescent probe in the deeper layers of the stratum corneum, the fluorescent signal was not associated with any vesicle-like shape. The authors concluded that it was the flexible vesicle formulation components that contributed to permeation enhancement and that vesicle permeation reported in earlier studies may have been due to the use of mouse skin with its thinner stratum corneum. Regardless of the mechanism, flexible vesicles have been shown to enhance skin permeation of many compounds, including photosensitizers for topical photodynamic therapy [111], drugs for targeting acne [96, 112], and even siRNA [103, 104].

SLNs and NLCs are colloidal dispersions composed of lipids that are solid (SLN) or liquid (NLC) at room temperature and stabilized as a nanodispersion by a surface covering of surfactant(s) [113]. They increase the solubility and stability of lipophilic compounds such as retinol that are prone to decomposition in the presence of light and oxygen [114] and increase the delivery into the stratum cornuem [115]. The NLC lipids' spatial structure allows greater drug loading and better stability compared to SLN, resulting in greater skin deposition [116–118]. Their mechanism of permeation enhancement is attributed to (1) prolonged contact with the skin surface; (2) their occlusive nature due to formation of a film on the skin surface that combines with the skin lipid film to reduce water loss, thus hydrating the skin [119]; and (3) interaction between the formulation lipids and stratum corneum lipids, facilitating permeation of lipid-soluble compounds [120].

17.8   CONTROLLED/PROLONGED DELIVERY: TRANSDERMAL PATCHES

Whereas most topical formulations (creams, gels, ointments, foams, etc.) are applied to the skin, often with rubbing or massage, for delivery to the skin layers or deeper tissues, transdermal patches are intended to deliver drug via the cutaneous circulation for a systemic effect and may remain in place for a prolonged period of up to seven days. There are three main types of transdermal patches: drug in adhesive, drug in a matrix, and drug in a reservoir, with the latter being the original patch design but largely superseded due to a greater risk of product failure and dose dumping. There are currently about 20 drugs available as transdermal patches used in the management of a wide range of conditions, including angina, hormone replacement, smoking cessation, attention deficit hyperactivity disorder, depression, Alzheimer disease, and Parkinson disease [121]. A detailed history of the development of transdermal patches and their formulation design principles was provided by Pastore and co-authors [121]. Patches benefit from occlusion and may incorporate permeation enhancers such as alcohols, glycols, surfactants, pyrrolidones, and fatty acids that also function to solubilize the drug present. However, as seen from the currently marketed patches, the drugs included are typically potent and have physicochemical properties that make them favorable for percutaneous absorption.

17.9   CONCLUSION

It is clear that the formulation in which a permeant is applied to the skin can profoundly affect the percutaneous absorption of both hydrophilic and lipophilic permeants. Indeed, it is important to note that the wide range of components in a formulation often work in combination to influence skin delivery. This is particularly the case with components that act by different mechanisms; thus, the rational design of a topical formulation must apply this knowledge to optimize a topical formulation for efficacy, stability, cosmetic elegance, and patient acceptance.

REFERENCES

1. Otto, A., et al., *Formulation effects of topical emulsions on transdermal and dermal delivery.* Int J Cosmet Sci, 2009. **31**(1): p. 1–19.
2. Otto, A., et al., *Effect of emulsifiers and their liquid crystalline structures in emulsions on dermal and transdermal delivery of hydroquinone, salicylic acid and octadecenedioic acid.* Skin Pharmacol Physiol, 2010. **23**(5): p. 273–82.
3. Roberts, M.S., et al., *Epidermal permeability-penetrant structure relationships. 1. An analysis of methods of predicting permeation of monofunctional solutes from aqueous solutions.* Int. J. Pharm., 1995(2): p. 219–33.
4. Magnusson, B.M., et al., *Molecular size as the main determinant of solute maximum flux across the skin.* J Invest Dermatol, 2004. **122**(4): p. 993–99.
5. Anderson, B.D., et al., *Heterogeneity effects on permeability-partition coefficient relationships in human stratum corneum.* Pharm Res, 1988. **5**(9): p. 566–73.

6. Wenkers, B.P. and B.C. Lippold, *Prediction of the efficacy of cutaneously applied nonsteroidal anti-inflammatory drugs from a lipophilic vehicle.* Arzneimittelforschung, 2000. **50**(3): p. 275–80.

7. Megwa, S.A., et al., *Ion-pair formation as a strategy to enhance topical delivery of salicylic acid.* J Pharm Pharmacol, 2000. **52**(8): p. 919–28.

8. Megwa, S.A., et al., *Effect of ion pairing with alkylamines on the in-vitro dermal permeation and local tissue disposition of salicylates.* J Pharm Pharmacol, 2000. **52**(8): p. 929–40.

9. Valenta, C., et al., *The dermal delivery of lignocaine: influence of ion pairing.* International Journal of Pharmaceutics, 2000. **197**(1-2): p. 77–85.

10. Watkinson, R.M., et al., *Influence of ethanol on the solubility, ionization and permeation characteristics of ibuprofen in silicone and human skin.* Skin Pharmacol Physiol, 2009. **22**(1): p. 15–21.

11. Kushla, G.P. and J.L. Zatz, *Correlation of water and lidocaine flux enhancement by cationic surfactants in vitro.* J Pharm Sci, 1991. **80**(11): p. 1079–83.

12. Obata, Y., et al., *Effect of ethanol on skin permeation of nonionized and ionized diclofenac.* Int J Pharm, 1993. **89**: p. 191–98.

13. Yalkowsky, S.H., Techniques of Solubilization of Drugs. 1981, New York: Marcel Dekker.

14. Rubino, J.T. and S.H. Yalkowsky, *Cosolvency and cosolvent polarity.* Pharm Res, 1987. **4**(3): p. 220–30.

15. Hildebrand, J.H. and R.L. Scott, *The entropy of nonelectrolytes.* J Chem Phys 1952. **20**(10): p. 1520–1521.

16. Hansen, C.M., The Three Dimensional Solubility Parameter and Solvent Diffusion Coefficient: Their Importance in Surface Coating Formulation. 1967, Copenhagen: Danish Technical Press.

17. Hansen, C.M., Hansen Solubility Parameters: a User's Handbook. 2nd ed. 2007, Boca Raton: CRC Press.

18. Hossin, B., et al., *Application of Hansen Solubility Parameters to predict drug-nail interactions, which can assist the design of nail medicines.* Eur J Pharm Biopharm, 2016. **102**: p. 32–40.

19. Vay, K., et al., *Application of Hansen solubility parameters for understanding and prediction of drug distribution in microspheres.* Int J Pharm, 2011. **416**(1): p. 202–09.

20. Sloan, K.B., et al., *Use of solubility parameters of drug and vehicle to predict flux through skin.* J Invest Dermatol, 1986. **87**(2): p. 244–52.

21. Ursin, C., et al., *Permeability of commercial solvents through living human skin.* Am Ind Hyg Assoc J, 1995. **56**(7): p. 651–60.

22. Hansen, C.M. and B.H. Andersen, *The affinities of organic solvents in biological systems.* Am Ind Hyg Assoc J, 1988. **49**(6): p. 301–88.

23. Abbott, S., *An integrated approach to optimizing skin delivery of cosmetic and pharmaceutical actives.* Int J Cosmet Sci, 2012. **34**(3): p. 217–22.

24. Ezati, N., et al., *Measurement of Hansen solubility parameters of human stratum corneum.* Ir. J. Pharm. Res, 2020. 19(3): p. 572–78.

25. Lee, C.K., et al., *Skin permeation enhancement of tegafur by ethanol/panasate 800 or ethanol/water binary vehicle and combined effect of fatty acids and fatty alcohols.* J Pharm Sci, 1993. **82**(11): p. 1155–59.

26. Lee, P.J., et al., *Evaluation of chemical enhancers in the transdermal delivery of lidocaine.* Int J Pharm, 2006. **308**(1-2): p. 33–39.

27. Abd, E., et al., *Synergistic skin permeation enhancer and nanoemulsion formulations promote the human epidermal permeation of caffeine and naproxen.* J Pharm Sci, 2016. **105**(1): p. 212–20.

28. Kuswahyuning, R., et al., *Formulation effects in percutaneous absorption*, in *Percutaneous Permeation Enhancers*. Chemical Methods in Permeation Enhancement: Drug Manipulation Strategies and Vehicle Effects., N. D'ragicevic and H.I.A. Maibach, K., Editors. 2015, Springer-Verlag: Berlin Heidelberg. p.109–134.

29. Twist, J.N. and J.L. Zatz, *Influence of solvents on paraben permeation through idealized skin model membranes* J Soc Cosmet Chem, 1986. **37**: p. 429–444.

30. Twist, J.N. and J.L. Zatz, *Characterization of solvent enhanced permeation through a skin model membrane.* J Soc Cosmet Chem, 1988. **39**: p. 324.

31. Barry, B.W., et al., *Vapour and liquid diffusion of model penetrants through human skin; correlation with thermodynamic activity.* J Pharm Pharmacol, 1985. **37**(4): p. 226–36.

32. Barry, B.W., et al., *Correlation of thermodynamic activity and vapour diffusion through human skin for the model compound, benzyl alcohol.* J Pharm Pharmacol, 1985. **37**(2): p. 84–90.

33. Megrab, N.A., A.C. Williams, and B.A. Barry, *Oestradiol permeation through human skin and silastic membrane: effects of propylene glycol and supersaturation.* J Control Release, 1995. **36**: p. 277–94.

34. Iervolino, M., et al., *Permeation enhancement of ibuprofen from supersaturated solutions through human skin.* Int J Pharm, 2001. **212**(1): p. 131–41.

35. Pellett, M.A., et al., *Supersaturated solutions evaluated with an in vitro stratum corneum tape stripping technique.* Int J Pharm, 1997. **151**: p. 91–98.
36. Pellett, M.A., et al., *Effect of supersaturation on membrane transport. 2. Piroxicam.* Int J Pharm, 1994. **111**: p. 1–6.
37. Kemken, J., et al., *Influence of supersaturation on the pharmacodynamic effect of bupranolol after dermal administration using microemulsions as vehicle.* Pharm Res, 1992. **9**(4): p. 554–58.
38. Reid, M.L., et al., *Transient drug supersaturation kinetics of beclomethasone dipropionate in rapidly drying films.* Int J Pharm, 2009. **371**(1-2): p. 114–19.
39. Jones, S.A., et al., *Determining degree of saturation after application of transiently supersaturated metered dose aerosols for topical delivery of corticosteroids.* J Pharm Sci, 2009. **98**(2): p. 543–54.
40. Reid, M.L., et al., *Topical corticosteroid delivery into human skin using hydrofluoroalkane metered dose aerosol sprays.* Int J Pharm, 2013. **452**(1-2): p. 157–65.
41. Wiechers, J.W., et al., *Formulating for fast efficacy.* J Cosmet Sci, 2006. **57**(2): p. 191–92.
42. Wiechers, J.W., et al., *Formulating for efficacy.* Int J Cosmet Sci, 2004. **26**(4): p. 173–82.
43. Wiechers, J.W., et al., *Predicting skin permeation of actives from complex cosmetic formulations: an evaluation of inter formulation and inter active effects during formulation optimization for transdermal delivery.* Int J Cosmet Sci, 2012. **34**(6): p. 525–35.
44. Barry, B.W., *Lipid-protein-partitioning theory of skin permeation enhancement.* J Control Rel, 1991. **15**: p. 237–48.
45. Williams, A.C. and B.W. Barry, *Skin absorption enhancers.* Crit Rev Ther Drug Carrier Syst, 1992. **9**(3-4): p. 305–53.
46. Williams, A.C. and B.W. Barry, *Permeation enhancers.* Adv Drug Deliv Rev, 2004. **56**(5): p. 603–18.
47. Dragicevic, N. and H.I. Maibach, Percutaneous Permeation Enhancers, Chemical Methods in Permeation Enhancement; Modification of the Stratum Corneum. 2015, Berlin: Springer-Verlag.
48. van Smeden, J., et al., *The important role of stratum corneum lipids for the cutaneous barrier function.* Biochim Biophys Acta, 2014. **1841**(3): p. 295–313.
49. Blank, I.H., *Factors which influence the water content of the stratum corneum.* J Invest Dermatol, 1952. **18**: p. 433–40.
50. Feldmann, R.J. and H.I. Maibach, *Permeation of 14c hydrocortisone through normal skin: the effect of stripping and occlusion.* Arch Dermatol, 1965. **91**: p. 661–66.
51. Scheuplein, R.J., *Mechanism of percutaneous adsorption. I. Routes of permeation and the influence of solubility.* J Invest Dermatol, 1965. **45**(5): p. 334–46.
52. Blank, I.H., *Further observations on factors which influence the water content of the stratum corneum.* J Invest Dermatol, 1953. **21**(4): p. 259–71.
53. Roberts, M.S., et al., *Skin hydration – A key determinant in topical absorption*, in Dermatologic, Cosmeceutic, and Cosmetic Development K.A. Walters and M.S. Roberts, Editors. 2008, Informa Healthcare: New York. p. 115–2 ACX8
54. Hikima, T. and H. Maibach, *Skin permeation flux and lag-time of steroids across hydrated and dehydrated human skin in vitro.* Biol Pharm Bull, 2006. **29**(11): p. 2270–73.
55. Alber, C., et al., *Effects of water gradients and use of urea on skin ultrastructure evaluated by confocal Raman microspectroscopy.* Biochim Biophys Acta, 2013. **1828**(11): p. 2470–78.
56. Benson, H., *Transdermal drug delivery: permeation enhancement techniques.* Curr Drug Deliv, 2005. **2**(1): p. 23–33.
57. Williams, A.C. and B.W. Barry, *Urea analogues in propylene glycol as permeation enhancers in human skin.* Int J Pharm, 1989. **56**(1): p. 43–50.
58. Kim, C.K., et al., *Effect of fatty acids and urea on the permeation of ketoprofen through rat skin.* Int J Pharm, 1993. **99**(2–3): p. 109–18.
59. Williams, A.C. and B.W. Barry, *Urea analogues in propylene glycol as permeation enhancers in human skin.* Int J Pharm, 1989. **36**: p. 43–50.
60. Feldmann, R.J. and H.I. Maibach, *Percutaneous permeation of hydrocortisone with urea.* Arch Dermatol, 1974. **109**(1): p. 58–59.
61. Barry, B.W., *Novel mechanisms and devices to enable successful transdermal drug delivery.* Eur J Pharm Sci, 2001. **14**(2): p. 101–14.
62. Zhai, H. and H.I. Maibach, *Occlusion vs. skin barrier function.* Skin Res Tech, 2002. **8**(1): p. 1.
63. Roberts, M.S., et al., *Skin hydration - a key determinant in topical absorption*, in Dermatologic, Cosmeceutic, and Cosmetic Development, K.A. Walters and M.S. Roberts, Editors. 2008, Informa Healthcare: New York. p. 115–28.

64. O'Flaherty, E.J., *Absorption, distribution, and elimination of toxic agents*, in Principles of Toxicology: Environmental and Industrial Applications, P.L. Williams, R.C. James, and M.S. Roberts, Editors. 2000, John Wiley and Sons: New York. p. 35–55.

65. Mathur, H.B., et al., *Analysis of pesticide residues in blood samples from villages of Punjab*. Centre of Science and Environment, CSE Report, 2005: p. 10–15.

66. Grandjean, P., Skin Permeation: Hazardous Chemicals at Work. 1990, London: Taylor & Francis.

67. Schalock, P.C. and K.A. Zug, *Protection from occupational allergens*, in Skin Protection: Practical Applications in the Occupational Setting, S. Schliemann and P. Elsner, Editors. 2007, Karger: Basel. p. 58–75.

68. Moghimi, H.R. and A. Shakerinejad, *Retardation effects of β-cyclodextrin and polyethylene glycol on percutaneous absorption of nitroglycerin*, in 6th International Conference on Perspectives in Percutaneous Permeation. 1998: Leiden, The Netherlands.

69. Shakerinejad, A., *Reduction of percutaneous absorption of toxic compounds*, in School of Pharmacy. 1998, Shahid Beheshti Medical University: Tehran, Iran.

70. Erfan, M., et al., Poly(CPP-SA) anhydride as a reactive barrier matrix against percutaneous absorption of toxic chemicals, U.S. Patent, Editor. 2015: USA.

71. Moghimi, H.R., et al., *Reduction of percutaneous absorption of toxic chemicals by dendrimers*. Cutan Ocul Toxicol, 2010. **29**(1): p. 34–40.

72. Kaushik, D., A. Costache, and B. Michniak-Kohn, *Percutaneous permeation modifiers and formulation effects*. Int J Pharm, 2010. **386**(1-2): p. 42–51.

73. Kaushik, D. and B. Michniak-Kohn, *Percutaneous permeation modifiers and formulation effects: thermal and spectral analyses*. AAPS Pharm Sci Tech, 2010. **11**(3): p. 1068–83.

74. Rhee, Y.-S., et al., *Effects of vehicles and enhancers on transdermal delivery of clebopride*. Arch Pharmacal Res, 2007. **30**(9): p. 1155–61.

75. Megrab, N.A., et al., *Oestradiol permeation across human skin, silastic and snake skin membranes: the effects of ethanol/water co-solvent systems*. Int J Pharm, 1995. **116**(1): p. 101–12.

76. Hatanaka, T., et al., *Effect of vehicle on the skin permeability of drugs: polyethylene glycol 400-water and ethanol-water binary solvents*. J Control Release, 1993. **23**(3): p. 247–60.

77. Obata, Y., et al., *Effect of ethanol on skin permeation of nonionized and ionized diclofenac*. Int J Pharm, 1993. **89**(3): p. 191–98.

78. Pershing, L.K., et al., *Mechanism of ethanol-enhanced estradiol permeation across human skin in vivo*. Pharm Res, 1990. **7**(2): p. 170–75.

79. Arellano, A., et al., *Influence of propylene glycol and isopropyl myristate on the in vitro percutaneous permeation of diclofenac sodium from carbopol gels*. Eur J Pharm Sci, 1999. **7**(2): p. 129–35.

80. Nicolazzo, J.A., et al., *Synergistic enhancement of testosterone transdermal delivery*. J Control Release, 2005. **103**(3): p. 577–85.

81. Grice, J.E., et al., *Relative uptake of minoxidil into appendages and stratum corneum and permeation through human skin in vitro*. J Pharm Sci, 2010. **99**(2): p. 712–18.

82. Zhang, Q., et al., *Skin solubility determines maximum transepidermal flux for similar size molecules*. Pharm Res, 2009. **26**(8): p. 1974–85.

83. Zhang, Q., et al., *Maximum transepidermal flux for similar size phenolic compounds is enhanced by solvent uptake into the skin*. J Control Release, 2011. **154**(1): p. 50–57.

84. Zhang, Q., et al., *Effect of vehicles on the maximum transepidermal flux of similar size phenolic compounds*. Pharm Res, 2013. **30**(1): p. 32–40.

85. Peltola, S., et al., *Microemulsions for topical delivery of estradiol*. Int J Pharm, 2003. **254**(2): p. 99–107.

86. Chen, H., et al., *Hydrogel-thickened microemulsion for topical administration of drug molecule at an extremely low concentration*. Int J Pharm, 2007. **341**(1-2): p. 78–84.

87. Valenta, C. and K. Schultz, *Influence of carrageenan on the rheology and skin permeation of microemulsion formulations*. J Control Release, 2004. **95**(2): p. 257–65.

88. Cross, S.E., et al., *Can increasing the viscosity of formulations be used to reduce the human skin permeation of the sunscreen oxybenzone?* J Invest Dermatol, 2001. **117**(1): p. 147–50.

89. Roberts, M.S., et al., *Topical and cutaneous delivery using nanosystems*. J Control Release, 2017. **247**: p. 86–105.

90. Nastiti, C.M.R.R., et al., *Topical nano and microemulsions for skin delivery*. Pharmaceutics, 2017. **9**(4).

91. Nastiti, C., et al., *Novel nanocarriers for targeted topical skin delivery of the antioxidant resveratrol*. Pharmaceutics, 2020. **12**(2).

92. Muzzalupo, R., et al., *A new approach for the evaluation of niosomes as effective transdermal drug delivery systems.* Eur J Pharm Biopharm, 2011. **79**(1): p. 28–35.

93. Manosroi, J., et al., *Potent enhancement of transdermal absorption and stability of human tyrosinase plasmid (pAH7/Tyr) by Tat peptide and an entrapment in elastic cationic niosomes.* Drug Deliv, 2013. **20**(1): p. 10–18.

94. Godin, B. and E. Touitou, *Ethosomes: new prospects in transdermal delivery.* Crit Rev Ther Drug Carrier Syst, 2003. **20**(1): p. 63–102.

95. Das, S.K., et al., *Ethosomes as novel vesicular carrier: an overview of the principle, preparation and its applications.* Curr Drug Deliv, 2018. **15**(6): p. 795–817.

96. Apriani, E.F., et al., *Formulation, characterization, and in vitro testing of azelaic acid ethosome-based cream against Propionibacterium acnes for the treatment of acne.* J Adv Pharm Technol Res, 2019. **10**(2): p. 75–80.

97. Cevc, G., *Transfersomes, liposomes and other lipid suspensions on the skin: permeation enhancement, vesicle permeation, and transdermal drug delivery.* Crit Rev Ther Drug Carrier Syst, 1996. **13**(3-4): p. 257–388.

98. De Marco Almeida, F., et al., *Physicochemical characterization and skin permeation of cationic transfersomes containing the synthetic peptide PnPP-19.* Curr Drug Deliv, 2018. **15**(7): p. 1064–71.

99. Manconi, M., et al., *Nanodesign of new self-assembling core-shell gellan-transfersomes loading baicalin and in vivo evaluation of repair response in skin.* Nanomedicine, 2018. **14**(2): p. 569–79.

100. Garg, V., et al., *Ethosomes and transfersomes: principles, perspectives and practices.* Curr Drug Deliv, 2017. **14**(5): p. 613–33.

101. Dragicevic-Curic, N., et al., *Temoporfin-loaded invasomes: development, characterization and in vitro skin permeation studies.* J Control Release, 2008. **127**(1): p. 59–69.

102. Shah, S.M., et al., *LeciPlex, invasomes, and liposomes: a skin permeation study.* Int J Pharm, 2015. **490**(1-2): p. 391–403.

103. Geusens, B., et al., *Flexible nanosomes (SECosomes) enable efficient siRNA delivery in cultured primary skin cells and in the viable epidermis of ex vivo human skin.* Adv Funct Mater, 2010. **20**(23): p. 4077–90.

104. Bracke, S., et al., *Targeted silencing of DEFB4 in a bioengineered skin-humanized mouse model for psoriasis: development of siRNA SECosome-based novel therapies.* Exp Dermatol, 2014. **23**(3): p. 199–201.

105. Mura, S., et al., *Permeation enhancer-containing vesicles (PEVs) as carriers for cutaneous delivery of minoxidil: in vitro evaluation of drug permeation by infrared spectroscopy.* Pharm Dev Technol, 2013. **18**(6): p. 1339–45.

106. Manconi, M., et al., *Ex vivo skin delivery of diclofenac by transcutol containing liposomes and suggested mechanism of vesicle-skin interaction.* Eur J Pharm Biopharm, 2011. **78**(1): p. 27–35.

107. Manca, M.L., et al., *Glycerosomes: Investigation of role of 1,2-dimyristoyl-sn-glycero-3-phosphatidylcholine (DMPC) on the assembling and skin delivery performances.* Int J Pharm, 2017. **532**(1): p. 401–07.

108. Dreier, J., et al., *Superresolution and fluorescence dynamics evidence reveal that intact liposomes do not cross the human skin barrier.* PLoS One, 2016. **11**(1): p. e0146514.

109. Brewer, J., et al., *Spatially resolved two-color diffusion measurements in human skin applied to transdermal liposome permeation.* J Invest Dermatol, 2013. 133 (5): p. 1260–68.

110. Cevc, G. and D. Gebauer, *Hydration-driven transport of deformable lipid vesicles through fine pores and the skin barrier.* Biophys J, 2003. 84 (2 Pt 1): p. 1010–24.

111. Dragicevic-Curic, N. and A. Fahr, *Liposomes in topical photodynamic therapy.* Expert Opin Drug Deliv, 2012. 9 (8): p. 1015–32.

112. Vasanth, S., et al., *Development and investigation of vitamin C-enriched adapalene-loaded transfersome gel: a collegial approach for the treatment of acne vulgaris.* AAPS Pharm Sci Tech, 2020. 21 (2): p. 61.

113. Muller, R.H., et al., *Solid lipid nanoparticles (SLN) and nanostructured lipid carriers (NLC) in cosmetic and dermatological preparations.* Adv Drug Deliv Rev, 2002. 54 (Suppl 1): p. S131–55.

114. Jenning, V., et al., *Vitamin A loaded solid lipid nanoparticles for topical use: occlusive properties and drug targeting to the upper skin.* Eur J Pharm Biopharm, 2000. 49 (3): p. 211–18.

115. Zhang, Y.T., et al., *An in vitro and in vivo comparison of solid and liquid-oil cores in transdermal aconitine nanocarriers.* J Pharm Sci, 2014. 103 (11): p. 3602–10.

116. Pople, P.V. and K.K. Singh, *Development and evaluation of colloidal modified nanolipid carrier: application to topical delivery of tacrolimus.* Eur J Pharm Biopharm, 2011. 79 (1): p. 82–94.

117. Pople, P.V. and K.K. Singh, *Development and evaluation of colloidal modified nanolipid carrier: application to topical delivery of tacrolimus, Part II–in vivo assessment, drug targeting, efficacy, and safety in treatment for atopic dermatitis.* Eur J Pharm Biopharm, 2013. 84 (1): p. 72–83.

118. Xia, Q., et al., *Nanostructured lipid carriers as novel carrier for sunscreen formulations.* Int J Cosmet Sci, 2007. **29**(6): p. 473–82.

119. Wissing, S.A. and R.H. Muller, *The influence of solid lipid nanoparticles on skin hydration and viscoelasticity–in vivo study.* Eur J Pharm Biopharm, 2003. 56 (1): p. 67–72.

120. Khurana, S., et al., *Preparation and evaluation of solid lipid nanoparticles based nanogel for dermal delivery of meloxicam.* Chem Phys Lipids, 2013. **175-176**: p. 65–72.

121. Pastore, M.N., et al., *Transdermal patches: history, development and pharmacology.* Br J Pharmacol, 2015. **172**(9): p. 2179–209.

18 *In Vitro* Release from Semisolid Dosage Forms
What Is Its Value?

Vinod P. Shah
VPS Consulting, LLC, North Potomac, Maryland

CONTENTS

18.1 INTRODUCTION

A key aspect of any new drug product is its safety and efficacy as demonstrated in controlled clinical trials. The time and expense associated with such trials make them unsuitable as routine quality control methods to reestablish comparability in quality and performance following a change in formulation or method of manufacture. Therefore, in vitro and in vivo surrogate tests are often used to assure that product quality and performance are maintained over time. The focus of this chapter is the application of in vitro release (IVR) approaches in the documentation of the performance of semisolid dosage forms. In vitro approaches, such dissolution, are standard methods used to assess performance characteristics of a solid oral dosage formulation. It has evolved as a critical test method in the field of drug development. In vitro dissolution is used specifically to guide formulation development, monitor manufacturing process, ensure batch-to-batch quality, and possibly predict in vivo performance. When used as a quality control procedure, in vitro dissolution testing can signal an inadvertent change in drug and/or excipient characteristics or in the manufacturing process. Dissolution tests are used to provide a biowaiver for drug products containing highly soluble, highly permeable drug substances with rapid dissolution characteristics (Biopharmaceutics Classification System [BCS]) and for lower-strength dosage forms under certain conditions. Extension of in vitro dissolution methodology to semisolid dosage forms (topical dermatological drug products such as creams, ointments, gels, and lotions) has been the subject of both substantial research efforts and debate. A simple, reliable, reproducible, relevant, and generally acceptable in vitro method to assess drug release from a semisolid dosage form is highly valuable for the same reasons that such methodology has proved valuable in the development, manufacture, and batch-to-batch quality control of solid oral dosage forms. The quality control tests for semisolid dosage forms include identification, assay, strength, quality, purity, potency, homogeneity, viscosity, specific gravity, particle size, microbial limits, and impurity profile. These tests do not provide any information about drug release properties of the product, stability of the product, or effects of manufacturing and processing variables on the performance of the finished dosage form.

18.2 IN VITRO RELEASE TESTING

IVR is one of several methods used to characterize performance characteristics of a finished topical dosage form. Important changes in the characteristics of a drug product or in the thermodynamic properties of the drug substance in the dosage form should be manifested as a difference in drug release. Drug release of semisolid dosage form is theoretically proportional to the square root of time when the drug release from the formulation is rate limiting. A plot of the amount of drug released per unit area (mcg/cm^2) against the square root of time yields a straight line, the slope of which represents the release rate. This release rate measure is formulation specific and can be used to monitor product quality. The IVR methodology for semisolid dosage forms is very well summarized in the Scale-Up and Post-Approval Changes (SUPAC-SS) guidance document of U.S. Food and Drug Administration (FDA) (1). The drug release methodology uses a vertical diffusion cell system (VDC) and is described briefly here.

- *Diffusion cell system*: A static diffusion cell system with a standard open-cap, ground-glass surface with 15-mm-diameter orifice and total diameter of 25 mm.
- *Synthetic membrane*: Appropriate inert, porous, and commercially available synthetic membranes such as polysulfone or cellulose acetate/nitrate mixed ester of appropriate size to fit the diffusion cell diameter (e.g., 25 mm in the preceding case).
- *Receptor medium*: Appropriate receptor medium such as aqueous buffer for water-soluble drugs or a hydroalcoholic medium for sparingly water-soluble drugs or another medium with proper justification.
- *Number of samples*: A minimum of six samples is recommended to determine the release rate (profile) of the topical dermatological product.
- *Sample applications*: About 300 mg of the semisolid preparation is placed uniformly on the membrane and kept occluded to prevent solvent evaporation and compositional changes. This corresponds to an infinite-dose condition.
- *Sampling time*: Multiple sampling times (at least five times) over an appropriate period to generate an adequate release profile and to determine the drug release rate (a six-hour study period with no fewer than five samples, i.e., at 30 minutes and one, two, four, and six hours) are suggested. The sampling times may have to be varied depending on the formulation. An aliquot of the receptor phase is removed at each sampling interval and replaced with fresh aliquot so that the lower surface of the membrane remains in contact with the receptor phase over the experimental period.
- *Sample analysis*: An appropriate validated, specific, and sensitive analytical procedure, generally high-pressure liquid chromatography (HPLC), is used to analyze the samples and to determine the drug concentration and the amount of drug released.
- *IVR rate*: A plot of the amount of drug released per unit membrane area (mcg/cm^2) versus square root of time should yield a straight line. The slope of the line (regression) represents the release rate of the product.

The relationship between drug release and square root of time has been shown to be linear and valid for topical formulations as long as the percentage of drug release is less than 30% of the drug applied in the donor chamber. This relationship holds true for topical formulations with either fully dissolved or suspended drug. An X-intercept typically corresponding to a small fraction of an hour is a normal characteristic of such plots.

18.3 DISCUSSION

When drugs are applied topically, a pharmacologically active agent must be released from its carrier (vehicle) before it can contact the epidermal surface and be available for penetration in the stratum corneum and lower layers of the skin. A topical formulation is a complex drug delivery system, and the dynamics of drug release from a vehicle have been a subject of debate and investigation for many years. A simple and reproducible method, generally applicable to all topical dermatological dosage forms, has been developed to measure in vitro drug release from the dosage form using a VDC and a synthetic membrane, as described in SUPAC-SS guidance (1).

The IVR test is gaining importance as a product performance and quality control test. Scientific workshops on scale-up of a semisolid disperse system (2) and on the value of in vitro drug release (3) have resulted in recommendations on the use of IVR tests as a measure of in-process control and also as a finished product specification for creams, ointments, and gels. In addition, the cited workshop report recommends the use of an IVR test for monitoring product reproducibility during component and compositional changes, manufacturing equipment and process changes, scale-up, and/or transfer to another manufacturing site (2, 3). These recommendations (use of IVR test) are the basis of assuring product sameness after SUPAC (1).

18.4 PRODUCT PERFORMANCE TEST

Following regulatory approval of a drug product by the regulatory authority, e.g., FDA, the product performance test becomes the sole means of directly monitoring the ongoing performance of the dosage form. Two categories of tests are performed with drug products: (1) product quality tests and (2) product performance tests. Product quality tests are intended to assess attributes of the dosage form such as identification, assay (strength), impurities, physicochemical properties, uniformity of dosage units, pH, apparent viscosity, microbial limits, antimicrobial preservative content, antioxidant content, sterility (if applicable), and other tests that may be product specific that are part of a compendial monograph. Product performance tests are designed to assess the performance of the dosage form that in many cases is related to drug release from the finished drug product.

USP General Chapter <1724> provides procedures for determining product performance test/drug release from semisolid dosage forms (4). The product performance tests do not directly measure bioavailability and relative bioavailability (bioequivalence), although they can detect product changes that may correspond to altered in vivo performance of the dosage form. These changes may arise from changes in physicochemical characteristics of the drug substance and/or excipients or to the formulation itself, changes in the manufacturing process, shipping and storage effects, aging effects, and other formulation and/or process factors.

The VDC system is the most common in vitro drug release system. It is a reliable and reproducible means of measuring drug release from semisolid dosage forms. In addition to the VDC system, an immersion cell and modified flow-through cell system can be used to assess drug release from semisolid dosage forms.

18.5 APPLICATIONS OF THE IN VITRO RELEASE TEST

Application of IVR testing in drug development and its value in topical drug products quality assurance was discussed extensively in scientific workshop entitled "Assessment of Value and Applications of In Vitro Testing of Dermatological Drug Products" (3). The report indicates that the IVR methodology is based on sound scientific principles and is of value in assessing product quality. It also indicates that the IVR should not be used to compare fundamentally different types of topical formulations such as creams, ointments, and gels. IVR testing may find a future use as a quality control tool to assure batch-to-batch uniformity, just as the dissolution test is used to assure quality and performance of solid oral dosage forms.

18.5.1 SUPAC-SS

In May 1997, the FDA released a guidance for industry entitled "SUPAC-SS—Nonsterile Semisolid Dosage Forms—Scale-Up and Post-approval Changes: Chemistry, Manufacturing, and Controls; In Vitro Release Testing and In Vivo Bioequivalence Documentation" (1). The guidance relies on IVR testing to assure product sameness between pre-change (approved, reference) product and post-change (SUPAC-related changes, test) product. Release rates are considered similar when the ratio of the median release rate for the post-change (test) product over the median release rate for the pre-change (reference) product is within the 90% confidence interval limits of 75% to 133.33%. The product performance IVR test is used to assess product sameness for the product after SUPAC. The release rate is regarded as a "final quality control" test that can signal possible inequivalence in performance, thus comprising in the aggregate a number of physicochemical tests that might be performed individually.

18.5.2 WAIVERS FOR LOWER STRENGTH

For solid oral dosage forms, biowaivers for generic products are generally granted in situations where the formulations of lower-strength product(s) are proportionately similar and the dissolution profile is also similar [21 CFR 320.22 (d) (2)]. Using these same principles, bioequivalence waivers for lower strengths of topical dermatological drug products might also be granted based on IVR rate measurements. To request a biowaiver for lower strength, the product must meet the following criteria: Formulations of the two strengths should differ only in the concentration of the active ingredient and equivalent amount of the diluent. No differences should exist in manufacturing process and equipment between the two strengths. For a generic application, that is, an abbreviated new drug application (ANDA) the reference listed drug (RLD) should be marketed at both higher and lower strengths. In vitro drug release rate studies should be measured under the same test conditions for all strengths of both the test and RLD products. The IVR rate ratio of the two strengths of reference product and the two strengths of the test product should be similar.

18.5.3 REGULATORY APPLICATION OF IN VITRO DRUG RELEASE

Another important application of IVR testing is the biowaiver for generic drug products. Recently, the FDA released several product-specific draft guidelines for topical drug products that utilize microstructure determination and IVR as a measure of bioequivalence, for example, guidance for acyclovir ointment 5% (5) and for cyclosporine ophthalmic emulsion (6). These developments may result in the use of IVR tests as a routine product performance test for semisolid dosage forms as the dissolution test is for oral dosage forms and may also be used for biowaiver under certain conditions.

18.5.4 TOPICAL DRUG CLASSIFICATION SYSTEM

The Topical Drug Classification System (TCS) is a science-based approach to simplifying the regulatory pathway for topical drugs (7). TCS classification is similar to the well-established BCS. TCS considers the qualitative (Q1) and quantitative (Q2) composition of inactive ingredients between the test (generic) product and reference (brand name) product and the microstructure arrangement with rheological properties (Q3) of topical semisolid products. The IVR reflects the combined effects of several physicochemical characteristics, particle or droplet size, viscosity, the microstructure arrangement of the matter (Q3), and the state of aggregation of the dosage form (1). Based on composition (Q1 and Q2) and IVR similarity, the topical drug products are classified as TCS class 1, 2, 3, or 4. Under the proposed classification, topical drug products under TCS class 1 and TCS class 3 are eligible for biowaiver; topical drug products under TCS class 2 and TCS class 4 are not eligible for biowaiver and will require appropriate in vivo bioequivalence (BE) studies for drug

Topical Drug Classification System - TCS

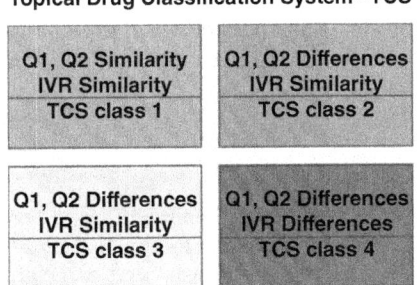

Q1, Q2 Similarity IVR Similarity **TCS class 1**	Q1, Q2 Differences IVR Similarity **TCS class 2**
Q1, Q2 Differences IVR Similarity **TCS class 3**	Q1, Q2 Differences IVR Differences **TCS class 4**

FIGURE 18.1   Topical Drug Classification system (TCS). (Modified from Shah et al. 7.)

- **TCS Class 1:** If the test product is Q1 and Q2 with the reference product and if it meets IVR comparison criteria and the confidence interval identified in SUPAC-SS, a biowaiver can be provided. This corresponds to the definition of Level 1 changes in the SUPAC-SS guidance. There is no reason to expect the generic product to perform differently than the reference product under such a scenario.
- **TCS Class 2:** If the test product is Q1 and Q2 but has different IVR and different Q3 compared to the reference product, then a biowaiver cannot be granted and an appropriate BE study should be required for drug approval.
- **TCS Class 3:** If the test product is not Q1 and Q2 with the reference product, then it necessitates evaluation of the excipients to determine if they are inert or not. Excipients can influence drug penetration and may have an effect on in vivo performance of the product, thereby changing the safety and efficacy profiles. It is likely that different excipients may exhibit similar functional properties. If the excipients are inert and IVR is the same as the reference product and meets the confidence interval criteria, then the dosage form can be provided a biowaiver.
- **TCS Class 4:** If the test product is not Q1 and Q2 with the reference product and the IVR is different, then a biowaiver cannot be granted and an appropriate in vivo study will be required for topical drug product approval.

The TCS concept is shown in Figure 18.1. In all our studies we have found IVR reflects Q3 measurements. There is also a good similarity between BCS and TCS. In both cases, the biowaiver is based on dissolution/IVR comparison (8). In both cases, Class 1 drug products are eligible for biowaiver and Class 3 drug products require additional testing or stricter criteria for biowaiver.

approval. The nature and type of in vivo BE study will depend on the therapeutic class and dosage form category. The TCS simplifies the regulatory requirements for certain classes of drug products and reduces the regulatory burden but maintains the drug product quality. It will make the drug products more affordable to consumers.

18.6   CONCLUSION

IVR rate methodology for topically applied, locally acting drug products is slowly gaining importance in the same manner as the dissolution for the oral dosage forms. It can reflect the combined effect of several physical and chemical parameters, including solubility and particle size of the active ingredient and rheological properties of the dosage form. In most cases, IVR rate is a useful test to assess product sameness between pre-change and post-change semisolid products. The TCS classification can help in reducing regulatory burden and help ease approval of generic drug products.

REFERENCES

1. Guidance for Industry: SUPAC-SS Nonsterile Semisolid Dosage Forms. Scale-Up and Post-approval Changes: Chemistry, Manufacturing, and Controls; In Vitro Release Testing and In Vivo Bioequivalence Documentation. US Department of Health and Human Services, Food and Drug Administration, Center for Drug Evaluation and Research, May 1997.
2. Van Buskirk GA, Shah VP, Adair D, et. al., Workshop report: scale-up of liquid and semisolid disperse systems. Pharm Res 1994; 11:1216–1220.
3. Flynn GL, Shah VP, Tanjarla SN, et. al., Workshop report: assessment of value and applications of in vitro testing of topical dermatological drug products. Pharm Res 1999; 16:1325–1330.
4. USP General Chapters <3>; <1724> and <724>.
5. FDA Draft Guidance on Acyclovir Ointment 0.05%, March 2012.
6. FDA Draft Guidance on Cyclosporine Emulsions/Ophthalmic, June 2013.
7. VP Shah, A Yacobi, FS Radulescu, et. al.. A science based approach to topical drug classification system (TCS). Int J Pharmaceutics 2015; 491:21–25.
8. VP Shah, FS Radulescu, DS Miron, et. al.. Commonality between BCS and TCS. Int J Pharmaceutics 2016; 509:35–40.

19 Understanding Skin Metabolism–Effect on Altering *In Vitro* Skin

Absorption and Bioavailability of Topically Applied Chemicals

Jeffrey J. Yourick and Margaret E.K. Kraeling
Office of Applied Research and Safety Assessment,
Food and Drug Administration, Laurel, Maryland

CONTENTS

Disclaimer: This book chapter reflects the views of the authors and should not be construed to represent FDA's views or policies.

19.1 INTRODUCTION

The skin is the largest organ of the body. The skin can also be considered a barrier from environmental factors, as well as a route of exposure for local and systemic absorption of chemicals. Skin possess the capacity to metabolize chemicals that diffuse through the protective stratum corneum barrier. Ideally, metabolism can be viewed as a protective measure for chemicals that are absorbed to guard against toxins having an adverse systemic effect. However, we must also be cognizant that skin metabolism can transform dermally applied nontoxic chemicals to toxic metabolites that would subsequently be available for systemic absorption (1).

Early studies found that benzo[a]pyrene could be metabolized by mouse skin floating in tissue culture media, which indicated the potential importance of the metabolism of compounds during skin absorption (2). In 1984, a skin permeability chamber was developed to be easy to use, maintain metabolic integrity, and measure penetration (3). This study found that in vitro skin absorption can be affected by metabolism. Therefore, characterization of chemical skin absorption is a function of both skin metabolism and diffusional properties.

Skin has long been known to have a reduced level of metabolic capacity when compared with the liver. Human skin expresses basal levels of messenger RNA (mRNA) for many of the cytochrome

P450 enzymes that are also found in the liver (4). Skin protein expression levels of alcohol dehy-drogenase, aldehyde dehydrogenase, oxidases, hydrolases, carboxylesterase, and glutathione S-transferase were generally fourfold to tenfold lower than in the liver. Skin cytochrome P450 pro-tein levels were nearly 300-fold lower than those measured in liver. This indicates that cytochrome P450 enzymes will minimally affect chemical metabolism during skin absorption (5).

As alternative methods are developed to reduce animal usage for toxicity testing, in vitro human skin and animal skin models are being increasingly utilized for skin absorption and biochemi-cal function studies. It is important to understand how similar in vitro human skin models are to intact human skin for barrier function and metabolic capacity. Understanding the pathways of chemical metabolism and the metabolic capacity of human skin is needed given the increased use of alternative methods. In EpiSkin it was found that 61 phase I and II enzyme mRNA expression levels were similar to the human epidermis (6). There was reduced expression of cytochrome P450s and flavin monooxygenase in EpiSkin, whereas phase II enzyme expression was present at higher background levels. A proteomics method was used to further characterize the profile of chemical metabolizing enzymes in human skin and other in vitro skin models (5). Four in vitro human skin models (EpiDerm, EpiSkin, an in vitro reconstructed human epidermis [RHE], and the HaCaT cell line) have metabolic protein expression profiles that are comparable to enzyme activities found in intact human skin. Furthermore, when the expression of 139 genes related to metabolic enzymes were compared in EpiDerm and intact human skin, it was found that there was an 87% homology of expressed genes (7). Even though there was low expression of cytochrome P450s in both intact human skin and EpiDerm, it is possible to induce cytochrome P450 expression and activity with 3-methylcholanthrene (7). Animal skin metabolic capacity will be discussed further later.

19.2   SKIN VIABILITY

The use and maintenance of viable skin in absorption studies is a requirement for studying metabo-lism of compounds diffusing through skin. In fact, it is stated in the Organisation for Economic Co-operation and Development (OECD) guideline for in vitro skin absorption studies that "if metabolism is being studied, the receptor fluid must support skin viability throughout the experi-ment" (8). Early on it was demonstrated that benzo[a]pyrene mouse skin penetration was increased after induction of epidermal oxidase activity and was reduced using previously frozen skin, which had decreased viability (3).

Several improvements and advances have been developed to better maintain in vitro skin disc viability over the years. For example, pig skin viability was maintained using an oxygenated (95% O_2:5% CO_2) tissue culture medium as the receptor fluid for 50 hours (9). As an indirect way to prove viability, the pig skin discs were removed from the in vitro penetration-evaporation cells after 50 hours and were successfully grafted onto athymic nude mice.

The viability of skin in flow-through diffusion cells was thoroughly examined (10). Skin viability can be determined by measuring lactate found in the receptor fluid as a measure of skin glucose uti-lization. Skin viability can be assessed in this manner throughout the time course of an experiment. Many different tissue culture media or water/solvent mixes have been used by different investigators for receptor fluids. It was shown that a HEPES-buffered Hanks' balanced salt solution (HHBSS) was equivalent to minimal essential media in maintaining skin viability for at least 24 hours after mounting a skin disc in a diffusion cell. Skin viability was also confirmed by examining the cellular ultrastruc-ture by electron microscopy and by the maintenance of estradiol and testosterone skin metabolism.

The use of the 3-[4,5- dimethylthiazol-2yl]-2,5-diphenyltetrazolium bromide (MTT) assay for determining skin viability has been defined. Sometimes it is necessary to add bovine serum albu-min (BSA) to the receptor fluid to enhance chemical partitioning from skin into the receptor fluid. However, the addition of 4% BSA to an HHBSS-based receptor fluid interfered with the lactate assay (11). Therefore, the MTT assay was adapted to assess skin viability during this in vitro absorption study. The viability of human, fuzzy rat, and hairless guinea pig skin was found to be maintained for 24 hours in flow-through diffusion cells. However, a limitation of using the MTT assay is that it is a terminal assay and can only be conducted at the end of a study when the skin disc is removed from the diffusion cell. As previously noted, glucose utilization monitored by lactate formation and measurement can be conducted throughout the course of an experiment.

19.3   SKIN ENZYME LEVELS

Absolute levels of skin metabolic capacity often differ from liver metabolic capacity for specific enzymes and differ across species. Since many different animal species and in vitro skin models are currently being used for penetration/absorption studies, it is important to understand the differences when attempting to promote the use of a specific model as a replacement for intact human skin for dermal safety assessments. There are four detailed reviews pertaining to this subject that compare species and model differences in skin metabolic conversion capacity (1, 12–14). The cytochrome P450 activity in skin is only a small fraction of liver activity. This is true for pig, guinea pig, mouse, rat, and human skin. Therefore, there is less chance for reactive metabolite formation due to cytochromes P450 activity in skin when compared to other non–cytochrome P450 hydrolytic activity and phase II metabolic levels.

When comparing in vitro human skin models, cytochrome P450 activity is still low compared to liver activity (1). The in vitro human skin models are generally similar in cytochrome P450 activity compared with animal skin models. The activity of NADH/NADPH quinone reductase in intact human skin is similar to that of primary human keratinocytes, EpiDerm and EpiSkin. When comparing esterase activity between species, human and pig skin have similar esterase activity, while rat skin has lower esterase activity (1). Other early work found that diethyl malonate was metabolized during skin absorption using pig skin mounted in a penetration cell (15). The almost total metabolism of diethyl malonate was determined to be mainly due to esterases in the skin. Heat treatment of the skin to destroy esterase activity resulted in much more of the parent compound being absorbed unmetabolized through skin.

Comparing phase II conjugating enzyme activity across animal species is difficult due to a lack of data. However, comparison can be made across in vitro human skin models. Phase II conjugating activity is similar in human skin, primary human keratinocytes, and the HaCaT cell line. The activity of glutathione S-transferase was found to be either lower or higher in EpiDerm, EpiSkin, and SkinEthik than in intact human skin but was within tenfold for glutathione S-transferase activity across whole skin and the in vitro human skin models (1).

N-acetyltransferase activity in EpiDerm, EpiSkin, and SkinEthik are either lower or higher than the activity of intact human skin but are generally within twofold to threefold activity when compared with intact human skin (1). N-acetyltransferase activity in whole skin, measured by gene expression levels, is an enzyme where there is many-fold higher activity in skin compared with liver (16).

The use of animal skin or in vitro human skin models (e.g., cell lines or reconstructed models) should have enzymatic activity like that of intact human skin to be a good predictive model for chemical skin absorption. It is important to be cognizant of enzyme activity differences in these animals and models when choosing to use a specific model. Specific chemical toxicity after dermal contact is dependent upon the extent of skin absorption, which is a function of (1) chemical-specific physiochemical properties that influence diffusion properties and (2) the extent of chemical metabolism while diffusing through the skin layers.

19.4   EXAMPLES OF SPECIFIC CHEMICAL SKIN ABSORPTION AND METABOLISM STUDIES

The following skin absorption and metabolism studies were selected as examples to illustrate the types of compounds that are metabolized in skin upon penetration/absorption. In many cases, the metabolites formed from the parent compounds have been identified, and important metabolic reactions in skin have been elucidated.

In early studies, the penetration and metabolism of estradiol and testosterone (10), acetyl ethyl tetramethyl tetralin and butylated hydroxytoluene (17), benzo[a]pyrene and 7-ethoxycoumarin (18), and azo colors (19) were examined by using viable, dermatomed, split-thickness skin discs from mice, rats, hairless guinea pigs, and humans. These early studies will not be discussed here but are noted for the interested reader.

The skin absorption and metabolism of three structurally related compounds—benzoic acid, p-aminobenzoic acid (PABA), and ethyl aminobenzoate (benzocaine)—were measured using hairless guinea pig and human skin in vitro (20). Approximately 7% of absorbed benzoic acid was conjugated with glycine to form hippuric acid. It was found that both benzocaine and PABA were extensively N-acetylated during diffusion through the skin. However, when distilled water was used as the receptor fluid to render the skin nonviable, only minimal N-acetylation of PABA or benzocaine was found.

The extent of metabolism of radiotracer doses of benzocaine in the previous study was compared with the metabolism of much larger doses of benzocaine in formulations simulating exposure from the use of topical benzocaine anesthetic products (21). When a 2 μg/cm^2 dose of benzocaine was applied, approximately 80% of the benzocaine was metabolized by N-acetyltransferase to acetylbenzocaine. As the dose was increased to a therapeutic dose of 200 μg/cm^2, the fraction of benzocaine metabolized by N-acetyltransferase decreased to 34%, which suggested saturation of N-acetyltransferase activity at the higher dose.

Alcohol dehydrogenase and esterase activity were characterized in hairless guinea pig skin using methyl salicylate and benzyl alcohol (22). It was determined that hairless guinea pig skin contains the enzymatic capacity to metabolize esters to alcohols and can oxidize alcohols to acids. The skin absorption and metabolism of retinyl palmitate were determined in vitro using hairless guinea pig and human skin (22). Skin absorption of retinyl palmitate (i.e., an ester of retinol) was characterized as the sum of the amount of penetrated retinyl palmitate in skin plus the amount of retinyl palmitate in receptor fluid within 24 hours. The majority of penetrated radiolabel remained in the skin. All the retinyl palmitate (ester) was hydrolyzed to retinol (alcohol) when receptor fluid fractions were analyzed, but there was no oxidation of the retinol (alcohol) to retinoic acid.

Absorption values from in vitro studies with viable hairless guinea pig skin have been found to compare closely with in vivo results for phenanthrene, pyrene, and benzo[a]pyrene (23). Also, significant metabolism was observed in vitro during the absorption of all three compounds. For example, phenanthrene was metabolized in vitro to 9,10-dihydrodiol, 3,4-dihydrodiol, 1,2-dihydrodiol, and traces of hydroxy phenanthrenes (23). After topical administration of phenanthrene, approximately 7% of the percutaneously absorbed material was metabolized to dihydrodiol metabolites.

Benzo[a]pyrene was found to be metabolically activated during skin absorption studies using hairless guinea pig skin (24). A benzo[a]pyrene metabolite, benzo[a]pyrene 7,8,9,10-tetrahydrotetrol, was measured in diffusion cell receptor fluid fractions. This metabolite is a hydrolysis metabolite of the DNA-reactive carcinogen, benzo[a]pyrene-7,8- dihydrodiol-9,10-epoxide. This is an example of how skin metabolism can metabolically activate a chemical during skin absorption to a toxic metabolite.

The skin absorption and metabolism of trinitrobenzene was examined in human, rat, and hairless guinea pig skin (25). Rapid absorption of nitrobenzene was observed through human and animal skin. The two major metabolites found were 1,3,5-benzene triacetamide and 3,5-dinitroaniline. It appears that nitro groups on trinitrobenzene can be reduced in skin to amino groups, which are sometimes further metabolized by acetylation to an acetamide derivative.

The metabolism of 2-nitro-p-phenylenediamine (2NPPD) absorbed by rat skin and rat intestine was determined in receptor fluid fractions using a high-performance liquid chromatography (HPLC) method (26). More than 50% of the 2NPPD applied to rat skin remained unmetabolized, while only 40% of 2NPPD was unmetabolized by rat intestine. Substantially more acetylation of 2NPPD to N4-acetyl-2NPPD occurred during absorption through the skin. However, triaminobenzene was formed to a greater extent in the intestine. The amount of sulfated 2NPPD and other metabolites was also greater in effluent from intestinal tissue. The extent of metabolism of 2NPPD in human skin (in a semipermanent hair dye vehicle) was also determined. Approximately 60% of the absorbed radiolabeled dose was metabolized to equal amounts of triaminobenzene and N4-acetyl-2NPPD. No sulfated compounds were found in effluents from human skin. Significant differences in 2NPPD metabolism were found during penetration through human and rat skin, as well as differences in metabolism through rat skin and intestinal tissue.

The importance of skin metabolism has been highlighted with the conversion of butoxyethanol by alcohol dehydrogenase and parabens by carboxyesterases (27). Butoxyethanol was converted by alcohol dehydrogenase to butoxyacetic acid in human and rat skin homogenates and subcellular fractions. In cultured HaCaT cells, methylparaben was hydrolyzed by carboxylesterase to p-hydroxybenzoic acid. When paraben esters were applied to skin discs in flow-through cells, little metabolism was found. It was concluded that it is more difficult to observe metabolism in in vitro diffusion cell studies due to the rapid diffusion that limits exposure of the chemicals to metabolic enzymes (27).

Local skin metabolism of penetrated chemicals is also important for adverse biological processes such as allergic contact dermatitis. The potency of contact sensitizers such as trans-cinnamaldehyde and trans-cinnamic alcohol can be altered by metabolic activation or metabolic deactivation. Trans-cinnamaldehyde is detoxified by aldehyde dehydrogenase to cinnamic acid and is further metabolized to cinnamic alcohol by alcohol dehydrogenase. Trans-cinnamic alcohol is metabolically activated to a reactive hapten by skin oxidoreductases. When skin homogenates were further isolated into subcellular fractions, the majority of cinnamic alcohol and cinnamaldehye metabolism was found in the cytosolic fraction (28).

Recently, Géniès et al. (29) compared skin penetration and metabolism across human and pig skin explants for 10 chemicals. Most of the chemicals were metabolized by phase I and phase II pathways in both human and pig skin. However, 3 of the 10 chemicals were not metabolized by human or pig skin. One chemical, caffeine, is metabolized by CYP1A2 in liver slices and microsomes (30) but not by rat skin (17). There is a low level of CYP activity in skin, which may be 300-fold lower than in the liver (5). A species difference was found when examining phase II sulfation pathways in human and pig skin for resorcinol and 4-amino-3-nitrophenol (29). Human skin metabolism has a higher level of sulfated metabolites, while sulfated metabolites in pig skin were limited. Pig tissue is known to have reduced levels of aryl sulfotransferase activity (31).

The skin absorption and metabolism of 7-ethoxycoumarin was investigated using an ex vivo pig ear skin model (32). Skin absorption was followed, as well as the metabolic conversion of ethoxycoumarin by phase I and phase II enzymes. Absorption of 7-ethoxycoumarin into pig ear skin was extensive 48 hours after application. Approximately 25% of the absorbed 7-ethoxycoumarin was initially metabolized to 7-hydroxycourmarin and further converted to glucuronide and sulfated conjugates. This study provides further evidence of pig skin phase I and phase II metabolism during skin absorption.

The use of EpiSkin S9 fractions is suggested as a metabolism screening assay to provide an initial indication of the metabolic stability of a chemical that is topically applied. Chemicals that are not metabolized by EpiSkin S9 fractions can be tested in longer-term incubations with in vitro human explant skin to determine whether a chemical is slowly metabolized or not metabolized at all. These data support the use of EpiSkin S9 fractions as a metabolism screening assay, while in vitro skin explants are more comprehensive and integrate metabolism with cutaneous distribution of the parent compound and metabolites (33).

19.5 CONCLUSION

In vitro and in vivo studies indicate that significant chemical metabolism can occur while a chemical diffuses through the skin. The effect of skin metabolism on the biological response to a parent chemical or one of its metabolites, either local in the skin or after systemic absorption, must be considered for safety. There are species-specific differences in metabolic pathway capacity that must be considered, as pig skin is increasingly being recommended by regulatory agencies and industry worldwide for in vitro skin absorption studies. Specific metabolic pathways in skin, such as cytochrome P450, have relatively low activity when compared with the liver. Pig skin metabolism may not always equate to human skin metabolism. Pig skin (29), human-derived EpiSkin S9 (33) fractions, and other in vitro human skin models have utility for initial chemical screening in a qualitative manner. However, if metabolism is deemed important as it relates to skin absorption, there may not be a completely acceptable skin model substitute for viable intact human skin use in a human safety assessment (29).

REFERENCES

1. Oesch F, Fabian E, Landsiedel R. Xenobiotica-metabolizing enzymes in the skin of rat, mouse, pig, guinea pig, man, and in human skin models. Arch Tox 2018; 92:2411–2456.
2. Smith LH, Holland JM. Interaction between benzo[a]pyrene and mouse skin in organ culture. Toxicology 1981; 21:47–57.
3. Holland JM, Kao JY, Whitaker MJ. A multisample apparatus for kinetic evaluation of skin penetration in vitro: the influence of viability and metabolic status of skin. Toxicol Appl Pharmacol 1984; 72:272–280.
4. Yengi LG, Xiang Q, Pan J, Scatina J, Kao J, Ball SE, Fruncillo R, Ferron G, Wolf CR. Quantitation of cytochrome P450 mRNA levels in human skin. Analytical Biochemistry 2003; 316:103–110.
5. van Eijl S, Zhu Z, Cupitt J, Gierula M, Götz C, Fritsche E, Edwards RJ. Elucidation of xenobiotic metabolism pathways in human skin and human skin models by proteomic profiling. PLoS ONE 2012; 7(7):e41721.
6. Luu-The V, Duche D, Ferraris C, Meunier JR, Leclaire J, Labrie F. Expression profiles of phases 1 and 2 metabolizing enzymes in human skin and the reconstructed skin models Episkin™ and full thickness model from Episkin™. J Steroid Biochem Mol Biol 2009; 116:178–186.
7. Hu T, Khambatta ZS, Hayden PJ, Bolmarcich J, Binder RL, Robinson MK, Carr GJ, Tiesman JP, Jarrold BB, Osborne R, Reichling TD, Nemeth ST, Aardema MJ. Xenobiotic metabolism gene expression in the EpiDerm™ in vitro 3D human epidermis model compared to human skin. Toxicol in Vitro 2010; 24: 1450–1463.
8. OECD. Test No. 428: Skin Absorption: In Vitro Method. OECD Guidelines for the Testing of Chemicals, Section 4, OECD Publishing, Paris, 2004.
9. Hawkins GS, Reifenrath WG. Influence of skin source, penetration cell fluid, and partition coefficient on in vitro skin penetration. J Pharm Sci 1986; 75:378–381.
10. Collier SW, Sheikh NM, Sakr A, Lichtin JL, Stewart RF, Bronaugh RL. Maintenance of skin viability during in vitro percutaneous absorption/metabolism studies. Toxicol Appl Pharmacol 1989; 99:522–533.
11. Hood HL, Bronaugh RL. A comparison of skin viability assays for in vitro skin absorption and metabolism studies. In Vitro Mol Toxicol 1999; 12:3–9.
12. Oesch F, Fabian E, Oesch-Bartlomowicz B, Werner C, Landsiedel R. Drug-metabolizing enzymes in the skin of man, rat, and pig. Drug Metab Rev 2007; 39:659–698.
13. Pyo SM, Maibach HI. Skin metabolism: relevance of skin enzymes for rational drug design. Skin Pharmacol Physiol 2019; 32:283–293.
14. Kazem S, Linssen EC, Gibbs S. Skin metabolism phase I and phase II enzymes in native and reconstructed human skin: a short review. Drug Discov Today 2019; 24(9):1899–1910.
15. Chellquist EM, Reifenrath WG. Distribution and fate of diethyl malonate and diisopropyl fluorophosphate on pig skin in vitro. J Pharm Sci 1988; 77:850–854.
16. Wiegand C, Hewitt NJ, Merk HF, Reisinger K. Dermal xenobiotic metabolism: a comparison between native human skin, four in vitro skin test systems and a liver system. Skin Pharmacol Physiol 2014; 27:263–275.
17. Bronaugh RL, Stewart RF, Storm JE. Extent of cutaneous metabolism during percutaneous absorption of xenobiotics. Toxicol Appl Pharmacol 1989; 99:534–543.
18. Storm JE, Collier SW, Stewart RF, Bronaugh RL. Metabolism of xenobiotics during percutaneous penetration: role of absorption rate and cutaneous enzyme activity. Fund Appl Toxicol 15:132–141, 1990.
19. Collier SW, Storm JE, Bronaugh RL. Reduction of azo dyes during in vitro percutaneous absorption. Toxicol Appl Pharmacol 1993; 118:73–79.

20. Nathan D, Sakr A, Lichtin JL, Bronaugh RL. In vitro skin absorption and metabolism of benzoic acid, p-aminobenzoic acid, and benzocaine in the hairless guinea pig. Pharm Res 1990; 7:1147–1151.
21. Kraeling MEK, Lipicky RJ, Bronaugh RL. Metabolism of benzocaine during percutaneous absorption in the hairless guinea pig: acetylbenzocaine formation and activity. Skin Pharmacol 1996; 9:221–230.
22. Boehnlein J, Sakr A, Lichtin JL, Bronaugh RL. Characterization of esterase and alcohol dehydrogenase activity in skin. Metabolism of retinyl palmitate to retinol (vitamin A) during percutaneous absorption. Pharm Res 1994; 11:1155–1159.
23. Ng KME, Chu I, Bronaugh RL, Franklin CA, Somers DA. Percutaneous absorption/metabolism of phenanthrene in the hairless guinea pig: comparison of *in vitro* and *in vivo* results. Fund Appl Toxicol 1991; 16:517–524.
24. Ng KME, Chu I, Bronaugh RL, Franklin CA, Somers DA. Percutaneous absorption and metabolism of pyrene, benzo[a]pyrene, and di(2-ethylhexyl)phthalate: comparison of *in vitro* and *in vivo* results in the hairless guinea pig. Toxicol Appl Pharmacol 1992; 115:216–223.
25. Kraeling MEK, Reddy G, Bronaugh RL. Percutaneous absorption of trinitrobenzene: animal models of human skin. J Appl Toxicol 1998; 18:387–392.
26. Yourick JJ, Bronaugh RL. Percutaneous penetration and metabolism of 2-nitro-*p*-phenylenediamine in human and fuzzy rat skin. Toxicol Appl Pharmacol 2000; 166:13–23.
27. Williams FM. Potential for metabolism locally in the skin of dermally absorbed compounds. Human Experimental Toxicol 2008; 27: 277–280.
28. Cheung C, Hotchkiss SAM, Pease CKS. Cinnamic compound metabolism in human skin and the role metabolism may play in determining relative sensitisation potency. J Dermatol Sci 2003; 31:9–19.
29. Géniès C, Jamin EL, Debrauwer L, Zalko D, Person EN, Eilstein J, Grégoire S, Schepky A, Lange D, Ellison C, Roe A, Salhi S, Cubberley R, Hewitt NJ, Rothe H, Klaric M, Duplan H, Jacques-Jamin C. Comparison of the metabolism of 10 chemicals in human and pig skin explants. J Appl Toxicol 2018; 39(2):385–397.
30. Berthou F, Ratanasavanh D, Riche C, Picart D, Voirin T, Guillouzo A. Comparison of caffeine metabolism by slices, microsomes and hepatocyte cultures from adult human liver. Xenobiotica 1989; 19(4):401–417.
31. Saengtienchai A, Ikenaka Y, Nakayama SMM, Mizukawa H, Kakehi M, Bortey-Sam N, Darwish WS, Tsubota T, Terasaki M, Poapolathep A, Ishizuka M. Identification of interspecific differences in phase II reactions: determination of metabolites in the urine of 16 mammalian species exposed to environmental pyrene. Environ Toxicol Chem 2014; 33(9):2062–2069.
32. Jacques C, Perdu E, Dorio C, Bacqueville D, Mavon A, Zalko D. Percutaneous absorption and metabolism of [14C]-ethoxycoumarin in a pig ear skin model. Toxicol In Vitro 2010; 24:1426–1434.
33. Géniès C, Jacques-Jamin, C, Duplan H, Rothe H, Ellison C, Cubberley R, Schepky A, Lange D, Klaric M, Hewitt NJ, Grégoire S, Arbey E, Fabre A, Eilstein J. Comparison of the metabolism of 10 cosmetics-relevant chemicals in EpiSkin™ S9 subcellular fractions and *in vitro* human skin explants. J Appl Toxicol 2020; 40(2):313–326.

20 Phenomenon of Lateral Spread in Percutaneous Penetration

Rebecca M. Law
Memorial University of Newfoundland, St. John's,
Newfoundland and Labrador, Canada

Howard I. Maibach
University of California, San Francisco, California

CONTENTS

20.1 INTRODUCTION

Lateral spread, a factor that may affect percutaneous penetration of drugs or chemicals, is sometimes overlooked. For a discussion of many other factors, please refer to Chapter 21 and to Law et al. [1].

20.2 DEFINITION

In simplest terms, lateral spread describes the phenomenon of something flowing out in all directions from an original location and has been used to describe an earthquake's spread from its epicenter with landslide phenomena [2], as well as to describe the depth of freeze in cryotherapy of cancer [3]. From a skin perspective, lateral spread refers to the spreading behavior of a topically applied formulation beyond its original site of application [4]. It is this definition of lateral spread being considered here.

20.3 OTHER TERMINOLOGY

Lateral spread is a competitive process to the drug or chemical penetrating into and through skin. This effect has been quantified [5–7] but has also been an incidental finding in percutaneous penetration research [8]. Other terminology has been used to describe lateral spread, including lateral diffusion [7, 9, 10] and transverse diffusion [11].

20.4 FACTORS AFFECTING LATERAL SPREAD OF DRUGS OR CHEMICALS

Lateral spread may be dependent on the innate spreadability of the drug or chemical, which may vary based on physicochemical factors specific to the drug or chemical. These factors include the drug's pKa, solubility, hydrophilicity, lipophilicity, lipid/water partition coefficient, size, charge, polarity, molecular weight, and possibly others. Research on percutaneous penetration of drugs and chemicals with differing physicochemical properties reflect these differences [7, 8, 12]. Two pivotal studies have found penetration differences between the following drugs and chemicals: Gee et al. [7]—caffeine, hydrocortisone, and ibuprofen—and Feldmann and Maibach [8]—dinitrochlorobenzene, caffeine, benzoic acid, p-aminobenzoic acid, salicylic acid, acetylsalicylic acid, butter yellow, methylcholanthrene, diethyltoluamide, nicotinamide, potassium thiocyanate, malathion, urea, phenol, colchicine, hexachlorophene, chloramphenicol, nitrobenzene, thiourea, nicotinic acid, and hippuric acid.

While Gee et al. also specifically assessed lateral spread and found differences among the three drugs studied [7], Feldmann and Maibach [8] found incomplete absorption for all substances studied and slow penetration for some substances, noting that for most compounds, the surface loss rate must exceed the absorption rate (mostly <50%), implying the influence of other factors such as lateral spread, reservoir in the skin, etc.

Jacobi et al. [6] assessed the lateral spread and local penetration of two ultraviolet (UV) filter substances with different polarity and lipophilicity but similar in molar mass and volume and found identical results for both substances ($R^2 = 0.99$), noting that other factors such as emulsion differences may be at play.

Lateral spread may also be dependent on the formulation of the drug or chemical, including its viscosity, pH, and other excipients present [5, 11, 12]. Viscosity values often differ between types of formulations (ointments, creams, lotions, foams, etc.), and viscosity may differ even between a specific type of formulation, for example, ointments of different bases [5] or oil-in-water emulsions. The spreadability behavior of a formulation on the skin surface must be considered, as this affects lateral spread [13].

Lateral spread is affected by the type and location of the skin as well. Wrinkles and primary furrows produce opposite effects on lateral spread. Primary furrows such as fingerprints can act as conduits for drugs or chemicals, thus enhancing lateral spread [14]. However, wrinkles can act as reservoirs for drugs or chemicals, thus retarding lateral spread. In addition, there may be differences in lateral spread for drugs or chemicals applied to different locations of the body [14]. Hairy versus hairless locations may demonstrate differences, as the hair follicle may be a reservoir for drugs or chemicals [14].

Environmental factors such as heat or humidity may affect lateral spread. Exercise leading to sweating may also affect lateral spread. In addition, there may be numerous other factors that affect lateral spread, such as diseased skin (e.g., dermatitis skin, psoriatic skin) or other medical conditions.

Lateral spread may also occur as drugs or chemicals are penetrating through the stratum corneum to reach deeper layers [15]. However, not much is known about deeper lateral spread occurring in the viable epidermis, dermis, and possibly subcutaneous fat.

20.5   GRAPHIC DEPICTION OF LATERAL SPREAD

A schematic of the lateral spread phenomenon is reproduced here [16] (Figure 20.1).

20.6   SUMMARY

In summary, how might lateral spread affect percutaneous penetration of drugs or chemicals?

1. Lateral spread may result in less drug or chemical being absorbed systemically. This may reduce bioavailability.
2. Lateral spread may reduce the rate of absorption of the drug or chemical. This may prolong the onset of action.
3. Lateral spread may result in less drug or chemical remaining at the original site of application. This may affect the accuracy of quantification studies of the drug's or chemical's penetration into skin.

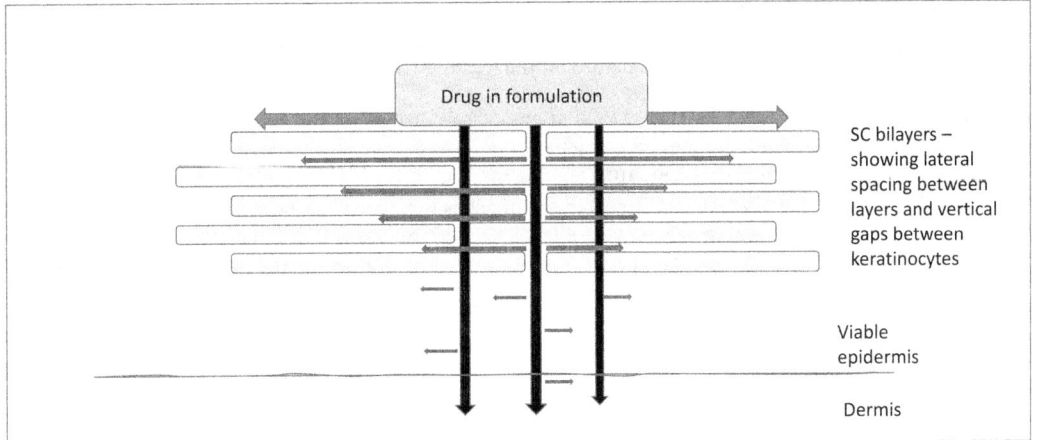

Horizontal arrows = potential pathways of lateral spread (on skin surface and along SC bilayers, possibly
in viable epidermis and dermis)
Vertical arrows = percutaneous penetration (a competitive process)

FIGURE 20.1 Lateral Spread and Percutaneous Penetration after Topical Drug Application. (Reprinted with
permission from Copyright Clearance Center on behalf of Elsevier's *International Journal of Pharmaceutics*:
Law RM and Maibach HI (2020) 588:119765 https://doi.org/10.1016/j.ijpharm.2020.119765 [License ID
1070153-1].)

4. Percutaneous penetration research of drugs or chemicals should incorporate a "correction
   factor" to estimate the effect of lateral spread on the results of quantitation studies.
5. Lateral spread may be a key factor in determining bioequivalence between innovator and
   generic topical formulations.

For a more in-depth discussion of lateral spread, the reader is referred to [16].

REFERENCES

1. Law RM, Ngo M, Maibach HI. Twenty clinically relevant factors/observations for percutaneous absorption in humans. Am J Clin Dermatol 2020;21(1):85–95.
2. Lateral Spread or Flow. Earthquake Glossary. Earthquake Hazards Program. https://earthquake.usgs.
   gov/learn/glossary/?term=lateral%20spread%20or%20flow#:~:text=Lateral%20spread%20or%20
   flow%20are,Photo%20courtesy%20of%20Geomatrix). Accessed June 6, 2020.
3. Torre D. Understanding the relationship between lateral spread of freeze and depth of freeze. J Dermatol
   Surg Oncol 1979;5(1):51–53.
4. Vieille-Petit A, Blickenstaff N, Coman G, et al. Metrics and clinical relevance of percutaneous penetration and lateral spreading. Skin Pharmacol Physiol 2015;28:57–64.
5. Ashworth J, Watson WS, Finlay AY. The lateral spread of clobetasol 17-propionate in the stratum corneum *in vivo*. Br J Dermatol 1988;119:351–358.
6. Jacobi U, Weigmann H-J, Baumann M, et al. Lateral spreading of topically applied UV filter substances
   investigated by tape stripping. Skin Pharmacol Physiol 2004;17(1):17–22.
7. Gee CM, Nicolazzo JA, Watkinson AC, et al. Assessment of the lateral diffusion and penetration of topically applied drugs in humans using a novel concentric tape stripping design. Pharm Res
   2012;29(8):2035–2046.
8. Feldmann RJ, Maibach HI. Absorption of some organic compounds through the skin in man. J Invest
   Dermatol 1970;54:399–404.
9. Schicksnus G, Muller-Goymann CC. Lateral diffusion of ibuprofen in human skin during permeation
   studies. Skin Pharmacol Physiol 2004;17:84–90.

10. Johnson ME, Berk DA, Blankschtein D, et al. Lateral diffusion of small compounds in human stratum corneum and model lipid bilayer systems. Biophysical J 1996;71(5):2656–2668.
11. Lieb WR, Stein WD. Non-stokesian nature of transverse diffusion within human red-cell membranes. J Membrane Biol 1986;92(2):111–119.
12. Gee CM, Watkinson AC, Nicolazzo JA, et al. The effect of formulation excipients on the penetration and lateral diffusion of ibuprofen on and within the stratum corneum following topical application to humans. J Pharm Sci 2014;103:909–919.
13. Gore E, Picard C, Savary G. Complementary approaches to understand the spreading behavior on skin of O/W emulsions containing different emollients. Colloids Surfaces B: Biointerfaces 2020;193:111132.
14. Jacobi U, Schanzer S, Weigmann H-J, et al. Pathways of lateral spreading. Skin Pharmacol Physiol 2011;24:231–237.
15. Johnson ME, Blankschtein D, Langer R. Evaluation of solute permeation through the stratum corneum: Lateral bilayer diffusion as the primary transport mechanism. J Pharm Sci 1997;86(10):1162–1172.
16. Law RM, Maibach Hi. Lateral spread and percutaneous penetration: an overview. Int J Pharm 2020;588:119765.

21 Clinically Pertinent Factors/Observations Affecting Percutaneous Absorption in Humans

Rebecca M. Law
Memorial University of Newfoundland,
St. John's, Newfoundland and Labrador, Canada

Mai A. Ngo
California Department of Toxic Substances Control,
Sacramento, California

Howard I. Maibach
University of California, San Francisco, California

CONTENTS

21.1 INTRODUCTION

Clinicians routinely use the topical route to administer medications with minimal consideration of details: If there is an approved topical formulation, then obviously absorption through the skin should work. But is percutaneous absorption that simple? What factors are involved for a medication—or for that matter, for any chemical—to be percutaneously absorbed? What can enhance or reduce topical absorption? We consider these factors when using the topical administration route as they may affect drug efficacy and/or toxicity and hence patient outcome. A discussion about these factors was recently published in the January 2020 issue of the *American Journal of Clinical Dermatology* [1] and has been updated for this chapter, with permission. What follows is evidence-based; the interested reader is encouraged to access the reference citations for the evidence behind this discussion of skin penetration and absorption (not mucous membranes). In addition, the chapter on lateral spread in this textbook (Chapter 20) provides a detailed discussion of this often -overlooked phenomenon and complements this chapter. Furthermore, other textbooks providing in-depth discussions of percutaneous absorption are available as reference sources. The reader is also referred to the extensive literature on percutaneous penetration enhancers in the five-volume series by Dragicevic and Maibach entitled *Percutaneous Penetration Enhancers: Chemical Methods in Penetration Enhancement* in addition to other chapters in this textbook. (See Further Reading section for details).

21.2 FACTORS IN PERCUTANEOUS ABSORPTION

What questions should we ask when using a topical medication? At least 20 factors should be considered. In 1983, Wester and Maibach [2] suggested a 10-factor guide in percutaneous absorption based on observations from *in vitro* and *in vivo* comparisons; in 2012, Ngo and Maibach [3] expanded this to 15 factors in reference to pesticides; in 2013, Hui and Maibach modified the information based on further *in vitro* research [4, 5]; and in 2017, Li et al. [6] added a discussion of clinical relevance and complexities. In this latest update, factors and observations affecting topical absorption are presented in simple and practical terms, including clinical implications. The questions/headings outlined in Sections 2.1 to 2.20 relate to the *most known* factors/observations for percutaneous absorption (not mucous membranes).

21.2.1 Relevant Physicochemical Properties of the Medication/Chemical

21.2.1.1 Particle Size/Molecular Weight

Smaller molecules are often more easily absorbed; most topical and transdermal medications are less than or around 500 Da in size/molecular weight (MW), with a few exceptions [6]. Li et al. [6] also noted that the MW of most haptens used in the ICDRG International Standard Series of contact allergens are <500 Da, with neomycin being an exception (MW 712 Da). Topical calcineurin inhibitors are efficacious despite larger particle sizes (tacrolimus [Protopic] at MW 822 Da and pimecrolimus [Elidel] at MW 810 Da) [6].

Intracutaneous diffusion and percutaneous absorption become problematic at higher MWs. This was shown in an animal study (male Wistar rats) [7]. Six water-soluble substances with a range of MW from 160 to 39,200 (sodium salicylate [SA, MW 160], sodium calcein [CAL, MW 580], fluorescein isothiocyanate–labeled dextran [FD-4, MW 2,820; FD-10, MW 10,095; FD-20, MW 19,800; FD-40, MW 39,200]) were injected intracutaneously (*in vitro* [excised rat abdominal skin] and *in vivo* [rat abdomen]) versus intravenously (rat jugular vein) to determine apparent diffusion coefficients and bioavailability [7]. Recognizing that rat skin differs from human skin, the *in vitro* study showed SA diffusing most rapidly, and progressively slower diffusion rates were seen as MW increases. Diffusion coefficients ranged from 10^{-4} (SA) to 10^{-5} (FD-40) cm^2/min. *In vivo* studies showed the most rapid elimination rate from the skin for SA and CAL (10% dose remaining after about 60 minutes), followed by FD-4 (10% dose remaining after 180 minutes). For FD-10, FD-20, and FD-40, elimination rates were slow (80% dose of FD-40 still remaining after 8 hours) and bioavailability as per plasma concentrations and area under the curve (AUC) was minimal to nonexistent [7]. Thus, there are *in vivo* animal data corroborating the effect of particle size/MW on percutaneous absorption.

21.2.1.2   Lipophilicity

The outer skin layer (stratum corneum [SC]) are overlapping corneocytes with cell membranes consisting of lipids, with proteins and water. Lipophilic drugs (and lipophilic chemicals) will be more readily absorbed than hydrophilic substances [4, 8]. However, highly lipophilic substances may be less well absorbed than moderately lipophilic compounds.

21.2.1.3   Solubility in Water

It follows from Section 2.1.2 that highly water-soluble drugs and chemicals would penetrate poorly through the SC, sometimes requiring the presence of porin channels for transport through the epithelium. An example is glyphosate, a broad-spectrum herbicide potentially hazardous to humans but is highly water soluble (for both the base and its mono isopropylamine salt used commercially). An *in vivo* study in the rhesus monkey found only 1.5% glyphosate being systemically absorbed over a 12-hour abdomen skin application period and that residual amounts left on the skin could be easily washed off with soap and water or water only [9].

Note that a prewetted i.e. better hydrated SC may affect penetration of substances with high water solubility [4]. This is discussed in Section 2.7.

21.2.1.4   Polarity

Polarity is defined by the distribution of electrical charge over the atoms of a molecule joined by chemical bonding. Although constant, the effect that a drug or chemical's polarity has on percutaneous absorption is potentially altered by many factors. These include type of solution (ethanolic differs from aqueous differs from PEG, etc.), pH of the formulation/environment, and even skin factors. Drugs or chemicals preferentially penetrate in a dissoluted and electrically neutral state; thus formulation plays a big role.

Although one expects the opposite effect to lipophilicity with respect to percutaneous absorption: i.e. the greater the polarity, the less readily the drug or chemical will diffuse through the phospholipid bilayers of the SC, the converse has also been documented [10, 11]. For example, *in vitro* percutaneous penetration of five corticosteroids, using a consistent dose of 25 uL of a 0.1% drug in ethanolic solution, showed *decreasing* penetration correlated with *decreasing* polarity: hydrocortisone (the most polar) > hydrocortisone-17-butyrate = triamcinolone acetonide > clobetasol-17-propionate > clobetasone butyrate (the least polar) [11].

However, in an *in vivo* study of percutaneous application of different corticosteroids in humans and using vasoconstrictor activity as a measure that drug has penetrated through the SC, McKenzie et al. found *increasing* vasoconstrictor activity with *decreasing* polarity, with hydrocortisone acetate (the most polar) being least active and fluocinolone acetonide (much less polar) being the most active [12, 13]. Recognizing that potency differences may play a role, they also found the highest corticosteroid potency with fluocinolone acetonide and the lowest with hydrocortisone acetate [13].

In an effort to eliminate the complex situation of SC penetration (which would also tease out the seemingly opposing effects of potency and polarity, as seen by McKenzie et al.), Sutton et al. [14] used the intradermal injection route instead of topical application and confirmed that intradermal injection is a feasible and practical method for testing corticosteroid potency via vasoconstrictive activity and that taking SC penetration out of the equation made a difference—as they compared their results to McKenzie's [14]. Questions remain about exactly how polarity affects percutaneous penetration and deeper/systemic absorption.

21.2.1.5 pH

The pH of the environment will determine the proportion of drug or chemical that is ionized versus un-ionized. Skin membrane proteins are basic in nature. It is the un-ionized form of a drug or chemical that passes through membranes. Thus, drugs and chemicals which are primarily in their un-ionized form in a basic pH environment will be optimally absorbed. Basic drugs will have a greater proportion in un-ionized form than acidic drugs; therefore, in a basic environment, basic drugs will be absorbed better than acidic drugs. Less ionization leads to increased lipid solubility and passage through membranes [15].

pH can also affect drug or chemical volatility. Salocks et al. [16] demonstrated the role of pH on methamphetamine: (1) increasing the solvent pH above 4 or so changes methamphetamine from a nonvolatile salt to a volatile base, and the higher the solvent pH, the greater the volatility and the less drug remains i.e., there is an inverse parabolic relationship; and (2) when applied to *in vitro* human skin, the amount of methamphetamine evaporated is significantly higher at a skin pH of 7 than at a skin pH of 4 [16]. Volatility is further discussed in Section 2.15.

21.2.1.6 Acid Dissociation Constant (pK$_a$)

The acid dissociation constant (pK$_a$) is a measure of a chemical's acid strength and provides details of the dissociation of an acid in aqueous solution. Since there is a specific pK$_a$ for each substance that relates to pH, knowing the pK$_a$ of a drug becomes a useful predictor of percutaneous drug absorption [15].

21.2.1.7 Partition coefficient (P)

The partition coefficient is the ratio of concentrations of a substance in a mixture of two immiscible phases at equilibrium. This ratio is therefore a measure of the difference in solubility of the substance in these two phases. There are two partition coefficients of relevance to percutaneous absorption: the oil to water partition coefficient (i.e. octanol:water P) and the partition coefficient for cream or ointment to the SC (i.e. formulation:skin P). Hydrophobic drugs or chemicals will have a high octanol:water P and will be mainly distributed to hydrophobic areas such as the lipid bilayers of cell membranes, whereas hydrophilic drugs or chemicals (with low octanol:water Ps) will penetrate SC poorly, and once absorbed systemically, will be mainly distributed to aqueous areas such as serum. The partition coefficient between a cream/ointment and the SC will depend on the product formulation. Thus, knowing the partition coefficients of a drug or chemical, for various immiscible phases, may be a useful predictor of percutaneous drug absorption and/or drug partitioning between biologic systems, which can include solids such as bone (i.e. blood:bone P).

Partitioning can also occur between environmental substances and SC or its components. This is an important consideration for hazardous chemicals found in our environment that may come into contact with human skin. For example, some polycyclic aromatic hydrocarbons (PAH) formed by incomplete combustion of organic materials (such as coal or crude oil processing or forest fires or vehicle exhaust fumes, etc.) may have genotoxic or carcinogenic potential [17]. A study assessing the soil:sebum partition coefficients of high MW PAH, using soil samples collected from former UK gasworks and artificial sebum, found that partitioning varied with the soil type and, not surprisingly, PAH properties (e.g. MW, octanol:carbon P) [17].

21.2.2   Effects of Vehicle/Formulation of the Product on Drug Absorption

Occlusive vehicles often aid absorption by increasing hydration [18]. Water-based vehicles are non-occlusive and are less helpful for topical drug absorption but they allow water-soluble drugs to dissolve in higher concentrations, which may offset the nonocclusive aspect. However, occlusion does not always increase absorption, and this is discussed in Section 2.7.1.

Oil-based vehicles provide occlusion and act as humectants to enhance drug penetration. Thus, for example, a betamethasone dipropionate 0.1% ointment will generally have a greater potency than a betamethasone dipropionate 0.1% cream. (Note that changing salt forms may affect potency—for example, betamethasone dipropionate 0.1% cream is more potent than betamethasone valerate 0.1% cream).

Although alcohol-based or acetone-based vehicles are less occlusive and have a skin-drying effect, they may enhance solubility of some drugs and thereby augment dermal absorption. Zhang et al. [19] assessed *in vitro* SC penetration by benzoic acid (MW 122, Log P1.98) and butenafine HCl (MW 354, Log P 6.6) and compared the vehicles ethanol (EtOH), isopropyl alcohol (IPA), and isopropyl myristate (IPM). Although all three are commonly used as penetration enhancers in formulations, IPA allowed the greatest SC penetration for both benzoic acid and butenafine HCL. Of course, there were significant differences in the penetration amount between the two drugs, reflecting their different physicochemical properties [19].

The pH of the vehicle may alter the un-ionized:ionized drug ratio, thus affecting drug absorption, since it is the un-ionized form of the drug which most efficiently crosses through the skin. Vehicle pH may affect volatility of some drugs or chemicals (as discussed in Section 2.1.5 regarding methamphetamine), hence affecting penetration and absorption [16]. Other excipients (i.e. inactive ingredients) in the vehicle such as surfactants may have been purposely added to enhance solubility and hence drug absorption.

In addition, there are formulations such as transdermal patches and intradermal depot implants that are formulated for prolonged drug release over time; specifics of how they affect percutaneous absorption is beyond the scope of this chapter [20, 21].

21.2.3   Effects of Conditions of Drug Exposure (Dose, Duration, Surface Area, and Frequency of Exposure) on Drug Absorption

Intuitively, greater dose, longer treatment duration, larger surface area of application, and greater frequency of reapplication (once up to three or four times a day) should all increase the amount of drug absorbed, and they generally do. However, although the experimental data remain sparse, with corticosteroids, a high single exposure (hydrocortisone 40 ug/cm^2) substantially increases absorption over one-third of the dose (13.3 ug/cm^2) applied either once or three times in 1 day—there was no statistically significant difference seen with increasing frequency of reapplication [22]. With multiple dosing over many days, there is currently insufficient experimental data to provide a general predictive statement.

In addition, the body surface area (BSA) to body weight (BW) ratio (BSA:BW) is important, as this may affect drug toxicity, since drug doses are usually based on BW (with a few exceptions such as in oncology). In particular, newborns have a BSA:BW ratio at least twice that of adults, so that topical drug doses—even when adjusted for body weight—will still cover a larger percentage of BSA than in adults. Thus, newborns are at greater risk of systemic drug toxicity from topical application of drugs or chemicals. It is partially for this reason that sun protection in newborns less than 6 months of age DOES NOT routinely include the use of sunscreens/sunblocks, even the physical (mineral-based) sunblocks like titanium dioxide. (Recommendations by the American Academy of Pediatrics for sun protection in this population include sun avoidance, using a stroller cover, wearing lightweight clothing that covers the arms and legs, and hats with wide brims that shade the neck. Only when adequate clothing and shade are not available, should parents apply a minimal amount of sunscreen to small areas such as the infant's face and the back of the hands [23].)

Also, note the following: (1) there may be residual drug remaining on and in the skin even if the dose is wiped off, i.e. treatment duration may be unknowingly extended; (2) repeated exposure over time may lead to chronic toxicity manifestations, such as corticosteroid-induced skin atrophy; (3) inadvertent chemical/drug exposure may occur via transfer from one person to another, e.g. a mother wearing sunscreen and holding her infant with bare arms. (This is discussed further in Section 2.14.)

21.2.4 WHAT ROLES DO SKIN APPENDAGES (HAIR FOLLICLES, SEBACEOUS GLANDS, AND APOCRINE AND ECCRINE SWEAT GLANDS) HAVE IN TOPICAL DRUG ABSORPTION?

The answer to the question of whether skin appendages have a role in topical drug absorption is yes, although much of the specifics is unknown. Skin appendages, which originate in the dermis, are subanatomical pathways whereby drugs and chemicals can be transported through the skin. Diffusion of chemicals through skin appendages is termed "shunt diffusion." Hair follicles can contribute to the total skin surface area for drug absorption and have also been shown to be reservoirs for drugs or chemicals.

The SC has a reservoir function for topically applied substances [24–26]. SC concentration of a chemical ultraviolet (UV) filter increased with increasing amounts of UV filter applied *in vivo* to human skin (flexor forearms of four females and one male); however, there was a saturation point where additional increased amounts did not further increase SC concentration, but were recovered as excess [24]. This indicated a storage function for SC which is saturable.

Using nanoparticle distribution studies, Ladermann et al. [25] demonstrated a 10 times longer reservoir storage duration within hair follicles than within the SC, with nanoparticles penetrating deeply into the infundibulum versus nanoparticle storage on the skin surface and in intercellular spaces around the corneocytes in the upper two cell layers of the SC. Nanoparticles were stored for 24 hours in SC versus at least 10 days in hair follicles. However, the amount of nanoparticles in SC were eight times higher than the concentration in hair follicles [25].

Using red marker dye to visualize lateral spread *in vivo* in humans (seven females, five males), Jacobi et al. observed that hair follicles retained dye 1 hour and 24 hours after application, even when the skin had been washed or had been in contact with clothing [26]. Lateral spread is discussed in Section 2.19.

Skin appendages are especially important for the penetration and skin storage of larger molecules (e.g. proteins), as discussed in Section 2.9. Little data exist regarding transport through the eccrine, apocrine, and sebaceous glands.

21.2.5 HOW DO THE SKIN SITES OF APPLICATION AFFECT ABSORPTION?

There is marked regional variability in absorption: absorption rates vary at different anatomical skin sites [20, 27–29]. In general, faster/greater absorption occurs if hair follicles are present in large numbers and somewhat slower if the SC is thick [27].

More specifically, the scrotum has the highest rate of topical absorption due to having both a very thin SC and a rich blood supply. Feldmann and Maibach [27] assessed the percutaneous absorption of hydrocortisone from various skin sites by analyzing urinary excretion of ^{14}C hydrocortisone applied to the forearm (ventral and dorsal), foot arch (plantar), ankle (lateral), palm, back, scalp, axilla, forehead, jaw angle, and scrotum [27]. They found a significantly faster excretion rate and a 42 times greater percentage of the dose excreted in the urine for the dose applied to the scrotum compared to the ventral forearm [27]. Farahmond reported that the scrotum had a fivefold greater permeability to transdermal testosterone than other skin sites [20].

Feldmann and Maibach found the next highest body areas for ^{14}C hydrocortisone absorption were the jaw angle (13 times greater than ventral forearm), the forehead (6 times greater than ventral forearm), axilla, and scalp (3.6 and 3.5 times greater, respectively) [27]. These regional differences may partially relate to skin thickness and the number of cell layers in the SC. Body areas with the lowest topical absorption rates include the palms and soles (plantar foot arch < lateral ankle) [27]. Absorption of ^{14}C hydrocortisone from the back was 1.7 times greater than the ventral forearm [27].

Rougier et al. [28] assessed the *in vivo* penetration of benzoic acid, benzoic acid sodium salt, caffeine, and acetylsalicylic acid in male volunteers and found this general order of skin permeability: forehead > postauricular > abdomen > arm. Roberts et al. [29] assessed cumulative urinary salicylate recovery after topical application of methyl salicylate to different skin sites and found the skin permeability coefficient and percentage of salicylate absorption to be in the rank order of abdomen > forearm > instep > heel > plantar.

Changing the formulation or type of application adds complexity. Maximal plasma drug concentration from transdermal drug patches vary not only with skin sites of application but also with drug physicochemical characteristics (MW, lipophilicity, partition coefficient, etc.) and other interindividual differences [20]. The interested reader is referred to empiric predictive models developed by Farahmand and Maibach [20].

21.2.6   POPULATION VARIABILITY FACTORS AFFECTING TOPICAL ABSORPTION

21.2.6.1   Ethnicity/Pluralistic Societies

Although the skin is approximately equally thick in persons of different pluralistic societies, the SC in blacks has more cell layers and a higher lipid content than in whites [30]. These differences may lead to absorption differences. In addition, blacks and Hispanics have stronger irritant reactions than whites to sodium lauryl sulfate [31, 32], a surface active agent often found in nonmedicated and medicated shampoos. (Note that experimental data in comparing blacks and Hispanic skin are limited, and there are conflicting data. The interested reader can obtain more information from two editions of a textbook detailing these points by Berardesca et al. (See Further Reading section for details.) Skin irritation may lead to inflammation and enhanced absorption of topical agents.

21.2.6.2   Age

Age can significantly affect topical absorption. Aged skin is drier with less skin surface lipids [33]. It is also thinner and more friable—skin aging is associated with progressive dermal atrophy, including atrophy of the skin's capillary network, resulting in a gradual reduction of blood supply to the skin [33]. All of these changes may potentially affect topical absorption. Overall, it paradoxically appears that the *permeability barrier function* of the skin is increased as we age. In particular, percutaneous absorption of less lipophilic substances (e.g. hydrocortisone, benzoic acid, acetylsalicylic acid, caffeine) are reduced, while more lipophilic substances (e.g. testosterone, estradiol) are not [33]. However, increased friability may result in broken skin, resulting in the loss of permeability barrier function and increased percutaneous absorption.

At the other end of the age spectrum i.e. infants and children, topical absorption may be increased. In the preterm baby, the permeability barrier function of the skin is not yet intact. Prenatal skin undergoes developmental stages in utero (including permeability barrier development e.g. proteolipid layer and pilosebaceous units), but some functions are not fully developed even in the neonate [34]. Importantly, the acid mantle is developed in the first 4 weeks after birth, and skin surface pH of both term newborns and premature neonates is less acidic than that of children and adults [35]. Newborn skin has higher permeability to topical agents. Pediatric skin is thinner, potentially allowing for an increase in the rate and amount of drug absorbed. In fact, pediatric and in particular neonatal and infant skins have skin surface conditions different from adult skin surface conditions, which may enhance absorption [36]. However, the dynamic nature of pediatric and especially neonatal skin and their respective skin barrier functions must be appreciated [37, 38] and taken into consideration when assessing percutaneous absorption or toxicity studies.

Skin hydration naturally differs with age. Although at birth the skin surface is rougher and drier compared with older children, within the first 30 days the skin smoothens and skin hydration increases [36, 39]. During the next 3 months, skin hydration continues to increase and then exceeds that found in adults [39–41]—perhaps relating to sweat gland maturation in terms of function [42]. The SC in infants 3 to 12 months of age is significantly more hydrated compared to adult skin [36, 39]. These factors may increase the potential for drug and chemical toxicities in neonates, infants, and children, and this should be kept in mind whenever the topical route is used. For example, increased topical absorption and toxicity have been reported in infants with the use of rubbing alcohol [43, 44]; boric acid powders [45]; and hexachlorophene baths, emulsions, and soaps [46, 47]—thus their use should be minimized. The evidence that rubbing enhances percutaneous penetration has recently been reviewed [48]. The preterm infant may be at even greater risk—even medications that are not normally administered topically due to their physicochemical characteristics may be absorbed enough to be efficacious or cause toxicity. For example, a theophylline gel (17 mg spread over an area 2 cm in diameter) applied to the abdomens of premature infants produced therapeutic serum theophylline concentrations [49].

21.2.7 SKIN SURFACE CONDITIONS AFFECTING TOPICAL DRUG ABSORPTION

21.2.7.1 Hydration

Hydration is crucial (as discussed in Section 2.6.2 with age comparisons). Well-hydrated skin often promotes topical absorption, and it is for this reason that occlusion is often intentional in product formulation, e.g. ointments are often more potent than creams or lotions, also mentioned earlier, since occlusion creates a humectant effect. Formulation or application changes resulting in potency differences should be remembered when prescribing (e.g. clobetasol or hydrocortisone). For example, a tenfold increase in hydrocortisone absorption was seen when occlusion was applied for 24 hours after topical administration [3, 50].

However, an unexpected observation was found when powdered SC was prewetted with water: substances with high water solubility and low oil:water partition coefficient (Log $P_{o/w}$), such as hydrocortisone (Log $P_{o/w}$ 1.61) and malathion (Log $P_{o/w}$ 2.36), partitioned *significantly less well* into the SC ($p < 0.05$). This prewetting effect is negated as Log $P_{o/w}$ increases and/or water solubility decreases [4]. The lipophilic drug acitretin (Log $P_{o/w}$ 6.40) partitioned well into powdered SC, and the SC:water partition coefficient is not altered with SC water prewetting for 30 minutes [4]. Thus, at least into powdered SC, it appeared that penetration of highly water-soluble drugs and chemicals was *reduced* by increased hydration status of the SC but unaffected for highly lipid-soluble drugs. Occlusion also increases hydration status of the SC, and Bucks and Maibach [51] confirmed that occlusion did not always increase percutaneous absorption of several steroids *in vivo* in humans, with hydrocortisone (water soluble) being unaffected.

21.2.7.2 Skin Temperature

Skin temperature also affects topical absorption: an increase in skin temperature—such as a febrile state or sometimes even when a heating pad is present—may increase topical absorption. For example, skin temperature at 40°C increases the transdermal delivery of testosterone and fentanyl [52].

21.2.7.3 Skin pH

The skin pH may affect topical absorption: a less acidic skin pH may enhance absorption. The normal SC is typically acidic and hence favors transport of chemicals and drugs whose pK_a values allow for greater un-ionized forms in an acidic environment. Abnormal SC frequently has higher a pH (i.e. a more basic environment), and this would favor the penetration of chemicals and drugs whose pK_a allows for greater un-ionized forms in a basic environment. Thus, the acid mantle of the intact adult skin (pH 4 to 5) would be an absorption barrier to most basic drugs and some acidic drugs.

Skin pH elevations can occur with occlusion [53] or with a change in the skin microbiome (e.g. caused by prolonged occlusion [53]). Even 1 day of occlusion (with plastic wrap) can cause a 10^4

increase in bacterial count (most significantly with coagulase-negative *Staphylococci*), resulting in a corresponding increase in skin pH [53]. With 4 days of occlusion the skin pH can change from acidic to neutral (4.38 to 7.05) [53].

As discussed earlier, changes in skin pH also affect volatile substances such as methamphetamine [16].

21.2.7.4   Skin Surface Topography

The skin surface topography can also affect topical absorption, since it affects lateral spread of the drug or chemical. (See Section 2.19.)

21.2.8   How Do Skin Health and Skin Integrity Affect Topical Absorption?

Be cognizant that *any skin damage or trauma*—be it mechanical, chemical, biocidal, or clinical disease—may potentially enhance topical absorption [6, 54], and the effects may be more significant for hydrophilic (water-soluble) substances than lipophilic (oil-soluble) substances [54]. These effects are not only demonstrated in *in vivo* human studies measuring penetration through damaged or diseased skin [54], but enhanced absorption has also been shown in *in vitro* studies using human models of damaged or diseased skin [55]. Even mild skin trauma such as adhesive tape stripping (which removes SC layers) may significantly enhance absorption. For example, penciclovir absorption was increased by 1300-fold and acyclovir absorption by 440-fold through tape stripping (to glistening but not broken skin) [56]. Skin compromised by sodium lauryl sulfate (a surfactant) was more permeable to various polyethylene glycols of different molecular weights [57].

Skin diseases (e.g. psoriasis, atopic dermatitis [58]) also compromise skin integrity, and topical drugs and chemicals may be absorbed faster and in greater amounts. There is some complexity, though. For example, in atopic dermatitis (AD) patients, when compared to healthy individuals, increased absorption occurred not only through lesional skin but also through nonlesional skin [58–60]. Although nonlesional AD skin is "normal-appearing," it still responds to petrolatum applied to it by increasing SC thickness, reducing T-cell infiltrates, upregulating antimicrobial peptides, etc. [58]. And both lesional and nonlesional skin of AD patients have higher *Staphylococcus aureus* levels than healthy controls, which correlates with disease severity [61]. However, it is AD patients with clinically active disease who demonstrated increased skin absorption in both lesional and nonlesional skin—patients with clinically inactive disease did not [59, 62, 63]. Furthermore, skin absorption increases significantly with the severity of AD [59, 64, 65].

Practically, this means that topical medications are better absorbed during dermatologic disease flare-ups, thus (1) becoming more effective at that time—a useful phenomenon; (2) being potentially less effective when used as maintenance therapy, especially if intermittent (twice weekly) regimens are used, thus patient monitoring and follow-up during periods of inactive disease would be important; and (3) systemic toxicity from topical medications may be significantly increased during disease flare-ups, especially if higher-potency agents within a class of medications are used (e.g. corticosteroids). Furthermore, absorption of and potential systemic toxicity of *any* chemical touching the skin may be similarly increased during a skin disease flare-up, such as in AD.

21.2.9   How Do Substantivity and Binding to the Different Skin Components Affect Topical Absorption?

Substantivity can be defined as the adherence of chemicals to the SC, i.e. more like adsorption. In practical terms, the substantivity of a sunscreen (as an example) would be that sunscreen's ability to remain effective during prolonged exercise, sweating, or swimming, and this may be a property of the active ingredient, the vehicle, or both. Obviously, the greater the substantivity, the greater the potential efficacy and systemic toxicity of a topical formulation that is meant for local/topical treatment or prevention (e.g. sunscreens, antibacterials, antifungals). Substantivity should be considered in topical dosing strategies and new drug development [66].

Binding can occur to various other skin proteins, lipids, or other substances, which have differing binding sites and chemical affinities [4]. Thus, binding is drug or chemical specific. Binding can significantly affect dermal penetration. Theophylline binding to SC is so substantial that at equilibrium there is more bound than free theophylline in one *in vitro* study [67], confirming that the topical route is less than ideal for theophylline, as systemic therapeutic drug levels must be reached for clinical efficacy. Potential bindings to different skin components (such as eccrine and apocrine sweat glands and hair follicles) are also important to consider, as the bound drug or chemical may serve as a skin reservoir. Further, drugs or chemicals stored in skin reservoirs may be absorbed systemically, potentially causing prolonged pharmacologic effect or toxicity. This is an area of current decontamination research, as bound substances may not be easily washed off or otherwise removed [4, 5]. (Washing is further discussed in Section 2.12.)

21.2.10   How Does Topical Application Result in Systemic Distribution of the Drug or Chemical?

21.2.10.1   Systemic Distribution

Systemic distribution is caused by topical application of a drug or chemical in three ways. First, drugs or chemicals are adsorbed to the superficial skin surface (substantivity being an issue here). Second, drugs or chemicals may penetrate and bind to various skin proteins, lipids, skin appendages, and other substances (binding affinity being an issue here). Third, drugs or chemicals penetrate deeper into the lower dermis, where there is a vascular blood supply, and partition into the bloodstream for systemic circulation [15]. The important issues here are affinity for blood components such as albumin or other plasma proteins (plasma protein binding) and local blood flow [15].

Vasodilatation enhances blood flow and may promote systemic distribution of a topically administered medication. Of note, some medications may have vasodilating properties; for example, transdermal nitroglycerin (NTG, a venodilator) acts within minutes and may be a temporary measure to provide sustained NTG blood concentrations before intravenous (IV) line insertion can be done to administer an IV NTGinfusion.

The converse should also be noted—some medications have vasoconstrictive effects (such as corticosteroids) and may inhibit systemic absorption. In addition to skin surfaces, drugs or chemicals may be applied to (or otherwise be in contact with) mucosal surfaces such as the eyes or nose—the nose has a highly vascular mucosa that almost guarantees systemic absorption.

21.2.10.2   Systemic Toxicity

Thus, there is potential for systemic toxicity from topical administration. As exposure from use of ophthalmic drops is to both the eye and surrounding skin, ophthalmic beta-blockers have caused bronchospasm, congestive heart failure and pulmonary edema, bradyarrhythmias and sinus arrest, central nervous system (CNS) toxicity, impotence, and dyslipidemias [68–70]. Ophthalmic sulfonamides have induced Stevens-Johnson syndrome [71]. Topical corticosteroids have caused systemic side effects, including hypothalamic–pituitary–adrenal (HPA) axis suppression and adrenal insufficiency, Cushing syndrome, and hypertension [68]. Topical salicylates have caused a refractory hypoglycemia [72] by increasing glucose metabolism and reducing gluconeogenesis [68]. Significant systemic absorption of topical salicylates has resulted in systemic salicylate toxicity: tinnitus, hearing loss, blurred vision, sweating, tachypnea, diarrhea, nausea/vomiting, and weakness. [68]. Topical minoxidil 2% applied to the scalp may have caused cardiovascular adverse effects, including palpitations, dizziness, hypotension, tachycardia, paroxysmal atrial fibrillation, and sinus arrhythmia

[68]. There are many other drugs and chemicals applied topically that may have increased systemic toxicity as skin barrier properties change.

Inadvertent systemic toxicity from cosmeceuticals and other products have occurred. For example, phenol can be cardiotoxic: a phenol and croton oil solution used in deep chemical peels caused cardiac arrhythmias, including atrial and ventricular tachycardia, premature ventricular beats, and bigeminy; people with diabetes mellitus, hypertension, and depression may be at higher risk [68]. There is also concern about mercury-containing skin care products (such as skin-lightening creams and soaps, local antiseptics, etc.), and their potential to cause neurotoxicity or nephrotoxicity with enough systemic absorption [68]. Arsenic is another toxic metal that is used (or is a contaminant) in cosmetics, medications, pigments, and natural health products that when applied onto skin over time or in sufficient amounts can result in systemic toxicity effects, including psychoses, seizures, multiorgan failure and death [68]. Be cognizant that *any* drug or chemical that touches the skin has the potential for percutaneous absorption that may result in systemic distribution and possible systemic toxicity.

21.2.11   Does Exfoliation Affect Topical Absorption?

Exfoliation is part of a natural skin cell renewal process: keratinocytes begin as boxlike basal cells at the base of the epidermis, then migrate up towards the skin surface, flattening out to become a layer of overlapping corneocytes which have no nuclei—thus termed dead skin cells—which are then "sloughed off" i.e. exfoliated. Drugs or chemicals bound to skin cells could either be lost by the exfoliation process or be absorbed deeper into the dermis; thus, exfoliation can affect drug bioavailability after topical administration. Urea, which is minimally absorbed topically, can be used as an exfoliation marker [73].

21.2.12   Does Washing Affect Topical Absorption?

There are two opposing wash effects that can affect topical absorption of drugs and chemicals. Loss by exfoliation can be enhanced by washing [3] even hours after application [73] if there is drug remaining in the SC, and this would be a "*washing-off*" effect. Note that for highly lipid-soluble drugs or chemicals (e.g. pesticides), washing with soap and water may not be sufficiently effective in removing them [74].

In fact, the opposite may happen: washing the site of application in between doses may actually enhance topical absorption/penetration, and this would be a "*wash-in*" effect [75–77]. (See also Section 2.13.) Be aware that washing may promote drug or chemical penetrance through the skin, leading to toxicity, e.g. with insect repellents [75–77]. Care should be taken when insect repellents are used, especially in children. The U.S. Environmental Protection Agency (EPA) recommends that instructions on the label be followed [6] for insect repellent products, and they should be used according to the time of day when mosquitoes are most active, which may vary for the species and type of diseases transmitted [6]. Care should also be taken in the work environment if there is occupational exposure to chemicals: workers should be counseled to wear protective clothing and use protective equipment and be warned about the "wash-in" phenomenon [6]. They should be aware that the mechanical friction from handwashing may increase percutaneous absorption, in particular of inorganic compounds [75].

21.2.13   Does Rubbing or Massaging Affect Topical Absorption?

There are two important concepts regarding whether rubbing or massaging affect topical absorption: *rub enhancement* and *rub resistance,* both of which occur with rubbing/massaging. One example of rub enhancement relates to sunscreen application and washing: the mechanical stress of skin washing can massage the sunscreen deeper into the hair follicle [78], and this washing/massaging may enhance transfollicular sunscreen absorption [75]. Massaging may also increase the follicular penetration depth of liposomes used as drug carriers [79, 80]. Massaging/rubbing reduces skin barrier function to facilitate penetration [80]. However, this effect differs between hydrophilic and lipophilic substances—lipophilic/organic substances are less affected, if at all.

With regard to rub resistance, this is a term used to describe whether a substance applied topically will still be effective after being rubbed with a textile (clothing, towel, etc.). Rub resistance would be an important factor for a sunscreen or a topical medication to possess, and a Rub Resistance Factor (RRF) can be calculated to allow comparisons between products of the same class (e.g. sunscreens) [81]. Parameters that influence RRF include rubbing pressure, rubbing duration, rubbing speed, and the textile (composition, thickness, etc.) [81]. Obviously, the higher the RRF, the greater the amount of drug or chemical remaining on the skin and the greater the likelihood for percutaneous absorption.

21.2.14   CAN MEDICATIONS OR CHEMICALS BE TRANSFERRED FROM ONE PERSON TO ANOTHER THROUGH SKIN CONTACT, CLOTHING, OR CONTACT WITH AN INANIMATE SURFACE?

As briefly mentioned in Section 2.3, inadvertent drug or chemical exposure can occur via transfer from one person to another—such as a mother wearing sunscreen and holding her baby with bare arms. Drug transfer can sometimes have serious consequences: a father who used testosterone cream without routine handwashing after application transferred enough testosterone over time to his infant son to cause precocious puberty—pronounced virilization in a two-year-old boy [82]. The skin-to-skin contact time need not be lengthy: a controlled 15-minute ventral forearm–to–ventral forearm rub/contact time transferred sufficient estradiol from donor volunteers to recipient volunteers for estradiol to be detected in the recipients' urine [83]. There was also enough estradiol left on the sleeve of the donors for the possibility of transfer from clothing to occur [83]. Using a hair follicle drug screening test, a Department of Health and Human Services study detected methamphetamine in newborns and young children—postulating that "sweat glands glom onto meth which can then be transferred through skin-to-skin contact, like coddling an infant" [84]. However, besides sweat, other possibilities were children picking it up "from the environment, from the smoke or residue" [84]. Methamphetamine can be readily transferred to skin from inanimate objects such as vinyl tile even with very brief contact times (5 seconds and 5 minutes) [85]. Other examples include additional controlled studies confirming that skin-to-skin drug transfers exist [86, 87]. Skin-to-skin transfer can also occur in the same individual [87].

Practically, what does this mean? Anytime that a topical medication or chemical substance is used, we should be aware that transfer may occur from one person to another, including to infants who may be at greater risk of systemic toxicity, unless the substance is inert. Obviously, the other factors of percutaneous absorption would also apply to the transferred drug or chemical, and those factors would ultimately determine the clinical significance of the drug or chemical transfer.

21.2.15   HOW IS TOPICAL ABSORPTION AFFECTED IF A DRUG OR CHEMICAL IS VOLATILE?

Volatility means that a substance has the ability to spontaneously vaporize into the air, or, in the case of a topical agent applied on skin, to evaporate from skin over time. Medications or chemicals applied to skin are often in product formulations that are a mixture of active and inactive ingredients, some of which may be volatile and others are not. For volatile substances, the degree of volatility may vary from substance to substance and may be affected by other factors such as formulation (pH etc.), environment (humidity, temperature, etc.), and skin characteristics (pH, hydration, skin temperature, etc.). Some substances may be volatile only when certain conditions are met. As discussed in Section 2.1.5, methamphetamine HCl (a basic drug with a pK_a of 9.9) in aqueous solution can change from a nonvolatile salt to a volatile-free base when the pH of the solution exceeds 4 or 5 [16].

What implications does volatility of a drug or chemical have on percutaneous absorption? Important issues include the following:

1. For a multiingredient product, the contents of what is left behind may alter the function of the applied product, which may have implications for efficacy and safety [88].
2. If the vehicle and not the active ingredient is volatile, over time there will be a concentrating effect as more and more of the vehicle evaporates, potentially increasing the potency and/or toxicity of the active ingredient. This is important, as volatile solvents are commonly used in drug and other formulations (cosmetic, patch test [89], etc.), for example, an acetone-based benzoyl peroxide product or an acetone-based patch test chemical [89].
3. Skin patch testing detects contact irritants and allergens, and volatility can lead to false positives and false negatives, with test vehicle evaporation leading to too high a test chemical concentration causing a false-positive result [89] and test chemical evaporation leading to too low a test chemical concentration, causing a false-negative result [89, 90]. For example, fragrance chemicals are usually volatile substances and are common contact allergens often patch-tested as "Fragrance mix 1" and "Fragrance mix 2." A study of two radiolabeled fragrance chemicals (geraniol and citronellol) detected that, due to evaporation, within 40 minutes geraniol lost up to 39% of its dose and citronellol up to 26% of its dose [90].
4. Rapid volatilization reduces the dose and prevents oversaturation of skin's absorptive capacity. This allows for a direct relationship between dose and percutaneous absorption for volatile substances that is calculable (i.e. predictable). Two equations have been developed to correlate the relationship between volatilization and absorption for a small dose vs. a large dose [91]. These equations may be useful in assessing the risk of topical products and their pharmacokinetics, pharmacodynamics, and toxicities. An in-depth discussion of these equations is beyond the scope of this paper, and the interested reader should review the reference indicated [91].

Volatility is important in other ways. Mosquito repellents depend on volatility for their effects, and volatility remains a limiting efficacy factor (i.e. in providing sufficient biting protection from mosquitos). Traditional contact repellents such as *N,N*-diethyl-*meta*-toluamide (DEET) applied on human skin require frequent reapplication and may carry a risk of systemic absorption [92]. However, spatial repellents may prevent mosquito entry into particular areas or into a home and may be particularly useful in areas endemic to mosquito-borne disease [92]. For example, metofluthrin-impregnated latticework plastic strips were capable of preventing the resting of *Aedes aegypti* (L.) within residences in Vietnam for a minimum of 8 weeks after they were introduced [92, 93].

21.2.16 DOES METABOLIC TRANSFORMATION OCCUR DURING TOPICAL ABSORPTION AND, IF SO, HOW AND WHAT? DOES CUTANEOUS METABOLISM OCCUR?

Depending on the drug or chemical, metabolic transformation can occur in skin prior to systemic absorption, since there are metabolizing enzymes in skin. Both phase I (e.g. CYP450 enzymes) and phase II (e.g. N-acetyltransferase) enzymes have been found in skin—with the messenger RNA (mRNA) and protein being detected more often than the quantified enzyme activity (being much lower than in the liver and often at the limit of detection) [94]. Sometimes, UV light is required for transformation (see Section 2.17).

Biotransformation changes the drug or chemical. This change can be in the drug's physicochemical properties or in its pharmacodynamic activity, or it may be both. This can result in (1) the active agent becoming inactive (a degradation process); (2) the inactive agent becoming active (an activation process for a pro-drug); or (3) a lipophilic agent becoming more water soluble (via various metabolic pathways e.g. oxidation, hydroxylation, acetylation, etc.). These changes can affect the drug's penetration through skin.

For example, highly lipophilic compounds, often large, do not penetrate through skin well (a good thing). However, the highly lipophilic preservative butylparaben (one example) can be metabolized to p-hydroxybenzoic acid in skin—this metabolite is less lipophilic and thus more readily penetrates through skin [3, 95]. Cutaneous metabolism of endogenous substrates such as vitamin A and vitamin D also occurs [3].

There are many examples of cutaneous steroid metabolism. The sex steroid hormones testosterone, estradiol, and progesterone are all metabolized by skin, as is dehydroepiandrosterone and hydrocortisone [2]. Skin contains the enzymatic processes for not only steroid biotransformation but also for elimination of polar materials via sulfate conjugation [2].

21.2.17 DOES PHOTOCHEMICAL TRANSFORMATION OCCUR DURING TOPICAL ABSORPTION AND IF SO, HOW AND WHAT?

Similarly to Section 2.16, the effect of UV light on a drug or chemical applied to the skin can cause a photochemical transformation (degradation or activation, etc.) In particular, photochemical changes to a drug or chemical can induce a phototoxic or photoallergic reaction.

A *phototoxic* reaction is caused by a drug or chemical absorbing UVA and causing direct damage to sun-exposed skin, whereas a *photoallergic* reaction requires the drug or chemical to be changed by UVA into an allergen—with skin damage occasionally spreading beyond the sun-exposed skin areas.

Photosensitivity—an adverse cutaneous response to normally harmless doses of UV radiation—is a property related to the drug chemistry and can be seen with topical or systemic administration. Examples of phototoxic agents include amiodarone, tetracyclines (e.g. doxycycline), coal tar, psoralens, and sulfonamides. Examples of photoallergic agents include sulfonamides, sulfonylureas, thiazides, chloroquine, carbamazepine, etc. Practically, if a drug or chemical is known to cause photosensitivity, sun protection is recommended if used during the day; application/dosing at night rather than in more sunlit hours may minimize photosensitivity.

21.2.18 HOW DOES METABOLISM AFFECT EXCRETION PHARMACOKINETICS OF THE DRUG OR CHEMICAL? AND HOW DO EXCRETION PHARMACOKINETICS RELATE TO TOPICAL ABSORPTION?

A drug or chemical can be excreted from the body unchanged, or it may undergo metabolic changes before excretion. Thus, the factors discussed in Sections 2.16 and 2.17 regarding biotransformation in the skin will affect excretion pharmacokinetics. For example, a highly lipophilic drug or chemical that is biotransformed into a more water-soluble metabolite will not only be more easily absorbed through the skin, it will also be more easily excreted in the urine. Water-soluble drugs often do not require metabolic changes for urinary excretion, and a greater proportion of the administered dose may be excreted unchanged.

Metabolism and excretion are two mechanisms for elimination of drug or chemical, which can be affected by numerous factors [15]. Note that metabolism and excretion pharmacokinetics can differ greatly between structurally similar drugs or chemicals. Thus, depending on the substance, elimination (i.e. drug clearance) may or may not be in proportion to the dose absorbed. For researchers conducting *in vivo* studies, the clearance rate of the drug or chemical must be considered when estimating percutaneous absorption from blood or tissue samples [15].

21.2.19   How Does Lateral Spread Affect Percutaneous Absorption?

A detailed discussion about lateral spread is found in Chapter 20 and in reference 96, as this factor is often overlooked. Lateral spread is the ability of a topical agent to spread beyond the site of application, i.e. the drug or chemical "flows" laterally on the skin surface from the application area to outside of it [97]. (Note that lateral spread is also more commonly used in describing earthquake phenomena.) Lateral spread of a topically applied drug or chemical is a competitive process to drug or chemical penetration into the SC [26, 97]. The spreading can reduce the amount of drug substance within the area of application, which can modify the desirable effect expected in the treated area [97].

Time is a factor: for example, a 10% urea in water solution applied to skin provided a 90.4% recovery rate at the site of application after 1 hour versus a 79.6% recovery rate after 6 hours [97]. Why is there less urea remaining at the site of application after 6 hours than after 1 hour? The cause is lateral spread and not percutaneous absorption, as less than 1% of urea penetrates *in vivo* in humans [98]. Thus, lateral spread is time dependent.

Furthermore, *skin surface topography* can affect the degree of lateral spread: primary furrow networks such as fingerprints and palm prints can function as pathways for lateral spreading [26], whereas follicles and wrinkles can be reservoirs for drugs or chemicals [25, 26], and little is known about lateral spread in these areas. Although there appears to be no difference in lateral spread between the forearm and back [26], little is known about other anatomical sites.

Practically, we should be aware that lateral spread happens, and the lengthier the time from the time of application, the greater the effect of lateral spread, resulting in less and less drug or chemical remaining at the site of application for percutaneous absorption.

21.2.20   For Investigators, Does the Method of Determining Percutaneous Absorption Influence the Results and the Interpretation of Study Results?

Based on what has been discussed from the numerous factors earlier, many issues can influence percutaneous absorption and, if not controlled for, can be confounders to study results. In particular, *in vivo* studies would be subject to many more confounding variables than *in vitro* studies. *In vitro* experiments can sometimes be better controlled than *in vivo* studies. Also, differences in experimental parameters such as animal species, anatomical site, vehicle, preparation of skin samples (*in vitro* studies), and other exposure conditions may affect the interpretation of and comparison between studies [3]. Furthermore, there are limits of quantification and limits of detection that must be kept in mind when interpreting study results.

21.3   CONCLUSION

Percutaneous absorption is complex and requires more thought than just simply applying a topical formulation on the skin and assuming that it works. Many factors—at least the ones that have been discussed here (Table 21.1)—need to be considered, as they may affect the efficacy and/or toxicity of the medications, and hence patient outcome.

ACKNOWLEDGEMENT

Reprinted and updated by permission from Copyright Clearance Center's RightsLink service on behalf of Springer Nature's *American Journal of Clinical Dermatology*: Law et al. (2020) 21:85–95. https://doi.org/10.1007/s40257-019-00480-4 (License No. 4773720663838).

TABLE 21.1

Clinically Pertinent Factors of Percutaneous Absorption

1	Relevant physicochemical properties (particle size/molecular weight, lipophilicity, water solubility, polarity, pH, pK_a, partition coefficient)
2	Vehicle/formulation
3	Conditions of drug exposure (dose, duration, surface area, exposure frequency)
4	Skin appendages (hair follicles, glands) as subanatomical pathways
5	Skin application sites (regional variation in penetration)
6	Population variability (prematurity, infants, and aged)
7	Skin surface conditions (hydration, temperature, pH)
8	Skin health and integrity (trauma, skin diseases)
9	Substantivity and binding to different skin components
10	Systemic distribution and systemic toxicity
11	Exfoliation
12	Washing-off and washing-in
13	Rubbing/massaging
14	Transfer to others (from human to human and hard surface to human)
15	Volatility
16	Metabolic biotransformation/cutaneous metabolism
17	Photochemical transformation and photosensitivity
18	Excretion pharmacokinetics
19	Lateral spread
20	Chemical method of determining percutaneous absorption

REFERENCES

1. Law RM, Ngo MA, Maibach HI. Twenty clinically pertinent factors/observations for percutaneous absorption in humans. Am J Clin Dermatol 2020;21(1):85–95.
2. Wester RC, Maibach HI. Cutaneous pharmacokinetics: 10 steps to percutaneous absorption. Drug Metab Rev 1983;14(2):169–205.
3. Ngo MA, Maibach HI. Chapter 6: 15 factors of percutaneous penetration of pesticides. ACS Symp. Ser. Volume 1099. Am. Chem. Soc 2012; 67–86. DOI:10.1021/bk-2012-1099.ch006
4. Hui X, Lamel S, Qiao P, et al. Isolated human/animal stratum corneum as a partial model for 15 steps in percutaneous absorption: emphasizing decontamination, Part I. J Appl Toxicol 2013;33:157–172.
5. Hui X, Lamel S, Qiao P, et al. Isolated human and animal stratum corneum as a partial model for the 15 steps in percutaneous absorption: emphasizing decontamination, part II. J Appl Toxicol 2013;33:173–182.
6. Li BS, Ngo MA, Maibach HI. Clinical relevance of complex factors of percutaneous penetration in man. Curr Top Pharmacol 2017;21:85–107.
7. Yoshida D, Todo H, Hasegawa T, et al. Effect of molecular weight on the dermatopharmacokinetics and systemic disposition of drugs after intracutaneous injection. Eur J Pharmaceut Sci 2008;35:5–11.
8. Keurentjes AJ, Maibach HI. Percutaneous penetration of drugs applied in transdermal delivery systems: An in vivo based approach for evaluating computer generated penetration models. Regul Toxicol Pharmacol 108 (2019); 104428.1–12.
9. Wester RC, Melendres J, Sarason R, et al. Glyphosate skin binding, absorption, residual tissue distribution, and skin decontamination. Fundamental App Toxicol 1991;16:725–732.
10. Osamura H. Penetration of topical corticosteroids through human epidermis. J Dermatol 1982;9:45–58.
11. Ponec M, Polano MK. Penetration of various corticosteroids through epidermis in vitro. Arch Dermatol Res 1979;265(1):101–104.
12. McKenzie AW, Stoughton RB. Method for comparing percutaneous absorption of steroids. Arch Dermatol 1962;86:608–610.
13. McKenzie AW. Percutaneous absorption of steroids. Arch Dermatol 1962;86:611–614.
14. Sutton PM, Feldmann RJ, Maibach HI. Vasoconstrictor potency of corticoids: intradermal injection. J Investigative Dermatol 1971;57(6):371–376.

15. Burton ME, Schentag JJ, Shaw LM, et al. Applied Pharmacokinetics and Pharmacodynamics: Principles of Therapeutic Drug Monitoring. 4th ed. Lippincott, Williams, and Wilkins, 2006.
16. Salocks CB, Hui X, Lamel S, et al. Dermal exposure to methamphetamine hydrochloride contaminated residential surfaces. Surface pH values, volatility, and *in vitro* human skin. Food Chem Toxicol 2012;50:4436–4440.
17. Beriro DJ, Cave M, Kim A et al. Soil-sebum partition coefficients for high molecular weight polycyclic aromatic hydrocarbons (HMW-PAH). J Hazard Mater 2020;398:122633. 3
18. Marechal Y. The water molecule in (bio)macromolecules. In: The Hydrogen Bond and the Water Molecule: The Physics and Chemistry of Water, Aqueous and Bio Media. Elsevier, 249–275, 2007.
19. Zhang A, Jung E-C, Zhu H, et al. Vehicle effects on human stratum corneum absorption and skin penetration. Toxicol Ind Health 2017;33(5):41–425.
20. Farahmand S, Maibach HI. Transdermal drug pharmacokinetics in man: Interindividual variability and partial prediction. Int J Pharmaceutics 2009;367:1–15.
21. Berner B, John VA. Pharmacokinetic characterisation of transdermal delivery systems. Clin Pharmacokinet 1994;26(2):121–134.
22. Wester RC, Noonan PK, Maibach HI. Frequency of application on percutaneous absorption of hydrocortisone. Arch Dermatol 1977;113:620–622.
23. Sun Safety and Protection Tips from the American Academy of Pediatrics. AAP. https://www.aap.org/en-us/about-the-aap/aap-press-room/news-features-and-safety-tips/Pages/Sun-Safety-and-Protection.aspx. Accessed July 6, 2020.
24. Teichmann A, Jacobi J, Weigmann H-J, et al. Reservoir function of the stratum corneum: Development of an in vivo method to quantitatively determine the stratum corneum reservoir for topically applied substances. Skin Pharmacol Physiol 2005;18:75–80.
25. Ladermann J, Richter H, Schaefer UF, et al. Hair follicles – a long-term reservoir for drug delivery. Skin Pharmacol Physiol 2008;19:232–236.
26. Jacobi U, Schanzer S, Weigmann H-J, et al. Pathways of lateral spreading. Skin Pharmacol Physiol 2011;24:231–237.
27. Feldmann RJ, Maibach HI. Regional variation in percutaneous penetration of ^{14}C cortisol in man. J Invest Dermatol 1967;48(2):181–183.
28. Rougier A, Lotte C, Maibach HI. In vivo percutaneous penetration of some organic compounds related to anatomic site in humans: Predictive assessment by the stripping method. J Pharm Sci 1987;76(6):451–454.
29. Roberts MS, Favretto WA, Meyer A, et al. Brief communication: Topical bioavailability of methyl salicylate. Aust NZ J Med 1982;12(3):303–305.
30. Berardesca E, Mariano M, Cameli N. Biophysical properties of ethnic skin. In Vashi NA, Maibach HI, editors. Dermatoanthropology of Ethnic Skin and Hair. Springer Nature, Springer International Publishing AG, 2017.
31. Berardesca E, Maibach HI. Racial differences in sodium lauryl sulfate induced cutaneous irritation: Black and white. Contact Dermatitis 1988;18:65–70.
32. Berardesca E, Maibach HI. Sodium-lauryl-sulfate-induced cutaneous irritation. Comparison of white and Hispanic subjects. Contact Dermatitis 1988;19:136–40.
33. Roskos KV, Maibach HI, Guy RH. The effect of aging on percutaneous absorption in man. J Pharmacokinet Biopharm 1989;17(6):617–630.
34. Hoath SB, Maibach HI. Neonatal skin. In Structure and Function, 2nd ed. CRC Press, 2003.
35. Mauro TM, Behne MJ. Chapter 3: Acid mantle. In Hoath SB, Maibach HI, editors. Neonatal Skin: Structure and Function, 2nd ed. CRC Press, 2003.
36. Nikolovski J, Stamatas GN, Kollias N et al. Barrier function and water-holding and transport properties of infant stratum corneum are different from adult and continue to develop through the first year of life. J Invest Dermatol 2008;128:1728–1736.
37. Karan A, Alikhan A, Maibach HI. Toxicologic implications of cutaneous barriers: A molecular, cellular, and anatomical overview. J Appl Toxicol 2009;29:551–559.
38. Yosipovitch G, Maayan-Metzger A, Merlob P, et al. Skin barrier properties in different body areas in neonates. Pediatrics 2000;106:105–108.
39. Oranges T, Dini V, Romanelli M. Skin physiology of the neonate and infant: Clinical implications. Advances in Wound Care 2015;4(10):587–595.
40. Hoeger PH, Enzmann CC. Skin physiology of the neonate and young infant: A prospective study of functional skin parameters during early infancy. Pediatr Dermatol 2002;19:256–262.

41. Visscher MO, Chatterjee R, Munson KA et al. Changes in diapered and non-diapered infant skin over the first month of life. Pediatr Dermatol 2000;17:45–51.
42. Saijo S, Tagami HJ. Dry skin of newborn infants: Functional analysis of the stratum corneum. Pediatr Dermatol 1991;8:155–159.
43. Brayer C, Micheau P, Bony C, et al. [Neonatal accidental burn by isopropyl alcohol]. Arch Pediatr 2004;11(8):932–935.
44. DeBellonia RR, Marcus S, Shih R, et al. Curanderismo: Consequences of folk medicine. Pediatr Emerg Care 2008;24(4):228–229.
45. George AJ. Toxicity of boric acid through skin and mucous membranes. Food Cosmet Toxicol 1965;3:99–101.
46. Martin-Bouyer G, Toga M, Lebreton R, et al. Outbreak of accidental hexachlorophene poisoning in France. Lancet (Public Health) 1982; 319(8263):91–95.
47. Mullick FG. Hexachlorophene toxicity – human experience at the Armed Forces Institute of Pathology. Pediatrics 1973;51(2):395–399.
48. Li BS, Cary JH, Maibach HI. Should we instruct patients to rub topical agents into skin? The evidence. J Dermatolog Treat 2019;30(4):328–332.
49. Evans NJ, Rutter N, Hadgraft J, et al. Percutaneous administration of theophylline in the preterm infant. J Pediatr 1985:107(2):307–311.
50. Zhai H, Maibach HI. Effects of skin occlusion on percutaneous absorption: An overview. Skin Pharmacol Appl Skin Physiol 2001;14(1):1–10.
51. Bucks D, Maibach HI. Chapter 5: Occlusion does not uniformly enhance penetration in vivo. In Bronaugh RL, Maibach HI, editors. Percutaneous Absorption: Mechanisms-Methodology-Drug Delivery, 3rd ed. Marcel Dekker, 1999;81–106.
52. Shomaker TS, Zhang J, Ashburn MA. A pilot study assessing the impact of heat on the transdermal delivery of testosterone. J Clin Pharmacol 2001;41(6):677–682.
53. Aly R, Shirley C, Cunico B, et al. Effect of prolonged occlusion on the microbial flora, pH, carbon dioxide and transepidermal water loss on human skin. J Invest Dermatol 1978;71(6):378–381.
54. Gattu S, Maibach HI. Modest but increased penetration through damaged skin: An overview of the in vivo human model. Skin Pharmacol Physiol 2011;24(1):2–9.
55. Gattu S, Maibach HI. Enhanced absorption through damaged skin: An overview of the in vitro human model. Skin Pharmacol Physiol 2010;23:171–176.
56. Morgan CJ, Renwick AG, Friedmann PS. The role of stratum corneum and dermal microvascular perfusion in penetration and tissue levels of water-soluble drugs investigated by microdialysis. Br J Dermatol 2003;148:434–443.
57. Jakasa I, Verberk MM, Bunge AL, et al. Increased permeability for polyethylene glycols through skin compromised by sodium lauryl sulfate. Exper Dermatol 2006;15:801–807.
58. Jacob SE. Percutaneous absorption risks in atopic dermatitis. Br J Dermatol 2017;177:11–12.
59. Halling-Overgaard AS, Kezic S, Jakasa I, et al. Skin absorption through atopic dermatitis skin: A systematic review. Br J Dermatol 2017;177(1):84–106.
60. Garcia OP, Hansen SH, Shah VP, et al. Impact of adult atopic dermatitis on topical drug absorption: Assessment by cutaneous microdialysis and tape stripping. Acta Derm Venereol 2009;89:33–38.
61. Tauber M, Balica S, Hsu CY, et al. Staphylococcus aureus density on lesional and nonlesional skin is strongly associated with disease severity in atopic dermatitis. J Allergy Clin Immunol 2016;137:1272–1274, e1–e3.
62. Jakasa I, de Jongh CM, Verberk MM, et al. Percutaneous penetration of sodium lauryl sulfate is increased in uninvolved skin of patients with atopic dermatitis compared with control subjects. Br J Dermatol 2006;155:104–109.
63. Jakasa I, Verbek MM, Esposito M, et al. Altered penetration of polyethylene glycols into uninvolved skin of atopic dermatitis patients. J Invest Dermatol 2007;127:129–134.
64. Hata M, Tokura Y, Takigawa M, et al. Assessment of epidermal barrier function by photoacoustic spectrometry in relation to its importance in the pathogenesis of atopic dermatitis. Lab Invest 2002;82:1451–1461.
65. Mochizuki J, Tadaki H, Takami S, et al. Evaluation of out-in skin transparency using a colorimeter and food dye in patients with atopic dermatitis. Br J Dermatol 2009;160:972–979.
66. Li BS, Cary JH, Maibach HI. Stratum corneum substantivity: Drug development implications. Arch Derm Res 2018;310:537–549.
67. Frasch HF, Barbro AM, Hettick JM, et al. Tissue binding affects the kinetics of theophylline diffusion through the stratum corneum barrier layer of skin. J Pharm Sci 2011;100:2989–2995.

68. Alikhan FS, Maibach HI. Topical absorption and systemic toxicity. Cutan Ocul Toxicol 2011;30(3):175–186.

69. Lewis PR, Phillips TG, Sassani JW. Topical therapies for glaucoma: What family physicians need to know. Am Fam Physician 1999;59:1871–1879,1882.

70. Goldberg I, Moloney G, McCluskey P. Topical ophthalmic medications: what potential for systemic side effects and interactions with other medications? Med J Aust 2008;189:356–357.

71. Rubin Z. Ophthalmic sulfonamide-induced Stevens-Johnson syndrome. Arch Dermatol 1977;113:235–236.

72. Raschke R, Arnold-Capell PA, Richeson R, et al. Refractory hypoglycemia secondary to topical salicylate intoxication. Arch Intern Med 1991;151:591–593.

73. Zheng Y, Vieille-Petit A, Chodoutard S, et al. Dislodgeable stratum corneum exfoliation: Role in percutaneous penetration? Cutan Ocul Toxicol 2011;30(3):198–204.

74. Zhu H, Maibach HI. Skin Decontamination: A Comprehensive Clinical Research Guide. Springer, 2020.

75. Rodriguez J, Maibach HI. Percutaneous penetration and pharmacodynamics: Wash-in and wash-off of sunscreen and insect repellent. J Dermatolog Treat 2016;27–11.

76. Moody RP. Letter to the editor: The safety of diethyltoluamide insect repellents. JAMA 1989:262:28–29.

77. Moody RP, Benoit FM, Riedel R, et al. Dermal absorption of the insect repellent DEET (N,N-diethyl-m-toluamide) in rats and monkeys: Effect of anatomical site and multiple exposure. J Toxicol Environ Health 1989;26:137–147.

78. Lademann J, Patzelt A, Schanzer S, et al. *In vivo* laser scanning microscopic investigation of the decontamination of hazardous substances from the human skin. Laser Phys Lett 2010;7:884–888.

79. Trauer S, Richter H, Kuntsche J, et al. Influence of massage and occlusion on the ex vivo skin penetration of rigid liposomes and invasomes. Eur J Pharm Biopharm 2014;86:301–306.

80. Phuong C, Maibach HI. Effect of massage on percutaneous penetration and skin decontamination: man and animal. Cutan Ocul Toxicol 2016;35(2):153–156.

81. Delamour E, Miksa S, Lutz D, et al. How to prove 'rub-resistant' sun protection. Cosmetics & Toiletries Science Applied. Published April 12, 2016. Available at: https://www.cosmeticsandtoiletries.com/testing/efficacyclaims/How-to-Prove-Rub-resistant-Sun-Protection-373779591.html. Accessed July 8, 2020.

82. Franklin SF, Geffner ME. Precocious puberty secondary to topical testosterone exposure. J Pediatr Endocr Metab 2003;16:107–110.

83. Wester RC, Hui X, Maibach HI. *In vivo* human transfer of topical bioactive drug between individuals: Estradiol. J Invest Dermatol 2006;126:2190–2193.

84. Linck M. Screens detect all: Mom, dad, kids, newborns all test positive for meth. Sioux City Journal. Published December 18, 2003. Available at: https://siouxcityjournal.com/news/screens-detect-all-mom-dad-kids-newborns-all-test-postive/article_5c9a48cf-4855-5308-ba83-c11bf1b44239.html. Accessed July 8, 2020.

85. Salocks CB, Hui X, Lamel S, et al. Dermal exposure to methamphetamine hydrochloride contaminated residential surfaces II. Skin surface contact and dermal transfer relationship. Food Chem Toxicol 2014;66:1–6.

86. Dmochowski RR, Newman DK, Sand PK, et al. Pharmacokinetics of oxybutynin chloride topical gel. Clin Drug Investig 2011;31(8):559–571.

87. Isnardo D, Vidal J, Panyella D, et al. Nickel transfer by gingers. Actas Dermo-Sifiliográficas (English Edition) 2015;106(5):e23–e26.

88. Rouse NC, Maibach HI. The effect of volatility on percutaneous absorption. J Dermatol Treat 2016;27(1):5–10.

89. Bruze M. Thoughts on how to improve the quality of multicentre patch test studies. Contact Dermatitis 2016;74:168–174.

90. Gilpin SJ, Hui X, Maibach HI. Volatility of fragrance chemicals: Patch testing implications. Dermatitis 2009;20(40):200–207.

91. Kasting GB, Miller MA. Kinetics of finite dose absorption through skin 2: Volatile compounds. J Pharm Sci 2006;95:268–280.

92. Norris EJ, Coats JR. Current and future repellent technologies: The potential of spatial repellents and their place in mosquito-borne disease control. Int J Environ Res Public Health 2017;14(2):124–168.

93. Kawada H, Temu EA, Minjas JN, et al. Field evaluation of field repellency of metofluthrin impregnated latticework plastic strips against *Aedes aegypti* (L.) and analysis of environmental factors affecting its efficacy in My Tho City, Tien Giang, Vietnam. Am J Trop Med Hyg 2006;75:1153–1157.

94. Kazem S, Linssen EC, Gibbs S. Skin metabolism phase I and phase II enzymes in native and recon-
     structed human skin: A short review. Drug Discovery Today. Published June 2019 ePub ahead of print.
     Available at: https://www.sciencedirect.com/science/article/pii/S1359644618302198.
95. Bando H, Mohri S, Yamashita F, et al. Effects of skin metabolism on percutaneous penetration of lipo-
     philic drugs. J Pharm Sci 1997;86(6):759–761.
96. Law RM, Maibach Hi. Lateral spread and percutaneous penetration: an overview. Int J Pharm
     2020;588:119765.
97. Vieille-Petit A, Blickenstaff N, Coman G, et al. Metrics and clinical relevance of percutaneous penetra-
     tion and lateral spreading. Skin Pharmacol Physiol 2015;28:57–64.
98. Feldman RJ, Maibach HI. Absorption of some organic compounds through the skin in man. J Invest
     Dermatol 1970;54:399–404.

FURTHER READING

Law RM, Maibach HI. Phenomenon of lateral spread in percutaneous penetration. In Bronaugh/Maibach Hi,
     editor. Percutaneous Absorption: Drugs-Cosmetics-Mechanisms-Methods 5th ed. Informa, 2021. (In
     press).
Dragicevic N, Maibach HI, editors. Percutaneous Penetration Enhancers: Chemical Methods in Penetration
     Enhancement. Springer, 2015.
Berardesca E, Leveque J-L, Maibach HI, editors. Ethnic Skin and Hair. CRC Press, 2006.
Berardesca E, Leveque J-L, Maibach HI, editors. Ethnic Skin and Hair. CRC Press, 2019.

22 Percutaneous Absorption of Chemical Mixtures

Jim E. Riviere
North Carolina State University, Raleigh, North Carolina

CONTENTS

22.1 INTRODUCTION

A primary route of occupational and environmental exposure to toxic chemicals is often through the skin. Although exposure to complex chemical mixtures is the norm, only mechanisms of absorption for single chemicals have been studied, and most risk-assessment profiles are based on the behavior of single chemicals. Effects of co-administered chemicals on the rate and extent of absorption of a topically applied systemic toxicant may determine whether toxicity is ever realized.

The application of risk assessment to dermal absorption by U.S. regulatory agencies (Environmental Protection Agency, Occupational Safety and Health Administration, Agency for Toxic Substance and Disease Registry) is varied and highly dependent upon available data (1–3). A similar concern over lack of data exists for overall risk assessment of chemical mixtures (4–7). A congressional Commission of Risk Assessment and Risk Management (8) recommended moving beyond individual chemical assessments and focusing on the broader issues of toxicity of chemical mixtures. Current approaches are based on assigning toxicological equivalent units to similar chemical congeners (e.g., dioxins) or assessing toxicity after exposure to the complete mixture. It is recognized (4) that the dose–response curves of individual mixture components should be characterized and then a "no interaction" hypothesis for these components in a mixture is tested. With complex mixtures of hundreds of components, these approaches become exceedingly complex. Finally, mixture component interactions that involve modulation of a known toxicant's absorption, and thus systemic bioavailability, have not been defined.

This problem is conceptually similar to that of dermatological formulations in the pharmaceutical arena. The primary difference is that most pharmaceutical formulation components are added for a specific purpose relative to the delivery, stability, or activity of the active ingredient. In the environmental and occupational scenarios, additives are a function of either their natural occurrence or presence in a mixture for a purpose related to uses of that mixture (e.g., a fuel performance additive) and not for their effects on absorption or toxicity of the potential toxicant. The same is true for cosmetics and topical botanical preparations, where ingredients are added for a purported effect and not for specifically modulating absorption. The appreciation of the importance of chemical mixture interactions to affect chemical and drug disposition, pharmacokinetics, and activity has been well recognized for many years and is extensively reviewed elsewhere (4, 5, 9–13). Despite the widespread knowledge base of the importance of drug–drug interactions and the importance of chemical interactions in systemic pharmacology and toxicology, very little attention outside of the dermatological and transdermal formulation arenas have been paid to interactions that may occur after topical exposure to complex mixtures. The focus of this chapter is to overview the potential mechanisms operative in topical chemical mixtures, as well as to illustrate these interactions with data from our laboratory.

22.2   RISK ASSESSMENT

Dermal risk assessment of individual chemicals is based on knowledge of the permeability characteristics of specific chemicals through skin, with extrapolations being made to potential absorption in humans (14). Numerous contributions in the present text discuss this field. A great deal of emphasis is appropriately placed on calculating potential exposure, with less attention focused on the actual permeability of the exposed compound through skin, which is required to estimate systemic exposure. Collection of this latter data is preferably done in a controlled and validated laboratory animal model, although one could argue that even quality data in a laboratory rodent might not be optimal for predicting human skin absorption due to well-known species differences. Unfortunately, very little human data exist to support these estimates, and it is unethical to expose humans to hazardous materials to generate these parameters. When data are not present, extrapolations of potential absorption are made based on physical chemical parameters (e.g., molecular volume and water solubility) or surrogates such as partition coefficient (PC) (concentration ratio between vehicle and membrane) that correlates to permeability of individual chemicals primarily through in vitro skin models. These models and analyses are called quantitative structure permeability relationships (QSPRs). A great deal of effort has been spent on developing these permeability estimates. However, it is evident from a close review of these approaches that the combination of dermal absorption and mixture guidelines has not yet routinely occurred, despite broad acceptance that the skin is a primary route of exposure for many chemicals and that most chemical exposure occurs in mixtures.

It is impossible to assess all potential combinations of chemicals in order to determine which have the greatest potential to modulate absorption of a known toxic entity topically exposed in a chemical mixture. The present state of knowledge in this area is particularly weak, since the significance of specific interactions has not been quantified, let alone in many cases even identified. In many ways, this same concern continues to define the very nature of chemical mixture toxicology (5, 9, 10, 12, 13). In cases where the potential toxicity of a specific mixture is of concern (e.g., at a specific toxic waste site), the complete mixture is often tested (15). However, how does one quantitate the absorption of a mixture consisting of 50 chemicals? How are markers selected? How are these data expressed? Unfortunately, even after a complete toxicological profile of a specific mixture (e.g., "standard" mixture of 50 environmentally relevant compounds, surrogate jet fuels, etc.) is defined using all the techniques modern toxicology and toxicogenomics has to offer, one cannot define the links between absorption and the effects seen. Could the observed toxicity be exerted because a specific toxicant was in the mixture, because two synergistic toxicants were absorbed, or was it exerted simply by the presence of a mixture component (e.g., alcohol, surfactant, and fatty acid) that enhanced the absorption of a normally minimally absorbed toxicant? In this latter scenario, if the enhancer were not present, absorption would have fallen below the toxicological threshold. We have demonstrated such an interaction with the putative toxins involved in the Gulf War syndrome, where systemic pyridostigmine bromide or co-exposure to jet fuel was shown to greatly enhance the dermal absorption of topical permethrin (16, 17). Would other pesticides be similarly affected? How does one take into account such critical interactions so that a proper risk assessment may be conducted?

One recently reported approach to address this problem assesses potential interactions in dermal absorption by fractionating the effects of a vehicle on drug penetration onto the two primary parameters describing permeation according to Fick's law: partitioning (PC) and diffusivity (D) [see later; permeability (K_p) = D × PC/membrane thickness] (18). Although this study only reported on four compounds, one (diazepam) was not predictable using this approach, as its physiochemical properties were already optimal for absorption, and only absorption enhancers were investigated. This study illustrates the difficulty of making broad generalizations across compounds solely on physical chemical properties.

A more inclusive approach to this problem is to define chemicals on the basis of how they would interact with other components of a mixture, as well as with the barrier components of the skin. What are the physical-chemical properties that would significantly modify absorption and potentiate systemic exposure to a toxicant? What are the properties of molecules susceptible to such modulation? Unlike pharmaceutical formulation additives in a dermal medication, chemical components of a mixture are not classified by how they could modulate percutaneous absorption of simultaneously exposed topical chemicals. They are either present functionally for specific purposes (e.g., performance additives, lubricants, and modulators of some biological activity), sequentially because they were applied to the skin independently at different times for unrelated purposes (cosmetic followed by topical insect repellent), accidentally because they were disposed of simultaneously as waste, or they are coincidentally associated as part of a complex occupational or environmental exposure.

22.3 MECHANISMS OF INTERACTIONS

Chemical interactions that may modulate dermal absorption can be conveniently classified according to physical location where an interaction may occur. The advantage of this approach is that potential interactions may be defined on the basis of specific mechanisms of action involved, as well as by the biological complexity of the experimental model required to detect it.

Surface of skin:

- Chemical-chemical (binding, ion-pair formation, etc.)
- Altered physical-chemical properties (e.g., solubility, volatility, and critical micelle concentration)
- Altered rates of surface evaporation
- Occlusive behavior
- Binding or interaction with adnexal structures or their products (e.g., hair, sweat, and sebum)

Stratum corneum:

- Altered permeability through lipid pathway (e.g., enhancer)
- Altered partitioning into stratum corneum
- Extraction of intercellular lipids

Epidermis:

- Altered biotransformation
- Induction of and/or modulation of inflammatory mediators

Dermis:

- Altered vascular function (direct or secondary to mediator release)

The first and most widely studied area of chemical-chemical interactions is on the surface of the skin. The types of phenomena that could occur are governed by the laws of solution chemistry and

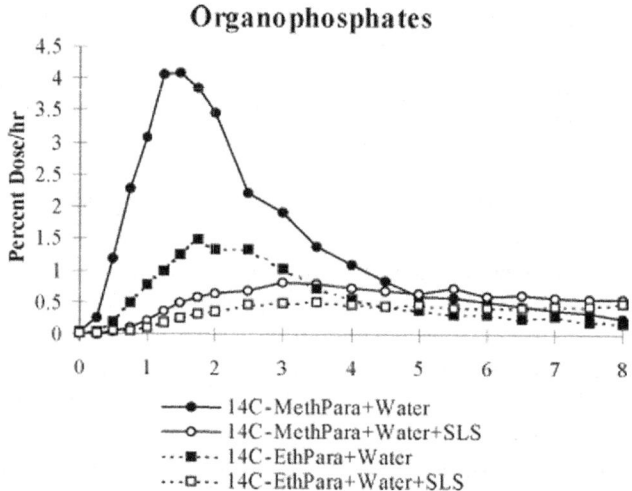

FIGURE 22.1 Effect of sodium lauryl sulfate (SLS) on mean absorption profiles of ethyl- and methyl-parathion in isolated perfused porcine skin.

include factors such as altered solubility, precipitation, supersaturation, solvation, or volatility, as well as physical-chemical effects such as altered surface tension from the presence of surfactants, changed solution viscosity, and micelle formation (19–22). For some of these effects, chemicals act independently of one another. However, for many, the presence of other component chemicals may modulate the effect seen.

Figure 22.1 illustrates the effects of the surfactant sodium lauryl sulfate (SLS) on the absorption of methyl and ethyl parathion in perfused porcine skin. Despite differences in the overall absorptive flux of both compounds administered in these aqueous vehicles, SLS decreased the absorption of both.

Chemical interactions may further be modulated by interaction with adnexal structures or their products such as hair, sebum, or sweat secretions. The result is that when a marker chemical is dosed on the skin as a component of a chemical mixture, the amount freely available for subsequent absorption may be significantly affected. The primary driving force for chemical absorption in skin is passive diffusion that requires a concentration gradient of thermodynamically active (free) chemical.

Second levels of potential interaction are those involving the marker and/or component chemicals with the constituents of the stratum corneum. These include the classic enhancers such as oleic acid, Azone or ethanol, widely reviewed elsewhere (22). These chemicals alter a compound's permeability within the intercellular lipids of the stratum corneum. Organic vehicles persisting on the surface of the skin may extract stratum corneum lipids that would alter permeability to the marker chemical (23, 24). Compounds may also bind to stratum corneum constituents, forming a depot.

The PC between the drug in the surface dosing vehicle and stratum corneum lipids may be altered if chemical components of the mixture also partition and diffuse into the lipids and thus alter their composition. This provides a potential mechanism to assess the effects of a mixture interaction on subsequent absorption. Figure 22.2 illustrates the PC of pentachlorophenol (PCP) into porcine stratum corneum administered in a series of six mixtures (water, water / ethanol / methyl nicotinate, water / ethanol, water / SLS, ethanol / methyl nicotinate, ethanol). Figure 22.3 compares PCP absorption in perfused porcine skin dosed in these same mixtures against PC, illustrating that PC determined from the mixture of concern does correlate to absorption across viable skin.

Another level of interaction would be with the viable epidermis. The most obvious point of potential interaction would be with a compound that undergoes biotransformation (25, 26).

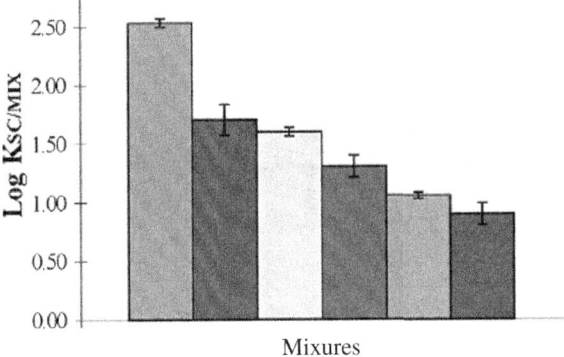

FIGURE 22.2 Isolated porcine stratum corneum/vehicle partiton coefficients (log KSC/MIX) for penta-chlorophenol (PCP) across six different chemical mixtures.

A penetrating chemical and mixture component could interact in a number of ways, including competitive or noncompetitive inhibition for occupancy at the enzyme's active site, or induction or inhibition of drug-metabolizing enzymes. Other structural and functional enzymes could also be affected (e.g., lipid synthesis enzymes), which would modify barrier function (27). A chemical could also induce keratinocytes to release cytokines or other inflammatory mediators (28–30), which could ultimately alter barrier function in the stratum corneum or vascular function in the dermis. Alternatively, cytokines may modulate biotransformation enzyme activities (31). The last level of potential interaction is in the dermis, where a component chemical may directly or indirectly (e.g., via cytokine release in the epidermis) modulate vascular uptake of the penetrated toxicant (32, 33). In addition to modulating transdermal flux of chemical, such vascular modulation could affect the depth and extent of toxicant penetration into underlying tissues.

22.4 IMPACT OF MULTIPLE INTERACTIONS

The complexity occurs when one considers that these interactions are all independent, making the observed effect in vivo a vectorial sum of all interactions. This allows so-called "emergent properties" of complex systems (34) to be observed when the individual interactions are finally summed in the intact system, in our case in vivo skin. For example, assume that mixture component A decreases absorption of a chemical across the skin due to increase binding to skin components. In contrast, mixture component B increases its absorption due to an enhancer effect on stratum corneum lipids. When the mixture components A and B are administered in combination, the transdermal flux of the chemical being studied may not differ from control. This is illustrated by the

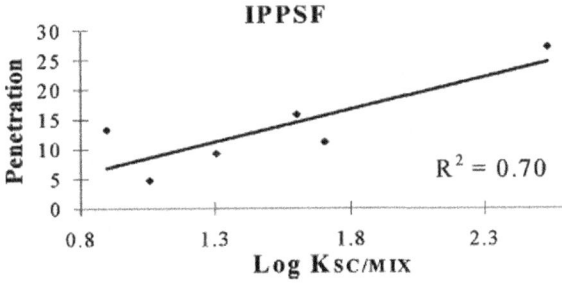

FIGURE 22.3 Correlation of pentachlorophenol (PCP) log KSC/MIX and absorption in isolated perfused procine skin.

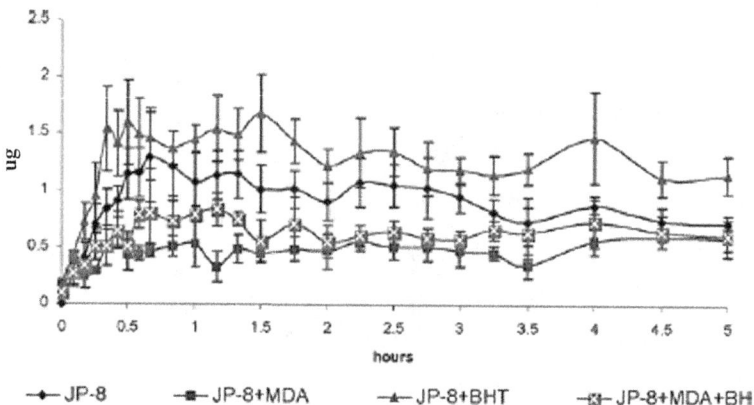

FIGURE 22.4 Effects of fuel performance additives butylated hydroxytoluene (BHT) and metal deactivator additive (MDA) on dermal absorption of naphthalene in isolated perfused porcine skin.

effect of two different jet fuel performance additives (metal deactivator additive [MDA] and butylated hydroxytoluene [BHT]) on dermal absorption of naphthalene administered from the base fuel JP-8 not containing these additives or in combination (Figure 22.4). In this case we hypothesize that MDA increases surface retention of naphthalene, thereby decreasing its absorption, while BHT functions more like a penetration enhancer. When both are present, flux returns to base levels. We have previously seen similar effects with other combinations of additives on absorption of jet fuel hydrocarbons (35, 36).

It may be a mistake to assume that these opposite effects simply cancel one another out and that the flux of chemical is now equivalent to it being applied alone. The mechanisms behind the similarity in control and competing additive mixture fluxes are different. Fick's first law of diffusion can be used to illustrate this. In the base situation (ø), compound flux would equal:

$$\text{Flux}_\phi = K_p \Delta C$$

where K_p is the permeability coefficient and ΔC is the concentration gradient driving the absorption process. We will consider ΔC the effective dermal dose, since increasing concentration on the surface of the skin effectively increases ΔC. In the presence of additives, we had two scenarios where additive A decreased absorption by retaining chemical on the surface, effectively reducing ΔC:

$$\downarrow \text{Flux}_A = K_p (\downarrow \Delta C)$$

and scenario B where flux increased due to an increased K_p:

$$\uparrow \text{Flux}_B = \left(\uparrow K_p \right) \Delta C$$

When both A and B are present, the flux is now back to base levels, but is governed by a fundamentally different set of diffusion parameters:

$$\text{Flux}_{A+B} \approx \text{Flux}_\phi = \left(\uparrow K_p \right) \left(\downarrow \Delta C \right)$$

One can appreciate how different factors that would interact with these altered parameters could drastically change dermal flux compared to the baseline scenario and potentially cause other chemical or biological interactions not seen under the control dosing scenario in the absence of absorption modulators.

Recently, our group has continued to develop mathematical models that attempt to account for the observed modulation of a mixture component on the transdermal flux of an applied compound. In most of these QSPR approaches, linear free energy relationships (LFERs) relate a compound K_p to the physical-chemical properties of the penetrating compound. In a mixture LFER model, the physical-chemical properties of the additives which modify the penetrant's absorption (e.g. refractive index, polar surface area, etc.) are now included in the model as a mixture factor (MF).

$$\text{Flux}_{mix} = K_p \Delta C \times MF$$

A number of mathematical approaches are used to accomplish this modulation depending on the variables being modeled (e.g. K_p, transdermal flux, or some other pharmacokinetic parameter) (37–43). Differences between these methods also relate to how the physical-chemical properties of both the penetrants and the additives are determined, how the interactions are mathematically modeled, and the complexity of the biological system being studied (e.g. in vivo versus ex vivo skin). In the cases where similar compounds are studied but the biological system is more complex, different MFs may be computed (44). As with any such analysis, the actual compounds being studied, which define the applicable chemical space of the analysis, are also important in that predictions only apply for new compounds (both penetrants and mixture additives) with similar physical-chemical properties. With the continued explosion of the ability to model ever increasingly large data sets, such analyses will continue to be more accurate and predictive of absorption from more complex mixtures.

22.5 CONCLUSION

This brief overview of mixture absorption illustrates the complexity involved when trying to extrapolate single interactions seen with binary mixtures onto absorption from more complex mixtures. However, strategies aimed at quantitating potential interactions in the framework of mechanisms of absorption would seem to be the most promising approach to put order into this complex problem. The data that indicate that measured stratum corneum PC correlates to subsequent absorption through intact skin is encouraging, as it provides an approach to experimentally assessing the effects of complex mixtures on K_p.

ACKNOWLEDGMENTS

The author would like to thank Dr. F. Muhammed for his help in analysis of the naphthalene data depicted in Figure 22.4 and NIOSH Grant R01-OH-07555 for supporting these mixture studies.

REFERENCES

1. Poet TS, McDougal JN. Skin absorption and human risk assessment. Chem Biol Interact 2002; 140:19–34.
2. EPA. Dermal Exposure Assessment: Principles and Applications. EPA/600/8-91/011B, 1995.
3. EPA. Risk Assessment Guidance for Superfund. Vol. 1: Human Health Evaluation Manual (Part E. Supplemental Guidance for Dermal Risk Assessment) Interim Guidance. Office of Emergency and Remedial Response, Washington, DC, 1999.
4. Borgert CJ, Price B, Wells CS, Simon GS. Evaluating chemical interaction studies for mixture risk assessment. Hum Ecol Risk Assess 2001; 7:259–306.

5. Pohl HR, Hansen H, Selene J, Chou CH. Public health guidance values for chemical mixtures: current practice and future directions. Regul Toxicol Pharmacol 1997; 26:322–329.
6. EPA. Guidelines for the health risk assessment of chemical mixtures. Fed Reg 1986; 5:34014–34025.
7. EPA. Technical Support Document on Risk Assessment of Chemical Mixtures. EPA/600/8-90/064, 1988.
8. CRARM (Commission on Risk Assessment and Risk Management). U.S. Congress, Washington, DC, 1997.
9. Bliss CI. The toxicity of poisons applied jointly. Ann Appl Biol 1939; 26:585–615.
10. Yang RSH. Toxicology of Chemical Mixtures. San Diego: Academic Press, 1994.
11. Haddad S, Charest-Tardif G, Tardif R, Krishnan K. Validation of a physiological modeling framework for simulating the toxicokinetics of chemicals in mixtures. Toxicol Appl Pharmacol 2000; 167:199–209.
12. Haddad S, Be´liveau M, Tardif R, Krishnan K. A PBPK modeling-based approach to account for interactions in the health risk assessment of chemical mixtures. Toxicol Sci 2001; 63:125–131.
13. Groten JP, Feron VJ, Sühnel J. Toxicology of simple and complex mixtures. Trends Pharmacol Sci 2001; 22:316–322.
14. Robinson PJ. Prediction: simple risk models and overview of dermal risk assessment. In: Roberts MS, Walters KA, eds. Dermal Absorption and Toxicity Assessment. New York: Marcel Dekker, 1998:203–229.
15. McDougal JN, Robinson PJ. Assessment of dermal absorption and penetration of components of a fuel mixture (JP-8). Sci Total Environ 2002; 288:23–30.
16. Baynes RE, Monteiro-Riviere NA, Riviere JE. Pyridostigmine bromide modulates the dermal disposition of C-14 permethrin. Toxicol Appl Pharmacol 2002; 181:164–173.
17. Riviere JE, Monteiro-Riviere NA, Baynes RE. Gulf War Illness-related exposure factors influencing topical absorption of 14C-permethrin. Toxicol Lett 2002; 135:61–71.
18. Rosada C, Cross SE, Pugh WJ, Roberts MS, Hadgraft J. Effect of vehicle pretreatment on the flux, retention, and diffusion of topically applied penetrants in vitro. Pharm Res 2003; 20:1502–1507.
19. Idson B. Vehicle effects in percutaneous absorption. Drug Metab Rev 1983; 14:207–222.
20. Barry BW. Novel mechanisms and devices to enable successful transdermal drug delivery. Eur J Pharm Sci 2001; 14:101–114.
21. Moser K, Kriwet K, Kalia YN, Guy RH. Enhanced skin permeation of a lipophilic drug using supersaturated formulations. J Control Release 2001; 73:245–253.
22. Williams AC, Barry BW. Chemical penetration enhancement: possibilities and problems. In: Roberts MS, Walters KA, eds. Dermal Absorption and Toxicity Assessment. New York: Marcel Dekker, 1998:297–312.
23. Monteiro-Riviere NA, Inman AO, Mak V, Wertz P, Riviere JE. Effects of selective lipid extraction from different body regions on epidermal barrier function. Pharm Res 2001; 18:992–998.
24. Rastogi SK, Singh J. Lipid extraction and transport of hydrophilic solutes through porcine epidermis. Int J Pharm 2001; 225:75–82.
25. Bronaugh RL, Stewart RF, Strom JE. Extent of cutaneous metabolism during percutaneous absorption of xenobiotics. Toxicol Appl Pharmacol 1989; 99:534–543.
26. Mukhtar H. Pharmacology of the Skin. Boca Raton: CRC Press, 1992.
27. Elias PM, Feingold KR. Lipids and the epidermal water barrier: metabolism, regulation, and pathophysiology. Semin Dermatol 1992; 11:176–182.
28. Allen DG, Riviere JE, Monteiro-Riviere NA. Induction of early biomarkers of inflammation produced by keratinocytes exposed to jet fuels Jet-A, JP-8, and JP-8(100). J Biochem Mol Toxicol 2000; 14:231–237.
29. Luger TA, Schwarz T. Evidence for an epidermal cytokine network. J Invest Dermatol 1990; 95:104S–110S.
30. Monteiro-Riviere NA, Baynes RE, Riviere JE. Pyridostigmine bromide modulates topical irritant-induced cytokine release from human epidermal keratinocytes and isolated perfused porcine skin. Toxicology 2003; 183:15–28.
31. Morgan ET. Regulation of cytochrome P450 by inflammatory mediators: why and how? Drug Metab Dispos 2001; 29:207–212.
32. Riviere JE, Williams PL. Pharmacokinetic implications of changing blood flow to the skin. J Pharm Sci 1992; 81:601–602.
33. Williams PL, Riviere JE. Model describing transdermal iontophoretic delivery of lidocaine incorporating consideration of cutaneous microvascular state. J Pharm Sci 1993; 82:1080–1084.
34. Bar-Yum Y. Dynamic of Complex Systems. Reading: Addison-Wesley, 1997.

35. Baynes RE, Brooks JD, Budsaba K, Smith CE, Riviere JE. Mixture effects of JP-8 additives on the dermal disposition of jet fuel components. Toxicol Appl Pharmacol 2001; 175:269–281.
36. Riviere JE, Monteiro-Riviere NA, Brooks JD, Budsaba K, Smith CE. Dermal absorption and distribution of topically dosed jet fuels Jet A, JP-8, and JP-8(100). Toxicol Appl Pharmacol 1999; 160:60–75.
37. Riviere JE, Brooks JD. Predicting skin permeability from complex chemical mixtures. Toxicol Appl Pharmacol 2005; 208:99–110.
38. Chittenden J, Brooks JD, Riviere JE. Development of a mixed-effect pharmacokinetic model for vehicle modulated in vitro transdermal flux of topically applied penetrants. J Pharm Sci 2014; 103:1002–1012.
39. Chittenden JT, Riviere JE. Quantification of vehicle mixture effects on in vitro transdermal chemical flux using a random process diffusion model. J Contr Release 2015; 217:74–81.
40. Muhammad F, Jaberi-Douraki M, de Sousa D P, Riviere J E. Modulation of topical chemical absorption by 14 natural compounds: A quantitative strcture permeation (QSPR) analysis of compounds often found in topical preparations. Cutan Ocul Toxicol 2017; 36:237–252.
41. Karadzovska D, Brooks JD, Monteiro-Riviere NA, Riviere JE. Predicting skin permeability from complex mixtures. Adv Drug Del Rev 2013; 65:265–277.
42. Xu G, Hughes-Oliver JM, Brooks JD, Baynes RE. Predicting skin permeability from complex chemical mixtures: incorporation of an expanded QSAR model. SAR QSAR Environ Res. 2013; 24:711–731.
43. Hughes-Oliver, J., Xu, G., Baynes RE. Skin permeation of solutes from metalworking fluids to build prediction models and test a partition theory. Molecules 2018; 23:3076.
44. Riviere JE, Brooks JD. Predicting skin permeability from complex chemical mixtures: Dependency of quantitative structure permeability relationships (QPSR) on biology of skin model used. Toxicol Sci 2011; 119:224–232.

23 Dermal Decontamination and Percutaneous Absorption

Howard I. Maibach
University of California, San Francisco, California

CONTENTS

Although decontamination of a chemical from the skin is commonly done by washing with soap and water, as it has been assumed that washing will remove the chemical, recent evidence suggests that often the skin and the body are unknowingly subjected to enhanced penetration and systemic absorption/toxicity because the decontamination procedure does not work or may actually enhance absorption. This chapter reviews some of the recent literature, then offers new in vitro and in vivo techniques to determine skin decontamination.

23.1 IN VIVO DECONTAMINATION MODEL

Figure 23.1 shows a skin decontamination model (1) where the time course of decontamination for several solvent systems can be tested. The illustration is for the abdomen of a rhesus monkey, but any large skin area can be used, including human. A grid of 1-cm^2 areas is marked on the skin. The illustration shows 24 separate blocks. As an example of use, the four blocks across the grid can represent four different decontaminating systems. The blocks down the abdomen can represent six time periods in which the skin is decontaminated. In our system, we use a cotton applicator laden with washing solvent to wash the skin block area. This is illustrated with the following data.

Figure 23.2 shows glyphosate, a water-soluble chemical, removed from rhesus monkey skin with three successive soap-and-water or water-only washes. Approximately 90% of the glyphosate is removed with the washes, most in the first wash. There is no difference between soap-and-water and water-only washing. Figure 23.3 shows alachlor, a lipid-soluble chemical, also decontaminated with soap-and-water and water-only washes. In contrast to glyphosate, more alachlor is removed with soap-and-water than with water-only washes. Although the first alachlor washing removed a majority of the chemical, successive washings contributed to the overall decontamination.

Figures 23.4 (glyphosate) and 23.5 (alachlor) illustrate skin decontamination with soap-and-water or water-only washes over a 24-hour dosing period, using the grid methodology from Figure 23.1. The three successive washes were pooled for each data time point. Certain observations are made. First, the amount recovered decreases over time. This is because this is an in

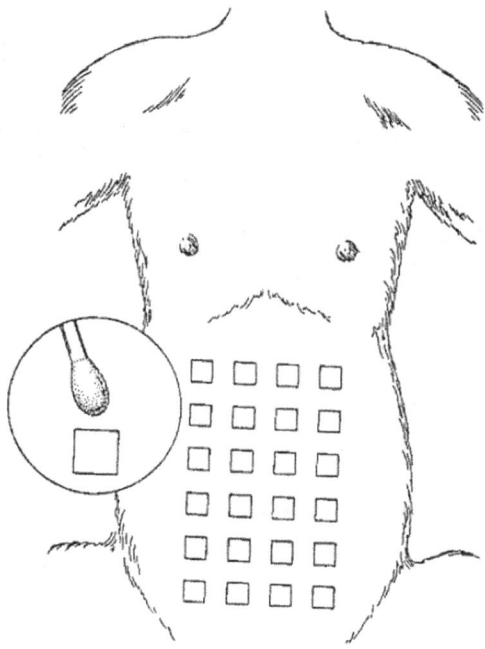

FIGURE 23.1 Illustration of grid method where multiple single doses are marked on rhesus monkey abdomen for skin decontamination with time using a cotton-tip applicator laden with appropriate solvent.

vivo system and percutaneous absorption is taking place, decreasing the amount of chemical on the skin surface. There also may be some loss due to skin desquamation. Note that alachlor is more readily absorbed across skin than is glyphosate. The second observation is, again, that soap-and-water and water-only washes removed equal amounts of glyphosate, but alachlor is

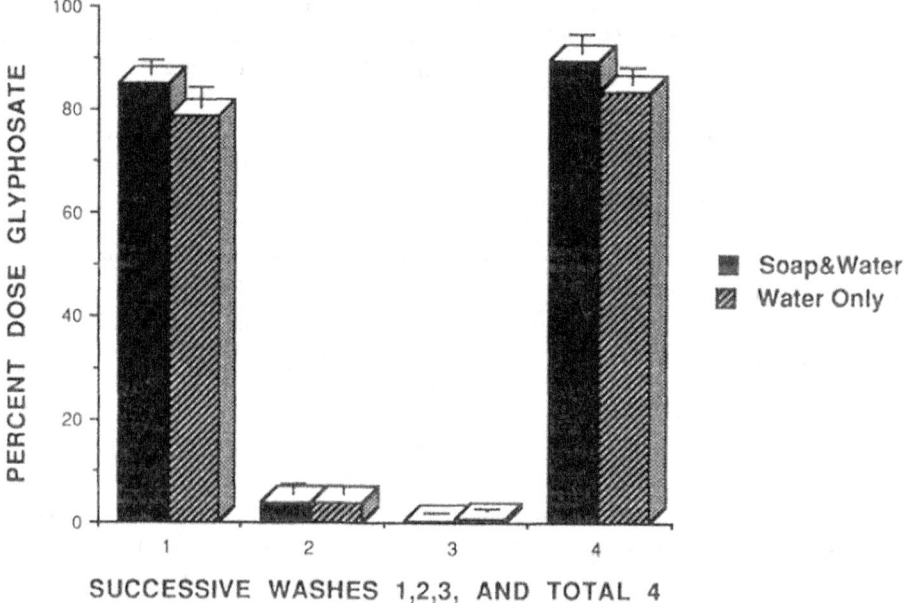

FIGURE 23.2 Glyphosate removal from rhesus monkey skin in vivo with successive washes. Note that water only and the addition of soap are equally effective. Glyphosate is water-soluble.

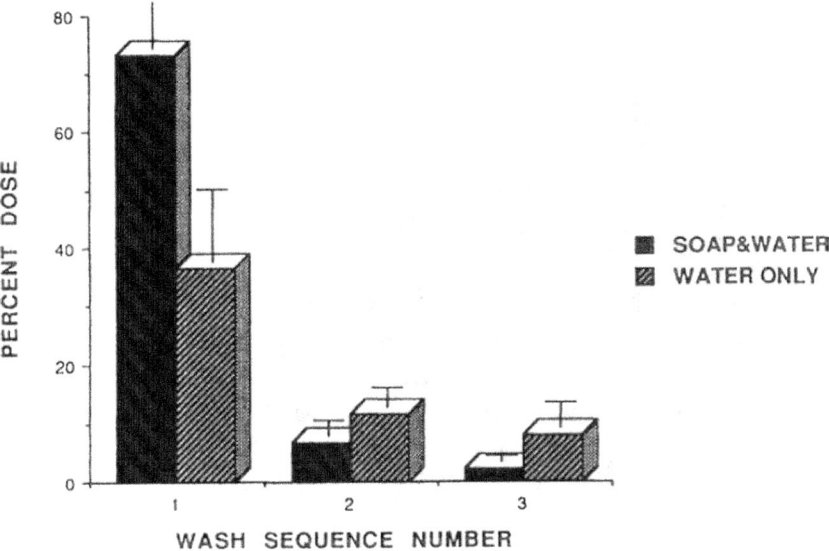

FIGURE 23.3   Alachlor removal from rhesus monkey skin in vivo with successive washes. Note that soap and water removes more alachlor than water only. Alachlor is lipid soluble.

more readily removed with soap-and-water washing than with water only. The reason is that glyphosate is water soluble; thus, water is a good solvent for it. Alachlor is lipid soluble and needs the surfactant system for more successful decontamination (1, 2).

Figure 23.6 shows alachlor skin decontamination at four dose concentrations washed with multiple successive soap-and-water applications. Most of the dose is removed with the first washing, and three successive washes are adequate to remove the dose.

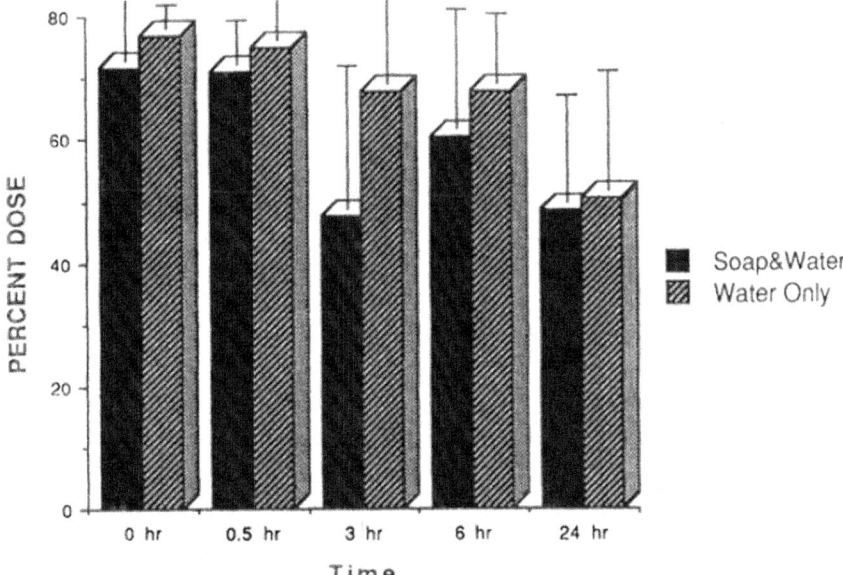

FIGURE 23.4   Time course, 0 to 24 hours, for in vivo glyphosate removal with skin washing. Over time, the ability to remove glyphosate decreases due to ongoing skin absorption. Soap-and-water and water-only washes were equally effective. Glyphosate is water-soluble.

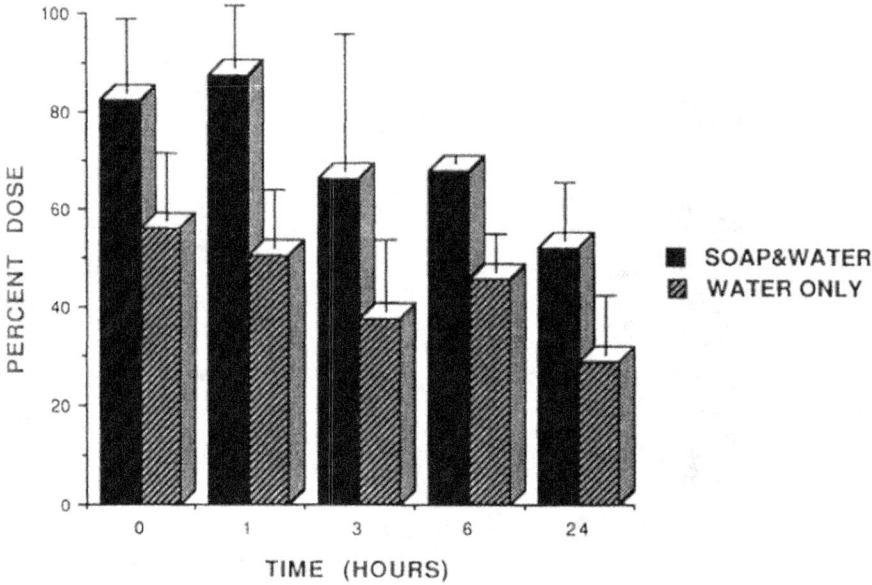

FIGURE 23.5 Time course, 0 to 24 hours, for in vivo alachlor removal with skin washing. Over time the ability to remove alachlor decreases due to ongoing skin absorption. Soap and water was more effective than water only. Alachlor is lipid-soluble.

Figure 23.7 shows 42% polychlorinated biphenyls (PCBs) applied in vivo in trichlorobenzene (TCB) or mineral oil (MO) to rhesus monkey skin and washed over a 24-hour period with soap and water. With time, the wash recovery of PCBs decreases due to the ongoing skin absorption. The PCBs can be removed from skin with soap and water if the decontamination is done soon enough after exposure (3).

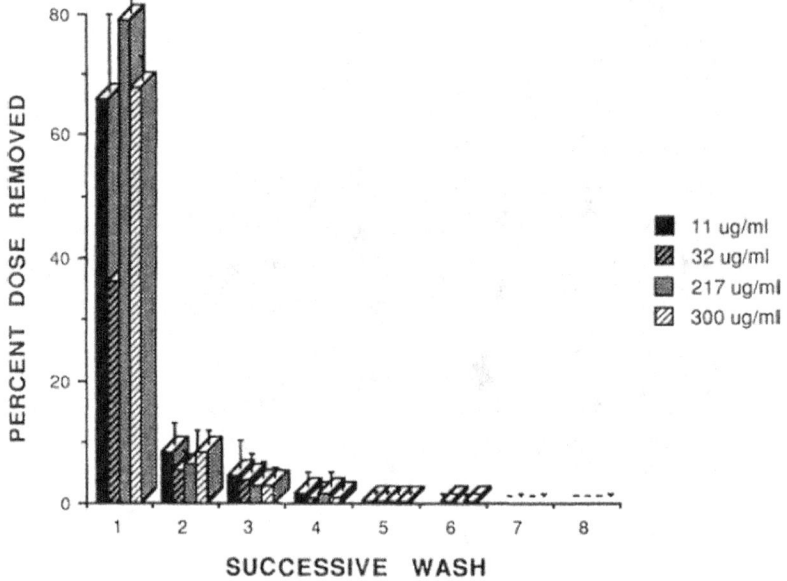

FIGURE 23.6 Alachlor soap-and-water skin decontamination with multiple successive washes. Three successive washes seem adequate for decontamination.

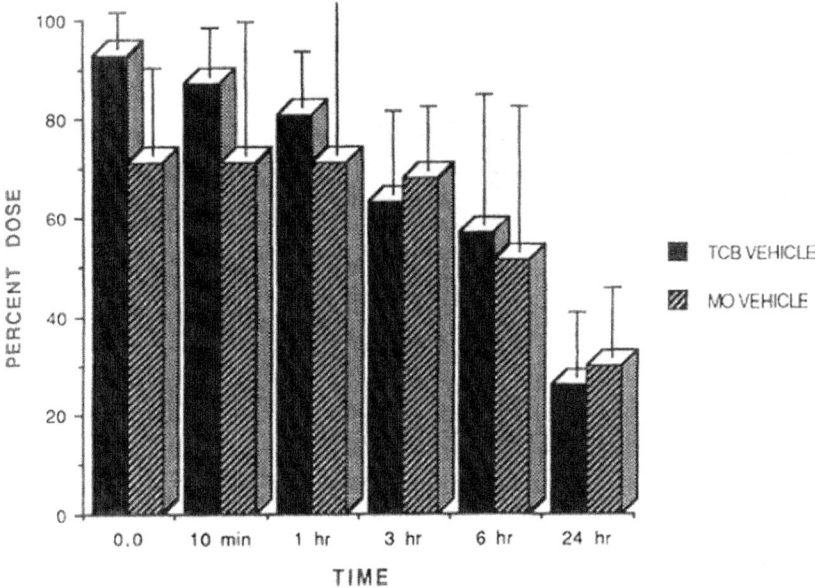

FIGURE 23.7 Polychlorinated biphenyls (PCBs) can be removed with soap and water; however, skin absorption of PCBs is high, and the chance to remove them from skin decreases with time. PCBs were applied to skin in either trichlorobenzene (TCB) or mineral oil (MO) vehicle.

The preceding discussion shows (Table 23.1) that there are two factors with in vivo skin decontamination. The first is the "rubbing effect" that removed loose surface stratum corneum due to natural skin desquamation. The second is the "solvent effect," which is related to chemical lipophilicity and was illustrated for glyphosate and alachlor.

23.2   IN VITRO DECONTAMINATION MODEL

In vitro skin mounted in diffusion cells can be decontaminated with solvents. A problem exists in that the mounted skin is fragile and cannot be rubbed, as naturally occurs with people washing their skin. Another in vitro technique that is easy to use for solvent efficiency in decontamination is with powdered human stratum corneum (PHSC). Figure 23.8 shows results when alachlor was added to PHSC and then partitioned against water only or against water with 10% and 50% soap. Alachlor stayed with the PHSC when partitioned against water-only; however, it readily partitioned to the solvents against 10% and 50% soap. These are the same confirming results shown in Figures 23.3, 23.5, and 23.6.

TABLE 23.1
In Vivo Skin Decontamination

1. *Rubbing effect*
    Removes "loose" surface stratum corneum
    "Loose" = natural desquamation
2. *Solvent effect*
    Water only
    Soap and water
    Related to chemical lipophilicity

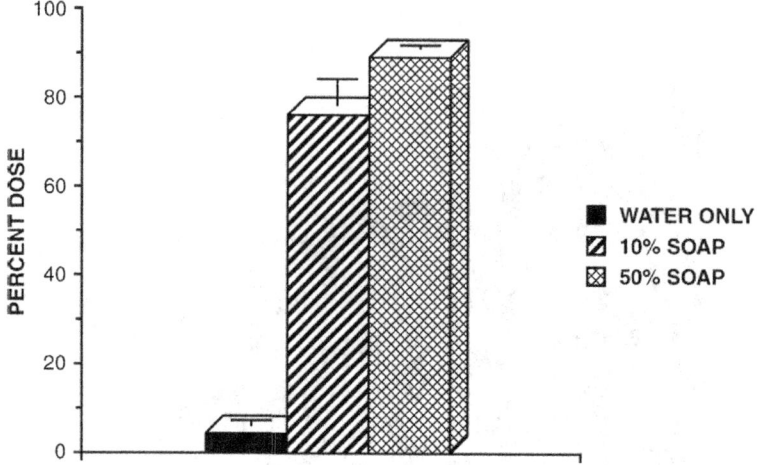

FIGURE 23.8 Alachlor was added to powdered human stratum corneum and then partitioned against water only or against water with 10% or 50% soap. Soap is required to remove alachlor, which is lipid soluble. This is a good in vitro model to screen potential decontamination vehicles.

The PHSC is made according to Wester et al. (4). It is then mixed with [^{14}C]alachlor in Lasso formulation, allowed to sit for 30 minutes, and then centrifuged. The alachlor, a lipid-soluble chemical, partitions ($90.3 \pm 1.2\%$) into the PHSC; $5.1 \pm 1.2\%$ remains in the Lasso formulation. Water-only wash (and subsequent centrifugation) removes only $4.6 \pm 1.3\%$ of the "bound" alachlor. However, when the bound alachlor–stratum corneum is washed with 10% and 50% soap and water (v/v), $77.2 \pm 5.7\%$ and $90.0 \pm 0.5\%$ of the alachlor is removed from the stratum corneum, respectively. Such a model would predict that alachlor in Lasso cannot be removed from the skin with water-only washing, but that the use of soap will decontaminate the skin. The "lipid" constituents of soap probably offer a more favorable partitioning environment for the alachlor.

23.3 EFFECTS OF OCCLUSION AND EARLY WASHING

Table 23.2 shows the effect of duration of occlusion on the rate of absorption of malathion (5). What is important from this table is that 9.6% of the applied malathion was absorbed during a zero-time duration. There was an immediate wash of the site of application with soap and water. Almost

TABLE 23.2
Effect of Duration of Occlusion on Percutaneous Absorption of Malathion in Humans

Duration (hr)	Absorption (%)
0[a]	9.6
0.5	7.3
1	12.7
2	16.6
4	24.2
8	38.8
24	6.8

[a] Immediate wash with soap and water.

TABLE 23.3

Short-Term Wash Recovery for Benzo[a]pyrene and DDT: 25-Minute Exposure vs. 24-Hour Exposure

	Percentage of dose		
Chemical	Short exposure (25 min), in vitro receptor fluid	Skin	Long exposure (24 hr), in vivo
Benzo[a]pyrene	0.00 ± 0.00	5.1 ± 2.1	51.0 ± 22.0
DDT	0.00 ± 0.00	16.7 ± 13.2	18.8 ± 9.4

Note: In vitro, the chemical in the acetone vehicle was dosed on human skin then washed with soap and water after a 25-minute period. The in vivo studies were 24-hour exposure with acetone vehicle dosing.

10% of the applied dose was not washed off, but, in fact, persisted on the skin through the wash procedure and was later absorbed into the body. Table 23.3 shows the short-term wash recovery for benzo[a]pyrene and DDT. Even when skin washing was initiated within 25 minutes of dosing, some benzo[a]pyrene and all of the DDT had absorbed sufficiently into the skin. Therefore, early washing after exposure is critical, but it may not provide complete decontamination (6).

Table 23.4 shows the effect of washing on the percutaneous absorption of hydrocortisone in a rhesus monkey. With a nonwashing sequence between dose applications, the percentage of the dose absorbed was $0.55 \pm 0.06\%$ of the applied dose. When a post-24-hour wash procedure was introduced, the percentage of dose absorbed statistically ($p < 0.05$) increased to $0.72 \pm 0.06\%$. The post-24-hour wash was supposed to remove the excess materials and thus decrease absorption. However, the soap-and-water wash hydrated the skin, and the rate of absorption of hydrocortisone increased.

Table 23.5 shows dermal washing efficiency for PCBs in the guinea pig. When 42% PCB was applied to guinea pig skin and immediately washed, only 58.9% of the applied dose could be

TABLE 23.4

Effect of Washing on Percutaneous Absorption of Hydrocortisone in Rhesus Monkey

Treatment	Absorption (% ± SD)
No wash	0.55 ± 0.06
Post-24-hr wash[a]	0.72 ± 0.06

[a] Soap-and-water wash.

TABLE 23.5

Dermal Wash Efficiency for Polychlorinated Biphenyls (PCBs) in Guinea Pig

PCB (%)	Wash Time[a]	Dose Removed (% ± SD)
42	Immediate	58.9 ± 7.5
42	Post-24-hr	0.9 ± 0.2
54	Post-24-hr	19.7 ± 5.5

[a] Wash procedure: twice with water, twice with acetone, and twice with water.

removed. The rest of the material was available for subsequent percutaneous absorption. When 42% PCB was applied to guinea pig skin and 24 hours later the site of application was washed, only 0.9% of the applied dose was removed. Thus, all the applied PCB was available for absorption or had already been absorbed into the body. When 54% PCB was applied to guinea pig skin and washed 24 hours post-application, 19.7% of the applied dose was removed. Thus, with 54% PCB, 80% of the applied dose could not be removed or had already been absorbed into the body. Subsequent examination of the rate of absorption of PCB showed that most was absorbed into the body. This study illustrates that the hypothesis that washing or bathing and any other application of water will remove all material from skin is wrong. Substantivity (the nonspecific absorption of material to skin) can be a strong force.

Figure 23.9 shows the percentage of dose absorbed per hour of an herbicide in the rhesus monkey (7). At 24 hours post-application, the site of absorption was washed with water and acetone sequentially. The time curve shows a "washing-in effect" following the 24-hour post-application wash. Thus, as we saw previously with hydrocortisone, there is definitely a washing-in effect. The application of water and acetone changed the barrier properties of skin and caused an increase in the rate of absorption of this herbicide. Moody and Nadeau (8) also recently showed the washing-in effect for 2,4-dichlorophenoxyacetic acid amine during in vitro percutaneous absorption studies in rat, guinea pig, and human skin.

It is generally assumed that pesticides and other chemicals can be easily removed from the skin. Another series of experiments by Feldman and Maibach (5) was designed to determine just how effective the removal is in terms of decreasing percutaneous absorption. The experimental variable was the removal of applied pesticide in different groups of subjects at varying times. Decontamination was attempted by a two-minute wash with soap and hot water. Data are presented in Table 23.6. Absorption of azodrin at a concentration of 4 µg/cm^2 on the human forearm was 14.7% if the site was not washed for 24 hours. Washing after four hours decreased absorption to

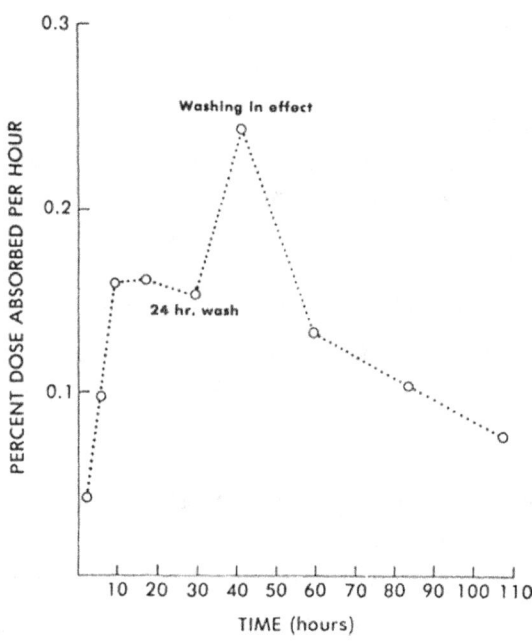

FIGURE 23.9   Effect of washing on absorption. Washing at 24 hours enhanced absorption, as shown by the peak effect at 48 hours.

TABLE 23.6
Effect of Washing on Percent Penetration

Compound, Dose (µg/cm2), and Site	Minutes				Hours				
	1	5	15	30	1	2	4	8	24
Soap and water									
Azodrin, 4, arm			2.3				8.6		14.7
Ethion, 4, arm			1.6				2.9		3.3
Guthion, 4, arm									
Malathion									
4, arm	1.2		4.3	4.5	6.1	8.3	12.1		6.8
40, arm			4.7				6.8		
400, arm			1.4		2.0		4.7		
Parathion									
4, arm	2.8		6.7		8.4		8.0	15.8	8.6
40, arm			3.1				6.9		9.5
400, arm			2.2		2.3		4.2		4.8
4, forehead	8.4		7.1	12.2	10.5	20.1	27.7		36.3
4, palm		6.2	13.6	13.3	11.7	9.4	7.7		11.8
Lindane, 4, arm		1.7	1.8	4.2	3.9	6.7	5.1		9.3
Baygon, 4, arm	1.2		4.7	4.5	4.7	11.8	15.5	11.3	19.6
2,4-D									
4, arm	0.5		0.7	1.8	1.2	3.7	3.7		5.8
40, arm			0.7				2.8		
Rubbing alcohol									
Malathion, 4, arm			17.7		5.8		16.8		
Parathion, 4, arm			8.2		7.0		10.3		

8% of the dose. Washing after only 15 minutes decreased penetration, but still 2.3% of the dose was absorbed. With similar experimental variables, ethion washing in 15 minutes decreased the penetration from the 24-hour time period from only 3.3% to 1.6%. Malathion decrease from the 24-hour to 15-minute wash was from only 6.8% to 4.3%.

A similar relationship was maintained when the applied concentration was greatly increased. For instance, at a concentration of 4 µg/cm^2 of parathion, the penetration after washing at 24 hours was 8.6%; this was only decreased to 6.7% by washing in 15 minutes.

The effect of the anatomic site was also studied. On the palm, the penetration of parathion was 11.8% with washing at 24 hours. There was no significant decrease in penetration washing in 15 minutes; in fact, there was a slight increase. Thus, the very potent pesticide parathion absorbs into skin despite washing and is absorbed into the body.

Experiments with rubbing alcohol had similar results. When used with malathion, alcohol washing at four hours allowed 16.8% penetration and at 15 minutes 17.7%. Penetration with parathion at four hours was 10.3% and at 15 minutes, 8.2%. These data suggest that a careful examination be made of recommendations given to consumers and workers about when they can remove these substances from their skin and what materials should be used. It is obvious that protection from washing and bathing is not what had been predicted.

It was questioned whether a whole-body exposure to a solvent such as water might not be more effective at removing pesticides. For this reason, a group of subjects was showered four hours after application instead of being washed locally with soap and water. The data for

TABLE 23.7

Effect of Shower on Different Types of Removal at Four Hours

Compound	Absorption (%) after Shower[a]		
	Arm	Forehead	Palm
Malathion	8.8 (12.1)	32.7	7.2
Parathion	16.5 (9.0)	41.9 (27.7)	13.4 (7.7)
Baygon	9.9 (15.5)	20.5	8.7

[a] Values in parentheses: after washing.

malathion, parathion, and Baygon are in Table 23.7. The shower was no more (and perhaps less) effective than the local application of soap and water. Showering does not appear to be a solution to the problem.

23.4 TRADITIONAL SOAP-AND-WATER WASH AND EMERGENCY SHOWER

In the home and workplace, decontamination of a chemical from skin is traditionally done with soap-and-water wash; some workplaces may have an emergency water shower. It has been assumed that these procedures are effective, yet workplace illness and even death occur from chemical contamination. Water or soap-and-water washing may not be the most effective means of skin decontamination, particularly for fat-soluble materials. This study was undertaken to help determine whether there are more effective means of removing methylene bisphenyl isocyanate (MDI), a potent contact sensitizer, from the skin. MDI is an industrial chemical for which skin decontamination using traditional soap-and-water washing and nontraditional polypropylene glycol, a polyglycol-based cleaner (DTAM), and corn oil was done in vivo in the rhesus monkey over eight hours. Water and soap-and-water (5% and 50% soap) washes were partially effective in the first hour, removing 51% to 69% of the applied dose. However, decontamination fell to 40% to 52% at four hours and 29% to 46% at eight hours (Figure 23.10). Thus, the majority of MDI was not removed by traditional soap-and-water wash; skin tape stripping after wash confirmed that

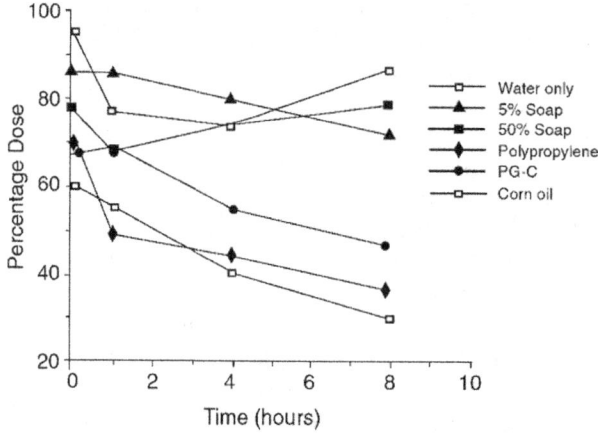

FIGURE 23.10 Mean percent applied dose of methylene bis phenyl isocyanate (MDI) removed with designated decontamination procedure at designated time period. Water and soap-and-water are the least effective, especially at four and eight hours.

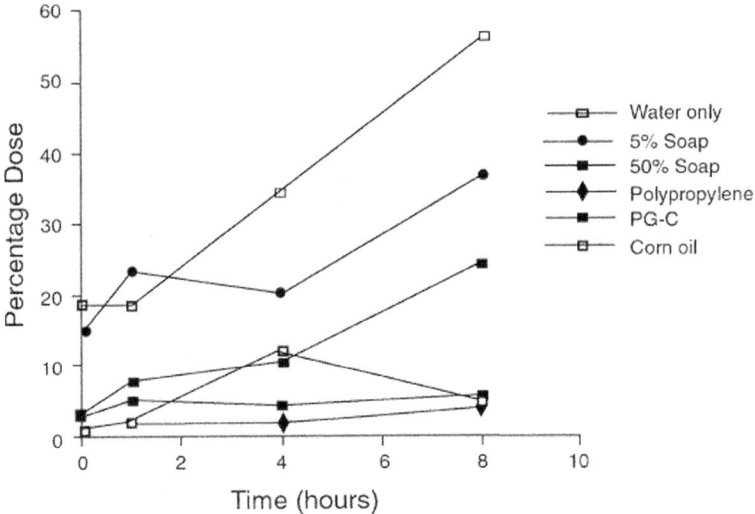

FIGURE 23.11 Mean percent applied dose of methylene bis phenyl isocyanate (MDI) removed by cellophane tape stripping following wash decontamination. This confirms that the MDI not removed by water and soap-and-water washes was still present on the skin.

MDI was still on the skin (Figure 23.11). In contrast, polypropylene glycol, DTAM, and corn oil removed 68% to 86% of the MDI in the first hour, 74% to 79% at four hours, and 72% to 86% at eight hours. Statistically, polypropylene glycol, DTAM, and corn oil were all better ($p < 0.05$) than soap and water at four hours and eight hours after dose application. These results indicated that traditional soap-and-water wash and the emergency water shower are relatively ineffective at removing MDI from the skin. More effective decontamination procedures, as shown here, are available.

23.5   CONCLUSION

Substantivity has been defined as the nonspecific absorption of material from skin. It is obvious that the standard washing procedures do not always readily remove materials from skin. How important is this in terms of occupational exposure? Kazen et al. (9) did hexane hand rinsings on occupationally exposed people. They analyzed the rinsings by electron capture and flame photometric/gas–liquid chromatography for pesticide residues to determine whether or not these chemicals persisted on the skin long after exposure. Chlordane and dieldrin apparently persisted on the hands of a former pest control operator for at least two years. Methoxychlor, captan, and malathion persisted for at least seven days on the hands of a fruit and vegetable grower. Parathion was found on the hands of one man two months after his last known contact with this pesticide. Endosulfan, dichlorodiphenyl-dichloroethane (DDD), kelthane, decthal, trithijon, imidan, and guthion have persisted on the hands of some exposed workers from less than a day to 112 days after exposure (10–15).

In conclusion, washing is generally good, but it does not prevent penetration of some chemicals. Surely, the understanding of the mechanism and the development of more efficient removal systems must be a high priority for research.

REFERENCES

1. Wester RC, Melendres J, Sarason R, McMaster J, Maibach HI. Glyphosate skin binding, absorption, residual tissue distribution, and skin decontamination. Fundam Appl Toxicol 1991; 16:725–732.
2. Wester RC, Melendres J, Maibach HI. *In vivo* percutaneous absorption of alachlor in Rhesus monkey. J Toxicol Environ Health 1992; 36:1–2.

3. Wester RC, Bucks DAW, Maibach HI. Polychlorinated biphenyls (PCBs): dermal absorption, systemic elimination, and dermal wash efficiency. J Toxicol Environ Health 1984; 12:511–519.

4. Wester RC, Mobayen M, Maibach HI. *In vivo* and *in vitro* absorption and binding to powdered stratum corneum as methods to evaluate skin absorption of environmental chemical contaminants from ground and surface water. J Toxicol Environ Health 1987; 21:367–374.

5. Feldmann RJ, Maibach HI. Systemic absorption of pesticides through the skin of man. Occupational Exposure to Pesticides: Report to the Federal Working Group on Pest Management from the Task Group on Occupation Exposure to Pesticides. 1974; Appendix B, 120–127.

6. Wester RC, Maibach HI, Bucks DAW, Sedik L, Melenderes J, Liao C, Di Zio S. Percutaneous absorption of [^{14}C]-DDT and [^{14}C]-benzo(a)pyrene from soil. Fundam Appl Toxicol 1990; 15:510–5106.

7. Wester RC, Maibach HI. Advances in percutaneous absorption. In: Drill VA, Lazar P, eds. Cutanous Toxicity. New York: Raven Press, 1983:29–40.

8. Moody RP, Nadeau B. *In vitro* dermal absorption of two commercial formulations of 2,4-dichlorophen-oxyacetic acid dimethylamide (2,4-D amine) in rat, guinea pig and human skin. Toxicol in vitro 1997; 11:251–262.

9. Kazen C, Bloomer A, Welch R, Oudbier A, Price H. Persistence of pesticides on the hands of some occupationally exposed people. Arch Environ Health 1974; 29:315–318.

10. Geno PW, Camann DE, Harding JH, Villalobos K, Lewis RG. Handwipe sampling and analysis procedure for the measurement of dermal contact with pesticides. Arch Environ Contam Toxicol 1996; 30:132–138.

11. Hewitt PG, Hotchkiss PG, Caldwell J. Decontamination procedures after in vitro topical exposure of human and rat skin to 4,4^l-methylenebis[2-chloroaniline] and 4,4^l-methyle-nedianiline. Fundam Appl Toxicol 1995; 26:91–98.

12. Kintz P, Tracqui A, Morgin P. Accidental death caused by the absorption of 2,4-dichlor-ophenol through the skin. Arch Toxicol 1992; 66:298–299.

13. Merrick MV, Simpson JD, Liddell S. Skin decontamination—A comparison of four methods. Br J Radiol 1982; 55:317–318.

14. Wester RC, Noonan PK, Maibach HI. Frequency of application of percutaneous absorption of hydrocortisone. Arch Dermatol 1997; 113:620–622.

15. Wester RC, Hui X, Landry T, Maibach HI. *In vivo* skin decontamination of methylene bisphenyl isocyanate (MDI): soap and water ineffective compared to polypropylene glycol, polyglycol-based cleanser, and corn oil. Toxicol Sci 1998; 48:1–4.

24 Skin Decontamination 2020 Update

Annick Roul
Ministry of Interior, Paris, France

Howard I. Maibach
University of California, San Francisco, California

CONTENTS

24.1   INTRODUCTION

Decontamination, aimed at eliminating the contaminant and its human consequences, should be as rapid as possibly for the most efficient process. We propose approaches for operational and societal objectives depending on the (1) hazardous chemical nature, (2) its persistence and cross contamination risk, and (3) event circumstances e.g. location and numbers involved.

Best practices in skin decontamination may emerge from such information, including a decision support tool to reach the lowest level of chemical concentration as a "chemical no contaminant level."

Time and concentration of decontamination solutions are necessary to reach efficient skin decontamination. Therefore products mustn't irritate skin to be operational.

24.2   CONTAMINATION

24.2.1   DEFINITION

Contamination results from chemical forms, such as vapor, steam, aerosol, dust, liquid, or solid contaminants, while gaseous products are considered noncontaminants because of their form. Gas mixed with water or other solvents, such as aerosols, become contaminants.

24.2.2   CONTAMINATION

The first, or direct, contamination results from direct contact with the hazardous substance. Secondary decontamination, also called cross contamination, results when an uncontaminated person, surface, or piece of equipment contacts them.

24.2.3   SKIN CONTAMINATION

Contaminants, i.e. liquids and solids, spread on the *stratum corneum* (SC) and diffuse through the layers; anatomic pathways may favor penetration and accumulation of chemicals, depending on their characteristics such as physicochemical properties (log P, hydrophilicity, lipophilicity, molecular weight [MW]), as outlined in tables 1 to 24 of the thesis (1). The complex heterogeneous skin structure provides several penetration routes through SC barrier: the intercellular, intracellular, and follicular pathways.

Penetration mechanisms deal with the control of the intercellular penetration of lipids and through skin appendages (follicular pathway) that appears to contribute more than previously thought (2).

24.2.4 PERCUTANEOUS PENETRATION

Although the SC plays a critical role in the function of the permeability barrier, there are many structures and components that interact before entering the body (3). The influence of water content on the cutaneous permeation of exogenous molecules is of primary importance in physiology and pharmacology (4). Sebum, electrolytes, and cutaneous flora form a relatively simple ecosystem that protects the skin. Chemicals able to dissolve this milieu diffuse through the SC. Kinetic transfer is boosted, according to the rule of five, especially for molecules of small size, low melting temperature, and appropriate partition coefficient (5).

Molecules passively diffuse through the SC, described as a brick-and-mortar model (6). Penetration pathways are essentially intercellular and intracellular. Penetration between SC corneocytes is the path by which most compounds penetrate the intracellular way (proteins), while the lipid bilayer intercellular route favors lipophilic compounds. The intrafollicular pathway is considered a nonpredominant route (7).

Systemic effects resulting from passage across the viable epidermis and dermis are recognizable, and the severity of toxidromes depends on chemicals factors (dose, physicochemical characteristics).

24.2.5 SKIN CONTAMINANTS

According to persistence and lethality, skin contaminant chemicals are arranged by families (see tables 1 to 24 in [1]). Variables affecting agent diffusion such as contamination time (residence time surface), temperature, and concentration (surface density per unit of surface area) are essential parameters to estimate potential effects. Dermal penetration increases its duration of contact.

Some chemicals may cause, by dermal absorption, inhalation, cutaneous, and ocular burns exacerbating systemic effects. Therefore, medical and/or surgical treatment may be required to complement decontamination (8, 9). Toxidromes must be considered after chemical events to provide treatment and therapeutics in case of systemic effects (10). In emergency situations, chemicals are considered for short-term toxicity and secondary contamination and the remaining capacity should be considered for long-term contamination risk. Persistence of the chemical agent, in the absence of active decontamination, presents a risk due to remaining capacity (11).

24.2.6 PRIORITIES AND OPPORTUNITIES

Skin decontamination after exposure to contaminants e.g. chemical warfare agents (CWAs), dangerous toxic industrial chemicals (TICs), or fine particles is a priority to save lives from terrorism, criminal attack, accidents, or accidental work exposure. Since the usage of chemical weapons caused as many deaths during wars, not only defense departments and but authorities exhort scientists to explore data on opportunity and risks of remaining contaminants in case of inefficient or inappropriate decontamination processes. The detection of low-level chemical contamination should be an indicator of decontamination efficiency and a way for further studies (12).

24.3 PREVENTION AND PROTECTION

Time post-exposure remains a key factor to prevent health effects. Saving time leads to reduced contact time between the skin and chemical after exposure; therefore individual and collective protection is essential. Collective protection is essentially based on three main principles: time, screen, and distance.

Personal protective equipment (PPE) appropriate for the risk is absolutely required before initiating rescue efforts and working closely with contaminated casualties (13). Security level is defined by the rules applicable in respective countries (14).

24.4 DECONTAMINATION

24.4.1 Definition

Decontamination usually consists of physical removal or neutralization of hazardous contaminants from personnel or material. New technologies suggest both removing and degrading agents. But washing with water and cleaning with or without surfactants are clearly the most intuitive decontamination methods.

Decontamination is an essential phase to avoid cross contamination, stop chemical percutaneous penetration, and save lives.

Decontamination success depends in particular upon the properties of the agent, environmental conditions, and skin surface. Both chemistry and engineering are required in decontamination design (15).

Instituting decontamination by universal methods is the priority, but an appropriate decontamination process should be set up immediately after contaminant identification to better target an acceptable level of health protection.

24.4.2 Decontaminants

Knowledge of the properties of the agent in decontamination, also called the decontaminant, are essential to preserve the skin and avoid percutaneous penetration. This highlights that the versatile decontaminants, such as dry sorbents, must be used quickly before an appropriate specific or technical decontamination (16).

Skin decontaminants must not be corrosive to prevent damage by the decontamination processes. Therefore decontamination of eyes (17) and wounds are treated specifically in the first aid of medical care.

24.4.3 Essential Decontaminant Properties

The decontaminant's characteristics such as solubility, stability in a medium, reactivity, nature, and lifespan of its breakdown products must be considered. Temperature, concentration, and pH may influence those parameters (1). An optimum medium dissolves the agents and promotes the desired reaction (18).

24.5 MANAGING DECONTAMINATION

24.5.1 Self-Care Decontamination

It is essential to prevent contamination by developing clean habits for citizens and rescuers, regarding awareness and contamination avoidance. Self-care includes (1) casualties moving away from the contamination source, (2) wiping contaminant off exposed skin and hair, and (3) disrobing to minimize chemical penetration into skin and thereby limit contaminant dose (19).

24.5.2 Assisted Decontamination

This concept occurs from practical and operational observations. In emergency situations, we tend to help each other. This instinctive reflex needs to be consolidated and developed. Assisted decontamination of chemical agents could serve as a forum for advanced teaching and learning and facilitate development in the emerging field of decontaminants. Therefore, some simple and fast manipulations could be taught as collaborative techniques from the earliest age.

24.5.3 Disrobing

Disrobing, also called cut out, is proposed in every case and is widely recognized among scientists. In contrast there will be a delay between initial chemical exposure and decontamination setup for civilians compared to the military response (20). It's a challenge for authorities to reduce the time required to deploy decontamination processes after chemical exposure and limit potential health impacts to citizens. Removing clothing is a simple and highly effective action to remove external contaminants in the first minutes after the incident. Disrobing can remove 80% to 90% of contamination and specfically the external layer of clothes (21). Disrobing needs an ethical approach which must be organized at the crime scene, in the hospitals for emergencies, and widely advised to individuals returning home after exposure.

24.5.4 FIRST DECONTAMINATION

The first decontamination process, also called emergency or early decontamination, must be immediately set up, preferably before the identification of the hazardous substance. In order to save victims and avoid cross contamination, first decontamination must be considered when contamination is suspected by the emergence of toxidromes e.g. clinical symptoms of vesicants, such as blistering and swelling, whereas cholinergic symptoms e.g. copious secretions and respiratory muscle paralysis are indicative of nerve agent exposure. This essential process of early decontamination allows a rapid setup of medical countermeasures (22); therefore, versatile decontaminants able to adsorb the largest part of hazardous chemicals may be used as the first line.

24.5.5 SECONDARY DECONTAMINATION

Secondary or technical decontamination may complete the first decontamination. In some cases, gross mass water decontamination could be required on the crime scene to rapidly aid all exposed people.

If first decontamination has been performed following a gross mass water decontamination process based on the channeling of water from firefighting trucks, a secondary decontamination may be set up in mobile units, providing mass showering facilities that allow more thorough decontamination with warm or lukewarm water and soap, and bleach if necessary (23). Caution should be practiced when skin is washed, as the wash-in (W-I) effect may increase local cutaneous and systemic toxicity (24).

Experimental data on various chemicals are urgently needed. In any case, decontaminants applied onto the skin must be harmlessness and efficient.

24.5.6 DECONTAMINATION CONTROL

Measuring the efficiency of decontamination procedures towards chemical agents, breakdown products, or degraded chemicals needs to be evaluated. Some techniques, such as skin wipes, are useful to measure toxicant levels on the skin surface, predict dermal absorption, and measure the potential systemic contamination level (25, 26).

The efficiency of Fuller earth towards 4-cyanophenol, as a chemical agent, was assessed ex vivo (27). Studies based on the application of nontoxic chemicals, also called simili, to measure the efficiency of water shower ladder pipe systems, underlined that under certain conditions, showering in the presence of contaminated clothing resulted in the transfer of chemicals to the skin surface (28). Quantitative comparison of different decontamination protocols were carried out by the topical application of an ultraviolet (UV) fluorescent compound onto human volunteers. This highlighted that performance of protocols is necessary to assess efficiency. Improved decontamination procedures is a priority to manage short- and long-term chemical incidents (29). Low-level chemicals require technologies able to detect low concentrations in the order at least of parts per million (ppm).

24.6 DESIGN OF THE DECONTAMINATION PROCESS

Decontamination methods could be developed following various concepts. They can be ranked in three categories: (1) physical removal, (2) washing, and (3) neutralization ranging from the simplest to the most elaborate process in reference to the mechanism of action described for the methods.

Highly specific and advanced techniques such as nanoparticle technologies, chelation, enzymatic actions, and gel formulations may offer opportunities to complement conventional techniques. Some of the devices physically remove, neutralize, and the degrade contaminants (three in one).

24.6.1 PHYSICAL REMOVAL

Physical removal consists of the mechanical action of removing a chemical agent from the skin. This is performed by adsorptive powders, free or fixed on a substrate, but also by wipes brushes and some impregnated adsorptive tissues or plain adsorbent. This process remains conventional and essentially dry.

Dry decontamination uses adsorptive properties of powders or fabrics to passively remove contaminants from the skin surface and is especially effective for liquid contaminants.

24.6.1.1 Adsorbent Powders

Adsorptive powders are largely used in decontamination due to their specific surface area ($m^2 \cdot g^{-1}$) leading to highly adsorptive chemicals. Bleaching powders, mostly combined with adsorbing materials, provide the basis for skin decontaminantion (30). Nevertheless, powders are inappropriate for decontamination of mucous membranes (eyes) and wounds and may cause serious damage. Fuller earth, carbonaceous, activated or not, resins polymers mixture (XE-555), and activated alumina (A-200) are absorbents with the capacity to encapsulate toxic agents (31).

24.6.1.2 Activated Alumina A-200/Sorbent Decon System (SDS)

Activated alumina is a potentially efficient adsorbent material for some chemicals because of its high adsorption capacity and removal efficiency at the implementation levels (32). The Sorbent Decon System is made of 65% aluminium oxide (33).

24.6.1.3 Fuller Earth (FE)

Fuller earth powder, an alumina silicate that is chemically inert, abundant in nature, and known for its adsorptive properties (35), provides decontamination opportunities for chemical, biological, radiological, and nuclear agents. Since prehistory there are indications that clays mixed with water have been used to cure wounds and soothe irritation as a method of skin cleansing (35). This might have been due to their mimicking animals e.g. pachyderms, many of which instinctively use minerals for these purposes. FE, recommended for skin decontamination, is provided as a powder in containers and prefilled gloves and may be applied onto skin after short chemical exposure (36). Clay minerals, consisting of hydrous layers of silicates, can be studied in tersm of the function of their structure and composition, introducing it as a classification support tool (37). More than 20 years later, FE powder is, among other options, considered as the reference (38) in skin decontamination for mass casualties, as described in official French and European documents, and recognized as exellent for overall casualty decontaminant i.e. adsorbent for CWA (39). FE has been assessed ex vivo for its adsorption capacity and decontamination efficiency, comparing four different formulations in skin decontamination (27).

24.6.1.4 American Kit M291 – Carbonaceous Resins XE-555

A solid sorbent, the M291 skin decontamination kit consists of six foil-packaged, nonwoven fiber pads filled with 2.8 g of XE-555 carbonaceous resins with a total water content of 25 wt%. This nontoxic sorbent of high adsorption capacity was formulated for use where rapid decontamination is essential (40). Ambergard is a nonirritating skin decontaminant proposed by the U.S. Army for soldiers in battlefied situations (27, 28) and depends on competition between an ion-exchange resin and adsorption within the carboneous resin. XE-555 efficiency results may differ. Resins, made of a styrene/divinyl benzene copolymer, are composed of a high surface area carbonized macroreticular styrene/divinylbenzene resin (the sorptive resin), a strong acid (sulfonic acid group) cation-exchange resin, and a strong base (tetralkylammonium hydroxide groups) anion-exchange resin. The sorptive resin rapidly absorbs liquid agents, and the reactive resins promote hydrolysis of physisorbed agents (18). Acidic and basic groups in Ambergard XE-555 resin promote the destruction of trapped chemical agents. The M291 SDK weighs 45 grams and measures $112 \times 112 \times 36$ mm, which is suggested for a coverage area of 1300 cm^2 at a challenge level of 2.5 g.m^{-2} of agent per individual decontamination packet and is used to decontaminate skin following exposure or contamination to liquid chemical agents (41). The M291 SDK is regulated by the Food & Drug Administration (FDA) as a medical device.

24.6.1.5   Activated Charcoal

Molecules such as drugs or poisons adsorbed onto the huge surface area of 800 to 1200 m^2.g^{-1} or more with superactivated charcoals 2800 to 3500 m^{2}g^{-1} (42) are held there by van der Walls forces (physiosorption). For some substances, this adsorption may provide a tightly bound chemisorption (4443)

24.6.2   ADSORBENT GLOVES

24.6.2.1   Adsorbent Glove FiberTect

This adsorption filter material provides high adsorption capacity (2.5 times its weight in liquid contaminant) and low breakthrough (25). FiberTect, a three-layer, inert, flexible, drapeable, nonwoven composite substrate is proposed for absorbing and adsorbing CWAs, TICs, and pesticides. The three layers of material include a top and bottom fabric and a center of fibrous activated carbon that is needle-punched into a composite fabric. Top and bottom layers (polyester and unbleached raw cotton) provide structural coherence, improving mechanical strength and abrasion resistance, while the center layer acts as the active decontaminant. The inner adsorbent layer, made of activated carbon (ACN-K), whose precursor material is phenolic carbon, is a nonwoven fabric structure (44). FiberTect does not present a health or safety hazard to personnel; the patented technology (US7, 516,525), with an indefinite shelf-life, is self-contained and packaged for easy use, storage, and transport.

24.6.2.2   Fuller Earth Glove

An emergency glove for decontamination, based on FE adsorptive properties, which was expected in the case of liquid contamination on skin or equipment was developed by French army in 1971. The patent for an individual decontamination apparatus, developed as a kit for military, contains an absorbent mitten capable of absorbing toxic agents and was granted in 1991 (45).

This type of powdered FE glove could present some disadvantages e.g. (1) a cloud of powder with the risk of contamination transfer, (2) glove form, and (3) adsorptive powder without destruction of the adsorbed toxic.[1]

24.6.3   BRUSHING/WIPING

Tools such as brushes, sponges, and wipes may be used in skin decontamination with adapted processes to limit spreading and skin damage. Wipers require minimal training and provide immediate decontamination capability and are effective in removing physical contaminants; therefore, they may systematically be used.

Wiping, FiberTect, industrial wipes, M291 kit, and FE prefilled gloves are essential tools in decontamination.

24.6.3.1   Wipes

24.6.3.1.1   *Impregnated Wipers*

CeBeR Multi-Purpose Wipe (CeBeR MPW), developed by Steris for the U.S. Army, may be used to avoid cross contamination (46). Those wipes, containing isopropyl alcohol and emollient, are recognized to facilitate physical removal (10-year shelf-life) and are intended for first responder and government use. It is a self-contained, low-cost chemical decontamination wipe, simple to use and carry, which has been proven efficiency for the removal of chemical contamination from surfaces.

24.6.3.1.2 Nonwoven Composite Pad

The nonwoven composite pad, formed of a three-layered, nonwoven composite pad, was developed at Hobbs Bonded Fibers (Waco, TX), using a manufacturing-scale needle-punching line, viscose fibers, polyester fibers, and nonwoven activated carbon fabric (33). The viscose fibers in the top were single-needle-punched (top to bottom) to provide liquid absorption capability. The middle porous activated carbon nonwoven fabric serves as the adsorbent. The bottom polyester fabric, prepared by single needle punching, like the top fabric, enhances the overall structural integrity and strength of the composite. These pads are robust and sufficiently flexible to conform to difficult shapes and spaces, absorb large quantities of liquids, adsorb toxic vapors, and are compatible with a wide range of toxic or hazardous chemicals, including bleach. Nowadays, composite nonwoven materials, attractive and versatile, are developed for a variety of applications, including hygiene and medicine. This technology should provide an opportunity in the decontamination of wounded or injured skin (24).

24.6.3.1.3 Wipe Spray Wipe

The decontamination process is broken down into three steps, commonly referred to as (1) wipe, with the initial physical removal; (2) spray, by application of a detergent as a decontamination solution (hypochlorite calcium, bleach solution, and/or dichoroisocyanurate); and (3) a wipe for the final removal and drying (47). Information is derived from the decontamination process guide and quick reference card set ©2016 Jeffrey J. Berrigan. The WSP, Wipe Spray Wipe, decontamination process is utilized with the permission of Strategic Response Solutions, LLC.

24.6.3.2 Managing Wipe Selection

Many common items that are considered absorbent demonstrate some degree of affinity for both water- and oil-based substances; their results may be presented in absorbency (grams of water or oil absorbed per grams of test product) (20).

Domestic wipes do not represent the best choice to adsorb hazardous chemicals and are limited to bleach solutions. Wipes as decontaminants require high technology for hazardous chemicals.

24.6.4 NEUTRALIZATION AND DEGRADATION TECHNIQUES

Neutralization is treated here because of the combination of support, adsorption, and degradation. The combined action of adsorption, neutralization, and degradation successfully destroys chemicals and represents a major issue in skin decontamination. A high-technology program targeting decontaminants able to treat the whole problem of contamination with a three-in-one solution is the goal.

Elsewhere, a major drawback has been identified with the possible inhalation of such adsorptive powders, depending essentially on their particle size (48). Therefore, skin decontaminants, which lack dangerous effects to mucous membranes and wounds, are being developed such as specific technology based on metal oxide nanoparticles (NPs), cerium oxide (CeO_2) NPs, enzymes, or specific chemical e.g. oximes for nerve agents. New generations of decontaminants, metal oxides NPs, and CeO_2 NPs in water degrade organophosphorous compounds e.g. nerve agents and pesticides (49, 50). Metal oxide nanoparticles (51), providing high surface area, allows adsorption and simultaneous destruction of toxic chemicals—1 g can have a surface area exceeding 200 m^2.

24.6.4.1 Metal Oxide Nanoparticles

Cerium oxide, CeO_2, is known for its biomedical application as a reactive sorbent for the degradation of organophosphates such as parathion and chlorpyrifos in solvent media (heptane, acetonitrile) under ambient conditions. Formulation of NPs (thickening aqueous dispersions of CeO_2) were tested for skin decontamination with encouraging results (50).

MgO, Al_2O_3, and CaO, nanosized particles, are promising potential reactive sorbent materials due to to their high surface area, strong adsorbability, and potential reactivity toward CWAs. Those NPs remove the agent rapidly from the contaminated surfaces, degrade them in situ, and hence render them nontoxic (52). If degradation may present clear benefits, we must be careful with their use on skin (53). Nanosized particles of MgO, Al_2O_3, and CaO, with at least one dimension reaching 100 nanometers or less have been developed for skin decontamination (54), but the regulation of NPs has to be considered with respect to the rules for health (55).

24.6.4.2   Magnesium Oxide Nanoparticles

Single metallic oxide, MgO, nanocrystals are highly reactive and adsorb, neutralize, and degrade chemical agents. MgO nanoparticles with sizes ranging from 10 to 30 nm have been incorporated in a polyvalent device DEC'POL.

Whereas nanosized particles of MgO are not recommended for a cutaneous application, incorporated in the structure of a "superabsorbent material," the DEC'POL device is proposed for skin decontamination by transfer, neutralization, and degradation due to its active material (56).

24.6.4.3   Cerium Oxide Water Formulation

Cerium oxide, CeO_2, is known for its biomedical application as a reactive sorbent for the degradation of nerve agents (57) and organophosphates such as parathion and chlorpyrifos in solvent media (heptane, acetonitrile) under ambient conditions. The formulation of NPs with thickening aqueous dispersions of CeO_2 were tested for skin decontamination with encouraging results (49, 50).

24.6.4.4   Dermal Decon Gel

Dermal Decon (DD) gel is a formulation created after advances in knowledge in chemical partition binding to stratum corneum proteins, lipids, and hydration effects (2625). DD gel, a rapidly drying gel with a peel-off film, is prepared with ingredients such as carboxy methyl cellulose for its water capacity adsorption, Lutrol for binding chemical properties, Kollidon SR for binding and absorption for polar and nonpolar compounds, and FE as an adsorbing agent. Decontamination efficiency has been compared to several decontaminants (58). The main advantages are that massage is unnecessary, and additional cleanup is unnecessary compared to the Reactive Skin Decontamination Lotion (RSDL). DD gel has been comparaed on hairy and nonhairy skin after 30 minutes dermal exposure to paraoxon (an organophosphorous pesticide). DD gel is proposed for absorbance, binding, extraction, and detoxification in skin decontamination. Acute toxicity has not been studied, but its components are used in pharmaceutical or cosmeceutical industries or as decontaminating absorbance with no or low toxicity (59).

24.6.5   Suspensions and Emulsions

24.6.5.1   Suspensions

Succesful decontamination of FE suspension, enabling a dramatic reduction of skin contamination after a brief exposure scenario, appears to be rapid and reliable and should be formulated in a new device ready to use for self-decontamination (27).

24.6.5.2   Pickering Emulsions

Pickering emulsions, i.e. solid-stabilized emulsions, containing silica (S-PE) or Fuller earth (FE-PE), with the determination based on the high specific surface area (63).

24.6.6   Washing

24.6.6.1   Water

Water decontamination is largely used in mass decontamination and has optionally added detergents or bleach solutions. Wash and rinse may be set up quickly and rinse a large part of the involved person's hair, body, and skin. The main advantage of this raw material (water) is the speed with which it can be initiated by the first responders using fire apparatus that is generally readily available. First responders are organized to prepare a channel of water as a ladder pipe system, with the major drawback being the unheated water (20, 28). Water is used in mobile units of decontamination (MUDs) and may be heated with adapted systems; the major drawback is that installation on the crime scene needs time (around 30 minutes), even for trained firefighters. Temperature and time to shower are standardized to an optimal decontamination method (20, 61). It is relevant to consider the issues after decontamination by water. Mechanical washing may more or less remove hydrophilic viscous products; however, viscous hydrophobic substances are more difficult to remove. Water helps with the physical removal of chemicals and hydrolysis, i.e. sulfur mustard (18). Water can exercerbate skin lesions caused by sulfur mustard. Viscous and oily substances, difficult to remove mechanically, may be wiped on the the surface of the skin before decontamination. Water may enhance the dermal absorption of certain chemicals, a phenomenon known as the W-I effect (62). In some regions of France, the formal process of wet (showering) decontamination is often preceded by dry decontamination of casualties using FE (*gant poudre*). This can more rapidly achieve the initial decontamination and may assist in reducing gross contamination prior to showering (63).

24.6.6.2 Detergents

Detergents and soaps decrease surface tension, increasing the solubility and viscosity of the agents (64, 65). Surfactants that affect the permeability characteristics of several biological membranes, including skin, may solubilize SC lipids. Despite the fact that surfactants are considered chemical-penetration enhancers, especially by the transdermal route (66, 67), they are used in skin decontamination (68). The European project, the ORCHIDS protocol, consists of a 1.5-minute shower with a mild detergent, Argos, supplemented by physical removal (69). This soap is composed of anionic substances, alkyl benzene sulfonate sodium alkyléthersulfate sodium, nonionic, diethanolamide de coprah, and adjuvants (48). The role of surfactants, largely developed in decontamination processes, must be evaluated before skin utilization (62, 65, 70). According to their nature—anionic, cationic, nonionic, or zwitterionic—their potential enhancement effects could be assessed (71). A surfactant is a chemical that mixes readily with both oil-like and water-like chemicals. This include soaps, detergents, emulsifiers, and wetting agents.

24.6.7 SPECIFIC TECHNOLOGIES

24.6.7.1 Neutralization

Neutralization is a process of chemically reacting an agent to form other, less toxic chemicals. Four main types of chemical reactions are involved in neutralization: (1) substitution, (2) oxidation, (3) chelation, and (4) enzymatic and biodegradation. Neutralization was initiated by Lewis in 1959, who recommended initial copious water skin decontamination followed by neutralization of acid skin splashes with a solution of weighed sodium bicarbonate (½ ounce; 14.2g.) or 1% of sodium citrate for alkaline skin splashes, followed by more copious amounts of water (72).

24.6.7.1.1 Neutralization by Substitution

Neutralization by substitution is essentially performed by water hydrolysis, with a nucleophilic active decontaminant developed in the reactive skin decontamination lotion (RSDL) (73).

24.6.7.1.2 Hydrolysis

Substitution by hydrolysis depends on pH, which may be increased by modification, depending on the agent and the media. Hydrolysis takes place at any pH, but some hydrolysis products are still dangerous but less toxic e.g. G agents hydrolysis leads to methylphosphonic acid and hydrogen fluorid (HF) (74). Sulfur mustard hydrolyzes slowly to form thiodiglycol (TDG) (75, 76). The products of hydrolysis must be considered in the decontamination process.

24.6.7.1.3 Nucleophilic Substitution

Rapid nucleophilic decontamination is efficient for decontamination but nonappropriate for skin (77). RSDL is based on a mechanism chemically similar to hydrolysis, but at a milder pH. The active ingredient, a nucleophilic compound (2,3 butanedione monoxime), also called diacetyl monoxime (DAM), is dissolved in a glycol solvent, which dissolves most agents and allows them to be rinsed off with water. Decontamination must be initiated within 5 to 10 minutes to be the most efficient (78). RSDL destroys CWAs without corrosive effects and conteracts the inflammatory process, especially against sulfur mustard (36). RSDL is a skin decontaminant that is FDA approved (2002) (79). This viscous yellow lotion impregnated in a polymer sponge (pH 10.5) is water soluble and therefore easy to eliminate after decontamination and presented in individual packets ready to use (five-year shelf-life). The sponge is applied in a overlapping circular motion to skin, requiring at least two minutes' contact to achieve neutralization of agents (nerve agents, pesticides). For safety DAM, the active ingredient of RSDL may be percutaneously absorbed (MW 101.10; log P [octanol-water] 1.740) (80). The acute toxic effects of DAM, observed after injection to rats and rabbits, appears due to the compound itself (81). RSDL is not approved for eyes or in wounds (79). Safety precautions are recommended for RSDL: short time application (less than 6 hours), rinsing after decontamination, and respect the incompatibility with solid bleaching.

24.6.7.1.4 Neutralization by Oxidation

Oxidation is a reaction of an agent with an oxidizing chemical, which breaks many types of bonds. The most common oxidizers used in decontamination processes are bleaches (hypochlorites) such as after World War II, bleaching powders, permanganate ($KMnO_4$), and peroxides (hydrogen peroxides and peroxy acids). By World War II, superchlorinated bleaches were the most common general-purpose decontaminants (18, 30). Oxidizers composed of hypochlorites proposed for skin decontamination are

- bleach 2% to 6wt % NaClO in water,
- dutch powder, $Ca(O\,Cl)_2$ + MgO,
- activated solution of hypochlorite (ASH), 0.5% $Ca(OCl)^2$ + O.5% sodium dihydrogen phosphate buffer + 0.05% detergent in water
- self-limiting activated solution of hypochlorite (SLASH) 0.5% $Ca(OCl)^2$ + 1% sodium citrate + 0.2% citrate acid + 0.05% detergent in water.

However, there are disadvantages to using bleach as a decontaminant, and the necessary extemporaneous preparation due to the active chlorine content of the bleach gradually decreases with storage and its corrosity for the skin surface.

Sodium dichloroisocyanurate (NaDCC) is considered an alternative to hypochlorites, generating pH-neutral bleach when added to water (18). Fichlor (sodium N-N dichloroisocyanurate) detoxifies VX effectively by simple oxidation, but the pH influences the nerve agent's degradation kinetics. Tablets of NaDCC offer the advantage of stability (three-year storage) and is easily mixed with surfactants.

Hypochlorite solutions are efficacious when used to topically decontaminate intact skin. However, few studies examined the efficacy of decontamination of chemically contaminated wounds. Observations were performed after HD contamination.The lesions induced following decontamination are presumed due to the mechanical flushing of HD onto the perilesional skin, or by chemical damage induced by the solution, or HD–solution interaction. Comparing the decontamination efficacy of sodium hypochlorite (0.5% and 2.5% solutions) and calcium hypochlorite (0.5% and 2.5% solutions) is essential to manage skin decontamination with bleaching oxidizers (82). In skin decontamination by oxidizers, it is recommended to prepare the bleach solution 0.5% from certified lots of 5% household bleach diluted 1 to 10 (73). Nevertheless, bleaching is not universal in skin decontamination. Hypochlorite, diluted tenfold from a household bleach solution (0.5% concentration), is ineffective for agents such as VX, which require a significantly higher amount of hypochlorite for effective decontamination, but at this concentration hypochlorite effective for VX is damaging to the skin (83).

The formula of dilution presented in Equation (24.1), C1. $V_i= C_2$. V_2, is applied for dilution of sodium hypochlorite. C_1 is the initial concentration of the bleach solution, V_1 the initial volume. C_2 is the desired concentration appropriate in this case for skin decontamination: 0.5%; therefore, V2 is calculated as a total volume of the bleach solution extemporaneously prepared.

$$C1 = 5\% \quad V1 = 1 \text{ L}$$

$$C2 = 0.5\% \quad V2 = 10 \text{ L} \tag{24.1}$$

$$V2 = \frac{C1.V1}{C2}$$

Decontamination by oxidation is restricted in skin decontamination, and the results of testing reinforce the difficulty associated with developing a universal decontamination technology for cleanup of CWAs in a civilian setting (84).

24.6.7.2 Chelation

24.6.7.2.1 Diphoterine

Diphoterine and Hexafluorine, developed by Laboratoire Prevor, are referenced as medical device class IIa for technical skin and eye decontamination (15).

Diphoterine consists of a custom-made molecule that effectively attracts and renders harmless, among others, both hydrogen ions (H+) and hydroxide ions (OH-) and is a water-soluble powder. The rinsing and diluting effects of an equal volume of water (in the commercial preparations) are most likely retained. It is a polyvalent (actively binds multiple substances), amphoteric, hypertonic, chelating molecule with active binding sites for acids, bases, oxidizing agents, reducing agent, vesicant, lachrymators, irritants, solvents, etc. It is effective in preventing or decreasing the severity of burns to rapidly decrease pain and has resulted in fewer requirements for medical or surgical burn care (8, 85).

24.6.7.2.2 Hexafluorine

Hexafluorine, a colorless, sterile, aqueous solution of pH 7.2 to 7.7 that is slightly hypertonic, is an amphoteric, hypertonic, polyvalent compound for decontaminating hydrofluoric acid (HF) eye and skin splashes within the first two minutes and is efficient in reducing burns and consequences (86)

24.6.7.3 Enzymatic Decontamination and Biodegradation

Enzymatic decontamination, specific of the chemical were developed from 1946, and more after the selection of organophosphorus anhydrase (OPA) was selected in 1987 as a generic name for all enzymes capable of catalytically hydrolyzing organophosphorous compounds (18). Two promising candidates in enzymatic decontamination are organophosphorus acid anhydrolase (OPAA) from a strain of *Alteromonas* obtained from Grantsville Warm Spring, Utah, and organophosphorus hydrolase (OPH) from *Pseudomonas diminuta* or Flaviobacterium. High specifity and restrictions on pH and temperature of those enzymes limits their use in mass decontamination, but they are potentially sufficiently benign to be used directly on the skin of personnel and casualties. Research demonstrates the considerable potential of bacteria to sequence cloned genes (87). Biodegradation of sulfur mustard is underway to decrease potential toxicity.

24.6.8 Prospectives

Decontaminating skin by capture and destruction of the contaminants is under research. Compared to liquid decontaminants, less is known concerning the interaction of agents with solid decontaminants. In order to enhance knowledge of the interactions of solid agents, high technology developed by scanning or transmission electron microscopy, diffraction high resolution, and infrared spectroscopy will be helpful. Synchrotron beamlines are available for a quick and efficient characterization and should offer opportunities to visualize bindings between molecules and the kinetics of those interactions.

24.6.9 CONCLUSION

In the case of decontamination for humans involved in a chemical exposure, physical removal compared to neutralization is by far easier to set up. It begins with the disrobing and personnel protection equipment. The goal is to remove bulk contamination and remove the user from a suit in a timely, efficient manner. Dry decontamination, based on powders, and adsorptive glove wipe systems should be first considered for chemicals to ensure efficient decontamination, manage the emergency response, and ensure immediate first aid and medical countermeasures.

Wet decontamination, by washing with detergent or not, and then a rinse, is a universal method with some constraints in the organization when mass exposure is involved.

Conversely, neutralization can be considered only after identification of the chemical. Some constraints limit neutralization as the first decontamination method, such as its time consumption, volume dependence, and hazardous potential.

24.7 BEST PRACTICES IN DECONTAMINATION

24.7.1 HOW THE PROJECT OF BEST PRACTICES TAKES PLACE

Skin decontamination has been widely studied, suggesting consideration of both decontaminants and application processes whose main objective is to reduce contact time with the chemical after exposure and therefore health consequences. These numerous systems cover practically all degrees of efficiency that one wants to achieve. However, fundamental criteria may be met in order to complete decontamination methods.

1. Most of the methods mentioned may be not applicable in the context of chemical incidents involving mass exposure because of expense. Therefore, basic decontaminants available on the world market and easy to execute are usually used or put forward first.
2. Define the expected level for skin decontamination utilizing rigorous methods and safe applications onto skin, including two main factors: the population involved i.e. children, elderly, disabled and the number involved.

A best practices guide, expected to assist the best option in skin decontamination, considering first, the targeted population e.g. soldiers in war position exposed to CWA, civilian exposed unintentionally to TICs, contaminated individuals in disorderly arrival in hospitals, could emerge.

This guide may treat initial crucial actions to prevent contamination of first responders and cross contamination and offer a decision tool to deal with key issues with minimal delay according to decontaminant benefits and drawbacks.

Preventing the extent of contamination is essential to achieve improvement in clean habits, awareness, and avoidance of contamination for responders and populations alike. We suggest criteria in the chronological actions performed before decontamination.

24.7.2 PREVENTION AND PERSONAL PROTECTIVE EQUIPEMENT

In order to enable them to initiate rescue efforts and work closely with contaminated casualties, responders have to be equipped with appropriate PPE. Adsorption filter material with high adsorption capacity and low breakthrough behavior is found in Patent US 7, 160,369 B2 (2007), 2.5 times its weight in liquid contaminant, with an infinite shelf-life. The adsorption layer has an inital activated carbon layer with granular or spherical activated carbon particles (88). Relatively new classes of crystalline solids with tunable properties such as porosity and pore size, known as metal organic frameworks (MOFs) may have great potential in future applications (89) and destruction of CWAs (90).

24.7.3 SELF-CARE DECONTAMINATION

Self-care includes casualties moving away from the contamination source, wiping the contaminant off exposed skin and hair, and disrobing in order to stop the contaminant from penetrating into the skin and thereby limit percutaneous penetration (19).

24.7.4 DISROBING

Disrobing is widely recommended. In contrast, there will be a delay between initial chemical exposure and decontamination setup for civilians compared to the military response (20). It is a challenge to reduce the time required to deploy decontamination processes after chemical exposure and limit potential health impacts. Therefore, removing clothing is considered a simple and highly effective action to remove external contaminants in the first minutes after the incident and is highly recommended. Disrobing can remove 80% to 90% of contamination (21). Nonetheless, it needs an ethical approach beforehand, organized both on the crime scene and in the hospitals (91).

24.7.5 DECONTAMINANTS

Which decontaminants and application processes are interchangeable depends on their mechanism of action: adsorption added or not of adsorbed toxics degradation. Components in most cases are powders that might settle in gloves or be included in pads. Skin decontaminants must not be corrosive, so that skin surfaces are not damaged by decontaminants. Therefore, decontamination of eyes and wounds are treated separately. Depending on the magnitude of the change(s) in components and composition, mechanism of action and/or method of application, tests should prove the intended skin decontamination. Criteria tools and level of decontamination could be expected to improve and standardize systematically before approval of both decontaminants and decontamination processes (application and removing); thus information is necessary for each one in terms of the necessary contact time to adsorb (1) liquid at the surface, (2) more or less in the first layers of SC depending on kinetics of adsorbents, (3) define the appropriate rate of decontamination efficiency, and (4) methods to detect low-level residual contaminant.

24.7.6 CONTRAINTS IN DECONTAMINATION

Analysis and evaluation of decontamination methods require evaluation in safety and in decontamination efficiency. Even if in vivo human skin is considered the best model, ethical, financial, and safety considerations require testing with animal models, the most common of which are pigs, monkeys, rats, and rabbits (92).

Propositions are limited to decontaminants attested to or in progress, when applied on skin, to treat militarian and civilian mass casualties exposed to CWA sor very dangerous TICS. Nevertheless, powders, which inappropriate for the decontamination of mucous membranes and wounds, may cause serious damage (30). New products intended for topical application to the skin must be proven safe and effective before marketing. Some are approved as medical devices, boosting user confidence. Therefore, the establishment of principles and test procedures to ensure safe manufacture and use of nanomaterials in the marketplace is urgently required and achievable. Quality means features and characteristics of a product, in this case to be applied to skin. Define a degree of confidence for the test outcome and demonstrate interchangeability for their products during the developmental process or after approval (93).

24.7.7 IMPROVING DECONTAMINATION MANAGEMENT

Improving management decontamination of any chemical incident requires, first, security in the choice of decontaminant because of skin contact. The label of the medical device should increase its attractiveness and boost the confidence of users. Then, reducing the contact time and introducing a scale to measure contamination residual level should increase the readability of decontamination efficiency. Perform in the design of decontamination methods no delay in emergency medical care and therapeutics administration, which is a crucial challenge to save as many people as possible (12).

24.7.8 MEDICAL DEVICES

Medical devices recognized in the European Union (EU) and the United States and now worldwide tend to guarantee great confidence in the decontamination materials. Qualification means that the FDA has evaluated the tool and concurs with the available supporting evidence that the tool produces scientifically plausible measurements and works as intended within the specified context of use, which depends on the tool or product area in which the tool is proposed for qualification. European Council 93/42/EEC of 14 June 1993 (94) concerning medical devices defines essential requirement e.g. time of use and proposes a classification based on the destination of the devices (95).

24.7.9 WHY SKIN DECON IS A SOCIETAL CHALLENGE

The societal challenge for skin decontamination concerns in an emergency relate to people after exposure to acute chemicals, including lifelong skin exposure and risk of chronic toxicity in relation to the exposome (96). The comprehensive clinical research guide in skin decontamination, offering an extensive bibliography, would help governments and specialists to manage solutions that will decrease mortality and morbidity (97).

24.7.10 SKIN: A POTENTIAL TARGET

Knowledge of the anatomical heterogeneity complexities of skin demands an adapted system that is more or less sophisticated and that further breaks down the diffusion and partitioning steps to limit systemic effects. Therefore immediate action to reduce the concentration of any substance onto and within the skin will subsequently reduce the amount available and the risk of entry into the systemic circulation. Correlation between the penetration level of chemicals and the SC essentially depends on the barrier function, which constitutes a crucial physical obstacle protecting underlying tissues from aggressive environmental influences. The consequences of percutaneous penetration are correlated both to the inherent activity of chemicals and individual factors such as age, racial differences, and more specifically anatomic site (98, 99). Therefore it is conceivable to partially explain the higher penetration in sites where sebaceous glands are more numerous and the thickness of the SC. However, disorganization in intercellular lipids and lamellar sheets may imply subsequent disordering of the intercellular SC and be a second reservoir of contamination (100). Epidermal cells play a role in protection, such as Langerhans cells involved in the cutaneous immune system through the activation of cytokines, melanocytes provide photoprotection and neutralize free radicals, and Merkell cells scattered in the basal layer play an important role in the sensory function.

Formation of a reservoir in the SC partly explains difficulties in decontamination methods and prediction of chemical penetration through it. The properties of the agent in skin decontamination are essential to preserve the skin and avoid percutaneous penetration and migration of toxic agents.

24.7.11 PSYCHOSOCIAL POTENTIAL CONSEQUENCES

The presence of an unusual product on the skin provokes an immediate reaction to clean it up or remove it. Chemical disasters are associated with a variety of psychological, psychosocial, and physiological distresses. The psychological dimension is an essential phase at least as significant as the physical removal (91).

Disasters involving chemicals may cause more devastating long-term effects compared to natural disasters (101). Psychophysiological responses and biochemicals correlate to disaster stress; therefore, the challenge is to prevent a chronic effect. Depending on the chemical's nature—sticky, viscous, heating, freezing, irritating–those must be physically removed. The barrier function of skin limits permeability and penetration. A survey requesting information on people's contamination impact could help to measure the individual stress factor as an indicator.

Even if the challenge, after chemical exposure, is to prevent immediate effects and preserve the skin of the people involved and the health consequences, social and long-term effects are at least of equal importance to prevent chronisization after exposure (102). Emotional charge linked to the evenment, both for casualties and rescuers, must be evaluated to assist, prevent the chronicization and help for the resilience. Depending of chemicals, toxidromes which irreversibility may cause long-term consequences are concerned in this part.

24.7.12   Highlights for Decontamination Methods

In the case of decontamination for humans involved in a chemical exposure, physical removal compared to neutralization is by far easier to execute. Along with disrobing and personnel protection, the goal is to remove mass contamination and remove the user from their clothing in a timely, efficient manner according to ethical considerations.

Dry decontamination, based on powders, adsorptive gloves, and wipe systems, has to be first considered to ensure efficient decontamination, manage the emergency response, and provide immediate first aid and medical countermeasures. Wet decontamination, by washing with detergent or not, followed by rinsing, is a universal method with some constraints in the organization for the target population, depending on the location. We have tools and methods appropriate to the target population—pediatric, elderly, diseased people, disabled persons, and ethnic populations.

Some constraints limit the neutralization, such as its time consumption and volume, and may be hazardous.

24.7.13   Conclusion

Best practices for decontamination should be strongly encouraged to share and develop standards of good practices. Decontamination profiles should be organized in order to obtain a desirable or appropriate level of quality to protect public health, considering the toxicity of contaminant chemicals. A guide of best practices will be helpful to compare and assess the quality of methods until the required low-level toxicity is being achieved, considering the current data of the science. Professional deontology, ethical considerations, and human rights should guide the development of appropriate and operational responses in decontamination until we obtain the necessary public confidence in the legitimacy of implemented measures.

NOTE

1   In the current state of science we've got in the data.

REFERENCES

1. Roul A. Exposition de la peau aux produits chimiques : méthodologie et évaluation de la décontamination par la terre de foulon, Ingénierie biomédicale. Université de Lyon, 2018. Français. (NNT : 2018LYSE1134).
2. Elias PM, Wakefield JS. Skin Barrier Function. In: Krutmann J, Humbert P, editors. Nutrition for Healthy Skin. Springer Berlin Heidelberg; 2011. p. 35–48.

3. Ngo MA, Maibach HI: 15 Factors of Percutaneous Penetration of Pesticides. Vol. 1099. ACS Symposium Series; 2012.

4. Pierre Agache, Philippe H. Measuring the Skin. Springer; 2004.

5. Zhang M-Q, Wilkinson B. Drug discovery beyond the 'rule-of-five.' Curr Opin Biotechnol. 2007; 18(6):478–88.

6. Michaels AS, Chandrasekaran SK, Shaw JE. Drug permeation through human skin: Theory and invitro experimental measurement. AIChE J. 1975; 21(5):985–96.

7. Falson-Rieg F, Faivre V, Pirot F. Nouvelles formes médicamenteuses. Lavoisier/Tec & Doc; 2004.

8. Palao R, Monge I, Ruiz M, Barret JP. Chemical burns: Pathophysiology and treatment. Burns. 2010; 36(3):295–304.

9. Greenhalgh DG. Management of Burns. N Engl J Med. 2019; 380(24):2349–59.

10. Henretig FM, Kirk MA, McKay CA. Hazardous Chemical Emergencies and Poisonings. N Engl J Med. 2019; 380(17):1638–55.

11. Hauschild V, Watson A, Bock R. Decontamination and management of human remains following incidents of hazardous chemical release. Am J Disaster Med. 2012; 7:5–29.

12. Harvilchuck J, Noort D, Lawson G, Kyburz K, Verschraagen M, Director-Myska A. Decontamination of Chemically Contaminated Remains. In: Skin Decontamination. Springer International Publishing (ISBN 978-3-030-24009-7); 2020. p. 53–75.

13. Hick JL, Hanfling D, Burstein JL, Markham J, Macintyre AG, Barbera JA. Protective equipment for health care facility decontamination personnel. Ann Emerg Med. 2003; 42(3):370–80.

14. Regulation (EU) 2016/425 of the European Parliament and of the Council - of 9 march 2016 - on Personal Protective Equipment and Repealing Council Directive 89/686/eec.: 48.

15. Lewis CJ, Al-Mousawi A, Jha A, Allison KP. Is it time for a change in the approach to chemical burns? The role of Diphoterine® in the management of cutaneous and ocular chemical injuries. J Plast Reconstr Aesthet Surg. 2017;70(5):563–7.

16. Capoun T, Krykorkova J. Comparison of selected methods for individual decontamination of Chemical Warfare Agents. Toxics. 2014; 2(2):307–26.

17. Lynn DD, Zukin LM & Dellavalle R. The safety and efficacy of Diphoterine for ocular and cutaneous burns in humans. Cutan Ocul Toxicol. 2017;2:185–92.

18. Yang YC, Baker JA, Ward JR. Decontamination of chemical warfare agents. Chem Rev. 1992; 92(8):1729–43.

19. Raymond G. (RAY) Monteith Validation of a hazmat CBRN decontamination protocol with the Canadian context; Report Royal Roads University, Nov. 2013.

20. Chilcott RP. Managing mass casualties and decontamination. Environ Int. 2014; 72:37–45.

21. Clarke SFJ, Chilcott RP, Wilson JC, Kamanyire R, Baker DJ, Hallett A. Decontamination of multiple casualties who are chemically contaminated: A challenge for acute hospitals. Prehospital Disaster Med. 2008; 23(02):175–81.

22. Nambiar MP, Gordon RK, Rezk PE, Katos AM, Wajda NA, Moran TS, et al. Medical countermeasure against respiratory toxicity and acute lung injury following inhalation exposure to chemical warfare nerve agent VX. Toxicol Appl Pharmacol. 2007; 219(2–3):142–50.

23. Circular 27 2017. 700 n° 700/SGDN/PSE/PPS du 7 novembre 2008. Circulaire relative à la doctrine nationale d'emploi des moyens de secours et de soins face à une action terroriste mettant en œuvre des matières chimiques; SGDSN, FR. Roul A, Le CA, Gustin MP, Clavaud E, Verrier B, Pirot F, Falson F. Comparison of four different fuller's earth formulations in skin decontamination. J Appl Toxicol. 2017 Dec;37(12):1527-1536. doi: 10.1002/jat.3506. Epub 2017 Jul 26. PMID: 28745436.

24. Das D, Pourdeyhimi B. Composite Nonwoven Materials. Elsevier; 2014.

25. Gulson B, Anderson P, Taylor A. Surface dust wipes are the best predictors of blood leads in young children with elevated blood lead levels. Environ Res. 2013; 126:171–8.

26. Phuong C, Maibach HI. Recent knowledge: Concepts of dermal absorption in relation to skin decontamination: Dermal absorption related to skin decontamination. J Appl Toxicol. 2016; 36(1):5–9.

27. Roul A, Le C-A-K, Gustin M-P, Clavaud E, Verrier B, Pirot F, et al. Comparison of four different fuller's earth formulations in skin decontamination. J Appl Toxicol. 2017;

28. Matar H, Larner J, Kansagra S, Atkinson KL, Skamarauskas JT, Amlot R, et al. Design and characterisation of a novel in vitro skin diffusion cell system for assessing mass casualty decontamination systems. Toxicol Vitro Int J Publ Assoc BIBRA. 2014; 28(4):492–501.

29. Amlôt R, Larner J, Matar H, Jones DavidR, Carter H, Turner EA, et al. Comparative Analysis of Showering Protocols for Mass-Casualty Decontamination. Prehospital Disaster Med. 2010; 25(05):435–9.

30. Szinicz L. History of chemical and biological warfare agents. Toxicology. 2005; 214(3):167–81.

31. Yenisoy-Karakaş S, Aygün A, Güneş M, Tahtasakal E. Physical and chemical characteristics of polymer-based spherical activated carbon and its ability to adsorb organics. Carbon. 2004; 42(3):477–84.

32. Camacho LM, Torres A, Saha D, Deng S. Adsorption equilibrium and kinetics of fluoride on sol–gel-derived activated alumina adsorbents. J Colloid Interface Sci. 2010; 349(1):307–13.

33. Prasad GK, Ramacharyulu PVRK, Batra K, Singh B, Srivastava AR, Ganesan K, et al. Decontamination of Yperite using mesoporous mixed metal oxide nanocrystals. J Hazard Mater. 2010; 183(1–3):847–52.

34. Parsons CL. Fuller's earth. Bureau of Mines. Washington, DC: G.P.O.; 1913.

35. Carretero MI. Clay minerals and their beneficial effects upon human health. A review. Appl Clay Sci. 2002; 21(3–4):155–63.

36. Taysse L, Daulon S, Delamanche S, Bellier B, Breton P. Skin decontamination of mustards and organo-phosphates: comparative efficiency of RSDL and Fuller's earth in domestic swine. Hum Exp Toxicol. 2007; 26(2):135–41.

37. Millot G. Geology of Clays: Weathering · Sedimentology · Geochemistry. Springer Science & Business Media; 2013.

38. Cox RD. Decontamination and management of hazardous materials exposure victims in the emergency department. Ann Emerg Med; 1994; 23(4):761–70.

39. Ganesan K, Raza SK, Vijayaraghavan R. Chemical warfare agents. J Pharm Bioallied Sci. 2010; 2(3):166.

40. Wagner GW, Bartram PW. 31P MAS NMR study of the hydrolysis of O,S-diethyl phenylphosphonothioate on reactive sorbents. J Mol Catal Chem. 1995; 99(3):175–81.

41. Harvey SP, Kutchey CM, Whally CE. Evaluation of the efficacy of Rohm and Haas Ambergard XE-555 resin for decontamination of a biological simulant. Final report, Apr-Jul 91. Chemical Research, Development and Engineering Center, Aberdeen Proving Ground, MD (United States); 1992.

42. Olson KR. Activated charcoal for acute poisoning: one toxicologist's journey. J Med Toxicol. 2010; 6(2):190–8.

43. Chilcott RP, Jenner J, Hotchkiss SAM, Rice P. In vitro skin absorption and decontamination of sulphur mustard: comparison of human and pig-ear skin. J Appl Toxicol. 2001; 21(4):279–83.

44. Sata U, Wilusz E, Mlynarek S, Coimbatore G, Kendall R, Ramkumar SS. Development of cotton non-woven composite fabric for toxic chemical decontamination and characterization of its adsorption capabilities. J Eng Fibers Fabr. 2013; 8(1).

45. Miaud P, A GS. Individual decontamination apparatus. 1992. Citation patent registration US5368158 A.

46. Lalain T, Brickhouse MD, Pfarr J, Lloyd J, Flowers J, Mantooth B, et al. Evaluation of the Steris Sensitive Equipment Decontamination (SED) Apparatus on a 463L Pallet. Edgewood Chemical Biological Center Aberdeen Proving Ground, MD; 2007.

47. Wipe spray wipe. R Wipe /spray/wipe® decon process Strategic Responses Solutions. US20180333009A1.pdf

48. Gibbs AR, Pooley FD. Fuller's earth (montmorillonite) pneumoconiosis. Occup Environ Med. 1994; 51(9):644–646.

49. Salerno A, Devers T, Bolzinger M-A, Pelletier J, Josse D, Briançon S. In vitro skin decontamination of the organophosphorus pesticide Paraoxon with nanometric cerium oxide CeO_2. Chem Biol Interact. 2017 Apr 1;267:57-66. doi: 10.1016/j.cbi.2016.04.035. Epub 2016 Apr 26. PMID: 27129420.

50. Salerno A, Pitault I, Devers T, Pelletier J, Briançon S. Model-based optimization of parameters for degradation reaction of an organophosphorus pesticide, paraoxon, using CeO_2 nanoparticles in water media. Environ Toxicol Pharmacol. 2017; 53:18–28.

51. Kumar R J.Praveen, Ramacharyulu P.V.R.K., Prasad G.K., Singh B. Montmorillonites supported with metal oxide nanoparticles for decontamination of sulfur mustard. Appl Clay Sci. 2015; 116–117:263–72.

52. Prasad GK, Mahato TH, Singh B, Ganesan K, Srivastava AnchalR, Kaushik MP, et al. Decontamination of sulfur mustard and sarin on titania nanotubes. AIChE J. 2008; 54(11):2957–63.

53. Hoet PH, Brüske-Hohlfeld I, Salata OV. Nanoparticles – known and unknown health risks. J Nanobiotechnology. 2004; 15.

54. Nel A, Xia T, Mädler L, Li N. Toxic potential of materials at the nanolevel. Science. 2006; 311(5761):622–7.

55. Working Guidance on EPA's Section 8(a) Information Gathering Rule on Nanomaterials in Commerce. https://www.epa.gov/reviewing-new-chemicals-under-toxic-substances-control-act-tsca/working-guidance-epas-section-8a

56. Sellik A, Pollet T, Ouvry L, Briançon S, Fessi H, Hartmann DJ, et al. Degradation of paraoxon (VX chemical agent simulant) and bacteria by magnesium oxide depends on the crystalline structure of magnesium oxide. Chem Biol Interact. 2017; 267:67–73.

57. Janoš P, Henych J, Pelant O, Pilařová V, Vrtoch L, Kormunda M, et al. Cerium oxide for the destruction of chemical warfare agents: A comparison of synthetic routes. J Hazard Mater. 2016; 304:259–68.

58. Cao Y, Elmahdy A, Zhu H, Hui X, Maibach H. Binding affinity and decontamination of dermal decontamination gel to model chemical warfare agent simulants. J Appl Toxicol. 2018 May;38(5):724–33. doi: 10.1002/jat.3580. Epub 2018 Jan 7. PMID: 29315700.

59. Cao Y, Hui X, Zhu H, Elmahdy A, Maibach H. In vitro human skin permeation and decontamination of 2-chloroethyl ethyl sulfide (CEES) using Dermal Decontamination Gel (DDGel) and Reactive Skin Decontamination Lotion (RSDL). Toxicol Lett. 2018; 291:86–91.

60. Salerno A, Bolzinger M-A, Rolland P, Chevalier Y, Josse D, Briançon S. Pickering emulsions for skin decontamination. Toxicol In Vitro 2016; 34:45–54.

61. Jones DR, Larner J, Price SC, Chilcott RP. Optimisation of mass casualty decontamination procedures in vitro. Toxicology. 2010; 278(3):363.

62. Moody RP, Maibach HI. Skin decontamination: Importance of the wash-in effect. Food Chem Toxicol. 2006; 44(11):1783–8.

63. Josse D, Wartelle J, Cruz C. Showering effectiveness for human hair decontamination of the nerve agent VX. Chem Biol Interact. 2015; 232:94–100.

64. Lee S-W, Tettey KE, Yarovoy Y, Lee D. Effects of anionic surfactants on the water permeability of a model stratum corneum lipid membrane. Langmuir ACS J Surf Colloids. 2014; 30(1):220–6.

65. Zhu H, Jung E-C, Phuong C, Hui X, Maibach H. Effects of soap-water wash on human epidermal penetration: Effects of soap-water wash on human epidermal penetration. J Appl Toxicol. 2016; 36(8):997–1002.

66. Thong H-Y, Zhai H, Maibach HI. Percutaneous penetration enhancers: an overview. Skin Pharmacol Physiol. 2007; 20(6):272–82.

67. Dragicevic N, Maibach HI. Percutaneous penetration enhancers chemical methods in penetration enhancement. Nina Dragicevic, Howard I. Maibach. Springer Berlin Heidelberg; 2016.

68. Som I, Bhatia K, Yasir Mohd. Status of surfactants as penetration enhancers in transdermal drug delivery. J Pharm Bioallied Sci. 2012; 4(1):2–9.

69. Misik J, Pavlik M, Novotny L, Pavlikova R, Chilcott RP, Cabal J, et al. In vivo decontamination of the nerve agent VX using the domestic swine model. Clin Toxicol. 2012; 50(9):807–11.

70. Chan HP, Zhai H, Hui X, Maibach HI. Skin decontamination: principles and perspectives. Toxicol Ind Health. 2013; 29(10):955–68.

71. Lane ME. Skin penetration enhancers. Int J Pharm. 2013; 447(1–2):12–21.

72. Lewis Concept of Acids and Bases. Available at https://chem.libretexts.org/. Accessed 2020, 8.

73. Braue EH, Smith KH, Doxzon BF, Lumpkin HL, Clarkson ED. Efficacy studies of Reactive Skin Decontamination Lotion, M291 Skin Decontamination Kit, 0.5% bleach, 1% soapy water, and Skin Exposure Reduction Paste Against Chemical Warfare Agents, Part 2: Guinea pigs challenged with soman. Cutan Ocul Toxicol. 2011; 30(1):29–37.

74. Barr et al. Quantitation of metabolites of the nerve agents sarin, soman, cyclohexylsarin, VX, and Russian VX in human urine using isotope-dilution gas chromatography-tandem mass spectrometry. J Anal Toxicol, 2004 Jul-Aug; 28(5):372–8. PMID: 15239858.

75. Dell'Amico E, Bernasconi S, Cavalca L, Magni C, Prinsi B, Andreoni V. New insights into the biodegradation of thiodiglycol, the hydrolysis product of Yperite (sulfur mustard gas). J Appl Microbiol. 2009; 106(4):1111–21.

76. Munro NB, Talmage SS, Griffin GD, Waters LC, Watson AP, King JF, et al. The sources, fate, and toxicity of chemical warfare agent degradation products. Environ Health Perspect. 1999; 107(12):933.

77. Wagner GW, Yang Y-C. Rapid nucleophilic/oxidative decontamination of chemical warfare agents. Ind Eng Chem Res. 2002; 41(8):1925–8.

78. Thors L, Lindberg S, Johansson S, Koch B, Koch M, Hägglund L, et al. RSDL decontamination of human skin contaminated with the nerve agent VX. Toxicol Lett. 2017; 269:47–54.

79. Worek F, Jenner J, Thiermann H. Chemical Warfare Toxicology: Volume 2: Management of Poisoning. Royal Society of Chemistry; 2016.

80. ChemIDplus Advanced – Chemical information with searchable synonyms, structures, and formulas. Available at https://chem.nlm.nih.gov. Accessed October 3, 2017.

81. Askew BM, Davies DR, Green AL, Holmes R. The nature of the toxicity of 2-Oxo-oximes. Br J Pharmacol. 1956; 11(4):424–27. doi:10.1111/j.1476-5381.1956.tb00010.x

82. Gold MB, Bongiovanni R, Scharf BA, Gresham VC, Woodward CL. Hypochlorite solution as a decontaminant in sulfur mustard contaminated skin defects in the euthymic hairless guinea pig. Drug Chem Toxicol. 1994; 17(4):499–527.

83. Ramkumar SS, Love AH, Sata UR, Koester CJ, Smith WJ, Keating GA, et al. Next-generation nonparticulate dry nonwoven pad for chemical warfare agent decontamination. Ind Eng Chem Res. 2008; 47(24):9889–95. doi: 10.1016/j.jhazmat.2011.09.005. Epub 2011 Sep 8. PMID: 21944706.

84. Love AH, Bailey CG, Hanna ML, Hok S, Vu AK, Reutter DJ, et al. Efficacy of liquid and foam decontamination technologies for chemical warfare agents on indoor surfaces. J Hazard Mater. 2011;

85. Brent J. Water-based solutions are the best decontaminating fluids for dermal corrosive exposures: A mini review. Clin Toxicol. 2013; 51(8):731–6.

86. Mathieu L, Nehles J, Blomet J, Hall AH. Efficacy of hexafluorine for emergent decontamination of hydrofluoric acid eye and skin splashes. Vet Hum Toxicol. 2001; 43(5):263–65.

87. Cho CM-H, Mulchandani A, Chen W. Bacterial cell surface display of organophosphorus hydrolase for selective screening of improved hydrolysis of organophosphate nerve agents. Appl Environ Microbiol. 2002; 68(4):2026–30.

88. Blücher H von, Ouvry L, Kämper S, Moskopp M, Ruiter E de, Böhringer B, et al. Adsorption filter material with high adsorption capacity and low breakthrough behavior. 2004.

89. De Koning MC, van Grol M, Breijaert T. Degradation of paraoxon and the chemical warfare agents VX, tabun, and soman by the metal–organic frameworks UiO-66-NH$_2$, MOF-808, NU-1000, and PCN-777. Inorg Chem. 2017; 56(19):11804–9.

90. Mondloch JE, Katz MJ, Iii WCI, Ghosh P, Liao P, Bury W, et al. Destruction of chemical warfare agents using metal–organic frameworks. Nat Mater. 2015; 14(5):512.

91. Carter H, Drury J, Amlô R. Understanding the impact of responders management strategies on public experiences. Springer Nat; 2020;199–210.

92. Jung EC, Maibach HI. Animal models for percutaneous absorption. J Appl Toxicol. 2015; 35(1):1–10.

93. Carter H, Drury J, Rubin GJ, Williams R, Amlôt R. Public experiences of mass casualty decontamination. Biosecurity Bioterrorism Biodefense Strategy Pract Sci. 2012; 10(3):280–9.

94. Regulation (EU) 2017/745 of the European Parliament and of the Council of 5 April 2017 on Medical Devices, Amending Directive 2001/83/EC, Regulation (EC) No 178/2002 and Regulation (EC) No 1223/2009 and Repealing Council Directives 90/385/EEC and 93/42/EEC (Text with EEA relevance). OJ L, 32017R0745, May 5, 2017.

95. Directive C. 93/42/EEC of 14 June 1993 Concerning Medical Devices. 1993.

96. Miller GW. The exposome: A primer. Academic Press; 2013.

97. Jiang A, Maibach H. Skin Decontamination. In: John SM, Johansen JD, Rustemeyer T, Elsner P, Maibach HI, editors. Kanerva's Occupational Dermatology. Springer International Publishing; 2018. p. 1–4.

98. HI Maibach et al. Regional variation in percutaneous penetration in man. Arch Environ Health Int J. 1971 Sep 1; 23(3):208–11.

99. Rougier A, Dupuis D, Lotte C, Roguet R, Schaefer H. In vivo correlation between stratum corneum reservoir function and percutaneous absorption. J Invest Dermatol. 1983; 81(3):275–78.

100. Elias PM, Friend DS. The permeability barrier in mammalian epidermis. J Cell Biol. 1975; 65(1):180–91.

101. Van Ommeren M, Saxena S, Saraceno B. Mental and social health during and after acute emergencies: emerging consensus? Bull World Health Organ. 2005; 83(1):71–5.

102. Prager EM, Pidoplichko VI, Aroniadou-Anderjaska V, Apland JP, Braga MFM. Pathophysiological mechanisms underlying increased anxiety after soman exposure: Reduced GABAergic inhibition in the basolateral amygdala. NeuroToxicology. 2014; 44:335–43.

41. G.W. Wagner, P.W. Bartramr; Reactions of the nerve agent simulant diisopropyl fluorophosphate with self-decontaminating adsorbents A[31] P MAS NMR study; J Mol Catal A-Chem. 1999; 144:419–24.

25 Chemical Warfare Agent VX Penetration through Military Uniform and Human Skin
Risk Assessment and Decontamination

Howard I. Maibach
University of California, San Francisco, California

CONTENTS

25.1 INTRODUCTION

Most well-known warfare chemicals have similar molecular structures as the organophosphorus compounds. One of these, parathion, has been shown to exhibit body regional variation in human skin absorption (1). The exposed head and neck region (×4), trunk (×3), and genital area (×12) absorb more chemical than the arms and hands and legs and feet. In agricultural use, parathion has caused human death. Permeability constants (K_p) (potential chemical absorbed through human skin per unit area and time) indexed to regional variation give the mass of chemical absorbed through a region of the human body and the total body absorption when summed over all regions. The further overlap of toxicity data to absorption can be used to estimate potential lethality.

Percutaneous absorption and regional variation form the final barrier between the "outside" and the "inside" of the body where toxicity occurs. Percutaneous absorption is influenced by moisture, and certainly a soldier or civilian will sweat, and it does rain. Clothing also affects percutaneous absorption because material can act as both a barrier and a skin delivery system (2). Sweating, clothing, and skin absorption are thus interrelated.

Our objective of this study was to determine the percutaneous absorption of parathion when applied to naked human skin and uniformed skin with and without sweat and to predict potential human absorption and lethality of the structurally related chemical warfare agent (CWA) VX. A discussion as to skin decontamination of CWAs follows the absorption study.

25.2 METHODOLOGY

A soldier wearing a standard field uniform will have both naked skin (head, neck, arms, and hands) and uniform-covered skin exposed during a chemical warfare incident. And in military encounters, the soldier has no choice but to wear that same uniform for an extended period.

The study design was to dose, in a single exposure, naked skin and uniform-protected skin to the CWA stimulant parathion and continue the exposure and absorption period over 96 hours. Uniforms can become wet from sweating and rain, so both wet and dry uniform material were included.

[^{14}C]parathion (specific activity 9.2 mCi/mmol) was obtained from Sigma (St. Louis, Missouri, USA). The uniform material was standard army issue coat, hot weather woodland camouflage, combat pattern, 50% nylon and 50% cotton (American Apparel, Inc.).

The in vitro assembly consisted of flow-through design glass skin diffusion cells (LG-1084-LCP, Laboratory Glass Apparatus, Inc., Berkeley, California, USA). Human cadaver skin was treated with dermatome to a thickness of 500 μm. Skin backs from two different donors (white male, age 71, and white male, age 60) were used. The skin specimens were mounted in the diffusion cells, with an available skin area of 1 cm^2. The excised skin used in this study is of similar thickness (dermatoned) and obtained from the donors within 24 hours postmortem. A visual barrier integrity check was performed prior to the study.

Uniform material was placed over the skin before the skin samples were clamped into the diffusion cell. The receiver side of the diffusion cell consisted of continuous-flow Eagles MEM-BSS with gentamicin at a 3mL/hr flow rate (3). A single dose of [^{14}C]parathion (4 μg containing 1 μCi) was applied to each naked skin or uniform-covered skin cell. Those uniformed cells that were wetted received a 20 μL water dose each of the 4-day experiment. The receiver cells were placed over magnetic stirrers, and all the absorption experiments were carried out at 37°C, using a recirculating constant-temperature water bath. At designated intervals, samples were automatically collected into scintillation vials (4).

25.2.1 SURROGATE MODEL

Parathion was the chemical of choice to use as a surrogate for VX. Actual data with VX would be the best; however, little exists in the literature. To obtain radiolabeled VX and study it in the public domain is highly improbable. Parathion is in the same chemical class as VX (organophosphorus) and has the same functional groups as VX. Table 25.1 gives the structures of parathion and VX and physicochemical data, which relate to percutaneous absorption. The partition coefficients (log P octanol/water), molecular weights, and molecular volumes are close. Similar structure, log P, and molecular weight/molar volume suggest the potential for similar percutaneous absorption.

25.2.2 DATA CALCULATIONS

Parathion percutaneous absorption and permeability coefficients for naked skin and uniform (dry and wet) were obtained by experimentation. The permeability coefficient for VX (1.6×10^{-3} cm/hr) was calculated from Potts and Guy (5). Relative differences in permeability due to wet and dry

TABLE 25.1
Structure and Physicochemical Comparisons of Parathion and VX

	Parathion	VX
Parathion coefficient (log P octanol/water)	3.83	2.22
Molecular weight	291.26	267.37
Molar volume	219.5 ± 3.0	262.5 ± 3.0

TABLE 25.2

Barrier Properties of Dry and Moist Military Uniform to Parathion In Vitro Human Skin Absorption

Treatments	Percent Dose Absorbed (Mean ± SD)	Permeability Coefficient (K_p, cm/hr)
Skin ($n = 4$)[a]	1.78 ± 0.41	1.89×10^{-4}
Skin + dry uniform ($n = 6$)[b]	0.29 ± 0.17	2.04×10^{-5}
Skin + wetted uniform ($n = 5$)[c]	0.65 ± 0.16	6.16×10^{-5}

[a] Versus[b,c] $p = 0.000$.
[b] Versus[c] $p = 0.007$.

uniforms were then applied to the volumetric solution (VS) permeability coefficient. These in turn were applied to regional differences in human skin absorption (6), and predicted VX systemic concentration by skin absorption for each body region and total body exposure were calculated. Toxic 50% lethality of VX was obtained from References 7 and 8.

25.3   RESULTS

Table 25.2 gives the in vitro percutaneous absorption of parathion through naked human skin and skin protected by dry uniform material and wetted uniform material. Following this single exposure and 96-hour absorption period, 1.78 ± 0.41% dose was absorbed through naked human skin and 0.29 ± 0.17% and 0.65 ± 0.16% doses through skin protected by dry and moist uniforms, respectively. The absorption was continuous through the total exposure period. Therefore, an infinite dose was available through the 96-hour dosing period. Statistically, naked skin absorption was greater than that protected by dry uniform ($p = 0.000$) and moist uniform ($p = 0.000$). Absorption through moist uniform was statistically ($p = 0.007$) greater than through dry uniform (statistics done only on percentage of absorbed dose—the raw data).

Table 25.3 gives calculated VX systemic absorption and toxicity to uniformed personnel. This is a one-time 4 μg/cm² VX exposure, and the resulting systemic dose occurs by skin absorption only (no respiratory and oral involvement). At 1 hour post-exposure 50% lethality occurs with full-body exposure to the compromised sweated uniform, although the dry uniform is right at the threshold. At 8 hours post-exposure to the head and neck only or the trunk only, lethality might occur with both wet and dry uniform material. At 96-hours post-exposure lethality occurs with exposure to any body part (4).

25.4   DISCUSSION

25.4.1   PERCUTANEOUS ABSORPTION

CWAs are easily and inexpensively produced and are a significant threat to military forces and to the public. VX, as well as the other CWAs sarin and soman, belong to the chemical class of organophosphorus compounds along with the well-known pesticides parathion, malathion, fenitrothion, chlorpyrifos, and diazinon. Parathion was used as a CWA simulant and by experimentation gave relative bioavailability permeability coefficients between naked skin and skin wearing sweated or dry uniform. Risk assessment for VX was then determined using the bioavailability relative to uniformed and naked skin and the regional variation of human percutaneous absorption. Since the risk

TABLE 25.3

The VX Systemic Absorption and Toxicity to Uniformed Military Personnel

Exposure Time	Body Exposure	Calculated VX Systemic Dose[a]	
		Compromised[b] (mg)	Protected[c] (mg)
1 hr	Head/neck[d]	4.16	4.16
	Arms and hands[d]	0.52	0.52
	Trunk	4.07	1.35
	Genital-s	0.45	0.15
	Legs	0.68	0.22
	Total	**9.87***	**6.40**
8 hr	Head/neck[d]	33.26*	33.26*
	Arms and hands[d]	4.16	4.16
	Trunk	32.52*	10.77*
	Genitals	3.61	1.2
	Legs	5.42	1.8
	Total	**78.98***	**51.18***
96 hr	Head/neck[d]	399.16*	399.16*
	Arms and hands[d]	49.90*	49.90*
	Trunk	390.29*	129.25*
	Genitals	43.37*	14.36*
	Legs	65.05*	21.54*
	Total	**947.76***	**614.21***

* Estimated systemic LD50 of VX is 6.5 mg (human, 70 kg). Systemic concentration is more than 50% lethality dose.

[a] 4 μg/cm^2 on whole body area (1.8 m^2).

[b] Uniform with perspiration.

[c] Dry uniform.

[d] Head/neck and arms and hands are unprotected.

is for clothed humans, these factors need to be included in the assessment. These absorption factors combined with an assessment of VX toxicity show how deadly VX can be from just skin exposure.

Risk assessment for chemicals requires a bioavailability component to determine how much of an exposure gets into the body. In vivo bioavailability is usually available for animals, and sometimes for man. In vitro data have been substituted for in vivo data. This normal course of events changes when dealing with VX and other CWAs. The deadly nature of the compounds precludes them from normal scientific inquiry, and any data that may be available from a government remain under the control of the government. However, risk potential for the military and the public is real, and risk assessment needs to be done with the information at hand.

The Potts–Guy equation provides estimates for the permeation of pure molecules. The condition is for infinite application, generally, but not necessarily, aqueous. Parathion (neat) was applied to the skin in an amount that would be infinite for 96 hours. The proof of an infinite dose is the ever-increasing cumulative amount of permeation (Figure 25.1), which would have reached a plateau if the dose were finite. Also, only 1.78%, 0.29%, and 0.65% of applied doses were absorbed for the three treatments (Table 25.2). The dosing vehicle was toluene, which will evaporate immediately upon contact (9). Some water would be available from the circulating receptor fluid (diffusion), and, of course, moisture was added as one of the experimental treatments. The K_p for parathion in this study was 1.89×10^{-4} cm/hr for dermatoned skin. The calculated K_p in epidermis (the Potts–Guy

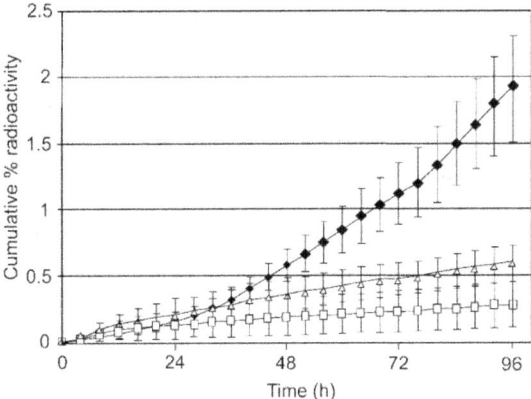

FIGURE 25.1   Percutaneous absorption of parathion across excised human skin (♦) without clothing; (■) with clothing; (▲) with clothing and sweat simulation. Values are means ± SD for each 4-hour time point.

equation) for parathion is 1.59×10^{-2} cm/hr. The calculated K_p for VX is 1.6×10^{-3} cm/hr (epidermis), which falls right between the two Kp (research-dermatoned skin and calculated-epidermis) for parathion.

Craig et al. (10) reported the percutaneous absorption of VX in subjects (U.S. Army enlisted men) using a cholinesterase inhibition assay. Subjects dosed on the forearm at 18°C room temperature for 6 hours had a penetration of $0.60 \pm 0.19\%$. Applying the Potts–Guy equation used in this study for a 4-μg dose over 6 hours gives a penetration of 0.96%, very similar to the empirical data of Craig et al. (10). They showed regional variation (cheek higher than forearm), justifying our use of regional variation for risk assessment. They also showed higher VX penetration with higher room temperature (46°C), suggesting sweat/moisture involvement, as with this current study.

Chemicals in cloth cause cutaneous effects. Hatch and Maibach (11) reported that chemicals added to cloth in 10 finish categories (dye, wrinkle resistance, water repellency, soil release, and so on) caused irritant and allergic contact dermatitis, atopic dermatitis exacerbation, and urticarial and phototoxic skin responses. This is qualitative information that chemicals will transfer from cloth to skin in vivo in humans. Quantitative data are lacking. Snodgrass (12) studied permethrin transfer from treated cloth to rabbit skin in vivo. Transfer was quantitative, but less than expected. Interestingly, permethrin remained within the cloth after detergent laundering. Wester et al. (2) showed in vitro percutaneous absorption of glyphosate and malathion through human skin decreased when added to cloth (the cloth was then placed on the skin). When water was added to glyphosate/cloth and water/ethanol to malathion/cloth, the percutaneous absorption increased (malathion to levels from solution). This perhaps reflects clinical situations where dermatitis occurs most frequently in human sweating areas (axilla and crotch).

One insecticide used widely in the Persian Gulf is the aliphatic chlorinated hydrocarbon permethrin. The military has done extensive studies on the use of permethrin-treated uniforms as a protective agent against insect-borne diseases. In the Gulf, military personnel were supplied cans of 0.5% permethrin and told to spray their own uniforms because the military did not have pretreated uniforms in stock. The dose recommended, 125 μg/cm², far exceeded the permethrin dose used in agriculture (i.e., 0.1 to 0.2 kg/ha or 2 μg/cm²). The result was that personnel who wore treated uniforms were subjected to dermal exposure via a massive dose of the insecticide for their entire period of service in the Gulf. This has been suggested as a contributing cause to the Gulf War syndrome (13).

This paper and that of Snodgrass (12) and Wester et al. (2) show that chemicals, including permethrin, can be absorbed into and through skin from cloth.

Time following exposure is most critical. Exposed clothing needs to be removed and skin decontaminated. It is imperative that the decontamination procedure not in itself enhance skin absorption (14). This applies to public as well as military situations. Society has a system of first responders for emergency incidents. Civilian CWA exposure has proved to be such an incident. First responders include police, firefighters, paramedics and other medical personnel, and good Samaritans. All but the firefighters will be wearing uniforms or civilian clothing similar in composition and design to that used in this bioavailability study. First responders have suffered the same fate as initial intended civilian targets, so their knowledge of this potential skin and clothing involvement is of importance.

These data refer directly to a model penetrant in an in vitro study and predicts in vivo toxicity for one of the CWAs. Although we do not wish to overgeneralize, the practical importance of this toxicological arena mandates broader study, such as model in vivo studies and examination of other fabrics and other CWA model compounds, as well as the agents themselves.

25.4.2 SKIN DECONTAMINATION

Recent events have brought forth concerns for weapons of mass destruction of which CWAs are included. The military has its protective and decontamination equipment, but little of this is privy to citizens. In the event of CWA civilian exposure, guidelines include:

1. Concern and essence of time following exposure
2. Remove contaminated clothing from victim
3. Hose (water) exposed skin
4. Transport to hospital facilities

From the percutaneous absorption and risk assessment presented here, numbers 1 and 2 are well justified. The essence of time is especially important. Number 3 presents a problem. Table 25.4 (15) shows in vivo human percutaneous absorption of parathion after soap and water wash. In a matter of minutes, certainly in the first hour, a large dose of parathion is absorbed. Time of effective response is very limited.

Table 25.5 (16) shows in vivo skin decontamination of methylene bisphenyl isocyamate (MDI). Water alone is fairly ineffective. This suggests that hosing victims of a CWA attack is limited in terms of effectiveness. Soap and water washing improved decontamination some, but as in Table 25.4, is not as effective as the public may believe. Two glycol-based cleaners were more effective than soap and water, as was off-the-shelf corn oil.

TABLE 25.4
Effect of Washing (Soap and Water) In Vivo Human Skin

	Percent Penetration							
	Minutes				Hours			
µg/cm²	1	5	15	30	1	2	48	24
Parathion, 4 arm	2.8		6.7		8.4		8.0 15.8	8.6
Parathion, 40			3.1				6.9	9.5
Parathion, 400 arm			2.2		2.3		4.2	4.8
Parathion, 4 forehead	8.4		7.1	12.2	10.5	20.1	27.7	36.3
Parathion, 4 palm		6.2	13.6	13.3	11.7	9.4	7.7	11.8

TABLE 25.5

Decontamination of [¹⁴C]-MDI as Percent Dose in Skin Washes Following Topical Administration in Rhesus Monkey

Washing Methods	Percent Dose Recovered [mean (±SD)]			
	5 min	1 hr	4 hr	8 hr
Water	60.0	56.7	40.2	29.2
	(11.1)	(10.1)	(8.9)	(9.7)
5% soap	71.2	51.1	46.1	36.6
	(5.2)	(14.1)	(8.2)	(12.8)
50% soap	67.3	68.6	54.4	45.7
	(9.6)	(16.0)	(5.2)	(6.6)
Polypropylene glycol	88.9	86.0	78.9	71.6
	(13.5)	(14.1)	(16.4)	(19.7)
PG-C	85.3	67.7	73.7	77.9
	(9.5)	(24.6)	(3.0)	(20.6)
Corn oil	95.1	77.2	73.2	86.2
	(9.0)	(24.2)	(17.4)	(10.0)

Abbreviations: MDI, methylene bisphenyl isocyanate.

REFERENCES

1. Maibach HI, Feldmann RJ, Milby TH, Sert WR. Regional variation in percutaneous penetration in man. Arch Environ Health 1971; 23:208–211.
2. Wester RC, Quan D, Maibach HI. In vitro percutaneous absorption of model compounds glyphosate and malathion from cotton fabric into and through human skin. Food Chem Toxicol 1996; 34:731–735.
3. Wester RC, Christoffel J, Hartway T, Poblete N, Maibach HI, Forsell J. Human cadaver skin viability for in vitro percutaneous absorption: storage and detrimental effects of heat-separation and freezing. Pharma Res 1998; 15:82.
4. Wester RM, Tanojo H, Maibach HI, Wester RC. Predicted chemical warfare agent VX toxicity to uniformed soldier using parathion in vitro human skin exposure and absorption. Toxicol Appl Pharmacol 2000; 168:149–152.
5. Potts RO, Guy RH. Predicting skin permeability. Pharm Res 1992; 9:663–669.
6. Guy RH, Maibach HI. Calculations of body exposure from percutaneous absorption data. In: Bronaugh R, Maibach HI, eds. Percutaneous Absorption. New York: Marcel Dekker, 1985:461–466.
7. Somani SM, Solana RP, Dube SN. Toxicology of nerve agents. In: Somani SM, ed. Chemical Warfare Agents. San Diego: Academic Press, 1992:76.
8. Sidell FR. Nerve agents. In: Sidell FR, Takafuji ET, Franz DR, eds. Medical Aspects of Chemical and Biological Warfare. Textbook of Military Medicine, Part I: Warfare, Weaponry, and the Casualty. Washington DC: Borden Institute, 1995:141.
9. Wester RC, Maibach HI. Benzene percutaneous absorption: dermal exposure relative to other benzene sources. Int J Occup Environ Health 2000; 6:122–126.
10. Craig FN, Cummings E, Sim VM. Experimental temperature and the percutaneous absorption of a cholinesterase inhibitor, VX. J Invest Dermatol 1977; 68:357–361.
11. Hatch KL, Maibach HI. Textile chemical finish dermatitis. Contact Dermatitis 1996; 14:1–13.
12. Snodgrass HL. Permethrin transfer from treated cloth to the skin surface: potential for exposure in humans. J Toxicol Environ Health 1992; 35:912–915.
13. Plapp FW. Permethrin and the gulf war syndrome. Arch Environ Health 1999; 54:312.
14. Wester RC, Maibach HI. Advances in percutaneous absorption. In: Drill V, Lazar P, eds. Cutaneous Toxicity. New York: Raven Press, 1984:29–40.
15. Maibach HI, Feldmann R. Systemic absorption of pesticides through the skin of man. Occupational Exposure to Pesticides. Federal Working Group on Pest Management. Washington, DC. Appendix B, 1974:120–127.
16. Wester RC, Hui H, Andry LT, Maibach HI. In vivo skin decontamination of MDI: soap and water ineffective compared to propylene glycol, polyglycol-based cleanser, and corn oil. Toxicol Sci 1999; 48:1–4.

26 Percutaneous Absorption of Hazardous Chemicals from Fabric into and through Human Skin

Howard I. Maibach
University of California, San Francisco, California

CONTENTS

26.1 INTRODUCTION

The treated surface that is in most contact with skin is fabric. Consider clothes worn day and night, sheets and blankets, and fabric in rugs and upholstery. The fabric environment may have been assumed safe in the following exposure problems. Brown (1) and Armstrong et al. (2) reported separate cases of phenolic disinfectants in a hospital laundry causing the death of infants and sickening in others. Toxic compounds in clothing such as diapers were spread over a large surface area on a skin site with potential absorption. Both parameters (large surface area and application to the urorectal area) enhance absorption (3). If the diaper were covered with rubber pants or more clothing, this could enhance absorption. Dermatitis is reported for chemical finish in textiles (possible pesticides in raw cotton, chemicals in the manufacturing process, chemicals added for correct color and sheen). These must involve chemical transfer from fabric to skin. The clothing of field workers is filled with pesticides from spraying, with the work of Snodgrass (4) suggesting that it may not launder out, but instead remain bioavailable. The pesticide "bomb" in the house settles on rugs, fabric chairs, etc., and the baby crawls over it. Finally, it should be noted that insecticide sprayed into the uniforms of Desert Storm personnel might have transferred from the fabric into and through the soldiers' skin. Both soldiers and civilians have the added threat of sprayed chemical warfare agents, which will settle on uniforms or clothing then diffuse to the skin and eventually into the body.

26.2 GLYPHOSATE (WATER-SOLUBLE HERBICIDE)

Tables 26.1 and 26.2 show the absorption profiles of 1% glyphosate through human skin and of glyphosate across cotton sheets into human skin. The 0-day treatment means that cotton sheets were treated with glyphosate and immediately added to the donor side while wet; the one- and

TABLE 26.1

Percutaneous Absorption Parameters of Glyphosate Across Cotton Sheets into Human Skin Under Different Donor Conditions

Donor Conditions	Treatment[a]	Flux (J) (μg/hr)	Permeability Constant (P) (cm/hr)	Lag Time (t) (hr)
1% glyphosate solution	None	4.12 ± 1.35	$4.59 \pm 1.56 \times 10^{-4}$	10.48 ± 1.23
Cotton–1% glyphosate solution	0 days	0.47 ± 0.08	$4.90 \pm 1.41 \times 10^{-5}$	5.00 ± 0.87
Cotton–1% glyphosate solution	1 day	0.05 ± 0.01	$5.21 \pm 0.69 \times 10^{-6}$	2.52 ± 0.53
Cotton–1% glyphosate solution	2 days	0.05 ± 0.01	$5.21 \pm 0.74 \times 10^{-6}$	1.31 ± 0.68
Cotton–1% glyphosate solution	Add water	0.23 ± 0.07	$2.40 \pm 0.54 \times 10^{-5}$	3.11 ± 1.02

Note: "Add water" means that the donor side included the treated cotton sheet and a certain amount of distilled water. Mean $\pm$ SEM ($n = 6$).

[a] A certain amount of 1% glyphosate aqueous solution was applied to cotton sheets, and the sheets were dried at room temperature for 0 to 2 days.

2-day treatment means that treated cotton sheets were dried for 1 or 2 days, and "add water" means that the donor side included the treated cotton sheet and 300 μL distilled water or aqueous ethanol. Clearly, when the glyphosate-treated cotton sheets were used as a donor side, the absorbed amount of glyphosate was less than that of glyphosate solution (control). Comparison of the three treatments showed that zero-day treatment caused two times higher skin absorption than did 1- or 2-day treatments. Table 26.1 gives the in vitro absorption parameters of glyphosate. The absorption of glyphosate under zero-day treatment showed about 10 times less than the control sample and 100 times less than 1- or 2-day treatments; the absorption (cm/hr) of the control sample or 0-, 1-, and 2-day treatments were 4.59×10^{-4}, 4.90×10^{-5}, 5.21×10^{-6}, and 5.21×10^{-6}, respectively. Adding water to treated cotton sheets in a donor side resulted in an increase in absorption compared with that of 1- or 2-day treatment. This result indicated that cotton sheets played a protective role. Decreases in the lag time of glyphosate were observed (Table 26.1) with the change of the donor-side conditions.

The residual amount of glyphosate in the skin or on the skin (after the cotton sheet is removed) after a 24-hour application is shown in Table 26.2. Note that 0-day treatment showed the highest residual amounts in the skin as well as on the skin (6.71% and 4.32%, respectively). A possible reason is that

TABLE 26.2

Comparison of Percutaneous Absorption Profiles of Glyphosate Across Cotton Sheets into Human Skin Under Different Donor Conditions

Donor Conditions	Treatment[a]	Absorbed Amount Across Skin (%)	Residual Amount on the Skin (%)	Residual Amount in the Skin (%)
1% glyphosate solution	None	1.42 ± 0.25	—	0.56 ± 0.13
Cotton–1% glyphosate solution	0 days	0.74 ± 0.26	6.71 ± 2.80	4.32 ± 1.95
Cotton–1% glyphosate solution	1 day	0.08 ± 0.02	0.69 ± 0.07	0.23 ± 0.13
Cotton–1% glyphosate solution	2 days	0.08 ± 0.01	0.42 ± 0.18	0.06 ± 0.01
Cotton–1% glyphosate solution	Add water	0.36 ± 0.07	—	0.23 ± 0.13

Note: "Add water" means that the donor side included the treated cotton sheet and a certain amount of distilled water. Mean $\pm$ SEM ($n = 6$).

[a] A certain amount of 1% glyphosate aqueous solution was applied to cotton sheets, and the sheets were dried at room temperature for 0 to 2 days.

TABLE 26.3

Percutaneous Absorption Parameters of Malathion Across Cotton Sheets Into Human Skin Under Different Donor Conditions

Donor Conditions	Treatment[a]	Flux (J)(μg/hr)	Permeability Constant (P)(cm/hr)	Lag Time (t)(hr)
1% malathion solution	None	2.40 ± 0.34	$2.03 \pm 0.65 \times 10^{-1}$	5.10 ± 1.24
Cotton–1% malathion solution	0 days	1.60 ± 0.18	$1.36 \pm 0.68 \times 10^{-1}$	4.26 ± 1.10
Cotton–1% malathion solution	1 day	0.26 ± 0.04	$2.20 \pm 0.71 \times 10^{-2}$	1.08 ± 0.28
Cotton–1% malathion solution	2 days	0.27 ± 0.01	$2.29 \pm 1.04 \times 10^{-2}$	1.12 ± 0.31
Cotton–1% malathion solution	Add solution	2.34 ± 0.54	$1.98 \pm 0.82 \times 10^{-1}$	5.60 ± 1.04

Note: "Add solution" means that the donor side included the treated cotton sheet and a certain amount of aqueous ethanol. Mean $\pm$ SEM ($n = 6$).

[a] A certain amount of 1% malathion-aqueous ethanol was applied to cotton sheets, and the sheets were dried at room temperature for 0 to 2 days.

when the cotton sheets were treated with glyphosate solution and immediately applied to the skin, the glyphosate was not yet bound to the cotton sheet and continued to separate onto the skin surface (5).

26.3 MALATHION (LIPID-SOLUBLE PESTICIDE)

The absorption profiles of malathion under different treatments are given in Tables 26.3 and 26.4. The 2-day treatment caused the lowest percutaneous absorption due to the cotton absorption of the compound. However, 0-day treatment and adding solution to treated cotton sheets caused higher absorption. All the in vitro absorption parameters are listed in Table 26.3. Note that there were no great differences in the skin absorption of malathion among the control, 0-day treatment and adding solution to cotton sheets treatment (0.20, 0.14, and 0.20 cm/hr, respectively). The skin absorption of malathion under 1- and 2-day treatment was approximately six times less than under 0-day treatment. It was found the lag time of malathion was shorter than glyphosate except for the "add solution" samples.

From Table 26.4, it can be seen that the residual amount of malathion in the skin increased with the following order (listed as the donor conditions): adding solution to treated cotton sheets (9.4%),

TABLE 26.4

Comparison of Percutaneous Absorption Profiles of Malathion Across Cotton Sheets into Human Skin Under Different Donor Conditions

Donor Conditions	Treatment[a]	Absorbed Amount Across Skin (%)	Residual Amount on the Skin (%)	Residual Amount in the Skin (%)
1% malathion solution	None	8.77 ± 1.43	—	7.63 ± 1.42
Cotton–1% malathion solution	0 days	3.92 ± 0.49	4.71 ± 1.27	4.43 ± 1.59
Cotton–1% malathion solution	1 day	0.62 ± 0.11	1.67 ± 0.77	2.68 ± 0.19
Cotton–1% malathion solution	2 days	0.60 ± 0.14	0.99 ± 0.08	0.85 ± 0.34
Cotton–1% malathion solution	Add solution	7.34 ± 0.61	—	9.40 ± 2.8

Note. "Add solution" means that the donor side included the treated cotton sheet and a certain amount of aqueous ethanol. Mean $\pm$ SEM (n = 6).

[a] A certain amount of 1% malathion-aqueous ethanol was applied to cotton sheets, and the sheets were dried at room temperature for 0 to 2 days.

no cotton (control, 7.63%) > 0-day treatment (4.43%) > 1-day treatment (2.68%) > 2-day treatment (0.85%). The residual amounts of malathion in the skin were higher than the corresponding amounts of glyphosate (5).

26.4 PARATHION (LIPID-SOLUBLE PESTICIDE)

Parathion was the chemical of choice to use as a surrogate for VX. Actual data with VX would be best; however, little exists in the literature. To obtain radiolabeled VX and study it in the public domain is highly improbable. Parathion is in the same chemical class as VX (organophosphorus) and has the same functional group as VX. The structures of parathion and VX and physicochemical data that relate to percutaneous absorption are similar. The partition coefficients (log P octanol/water), molecular weights, and molecular volumes are close. Similar structure, log P, and molecular weight/molar volume suggest the potential for similar percutaneous absorption.

Table 26.5 gives the in vitro percutaneous absorption of parathion through naked human skin and skin protected by dry uniform material and wetted uniform material. Following this single-exposure and 96-hour absorption period, $1.78 \pm 0.41\%$ dose was absorbed through naked human skin, and $0.29 \pm 0.17\%$ and $0.65 \pm 0.16\%$ doses were absorbed through skin protected by dry and moist uniforms, respectively. The absorption was continuous though the total exposure period. Therefore, an infinite dose was available through the 96-hour dosing period.

Statistically, naked skin absorption was greater than that protected by dry uniform ($p = 0.000$) and moist uniform ($p = 0.000$). Absorption through moist uniform was statistically ($p = 0.007$) greater than through dry uniform. Table 26.6 shows the total body surface area of a uniformed soldier. Head, neck, and arms (including hands) are unprotected naked skin. The other body areas are covered with uniform. VX systemic absorption and toxicity to uniformed personnel was calculated. This is a one-time $4\,\mu g/cm^2$ VX exposure, and the resulting systemic dose occurs by skin absorption only (no respiratory and oral involvement). At 1-hour post-exposure 50% lethality occurs with full-body exposure to the compromised sweated uniform, although the dry uniform is right at the threshold. At 8 hours post-exposure to the head and neck only or trunk only, lethality might occur with both wet and dry uniforms. At 96 hours post-exposure, lethality occurs with exposure to any body part (6).

26.5 ETHYLENE OXIDE (COLORLESS GAS AT ORDINARY ROOM TEMPERATURE AND PRESSURE)

Ethylene oxide is used as a fumigant for textiles and foodstuffs and to sterilize surgical instruments and hospital gowns. It is a highly reactive alkylating agent that can react directly with cellular macromolecules, including deoxyribonucleic acid (DNA), ribonucleic acid (RNA), and

TABLE 26.5
Barrier Properties of Dry and Moist Military Uniform to Parathion In Vitro Human Skin Absorption

Treatments	Percent Dose Absorbed (mean $\pm$ SD)	Permeability Coefficient (K_p, cm/hr)
Skin (n = 4)[a]	1.78 ± 0.41	1.89×10^{-4}
Skin + dry uniform (n = 6)[b]	0.29 ± 0.17	2.04×10^{-5}
Skin + wetted uniform (n = 5)[c]	0.65 ± 0.16	6.16×10^{-5}

[a] Versus[b,c] $p = 0.000$.
[b] Versus[c] $p = 0.007$.

TABLE 26.6

VX Systemic Absorption and Toxicity to Uniformed Military Personnel

		Calculated VX Systemic Dose[a]	
Exposure Time	Body Exposure	Compromised[b] (mg)	Protected[c] (mg)
1 hr	Head/neck[d]	4.16	4.16
	Arms and hands[d]	0.52	0.52
	Trunk	4.07	1.35
	Genitals	0.45	0.15
	Legs	0.68	0.22
	Total	**9.87**	**6.40**
8 hr	Head/neck[d]	33.26	33.26
	Arms and hands[d]	4.16	4.16
	Trunk	32.52	10.77
	Genitals	3.61	1.2
	Legs	5.42	1.8
	Total	**78.98**	**51.18**
96 hr	Head/neck[d]	399.16	399.16
	Arms and hands[d]	49.90	49.90
	Trunk	390.29	129.25
	Genital-s	43.37	14.36
	Legs	65.05	21.54
	Total	**947.76**	**614.21**

Note: 'Estimated systemic LD50 of VX is 6.5 mg (human, 70 kg). Systemic concentration is
more than 50% lethality dose.

a $4 \mu g/cm^2$ on whole body area ($1.8 \, cm^2$).

b Uniform with perspiration.

c Dry uniform.

d Head/neck and arms and hands are unprotected.

protein, without prior metabolic activation (7). Data have been collected on the genotoxicity of ethylene oxide in somatic and germ cells (8). Major et al. (9) have reported genotoxicological changes in nurses occupationally exposed to low-dose ethylene oxide. Studies to assess ethylene oxide risk use inhalation and intravenous (IV) routes of administration (10). As ethylene oxide exposure of humans can occur through exposure of fabric/skin in the workplace (5), a study was done to determine the percutaneous absorption of [¹⁴C] ethylene oxide from fabric into and through human skin. This study also serves as a model for exposure of fabric/skin to any potentially hazardous gas, be it under circumstances of war (5), the workplace, or some terrorist act, as recently occurred in Japan.

Table 26.7 gives the in vitro percutaneous absorption of [¹⁴C] ethylene oxide from fabric through human skin. In cells where the fabric/skin surface area was open to the air, 0.72% and 0.85% of the applied dose accumulated in the receptor fluid and 0.62% and 0.32% in the skin. This gives percutaneous absorption values of 1.34% (receptor fluid accumulation plus skin content) and 1.17% of the dose (average 1.3% of the dose). Less than 10% of the residual radioactivity was recovered in fabric and washings.

In cells where the fabric/skin was occluded with double latex material, 46.16% and 39.54% of the dose was recovered in receptor fluid and 3.25% and 3.12% was in the skin. This gives percutaneous absorption values of 49.41% and 42.66% (average 46.0%). Less than 5% of the residual radioactivity was recovered in fabric and washings. It is assumed that the remainder of the [¹⁴C] ethylene oxide was lost to the surrounding air.

TABLE 26.7

In Vitro Percutaneous Absorption of [¹⁴C] Ethylene Oxide from Fabric Through Human Skin

Surface	Item Assayed	Percentage of Dose	
		Skin Source 1	Skin Source 2
Open to air	Receptor fluid (RF)	0.72	0.85
	Fabric	7.65	5.65
	Skin wash	0.03	0.03
	Skin rinse	0.001	0.001
	Skin content	0.62	0.30
	Average absorbed (RF + skin)		1.3
Occluded	Receptor fluid (RF)	46.16	39.54
	Fabric	3.62	3.62
	Skin wash	0.07	0.05
	Skin rinse	0.01	0.02
	Skin content	3.25	3.12
	Average absorbed (RF + skin)		46.0

Figure 26.1 shows the accumulation of radioactivity in receptor fluid. Almost all of the skin-absorbed radioactivity was in the first 0- to 4-hour interval.

Some receptor fluid accumulations from a nonradioactive study were quickly frozen and shipped to NAmSA laboratories (Irvine, California, USA) for assay. At a dose of 600 ppm, no ethylene oxide, ethylene chlorohydrin, or ethylene glycol was detected. At 3892 ppm, ethylene oxide represented 4.5% to 8.3% of the dose in the receptor fluid; no ethylene chlorohydrin or ethylene glycol was detected. The potential loss of ethylene oxide during analysis is not known; however, ethylene oxide is able to be absorbed unchanged across human skin (11).

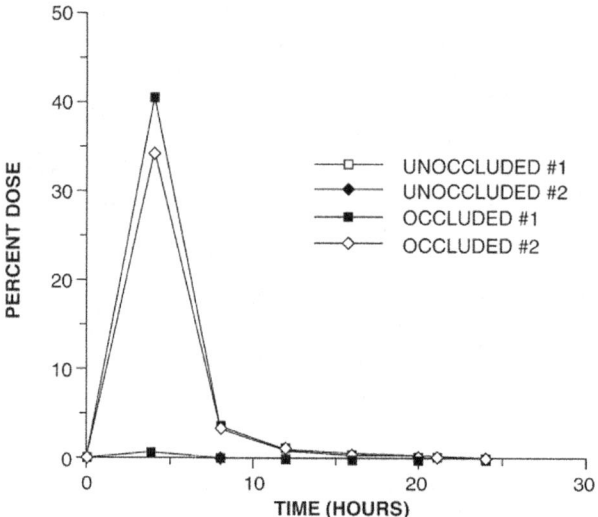

FIGURE 26.1   Ethylene oxide percutaneous absorption from fabric into human skin.

26.6   2-BUTOXYETHANOL (VAPOR)

Jones et al. (12) conducted a human in vivo study using 2-butoxyethanol to investigate the influence of temperature, humidity, and clothing on the dermal absorption of vapors. The extent of dermal absorption was determined by biological monitoring to measure the resultant body burden of the chemical. The study showed that clothing had a minimal effect on the dermal contribution to total body burden, with neither minimal clothing nor overalls having a significant effect on the amount absorbed through the skin. This could be because the rate of gas exchange through the clothing exceeds the absorption rate of 2-butoxyethanol through the skin.

Combining high temperature, high humidity, and the wearing of overalls had a significant impact on the percentage of dermal absorption, resulting in a mean dermal contribution to total body burden of 39% (range 33% to 42%). This may be due to the overalls generating a micro-climate next to the skin where the environment is significantly hotter and more humid than the ambient environment.

The work showed that dermal absorption of vapors can be significant and that environmental conditions may affect the absorption. Some types of protective clothing may not be suitable to reduce absorption. The possibility of dermal absorption of vapors should be considered, particularly for workers in high vapor concentration conditions where control of exposure relies on respiratory protection.

26.7   CONCLUSION

Chemicals are introduced to fabric at many steps during manufacture and use. Cotton plants are treated with pesticides. Many chemical dyes and finishes are added to fabric during manufacture, and these chemicals can cause human disease (13). The addition of chemicals (phenolic disinfectants) to fabric has caused human infant sickness and death (1, 2). There are implications that the "Gulf War syndrome" toxicity exhibited by soldiers may have been caused by interactions of insecticides and anti–nerve gas pills. The insecticides were impregnated into uniform fabric to ward off insects. This study and that of Snodgrass (4) show that chemicals in fabric will be absorbed from fabric into skin and then into the systemic circulation. Clothing and other fabric media (rugs and upholstery) must be considered repositories for hazardous chemicals, and these hazardous chemicals within fabric can be transferred to human skin. The threat of chemical warfare agents adds to the potential hazard of chemicals in clothing. Clothing seems to have minimal effect on vapors because the rate of gas exchange can exceed the rate of skin absorption.

REFERENCES

1. Brown BW. Fatal phenol poisoning from improperly laundered diapers. Am J Publ Health 1970; 60:901–902.
2. Armstrong RW, Eichner ER, Klein DE, Barthel WF, Bennett JV, Johnson V, Bruce H, Loveless LE. Pentachlorophenol poisoning in a nursery for newborn infants II. Epidemiologic and toxicologic studies. J Pediatr 1969; 75:317–325.
3. Wester RC, Maibach HI. Comparative percutaneous absorption. In: Maibach HI, Boisits E, eds. Neonatal Skin. New York: Marcel Dekker, 1982:137–147.
4. Snodgrass HL. Permethrin transfer from treated cloth to the skin surface: potential for exposure in humans. J Toxicol Environ Health 1992; 35:91–105.
5. Wester RC, Quan D, Maibach HI. In vitro percutaneous absorption of model compounds glyphosate and malathion from cotton fabric into and through human skin. Food Chem Toxicol 1996; 34:731–735.
6. Wester RM, Tanojo H, Maibach HI, Wester RC. Predicted chemical warfare agent VX toxicity to uniformed soldier using parathion in vitro human skin exposure and absorption. Toxicol Appl Pharmacol 2000; 168:149–152.
7. Brown CD, Wong BA, Fennell TR. In vitro and in vivo kinetics of ethylene oxide metabolism in rats and men. Toxicol Appl Pharmacol 1996; 136:8–19.

8. Preston RJ, Fennell TR, Leber AP, Sielken RL Jr, Swenberg RL. Reconsideration of the genetic risk assessment for ethylene oxide exposures. Environ Mol Mutagen 1995; 26:189–202.

9. Major J, Jakob MG, Tompa A. Genotoxicological investigation of hospital nurses occupationally exposed to ethylene oxide: 1. Chromosome aberrations, sister-chromatid exchanges, cell cycle kinetics, and UV-included DNA synthesis in peripheral blood lymphocytes. Environ Mol Mutagen 1996; 27:84–92.

10. Ehrenberg L, Törnquist M. The research background for risk assessment of ethylene oxide: aspects of dose. Mutat Res 1995; 330:41–54.

11. Wester RC, Hartway T, Serranza S, Maibach HI. Human Skin in vitro percutaneous absorption of gaseous ethylene oxide from fabric. Food Chem Toxicol 1997; 35:513–515.

12. Jones K, Cocker J, Dodd LJ, Fraser I. Factors affecting the extent of dermal absorption of solvent vapors: a human volunteer study. Ann Occup Hyg 2003; 47:145–150.

13. Hatch KL, Maibach HI. Textile chemical finish dermatitis. Contact Dermatitis 1986; 14:1–13.

27 Percutaneous Absorption of Chemicals from Fabric (Textile)[*]

Jordan L. Bormann
University of South Dakota, Sioux Falls, South Dakota

Ayse Sermin Filiz Acipayam
Bakirkoy Dr Sadi Konuk Training and Research Hospital,
Istanbul, Turkey

Howard I. Maibach
University of California, San Francisco, California

CONTENTS

27.1 STANDARD ABSTRACT

Percutaneous penetration of chemicals from clothing can result in both acute and chronic toxicities. Although personal protective equipment composed of nonwoven material can provide thorough protection, it is often uncomfortable under normal occupational conditions. Certain everyday textiles are often utilized as protective clothing due to their cost, comfort, and convenience. Although common textiles may cover most skin, certain regions remain exposed by such outfits. The body areas covered by the fabric are at risk for fabric permeation and percutaneous penetration of chemical, either immediately or over time, dependent on the fabric composition and the characteristics of the chemical used. *In vitro* and *in vivo* publications studied percutaneous penetration of chemicals from contaminated fabric and show that everyday textiles are superior to bare skin. The increased protection offered can be attributed to properties of the fabric such as weave, thickness, fabric finish, absorbency, and the overall barrier provided. Although common textiles do offer some protection, they remain inferior to nonwoven

---

[*] Reprinted with permission (pending) from Journal of Applied Toxicology.

personal protective equipment. Much remains unknown regarding percutaneous penetration and protection offered by everyday textiles.

27.2 INTRODUCTION

Percutaneous penetration of chemicals from fabric can occur when contaminated clothing comes in contact or in proximity with human skin. Such situations can range from sleeping in night clothes mercerized by a protective chemical to the battlefields where chemically treated military uniforms are utilized to defend against insect-vector diseases. Occupational exposure to pesticides in the agricultural industry extends itself to a high exposure risk, leading to chronic illness, or in more severe cases, acute toxicity and death. Here we review the literature and summarize what is known about the percutaneous penetration of chemicals from fabric in quantifiable terms. We also summarize dermal protection from pesticides and other chemicals, or lack thereof, offered by the many types of fabric worn for occupational use. It is imperative to consider the percutaneous penetration of pesticides and other toxins from textiles due to the local and systemic toxicities that may occur.

27.3 METHODS

We searched PubMed, Embase, Web of Science, and Google Scholar with extensive bibliographical review from January 1980 to May 2020, with the search words "textile," "fabric," "percutaneous penetration," "percutaneous absorption," "protection," "pesticides," "dermal absorption," "dermal penetration," "skin absorption," and "clothing." We included *in vitro* and *in vivo* studies (rabbit and human). The cutaneous barrier penetration results, along with description/use of the chemical and description of the fabric used in each study, are summarized in tables.

27.4 RESULTS

We found 22 publications pertaining to percutaneous penetration of chemicals from fabrics. Tables 27.1 and 27.2 present this limited experimental data. Table 27.1 includes *in vitro* data and Table 27.2 includes *in vivo* data.

TABLE 27.1

Summary of *In Vitro* Studies. Chemical Characteristics and Various Fabric Properties Influenced Percutaneous Absorption

Reference	Fabric Description	Chemical(s)	Cutaneous System	Findings
Liquids				
Wester et al. (2000)	Standard army issue coat, 50% cotton and 50% nylon	Parathion (pesticide)	Human skin	Parathion absorption was significantly less through uniformed skin when compared to naked skin. Dry uniform offered significantly more protection than moist uniform.
Wester et al. (1996)	100% cotton sheet	Glyphosate (herbicide), malathion (insecticide)	Human skin	Allowing fabric contaminated with chemical to dry before skin contact decreased amount of percutaneous penetration. Adding water to the dried contaminated cloth to simulate perspiration increased percutaneous absorption. Pesticides exhibit unique chemical properties, and their percutaneous absorption from fabric can vary.

TABLE 27.1 (*Continued*)
Summary of *In Vitro* Studies. Chemical Characteristics and Various Fabric Properties Influenced Percutaneous Absorption

Reference	Fabric Description	Chemical(s)	Cutaneous System	Findings
Liquids				
Obendorf et al. (2003)	Bleached and bleached/ mercerized: print fabric (102–107 g/m²) and denim (274 g/m²)	Methyl parathion (pesticide)	Model membrane	There was significantly less pesticide absorption through starched fabrics compared to nonstarched fabrics. Thicker fabric may increase absorption and decrease percutaneous penetration of pesticide.
Welch and Obendorf (1997)	Unfinished 100% cotton denim, 274 g/m²	Methyl parathion (pesticide)	Human skin	Denim fabric decreased pesticide transport through human skin.
Moore et al. (2014)	Cotton shirt material	Chlorpyrifos, dichlorvos (pesticides)	Human skin	Removing contaminated clothing after exposure can limit dermal absorption. Everyday clothing can protect against dermal absorption of pesticides in a variety of applicator formulations.
Iadaresta et al. (2018)	Textile fabric	Benzothiazole (many industrial uses)	Strat-M artificial membranes	Greater than 60% of the benzothiazole penetrated through the artificial membrane in 24 hours.
Gaseous Chemicals				
Wester et al. (1997)	100% polyester material	Ethylene oxide (fumigant)	Human skin	Ethylene oxide was rapidly absorbed through skin from contaminated fabric. Occlusion of the fabric by latex gloves resulted in increased percutaneous penetration.
Gaskin et al. (2013a)	100% cotton (denim)	Ammonia gas (HAZMAT)	Human skin	Denim material covering cutaneous barrier resulted in negligible systemic absorption of ammonia gas at a concentration of 2000 ppm.
Gaskin et al. (2013b)	100% cotton (denim)	Hydrogen cyanide, chlorine gases (HAZMAT)	Human skin	Hydrogen cyanide gas negligibly penetrated the cutaneous barrier with and without denim covering. Chlorine gas penetration significantly increased with denim fabric over the skin.
Gaskin et al. (2019)	100% cotton (denim)	Nitric oxide, nitrogen dioxide, sulfur dioxide gases (HAZMAT)	Human skin	Study showed no significant absorption of nitric oxide or nitrogen dioxide with or without denim covering. There was slightly increased absorption of sulfur dioxide in the presence of denim covering.
Gaskin et al. (2017)	100% polyester and 100% cotton (denim)	Methyl bromide, sulfuryl fluoride, and chloropicrin (pesticides)	Human skin	Clothing was protective against percutaneous penetration of methyl bromide. Percutaneous penetration of sulfuryl fluoride and chloropicrin were minimally affected by addition of cloth covering the skin.
Heath et al. (2017)	Denim fabric	Ethylene oxide gas (sterilant, fumigant)	Human skin	There were no significant differences in percutaneous penetration of ethylene oxide with or without denim covering the cutaneous barrier.

TABLE 27.2

Summary of *In Vivo* Studies. Various Pesticides, Organic Compounds, and HAZMAT Simulation Exposures Were Studied in Regard to Their Percutaneous Penetration Through Clothing

Reference	Fabric Description	Chemical	Subject	Findings
Liquids				
Blum et al. (1978)	Children's sleepwear	Tris(2,3-dibromopropyl) phosphate (tris-BP) (flame retardant)	Human	Sleepwear treated with tris-BP caused significantly elevated urinary excretion levels of 2,3-dibromopropanol.
Ulsamer et al. (1978)	Polyester cloth (3 oz/sq yd)	Radiolabeled tris(2,3-dibromopropyl) phosphate (tris-BP) (flame retardant)	Rabbit	Sweat- and urine-soaked cloth resulted in greater percutaneous penetration of chemical than from dry cloth over 96 hours.
Snodgrass (1992)	100% cotton military uniform (Type III) and 50% nylon/50% cotton military uniform (NYCO)	Permethrin (insecticide)	Rabbit	The study showed percutaneous absorption of permethrin from 100% cotton or 50/50 cotton and nylon fabric over 7-day study. Environment and fabric type were not significant variables.
Rossbach et al. (2010)	Battle dress uniforms	Permethrin (insecticide)	Human	Significantly higher levels of permethrin metabolites were found in the urine of soldiers wearing permethrin-impregnated uniforms.
Rossbach et al. (2016)	Forestry worker pants (2 separate distributors)	Permethrin (insecticide)	Human	Workers wearing permethrin-impregnated pants resulted in higher amounts of permethrin urinary metabolites compared to workers wearing nonimpregnated pants.
Rossbach et al. (2014)	Commercially available permethrin-impregnated forestry work clothing	Permethrin (insecticide)	Human	Increased physical workload, temperature, and humidity resulted in higher levels of urinary permethrin metabolites.
Meinke et al. (2009)	Polyester/cotton fabric (65/35)	Dianix Leuchtgelb 10G (textile dye)	Human	Sweat greatly increased chemical migration from fabric into skin.
Gaseous Chemicals				
Morrison et al. (2016)	Cotton clothing articles	Airborne phthalates (semi-volatile organic compound)	Human	Exposed cotton clothing led to increased dermal uptake of phthalates, while clean clothing protected against uptake.
Morrison et al. (2017)	100% cotton long-sleeve shirts	Airborne benzophenone-3 (UV light filter)	Human	Wearing clothing with previous exposure to airborne benzophenone-3 resulted in increased urinary levels of benzophenone-3.
Bekö et al. (2017)	Cotton clothing articles, unexposed or exposed to nicotine	Nicotine (drug)	Human	Wearing clean clothing resulted in 4 times less absorption of airborne nicotine than when wearing nicotine-exposed clothing.

27.4.1 PERCUTANEOUS PENETRATION: *IN VITRO* STUDIES

27.4.1.1 Liquids

Military personnel may be exposed to chemicals as a means of attack through chemical warfare. Chemicals in the organophosphate family, such as agent VX, are widely studied. Agent VX is a chemical warfare agent with lethal properties when dermally absorbed. Due to the lethality of agent VX, parathion, a common pesticide with similar chemical properties as VX, was used to estimate percutaneous penetration of the more lethal agent VX when transferred from clothing

(Wester et al. 2000). The standard army-issued coat, hot weather woodland camouflage, combat pattern; 50% nylon and 50% cotton (American Apparel, Inc.) was utilized as the uniform material. The arms, head, and neck were unprotected by the military uniform. Parathion absorption was measured at 1 hour, 8 hours, and 96 hours after contact with the contaminated fabric, or, in the case of naked skin, after chemical contamination with no uniform barrier.

A one-hour time frame simulated exposure and quick removal of the exposed clothing or decontamination. An 8-hour time frame simulated the average workday, and the 96-hour window reproduced the conditions experienced by military personnel in the field where a change of clothing may not be available for an extended time. Military uniform, both dry and wet, offered significantly more protection against parathion than naked skin alone ($p = 0.000$). The mean percentages of parathion absorbed after 96 hours by a military worker with no uniform, a wetted uniform, and a dry uniform were 1.8%, 0.7%, and 0.3%, respectively. Their study showed significant differences in chemical percutaneous penetration of dry clothing and moist clothing at 1, 8, and 96 hours after exposure ($p = 0.007$). The calculated VX systemic dose from their *in vitro* study showed total dermal absorption of 9.9 mg, 79.0 mg, and 947.8 mg at 1 hour, 8 hours, and 96 hours, respectively, in military workers wearing a moist uniform. In a military worker wearing a dry uniform, 6.4 mg, 51.2 mg, and 614.2 mg was absorbed at 1 hour, 8 hours, and 96 hours, respectively (Table 27.1).

In another *in vitro* study utilizing human skin, percutaneous absorption of the herbicides glyphosate (water-soluble) and malathion (water-insoluble) from solution were compared to their percutaneous absorption from contaminated 100% cotton fabric (Wester et al. 1996). The fabric was in contact with human skin on day 0, day 1, or day 2 after contamination occurred. By day 2, the contaminated cotton fabric had dried, and water was added to simulate wet conditions such as perspiration on a hot day.

Percutaneous absorption was measured for the wetted fabric, and 1.4% of the glyphosate 1% solution control was absorbed across the skin, while 0.7%, 0.1%, 0.1%, and 0.4% of the glyphosate was absorbed across the skin from cotton fabric on day 0, day 1, day 2, and day 2 with the addition of water, respectively. A reported 8.8% of the 1% malathion solution control was absorbed across the skin, while 3.9%, 0.6%, 0.6%, and 7.3% of the malathion was absorbed across the skin from cotton fabric on day 0, day 1, day 2, and day 2 with the addition of water, respectively. These results suggest that chemical drying decreased the absorption, but wetting the dried-on chemical increased its absorption. This study reinforces the increased protection offered by some fabrics against chemicals involved in occupational exposure and the importance of removing contaminated clothing as soon as feasible after contamination (Table 27.1).

The Franz diffusion cell technique was utilized to study percutaneous penetration of pesticide from contaminated textiles (Welch & Obendorf 1997). Using the pesticide methyl parathion and an unfinished 100% cotton denim, they observed a statistical difference in pesticide transferred through human skin between pesticide exposure without fabric compared to the same system with protection from denim fabric. A reported 0.08 mg of methyl parathion was transferred through skin with no fabric barrier, while only 0.01 mg was transferred when utilizing denim fabric during the primary exposure and 0.02 mg utilizing fabric under secondary exposure conditions (Table 27.1).

Obendorf et al. (2003) utilized a synthetic membrane system to determine absorption of the pesticide methyl parathion from dry cotton fabric. Cotton fabric in print cloth, simulating the thickness of shirt material, showed 2.1% absorption of the pesticide eight hours after fabric contamination. Bleached print cloth, mercerized print cloth, and carboxymethylated print cloth revealed 1.4%, 2.4%, and 2.6% absorption after eight hours, respectively. Bleached, mercerized, and carboxymethylated cloth were significantly decreased with the addition of starch to the fabric; absorption after eight hours was 0.8%, 0.6%, and 1.9%, respectively. In the second part of their study, they used a denim fabric, which was thicker than the print fabric, to simulate absorption through pant material. They compared pesticide penetration through human skin from the denim fabric to pesticide penetration through human skin with no fabric barrier. At 50 hours post-exposure, ~4% of the pesticide had transported through human skin with no fabric, while only ~1% of the pesticide transported through human skin protected by denim fabric. Their results suggest that thickness and weave of fabric can significantly affect pesticide percutaneous penetration. They also suggest that starching aids in absorbing pesticide, which reduces pesticide exposure and subsequent penetration (Table 27.1).

Moore et al. (2014) measured percutaneous penetration of chemicals from clothing using chlorpyrifos and dichlorovos to contaminate fabric. Dichlorvos is a moderately lipophilic liquid, while chlorpyrifos is a lipophilic solid. Pesticides were applied in two different vehicles: isopropranolol (IPA) and propylene glycol (PG). Fabrics contaminated with chlorpyrifos in both IPA and PG solutions showed significantly reduced cutaneous penetration compared to contaminated unclothed human skin. There was no statistical significance in chlorpyrifos cutaneous penetration between the 4-hour and 24-hour periods between fabric removal and skin decontamination in the IPA solution, while there was a statistical difference in the PG vehicle between those two time points. Percentages of absorbed chlorpyrifos in IPA with clothing decontamination at 4 hours, clothing decontamination at 24 hours, and unclothed decontamination at 4 hours were 2.3%, 1.0%, and 1.0%, respectively. There was, however, a statistical difference in percutaneous penetration of chlorpyrifos in the PG solution when decontamination occurred at 4 hours instead of 24 hours. Percentages of absorbed chlorpyrifos in PG with clothing decontamination at 4 hours, clothing decontamination at 24 hours, and unclothed decontamination at 4 hours were 2.2%, 0.6%, and 1.1%, respectively. Percentages of absorbed dichlorvos in IPA solution were 1.3%, 2.6%, and 10.1% for decontamination at 30 minutes, decontamination at 24 hours, and unclothed decontamination at 30 minutes, respectively. Percentages of absorbed dichlorvos in PG solution were 1.2%, 2.0%, and 6.4% for decontamination at 30 minutes, decontamination at 24 hours, and unclothed decontamination at 30 minutes, respectively. This study reveals that significant reduction of pesticide cutaneous absorption can occur with swift removal of contaminated clothing. Different chemicals absorb into the skin at different rates, and it is imperative to remove the contaminated clothing as soon as possible (Table 27.1).

Keeble et al. (1993) utilized an *in vitro* test system to determine percutaneous absorption of azinphos-methyl, paraoxon, and malathion from glove fabrics. Absorption was quantified as the amount of acetyl cholinesterase inhibition that occurred within the *in vitro* test system. Out of the fabrics tested, 100% cotton in 13-cut and 7-cut displayed the lowest rates of acetyl cholinesterase inhibition through the *in vitro* system, therefore providing the best protection against the organophosphate pesticides (Keeble et al. 1993). A later study by Keeble et al. (1996) used *in vitro* test systems to study the effect of laundering on the permeation properties of fabric and subsequent percutaneous penetration. They found that fabric contaminated with azinphos-methyl in petroleum distillates provided protection regardless of fabric laundering status, whereas fabric contaminated with paraoxon in ethanolic solution displayed decreased protection against percutaneous absorption when the fabric had been laundered (Table 27.1).

Iadaresta et al. (2018) studied the penetration of benzothiazole with a Strat-M artificial membrane system utilizing a flow-through diffusion cell method. Fifty microliters of benzothiazole solution (0.228 mg/mL in H_2O:EtOH, 50:50 v:v) was applied to 0.5 cm^2 t-shirt material over the membrane. After 24 hours, 56.9% ± 3.2% of the chemical applied to the textile was recovered with 26.9% ± 1.9% having penetrated through the artificial membrane into the receiving chamber. The textile contained 13.3% ± 4.6% of the recovered chemical, and the artificial membrane contained 16.7% ± 2.4% of chemical recovered (Table 27.1).

27.4.1.2 Gaseous Chemicals

Gaskin et al. (2013a) simulated a hazardous material (HAZMAT) incident scenario with ammonia gas at 2000 ppm to determine percutaneous penetration through a human abdominal skin/Franz diffusion cell system with denim fabric as protection. They found negligible absorption; however, the fabric acted a reservoir with potential for secondary exposure. Systemic absorption was also negligible with addition of a post-exposure ventilation period, but there was a significant reduction in the amount of ammonia contained within the denim fabric compared to no post-exposure ventilation period (Table 27.1). In an additional study by Gaskin et al. (2013b), similar protocols were followed utilizing chlorine and hydrogen cyanide gases. A significant increase in chlorine gas penetration at 500 ppm occurred in the presence of denim fabric. Elevated levels of hydrogen cyanide gas (800 ppm) resulted in marginal percutaneous penetration; however, the presence of the denim covering slightly increased penetration compared to no denim covering (Table 27.1).

Gaskin et al. (2019) performed a similar study with nitrogen and sulfur gases. Nitrogen dioxide, nitric oxide, and sulfur dioxide gases were exposed to denim covering a human abdominal skin/Franz diffusion cell system. Nitrogen dioxide and nitric oxide were minimally absorbed with or without the presence of denim. Only sulfur dioxide absorption slightly increased in the presence of fabric; there were similar findings in the setting of a post-exposure ventilation period (Table 27.1). An additional study by Gaskin et al. (2017) found clothing protected skin from percutaneous penetration of methyl bromide, while textiles minimally affected the penetration of chloropicrin and sulfuryl fluoride (Table 27.1).

Heath et al. (2017) simulated a HAZMAT incident with ethylene oxide gas exposure. Negligible dermal penetration occurred at 800 ppm, and increased penetration occurred at concentrations of 3000 ppm. Denim present on the skin resulted in increased percutaneous penetration, but the values were insignificant. There was, however, a more than five times increase in chemical residue in fabric and human skin at the 3000 ppm concentration, potentially acting as a reservoir for further future penetration (Table 27.1).

Wester et al. (1997) created an *in vitro* model to determine hazardous gas percutaneous penetration from contaminated fabric. One hundred percent polyester material was contaminated with ethylene oxide, an alkylating agent. The contaminated fabric was placed in contact with human skin in the *in vitro* system. A portion of the fabric was left exposed to normal air conditions, while another portion was occluded with a double layer of latex glove material. Results revealed expeditious absorption through skin in under four hours; 1.3% of the ethylene oxide was percutaneously absorbed under nonoccluded conditions, while 46.0% of the ethylene oxide was absorbed under occluded conditions (Table 27.1)

27.4.2 Percutaneous Penetration: *In Vivo* Studies

27.4.2.1 Liquids

A pioneering study regarding percutaneous penetration from fabrics performed by Blum et al. (1978) investigated the flame retardant tris(2,3-dibromopropyl)phosphate (tris-BP), used on children's sleepwear from 1973 until its banning in 1977. Morning urine collection from a seven-year-old female with a history of wearing well-worn tris-BP–treated sleepwear was performed for 12 days. On the first two mornings, the level of 2,3-dibromopropanol in the urine was 0.4 ng/mL. On the second through sixth night, the subject wore new pajamas treated with tris-BP, and dibromopropanol levels in the female's urine increased significantly; measurements showed 11, 29, 21, and 18 ng/mL on nights 2, 3, 5, and 6, respectively. Urine collection was lost from night 4.

Five months after banning the sale of tris-BP–treated sleepwear, Blum et al. (1978) tested the urine of 10 children and one adult. No urinary excretion of 2,3-dibromopropanol was detected a child or adult; both reported no past use of tris-BP–treated sleepwear. Seven of the children who reported wearing washed tris-BP–treated sleepwear had levels of about 0.5 ng/mL in their urine, while an additional child's urine revealed 5 ng/mL of 2,3-dibromopropanol. The last child stopped wearing tris-BP–treated sleepwear around six months prior to the study, and his urine demonstrated only trace amounts of 2,3-dibromopropanol (Table 27.2).

Ulsamer et al. (1978) also studied percutaneous absorption of tris-BP from radiolabeled polyester cloth. A gauze patch was used to secure the cloth in place on white rabbits over a 96-hour study period. When controlling for exhaled radiolabel in the form of CO_2, dry cloth led to 4.31% absorption, sweat-treated cloth resulted in 4.79% absorption, and human urine–soaked cloth caused the greatest amount of absorption: 15.84%. The increased absorption may have resulted from a dermatitis-like reaction that developed on cloth-covered areas of the urine-soaked cloth group. Absorption was measured from the dose remaining in the body, urine, and feces (Table 27.2).

Although organophosphates can be used as chemical warfare agents against military personnel, similar agents may be used to the military's benefit in uniforms as protection against insect-vector diseases. A widely used clothing insect repellant is permethrin. Snodgrass (1992) used permethrin-treated military uniform fabric and measured the absorption of the pesticide from fabric through rabbit skin. One hundred percent cotton or a 50/50 blend of cotton and nylon military uniform fabric swatch contaminated with permethrin was attached to the hairless back of a rabbit for seven days. Percentage absorbed was measured by the amount of radiolabeled permethrin excreted in both urine and feces. The 100% cotton fabric contamination led to 0.9% percutaneous absorption under a temperate environment (no sweat), while a subtropical environment (sweat present) increased absorption to 3.2%. The 50/50 blend of cotton and nylon fabric contamination led to 1.7% percutaneous absorption in the temperate environment and 2.0% absorption in the subtropical environment. The authors suggest the absorption percentages may be higher in their study compared to those found when wearing a military uniform because uniforms are more loosely fitting than the apparatus applied to the rabbits in their study. The exposure dose to humans from wearing permethrin-treated (0.125 mg/cm^2) military clothing is predicted to be 6×10^{-4} mg/kg/d. They did not find environment or type of fabric to be statistically significant variables (Table 27.2).

Rossbach et al. (2010) studied percutaneous absorption of permethrin from military uniforms in a study comprising 187 participants who wore permethrin-impregnated or nonimpregnated uniforms for 40 to 72 hours per week for four weeks. Urine was collected and analyzed for permethrin metabolites at set time points throughout the study, which revealed significantly higher metabolite levels in the soldiers wearing permethrin-impregnated clothing compared to collection at initiation of the study. Of note, permethrin metabolites were still present four weeks after the study concluded (Table 27.2).

Rossbach et al. (2016) showed similar findings of increased permethrin uptake from permethrin-impregnated work pants in forestry workers, with the highest levels of permethrin urinary metabolites found 1 week into the 16-week study period. It was suggested that washing the pants throughout the study may have resulted in decreased permethrin concentrated within the pants, in turn resulting in decreased percutaneous penetration. Interestingly, there were significant differences in permethrin percutaneous penetration between two different brands of pants used in the study, although concentrations of chemical were advertised as similar (Table 27.2). Rossbach et al. (2014) measured urinary metabolites of permethrin from commercial work outfits under different environmental and work conditions, finding that increased physical workload, temperature, and humidity resulted in higher levels of urinary permethrin metabolites (Table 27.2).

Meinke et al. (2009) approached the measurement of chemical migration into and through the cutaneous barrier differently, using tape stripping and tape extraction. Twelve volunteers wore a piece of cloth treated with textile dye on their lower backs for 12 hours; six of the participants performed no sport activity during the study, while the other half of the cohort performed 30 minutes of physical activity while wearing the textile dyed clothing. Level of activity more significantly affected dye migration than did the time elapsed from first contact with the dyed material (Table 27.2). *In vitro* studies performed by Meinke et al. (2009) correlated with the *in vivo* results described here.

27.4.2.2 Gaseous Chemicals

Several volatile organic compounds are encountered in the workplace, and percutaneous absorption of such compounds can occur (Rehal & Maibach 2011). Morrison et al. (2016) studied dermal absorption of airborne phthalates under conditions of bare skin, clean cotton clothing, and cotton clothing exposed to phthalates for at least one week. Individuals wearing cotton clothing exposed to phthalates (diethylphthalate and di-n-butylphthalate) for at least one week exhibited increased excretion of chemical metabolites in their urine, while clean cotton clothing was protective against dermal absorption. Compared to bare skin, exposed clothing led to 6.5 and 3.3 times higher absorption of diethylphthalate and di-n-butylphthalate, respectively. Clean clothing resulted in 5.6 and 3.2 times lower dermal uptake of diethylphthalate and di-n-butylphthalate, respectively, compared to bare skin (Table 27.2). A similar study by Morrison et al. (2017) found significantly higher levels of benzophenone-3 in the urine of individuals wearing clothing with previous exposure to airborne benzophenone-3 compared to that of urine samples from the same individuals before contact with the contaminated clothing (Table 27.2).

Bekö et al. (2017 determined dermal uptake of nicotine from air under conditions of bare skin, cotton clothing, and exposed cotton clothing by urinary measurements of nicotine and its metabolites. Two bare-skinned individuals wearing only shorts were exposed to nicotine for 3 hours (estimated nicotine air concentration 420 ug/m^3); urinary excretion of nicotine and its metabolites were measured for 60 hours after removal from the airborne nicotine chamber. A third individual wearing clean cotton clothing entered and left the chamber at the same time points as the two bare-skinned individuals, and urinary excretion was measured for 24 hours. At 24 hours after exiting the chamber, that individual reentered the chamber wearing clean clothing except for a nicotine-exposed shirt (five-day exposure at estimated >200 ug/m^3) for an additional 3 hours. Urinary excretion of nicotine and its metabolites were measured for 60 hours after his exit from the chamber. Both exposed and unexposed clothing resulted in decreased dermal uptake of nicotine compared to bare skin; however, clean clothing resulted in four times less absorption than exposed clothing (Table 27.2).

27.5   CONCLUSION

Percutaneous penetration of pesticides from clothing in the occupational worker is a nearly inevitable process unless full personal protective equipment is worn. Depending on the chemical being used, exposure can result in chronic illness or acute toxicity. Such exposure over the course of decades of work may be related to increased incidence of cancer and other health conditions. Oftentimes, environmental conditions, such as heat and humidity, limit the practicability of full personal protective equipment use. Continuous innovation and modification of everyday clothing materials to create protective gear that is user friendly while still preventing penetration of chemicals is imperative.

It is necessary to consider the variable properties of protective fabrics when choosing clothing for occupational workers. Fabrics that decrease the penetration of pesticide ultimately result in less pesticide reaching the skin and therefore decreased opportunity for dermal penetration. Tyvek, a 100% olefin spun-bonded nonwoven material, exhibited the lowest transmission level, followed by 100% cotton and cotton/polyester blend fabrics, whereas woven fabrics made of 100% synthetic fibers exhibited high levels of pesticide transmission (Raheel 1991). Tyvek provided more protection than cotton with azinphos-methyl exposure (Orlando et al. 1981). In a study by Lillie et al. (1981), chlordane, diazinon, carbaryl, and prometon penetrated 100% polyester more than 100% cotton. In addition to the type of fabric, motion of the worker in contaminated clothing while performing occupational duties could transfer up to 12% of the pesticide to human skin through friction (Yang & Li 1993).

Oftentimes the comfort of occupational clothing is inversely related to the protection it provides. A full personal protective equipment outfit revealed penetration factor values of 0.0% to 2.1%, while average work clothing of a cotton shirt, pants, and tennis shoes or rubber boots yielded penetration factor values of 0.0% to 24.0% (Protano et al. 2009). Certain body regions are more likely to be contaminated with pesticides than others (Guy & Maibach, 1985). Certain pesticide application methods also yield increased deposition of pesticide contamination compared to an alternative method (Chan et al. 2010). More data are needed to determine which common textiles afford the best protection, as occupational workers will most likely choose comfort and convenience over the increased efficacy of the personal protective equipment available today.

To understand percutaneous penetration from contaminated fabric, more *in vitro* and *in vivo* studies must be performed. The limited data summarized here show that the type of fabric influences the pesticide's transfer from fabric to human skin or to a model membrane. Certain properties such as weave, thickness, starch, carboxymethylation, and mercerization can influence the fabric's ability to either allow permeation of the pesticide or to absorb the pesticide to prevent transfer to the skin surface (Obendorf et al. 2003). Other environmental conditions such as heat, humidity, and worker perspiration can also affect transfer of pesticide from clothing to skin (Wester et al. 2000).

Absorption and permeability of fabric can be influenced by how the pesticide distributes within the fabric itself. In a study by Solbrig and Obendorf (1985), both cotton and polyester fabrics revealed malathion distributed on the surface of the fibers; however, only the cotton fabric had malathion distributed within the fibers themselves. Information about the distributive properties of the pesticide could aid in creating more defensive clothing. Distributive information has the potential to determine which fabrics retain their protective qualities after multiple washings or uses. The hydrophilic or hydrophobic properties of each pesticide should also be considered.

Limited studies described percutaneous penetration from contaminated fabric utilizing an *in vivo* system. Of interest, one of the included studies utilized rabbits (Snodgrass 1992, Table 27.2). Rabbits display increased permeability of their skin compared to humans, rats, and pigs (Bartek et al. 1972). Further, Sidon et al. (1988) investigated the permeability of permethrin through monkey and rat skin. Although *in vivo* studies in man are not readily available due to the illness and toxicity that may ensue, future *in vivo* studies utilizing a myriad of pesticides and fabric conditions could lead to better understanding of the mechanisms involved in percutaneous penetration from fabrics. Law et al. (2020) provided detail as to the factors involved in cutaneous penetration; further investigation must be directed towards understanding the interplay between those factors and fabric permeability.

REFERENCES

Bartek, M. J., LaBudde, J. A., & Maibach H.I. (1972). Skin permeability in vivo: Comparsion in rat, rabbit, pig and man. Journal of Investigative Dermatology, 58, 114–123.

Bekö, G., Morrison, G., Weschler, C. J., Koch, H. M., Pälmke, C., Salthammer, T., Schripp, T., Toftum, J., & Clausen, G. (2017). Measurements of dermal uptake of nicotine directly from air and clothing. Indoor Air, 27, 427–433.

Blum, A., Gold, M. D., Ames, B. N., Jones, F. R., Hett, E. A., Dougherty, R. C., Horning, E. C., Dzidic, I., Carroll, D. I., Stillwell, R. N., & Thenot, J. P. (1978). Children Absorb tris-BP flame retardant from sleepwear: urine contains the mutagenic metabolite, 2,3-dibromopropanol. Science, 201, 1020–1023.

Chan, H. P., Honbo, Z., Wester, R. C., & Maibach, H. I. (2010). Agricultural chemical percutaneous absorption and decontamination. In R. I. Krieger (Ed.), Hayes' handbook of pesticide toxicology (pp. 683–700). New York, NY: Marcel Dekker.

Gaskin, S., Pisaniello, D., Edewards, J. W., Bromwich, D., Reed, S., Logan, M., & Baxter, C. (2013a). Application of skin contamination studies of ammonia gas for management of hazardous material incidents. Journal of Hazardous Materials, 252–253, 338–346.

Gaskin, S., Pisaniello, D., Edwards, J. W., Bromwich, D., Reed, S., Logan, M.,& Baxter, C. (2013b). Chlorine and hydrogen cyanide gas interactions with human skin: In vitro studies to inform skin permeation and decontamination in HAZMAT incidents. Journal of Hazardous Materials, 262, 759–763.

Gaskin, S., Heath, L., Pisaniello, D., Edwards, J. W., Logan, M. Baxter, C. (2017). Dermal absorption of fumigant gases during HAZMAT incident exposure scenarios-Methyl bromide, sulfuryl fluoride, and chloropicrin. Toxicology and Industrial Health, 33, 547–554.

Gaskin, S., Heath, L., Pisaniello, D., Logan, M., & Baxter, C. (2019). Skin permeation of oxides of nitrogen and sulfur from short-term exposure scenarios relevant to hazardous material incidents. Science of the Total Environment, 665, 937–943.

Guy, R. H., & Maibach, H. I. (1985). Calculations of body exposure from percutaneous absorption data. In R. Bronaugh & H. I. Maibach (Eds.), Percutaneous Absorption (4th ed., pp. 461–466). New York, NY: CRC Press.

Heath, L., Gaskin, S., Pisaniello, D., Crea, J., Logan, M., & Baxter, C. (2017). Skin absorption of ethylene oxide gas following exposures relevant to HAZMAT incidents. Annals of Work Exposures and Health, 61, 589–595.

Iadaresta, F., Manniello, M. D., Östman, C., Crescenzi, C., Holmbäck, J., Russo, P. (2018). Chemicals from textiles to skin: an in vitro permeation study of benzothiazole. Environmental Science and Pollution Research, 25, 24629–24638.

Keeble, V. B., Corell, L., & Ehrich, M. (1993). Evaluation of knit glove fabrics as barriers to dermal absorption of organophosphorus insecticides using an in vitro test system. Toxicology, 81, 195–203.

Keeble, V. B., Corell, L., & Ehrich, M. (1996). Effect of laundering on ability of glove fabrics to decrease the penetration of organophosphate insecticides through in vitro epidermal systems. Journal of Applied Toxicology, 16, 401–406.

Law, R. M., Ngo, M. A., & Maibach H. I. (2020). Twenty clinically pertinent factors/observations for percutaneous absorption in humans. American Journal of Clinical Dermatology, 21, 85–95.

Lillie, T. H., Livingston, J. M., & Hamilton, M.A. (1981). Recommendations for selecting and decontaminating pesticide applicator clothing. Bulletin of Environmental Contamination and Toxicology, 27, 716–723.

Meinke, M., Abdollahnia, M., Gähr, F., Platzek, T., Wolfram, S., Lademann, J. (2009). Migration and penetration of a fluorescent textile dye into the skin - in vivo versus in vitro methods. Experimental Dermatology, 18, 789–792.

Moore, C. A., Wilkinson, S. C., Blain, P. G., Dunn, M., Aust, G. A., & Williams, F. M. (2014). Use of a human skin in vitro model to investigate the influence of 'every-day' clothing and skin surface decontamination on the percutaneous penetration of organophosphates. Toxicology Letters, 229, 257–264.

Morrison, G. C., Weschler, C.J., Bekö, G., Koch, H. M., Salthammer, T., Schripp, T., Toftum, J., & Clausen, G. (2016). Role of clothing in both accelerating and impeding dermal absorption of airborne SVOCs. Journal of Exposure Science and Environmental Epidemiology, 26, 113–118.

Morrison, G. C., Bekö, G., Weshcler, C., Schripp, T., Salthammer, T., Hill, J., Andersson, A-M., Toftum, J., Clausen, G., & Frederiksen, H. (2017). Dermal uptake of benzophenone-3 from clothing. Environmental Science and Technology, 51, 11371–11379.

Obendorf, S. K., Csiszár, E., Maneefuangfoo, D., & Borsa, J. (2003). Kinetic transport of pesticide from contaminated fabric through a model skin. Archives of Environmental Contamination and Toxicology, 45, 283–288.

Orlando, J., Branson, D., Ayres, G., & Leavitt, R. (1981). The penetration of formulated guthion spray through selected fabrics. Journal of Environmental Science & Health, Part B, 16, 617–628.

Protano, C., Guidotti, M., & Vitali, M. (2009). Performance of different work clothing types for reducing skin exposure to pesticides during open field treatment. Bulletin of Environmental Contamination and Toxicology, 83, 115–119.

Raheel, M. (1991). Pesticide transmission in fabrics: Effect of particulate soil. Bulletin of Environmental Contamination & Toxicology, 46, 845–851.

Rehal, B. & Maibach, H. (2011). Percutaneous absorption of vapors in human skin. Cutaneous and Ocular Toxicology, 30, 87–91.

Rossbach, B., Appel, K. E., Mross, K. G., & Letzel, S. (2010). Uptake of permethrin from impregnated clothing. Toxicology Letters, 192, 50–55.

Rossbach, B., Kegel, P., Süß, H., & Letzel, S. (2016). Biomonitoring and evaluation of permethrin uptake in forestry workers using permethrin-treated tick-proof pants. Journal of Exposure Science and Environmental Epidemiology, 26, 95–103.

Rossbach, B., Niemietz, A., Kegel, P., & Letzel, S. (2014). Uptake and elimination of permethrin related to the use of permethrin treated clothing for forestry workers. Toxicology Letters, 231, 147–153.

Sidon, E. W., Moody, R. P., & Franklin, C.A. (1988). Percutaneous absorption of cis- and trans-permethrin in rhesus monkeys and rats: anatomic site and interspecies variation. Journal of Toxicology and Environmental Health, 23, 207–216.

Snodgrass, H. L. (1992). Permethrin transfer from treated cloth to the skin surface: potential for exposure in humans. Journal of Toxicology and Environmental Health, 35, 91–105.

Solbrig, C. M. & Obendorf, S. K. (1985). Distribution of residual pesticide within textile structures as determined by electron microscopy. Textile Research Journal, 55, 540–546.

Ulsamer, A. G., Porter, W. K., & Osterberg, R. E. (1978). Percutaneous absorption of radiolabeled TRIS from flame-retarded fabric. Journal of Environmental Pathology and Toxicology, 1, 543–549.

Welch, O. & Obendorf, S.K. (1997). Limiting dermal exposure of workers to pesticides from contaminated clothing. In J. Still & A. Schwope (Eds.), Performance of Protective Clothing (6th vol.). West Conshohocken, PA: American Society for Testing and Materials.

Wester, R. C., Hartway, T. Serranzana, S., & Maibach, H. I. (1997). Human skin in vitro percutaneous absorption of gaseous ethylene oxide from fabric. Food and Chemical Toxicology, 35, 513–515.

Wester, R. C., Quan, D., & Maibach, H. I. (1996). In vitro percutaneous absorption of model compounds glyphosate and malathion from cotton fabric into and through human skin. Food and Chemical Toxicology, 34, 731–735.

Wester, R. M., Tanojo, H., Maibach, H. I., & Wester, R. C. (2000). Predicted chemical warfare agent VX toxicity to uniformed soldier using parathion in vitro human skin exposure and absorption. Toxicology and Applied Pharmacology, 168, 149–152.

Yang, Y. & Li, S. (1993). Frictional transition of pesticides from protective clothing. Archives of Environmental Contamination and Toxicology, 25, 279–284.

28 The Fate of Material Remaining in Skin in *In Vitro* Absorption Studies

Margaret E.K. Kraeling and Jeffrey J. Yourick
Food and Drug Administration, Laurel, Maryland

Disclaimer: This book chapter reflects the views of the authors and should not be construed to represent FDA's views or policies.

CONTENTS

28.1 INTRODUCTION

When conducting *in vitro* studies to determine the percutaneous absorption of chemicals, it has been recognized that lipophilic compounds and compounds that bind in the skin can present a problem in the *in vitro* measurement of percutaneous absorption. The skin reservoir is defined as the amount of applied chemical that remains in the skin (i.e., in the stratum corneum, epidermis, and dermis) at the end of an *in vitro* absorption study. The skin reservoir may be considered part of the material available for systemic absorption. However, when the skin reservoir is significant compared to levels measured in the receptor fluid, the contribution of the skin reservoir to systemic absorption should be examined. Compounds that are insoluble in water may not partition freely from excised skin into an aqueous receptor fluid. The problem was alluded to by Franz (1), who in selecting compounds for the study, omitted highly water-insoluble compounds to avoid results that were limited due to insolubility. The methodological problem that a skin reservoir creates may not be limited to lipophilic compounds. Studies with alpha hydroxy acids (AHAs), such as glycolic acid and lactic acid, have shown that very polar compounds can still be substantially retained in skin at the end of a 24-hour absorption study (2).

28.2 MODIFICATION OF RECEPTOR FLUID

The receptor fluid used in *in vitro* dermal absorption studies is important and should not act as a rate-limiting step in the permeation process due to the limited solubility of the test compound in the receptor medium (3). A buffered salt solution, such as HEPES-buffered Hanks' balanced salt solution (HHBSS), or saline solution may be an appropriate receptor fluid for determining skin absorption for hydrophilic compounds, but it is not likely to be applicable for lipophilic compounds. Attempts have been made to overcome the solubility problem by modifying the receptor fluid composition. Bovine serum albumin (BSA) is sometimes added to the receptor fluid to increase the solubility of lipophilic compounds. Brown and Ulsamer (4) found that the skin permeation of the hydrophobic compound hexachlorophene increased twofold when normal saline was replaced with 3% BSA in a physiological buffer in the diffusion cell receptor fluid. Various receptor fluids with different solubility properties have been investigated to increase the partitioning of lipophilic chemicals into the receptor fluid that have penetrated skin during *in vitro* absorption studies. Increasing the lipophilicity of receptor fluids used in *in vitro* absorption studies with chemicals such as Volpo 20, ethanol, methanol, BSA, or cyclomethicone can increase the partitioning of a lipophilic chemical from skin into the receptor fluid (5–7). In an *in vitro* percutaneous absorption study of azo pigment 1-[4-phenylazophenylazo]-2-naphthol (PAN) (the color component of the certified color D&C Red No. 17), low absorption of PAN occurred in human and porcine skin exposed to consumer products containing this certified color additive (8). For the suntan product studied, most of the applied PAN was washed off the surface of the skin as unpenetrated color. The majority of PAN that penetrated remained in the skin after 24 hours, and typically a very small amount (0.02% to 0.33% of the applied dose) was found in the receptor fluid after 24 hours for both human cadaver and porcine skin. Extended absorption studies (72 hours) showed that PAN, which penetrated skin within 24 hours, remained in the skin, with little PAN diffusing out into the receptor fluid over 72 hours. These results suggest that little of the PAN remaining in skin after 24 hours is available for systemic absorption. Since there were high levels of PAN found remaining in skin after 24 and 72 hours in human skin—12.6% and 15.3% of the applied dose, respectively—an investigation was conducted testing different lipophilic receptor fluids to determine if they increased the partitioning of PAN out of the skin into the receptor fluid. Four lipophilic receptor fluids were tested in addition to HHBSS with 4% BSA, which included 1%, 3%, and 6% Volpo 20 as weight % in deionized water and ethanol:water (50:50). These studies were conducted using human cadaver skin (8). The solubility of PAN in 6% Volpo 20 (0.26 mg/mL) was approximately 37% higher than in HHBSS + 4% BSA (0.19 mg/mL). However, no significant differences were observed in the penetration and subsequent partitioning of PAN from the skin into the two receptor fluids. The lowest solubility of PAN was observed in the ethanol:water (50:50; 0.04 mg/mL) receptor fluid, and yet absorption was found to significantly increase when this receptor fluid was used in the penetration studies. However, care must be taken not to damage the barrier integrity of skin with the receptor fluid selected for an *in vitro* study. It has been shown that a methanol:water (50:50) solution caused damage to rat skin during an *in vitro* absorption study (5). Therefore, the likely reason for the enhanced absorption of PAN with the ethanol:water (50:50) receptor fluid in the skin penetration study is probably due to skin damage.

It is preferable to use a physiological buffer to maintain viability of skin even when metabolism is not measured to simulate *in vivo* conditions. The viability of skin can be maintained by using a balanced salt solution or a tissue culture medium. Addition of 4% BSA may be enough in some cases to enhance receptor fluid levels of applied compound without altering skin viability (9).

28.3   SYSTEMIC ABSORPTION

In *in vitro* skin absorption/penetration studies, definitions of absorption and penetration must be clearly defined. Skin/dermal/percutaneous *absorption* represents the amount of topically applied chemical that is ultimately determined to be systemically available. This usually constitutes receptor fluid contents at the end of an *in vitro* study. However, if a substantial amount of test compound remains in the skin (skin reservoir), *absorption* would constitute receptor fluid content plus skin content if it is determined that material remaining in the skin ultimately diffuses and partitions into the receptor fluid. Therefore, it must be determined for an individual study whether the stratum corneum and/or viable epidermal/dermal content should be considered systemically available. Skin/dermal/percutaneous *penetration* represents the total amount of topically applied chemical that is found in the receptor fluid plus the skin at the end of a study. However, not all of this material may be systemically available for absorption.

The guideline for skin absorption studies recommended by the European Union's Scientific Committee for Consumer Products (SCCP) requires that material remaining in the viable skin levels (exclusive of stratum corneum) be considered as systemically absorbed (10). The Organization for

Economic and Cultural Development (OECD) guideline for *in vitro* skin absorption studies states that all material remaining in skin (including the stratum corneum) may need to be considered as systemically absorbed unless additional studies show that there is no eventual absorption (3, 10).

28.4 EXAMPLES OF SPECIFIC SKIN ABSORPTION STUDIES ADDRESSING THE FATE OF ABSORBED MATERIAL IN SKIN

In *in vitro* percutaneous absorption studies, where a substantial amount of test chemical remains in the skin at the end of a 24-hour study, it is important to determine the systemic fate or potential bioavailability of this material remaining in skin before an estimation of systemic absorption is determined. Failure to make this determination may result in an inaccurate estimation of skin absorption. Extended absorption studies (72-hour studies) can help determine if a compound will subsequently diffuse into the receptor fluid. The fate of test compounds that are extensively retained in skin after a 24-hour exposure in *in vitro* diffusion cell studies has been examined in the following studies.

The safety of lawsone as a coloring agent in hair dye products was evaluated by the Scientific Committee on Cosmetics and Non-Food Products (SCCNFP) (now Scientific Committee for Consumer Products [SCCP]) and concluded that lawsone was mutagenic and not suitable for use as a hair coloring agent. *In vitro* diffusion cell skin absorption studies were conducted to measure the extent of lawsone absorption through human skin (11). Lawsone skin absorption was determined from two hair coloring products and two shampoo products, all containing henna. Products remained on the skin for 5 minutes (shampoos) and 1 hour (hair color paste). For one of the henna hair paste products, 0.3% of the applied dose was absorbed into the receptor fluid in 24 hours, while 2.2% remained in the skin (Table 28.1). For one of the henna shampoo products, 0.3% of the applied dose was absorbed into the receptor fluid at 24 hours, while 3.6% remained in the skin (Table 28.2). Extended absorption studies conducted for 72 hours showed that a small but significant increase in lawsone levels occurred in the receptor fluid values, while all skin levels (stratum corneum,

TABLE 28.1

Penetration of Lawsone from a Commercial Henna Hair Paste (Product A) in 24 and 72 Hours

	% of Applied Dose Penetrated	
	24 Hours[1]	72 Hours[2]
Receptor fluid	0.3 ± 0.1^a	0.5 ± 0.1^a
Stratum corneum	1.6 ± 0.2^a	0.5 ± 0.1^a
Epidermis and dermis	0.6 ± 0.1^a	0.3 ± 0.03^a
Total in skin	2.2 ± 0.3^a	0.8 ± 0.1^a
Total penetration	2.5 ± 0.3^a	1.3 ± 0.1^a
Wash	102.0 ± 3.3	93.1 ± 2.2

Source: From Reference 11.

[1] Values are the mean ± SEM of 11 replicates (two donors). Other 24-hour values are the mean ± SEM of six replicates (two donors). Lawsone applied dose was 1.51 ± 0.22 µg/cm^2.

[2] Values are the mean ± SEM of five replicates (one donor). Lawsone applied dose was 1.36 ± 0.03µg/cm^2.

[a] Significantly different between the 24-hour and 72-hour values (*t*-test, $p < 0.05$).

TABLE 28.2

Penetration of Lawsone from a Commercial Henna Shampoo (Product C) in 24 and 72 Hours

	% of Applied Dose Penetrated	
	24 Hours[1]	72 Hours[2]
Receptor fluid	0.3 ± 0.02^a	0.4 ± 0.04^a
Stratum corneum	2.4 ± 0.3^a	1.4 ± 0.2^a
Epidermis and dermis	1.2 ± 0.2^a	0.5 ± 0.1^a
Total in skin	3.6 ± 0.5^a	1.9 ± 0.2^a
Total penetration	3.9 ± 0.5^a	2.3 ± 0.3^a
Wash	90.3 ± 3.0	82.0 ± 3.2
Recovery	94.7 ± 3.1	84.7 ± 3.4

Source: From Reference 11.

[1] Receptor fluid values are the mean ± SEM of 24 replicates (three donors). Other 24-hour values are the mean ± SEM of 12 replicates (three donors). Lawsone applied dose was 1.08 ± 0.07 μg/cm².

[2] Values are the mean ± SEM of 12 replicates (three donors). Lawsone applied dose was 0.79 ± 0.14 μg/cm².

[a] Significantly different between the 24-hour and 72-hour values (*t*-test, $p < 0.05$).

epidermis, and dermis) significantly decreased. It was found that the majority of the lawsone still remained in the skin, with only slight amounts found in the receptor fluid contents. Therefore, this is an example of when receptor fluid values would be a good estimate of lawsone systemic absorption and lawsone skin levels should not be included.

The skin absorption of diethanolamine (DEA) was determined from cosmetic formulations using excised human skin in diffusion cells (12). When ¹⁴C-DEA was applied to skin in a commercially available lotion, only 0.7% of the applied dose was found in the receptor fluid at the end of the 24-hour studies (Table 28.3). Most of the absorbed compound was found in the skin, with the greatest amounts penetrating through the stratum corneum into the deeper epidermal and dermal regions. An extended

TABLE 28.3

Diethanolamine (DEA) Penetration in Viable Human Skin from a Lotion (3 mg/cm2; DEA dose 1.0 μg/cm²) for 72 Hours[1]

	% of Applied Dose Penetrated		
Time of Skin Study	24 h	48 h	72 h
Receptor fluid	0.7 ± 0.1	1.2 ± 0.1	1.7 ± 0.5
Stratum corneum	4.2 ± 0.2	3.3 ± 0.1	3.7 ± 0.3
Epidermis and dermis	7.7 ± 0.9	7.4 ± 1.3	7.4 ± 0.9
Total in skin	11.9 ± 0.7	10.7 ± 1.3	11.1 ± 0.6
Total penetration	12.5 ± 0.5	11.9 ± 1.3	12.8 ± 1.1
Recovery	95.2 ± 3.0	93.3 ± 3.4	96.6 ± 3.0

Source: From Reference 12.

[1] Values are the mean ± SEM of three replicates in each of three subjects.
Corresponding values at the different study times are not significantly different (ANOVA, $p < 0.05$).

absorption study conducted for an additional 48 hours showed that no significant increases occurred in the DEA receptor fluid levels after 72 hours. The lack of additional partitioning of DEA from skin into the receptor fluid could not be explained by poor water solubility. It appeared that DEA was binding to the skin, and therefore the DEA in the skin reservoir was not available for systemic absorption. Therefore, this is another example of when receptor fluid values would be a good estimate of DEA systemic absorption and DEA skin levels should not be included due to binding to skin components.

The percutaneous absorption of Disperse Blue 1 (DB1) was determined through human skin from a semi-permanent hair dye vehicle (13). Only a small amount of the absorbed compound (0.2% of the applied dose) was found in the receptor fluid at the end of 24 hours (Figure 28.1). The amount of penetrated DB1 in skin at 24 hours was 2.6% of the applied dose, with most of the compound in the stratum corneum (Figure 28.1). The unabsorbed material was removed from the skin surface with soap and water from some diffusion cells, and the studies were continued for an additional 48 hours (total 72 hours). Only a small amount of additional DB1 was found in the receptor fluid. It appeared that the DB1 in the skin reservoir was not available for significant percutaneous absorption. Because little additional DB1was absorbed into the receptor fluid, skin levels should not be considered as absorbed material for DB1.

The percutaneous absorption of retinol (vitamin A) from cosmetic formulations was studied in fuzzy rat and human skin to predict systemic absorption and to understand the significance of the skin reservoir in *in vitro* absorption studies (14). *In vivo* absorption studies using fuzzy rats were performed to compare with the *in vitro* studies. Retinol (0.3%) formulations (hydroalcoholic gel and oil-in-water emulsion) containing ^{3}H-retinol were applied, and absorption was measured at 24 or 72 hours. *In vitro* studies using human skin with the gel and emulsion vehicles found 0.3% and 1.3% of the applied retinol, respectively, in receptor fluid at 24 hours. Levels of retinol absorption in the receptor fluid increased over 72 hours with both vehicles. Using the gel vehicle, *in vitro* rat skin studies found 23% in skin and 6% of the applied retinol in receptor fluid at 24 hours, while 72-hour studies found 18% in skin and 13% in receptor fluid. Significant amounts of retinol remained in rat skin at 24 hours and decreased over 72 hours, with proportional increases in receptor fluid. *In vivo* rat studies with the gel found 4% systemic absorption of retinol after 24 hours, and systemic absorption did not increase at 72 hours. Retinol remaining in rat skin after *in vivo* application was 18% and 13% of the applied dermal dose after 24 and 72 hours, respectively. Similar observations were made with the oil-in-water

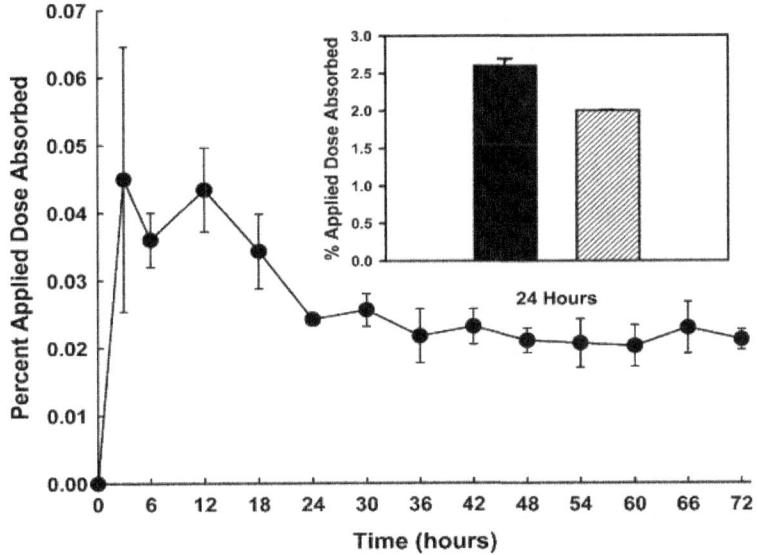

FIGURE 28.1 Time course of percutaneous absorption of DB1 into the receptor fluid. Inset: Skin levels of DB1, Bar 1 total skin. Bar 2 stratum corneum. Values are the mean ± SEM of determinations in two rat studies (13).

emulsion vehicle in the rat. Retinol formed a reservoir in rat skin both *in vivo* and *in vitro*. Little additional retinol was bioavailable after 24 hours. Comparison of these *in vitro* and *in vivo* results for absorption through rat skin indicates that the 24-hour *in vitro* receptor fluid value accurately estimated 24-hour *in vivo* systemic absorption. Therefore, based on the rat studies, the best single estimate of retinol systemic absorption from *in vitro* human skin studies is the 24-hour receptor fluid value. In this case, *in vivo* skin absorption studies were useful in determining whether to include material in the *in vitro* skin reservoir as absorbable material in estimates of systemic absorption.

28.5   CONCLUSION

It is important to fully understand the fate of compounds that form a reservoir in skin during percutaneous absorption studies. The OECD guideline for *in vitro* skin absorption studies states that all material remaining in skin (including the stratum corneum) may need to be considered as systemically absorbed unless additional studies show that there is no eventual absorption (3, 10). The skin reservoir is likely formed in skin by lipophilic compounds and chemicals, both polar and nonpolar, that bind to skin components during the absorption process. An estimate of systemic absorption should no longer be obtained simply by measuring receptor fluid levels; remaining skin levels must be measured and addressed to come up with a realistic dermal exposure estimate for a compound. Systemic absorption values should include absorbed material in the skin reservoir at the end of a study unless extended experiments have been conducted to determine the fate of that material remaining in the skin.

REFERENCES

1. Franz TJ. Percutaneous absorption. On the relevance of *in vitro* data. J Invest Dermatol 1975; 64:190–195.
2. Kraeling MEK, Bronaugh RL. *In vitro* percutaneous absorption of alpha hydroxy acids in human skin. J Soc Cosmet Chem 1997; 48:187–197.
3. OECD, Test No. 428: Skin Absorption: *In Vitro* Method, OECD Guidelines for the Testing of Chemicals, Section 4, OECD Publishing, Paris.
4. Brown DWC, Ulsamer AG. Percutaneous penetration of hexachlorophene as related to receptor solutions. Food Chem Toxicol 1975; 13:81–86.
5. Bronaugh RL, Stewart RF. Methods for *in vitro* percutaneous absorption studies III. Hydrophobic compounds. J Pharm Sci 1984; 73:1255–1258.
6. Bronaugh RL, Stewart RF. Methods for *in vitro* percutaneous absorption studies VI. Preparation of the barrier layer. J Pharm Sci 1986; 75:487–491.
7. Hood HL, Wickett RR, Bronaugh RL. The *in vitro* percutaneous absorption of the fragrance ingredient musk xylol. Food Chem Toxicol 1996; 34:483–488.
8. Yourick JJ, Sasik CT, Bronaugh RL. *In vitro* dermal absorption and metabolism of D&C red no. 17 in human and porcine skin. J Cosmet Sci 2007; 58(3):255–266.
9. Collier SW, Sheikh NM, Sakr A, Lichtin JL, Stewart RF, Bronaugh RL. Maintenance of skin viability during *in vitro* percutaneous absorption/metabolism studies. Tox Appl Pharmacol 1989; 99:522–533.
10. SCCP. Opinion Concerning Basic Criteria for the *In Vitro* Assessment of Percutaneous Absorption of Cosmetic Ingredients. Adopted by the Scientific Committee on Cosmetic Products and Non-Food Products Intended for Consumers During the 25th Plenary Meeting of 20 October 2003.
11. Kraeling MEK, Jung CT, Bronaugh RL. Absorption of lawsone through human skin. Cutan Ocul Toxicol 2007; 26:45–56.
12. Kraeling MEK, Yourick JJ, Bronaugh RL. Percutaneous absorption of diethanolamine in human skin *in vitro*. Food Chem Toxicol 2004; 42(10):1553–1561.
13. Yourick JJ, Koenig ML, Yourick DL, Bronaugh RL. Fate of chemicals in skin after dermal application: Does the *in vitro* skin reservoir affect the estimate of systemic absorption? Toxicol Applied Pharmacol 2004; 195(3):309–320.
14. Yourick JJ, Jung CT, Bronuagh RL. *In vitro* and *in vivo* percutaneous absorption of retinol from cosmetic formulations: significance of the skin reservoir and prediction of systemic absorption. Toxicol Applied Pharmacol 2008; 231:117–121.

29 Skin Absorption of Hair Dyes

Jeffrey J. Yourick and Margaret E.K. Kraeling
Food and Drug Administration, Laurel, Maryland

CONTENTS

Disclaimer: This book chapter reflects the views of the authors and should not be construed to represent FDA's views or policies.

29.1 INTRODUCTION

Consumer hair dye products can be divided into three product types: permanent, semipermanent, and temporary. Permanent or oxidation hair colors are the most widely used hair dye products. Oxidation hair dye products contain a solution of dye intermediates which form hair dyes by chemical reactions on the hair and preformed dyes that are added as toning agents to attain the intended shades. The dye solution and the hydrogen peroxide solution (developer) are mixed just prior to hair application. The applied mixture causes the hair shaft to swell. The dye intermediates and toning dyes penetrate the hair shaft to some degree before they have chemically reacted with the hydrogen peroxide to form the final colored hair dye. Semipermanent and temporary hair coloring products are typically solutions of several hair dyes that bind to the hair shaft to differing degrees. Temporary hair colors need to be reapplied after each shampooing.

The Food and Drug Administration (FDA) regulates cosmetic products under the authority of the Federal Food, Drug, and Cosmetic (FD&C) Act. This law is designed to assure that products under FDA jurisdiction are safe under intended conditions of use and properly labeled. The FDA, however, does not have the authority to approve cosmetic products, their formulations, or their labeling. Under the provisions of the FD&C Act, a cosmetic is deemed to be adulterated if, among other things, it bears or contains a poisonous or deleterious substance that may render it injurious to users under the conditions of use as prescribed in the labeling or under such conditions of use as are customary or usual. Coal-tar hair dyes are exempt from adulteration provisions of the FD&C Act, provided the product label bears the caution statement described in section 601(a) of the Act. Additional information regarding the safety and regulation of hair dyes can be found at https://www.fda.gov/cosmetics/cosmetic-products-ingredients.

Certain coal-tar hair dyes, such as 4-chloro-m-phenylenediamine, 2,4-toluenediamine, 2-nitro-p-phenylenediamine (2NPPD), 4-amino-2-nitrophenol, and Disperse Blue 1, have been reported to cause tumors in at least one animal species in lifetime feeding studies. The focus of this chapter will be to describe the skin absorption of certain hair dyes with potential safety issues.

The following definitions are used when referring to dermal/skin absorption and dermal/skin penetration. *Skin/dermal/percutaneous absorption* represents the amount of topically applied chemical that is ultimately determined to be systemically available. This would constitute receptor fluid content plus skin content if it is determined that material remaining in the skin ultimately partitions into the receptor fluid. Therefore, it must be determined individually whether the stratum corneum and/or viable epidermal/dermal content should be considered systemically available. *Skin/dermal/percutaneous penetration* represents the total amount of topically applied chemical that is found in the receptor fluid plus the skin at the end of a study. However, not all of this material may be systemically available for absorption.

29.2 SKIN ABSORPTION AND METABOLISM OF 2-NITRO-P-PHENYLENEDIAMINE

29.2.1 INTRODUCTION

2NPPD is a coal-tar dye used in semipermanent (nonoxidative) and permanent (oxidative) hair dye formulations. It is not an oxidation dye, but is present in oxidation formulations as a color tinting agent. The Cosmetic Ingredient Review Expert Panel concluded that 2NPPD is safe as a hair dye ingredient at current concentrations (up to 1%) of use (1). The mutagenicity and carcinogenicity of 2NPPD have been investigated in several different experimental systems. 2NPPD was mutagenic in Ames testing (2) and in several different mammalian tests (1, 3). Hair dye formulations containing 2NPPD are mutagenic to some strains of *Salmonella typhimurium* (1). The urine of rats was also found to be mutagenic when tested after topical application of hair dyes containing 2NPPD (1). In long-term carcinogenicity feeding studies with 2NPPD, mixed results have been found in rodents. An increase in hepatic carcinomas and adenomas was noted in female mice fed 2NPPD, but not male mice or rats (4). In a two-mouse strain chronic skin-painting study using a semipermanent hair dye formulation containing 2NPPD, there was a reduced time to tumor and an increased number of tumors noted in one strain of mice. In a chronic rat skin-painting study with a hair dye containing 1.1% 2NPPD, there was no increase in gross lesion numbers (1).

Because of the genotoxicity, potential for carcinogenicity reported for 2NPPD, and lack of skin metabolism information in previous studies, a study by Yourick and Bronaugh (5) investigated the in vitro skin absorption and metabolism of 2NPPD in human and fuzzy rat skin. Percutaneous absorption studies were done, as described in detail using flow-through diffusion cells (5). Barrier integrity of human skin discs were verified by using the 20-minute tritiated water test (6). 2NPPD and 2NPPD metabolites in receptor fluid or skin were determined by high-performance liquid chromatography (HPLC) using a modified method of Nakao et al. (7). A summary of the 2NPPD study (5) is presented next.

29.2.2 2NPPD RESULTS

29.2.2.1 Skin Penetration

The percutaneous absorption of radiolabeled 2NPPD through fuzzy rat skin into the receptor fluid with four dosing vehicles is depicted in Figure 29.1. 2NPPD rapidly penetrated rat skin, with the

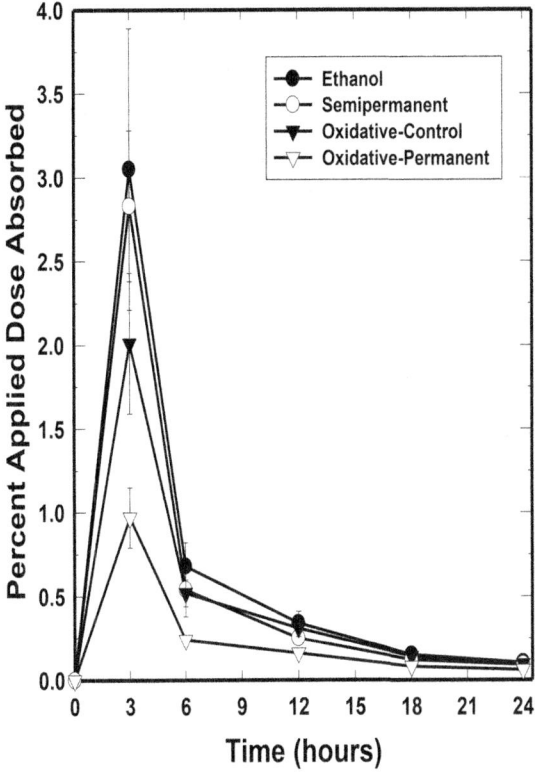

FIGURE 29.1   Percentage of applied 2NPPD dose absorbed over 24 hours in receptor fluid from fuzzy rat skin. Absorption values are the mean ± SE from three individual rat studies ($n = 3$). Each single absorption value was determined by averaging four to five replicate measurements for each time interval point and dosing solution. (From Reference 5.)

peak in absorption noted at the three-hour time point with all vehicles tested (percentage of applied dose absorbed ranged from approximately 0.9 to 3.1). When comparing the four vehicles tested for 2NPPD absorption, there were no significant differences between the various vehicles over the time points examined. However, it is interesting to note that absorption of 2NPPD from the oxidative-permanent hair dye formulation tended to be lower than the other dosing vehicles.

Table 29.1 summarizes 2NPPD percutaneous absorption in fuzzy rat skin 24 hours after application. No difference was seen in the amount of 2NPPD absorbed over 24 hours into the receptor fluid from the different dosing vehicles tested. A similar amount of 2NPPD remained in the skin (2.9 to 2.2 percent of the applied dose absorbed) for all the hair product formulations, although a higher amount of 2NPPD was found in skin dosed with an ethanol vehicle. When considering the total (receptor fluid + skin) percentage of applied dose absorbed after 24 hours, a similar amount of 2NPPD was absorbed from both the hair product formulations. A significantly higher amount of 2NPPD was absorbed with the ethanol vehicle than with the permanent (oxidative) formulation. After 30 minutes, approximately 67% (range 59.1% to 72.8%) of the 2NPPD was recovered in the washes for all vehicles tested. The average recovery of 2NPPD at the end of the experiment (after 24 hours) was 73.2% (range: 68.4% to 78.8%) of the total percentage of the applied dose. These low recovery values were potentially due to 2NPPD binding to the wooden stick of the applicators. Recovery values were improved by changing the applicator type from a wooden stick with a cotton swab to a plastic stick with a cotton swab. Since 2NPPD is not a volatile chemical, we would not

TABLE 29.1
Summary of 2NPPD Absorption in Fuzzy Rat Skin[1]

	Percentage of Applied Dose			
	Ethanol	**Semipermanent**	**Control-Permanent**	**Permanent**
Receptor Fluid	4.3 ± 1.07[2]	3.8 ± 0.98	3.1 ± 0.52	1.53 ± 0.19
Skin Content	$4.9 \pm 0.47^*$	2.9 ± 0.61	2.2 ± 0.21	2.7 ± 0.14
Total Applied Dose Penetrated	$9.3 \pm 1.17^\dagger$	6.9 ± 1.15	5.3 ± 0.53	4.2 ± 0.08
Wash	59.1 ± 2.69	72.8 ± 7.00	66.3 ± 10.30	69.8 ± 8.30
Recovery	68.4 ± 3.69	78.8 ± 6.69	71.6 ± 9.90	74.0 ± 8.70

[1] All values represent data 24 hours after 2NPPD application.

[2] Values are the means $\pm$ SE of four to five replicate measurements for three rats.

* Ethanol vehicle group is significantly (ANOVA followed by Tukey test, $p < 0.05$) greater than all other skin receptor fluid groups.

† Ethanol vehicle group is significantly (ANOVA followed by Tukey test, $p < 0.05$) greater than the permanent vehicle group.

Source: Reference 5.

predict that the lower recoveries were due to evaporative loss of 2NPPD. It is possible that 2NPPD was bound to the walls of the diffusion cell.

Absorption of 2NPPD through human skin for a 30-minute application of the dosing vehicles is shown in Figure 29.2. Percutaneous absorption of 2NPPP peaked at three hours in the receptor fluid for both the ethanol and semipermanent vehicles tested. There was no difference in the absorption measured between the two vehicles. Similar to the results in fuzzy rat skin, human skin

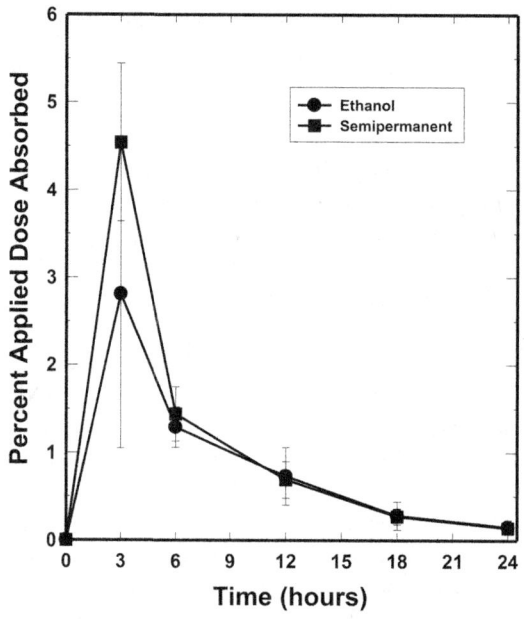

FIGURE 29.2   Percentage of applied 2NPPD dose absorbed over 24 hours in receptor fluid from human skin. Absorption values are the mean $\pm$ SD from two individual human donor studies ($n = 2$). Each single absorption value was determined by averaging four to five replicate measurements for each time interval point and dosing solution. (From Reference 5.)

TABLE 29.2

Summary of 2NPPD Absorption in Human Skin Using an Ethanol and Semipermanent Hair Dye Formulation[1]

	Percentage of Applied Dose	
	Ethanol	**Semipermanent Formulation**
Receptor Fluid	5.3 ± 2.57^2	7.1 ± 1.56
Skin Content	3.9 ± 3.17	2.5 ± 1.6
Total Applied Dose Absorbed	9.2 ± 5.75	9.5 ± 3.16
Wash	63.4 ± 4.44	54.2 ± 3.47
Recovery	72.6 ± 1.27	63.8 ± 0.31

[1] All values represent data 24 hours after 2NPPD application.

[2] Values are the means ± SD of four to five replicate measurements for two human subjects.

Source: Reference 5.

2NPPD absorption was rapid, peaked at three hours, and there was no difference between the dosing vehicles.

A summary of 2NPPD absorption in human skin using an ethanol or semipermanent hair dye formulation is presented in Table 29.2. No significant differences between the absorption were noted when the two vehicles were compared across the categories listed in Table 29.2. The total percentage of applied 2NPPD dose absorbed was 9.2 ± 5.75 and 9.5 ± 3.16 for the ethanol and semipermanent formulations, respectively. The approximate total penetration of 9% of the applied dose absorbed is represented by about 6% absorption into the receptor fluid and approximately 3% 2NPPD remaining in the skin.

29.2.2.2   Human and Rat Skin Metabolism of 2NPPD

The extent of 2NPPD metabolism and the metabolic profile changed dependent upon the tissue and dosing vehicle used in the fuzzy rat studies (Figure 29.3). When an ethanol dosing vehicle was used on rat skin, 2NPPD was approximately 85% metabolized. The majority (65%) of 2NPPD was metabolized to N4-acetyl-2NPPD, while lesser amounts were metabolized to triaminobenzene (17%) and a potential sulfated metabolite (3%). When a semipermanent hair dye formulation was used as the dosing vehicle, approximately 47% of the 2NPPD was metabolized upon absorption. Approximately 20% of the absorbed 2NPPD was metabolized to N4-acetyl-2NPPD and triaminobenzene and about 6% was potentially sulfated. The profile of metabolism in skin was altered by the dosing vehicle. When comparing the dosing vehicles in skin, greater metabolism of 2NPPD was noted with the ethanol dosing vehicle, and the major metabolite formed was the acetylated metabolite. Less 2NPPD was metabolized with the product vehicle and a smaller amount of acetylated 2NPPD was formed, while a larger percentage of metabolized 2NPPD was pushed toward the formation of triaminobenzene and the sulfated metabolite.

The in vitro metabolism of 2NPPD in human skin was also investigated (Figure 29.4). When 2NPPD was applied to human skin in ethanol, almost complete metabolism of the absorbed material to N4-acetyl-2NPPD (90%) was seen. A small amount (7%) of triaminobenzene was formed, and a smaller amount (3%) of unmetabolized 2NPPD was also found. When 2NPPD was applied to human skin in a semipermanent formulation, less 2NPPD (60%) was metabolized and approximately equal amounts of N4-acetyl-2NPPD and triaminobenzene were formed (Figure 29.4). In human skin, unlike the rat, there was no sulfation of 2NPPD.

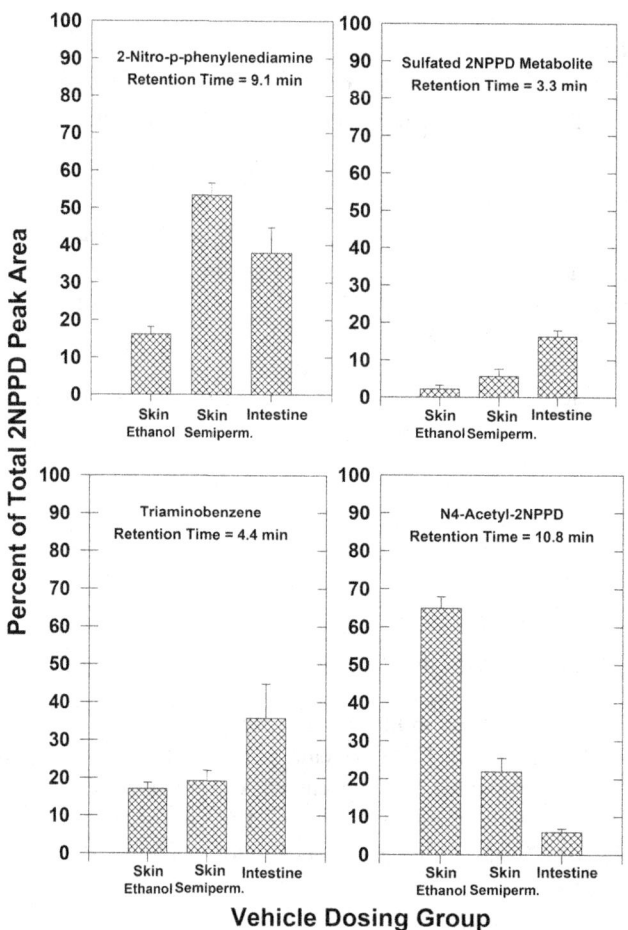

FIGURE 29.3 Metabolism of 2NPPD upon absorption through rat skin and intestinal tissue. 2NPPD and metabolites were determined in receptor fluid fractions from three-hour skin and one-hour intestinal samples. Total ^{14}C-peak area was determined for each chromatogram. Then a percentage of the total ^{14}C-peak area was calculated for each peak. Percentage of peak areas reported are the mean ± SE from three individual rat studies ($n = 3$). Each single percentage of peak area value was determined by averaging four to five replicate cell fractions from each rat study. (From Reference 5.)

29.2.3   2NPPD DISCUSSION

The in vitro percutaneous absorption and metabolism of the hair dye ingredient 2NPPD were determined in human and fuzzy rat skin. 2NPPD was applied to skin for 30 minutes, then removed to simulate consumer exposure to a typical hair dye product. Thus, the extent of absorption was limited by the relatively short application (i.e., exposure) time. Ethanol, when used as the dosing vehicle, can be considered as a test condition free from formulation constituent and other dye interactions. When ethanol was used as the dosing vehicle, a significant portion of the 2NPPD was absorbed and found in the receptor within three hours. The rapid percutaneous penetration of 2NPPD can be explained by its solubility properties. The extent of percutaneous penetration for a chemical is determined by its inherent physicochemical properties (8). Partition coefficients for 2NPPD have been reported in octanol/water and stratum corneum/water of 3.4 and 13.0, respectively (9). When an infinite dose of 2NPPD was applied in aqueous solution, a permeability constant of 5.0×10^{4} cm/h was determined (9). 2NPPD has both lipophilic and hydrophilic solubility properties and a relatively low molecular

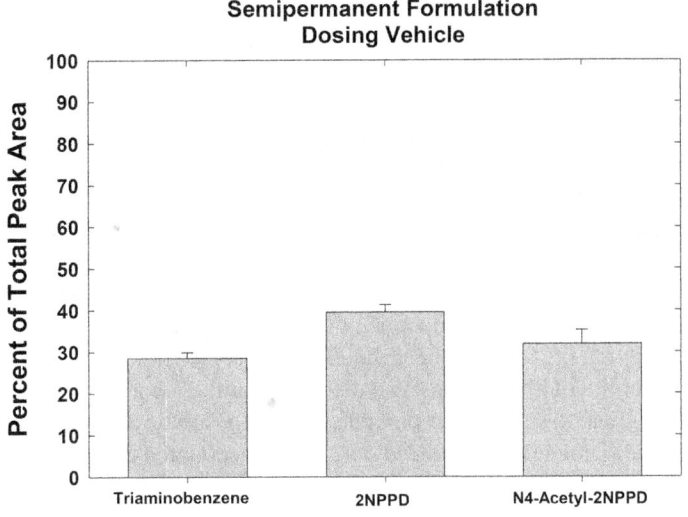

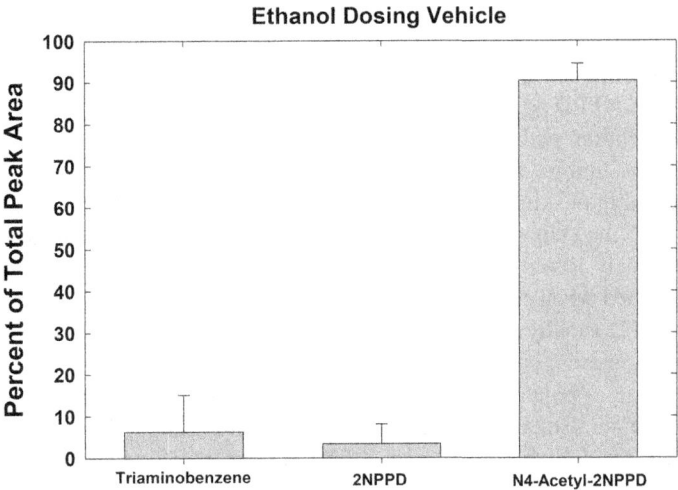

FIGURE 29.4   Metabolism of 2NPPD upon absorption through human skin using ethanol and a semipermanent dosing vehicle. 2NPPD and metabolites were determined in receptor fluid fractions from the three-hour time point. Total ^{14}C-peak area was determined for each chromatogram. Then a percentage of the total ^{14}C-peak area was calculated for each peak. Percentage of peak areas reported are the mean ± SD from two human studies ($n = 2$). Each single percentage of peak area value was determined by averaging four to five replicate cell fractions from each human study. (From Reference 5.)

weight of 153.1 g, which all contribute to its rapid skin penetration properties. Also, small, rapidly penetrating molecules may result in similar absorption values between human and rat skin, as found in this study with 2NPPD.

The absorption of 2NPPD from the semipermanent and permanent formulations was reduced by the presence of several dyes and dye intermediates—2-methylresorcinol, 4-amino-2-hydroxytoluene, N,N-bis(2-hydroxyethyl)-p-phenylenediamine sulfate, p-aminophenol, p-phenylenediamine, resorcinol—in the product and further reduced in the oxidative-permanent formulation by the addition of hydrogen peroxide. One explanation for the lower 2NPPD absorption from this formulation is that 2NPPD is chemically changed by oxidation due to the hydrogen peroxide. For example, the extent of HC Yellow No. 4 absorption was reduced if a dosing vehicle was applied that contained a formulation with seven other semipermanent hair dyes when compared with a formulation containing solely HC Yellow No. 4 (10). Mixtures of several dyes contained in one product formulation may change the solubility properties of the individual dyes. Furthermore, mixtures of dyes in formulations may result in the formation of dye aggregates through hydrogen bonding that could change the partition coefficient and molecular volume of the individual dyes (11). These dye-to-dye interactions are expected to slow the percutaneous penetration of an individual dye component.

The metabolism of 2NPPD after dermal application to human and rat skin can currently be summarized by Figure 29.5. In human and rat skin, it appears that 2NPPD is being metabolized via two pathways. The major pathway consists of N4-acetylation of the corresponding amine group. The second pathway consists of nitro reduction of the 2-nitro group to an amine. This was demonstrated by the presence of 1,2,4-triaminobenzene in the receptor fluid. In rat skin, but not human skin, a sulfated metabolite of 2NPPD was also detected, but the identity of the metabolite was not pursued. There is evidence to suggest it is possible to directly sulfate amine groups (12), indicating that sulfation potentially could have occurred on 2NPPD, acetylated-2NPPD, and/or triaminobenzene in rat skin.

The percutaneous absorption of 2NPPD obtained in the Yourick and Bronaugh study (5) was compared with another in vivo study (13). Results indicated that 5.4 µg 2NPPD per cm^2 was absorbed (based on 48.2 g of a semipermanent hair dye formulation containing 0.7% 2NPPD, 9.5% absorption, scalp skin surface area of 650 cm^2, and 10% of the applied formulation contacts the scalp skin) after a 30-minute application over 24 hours (5). In the Wolfram and Maibach study (13), approximately 3.4 µg 2NPPD per cm^2 was absorbed (based on 48.2 g formulation containing 1.36% 2NPPD, 0.143% absorption, and scalp surface area of 650 cm^2). The value of 3.4 µg/cm^2 2NPPD absorbed in the in vivo human application study (13) compares well with the value of 5.4 µg/cm^2 found in the in vitro human skin study (5), even though different hair dye formulations were used. The amount applied to the skin was based on the estimated amount that would actually contact the scalp skin (approximately 10% of the product applied). This resulted in a higher relative percentage of applied dose absorbed when compared with the Wolfram and Maibach study (13).

In summary, 2NPPD rapidly penetrates both human and fuzzy rat skin. Under conditions that simulate normal consumer use conditions, approximately 5% to 10% of the 2NPPD that contacts the skin would be expected to be absorbed. There was extensive metabolism of 2NPPD upon absorption. The extent of metabolism and the metabolic profile were found to be both species and dosing vehicle dependent. Even though no sulfation of 2NPPD was seen in human skin, unmetabolized

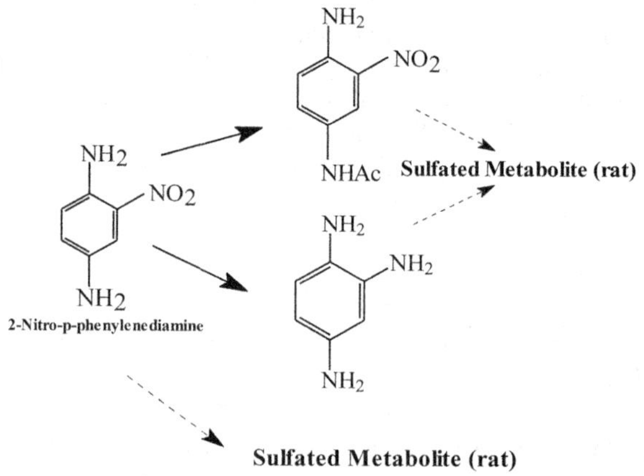

FIGURE 29.5 A proposed pathway for the metabolism of 2NPPD upon percutaneous absorption through human and rat skin. Metabolism of 2NPPD to sulfated metabolites was only observed in the rat. (From Reference 5.)

2NPPD that is systemically absorbed after dermal application could potentially be sulfated in other tissues (e.g., liver). The metabolism information will be useful in predicting the extent of 2NPPD and/or metabolite systemic absorption relative to a dermal exposure.

29.3 SKIN ABSORPTION OF DISPERSE BLUE 1

29.3.1 INTRODUCTION

Disperse Blue 1 (DB1; 1,4,5,8-tetraaminoanthraquinone) is a dye with a tetraaminoanthraquinone structure possessing a blue-black color. DB1 is used in temporary and semipermanent (nonoxidative) hair dyes, colors, and rinses. It is mutagenic in certain strains of *S. typhimurium* both with and without S9 activation (14). Positive tests are also noted with DB1 using several different mammalian mutagenicity assays (15). In a National Toxicology Program (16) rodent carcinogenicity feeding study with DB1, there was "clear evidence of carcinogenicity for male and female F344/N rats." DB1 administration resulted in "equivocal evidence of carcinogenicity in male B6C3F1 mice" and "no evidence of carcinogenicity in female B6C3F1 mice." Due to the carcinogenicity of DB1 in rodents after oral administration, the potential for DB1 skin absorption was investigated.

A study by Yourick et al. (17) investigated the in vitro skin absorption and metabolism of DB1 in human and fuzzy rat skin. The skin absorption of DB1 and the fate of the material remaining in the skin at the end of a 24-hour in vitro absorption study were investigated. An extended absorption study was conducted with DB1 to more thoroughly determine systemic availability of the dye. A summary of the DB1 study (17) is presented next.

29.3.2 DB1 RESULTS

29.3.2.1 Skin Absorption of Disperse Blue 1

The percutaneous absorption of DB1 through human skin into the receptor fluid with ethanol and the semipermanent dosing vehicles is depicted in Figure 29.6. DB1 slowly penetrated human skin

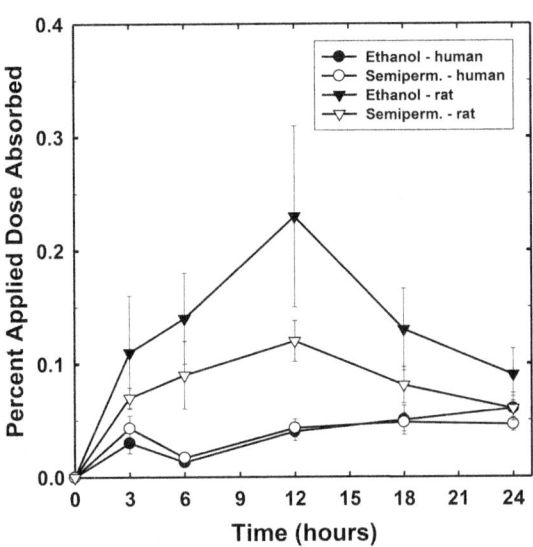

FIGURE 29.6 Percentage of applied DB1 dose absorbed over 24 hours in receptor fluid from human and rat skin. Absorption values are the X ± SE from four separate human studies (*n* = 4) and three individual rat studies (*n* = 3). Each individual absorption value within a study was determined by averaging four to five replicate diffusion cell measurements for each time interval point and dosing solution. (From Reference 17.)

with relatively constant absorption over the course of 24 hours. In human skin ($n = 4$), the percentages of applied dose absorbed over 24 hours into the receptor fluid were 0.2 ± 0.04 (mean $\pm$ SE) and 0.2 ± 0.02 for the ethanol and semipermanent vehicles, respectively, with approximately 11% and 3% remaining in skin, respectively (Table 29.3). There was no effect of the vehicle on the absorption of DB1 into the receptor fluid; however, there was a significant increase in the amount of DB1 that remained in the skin in an ethanol vehicle compared to the semipermanent formulation vehicle. This resulted in a significantly lower total penetration of DB1 into human skin when the semipermanent hair dye vehicle was compared to the ethanol vehicle. The amount of DB1 that was absorbed into the receptor fluid was significantly lower in human skin when compared with rat skin (Table 29.3). In addition, no human skin metabolism of DB1 was found by HPLC analysis of skin or receptor fluid.

Dermal absorption of DB1 through fuzzy rat skin into the receptor fluid over 24 hours is shown in Figure 29.6. DB1 also slowly diffused across fuzzy rat skin, similar to human skin, with relatively constant absorption over the course of 24 hours. In rat skin ($n = 3$), the percentages of applied dose absorbed over 24 hours into the receptor fluid were 0.7 ± 0.23 and 0.4 ± 0.07 for the ethanol and product vehicles, respectively, with approximately 9% and 3% remaining in skin, respectively (Table 29.3). The localization of the substantial amount of DB1 remaining in skin was investigated. The majority of DB1 (approximately 80%) was found in the stratum corneum, with the remainder

TABLE 29.3
Summary of Disperse Blue 1 Penetration in Human and Fuzzy Rat Skin[1]

	Percentage of Applied Dose	
	Dosing Vehicle	
	Ethanol	Semipermanent
Receptor Fluid		
Rat	0.7 ± 0.23[2]	0.4 ± 0.074
Human	0.2 ± 0.04[+]	0.2 ± 0.02[+]
Skin Content		
Rat	8.8 ± 1.64	2.6 ± 0.13*
Human	11.1 ± 1.30	3.1 ± 0.28*
Total Penetrated		
(Receptor Fluid + Skin)		
Rat	9.5 ± 1.55	3.0 ± 0.20*
Human	11.3 ± 1.34	3.3 ± 0.30*
Wash		
Rat	74.2 ± 3.37	80.9 ± 8.62
Human	76.1 ± 5.37	88.2 ± 2.21
Recovery		
Rat	83.5 ± 1.95	83.9 ± 8.82
Human	87.4 ± 5.83	91.5 ± 2.50

[1] All values represent data 24 hours after Disperse Blue 1 application.
[2] Values are the $X \pm SE$ for rat ($n = 3$) and human ($n = 4$) skin.
* Significantly different from the ethanol dosing vehicle.
[+] Significantly different from rat skin.
Source: Reference 17.

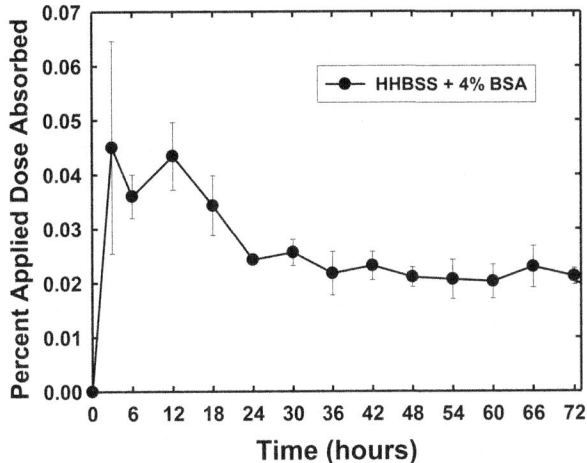

FIGURE 29.7 Extended DB1 absorption study in fuzzy rat skin. Absorption values are the X ± SE from two separate rat studies. Each individual absorption value within a study was determined by averaging three to four replicate diffusion cell measurements for each time interval point. (From Reference 17.)

contained in the viable epidermis/dermis layer (data not shown). To examine the fate of DB1 from the skin reservoir, an absorption study in rat skin was extended to 72 hours (Figure 29.7). The extended absorption study (skin washed after 24 hours) revealed that little (0.16% of the applied dose) of the DB1 that penetrated skin within 24 hours (2.6% of the applied dose; Table 29.3) moves through the skin to be absorbed into the receptor fluid over 72 hours. No rat skin metabolism of DB1 was found by HPLC analysis of skin or receptor fluid.

29.3.3   DB1 DISCUSSION

In summary, the skin reservoir can often contribute to the amount of material considered absorbed in diffusion cell studies. When the skin reservoir is significant compared to levels in receptor fluid, the contribution of the skin reservoir to systemic absorption should be examined. Therefore, it is important to determine the fate of chemicals remaining in the skin at the end of a typical 24-hour in vitro absorption study. An extended (72 hours) absorption study demonstrated that the DB1 remaining in the skin did not appreciably move into the receptor fluid beyond the extent measured after 24 hours. The barrier property of skin in diffusion cell studies has been shown to remain intact for 72 hours (18). Therefore, it seems reasonable to disregard the skin content as absorbed material. For exposure assessment purposes, the amount of DB1 considered systemically bioavailable would simply be the DB1 absorbed in the receptor fluid at 24 hours. With further investigation of the skin reservoir, it was determined not appropriate to add the skin levels of DB1 to the receptor fluid levels to characterize the total of absorbed material. This essentially reduced the percentage of applied dose absorbed being considered for exposure estimates from 3.3% to 0.2% for DB1.

29.4   HAIR DYE ABSORPTION: CORRELATION WITH PARTITION COEFFICIENTS

Percutaneous absorption through human skin of a homologous series of hair dyes was investigated (9). The hair dyes studied were p-phenylenediamine, o-phenylenediamine, 2-nitro-p-phenylenediamine, 2-amino-4-nitrophenol, 4-chloro-m-phenylenediamine, and 4-amino-2-nitrophenol. A compound's oil and water solubility properties affect its ability to diffuse across the epidermal membrane. The permeability constants for these dyes were compared to the octanol/water and

TABLE 29.4

Percutaneous Absorption of Hair Dyes and Correlation with Partition Coefficients

Compound	pKa	Octanol/Water Partition Coefficient	Stratum Corneum/Water Partition Coefficient	Permeability Constant (cm/hr[1])
p-Phenylenediamine	6.3	0.5	ND	2.4×10^{-4}
o-Phenylenediamine	4.8	1.4	6.9	4.5×10^{-4}
2-Nitro-p-phenylenediamine	3.9	3.4	13.0	5.0×10^{-4}
2-Amino-4-nitrophenol	7.1	13.5	ND	$<3.0 \times 10^{-5}$ (6.6×10^{-4})
4-Chloro-m-phenylenediamine	4.1	7.0	ND	2.1×10^{-3}
4-Amino-2-nitrophenol	7.8	9.1	13.0	8.6×10^{-5} (2.8×10^{-3})

[1] Values were obtained with a borate buffer (pH 9.7) as the vehicle. Numbers in parentheses were obtained in water to prevent ionization. Results are the mean of three to seven determinations.

ND = not determined.

Source: Reference 9.

skin membrane/water partition coefficients (Table 29.4). The permeability constants determined for these dyes were in the same rank order as the octanol/water partition coefficients, except for 4-chloro-m-phenylenediamine. Stratum corneum/water partition values correlated in a reverse order when compared with skin permeability constant values. It was apparent that once binding of the hair dye to the membrane was saturated, the partition coefficients more closely correlated with the rank order of the permeability constants. It was concluded that the prediction of percutaneous absorption of the homologous series of hair dyes was most closely associated with the oil/water partition coefficient, but this may be confounded by the capacity of the dye to bind to skin components.

29.5   EXAMPLES OF SPECIFIC HAIR DYE SKIN ABSORPTION STUDIES

29.5.1   Lawsone

Lawsone (2-hydroxy-1,4-naphthoquinone) is the principal color ingredient in henna, a color additive approved with limitations for coloring hair by the FDA under 21 CFR 73.2190. In 2004, the Scientific Committee on Cosmetics and Non-Food Products (SCCNFP) (19) concluded that lawsone was mutagenic and not allowable as a hair coloring dye. Studies were done to determine the extent of lawsone absorption through human skin. Lawsone skin absorption was determined from two hair coloring products and two shampoo products, all containing henna (20). It was found that the majority of the lawsone remained in the skin, with only slight amounts found in the receptor fluid contents. Therefore, for exposure assessment purposes, receptor fluid values would be a good estimate of lawsone systemic absorption, and lawsone skin levels should not be included.

In 2013, the Scientific Committee on Consumer Safety (SCCS) released an opinion on an assessment based on henna batches numbers 1271 and 830.72 (21) that contained a maximum concentration of 1.4% lawsone. For example, when 100 g henna powder is mixed with 300 mL boiling water, put into a formulation, and applied as indicated under functions and uses, henna was considered safe for use by the SCCS under these consumer conditions of use. This assessment of henna powder safety does not pertain to other henna extracts, other compositions, or higher use concentrations. The SCCS also asked for a reassessment of the genotoxicity testing of lawsone.

29.5.2   Catechol: An Oxidative Hair Dye Coupler

The Cosmetic Ingredient Review Expert Panel could not conclude that catechol could be safely used in permanent hair dye products (22). Catechol has been used as a coupler in oxidative hair dye formulations, but its current use is limited in formulations. The Expert Panel stated that there was a lack of information regarding the extent of catechol skin absorption and the extent of catechol remaining after undergoing oxidative reactions during the hair dyeing process. Therefore, Jung et al. (23) measured catechol skin absorption after application of a spiked consumer permanent hair dye product using an in vitro flow-through skin absorption system using human and rat skin and in vivo in the rat. Catechol was quickly absorbed from an ethanol vehicle when measured in vitro and in vivo using rat skin. However, only approximately 0.5% of the applied catechol dose was absorbed using in vitro human skin. An extended in vitro absorption study found that little of the catechol found in skin layers after 24 hours diffused into the receptor fluid after 72 hours. For catechol, the authors concluded that the skin reservoir of catechol did not contribute to the total absorption through skin, and systemic exposure is best characterized by catechol located in the receptor fluid (in vitro) or in the body (in vivo).

29.5.3   Aromatic Amine Hair Dyes and Metabolism

Manwaring et al. (24) explored an approach to better refine and estimate aromatic amine hair dye systemic absorption after dermal application using a combination of skin penetration, epidermal metabolism, and systemic metabolism. They investigated these properties using human skin explants, human keratinocyte (HaCaT) cell cultures, and liver cell cultures. It was shown that the major metabolic pathway for aromatic amine hair dyes in both HaCaT cells and the human skin explants was the phase II metabolic pathway of N-acetylation. The amount of aromatic hair dye chemical being absorbed intact is a function of the rate of skin penetration, pertinent metabolic pathways, and the length of resident time in the skin layers (i.e., mainly the epidermis). A pharmacokinetic modeling approach was used after data collection for the hair dye chemicals. Parameters such as systemic exposure, internal dose, hepatic clearance, and C_{max} were estimated from the toxicokinetic modeling. After generating in vitro skin absorption and metabolism parameters for p-phenylenediamine and running these parameters through the model, it was found that systemic predicted levels of parent hair dye chemical and metabolites were similar to systemic levels directly measured from human volunteers. These data and concepts are being used to build more refined physiologically based pharmacokinetic (PBPK) models to better describe exposure of chemicals, especially aromatic amine hair dyes, which are dermally applied and ultimately are systemically absorbed.

Nohynek et al. (25) studied the metabolism of an oxidative arylamine hair dye chemical in a reconstructed human cell epidermis model (EpiSkin) and in human liver cell cultures. A difference was found between the primary metabolic pathways in human epidermis when compared to liver cells. Human epidermis primarily metabolized para-aminophenol to its N-acetylated metabolite, but liver cells primarily metabolized para-aminophenol to its glucuronic acid or sulfated metabolites. However, another related hair dye chemical, para-phenylenediamine, was metabolized primarily to N-acetylated metabolites in both reconstructed human epidermis and human liver cells. Interestingly, liver cells had several-fold higher metabolic capacities for processing arylamine hair dyes to N-acetylated metabolites when compared to the reconstructed human epidermal model. Neither para-aminophenol nor para-phenylenediamine were metabolically hydroxylated by either epidermal or liver cells. It was concluded by Nohynek et al. (25) that human exposure to para-aminophenol or para-phenylenediamine after dermal exposure is mainly to the N-acetylated metabolites of those parent hair dyes. They also promote the idea that it is therefore important to include such metabolic data in the safety assessment of these types of hair dye chemicals.

Nohynek et al. (26) investigated the systemic exposure of para-phenylenediamine from commercially available dark-shade oxidative hair dye products when applied to hair by professional hairdressers. This study examined two different use concentrations of ^{14}C-para-phenylenediamine in hair dye products of 1% and 2%. Most hair dye products use para-phenylenediamine at a concentration of 1% in commercial products. The hair was dyed for 30 minutes as per use conditions. For sampling, all hair was shaved from the scalp and the hair rinsing liquid was collected. In addition, systemic absorption was measured by collecting blood plasma and urine for 48 hours after hair dye application. Approximately 0.7% to 0.88% of the applied radioactivity was excreted in the urine within 24 hours of hair dyeing. The plasma and urine were also analyzed by liquid chromatography–mass spectrometry (LC-MS) for para-phenylenediamine and its metabolites. The N,N'-diacetylated-para-phenylenediamine metabolite of para-phenylenediamine was the only related chemical species found in urine or plasma in the human subjects. The authors concluded that since N,N'-diacetylated-para-phenylenediamine is a detoxified metabolite of para-phenylenediamine, there is less risk to consumers using hair dye products containing para-phenylenediamine at current concentrations.

The use of in vitro flow-through diffusion cell systems was further evaluated for determining hair dye chemical absorption by Steiling et al. (27) using porcine skin. Two representative permanent hair dyes, para-phenylenediamine and bis-(5-amino- 1-hydroxyphenyl)-methane, were tested under realistic consumer use conditions for oxidative formulations. It was found that less than 1% of the applied dose of the hair dyes penetrated the skin. The authors compared this level of skin absorption with previously published information and concluded that there was good agreement between these in vitro and in vivo results.

There is a skin reservoir for chemicals upon penetration that must be investigated as to whether these amounts left remaining in the skin will ultimately contribute to systemic bioavailability. Lademann et al. (28) investigated whether levels of the direct hair dye hydroxyanthraquinone–aminopropyl methyl morpholinium methosulphate (HAM) remaining in the skin should be considered absorbed for exposure assessment purposes. They determined the absorption of HAM in both in vitro and in vivo human skin from a consumer hair product. Levels of HAM were found to be similar in the epidermis and dermis of in vitro studies with that measured in the stratum corneum of in vivo studies. However, stratum corneum residues of HAM would be lost due to desquamation and not available for absorption. Therefore, the authors concluded that skin levels remaining at the end of an in vitro penetration study might or might not need to be considered systemically bioavailable. They suggested that a "Threshold of Skin Absorption (TSA)" for low to negligible levels of chemicals measured remaining in the skin would have little effect on systemic absorption and therefore exposure to hair dyes like HAM.

29.6   CONCLUSION

In summary, the skin absorption of several representative hair dye chemicals is presented in this chapter. It was demonstrated that 2NPPD rapidly penetrated both human and rat skin. Also, there was extensive metabolism of 2NPPD upon absorption. The extent of metabolism and the metabolic profile were found to be both species and dosing vehicle dependent. DB1 slowly penetrated human and rat skin and was not metabolized. An extended (72 hours) DB1 absorption study demonstrated that DB1 remaining in the skin did not appreciably move into the receptor fluid beyond the extent measured after 24 hours. It was also shown with a series of homologous hair dyes that prediction of dermal absorption is most closely associated with the oil/water partition coefficient, but skin binding must also be considered. Extended absorption studies in conjunction with additional information on skin localization, skin binding studies, and vehicle effects can help determine the fate of hair dye ingredients in skin. Results were also summarized for several other representative hair dye chemicals and couplers that penetrate skin. In addition, the use of skin absorption data, the fate of the skin reservoir, and skin metabolism were considered as they relate to conducting a realistic exposure assessment for hair dye chemicals.

REFERENCES

1. Elder RL. Final report on the safety assessment of 2-nitro-p-phenylenediamine and 4-nitro-o-phenylenediamine. J Amer Coll Toxicol 1985; 4:161–197.
2. Ames BN, Kammen HO, Yamasaki E. Hair dyes are mutagenic: identification of a variety of mutagenic ingredients. Proc Nat Acad Sci USA 1975; 72:2423–2427.
3. IARC. IARC Monographs on the Evaluation of the Carcinogenic Risk of Chemicals to Humans. 1,4-Diamino-2-nitrobenzene (2-nitro-para-phenylenediamine) 1993; 57:85–200.
4. National Cancer Institute (NCI). *Bioassay of 2-Nitro-p-Phenylenediamine for Possible Carcinogenicity (CAS No. 5307-14-2).* Technical Report Series No. 169. NCI Publication NCI-CG-TR-169. US Department of Health and Human Services, Public Health Services, National Institutes of Health, 1979.
5. Yourick JJ, Bronaugh RL. Percutaneous penetration and metabolism of 2-nitro-p-phenylenediamine in human and fuzzy rat skin. Toxicol Applied Pharmacol 2000; 166:13–23.
6. Bronaugh RL, Stewart RF, Simon M. Methods for *in vitro* percutaneous absorption studies VII: use of excised human skin. J Pharm Sci 1986; 75:1094–1097.
7. Nakao M, Gotoh Y, Matsuki Y, Hiratsuka A, Watabe T. Metabolism of the hair dye component, nitro-p-phenylenediamine, in the rat. Chem Pharm Bull 1987; 35:785–791.
8. Flynn GL. Mechanism of percutaneous absorption from physicochemical evidence. In: Bronaugh RL, Maibach HI, eds. Percutaneous Absorption: Mechanisms-Methodology-Drug Delivery, New York: Marcel Dekker, 1985:17–42.
9. Bronaugh RL, Congdon ER. Percutaneous absorption of hair dyes: correlation with partition coefficients. J Invest Dermatol 1984; 83:124–127.
10. Dressler WE, Azri-Meehan S, Grabarz R. Utilization of *in vitro* percutaneous penetration data in the safety assessment of hair dyes. In: Lisanski SG, Macmillan R, Dupris J, eds. Alternatives to Animal Testing. Proceedings of an International Scientific Conference, Newbury UK: CPL Press, 1996:269.
11. Dressler WE. Percutaneous absorption of hair dyes. In: Roberts MS, Walters KA, eds. Dermal Absorption and Toxicity Assessment. 2d ed. Boca Raton FL: CRC Press, 2008:635–650.
12. Parkinson A. Biotransformation of xenobiotics. In: Klaassen CD, ed. Casarett & Doull's Toxicology: The Basic Science of Poisons. 5th ed. New York: McGraw-Hill, 1996:168–170.
13. Wolfram LJ, Maibach, HI. Percutaneous penetration of hair dyes. Arch Dermatol Res 1985; 277:235–241.
14. Zeiger E, Anderson B, Haworth S, Lawlor T, Mortelmans K. Salmonella mutagenicity tests. IV. Results from the testing of 300 chemicals. Environ Molec Mutagen. 1988; 11(Suppl 12):1–158.
15. Pang SNJ. Final Report on the Safety Assessment of Disperse Blue 1. J Am Coll Toxicol 14(6):433–451, 1995.
16. NTP-TR- 299. National Toxicology Program. Technical Report Series No. 299. Toxicology and Carcinogenesis Studies of C.I. Disperse Blue 1 (CAS No. 2475-45-8) in F344/N Rats and B6C3F$_1$ Mice (Feed Studies). NIH Publication No. 86-2555. 241 pp. National Toxicology Program, Research Triangle Park, NC, and Bethesda, MD, 1986.
17. Yourick JJ, Koenig ML, Yourick DL, Bronaugh RL. Fate of chemicals in skin after dermal application: Does the *in vitro* skin reservoir affect the estimate of systemic absorption? Toxicol Applied Pharmacol 2004; 195(3):309–320.
18. Kraeling MEK, Yourick JJ, Bronaugh RL. Percutaneous absorption of diethanolamine in human skin *in vitro*. Food Chem Toxicol 2004; 42(10):1553–1561.
19. The Scientific Committee for Cosmetics and Non-Food Products (SCCNFP): Opinion of the SCCNFP Concerning Lawsone. COLIPA n° C146. SCCNFP/0798/04, 2004.
20. Kraeling MEK, Bronaugh, RL, Jung CT. Absorption of lawsone through human skin. Cutaneous Ocular Toxicol 2007; 26(1):45–56.
21. Scientific Committee on Consumer Safety (SCCS). Opinion on *Lawsonia inermis* (Henna), Colipa no. C169. SCCS/1511/13, 19/09/2013.
22. Andersen FA. Cosmetic Ingredient Review. Amended final report on the safety assessment of pyrocatechol. Int J Toxicol 1997; 16(S1):11–58.
23. Jung CT, Wickett RR, Desai PB, Bronaugh RL. *In vitro* and *in vivo* percutaneous absorption of catechol. Food Chem Toxicol 2003; 41:885–895.
24. Manwaring J, Rothe H, Obringer C, Foltz DJ, Baker TR, Troutmana JA, Hewitt NJ, Goebel C. Extrapolation of systemic bioavailability assessing skin absorption and epidermal and hepatic metabolism of aromatic amine hair dyes *in vitro*. Toxicol Appl Pharmacol 2015; 287:139–148.
25. Nohynek GJ, Duche D, Garrigues A, Meunier PA, Toutain H, Leclaire J. Under the skin: biotransformation of para-aminophenol and para-phenylenediamine in reconstructed human epidermis and human hepatocytes. Toxicol Lett 2005; 158:196–212.

26. Nohynek GJ, Skare JA, Meuling WJA, Wehmeyer KR, de Bie ATHJ, Vaes WHJ, Dufour EK, Fautz R, Steiling W, Bramante M, Toutain H. Human systemic exposure to [14C]-paraphenylenediamine-containing oxidative hair dyes: absorption, kinetics, metabolism, excretion and safety assessment. Food Chemical Toxicol 2015; 81:71–80.
27. Steiling W, Kreutz J, Hofer H. Percutaneous penetration/dermal absorption of hair dyes *in vitro*. Toxicol In Vitro 2001; 15:565–570.
28. Lademann J, Richter H, Jacobi U, Patzelt A, Hueber-Becker F, Ribaud C, Benech-Kieffer F, Dufour EK, Sterry W, Schaefer H, Leclaire J, Toutain H, Nohynek GJ. Human percutaneous absorption of a direct hair dye comparing *in vitro* and *in vivo* results: implications for safety assessment and animal testing. Food Chem Toxicol 2008; 46:2214–2223.

30 Hair Dye Penetration in Monkeys and Human Beings

Nadia Kashetsky
Memorial University of Newfoundland,
St. John's, Newfoundland, Canada

Rebecca M. Law
Memorial University of Newfoundland,
St. John's, Newfoundland and Labrador, Canada

Leszek J. Wolfram
Clairol, Inc., Stamford, Connecticut

Howard I. Maibach
University of California, San Francisco, California

CONTENTS

30.1 INTRODUCTION

Hair dyes have been in use for decades, yet even recent studies about their skin penetration potential have been restricted primarily to their evaluation in rats and dogs (1–6). Although useful, the results of these experiments are difficult to extrapolate to humans and to relate to the percutaneous absorption that occurs under conditions of practical usage of fully formulated products. Sporadic attempts have been made to single out individual ingredients for studies in humans (7, 8), but these could not be readily quantitated.

A thorough study by Wester et al. (9), comparing the percutaneous absorption in humans and different animal species, while pointing to the experimental advantages of using animal models, stresses the need for frequent checks at each stage of the penetration process. The authors conclude that both *in vivo* and *in vitro* studies of the rhesus monkey skin approximate the permeability characteristics of human skin.

This chapter summarizes the current literature on *in vivo* percutaneous absorption of hair dyes. The studies focus on humans, however the study by Wolfram and Maibach carries out a comparison using the rhesus monkey as the animal model (10).

The methodology for this chapter is as follows. Several sources of information were used. A general Google search was completed. Then, databases were searched, including MEDLINE, PubMed, Embase, Scopus, Web of Science, and Google Scholar. The journal *Cosmetics & Toiletries* was also searched. The search terms used included "hair dye*" or "hair colour*", "hair color*" and "percutaneous" or "absorp*" or "penetrat*" or "permeab*". The searches were performed to include papers published starting from 2004 through October 2019. The specific parameters for the literature search necessary to make the project feasible include only articles published from 2004 through October 2019, and *in vivo* percutaneous absorption of hair dyes. Initially, there were 29 hits from this search. All thirty abstracts were reviewed. After abstract review, 16 articles were retrieved to read the entire papers. The exclusion and inclusion criteria for full retrieval of the individual papers are as follows. Inclusion criteria are: studies published from 2004 through October 2019, studies must have *in vivo* human data and studies must discuss experimental methodology. Exclusion criteria included studies not published in the English language. Further, references of articles that were retrieved were scanned. Also, the Cosmetic Ingredient Review was contacted to ask for clarification on certain references that were included in particular papers with unpublished data to review the unpublished primary research.

30.2   THE WOLFRAM AND MAIBACH STUDY (10)

The methodology is, in general, patterned after the procedure developed by Feldmann and Maibach (11) for measurement of percutaneous absorption in human beings. This method involves quantifying absorption on the basis of the percentage of radioactivity excreted in the urine following application of a known amount of the labeled compound.

Commercially available hair dye products, representatives of permanent and semi-permanent hair color categories (Nice'n Easy and Loving Care formulations, respectively) were individually labeled with radioactive materials. The radioactively labeled dyes together with their urinary recoveries following parenteral (P) or oral (O) administration are listed in Table 30.1.

Process instructions, specific for each hair color product, were followed. Net weights of single-application hair coloring products vary between 3 (semi-permanent dyes) and 4 fl oz (oxidative and permanent dyes). While this is sufficient to color up to 120 g of hair, the average weight of female scalp hair 4-in long is about 60 g. The ratio of lotion to hair commonly operative during hair coloring is thus 1.5–2.0, and the latter value was chosen to arrive at the quantity of the dye mixture that was used in the studies with rhesus monkey.

The coloring was performed with one subject at a time. The subject was seated in a chair having his head rested on a specially constructed sink support for comfort and easy collection of rinse water. The dye mixture was applied to dry hair and worked gently into the hair mass over a period of 5–8 minutes and left on the hair for additional 20 (permanent color) or 30 (semi-permanent color) minutes. In the latter case, a plastic turban was wrapped around the hair for the dyeing period. The dyed hair was thoroughly rinsed, towel blotted, dried, and either clipped with an electric clipper or left on.

Animals were tranquilized with 0.2 ml of ketamine and placed comfortably in a supine position on a laboratory bench top. The head of each monkey was rested on a specially designed sink support to facilitate the coloring process and to assure quantitative collection of the rinse water. The dye lotion (total of 5 g in the case of oxidative dyes consisting of 2.5 g of the dye solution and 2.5 g of 6% aqueous hydrogen peroxide) was worked into the dry scalp hair until all the dye mixture was used (~3 minutes). The operator wore vinyl disposable gloves. Twenty minutes time was allowed for the dyeing process in the case of permanent color (30 minutes in the case of semi-permanent dye, where a plastic turban was also used). After dyeing, the hair was rinsed with a microshower until the rinsing water was free of color. The excess water remaining on the hair was blotted with a paper towel and dyed hair was cut off with electric clippers.

The subjects were given plastic urine containers for each time period: 0–4, 4–8, 8–12, and 12–24 hour and then for every 24-hour period for as long as required.

TABLE 30.1
Dyes Studied in this Work

Dye Structure	Dye	Species and Yield of Urinary Recovery from Parenteral (P) or Oral (O) Administration
	p-Phenylenediamine (PPD)	Man, 72% (P)
	Resorcinol	Rhesus monkey, 79% (P)
	4-Amino-2-hydroxytoluene	Man, 94% (O)
	2,4-Diaminoanisole (DAA)	Rhesus monkey, 61% (P)
	2-Nitro-PPD	Rhesus monkey, 56% (P)
	2-Nitro-4-aminophenol	Rhesus monkey, 68% (P)
	HC Blue No. 1	Man, 94% (O)
	HC Blue No. 2	Man, 51% (O)

After the dyeing procedure was completed, all the monkeys were restrained in ophthalmological chairs, thus preventing the animals from touching the scalp area. Urine samples were collected at 6, 12, and 24 hours and from then on at 24-hour intervals for 7 days. For both species and for each time period, total urine weights were recorded and an aliquot was removed for analysis.

All urine samples were filtered and assayed in para-phenylenediamine (PPD)/Triton/toluene with a liquid scintillation spectrometer. A [14C]toluene internal standard (100,000 cpm) was added to each counting vial to determine the extent of quenching. The counting cocktail was 81% efficient and the background was 22 cpm. Most specimens were also counted by the wet ashing method (11). The assay values listed in the tables have been corrected for incomplete excretion from internal application. For the latter, see Table 30.1.

Samples of hair or of the horny layer were digested overnight in counting vials, each containing 1 ml of Unisol. The digested samples were decolorized by the addition of 50% hydrogen peroxide and each was diluted with 15 ml of Unisol complement. Clear samples were equilibrated in the counting chamber at 4C before counting on a Packard Tricarb liquid scintillation spectrometer. Three samples were analyzed for each hair lot and one of the stratum corneum, with three radioactivity determinations for each sample.

Two methodological approaches (denoted "Application Only" and "Application and Wear"), reflecting different experimental objectives, have been developed in the course of this study. In the first one, the hair was removed immediately following the completion of the coloring procedure; in the other, the hair was left on. The first approach allowed us to evaluate the extent of skin penetration by hair dyes resulting from the hair coloring procedure alone. The second approach recognized that (a) people color their hair to wear it as such, and (b) the dyed hair represents a reservoir of dye moieties that, through a variety of routes, may become bioavailable.

The data on total excretion of radiolabeled dye ingredients are given in Table 30.2. In most cases, they reflect the counts obtained over 144 hours following application of the dye; occasionally a time span of 96 hours was used if the counts at longer times were at the background level.

Two entries of Table 30.2, namely (T1/2) and total dose excretion, should be clarified. It was found that the urinary excretion followed satisfactory first-order kinetics and thus, time required for 50% excretion (T1/2) was employed as an additional quantifying parameter. Regarding the dose, bear in mind that in the process of hair coloring, the product is usually applied in the form of a viscous lotion and uniformly distributed within the hair mass. Clearly, only the product that is in contact with the scalp serves as a dye reservoir available for skin penetration. The quantity available depends on the

TABLE 30.2
Parameters of Percutaneous Absorption of Hair Dyes

Hair Color Category	Labeled Ingredient	Species	Number of Subjects	Total Dose Excretion [% (#SD)]	T1/2 of Urinary Excretion (hr)
Permanent (oxidative)	2,4-Diaminoanisole (DAA)	Man	3	0.022 (0.01)	18
		Rhesus monkey	2	0.032	20
	Resorcinol	Man	3	0.076 (0.03)	31
		Rhesus monkey	3	0.177 (0.03)	31
	4-Amino-2-hydroxytoluene	Man	3	0.20 (0.10)	24
	p-Phenylenediamine (PPD)	Man	5	0.190 (0.06)	16
		Rhesus monkey	3	0.182 (0.06)	22
Semipermanent	2-Nitro-PPD	Man	3	0.143 (0.04)	24
		Rhesus monkey	3	0.551 (0.10)	24
	4-Amino-2-nitrophenol	Man	3	0.235 (0.08)	10
	HC Blue No. 1	Man	5	0.151 (0.12)	18
		Rhesus monkey	3	0.127 (0.03)	40

retention of the product by hair, which in turn is a function of total surface area of the hair mass and the viscosity of the product. Unless the product is applied sparingly (product/hair ratio much less than one—a situation that is unlikely to be encountered in hair dyeing), the thickness of the product film present on the scalp is at least 5–10 times that of the horny layer of the scalp; and under such conditions, the quantity of the absorbed dye reaches a limiting value and is independent of the quantity of lotion used (6). Throughout this work, every attempt was made to maintain a constant ratio of product to hair weight ("2) and thus to make the dose excretion values intercomparable.

From the five dyes that were concurrently evaluated on both humans and the rhesus monkey, three of them (DAA, PPD, and HC Blue No. 1) show striking equivalence in cutaneous absorption between these two species. This parallels the earlier finding of Wester et al. (9) and Bartek and LaBudde (12), who noted a similar pattern for absorption of benzoic acid, testosterone, and hydrocortisone. Two remaining dyes (2-nitro-PPD and resorcinol), representing the semi-permanent and permanent categories, respectively, do not follow this pattern. Both dyes show greater absorption for rhesus monkey than humans, although the T1/2 values are identical in both species.

The results also indicate that except for DAA, the dyes appear to penetrate the skin to a similar extent. This is in spite of substantial differences in the chemical structure of the dyes, in the nature of the dye bases, and in the reaction pathways responsible for color formation. The observed effect is, however, somewhat fortuitous because the various dyes are present in their respective formulations at different concentrations. A better perception of their penetration potential can be deduced from the flux values which were calculated for individual dyes from the 24-hour excretion data, normalizing the quantity applied in each case to 10 mM/cm^2 (Table 30.3).

There is approximately a 10-fold spread in the flux, with DAA being at the low end of the scale and 4-amino-2-nitrophenol exhibiting the highest potential. No apparent correlation to either molecular weight or the chemical structure is evident, but the spread in molecular weight is relatively small (it varies between 100 and 250), and all the dyes are unchanged under dyeing conditions. It is also interesting that the flux ranking of dyes is not reciprocated by their solubility characteristics. The membrane/vehicle partition coefficients (which reflect the solubility properties of materials in media of differing polarities) are considered to be important factors in determining the flux of materials through the stratum corneum but, surprisingly, their utility in this case is minimal (Table 30.4).

The octanol/water partition coefficients seem to be at odds as well with those determined for stratum corneum/water with no evidence of a pattern that could be persuasively interpreted. The data all but imply that the lipid domains in the horny layer are the unlikely sites for retention of lipophilic dyes. That the distribution of dyes in the stratum corneum is highly complex is further evidenced by the fact that the delipidization of stratum corneum by chloroform/methanol increases the values of partition coefficients of dyes irrespective of whether they are hydrophilic or prefer a nonpolar environment. Clearly, the removal of lipids augments the reservoir capacity of the horny layer. It would be presumptuous, however, to assume that such an increase would simply translate into faster or more extensive diffusion, since the latter is likely to be critically

TABLE 30.3
Flux of Hair Dyes Through Human Scalp

Dye	Flux (mol/cm^2 hr)		
DAA	9.2	$ 10	%11
Resorcinol	2.2	$ 10	%10
4-Amino-2-hydroxytoluene	4.5	$ 10	%10
2-Nitro-PPD	4.7	$ 10	%10
HC Blue No. 1	4.9	$ 10	%10
PPD	6.3	$ 10	%10
4-Amino-2-nitrophenol	8.3	$ 10	%10

TABLE 30.4

Partition Coefficients of Hair Dyes Between Octanol/Water and Guinea Pig Stratum Corneum/Water

Dye	Octanol/water	Intact Stratum Corneum/water	Delipidized Sratum Corneum/water
DAA	0.7	—	—
Resorcinol	7.0	3.6	7.7
4-Amino-2-hydroxytoluene	25.4	8.0	21.1
2-Nitro-PPD	3.6	13.2	28.9
HC Blue No. 1	10.8	2.8	7.3
PPD	0.2	4.0	7.3
4-Amino-2-nitrophenol	10.1	5.0	9.1

dependent on the binding of the dyes to the stratum corneum and there is no information about how delipidization affects the binding characteristics.

An additional and useful insight into the mechanism of scalp penetration by hair dyes can be gained from the T1/2 values of urinary excretions. The results of monitoring the urinary recoveries of dyes administered by parenteral injection or orally show that elimination of those materials from the organisms of either rhesus monkey or humans is rapid, yielding T1/2 values of 4 hours or less. That is clearly not the case with the urinary dye recoveries following hair dyeing, where T1/2 values vary from 10 to 40 hours, suggesting that only trivial amounts of dye penetrate the stratum corneum during the actual process of hair coloring. It follows that the bulk of the urine-recovered dye must have been taken up into the horny layer and then slowly released into the circulation. Some penetration from hair follicles and/or sweat ducts might also have occurred, but this shunt mechanism—judging again by high T1/2 values—seems to be of less importance. A direct experimental support for the magnitude of the horny layer reservoir has been obtained by applying a measured quantity of dye formulation to forearms of human volunteers, mimicking the dyeing procedure, and then removing sequential layers of stratum corneum all the way to the glistening layer by stripping with adhesive tape. The application areas were large enough to allow for stripping adjacent regions 16 or 18 hours after the color application. Figures 30.1 and 30.2 illustrate the results obtained in the case of PPD and HC Blue No. 1, respectively. The change in the concentration profiles of both dyes with time is a dramatic demonstration of their mobility in the horny layer and serves as an independent confirmation of the observed kinetics of scalp penetration. It is worth adding that the calculations based on the reservoir potential in both cases strongly suggest that the urinary excretion values, which are the measure of the extent of dye penetration, can be satisfactorily accounted for by the dye absorbed within the stratum corneum.

The hair coloring procedures employed in this study were identical to those described earlier, however, the collections of urine and their radioactive assays continued for as long as 30 days following the dye application. The results of the assays, both total and interim, are given in Table 30.5. The half-times (T1/2) of urinary excretions are also included as informative guides.

The results fall into a pattern that one would anticipate from the mechanism of hair coloring that is characteristic for a given class of dyes. In case of oxidative (permanent) dyes (based on PPD and its couplers), the color-forming reactions convert the small, mobile, and colorless molecules into much bulkier dye moieties trapped within the structure of the hair. There is little chance for these materials to diffuse out of the hair, even when it becomes fully swollen during

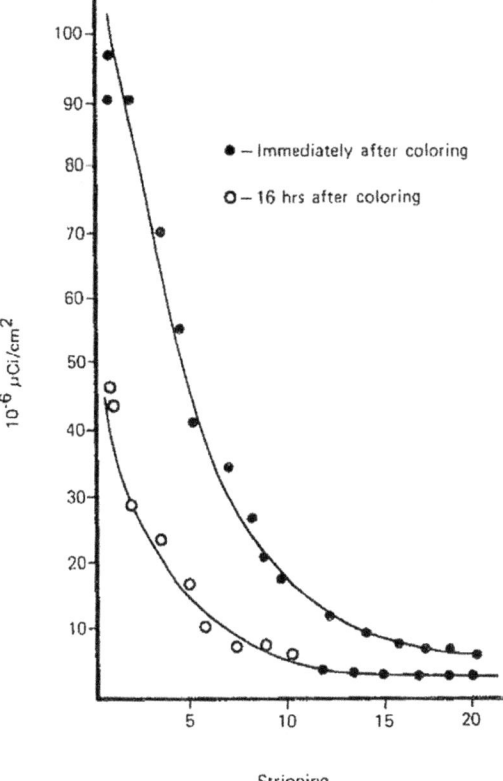

FIGURE 30.1   Distribution of radioactive PPD in the horny layer.

shampooing. On the other hand, the semi-permanent dyes do not undergo any changes in size upon their deposition in the fiber, and they retain a high degree of mobility which translates into a potential for outward diffusion. Thus, while the hair acts as a repository for both types of dye, their bioavailabilities are clearly different. The latter finds its experimental verification in the urinary excretion data. There is only a marginal increase in the dosage absorption of PPD when compared to the "Application Only" values, with most of the increase generated within 2 days of color application. HC Blue No. 1 and 2-nitro-PPD, on the other hand, register a four- to fivefold increase with measurable absorption values spread over several weeks. This trend is also reflected in the T1/2 values of urinary excretion—a trivial change for PPD, but a substantial increase for both HC Blue No. 1 and 2-nitro-PPD.

The excretion data of Table 30.5 reflect not only scalp penetration but also include dye that has become bioavailable through other ports of entry (dermal as well as oral)—a real-life situation. In this sense, the T1/2 values do not have the same meaning as those of Table 30.2, where they referred exclusively to scalp permeation.

The higher mobility of semi-permanent dyes when compared to their oxidative counterparts implies faster depletion of the hair "reservoir." This is fully attested to by the results of the radioactive assays of the dyed hair. Over the 30-day wear period, the hair colored with permanent dyes lost approximately 10% of its original dye content, while losses of well over 60% were recorded for hair dyed with semi-permanent dyes.

Table 30.5 contains one entry (HC Blue No. 2) that appears to be at odds with the remainder of the data. This dye is strikingly similar in its chemical structure to HC Blue No. 1; it remains

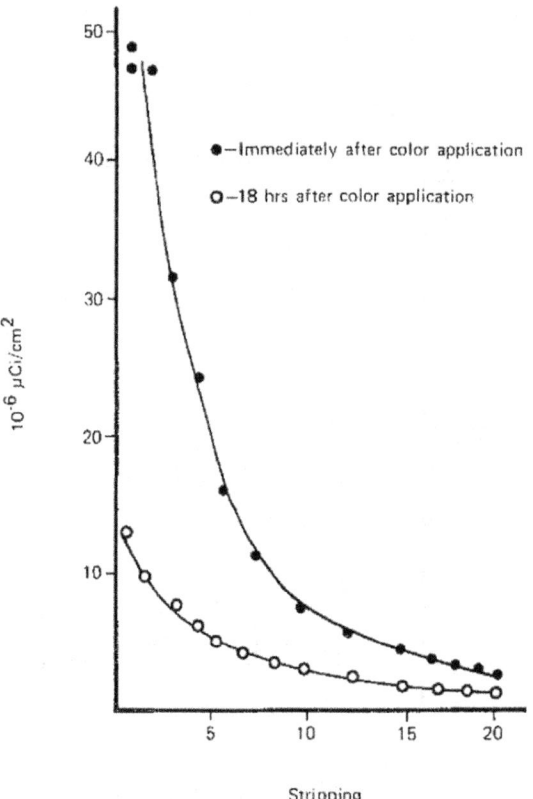

FIGURE 30.2   Distribution of radioactive HC Blue No. 1 in the horny layer.

unaltered during the dye-out, yet in its skin permeation characteristics it does not behave like a semi-permanent. The octanol/water partition coefficient for HC Blue No. 2, at 1.6, is much lower than that of HC Blue No. 1, and the dye partitions poorly into the stratum corneum from water. A clue to the unusual behavior of this dye was furnished by the skin stripping experiments. Figures 30.3 and 30.4 are the dye content profiles of human stratum corneum stripped from the forearms dyed with components containing either HC Blue No. 1 or No. 2. The stripping was done immediately upon dyeing and again 6 hours later. The radioactivities of the dye lotions were almost identical and so

TABLE 30.5

Dose Absorption of Hair Dyes in Man Under Conditions of Use (Application þ30 Days Wear)

Dye	Number of Subjects	Cumulative Dose Absorption (%)					
		1st day	10th day	20th day	30th day	T (#SD)	1/2 (h)
PPD	3	0.19	0.31	0.34	0.34	(0.12)	26
2-Nitro-PPD	4	0.19	0.42	0.62	0.75	(0.30)	150
HC Blue No. 1	4	0.15	0.28	0.30	0.50	(0.15)	138
HC Blue No. 2	4	0.01	0.07	0.094	0.094	(0.02)	52

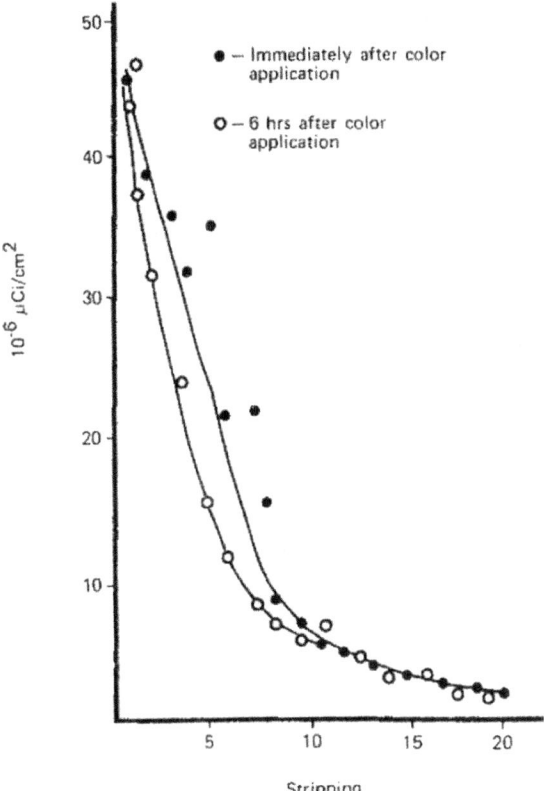

FIGURE 30.3   Distribution of radioactive HC Blue No. 1 in the horny layer.

were the assays of stratum corneum strips harvested right after dyeing (29.7 × 10⁻⁴ µCi for HC Blue No. 1, and 30.3 × 10⁻⁴ µCi for HC Blue No. 2). Obviously, both dyes were diffusing at comparative rates while the dye lotions were on. The assays of the 6-hour strips revealed, however, that while the activity of the skin dyed with HC Blue No. 1 decreased to 24.5 × 10⁻⁴ µCi (16% loss), that of tissue dyed with HC Blue No. 2 remained unchanged. The HC Blue No. 2 is thus obviously bound much more strongly to the stratum corneum than HC Blue No. 1, yet such a conclusion would hardly be arrived at on the basis of its partition coefficient.

There is little doubt that an increase in the tenacity of binding is inversely related to the dye mobility within the horny layer and thus adversely affects the diffusion of the dye into viable epidermis. With the diffusion process markedly slowed down, the natural process of desquamation attains an important role. The bulk of the dye reservoir is located in a few uppermost layers of the stratum corneum, and their loss by desquamation can lead to a rapid and precipitous drop in the quantity of the bioavailable dye, hence in the total extent of skin penetration. It appears from the results presented here that HC Blue No. 2 exemplifies such a behavior.

30.3   ADDITIONAL STUDIES

30.3.1   Study 1

Subsequent to this study, Nohynek et al. (2004) investigated urinary metabolites *in vivo* by applying [14C]-PPD containing oxidative hair dye to human subjects and attempting to correlate their metabolite profile with their respective N-acetyltransferase 2 (NAT2) genotypes (13).

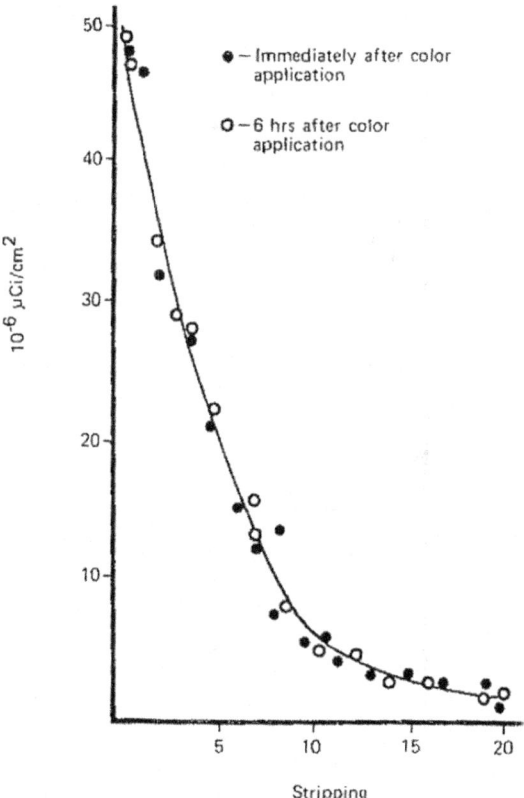

FIGURE 30.4 Distribution of radioactive HC Blue No. 2 in the horny layer.

Dark-shade oxidative hair dye containing [14C]-PPD was used. PPD and bi-acetylated PPD were purchased for use.

Seventy ml of the dark shade oxidative hair dye, with 1.31 ± 0.05 geq. [14C]-PPD was applied per subject. The [14C]-radioactivity of the formulation applied was a mean total of 7.14 ± 0.26 × 107 DPM per subject.

Eight healthy male volunteers from 18 to 42 years participated in the study. Oxidative hair dye was applied for 30 minutes, followed by rinsing and washing with water and 20 ml of shampoo. Drying was completed with paper towel and air drying.

Urine was collected for 120 hours following hair dye treatment, at 4-hour intervals, up to 12 hours, followed by collection every 12 hours. Urine samples were stored at +4°C until determination of radioactivity. Remaining urine was stored at −20°C. Pooled urine samples of the 0–24-hour period were stored at −20°C. 100 ml portions from the 0–24 hour period were used for determination of [14C]-PPD metabolites.

As described by Nohynek et al. (2004), urine sample analysis was completed with High-Performance Liquid Chromatography (HPLC) with the following parameters: the flow rate was 0.8 ml/minute, the UV detector was 230 nM, and the scintillator flow was 3.0 ml/minute. Urinary metabolite retention times were compared with standards.

Table 30.6 shows the urinary radioactivity and respective recovery rates per human subject. Loss of radioactivity in the SPE column ranged 3–19% during sample concentration and clean-up in the SPE column. Mean recovery rate was 87.3 ± 5.4%. Five metabolites were identified and labeled

TABLE 30.6
Subject Urinary Excretion of Radioactivity Over First 24 Hours

Subject Number	Recovery (%)	Excretion (%[^{14}C])	Radioactivity Urine$_{0-24h}$ (DPM x 10^4)	Radioactivity Extract (DPM x 10^3)
01	85.4	0.60	2.76	23.6
02	80.5	0.24	1.42	11.4
03	85.9	0.27	1.58	13.6
04	86.8	0.30	1.69	14.7
05	87.9	0.31	1.24	10.9
06	81.9	0.52	2.98	24.4
07	93.1	0.27	0.84	7.8
08	96.9	0.91	3.65	35.4
Mean ± SD	83.9 ± 6.8	0.43 ± 0.24	2.02 ± 0.98	17.7 ± 0.93

Adapted from Nohynek et al. (2004).

U1–U5. The presence of [14C]-urinary metabolites and their respective retention times are shown in Table 30.7. See original study for HPLC chromatograms of urine extract.

For metabolite identification, retention times of the analytical standards were in the range of 19.4–19.5 minutes for N,N′-diacetyl-PPD, 12.6–13.2 minutes for N-mono-acetyl-PPD, and 7.1–8.1 minutes for PPD. Identity of metabolites could not be definitely identified. However, when compared with the results of Goetz et al. (14), U4 and U5 correspond with N-mono- and N,N′-diacetylated PPD, respectively. Analytical standards and U2, U4, U5, and U3 were stable to acidic or basic hydrolysis.

TABLE 30.7
Urinary Metabolites in the First 24 Hours (% of total radioactivity) and Respective Peak Retention Times

Subject Number	U1 3.8–5.6 min	U2 10.5 min	U3 14.4 min	U4 12.2–15.8 min	U5 14.8–18.7 min
08	5.0	4.9	3.6	32.4	54.2
07	BLD	BLD	BLD	48.4	51.6
06	5.1	BLD	BLD	43.5	51.4
05	5.9	BLD	BLD	31.5	62.7
04	9.7	BLD	BLD	46.3	44.0
03	13.5	BLD	BLD	57.3	29.3
02	BLD	BLD	BLD	51.7	48.3
01	5.0	BLD	BLD	45.5	49.6
Mean ± SD	7.4 ± 3.5	Not calculated	Not calculated	44.6 ± 8.9	48.9 ± 9.6

BLD, below limit of detection.
Adapted from Nohynek et al. (2004).

U1 may be a conjugate of U3 as U1 disappeared after acidic hydrolysis and reappeared at the time of U3. The metabolite identity of U2 is unknown. NAT2 genotype results found three subjects classified as slow acetylators and five as intermediate acetylators.

Radioactivity suggests that only PPD-related metabolites were present in the urine of human subjects exposed to oxidative hair dye containing [14C]-PPD. There was no evidence of systemic absorption of reaction products of the oxidative hair dye process via high molecular weight. Also, that NAT2 genotype is independent of PPD metabolism after topical application of hair dye containing PPD. The possible association of NAT2 slow acetylator genotype and higher bladder cancer risk from exposure of PPD is not supported by this data.

30.3.2 Study 2

Skare and Nohynek et al. (15) completed an abstract on the overview of *in vitro*, *in vivo*, and clinical studies on the metabolism of oxidative hair dyes. In regards to *in vivo* percutaneous absorption of hair dye in humans, the abstract discusses metabolism studies with *in vivo*, widely used hair dye aromatic amines via the oral or dermal route. Results demonstrate that the aromatic amines are N-acetylated in the skin by NAT1, a detoxification pathway. N-acetylation is also a major hepatic pathway and there is no evidence of hepatic metabolic activation. Hepatic phase II conjugation reactions are also indicated as main pathways for the metabolism of some hair dyes. After hair dye use in human subjects, NAT2 NAT2 genotype does not influence urinary profile of PPD. This is inconsistent with the theory that hair dye may be linked to an increased bladder cancer risk in NAT2 slow acetylators.

30.3.3 Study 3

Subsequent to this study, Gube et al. (2011) investigated whether biological monitoring of aromatic diamines can quantify the occupational exposure of hairdressers to permanent hair dyes. Level were compared to levels in people after recent application of hair dyes (16).

Permanent hair dyes were used. Substances, 2,5-toluylene diamine (2,5-TDA) and p-phenylene diamine (p-PDA) are predominantly the active constituents of permanent hair dyes.

All operations associated with potential exposure to hair dyes were documented, including mixing color, applying color, washing hair after dyeing, and cutting freshly colored hair. Participants recorded whether or not they were wearing gloves.

This study involved 52 hairdressers, aged 16–63 years, 40 female and 12 male, from 16 salons. A control group of 19 people from the general population, aged 22–64 years old, 10 males and 9 females, was also included. All included participants stated no use of personal hair dyes 4 days prior to the study.

Urine samples were at the following times: the morning before the first shift of the work week, pre- and post-shift at the third day of the week, and pre- and post-final day of the work week. Hairdressers were asked to wash hands before handling urine samples to avoid external contamination. For the control group, spot urine samples were taken. Urine samples were frozen at −18°C immediately after collection; if this was not possible these were stored at 4–8°C overnight.

Gas chromatography-mass spectrometry (GC/MS) was used for determination of 2,5-TDA and p-PDA. Mean accuracy for 2,5-TDA was 97.3% and for p-PDA it was 93.8%. A 96-well plate photometer was used to determine urinary creatinine concentrations. Internal quality controls and biannual participation in round robins ensured quality of the urinary creatinine assay. Corrections for creatinine were always done for concentrations of urinary diamines.

For statistical analysis, calculations were done to obtain the medians of all individual values of each participant of both 2,5-TDA and p-PDA and the 95th percentile. An analysis of variance was conducted to detect whether there was an intra-shift effect, an effect across a working week, or a dependency on performing with or without protection gloves. The analysis of variance was completed by calculating a linear model. 2,5-TDA and p-PDA were the dependent variables and parameters of exposure were the independent variables.

2,5-TDA was quantified in urine samples of 40 out of 52 subjects during the working week. An elevated 2,5-TDA concentration was found in the urine sample of one subject in the control group. Two more people in the control group were slightly above the limit of 2,5-TDA. One person in the hairdresser group and one from the control group had highly elevated levels of 2,5-TDA and stated they had used personal hair dyes within 4 days of the start of the study. They were excluded from data analysis.

Data for median values for urinary 2,5-TDA are as follows. In the hairdresser group, they ranged from <0.2 µg/g creatinine before to the first shift to 1.7 µg/g creatinine post-shift on the last day of the work week with 95th percentiles of 6.9 µg/g creatinine up to 16.3 µg/g creatinine and maximums of 9.4 µg/g creatinine up to 155.8 lg/g creatinine. In the control group, median value was 0.2 µg/g creatinine with a 95th percentile of 0.9 and a maximum of 3.33 µg/g creatinine. Table 30.8 shows median, 95th percentile, and maximum concentrations of urinary 2,5-TDA and p-PDA in hairdressers and controls.

Four of 51 hairdressers showed urinary p-PDA concentrations above the limit of detection. p-PDA could not be detected in urine samples of the control group. Median value for p-PDA was <1 µg/g creatinine both in the hairdressers and in the controls at all points in time investigated. 95th percentile was <1 µg/g creatinine up to 2.3 µg/g creatinine in hairdressers. Maximum was 2.3 µg/g creatinine up to 36.6 µg/g creatinine in hairdressers. For controls, the 95th percentile and maximum were <1 µg/g creatinine. Chromatograms in the original article show medians of 2,5-TDA eliminated over the work week and medians of p-PDA elimination for each hairdresser's salon over the period of a work week. There were 2 participants with detectable p-PDA values in urine samples in salon number 14, 1 in salon number 8, and 1 in salon number 16.

Data analysis found there was neither intra-shift effect nor a cumulation of excretion after a complete work week. A slight but not statistically significant pre-shift to post-shift difference by the last day of the week was found. Lowest values of the working week were prior to the first shift of the week. It may be indicated that mixing hair dye had the highest excretion of 2,5-TDA. Median levels of urinary 2,5-TDA detected in the participating hairdressers was about 200 times lower than in the case of personal use of hair dyes. While the maximum level of 2,5-TDA found in this study was 155.8 µg/g in urine in the group of hairdressers, the maximum level in personal hair dye use is up to 2000 µg/g in urine 4–5 hours after application.

TABLE 30.8
Concentrations of Urinary 2,5-TDA and p-PDA in Controls and Hairdressers

	2,5-TDA (µg/g crea)			p-PDA (µg/g crea)		
	Median	95th Percentile	Maximum	Median	95th Percentile	Maximum
Controls	<0.2	0.9	3.3	<1	<1	<1
Hairdressers (n= 51)						
Before first shift	<0.2	6.9	9.4	<1	<1	2.3
Before third day shift	1.4	14.1	46.4	<1	<1	4.3
After third day shift	1.2	13.0	50.9	<1	<1	6.4
Before last shift of the week	1.2	16.3	155.8	<1	2.3	36.6
After last shift of the week	1.7	15.1	109.6	<1	1.4	27.5

Adapted from Gube et al. (2011).

This study (16) concludes 2,5-TDA was detectable in 39 of the hairdressers. Two controls also had elevated 2,5-TDA in urine samples, however they used personal hair dye more than 4 days before they provided urine samples which shows elimination may take more than 4 days. P-PDA was detectable in urine samples of four hairdressers. Also, use of gloves was found to have no influence on internal exposure of hairdressers.

30.3.4 STUDY 4

Nohynek et al. (2015) (17) measured systemic exposure after hair dyeing with oxidative hair dyes containing 2.0 or 1.0% [14C]-PPD in humans. This study is the first complete investigation of absorption, plasma kinetics, metabolism, and excretion of oxidative hair dyes in humans following a hair coloring procedure under conditions of a hairdresser salon.

Studies A (2.0% PPD) and B (1.0% PPD) used PPD with radioactivities of 4.40 or 4.44 GBq/mmol with a radiochemical purity of 97.6 or 98.7%, respectively. PPD concentration at application was 2.0% in study A after mixing the contents of the two bottles. PPD concentration at application was 1.0% in study B, after mixing the contents of the two bottles. In study A, the mean amount of PPD applied was 1.20 ± 0.16 g (0.86 to 1.41 g). In study B, the mean amount was 0.65 ± 0.11 g (0.45–0.95 g).

Thirty-two subjects, aged 20–34 years, 4 females and 28 males, participated in this study. Subjects had a similar approximate hair length of 5 cm.

Participants were divided into four groups with four people per group for each study. Over the course of a 3-day period, each group completed hair dye application and biological sampling. Radioactivity was measured in two samples of 200 µl by scintillation counting. Mean quantity of radioactivity in the four vials used in each study was 16.9 (range: 15.0–18.5) MBq for Study A and 26.0 (range: 24.6–27.4) MBq for study B. Hairdressers used their professional judgment along with the hair length and density of each subject to determine the amount of hair dye individually applied. The oxidative hair dye (30–50 g) with either 4% PPD (Study A) or 2% PPD (Study B) was weighed and [14C]-PPD tracer was added. Then an equal weight of developer was added. Contents were mixed with a brush in coded mixing bowls. To determine the amount applied to the study subjects, the amount remaining in the bowls and brush was subtracted by the amount prepared. The mean amount of radioactivity applied was 3.12 ± 0.60 MBq (2.08–4.33) in Study A and 3.30 ± 0.56 MBq (2.22–4.03) in Study B. The final specific activity was 155.9 ± 28.4 dpm/µg PPD in Study A and 306.6 ± 42.8 dpm/µg PPD in Study B.

Hair dye was applied to each subject by an experienced hairdresser with standard tools and utensils of professional hair salons. Hair dye was applied to hair with within 15–20 minutes, left for 30 minutes, rinsed with water, and washed twice with shampoo. Hair conditioner was put into hair for 5 minutes, rinsed with water, and dried via blotting with towels. All used materials were collected for determination of radioactivity including all water used for washing and rinsing. Hair was dried with an electric hair dryer and clipped using an electric clipper. Remaining hair was shaved with an electric razor. Ten successive adhesive tape strippings were used to collect stratum corneum in an area of 2×10 cm^2 on the right side of the scalp. Blank tape strips were taken from the forearm. A protective cap was worn after tape stripping overnight to obtain shed skin. Twenty-four hours after hair dying, a second set of 10 successive tape strippings were collected from the left side on the scalp. Strippings were cut into two parts: one part was used for radioactivity analysis and the other for chemical analysis (only study B). Tape strippings of each group were pooled for analysis. All materials were stored for radioactivity analysis.

As described by Nohynek et al. (17), urine samples were collected before treatment and over the intervals 0–12, 12–24, and 24–48 hours after the start of hair dye application. Blood samples were collected by arm vein puncture 30 minutes before hair dye application, and 2, 4, 6, 10, 24, 48 hours after the start of hair dye application.

To determine radioactivity, liquid scintillation counting (LSC) was used. Scintillation counting was done with Ultima Gold XR™ scintillation liquid, except plasma samples, skin strips, and

TABLE 30.9

Lower Limits of Quantification of the Analytical Methods of Skin Strippings, Plasma, and Urine for PPD, N-monoacetyl PPD, and N,N'-diacetyl PPD

	PPD	N-monoacetyl PPD	N,N'-diacetyl PPD
Skin tape strippings (ng/g)	0.49	Not determined	Not determined
Plasma (ng/ml)	0.5	1.0	0.5
Urine (ng/ml)	1.28	1.0	10.0

Adapted from Nohynek et al. (2015).

protective caps where Hionic Fluor® was used. All analyses were duplicated except for plasma and skin tape strip samples. Limit of detection was defined as three times the standard deviation of a blank matrix. For plasma it was 4.0 (Study A) and 4.7 (Study B) ng PPD eq/ml and for urine, it was 4.9 (Study A) and 6.1 (Study B) ng PPDeq/mL. Lower limit of quantification for plasma was 13.3 (Study A) and 15.8 ng (Study B) PPDeq/ml and for urine 16.4 (Study A) and 20.3 (Study B) ng PPDeq/ml. GraphPad Prism® Version 4 Software was used to calculate the plasma kinetic parameters such as C_{max}, T_{max}, Ke, T1/2, and AUC.

As described by Nohynek et al. (17), methods used for the analysis of PPD, N-monoacetylated PPD, and N,N'- diacetylated PPD from plasma, urine, and tape strips and for the analysis of only PPD in plasma and tape strips was the stable-isotope dilutive-based gradient reversed-phase HPLC with tandem mass spectrometry (LC-MS/MS) Table 30.9.

In washing water, hair, and study materials, the recovery of [14C]-PPD is summarized in Table 30.10. Urine analysis results are summarized in Table 30.11.

TABLE 30.10

Recovery of Radioactivity in Study Materials of Study A and Study B

	Study A 2.0% [^{14}C]-PPD			Study B 1.0% [^{14}C]-PPD		
	Mean of 16 Study Subjects (% of Applied [^{14}C])	SD	Range	Mean of 16 Study Subjects (% of Applied [^{14}C])	SD	Range
First Day						
Scalp tape strippings	0.007	0.002	0.005–0.011	0.007	0.003	0.003–0.014
Cut Hair	31.74	4.72	25.77–43.36	30.25	4.58	19.92–36.12
Hair drying	0.174	0.097	0.084–0.46	0.21	0.10	0.11–0.43
Washing water	61.50	6.23	48.29–67.84	64.71	4.63	58.12–74.65
Second day						
Scalp Tape strippings	0.006	0.002	0.004–0.010	0.005	0.003	0.002–0.016
Protective cap	0.02	0.005	0.02–0.03	0.017	0.012	0.001–0.06
Scalp rinse	0.15	0.04	0.08–0.21	0.14	0.006	0.06–0.26
Total unabsorbed	93.58	3.03	89.46–99.25	95.33	1.51	92.31–97.78
Urine 0–48 hours	0.72	0.25	0.31–1.43	0.88	0.46	0.40–2.06
Total recovery	94.30	3.01	89.88–100.01	96.21	1.57	93.59–98.59

Adapted from Nohynek et al. (2015).

TABLE 30.11

Recovery of [^{14}C]-PPD$_{eq}$ in Urine

	Study A 2.0% [^{14}C]-PPD		Study B 2.0% [^{14}C]-PPD	
	mg PPD$_{eq}$ ± SD	Mean ± SD of 16 subjects (% of applied radioactivity)	mg PPD$_{eq}$ ± SD	Mean ± SD of 16 subjects (% of applied radioactivity)
Total	0.72 ± 0.25	8.62 ± 2.96	0.88 ± 0.46	5.77 ± 3.23
0–12 hours	0.49 ± 0.15	5.99 ± 2.07	0.61 ± 0.34	4.02 ± 2.38
12–24 hours	0.15 ± 0.008	1.81 ± 0.81	0.19 ± 0.09	1.22 ± 0.64
24–48 hours	0.07 ± 0.03	0.82 ± 0.39	0.08 ± 0.05	0.53 ± 0.31

Adapted from Nohynek et al. (2015).

Majority of urinary excretion of [14C] occurred within first 24 hours after hair dyeing. In the 24–48 hour interval, less than 10% of the total amount excreted was recovered. Urinary excretion up to 48 hours was 0.72 ± 0.25% (Study A) or 0.88 ± 0.46% (Study B) of the applied radioactivity. This comes to 8.62 ± 2.96 (Study A) or 5.77 ± 3.23 mg [14C]-PPDeq (Study B). 117 ± 45 (Study A) and 69.2 ± 34.8 μg PPDeq/kg body weight (Study B) were the calculated mean systemic exposures. These were calculated from the total amount of urinary excretion.

Principal plasma pharmokinetic parameters are summarized in Table 30.12. Study A produced somewhat higher values for C$_{max}$ and AUC compared to Study B. However, this was not proportional to the differing concentrations of PPD in the hair dye formulations or the amount applied to the hair. As seen in Table 30.12, the mean elimination half-lives (T1/2) were similar for Study A and Study B.

In regards to the radioactivity in the scalp, for Study A, on the first day, for the 10 successive strips taken, the highest radioactivity was in the first strip. The value calculated to estimate the entire scalp surface was 23.2 ± 9.0 μg [14C]-PPDeq. The mean radioactivity decreased in successive tape strips. The 10th strip was used to estimate 4.8 ± 3.0 μg [14C]-PPDeq for the entire scalp. The second day produced similar findings except lower mean quantities of [14C]-PPDeq were calculated from 15.5 ± 8.2 (first strips) to 3.8 ± 1.9 μg [14C]-PPDeq (last strips). Total amount of [14C]-PPDeq

TABLE 30.12

Pharmacokinetic Parameters of Plasma [^{14}C]-PPD$_{eq}$

Parameter	Study A 2.0% [^{14}C]-PPD			Study B 2.0% [^{14}C]-PPD		
	Mean of 16 Study Subjects	SD	Range	Mean of 16 Study Subjects	SD	Range
T$_{1/2}$ (h)	7.8	2.1	4.5 to 12.5	7.8	5.1	3.5 to 25.8
C$_{max}$ (ng PPD$_{eq}$/ml)	132.6	52.0	46.0 to 219.5	97.4	61.5	20.9 to 234.0
T$_{max}$ (h)	2.0	—	—	2.0	—	—
Ke (h^{-1})	−0.095	0.025	−0.153 to −0.055	−0.109	0.044	−0.201 to −0.027
AUC$_{0-24h}$ (ng PPD$_{eq}$/ml*hrs)	1169	485	441 to 2182	762	401	410 to 1727
AU$_{0-\infty}$ (ng PPD$_{eq}$/ml*hrs)	1415	592	554 to 2716	966	575	228 to 1946

Adapted from Nohynek et al. (2015).

from both days together was approximately 0.013% of the applied radioactivity. Therefore, total radioactivity in the upper layers of the entire scalp stratum corneum on both days together was calculated to be approximately 0.38% of the applied radioactivity.

For Study B, radioactivity was highest in the first tape strip on the first day (15.2 ± 9.0 µg [14C]-PPDeq estimate for the entire scalp); it decreased in successive tape strips and was 2.2 ± 1.3 µg [14C]-PPDcq for the entire scalp for the last tape strip. On the second day, for the first strip the calculated estimate for the entire scalp was 7.0 ± 5.0 µg [14C]-PPDeq. For the last strip the calculated estimate for the entire scalp was 1.4 ± 0.8 µg [14C]-PPDeq. Total radioactivity for both days removed by the tape strippings was 0.012% of applied radioactivity. The total amount of radioactivity for both days in the stratum corneum of the entire scalp was approximately 0.35% of the applied radioactivity.

Plasma analysis provided the following results. Plasma levels were below the LLOQ for PPD (<500 pg/ml) and N-monoacetyl-PPD (<1000 pg/ml) after the exposure to hair dye. For 2 to 48 hours N,N′-diacetyl-PPD was found in all plasma. N,N′-diacetyl-PPD had a C_{max} of 118.2 ± 92.0 ng/ml at 2.50 ± 1.15 hours after beginning of hair dyeing and a $AUC0-\infty$ of 1170 ± 755 ng*hour/ml.

Urine analysis in Study B provided the following results which are shown in Table 30.13. There was trace levels of PPD (1.6–29.5 ng/ml) with a mean value of 6.91 ± 8.86 ng/ml in 9 out of 16 urine samples in the 0–12 hour collection. 2265 ± 1283 ng/mL was the highest concentration of N,N′-diacetyl-PPD and was found in the 0–12 hour samples, this was the main urinary metabolite. In the following 12–48 hour period the concentrations of N,N′-diacetyl-PPD were lower at 578.5 ± 348.8 ng/ml. In the 24–48 hour period it was 96.81 ± 83.86 ng/mL. Fourteen out of 16 subjects showed trace quantities of N-monoacetyl-PPD in the 0–12 hour period and 2 of 16 subjects showed trace quantities in the 12–24 hour period.

Tape strips were analyzed by for the presence of PPD in study B only. PPD was found in all tape strips on both days. First days mean values, after shaving, ranged from 684 ± 133 ng for the first strip to 77 ± 56 ng for the tenth strip for the entire scalp. For the second day, PPD values were lower and ranged from a value of 157 ng for the first strip to 52 ng for the tenth strip.

It is suggested that the recovery of the radioactivity applied was excellent based on the [14C]-based mass balance for studies A and B. For study A, it was 94.30 ± 3.01 with a range of 89.88–100.01, and for study B, it was $96.21 \pm 1.57\%$ with a range 93.59–98.59%. The dyed hair contained 30–32% of the applied radioactivity, while 62–65% was found in the washing water – of both studies. Mean urinary excretion of radioactivity was 0.72 ± 0.25 in Study A and $0.88 \pm 0.46\%$

TABLE 30.13
Urinary Concentrations in Study B of PPD, N,N′-diacetyl PPD and N-monoacetyl PPD

	PPD (ng/mL) Mean ± SD	N,N′-diacetyl PPD Mean ± SD	N-monoacetyl PPD Mean ± SD
Blank	<1.28	25.84 ± 9.86**	<1.0
0–12 hours	6.91 ± 8.86*	2265 ± 1283	3.50 ± 2.04†
12–24 hours	<1.28	578.5 ± 348.8	1.19 ± 0.06††
24–48 hours	<1.28	96.81 ± 83.86	<1.0

Adapted from Nohynek et al. (2015).

*calculated from 9/16 subjects.

**calculated from 8/16 subjects.

† calculated from 14/16 subjects.

†† calculated from 2/16 subjects.

in Study B. These values matched to a total absorbed dose of 8.62 ± 2.96 mg in Study A and 5.77 ± 3.23 mg [14C]-PPDeq in Study B.

Although mean plasma AUC and Cmax for [14C]-PPDeq values in Study A vs Study B were increased, this increase was not proportional to the concentrations of PPD applied. In both studies, human systemic exposure was mainly limited to 24 hours after hair dye exposure, then levels dropped to baseline

In study B, only N,N'-diacetyl-PPD was found in plasma. Complete first-pass metabolism in the skin by NAT1 may explain the lack of plasma unmetabolized PPD or N-monoacetylated PPD. N,N'-diacetyl-PPD was in the urine at 500 to 1000 more times concentration than of N-monoacetyl-PPD or PPD. Traces of N-monoacetyl-PPD or PPD were found in a few samples.

The results of this study suggest that there is human systemic exposure to low levels of N,N'-diacetyl-PPD with the use of oxidative hair dye products containing up to 2.0% PPD.

30.4   DISCUSSION AND STUDY LIMITATIONS

The study by Wolfram and Maibach investigates percutaneous absorption of hair dyes by quantifying absorption on the basis of the percentage of radioactivity excreted in the urine. This study assumes that all hair dye applied and absorbed will be excreted. However, there was no excretion control used. The excretion control compares excretion of substances by dermally applied hair dye versus excretion by intravenous, intraperitoneal, or intramuscular injection of hair dye substances (11). Without the excretion control, excretion, and therefore absorption, cannot be accurately measured. Also, radioactivity of washing water and materials was not measured to obtain all hair dye used. Further, distribution of hair dye in the body and metabolism of hair dye respectively were not investigated by Wolfram and Maibach. Another consideration is the amount of hair in the location of hair dye application. With more hair, it is expected that more will be absorbed by the hair and thus less may be bioavailable for the body. For example, the greater density of hair on the scalp would lead to decreased bioavailability compared to the forearm. Thus, conclusions made from the data obtained by applying hair dye to the forearm may not be applicable to hair dye applied to the scalp.

Nohynek et al. (2004) investigated metabolites excreted in urine (13). The study comments on systemic absorption of hair dyes based on metabolite radioactivity in urine excretion. Absorption of hair dye in the dermis was not measured, and it was assumed that the applied hair dye will be systemically absorbed, metabolized, and excreted. However, the distribution of hair dye was not investigated, thus it cannot be concluded that all of the hair dye was metabolized into all possible metabolites which in turn were excreted. Also, there was no excretion control. Another limitation in this study is that the authors did not comment on the density and length of participant hair. The same amount of hair dye was used for each participant; however, some participants may have had less or more bioavailability due to density and length of hair on the scalp.

The abstract by Skare and Nohynek et al. (15) comments on metabolism, absorption, and excretion of dyes. Distribution was not discussed.

Gube et al. (2011) measured active constituents of permanent hair dyes in urine to determine internal exposure of hairdressers to aromatic diamines. However, absorption was not directly measured. Furthermore, neither metabolism nor distribution was measured and there was no excretion control.

Finally, Nohynek et al. (2015) (17) measured systemic exposure in humans after dyeing hair with oxidative hair dyes investigating absorption, plasma kinetics, metabolism, and excretion of oxidative hair dyes in humans. Hair length and density for each participant was considered when applying amount of hair dye. The determination of radioactivity in hair washes, scalp rinsing water, materials, and caps thoroughly obtained all hair dye material involved. Tape strippings were taken from scalp for comparison with the forearm in the study by Wolfram and Maibach. However, since the tape strippings were taken from the scalp, this may have potentially decreased the systemic absorption and metabolism data from hair dye on the scalp. Also, the study did not measure distribution of hair dye in the body and no excretion control was completed.

Taken together, much has been learned about the percutaneous penetration of a few hair dye chemicals, as summarized in this chapter. Much remains to be learned about the penetration of the additionally commercially available over 200 hair dyes. A major void exists in data confirming or denying the completeness of excretion once absorbed.

REFERENCES

1. Frenkel EP, Brody F. Percutaneous absorption and elimination of an aromatic hair dye. Arch Envir Health 1973; 27:401–404.
2. Howes D, Black JG. Percutaneous penetration of 2-nitro-p-phenylenediamine. Int J Cosmet Sci 1983; 5:215–226.
3. Hruby E. The absorption of p-toluenediamine by the skin of rats and dogs. Cosmet Toxicol 1977; 15:595–599.
4. Hruby E. Cutaneous resorption of 2,4-diaminoanisole in the rat and dog. SGAE Report AOO37, March 1979.
5. Nakao M, Takeda Y. Body distribution, excretion and metabolism of p-phenylenediamine in rats. J Pharm Soc Japan 1979; 99:1149–1153.
6. Tsomi V, Kalopissis G. Cutaneous penetration of some hair dyes in the hairless rat. Tox-icol Eur Res 1982; 4:119–127.
7. Kiese M, Rauscher M. The absorption of p-toluenediamine through human skin in hair dyeing. Toxicol Appl Pharmacol 1968; 13:325–331.
8. Maibach HI, Leaffer MA, Skinner WA. Percutaneous penetration following use of hair dyes. Arch Dermatol 1975; 111:1444–1445.
9. Wester RC, Noonan P, Maibach HI. Recent advances in percutaneous absorption using the rhesus monkey model. J Soc Cosmet Chem 1979; 30:297–307.
10. Maibach HI, Wolfram LJ. Percutaneous penetration of hair dyes. J Soc Cosmet Chem 1981; 32:223–229.
11. Feldmann RJ, Maibach HI. Absorption of some organic compounds through the skin of man. J Invest Dermatol 1970; 54:399–404.
12. Bartek MJ, LaBudde JA. Animal models in dermatology: relevance to human dermatopharmacology and dermatotoxicology. In: Maibach HI, ed. London: Churchill-Livingstone, 1975:103–120.
13. Nohynek GJ, Skare JA Meuling WJA, Hein, DW, de Bie AThHJ, Toutain H. Urinary acetylated metabolites and N-acetyltransferase-2 genotype in human subjects treated with a para-phenylenediamine-containing oxidative hair dye. Food Chem Toxicol 2004; 42:1885–1891
14. Goetz N, Masserre P, Bore P, Kalopissis G. Percutaneous absorption of p-phenylenediamine during an actual hair dyeing process. J Cosmet Sci 1988; 10:63–73.
15. Skare J, Nohynek G, Powrie R, Goebel C, Pfuhler S, Duche D, Zeller A, Aardema M, Hu T, Meuling WJA. Metabolism of oxidative hair dyes: An overview of in vitro, in vivo, and clinical studies. Abstracts/Toxicol Lett 2007; 172:S1–S240.
16. Gube M, Heinrich K, Dewes P, Brand P, Kraus T, Schettgen T. Internal exposure of hairdressers to permanent hair dyes: a biomonitoring study using urinary aromatic diamines as biomarkers of exposure. Int Arch Occup Environ Health 2011; 84:287–292.
17. Nohynek GJ, Skare JA, Meuling W, Wehmeyer KR, Bie A, Vaes W, Dufour EK, Fautz R, Steiling W, Bramante M, Toutain H. Human systemic exposure to [14C]-paraphenylenediamine-containing oxidative hair dyes: Absorption, kinetics, metabolism, excretion and safety assessment. Food Chem Toxicol 2015; 81:71–80.

31 Percutaneous Absorption of Sunscreens

Heather A.E. Benson
Curtin University, Perth, Western Australia

Yousuf H. Mohammed
University of Queensland, Woolloongabba, Queensland

Kenneth A. Walters
An-Ex Analytical Services Ltd, Capital Business Park, Cardiff, Wales

Michael S. Roberts
University of Queensland, Woolloongabba, Queensland
University of South Australia, Adelaide, South Australia

CONTENTS

31.1 INTRODUCTION

Repeated long-term exposure to ultraviolet radiation causes skin aging and increased risk of skin cancer, whereas acute exposure can cause sunburn and significant discomfort. Strategies that have been demonstrated to protect the skin, including the regular use of efficient sunscreens [1–3], are heavily promoted by cancer prevention organizations and can provide better health outcomes for individuals and cost savings for health care systems [4, 5]. Consequently, sunscreen actives are present in many cosmetic and personal care products (moisturizers, lipsticks, hair conditioners), as well as "beach sunscreen" products (creams, lotions, foams, gels, sprays, sticks). In all cases the advice is to apply liberally, well before expected sun exposure.

Sunscreens are used to protect against solar ultraviolet radiation (UVR), with the first commercial sunscreen introduced by Eugène Schueller, the founder of L'Oréal, in 1936. Franz Greiter introduced the first specialized sunscreen product, called *Gletscher Crème* (Glacier Cream), in 1946, and formed the sunscreen manufacturing and marketing company Piz Buin, named in honor of the Alpine mountain where he received the sunburn that inspired his invention [6]. In 1962, Greiter introduced the "sun protection factor" (SPF), which became a worldwide standard for measuring the effectiveness of sunscreens.

Sunscreens with broad-spectrum UVA and UVB protection are now widely available. These include two inorganic (physical) sunscreen actives (zinc oxide and titanium dioxide) and a larger number of organic (chemical) sunscreen actives. The U.S. Food and Drug Administration (FDA) defines a sunscreen active ingredient as one that "absorbs, reflects, or scatters radiation in the ultraviolet range at wavelengths of 290–400 nm." Inorganic sunscreens reflect and scatter UVR to provide broad-spectrum protection. Most organic sunscreen actives absorb in the UVB spectrum (280 to 315 nm), though some absorb in both the UVA (315 to 400 nm) and UVB range. Examples of commonly used organic sunscreen actives approved for products throughout the world are shown in Table 31.1 [7]. The sunscreens approved for consumer use vary widely between countries, as shown in Table 31.1.

In recent years there have been two major developments that could greatly influence the commercial sunscreen market. First, environmental concerns have been raised about the prevalence of organic sunscreen actives in marine environments and their detrimental effects on marine ecology [8, 9]. Organic sunscreens enter the waterways by multiple mechanisms: (1) absorption via the skin and excretion in the urine, thus reaching wastewater treatment plants; (2) washed off the skin into shower or bath water, again reaching wastewater treatment plants; (3) waste runoff from factories manufacturing sunscreens, cosmetics, and personal care products; and (4) washed off the skin at recreational water sites. Wastewater treatment plants process wastewater prior to release to waterways, but these tend to be geared towards removal of particulate matter, and multiple studies in many countries have shown that organic sunscreens, including benzophenone-3 (oxybenzone), 4-methylbenzylidene, octinoxate, and octocrylene, are present in treated water [10, 11]. Of particular concern is the effect of sunscreens on coral reefs, with sunscreen being implicated in coral bleaching [12]. Of course, sunscreens are not the only environmental threat to the world's coral reefs, with ocean temperature increase the greatest threat, but pollutants are certainly adding to their global endangerment. Indeed, in May 2018 a law was passed in Hawaii to ban the sale or distribution of sunscreen products containing oxybenzone and octinoxate, starting in January 2021 [13]. This is highly controversial [14], and it is unclear if other jurisdictions will follow. Schneider and Lim provide an excellent review on the environmental effects of sunscreen active ingredients [15].

Second, a recent FDA *Federal Register* report expressed concerns about the potential misbranding of 16 currently marketed sunscreens and recommended that 12 of the organic sunscreen actives undergo further safety and efficacy testing. As of February 2019, the FDA classified only the two inorganic sunscreen actives, zinc oxide and titanium dioxide, as generally recognized as safe and effective (GRASE) [16]. The FDA also provides guidance as to how sunscreen products should be tested. Their November 2016 guidance titled "Guidance for Industry: Nonprescription Sunscreen Drug Products Safety and Effectiveness Data" [17] recommends an assessment of the human systemic absorption of sunscreen ingredients with a maximal usage trial [18] and a nonclinical safety assessment, including dermal carcinogenicity and embryofetal toxicity. They noted that some nonclinical toxicology studies may be waived based on favorable results of an adequately conducted human pharmacokinetic maximal usage trial that shows a steady-state blood level less than 0.5 ng/mL and no evidence of potential safety concerns during the trial.

TABLE 31.1
Organic Sunscreen Chemicals in Use Worldwide as of 2019

INCI Name	Soluble In	Chemical Structure	UVA or UVB	Max Wavelength	Max Permitted Levels %				
					EU	USA	Canada	Australia	Japan
Bis-ethylhexyloxyphenol methoxyphenyl triazine	Oil		UVA/UVB	341 nm	10	---	---	10	10
Butyl methoxydibenzoyl-methane	Oil		UVA	355 nm	5	3	3	5	10
Diethylamino hydroxy-benzoyl hexyl benzoate	Oil		UVA	354 nm	10	---	---	10	10
4-Methylbenzylidene camphor	Oil		UVB	303 nm	4	---	---	4	---
Benzophenone-3 (oxybenzone)	Oil		UVB/UVA	287 nm	10	.6	6	10	5

(Continued)

TABLE 31.1 (*Continued*)
Organic Sunscreen Chemicals in Use Worldwide as of 2019

INCI Name	Soluble In	Chemical Structure	UVA or UVB	Max Wavelength	Max Permitted Levels %				
					EU	USA	Canada	Australia	Japan
Benzophenone-4	Water		UVB/UVA	285 nm	5	10	10	10	10
Diethylhexyl butamido triazone	Oil		UVB	311 nm	10	---	---	---	---
Ethylhexyl methoxycinnamate	Oil		UVB	310 nm	10	7.5	7.5	10	20

Ethylhexyl salicylate	Oil		UVB	306 nm	5	5	5	5	10
Ethylhexyl triazone	Oil		UVB	312 nm	5	---	---	---	3
Octocrylene	Oil		UVB	302 nm	10	10	10	10	10
Phenylbenzimidazole sulfonic acid	Water (salt form)		UVB	307 nm	8	4	4	4	3

Source: Adapted from Reference 7.

31.2   SKIN PERMEATION OF ORGANIC SUNSCREENS

31.2.1   DATA FROM *IN VIVO* HUMAN STUDIES

Benzophenone-3 (oxybenzone) is a UVA/B sunscreen that is widely available for use in sunscreen products (Table 31.1). Following the topical application of a commercial sunscreen to the trunk and back of human volunteers, Hayden et al. [19] found between 1% and 2% of the applied benzophenone-3 was absorbed and excreted in the urine over the 12 hours after administration. Gustavsson Gonzalez et al. [20] reported approximately 0.4% of applied benzophenone-3 excreted in the urine over 48 hours following application of a commercial sunscreen lotion containing 4% benzophenone-3 to the whole body (except scalp and genital regions) of 11 human volunteers. In a subsequent study, this group investigated the total amount of benzophenone-3 excreted in the urine of 25 volunteers after repeated topical whole-body applications of the sunscreen product (morning and night for 5 days), and the effect of UV radiation [21]. The volunteers excreted 1.2% to 8.7% (mean 3.7%) of the total amount of benzophenone-3 applied during the 5-day application period and the 5 days following cessation. Benzophenone-3 metabolites were detected in the urine up to 5 days following sunscreen exposure. There was no significant difference between the group that received UV radiation and the unexposed group ($P < 0.99$, t-test).

The skin absorption and urinary excretion of benzophenone-3 are now sufficiently well established, such that Zamoiski et al. [22] used measurement of urinary excretion as a means of assessing the validity of self-reported frequency of sunscreen use in a representative sample of the general U.S. population, including in subgroups defined by age, sex, and race/ethnicity. They concluded that urinary benzophenone-3 levels measured by high-performance liquid chromatography (HPLC) were positively associated with self-reported frequency of sunscreen use in the general U.S. population, even in groups with overall low sunscreen use. There were some interesting trends in the use of sunscreens. First, across all the race/ethnic groups, men were more likely to report "never" using sunscreen, and women were more likely to report using sunscreen "most of the time" or "always." Second, there were no statistically significant differences in sunscreen use within each racial and ethnic group, within each sex, and within each age group. Third, with the exception of non-Hispanic white females, all ethnic groups and sexes were more likely to report "never" using sunscreen than "always." Given the extensive public health campaigns to raise awareness of the damaging effects of sun exposure to the skin, including skin cancer, and the promotion of sunscreens as part of a sun protection routine, this is a concerning trend. A fourth interesting trend reported was the statistically significant interaction between frequency of sunscreen use and age, with greater association in older participants.

Most sunscreen products contain multiple sunscreen actives to achieve a broad UV spectrum of activity. Treffel and Gabard [23] examined the permeation of benzophenone-3, 2-ethylhexyl-4-methoxycinnamate, and 2-ethylhexyl salicylate (octyl salicylate) from a commercial oil-in-water emulsion gel vehicle and petroleum jelly through human skin both *in vivo* and *in vitro*. Sunscreen formulations were applied to the skin surface at recommended topical application rates (2 mg/cm^2), and samples were taken at intervals up to a maximum exposure of six hours. For the *in vivo* study, tape stripping was applied to the site of application on the back at 0.5, 2, and 6 hours following application. Although there were no statistically significant differences in the amount of individual sunscreen agents in the stratum corneum tape strips following 0.5-hour exposure, there was a significant vehicle effect with higher amounts of all sunscreen agents recovered following administration of the emulsion gel compared to the petroleum jelly. This trend was confirmed in the *in vitro* study, where epidermal levels of the sunscreen agents were higher following application in the emulsion gel. It should be noted that with the exception of benzophenone-3, the levels in the dermis and receptor fluid were below the level of quantification. When applied in petroleum jelly, approximately 5% of the applied dose of benzophenone-3 permeated through human skin within six hours.

Using similar methods, they then compared the skin penetration *in vitro* and *in vivo* of five organic sunscreen actives (benzophenone-3, ethylhexyl methoxycinnamate, butyl methoxydibenzoyl methane, ethylhexyl salicylate, and homosalate) from the two vehicles (oil-in-water emulsion gel and petrolatum jelly), as well as the corresponding SPF *in vivo* [24]. Of the five sunscreens, only benzophenone-3 and ethylhexyl methoxycinnamate were found in the dermis at 30 minutes and 6 hours after application *in vitro*. *In vivo* there were no differences in the amount of individual sunscreen actives (as a percentage of the applied dose) in the stratum corneum tape strips taken 30 minutes after application of the formulations; however, the amount of all sunscreens present in the stratum corneum was significantly higher (around three times) with the emulsion gel than the petrolatum jelly vehicle. This correlated with the difference in the SPF measured *in vivo* at 30 minutes after product application (SPF 18 with the emulsion gel compared to SPF 10 with the petrolatum jelly). This study demonstrated that the choice of vehicle can assist in targeting the sunscreen actives to the stratum corneum, thereby minimizing unnecessary deeper skin permeation and optimizing sunscreen efficacy.

We evaluated commercial sunscreen products marketed for application to children and adults applied to human skin and showed that although the more lipophilic sunscreen actives penetrate the stratum corneum, they do not tend to permeate through into the viable epidermis [25] and therefore may eventually be lost by desquamation rather than eventually reaching deeper tissues or the systemic circulation. In contrast, the more polar benzophenone-3 is less tightly bound by the stratum corneum and can therefore permeate further [25], resulting in systemic absorption and urinary excretion, as seen in the *in vivo* human studies described earlier. These observations are pertinent to the interpretation of the data of Hagerdorn-Leweke and Lippold [26], who determined the human skin permeation of several sunscreen actives *in vivo*. Each active [octyl dimethyl PABA, 4-isopropyl-dibenzoylmethane, 3-(4-methyl-benzylidine), isoamyl-4-methoxycinnamate, and camphor and benzophenone-3] was applied as a saturated solution in 30% propylene glycol–water to the skin of the upper arm using glass chambers. Reduction of the permeant in the donor vehicle was assessed hourly for six hours. The calculated maximum flux ranged from 0.53 µg/cm^2/hour for octyl dimethyl PABA (log $P_{o/w}$ 5.75) to 4.93 µg/cm^2/hour for isoamyl-4-methoxycinnamate (log $P_{o/w}$ 4.83). There was a correlation between log P values and skin flux such that maximum flux decreased with increasing lipophilicity. These data were then used to estimate the amount of absorption of a saturated solution following total body exposure (surface area 1.8m^2) for one hour. It should be noted that these estimates were made using data obtained from repetitive infinite doses of sunscreen actives at maximum thermodynamic activity and under fully occluded conditions. These conditions constitute an unlikely scenario during actual consumer use of sunscreen products and are therefore of limited value in safety assessment.

Benech-Kieffer et al. [27] evaluated the systemic absorption of one of the more recently introduced UVA sunscreen actives, Mexoryl SX (terephthalylidine dicamphor sulphonic acid), following application to human skin in an emulsion formulation for 4 hours and reported a urine recovery of 0.014% of the topically applied dose. The corresponding *in vitro* absorption over a period of 24 hours after an application of 4 hours to excised human skin was 0.16% of the applied dose. In both sets of experiments most of the Mexoryl SX was recovered from washing the skin surface at completion of the 4-hour application period. The authors concluded that "under realistic exposure conditions, the human systemic exposure to this UVA filter is negligible and poses no risk to human health." In their review, D'Souza et al. [28] concluded that Mexoryl provides efficient UVA coverage, better photostability, and enhanced water resistance compared to older UVA sunscreens such as avobenzone (Parsol 1789).

In summary, data repeatedly show that of the sunscreen actives, benzophenone-3 exhibits the greatest skin absorption. This reflects the physicochemical properties of the organic sunscreen actives, with benzophenone-3 having a molecular weight and partition coefficient (MW 228 g/mol and XlogP 3.6) that are favorable for skin permeation. Other organic sunscreens are more lipophilic in nature; therefore, although they will readily absorb into the lipid domains of the stratum corneum, partitioning to the deeper skin tissues is more thermodynamically challenging.

Matta et al. [29] followed the FDA guidance documents [17, 18] in the design of their recently published clinical trial. They conducted a randomized clinical trial, applying 1 of 4 sunscreen products (two sprays, a lotion and a cream) to 24 healthy volunteers ($n = 6$) at a rate of 2 mg/cm^2 to 75% of their body surface area four times per day for 4 days. Blood samples were collected and analyzed for the sunscreens avobenzone, oxybenzone, octocrylene, and ecamsule. Systemic concentrations greater than 0.5 ng/mL were exceeded for all sunscreens, with mean maximum plasma concentrations ranging from approximately 170 to 210 ng/mL for oxybenzone and 2 to 8 ng/mL for the other sunscreens. The authors noted that one participant per sunscreen also reported an adverse event, commonly rash. The FDA's 2016 guidance for the assessment of nonprescription sunscreen drug products [17] states that sunscreen active ingredients with systemic absorption greater than 0.5 ng/mL or with safety concerns need further nonclinical toxicology assessment, including systemic carcinogenicity. The important outcome from this study was that all sunscreens tested under the FDA's maximal usage trial guidance [18] exceeded the 0.5 ng/mL plasma concentration threshold. Although the authors suggested the need for further studies to determine the clinical significance of their results, they clearly stated that their study does not indicate that individuals should stop using topical sunscreen products [29].

31.2.2   DATA FROM *IN VITRO* HUMAN SKIN STUDIES

Data from *in vitro* human skin studies should be interpreted carefully. Appropriate protocol design is critical for the accurate estimation of human skin permeation. In particular, when assessing highly lipophilic compounds, the choice of receptor conditions may greatly affect the observed extent of absorption. Infinite dosing is useful to assess formulation effects, but finite application better reflects *in-use* conditions. Similarly, the composition of the formulation vehicle may also significantly affect penetration, with applications in acetone or alcoholic vehicles not reflecting typical sunscreen product vehicles. For example, the *in vitro* skin penetration of padimate O (octyldimethyl p-aminobenzoate) from an alcoholic formulation was fourfold greater than from a lotion, most likely due to evaporation of the volatile components of the vehicle [30]. However, there is a considerable body of valuable *in vitro*–based experimental data that evaluates the effect of formulation vehicle on sunscreen active skin permeation.

Lazar et al. [31] evaluated the *in vitro* human skin permeation of octyl methoxycinnamate and butyl methoxydibenzoylmethane from a series of five emulsion vehicles (a conventional oil-in-water emulsion, an emulsifier-free oil-in-water preparation, a water-in-oil emulsion, a water-in-silicone emulsion, and an oil-in-water emulsion with lamellar liquid crystals). No sunscreen active was found in receptor solutions following 8-hour exposure to 2% butyl methoxy dibenzoylmethane irrespective of the application vehicle. However, when 8% octyl methoxycinnamate was applied, this sunscreen active was detected at varying amounts depending upon the vehicle: emulsifier-free oil-in-water preparation > oil-in-water emulsion containing lamellar liquid crystals > water-in-silicone formulation.

Sunscreen products are typically formulated to provide high skin substantivity (i.e., the sunscreen active is delivered preferentially to the skin surface, where it remains in or on the upper layers of the stratum corneum and resists washing off by sweat or bathing activities typical of common exposures for sunscreen products). It is therefore important that *in vitro* experiments are designed to assess both permeation through the skin and penetration into/retention in the skin over the time course of topical application.

Jiang et al. [25] evaluated the *in vitro* human skin penetration of sunscreen actives (benzophenone-3, octocrylene, octyl salicylate, octyl methoxycinnamate, and butyl methoxydibenzoylmethane) following application of a finite dose (2.0 to 2.5 mg formulation/cm^2) of commercial products marketed for use by either adults or children. Heat-separated human epidermal membranes (comprising stratum corneum and viable epidermis) were mounted in Franz-type diffusion cells, with 4% bovine serum albumin in phosphate buffered saline used as the receptor phase to ensure sink conditions of all actives. Only benzophenone-3 was detectable in the receptor phase, with approximately 10% of the applied dose permeated over the 8 hour application period. There was no significant difference in the penetration of benzophenone-3 through the skin for products marketed for adult or child use. Significant amounts (5 to 25 μg/cm²; 3% to 14% of the applied dose) of each of the sunscreen actives were recovered from the epidermal membranes at 8 hours.

Walters et al. [32] examined the *in vitro* human skin permeation of octyl salicylate from two vehicles deemed to be representative of commercial sunscreen products: an oil-in-water emulsion and a hydro-alcoholic lotion. Heat-separated human epidermal membranes were mounted in Franz-type diffusion cells, and the receptor phase consisted of phosphate buffered saline (pH 7.4) containing 6% Volpo N20 (polyoxyethylene-20-oleyl ether) to enhance solubility of the relatively lipophilic sunscreen active (logP 4.86). Permeation of 14C-labeled octyl salicylate to the receptor over 48 hours following administration of a finite dose (5 mg formulation/cm²) of each formulation was similar and less than 1% of the applied dose. The amount of applied octyl salicylate remaining in the epidermal membranes at 48 hours was slightly higher for the hydro-alcoholic lotion (32.8%) than the oil-in-water emulsion (17.2%). It should be noted that the surface rinsing procedure used here was not particularly rigorous, so this may not reflect a typical *in-use* scenario, particularly one involving extensive sweating or bathing.

Further confirmation of this pattern of skin permeation and penetration was provided by Potard et al. [33] who assessed an oil-in-water emulsion containing octyl methoxycinnamate, benzophenone-4, benzophenone-3, octyl triazone, and octocrylene. Only benzophenone-3 permeated across the skin to any extent, while greater than 94% of the applied sunscreen active was recovered in the first eight tape strips taken at 0.5 and 16 hours, with the amount recovered in the following order: octocrylene and octyl methoxycinnamate > octyl triazone and benzophenone-3 > benzophenone-4.

Cross et al. [34] demonstrated the importance of applying the sunscreen formulation under *in-use* conditions, in particular dosing at realistic amounts. The general advice for sunscreen application is that the product should be applied liberally and at least 20 minutes before sun exposure. The guideline for risk assessment for a UV sunscreen active in the European Union is based on the topical application of an amount of 2 mg formulation/cm² [33]. What Cross et al. [34] demonstrated is that a sunscreen product may perform quite differently, and changes to a sunscreen product formulation affect sunscreen active penetration differently under infinite and finite dosing protocols. They prepared oil-in-water emulsions of varied viscosity, each containing 2% w/w benzophenone-3, and applied to human skin mounted in Franz-type diffusion cells at *in-use* finite (3 to 4 mg/cm²) and infinite (1 mL/cm²) doses. Increasing the viscosity of the vehicle decreased benzophenone-3 penetration fluxes under infinite dosing conditions, whereas fluxes following finite dosing increased with higher viscosity. They suggested that the reduced penetration in the infinite dosing case reflects a diminished diffusivity of the sunscreen in the vehicle. In contrast, a high-viscosity product under *in-use* conditions promoted sunscreen penetration by greater hydration of the stratum corneum relative to the lower-viscosity vehicles. The results emphasized the need to conduct skin permeation studies under *in-use* conditions, not only for risk assessment, but also in product development.

31.2.3 ADVANCED FORMULATION TECHNOLOGIES FOR ORGANIC SUNSCREEN ACTIVES

Given the concern about potential skin penetration and toxicity of organic sunscreen actives, there have been a number of studies investigating formulation methods to reduce skin penetration and increase efficacy of topically applied sunscreens.

Advanced strategies have been investigated, including complexation and encapsulation of sunscreen actives within various polymer and lipid materials. Scalia's group at the University of Ferrara have published extensively on their investigations of complexation of a range of sunscreen actives with cyclodextrins, encapsulation into lipid nanoparticles and microparticles, and combining these techniques [35–59]. For example, they complexed butyl methoxybibenzoylmethane with hydroxypropyl-β-cyclodextrin (HP-β-CD) and loaded in lipid microparticles composed of tristearin with hydrogenated phosphatidylcholine as the surfactant [38]. Nonencapsulated butyl methoxybibenzoylmethane, its complex with HP-β-CD, the lipid microparticles loaded with sunscreen alone, or the sunscreen/HP-β-CD complex were introduced into oil-in-water emulsions applied to human volunteers and the skin permeation monitored by tape stripping followed by HPLC analysis. The amount of butyl methoxybibenzoylmethane in the stratum corneum was increased by the formulations containing the sunscreen/HP-β-CD complex and the microparticles loaded with butyl methoxybibenzoylmethane only (17.1 ± 3.2% and 15.1 ± 2.7% of the applied dose penetrated, respectively) compared to the sunscreen in emulsion (9.7 ± 2.5%). A significant decrease in butyl methoxybibenzoylmethane penetrated into the stratum corneum when applied as the microencapsulated sunscreen/HP-β-CD complex (6.0% ± 1.5%). Encapsulation in lipid and polymer-based nanoparticles has been shown to effectively increase the efficacy and improve the photostability of a range of common sunscreen actives [36, 60–63].

31.3 SKIN PERMEATION OF NANOPARTICULATE INORGANIC SUNSCREENS

Concern about the environmental impact of organic UV filters has further emphasized the need for alternative forms of photoprotection, and currently the best option is to recommend physical blockers as safe and effective photoprotection alternatives. For many years there was consumer reluctance to apply opaque sunscreens containing micronized forms of zinc oxide and titanium dioxide due to their unappealing appearance. This has been overcome by the development of transparent nanoparticle inorganic sunscreen aggregates, but has created its own problems, as a number of consumer advocate groups have suggested that these nanoparticle actives may not be safe [64]. This has led to a systematic examination of the skin permeation of nanoparticulate sunscreens that is summarized later. Figure 31.1 illustrates the aggregated nature of ZnO nanoparticles in a commercially available ZnO sunscreen product.

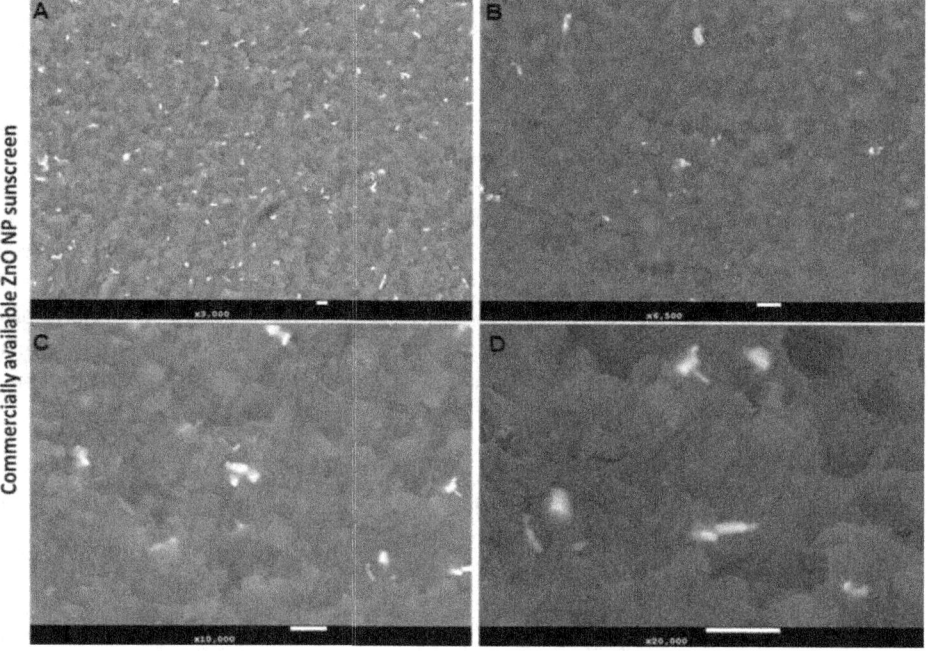

FIGURE 31.1 Characterization and distribution of coated ZnO nanoparticles within a commercial sunscreen formulation. (A–D) Representative CryoSEM images of coated ZnO nanoparticles over four magnifications in "over the counter" zinc sunscreen products. All scale bar 1 μm.

31.3.1 Data from Human Studies: Skin Permeation and Potential Toxicity

The safety of nanoparticle-based sunscreens has been a controversial issue due to studies in animals and humans that have reported elevated skin absorption of zinc following topical application of ZnO nanoparticle sunscreens [65]. For example, Gulson el al. [66, 67] reported small but significantly elevated zinc levels in the blood and urine following repeated applications of sunscreens containing ZnO nanoparticles that were more than 99% enriched with the stable isotope ^{68}Zn to the backs of human volunteers. Zn detection was by acid digestion followed by inductively coupled plasma mass spectrometry (ICP-MS); thus, it was not possible to determine if the Zn present in the blood and urine had been absorbed across the skin in a particulate or a soluble form. It should be noted that as this was conducted as a beach study, there was the likelihood of absorption of Zn ions due to their solubility in sweat.

Over recent years we have reported a series of studies that have systematically examined nanoparticle sunscreen penetration into human skin and the impact of a range of application procedures and lifestyle activities, including flexing and massage [68], occlusion and barrier impairment [69], and swimming [70]. We have consistently shown minimal skin penetration and a lack of cellular toxicity following application of zinc oxide nanoparticles (ZnO-NPs) to human volunteers. Key to these studies was the use of multiphoton tomography with fluorescence lifetime imaging microscopy (MPT-FLIM). This technology allows real-time imaging of ZnO nanoparticles throughout the epidermis of human volunteers following topical application to the skin surface [71]. In addition, it allows monitoring of metabolic changes in the skin tissues, thus identifying any potential toxic effects of penetrating substances. Nicotinamide adenine dinucleotide (NADH), NADH phosphate (NADPH), and flavine adenine dinucleotide (FAD) are the major autofluorescent metabolic species in human skin. NADH and NADPH share overlapping absorption, fluorescence, and lifetime properties and are therefore collectively referred to as NAD(P)H. They provide different measures of the oxidation state of a cell, altering in intensity with changes in the presence of oxygen. Changes in NAD(P)H and FAD intensities and fluorescence lifetimes are therefore linked to alterations in the cellular redox state [25] and can be monitored as a surrogate of metabolic change and thus toxic effects within the skin following topical administration and subsequent skin permeation. Figure 31.2 illustrates pseudo-colored images of human volunteer skin treated with uncoated (2A) and coated (2B) ZnO nanoparticles applied after pretreatment of the skin in four different ways [70]. In this case the skin was left dry or treated with water of a range of origins for 1 hour, simulating bathing activities in which sunscreens are commonly used. The nanoparticles can be clearly seen localized at the skin surface and concentrated at the skin furrows. The average NAD(P)H lifetime τm (ps) and the average metabolic ratio $\alpha 1/\alpha 2$ (au) for all treatment groups are plotted in Figure 31.2(C-F). Our imaging and analysis demonstrate how cellular indicators can be valuable to provide toxicological analysis based on comparison of skin post nanoparticle treatment.

We examined the effect of formulation, in particular coated and uncoated ZnO nanoparticles, applied to volunteer skin in a range of vehicles for up to 4 hours [72]. MPT-FLIM showed that the nanoparticles were localized predominantly within the stratum corneum and the skin furrows, with very limited penetration into the viable epidermis adjacent to the furrows. Significantly increased penetration compared to controls was detected only for the coated ZnO nanoparticles applied in a water-in-oil emulsion, but none of the formulations altered the redox state of the viable epidermis. The concentration of coated ZnO nanoparticles in the viable epidermis ranged from 0.51 to 1.12 mg/mL and contributes to the low but detectable levels of Zn ions reported following application of ZnO nanoparticles in *in vitro* [73] and *in vivo* studies [66, 67]. It is important to note that the ZnO nanoparticle signal was localized to the cell-furrow boundary, an area that is likely to have lipid boundaries. The triethoxycaprylylsilane coating that is applied to prevent the generation of reactive oxygen species (ROS) on exposure of the ZnO nanoparticles to sunlight may reduce agglomeration of nanoparticles and lead to a better dispersion on the skin surface. It may also lead to higher affinity of the coated nanoparticles to the lipid areas present in the skin furrows and thus

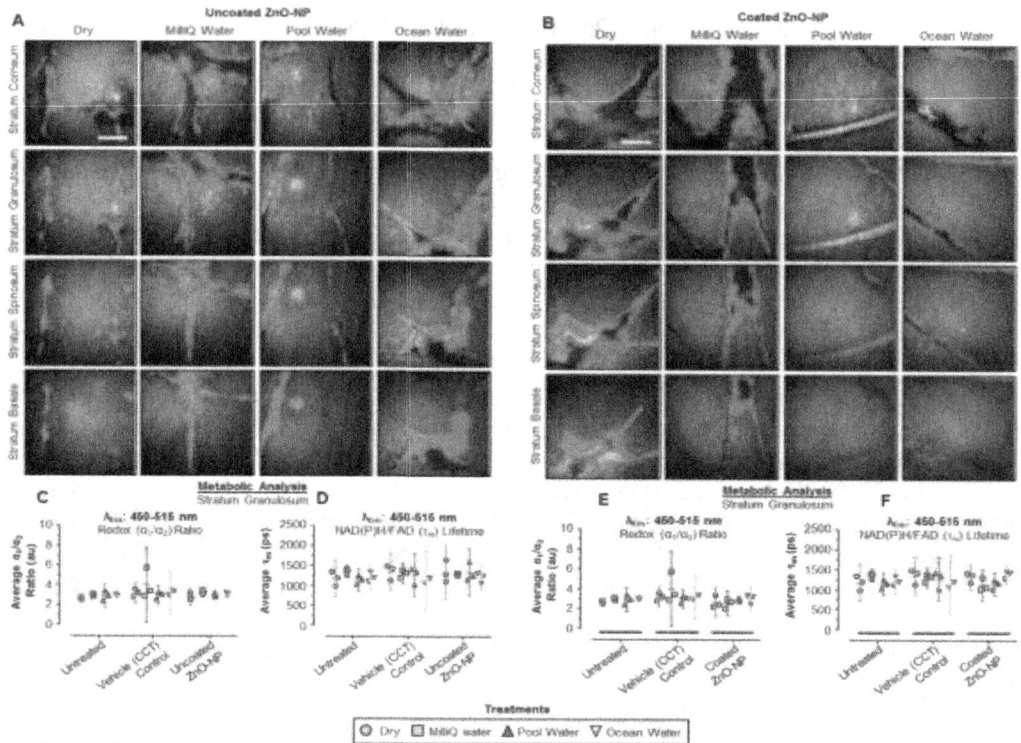

FIGURE 31.2 Penetration of uncoated and coated ZnO nanoparticles (ZnO-NP) in hydrated human skin *in vivo*. Hydration treatments include negative control, deionized, pool, and ocean water. (A) Representative pseudo-colored multispectral images (λEm: 370–390 nm [red]; λEm: 450–515 nm [green]; λEm: 515–620 nm [blue]) of different skin strata (SC, SG, SS, SB) following treatments (uncoated ZnO nanoparticles). (B) Representative pseudo-colored multispectral images (λEm: 370–390 nm [red]; λEm: 450–515 nm [green]; λEm: 515–620 nm [blue]) of different skin strata (SC, SG, SS, SB) following treatments (coated ZnO nanoparticles). The images are pseudo-colored to show cellular autofluorescence (green/blue) and ZnO-NP (red). The white bar represents a length of 40 μm. Metabolic and redox-associated changes in FLIM channel 2 (λ_{Em}: 450–515nm) within the SG following topical application of uncoated and coated ZnO nanoparticles to hydrated skin *in vivo*. Hydration treatments include negative control, deionized, pool, and ocean water. (C) Average α_1/α_2 ratios (a.u) following treatments with uncoated ZnO nanoparticles. (D) Average NAD(P)H/FAD weighted fluorescence lifetime (τm) following treatments with uncoated ZnO nanoparticles. (E) Average α_1/α_2 ratios (a.u) following treatments with coated ZnO nanoparticles. (F) Average NAD(P)H/FAD weighted fluorescence lifetime (τm) following treatments with coated ZnO NPs. Data represent mean lifetime (ps) or ratio ± 95% CI (*n* = 3). (Reprinted with permission from 70.)

promote localization and penetration in these regions. The authors also suggested that the presence of short-chain glycerides within the water-in-oil formulation, like caprylic/capric triglycerides, which are effective penetration enhancers [33, 34], may have reduced skin barrier resistance and thereby increased penetration from that formulation. However, in their measurements of transepidermal water loss (TEWL) they did not distinguish any differences following application of the formulations that would confirm barrier impairment.

Faunce et al [74] suggested that swimming could potentially facilitate absorption of TiO₂ and ZnO nanoparticles. We re-created water-based activities, such as swimming in a pool or ocean and the daily activity of showering, to determine their effects on ZnO nanoparticle distribution in the skin [70]. Following 1 hour soaking of test sites on the volar surface of the forearm of human volunteers with water from a swimming pool, the Pacific Ocean, or ultrapure water, coated ZnO nanoparticles were applied for a further hour. There was no direct permeation of coated ZnO nanoparticles through the stratum corneum to the viable epidermis and no evidence of metabolic changes following application to dry or soaked skin as assessed by MPT-FLIM (Figure 31.2).

In all of these studies the sunscreen was applied as a single application to the skin. However, in 2010 and 2012 Gulson et al. reported that following repeated topical application of ^{68}ZnO-NP sunscreen to human volunteers, ^{68}Zn ions were present in the blood and urine [66, 67]. They did not demonstrate the penetration of intact ZnO nanoparticles, as only the ions were measured. Given that sunscreens are applied on a daily basis, or indeed repeatedly through the day, where children or adults are engaged in play, sport, or work outdoors in sunny climates, this finding required further investigation. We used a dual experimental approach to further investigate this finding. First, we assessed the skin penetration and metabolic state of the viable epidermis by MPT-FLIM following repeated hourly (over 6 hours) and daily (over 5 days) topical application of uncoated and coated ZnO nanoparticles to human volunteers. We found that hourly or daily repeated topical applications of ZnO nanoparticles did not lead to significantly elevated nanoparticle penetration into the viable epidermis, and there was no evidence of metabolic change. The ZnO nanoparticles were concentrated on the skin surface and associated with the furrows, as had been seen previously in single applications under a range of application protocols. Second, to further explore the fate of nanoparticles that were localized on the skin surface, *in vitro* Franz cell–based studies were carried out with excised human skin using a labile zinc-specific probe, ZinPyr-1, to detect zinc ions in the skin. ZinPyr-1 is a specific chelating agent that permits mapping of the deposition of solubilized zinc species in ex vivo human skin so that the form of zinc penetrating through the skin is most likely to be the zinc ion and not insoluble zinc nanoparticles. This method has advantages over that used by Gulson et al. [66, 67], whereby detection was via acid digestion followed by ICP-MS and therefore does not permit determination of whether ^{68}Zn had been absorbed in a particulate or soluble form. Like Gulson, we saw an increase in labile zinc in the viable epidermis that we attributed to permeation of zinc ions liberated from the ZnO nanoparticles that accumulated on the skin surface and furrows, promoted by the hydrolysis of ZnO nanoparticles to Zn ions at the normal acidic pH of the skin. These zinc ions would then redistribute from the viable epidermis into the systemic circulation without adding significantly to the normal zinc ion concentrations in the body. This work demonstrates that repeated application of ZnO nanoparticle-based sunscreen products to the skin is safe.

There is now a clear body of evidence based on well-designed studies in human volunteers that demonstrate the safety of nanoparticle-based sunscreens in a wide range of *in-use* situations, including flexing [68], massage [68], occlusion [69], repeated hourly and daily application [75], and swimming/bathing. This provides confidence for health promotion organizations, health care professionals, teachers, and parents to recommend the use of effective nanoparticle-based sunscreens to protect children and adults from sunburn, skin cancer, and photoaging [65].

31.4   RISKS AND BENEFITS ASSOCIATED WITH TOPICAL SUNSCREEN USE

The most common adverse effects reported for topical products containing organic sunscreen chemicals are rashes resulting from allergy and photoallergy skin reactivity. Indeed in 2014, the American Contact Dermatitis Society listed benzophenones as the Allergen of the Year [12]. Oxybenzone appears to be of particular concern, potentially due to its inherent potential to elicit skin reactivity but also because it is the organic sunscreen chemical that is most readily penetrates the skin [19, 20, 29]. It has been consistently identified in patch-testing studies [76] and reviews of the scientific and clinical case-study literature as causing a range of forms of contact dermatitis, including contact urticaria [78].

Toxicity concerns regarding nanoparticle-based sunscreens have largely been based on cell culture studies that have reported cytotoxicity, oxidative stress, and DNA and metabolic damage when nanoparticles were applied to human liver cells (HepG2), epidermal cells (A431), keratinocytes (NCTC2544), and fibroblasts [78–82]. Although these studies may be an interesting academic exercise, they are not relevant to the real-life application of sunscreens if the nanoparticles do not actually come into contact with the cells. It is now clear, based on the evidence of many *in vivo* studies as discussed earlier, that nanoparticle-based sunscreens do not penetrate the skin to access the viable epidermis or deeper tissues; therefore, any potential damage that has been reported from direct application in cell culture is not relevant to their actual application as sunscreen products for human use.

REFERENCES

1. Waldman, R.A. and J.M. Grant-Kels, *The role of sunscreen in the prevention of cutaneous melanoma and nonmelanoma skin cancer.* J Am Acad Dermatol, 2019. **80**(2): p. 574–76 e1.
2. Seite, S., et al., *A broad-spectrum sunscreen prevents cumulative damage from repeated exposure to sub-erythemal solar ultraviolet radiation representative of temperate latitudes.* J Eur Acad Dermatol Venereol, 2010. **24**(2): p. 219–22.
3. Narbutt, J., et al., *Sunscreen applied at >/= 2 mg cm(-2) during a sunny holiday prevents erythema, a biomarker of ultraviolet radiation-induced DNA damage and suppression of acquired immunity.* Br J Dermatol, 2019. **180**(3): p. 604–14.
4. Gordon, L.G., et al., *Regular sunscreen use is a cost-effective approach to skin cancer prevention in subtropical settings.* J Invest Dermatol, 2009. **129**(12): p. 2766–71.
5. Mancuso, J.B., et al., *Sunscreens: an update.* Am J Clin Dermatol Clin, 2017. **18**: p. 643–50.
6. Cilag GmbH International, *OUR HERITAGE: A specialist sun care brand is born.* 2017. [Retrieved 30 October 2019]; Available from: https://www.pizbuin.com/en/our-heritage/.
7. Webster, Z., *Sunscreens*, in *Cosmetic Formulation Principles and Practice*, H.A.E. Benson, et al., Editors. 2019, CRC Press: Boca Raton. p. 279–308.
8. Downs, C.A., et al., *Toxicopathological effects of the sunscreen UV filter, oxybenzone (benzophenone-3), on coral planulae and cultured primary cells and its environmental contamination in Hawaii and the U.S. Virgin Islands.* Arch Environ Contam Toxicol, 2016. **70**(2): p. 265–88.
9. Kim, S. and K. Choi, *Occurrences, toxicities, and ecological risks of benzophenone-3, a common component of organic sunscreen products: a mini-review.* Environ Int, 2014. **70**: p. 143–57.
10. Ekpeghere, K.I., et al., *Distribution and seasonal occurrence of UV filters in rivers and wastewater treatment plants in Korea.* Sci Total Environ, 2016. **542**(Pt A): p. 121--8.
11. da Silva, C.P., E.S. Emidio, and M.R. de Marchi, *The occurrence of UV filters in natural and drinking water in Sao Paulo State (Brazil).* Environ Sci Pollut Res Int, 2015. **22**(24): p. 19706–15.
12. DiNardo, J.C. and C.A. Downs, *Dermatological and environmental toxicological impact of the sunscreen ingredient oxybenzone/benzophenone-3.* J Cosmet Dermatol, 2018. **17**(1): p. 15–9.
13. Moulite, M. *Hawaii bans sunscreens that harm coral reefs.* 2018. [Retrieved 30 October 2019]; Available from: https://edition.cnn.com/2018/07/03/health/hawaii-sunscreen-ban/index.html.
14. Sirois, J., *Examine all available evidence before making decisions on sunscreen ingredient bans.* Sci Total Environ, 2019. **674**: p. 211–12.
15. Schneider, S.L. and H.W. Lim, *Review of environmental effects of oxybenzone and other sunscreen active ingredients.* J Am Acad Dermatol, 2019. **80**(1): p. 266–71.
16. Administration, US Federal Drug. *Sunscreen Drug Products for Over-the-Counter Human Use.* 2019. [Retrieved 4 Sept 2019]; Available from: https://www.federalregister.gov/documents/2019/02/26/2019-03019/sunscreen-drug-products-for-over-the-counter-human-use.
17. U.S. FDA Center for Drug Evaluation and Research (CDER). *Guidance for Industry: Nonprescription Sunscreen Drug Products—Safety and Effectiveness Data,.* 2016. [Retrieved 11 Dec 2019]; Available from: https://www.fda.gov/regulatory-information/search-fda-guidance-documents/nonprescription-sunscreen-drug-products-safety-and-effectiveness-data.
18. U.S. FDA Center for Drug Evaluation and Research (CDER). *Maximal Usage Trials for Topically Applied Active Ingredients Being Considered for Inclusion in an Over-The -Counter Monograph: Study Elements and Considerations.* 2019. [Retrieved 11 Dec 2019]; Available from: https://www.fda.gov/regulatory-information/search-fda-guidance-documents/maximal-usage-trials-topically-applied-active-ingredients-being-considered-inclusion-over-counter.
19. Hayden, C.G., M.S. Roberts, and H.A.E. Benson, *Systemic absorption of sunscreen after topical application.* Lancet, 1997. **350**(9081): p. 863–4.
20. Gustavsson Gonzalez, H., A. Farbrot, and O. Larko, *Percutaneous absorption of benzophenone-3, a common component of topical sunscreens.* Clin Exp Dermatol, 2002. **27**(8): p. 691–4.

21. Gonzalez, H., et al., *Percutaneous absorption of the sunscreen benzophenone-3 after repeated whole-body applications, with and without ultraviolet irradiation.* Br J Dermatol, 2006. **154**(2): p. 337–40.

22. Zamoiski, R.D., et al., *Self-reported sunscreen use and urinary benzophenone-3 concentrations in the United States: NHANES 2003-2006 and 2009-2012.* Environ Res, 2015. **142**: p. 563–7.

23. Treffel, P. and B. Gabard, *Skin penetration and sun protection factor of ultra-violet filters from two vehicles.* Pharm Res, 1996. **13**(5): p. 770–4.

24. Chatelain, E., B. Gabard, and C. Surber, *Skin penetration and sun protection factor of five UV filters: effect of the vehicle.* Skin Pharmacol Appl Skin Physiol, 2003. **16**(1): p. 28–35.

25. Jiang, R., et al., *Absorption of sunscreens across human skin: an evaluation of commercial products for children and adults.* Br J Clin Pharmacol, 1999. **48**(4): p. 635–7.

26. Hagedorn-Leweke, U. and B.C. Lippold, *Absorption of sunscreens and other compounds through human skin in vivo: derivation of a method to predict maximum fluxes.* Pharm Res, 1995. **12**(9): p. 1354–60.

27. Benech-Kieffer, F., et al., *Percutaneous absorption of Mexoryl SX in human volunteers: comparison with in vitro data.* Skin Pharmacol Appl Skin Physiol, 2003. **16**(6): p. 343–55.

28. D'Souza, G., G.R. Evans, and C. Plastic Surgery Educational Foundation Technology Assessment, *Mexoryl: a review of an ultraviolet a filter.* Plast Reconstr Surg, 2007. **120**(4): p. 1071–5.

29. Matta, M.K., et al., *Effect of Sunscreen Application Under Maximal Use Conditions on Plasma Concentration of Sunscreen Active Ingredients: A Randomized Clinical Trial.* JAMA, 2019. **321**(21): p. 2082–91.

30. Kenney, G.K., et al., *In vitro skin absorption and metabolism of Padimate-O and a nitrosamine formed in Padimate-O-containing cosmetic products.* J Soc Cosmet Chem,, 1995. **46**: p. 117–27.

31. Lazar, G.M., et al., *Evaluation of in vitro percutaneous absorption of UV filters used in sunscreen formulations.* Drug and Cosmetic Industry, 1996(May): p. 50–62.

32. Walters, K.A., et al., *Percutaneous penetration of octyl salicylate from representative sunscreen formulations through human skin in vitro.* Food Chem Toxicol, 1997. **35**(12): p. 1219–25.

33. Potard, G., et al., *The stripping technique: in vitro absorption and penetration of five UV filters on excised fresh human skin.* Skin Pharmacol Appl Skin Physiol, 2000. **13**(6): p. 336–44.

34. Cross, S.E., et al., *Can increasing the viscosity of formulations be used to reduce the human skin penetration of the sunscreen oxybenzone?* J Invest Dermatol, 2001. **117**(1): p. 147–50.

35. Scalia, S., S. Battaglioli, and A. Bianchi, *In vivo human skin penetration of the UV filter ethylhexyl triazone: effect of lipid microparticle encapsulation.* Skin Pharmacol Physiol, 2019. **32**(1): p. 22–31.

36. Trotta, V., et al., *Influence of lipid microparticle encapsulation on in vitro efficacy, photostability and water resistance of the sunscreen agents, octyl methoxycinnamate and butyl methoxydibenzoylmethane.* Drug Dev Ind Pharm, 2014. **40**(9): p. 1233–9.

37. Scalia, S., M. Mezzena, and D. Ramaccini, *Encapsulation of the UV filters ethylhexyl methoxycinnamate and butyl methoxydibenzoylmethane in lipid microparticles: effect on in vivo human skin permeation.* Skin Pharmacol Physiol, 2011. **24**(4): p. 182–9.

38. Scalia, S., G. Coppi, and V. Iannuccelli, *Microencapsulation of a cyclodextrin complex of the UV filter, butyl methoxydibenzoylmethane: in vivo skin penetration studies.* J Pharm Biomed Anal, 2011. **54**(2): p. 345–50.

39. Scalia, S. and M. Mezzena, *Incorporation in lipid microparticles of the UVA filter, butyl methoxydibenzoylmethane combined with the UVB filter, octocrylene: effect on photostability.* AAPS PharmSciTech, 2009. **10**(2): p. 384–90.

40. Scalia, S. and M. Mezzena, *Incorporation of quercetin in lipid microparticles: effect on photo- and chemical-stability.* J Pharm Biomed Anal, 2009. **49**(1): p. 90–4.

41. Scalia, S. and M. Mezzena, *Co-loading of a photostabilizer with the sunscreen agent, butyl methoxydibenzoylmethane in solid lipid microparticles.* Drug Dev Ind Pharm, 2009. **35**(2): p. 192–8.

42. Vettor, M., et al., *Poly(D,L-lactide) nanoencapsulation to reduce photoinactivation of a sunscreen agent.* Int J Cosmet Sci, 2008. **30**(3): p. 219–27.

43. Iannuccelli, V., et al., *In vivo and in vitro skin permeation of butyl methoxydibenzoylmethane from lipospheres.* Skin Pharmacol Physiol, 2008. **21**(1): p. 30–8.

44. Tursilli, R., et al., *Solid lipid microparticles containing the sunscreen agent, octyl-dimethylaminobenzoate: effect of the vehicle.* Eur J Pharm Biopharm, 2007. **66**(3): p. 483–7.

45. Scalia, S., R. Tursilli, and V. Iannuccelli, *Complexation of the sunscreen agent, 4-methylbenzylidene camphor with cyclodextrins: effect on photostability and human stratum corneum penetration.* J Pharm Biomed Anal, 2007. **44**(1): p. 29–34.

46. Scalia, S., M. Mezzena, and V. Iannuccelli, *Influence of solid lipid microparticle carriers on skin penetration of the sunscreen agent, 4-methylbenzylidene camphor.* J Pharm Pharmacol, 2007. **59**(12): p. 1621–7.

47. Scalia, S., et al., *Encapsulation in lipospheres of the complex between butyl methoxydibenzoylmethane and hydroxypropyl-[beta]-cyclodextrin.* Int J Pharm, 2006. **320**(1-2): p. 79–85.

48. Scalia, S., et al., *Incorporation of the sunscreen agent, octyl methoxycinnamate in a cellulosic fabric grafted with beta-cyclodextrin.* Int J Pharm, 2006. **308**(1-2): p. 155–9.

49. Molinari, A., et al., *Influence of complexation with cyclodextrins on photo-induced free radical production by the common sunscreen agents octyl-dimethylaminobenzoate and octyl-methoxycinnamate.* Pharmazie, 2006. **61**(1): p. 41–5.

50. Iannuccelli, V., et al., *Influence of lipsosphere preparation on butyl-methoxydibenzoylmethane photostability.* Eur J Pharm Biopharm, 2006. **63**(2): p. 140–5.

51. Simeoni, S., S. Scalia, and H.A. Benson, *Influence of cyclodextrins on in vitro human skin absorption of the sunscreen, butyl-methoxydibenzoylmethane.* Int J Pharm, 2004. **280**(1-2): p. 163–71.

52. Scalia, S., et al., *Complexation of the sunscreen agent, phenylbenzimidazole sulphonic acid with cyclodextrins: effect on stability and photo-induced free radical formation.* Eur J Pharm Sci, 2004. **22**(4): p. 241–9.

53. Iaconinoto, A., et al., *Influence of cyclodextrin complexation on the photodegradation and antioxidant activity of alpha-tocopherol.* Pharmazie, 2004. **59**(1): p. 30–3.

54. Scalia, S., et al., *Influence of hydroxypropyl-beta-cyclodextrin on photo-induced free radical production by the sunscreen agent, butyl-methoxydibenzoylmethane.* J Pharm Pharmacol, 2002. **54**(11): p. 1553–8.

55. Scalia, S., et al., *Comparative studies of the influence of cyclodextrins on the stability of the sunscreen agent, 2-ethylhexyl-p-methoxycinnamate.* J Pharm Biomed Anal, 2002. **30**(4): p. 1181–9.

56. Perugini, P., et al., *Effect of nanoparticle encapsulation on the photostability of the sunscreen agent, 2-ethylhexyl-p-methoxycinnamate.* Int J Pharm, 2002. **246**(1-2): p. 37–45.

57. Scalia, S., *Determination of sunscreen agents in cosmetic products by supercritical fluid extraction and high-performance liquid chromatography.* J Chromatogr A, 2000. **870**(1-2): p. 199–205.

58. Scalia, S., S. Villani, and A. Casolari, *Inclusion complexation of the sunscreen agent 2-ethylhexyl-p- dimethylaminobenzoate with hydroxypropyl-beta-cyclodextrin: effect on photostability.* J Pharm Pharmacol, 1999. **51**(12): p. 1367–74.

59. Scalia, S., et al., *Complexation of the sunscreen agent, butyl-methoxydibenzoylmethane, with hydroxypropyl-b-cyclodextrin.* Int J Pharm, 1998. **175**: p. 205–13.

60. Ambrogi, V., et al., *Mesoporous silicate MCM-41 as a particulate carrier for octyl methoxycinnamate: Sunscreen release and photostability.* J Pharm Sci, 2013. **102**(5): p. 1468–75.

61. Bhuptani, R.S. and V.B. Patravale, *Starch microsponges for enhanced retention and efficacy of topical sunscreen.* Mater Sci Eng C Mater Biol Appl, 2019. **104**: p. 109882.

62. Suh, H.W., et al., *Biodegradable bioadhesive nanoparticle incorporation of broad-spectrum organic sunscreen agents.* Bioeng Transl Med, 2019. **4**(1): p. 129–40.

63. Barbosa, T.C., et al., *Development, Cytotoxicity and Eye Irritation Profile of a New Sunscreen Formulation Based on Benzophenone-3-poly(epsilon-caprolactone) Nanocapsules.* Toxics, 2019. **7**(4).

64. Berube, D.M., *Rhetorical gamesmanship in the nano debates over sunscreens and nanoparticles.* J Nano Res, 2008. **10**(Suppl 1): p. 23–37.

65. Wright, P.F.A., *Realistic Exposure Study Assists Risk Assessments of ZnO Nanoparticle Sunscreens and Allays Safety Concerns.* J Invest Dermatol, 2019. **139**(2): p. 277–78.

66. Gulson, B., et al., *Small amounts of zinc from zinc oxide particles in sunscreens applied outdoors are absorbed through human skin.* Toxicol Sci, 2010. **118**(1): p. 140–9.

67. Gulson, B., et al., *Comparison of dermal absorption of zinc from different sunscreen formulations and differing UV exposure based on stable isotope tracing.* Sci Total Environ, 2012. **420**: p. 313–8.

68. Leite-Silva, V.R., et al., *Effect of flexing and massage on in vivo human skin penetration and toxicity of zinc oxide nanoparticles.* Nanomedicine (Lond), 2016. **11**(10): p. 1193–205.

69. Leite-Silva, V.R., et al., *Human skin penetration and local effects of topical nano zinc oxide after occlusion and barrier impairment.* Eur J Pharm Biopharm, 2016. **104**: p. 140–7.

70. Mohammed, Y.H., et al., *Bathing does not facilitate the human skin penetration or adverse cellular effects of nanoparticulate zinc oxide sunscreens after topical application* J Invest Dermatol, 2020. **104**: p. 1656–9.

71. Lin, L.L., et al., *Time-correlated single photon counting for simultaneous monitoring of zinc oxide nanoparticles and NAD(P)H in intact and barrier-disrupted volunteer skin.* Pharm Res, 2011. **28**(11): p. 2920–30.

72. Leite-Silva, V.R., et al., *The effect of formulation on the penetration of coated and uncoated zinc oxide nanoparticles into the viable epidermis of human skin in vivo.* Eur J Pharm Biopharm, 2013. **84**(2): p. 297–308.

73. Cross, S.E., et al., *Human skin penetration of sunscreen nanoparticles: in vitro assessment of a novel micronized zinc oxide formulation.* Skin Pharmacol Physiol, 2007. **20**(3): p. 148–54.

74. Faunce, T.A., *Toxicological and public good considerations for the regulation of nanomaterial-containing medical products.* Expert Opin Drug Saf, 2008. **7**(2): p. 103–6.

75. Mohammed, Y.H., et al., *Support for the safe use of zinc oxide nanoparticle sunscreens: lack of skin penetration or cellular toxicity after repeated application in volunteers.* J Invest Dermatol, 2019. **139**(2): p. 308–15.

76. Warshaw, E.M., et al., *Patch test reactions associated with sunscreen products and the importance of testing to an expanded series: retrospective analysis of North American Contact Dermatitis Group data, 2001 to 2010.* Dermatitis, 2013. **24**(4): p. 176–82.

77. Verhulst, L. and A. Goossens, *Cosmetic components causing contact urticaria: a review and update.* Contact Dermatitis, 2016. **75**(6): p. 333–44.

78. Akhtar, M.J., et al., *Zinc oxide nanoparticles selectively induce apoptosis in human cancer cells through reactive oxygen species.* Int J Nanomedicine, 2012. **7**: p. 845–57.

79. Alarifi, S., et al., *Induction of oxidative stress, DNA damage, and apoptosis in a malignant human skin melanoma cell line after exposure to zinc oxide nanoparticles.* Int J Nanomed, 2013. **8**: p. 983–93.

80. Bakand, S., A. Hayes, and F. Dechsakulthorn. *Nanotoxicity and safety evaluation of nanoparticles in sunscreen products in vitro.* In *Australasian College of Toxicology and Risk Assessment 10th Annual Scientific Meeting.* 2017. Canberra, Australia.

81. Kocbek, P., et al., *Toxicological aspects of long-term treatment of keratinocytes with ZnO and TiO2 nanoparticles.* Small, 2010. **6**(17): p. 1908–17.

82. Sharma, V., D. Anderson, and A. Dhawan, *Zinc oxide nanoparticles induce oxidative stress and genotoxicity in human liver cells (HepG2).* J Biomed Nanotechnol, 2011. **7**(1): p. 98–9.

32 Sunscreen Percutaneous Penetration *In Vivo* in Man

Pranav Vasu
Case Western Reserve University, Cleveland, Ohio

Howard I. Maibach
University of California, San Francisco, California

CONTENTS

32.1 INTRODUCTION

Since World War II, an increased awareness of the harmful effects of sunlight exposure resulted in heightened sunscreen usage. Sunscreens, commonplace worldwide and with the exception of occasional instances of allergic contact dermatitis or photoallergic contact dermatitis, are generally regarded as relatively safe by most health care professionals.

In Europe, sunscreens are largely regulated as cosmetics and often have limited toxicological studies and do not have registries to document their potential involvement in extracutaneous organs. In the United States, however, sunscreens with medical claims are regulated as drugs and those without as cosmetics.

With increased sunscreen utilization, the safety and toxicity of the formulations have been questioned: Matta et al. [1] brought to the attention of the scientific world and the general public (when widely quoted by popular publications, including *The New York Times*) the lack of data regarding percutaneous absorption of sunscreens *in vivo* in man and provided data showing levels of absorption exceeding Food and Drug Administration (FDA) levels of concern. This manuscript documents experimental data, attempting to define one aspect of sunscreen dermatotoxicity: absorbed dose *in vivo* in man.

32.2 MATERIALS AND METHODS

We reviewed the following computer databases: PubMed, Embase, Google Scholar, Web of Science, and EBSCO host, utilizing the search queries "percutaneous penetration," "percutaneous absorption," "in vivo human," and "in vivo man," among others, from the initiation of the websites to April 2020.

Only articles written in English were studied. Seventy-five were reviewed, and from abstracts, all articles pertaining to the percutaneous penetration of FDA-approved sunscreens *in vivo* in man were formulated into table overviews. Since textbooks are not routinely indexed in these databases, we reviewed textbooks on dermatopharmacology, dermatotoxicology, and percutaneous penetration in the University of California, San Francisco Dermatology Department.

32.3 RESULTS

From the literature and FDA websites regarding percutaneous penetration *in vivo* in man, data for the following organic sunscreens were found: para-aminobenzoic acid (PABA), ethylhexyl dimethyl PABA, octinoxate, homosalate, octisalate, oxybenzone, sulisobenzone, avobenzone, ecamsule, and octocrylene.

Table 32.1 provides the organic and inorganic FDA-approved sunscreens and common nomenclature with ultraviolet (UV) categorization [2].

PABA data are available from Wester et al. in Tables 32.2 and 32.3 [3]. Table 32.2 provides percutaneous penetration data *in vivo* in man utilizing the Feldmann and Maibach [4] protocol. Dose of [^{14}C]-chemical was solubilized in 50 µl ethanol and spread over 10 cm^2 skin surface ventral forearm. Urinary excretion was $11.5 \pm 6.3\%$.

Table 32.3 provides the percutaneous absorption of PABA as a parenteral control to correct the topical administration, in which there was $74.9 \pm 18.2\%$ excretion, providing a calculation of 36.6% for the forearm. Although not directly comparable with data of Matta, the conclusion supports the high PABA percutaneous penetration.

TABLE 32.1
FDA-Approved Sunscreens, Their Common Nomenclature, and UV Protection Categorization

Sunscreen	Other Common Names	UV Protection
Organic		
PABA Derivatives		
Para-aminobenzoic acid	PABA	UVB
Padimate-O	Octyl dimethyl-p-aminobenzoate, Octyl dimethyl PABA, Ethylhexyl dimethyl PABA	UVB
Cinnamates		
Cinoxate		UVB
Octinoxate	Octyl methoxycinnamate	UVB
Salicylates		
Homosalate	Homomenthyl salicylate	UVB
Octisalate	2-ethylhexyl salicylate	UVB
Trolamine salicylate	Salicylic acid trolamine	UVB
Benzophenones		
Dioxybenzone	Benzophenone-8	UVB, UVA2
Oxybenzone	Benzophenone-3	UVB, UVA2
Sulisobenzone	Benzophenone-4	UVB, UVA2
Other		
Avobenzone	Butyl methoxydibenzoylmethane, Parsol 1789	UVA1
Ecamsule	Terephthalylidene dicamphor sulfonic acid	UVB, UVA2
Meradimate	Menthyl anthranilate	UVA2
Octocrylene		UVB
Inorganic		
Titanium dioxide		UVB, UVA2, UVA1
Zinc oxide		UVB, UVA2, UVA1

TABLE 32.2
Percutaneous Penetration *In Vivo* in Man from Wester et al.

This study used the Feldmann and Maibach protocol, which documents the urinary excretion over approximately seven
days. However, some chemicals such as highly lipophilic materials may not be completely excreted in urine, and hence a
parenteral (intravenous, subcutaneous, intramuscular, or intraperitoneal) control allows for an approximate correction of
incomplete urinary excretion in the topical study.
Approximately $11.5 \pm 6.3\%$ was excreted in the urine over seven days. Parenteral control in the rhesus monkey
(intravenous) (Table 32.2)—with urine for seven days revealed a $74.9 \pm 18.2\%$ excretion. Correcting the topical
administration with this $74.9 \pm 18.2\%$ excretion, the parenteral control provides an estimate of 36.6% for the forearm
data. The skin surface wash was $29.5 \pm 12.8\%$, suggesting that the study did not achieve a complete mass balance.
Objectives: Determine extent of percutaneous absorption *p*-Aminobenzoic Acid *in vivo*.

Methods:

- Five normal volunteers per group (males ages 18–55, and postmenopausal women ages 50–65).
- [^{14}C]-chemical was solubilized in 50 μl ethanol and spread over 10 cm^2 skin surface ventral forearm. Dose/cm^2 not available.
- Volunteers were instructed not to touch or wash the study area for 24 hours. Skin was unprotected during absorption
  period.
- Urine collected for seven days.
- At seven days after application, cellophane tape stripping was conducted 10 times for residual [^{14}C] chemical.
- Percutaneous absorption was determined from urine.

Results:

Urinary excretion, skin surface wash recovery, and tape strip recovery in man as a percentage of dose. Urine excretion
measured from 21.5 μg/cm^2 ethanol vehicle on ventral forearm. Skin surface wash measured 24 hours post-application.
Tape strip recovery measured seven days post-application with 10 consecutive tape strips. From Ref. 3.

Subject	Urine Excretion	Skin Surface Wash	Tape Strip
1	7.1	36.2	1.2
2	11.8	25.8	0.23
3	3.6	37.6	0.19
4	18.3	8.6	0.10
5	16.9	39.3	0.76
Mean ± SD	11.5 ± 6.3	29.5 ± 12.8	0.56 ± 0.47

Table 32.4 provides absorption data for sulisobenzone as a result of a tape stripping method [5],
but not that of the Rougier [6] method and is not readily interpreted. Similar to Table 32.4, data for
oxybenzone, octinoxate, avobenzone, and octisalate in Table 32.5 were retrieved by tape stripping
[7]; however, the aforementioned Rougier method was not used. Table 32.6 shows that approximately $9.68 \pm 1.51\%$ of avobenzone in an oil/water (O/W) emulsion and $16.65 \pm 2.99\%$ of compound
in lipospheres were found in tapes following 2 mg/cm^2 dose [8].
Urine and blood concentrations for oxybenzone and octinoxate after a 2 mg/cm^2 dose to body
surface area in a cream vehicle are in Table 32.7 [9]. In Table 32.8 [10], absorption quantities post-
application of a 2 mg/cm^2 dose to the forearm of ecamsule from a cream in blood and urine are more
readily compared to Matta.
Table 32.9 provides the plasma concentrations under maximal use conditions of avobenzone,
oxybenzone, octocrylene, and ecamsule. The dose was 2 mg/cm^2 over 75% of the body surface
area for four times daily over four days; the researchers concluded that it is likely that these sunscreens are absorbed beyond the FDA systemic absorption threshold. There was a 2.45% radioactivity in male urine and 1.18% in females found regarding the percutaneous absorption of ethylhexyl
dimethyl PABA (Table 32.10 [11]). The maximum plasma levels of avobenzone and octocrylene
following a 2 mg/cm^2 dose to body surface area were 11 μg/L and 25 μg/L, respectively, as found
by the studies of Hiller et al. indicated in Table 32.11 [12].

TABLE 32.3

Percutaneous Absorption of *p*-Aminobenzoic in Rhesus Monkey *In Vivo* as a Parenteral Control

Objectives: Determine extent of percutaneous absorption of *p*-aminobenzoic acid *in vivo*.

Methods:

- Parenteral control: [^{14}C]-PABA in 0.5 mL propylene glycol administered into the saphenous vein ($n = 4$).
- Urine samples collected over the seven days and 5-mL aliquots assayed for radioactivity.

Results:

Urinary excretion of PABA in rhesus monkeys after intravenous administration—used as a parenteral excretion control. From Ref. 3.

Time (days)	Percentage of Dose Excreted ± SD of Four Monkeys
1	72.0 ± 17.7
2	1.3 ± 0.2
3	0.4 ± 0.3
4	0.4 ± 0.4
5	0.3 ± 0.1
6	0.3 ± 0.2
7	0.2 ± 0.1
Total	74.9 ± 18.2

Studies utilizing only the tape stripping method (Tables 32.4, 32.5, and 32.6) all share the same conclusion—namely, the data imply that part of the sunscreen dose penetrated into the skin. However, it is not possible to quantify how much went into the skin, and there are no data on excretion from a parenteral dose.

TABLE 32.4

Data on 21 Adult Volunteers Utilizing Sulisobenzone (Benzophenone-4) at a Dose of 6.25 mg/cm² on the Forearm.

Note that this is approximately six times greater than the typical consumer dosage [16], and the endpoint consisted of stratum corneum tape stripping at one to seven hours post-dosing.

At seven hours, 45% remained in the first strip and 20% was unrecovered.

These data, as shown Figure 32.1, are not readily interpreted but do suggest that penetration occurred.

Objectives: Determine extent of percutaneous absorption of sulisobenzone (benzophenone-4)

Methods:

- Twenty-one healthy Caucasian women aged 22–34 (25 ± 3 years).
- 6.25 mg/cm² mg cream applied over a 4 cm² area on subject forearms. This is six times the typical consumer dosage.
- Skin strippings at one, two, five, and seven hours after treatment.
- Six strips removed stratum corneum and 10 mL of water added to each of the strips.
- Each sample shaken in a vortex mixer and sunscreen concentration determined.

Results:

- In first strip at one hour, 70% of sulisobenzone remained.
- After seven hours, 45% of the sulisobenzone remained in first strip and 20% remained unrecovered after all subsequent strips.

Parenteral excretion control: None

(Continued)

TABLE 32.4 (*Continued*)
Data on 21 Adult Volunteers Utilizing Sulisobenzone (Benzophenone-4) at a Dose of 6.25 mg/cm^2 on the Forearm.

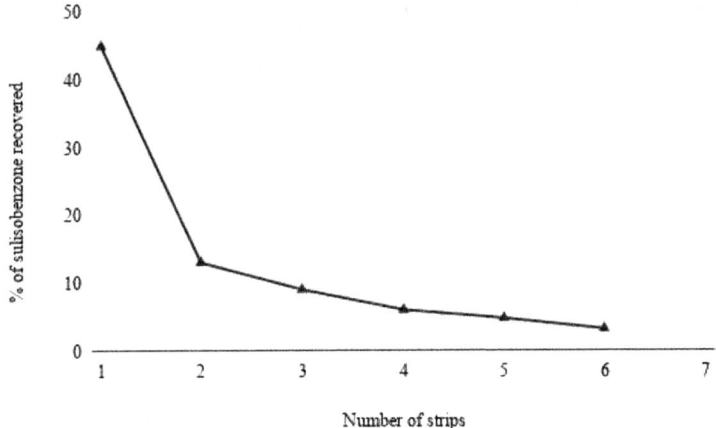

FIGURE 32.1 Percentage of recovered filter after seven hours according to number of strips. (Adapted from Reference 5.)

TABLE 32.5
Penetration of Oxybenzone, Octinoxate, Avobenzone, Octisalate, and Homosalate

The study compared the penetration from an emulsion system and petroleum jelly. Six volunteers were dosed at 2 mg/cm^2 of final formulation. Thirty minutes after application, the excess product was removed

As in the previous table, the data are difficult to interpret due to the lack of details. The interpretation was that there was a greater amount of all five sunscreens with the gel as compared to the petroleum jelly.

This does not appear to be the Rougier method of tape stripping—with washing at 30 minutes, which provides a reasonable estimate of what would appear in urine over four days.

Objectives: Comparing skin penetration in two vehicles: O/W emulsion and petroleum jelly, both *in vivo*.

Benzophenone-3 (BPH) (oxybenzone), ethylhexyl methoxycinnamate (EHM) (octinoxate), butyl methoxydibenzoylmethane (BMDM) (avobenzone), ethylhexyl salicylate (EHS) (octisalate), and homosalate (H).

Methods:

- Two emulsions were formulated: one in an oil/water emulsion and a petroleum jelly emulsion.
- Tape stripping method.
- Six healthy volunteers ages 25–53 years.
- A 2 mg/cm^2 dose of sunscreen applied to a 4 cm^2 area on the volar forearm. This is twice the typical consumer dosage.
- Thirty minutes after application, excess product was removed.
- Conducted 16 tape strips.
- Strip 1 measured separately 2–6, 7–11, and 12–16 were pooled and extracted with methanol.
- Extraction recovery was greater than 97%.

Results:

- Sunscreen penetration into dermis occurred in all tested sunscreens and was vehicle dependent.

Amount of UV filters present in tape strips 2–16 of the stratum corneum 30 minutes after application of µg/cm^2(% of applied dose). This is the tape method and is not readily interpreted.

(Continued)

TABLE 32.5 (*Continued*)
Penetration of Oxybenzone, Octinoxate, Avobenzone, Octisalate, and Homosalate

From Ref. 7.

UV Filter	Emulsion Gel	Petroleum
BPH	29.9 ± 6.6 (26.9)	9.8 ± 4.0 (10.7)
EHM	40.2 ± 8.9 (24.1)	13.8 ± 5.1 (10.0)
BMDBM	12.9 ± 3.5 (29.2)	3.9 ± 1.7 (10.6)
EHS	28.4 ± 6.6 (25.6)	10.1 ± 3.5 (11.0)
H	25.7 ± 6.4 (23.2)	8.3 ± 3.6 (9.0)

Conclusion:

- Both compounds detected in the dermis at 30 minutes after application. Penetration levels were vehicle dependent.

Parenteral excretion control: None

TABLE 32.6
Data for Avobenzone Penetration from Lipospheres

Volunteers received the compound at a dose of 2 mg/cm^2 and excess was material was removed. Approximately 9.68 ± 1.51% of BMDBM in an O/W emulsion (alone) and 16.65 ± 2.99% of compound in lipospheres were found in the tapes. This does not appear to be the Rougier method as described in the previous table description, and it is difficult to determine the absorbed quantity.

There was no parenteral control as expected for this method.

Objectives: Compare penetration of avobenzone in lipid microparticles (lipospheres) and avobenzone not in lipospheres *in vivo*.

Methods:

- Butyl methoxydibenzoylmethane (BMDBM) skin permeation determined with skin stripping technique.
- Caucasian volunteers (45.7 ± 12.3 years).
- BMDBM inside and out (free) of lipospheres prepared in O/W emulsion and applied 2 mg/cm^2 on 2 × 5 cm area for 30 minutes.
- Application site not stated.
- Remaining product removed from skin area and stratum corneum stripped 10 times.
- Maintained at 4°C and analyzed for BMDBM amounts.

Results:

- Tape strips 2–7 were considered the upper parts of the stratum corneum (SC) representing the unabsorbed BMDBM. Tape strips 8–10 were considered SC intermediate part.
- Average penetrated: 10% unencapsulated and 15% encapsulated.

Sunscreen distribution in the stratum corneum after 30 minutes *in vivo* (% of applied dose ± SD, $n = 6$).
From Ref. 8.

	BMDBM Alone	BMDBM in Lipospheres	P-value
Unabsorbed	81.30 ± 12. 34	85.27 ± 8.26	<0.05
Recovery in SC (tapes 2–10)	9.68 ± 1.51	16.65 ± 2.99	<0.05
Total Recovery	90.98 ± 5.67	101.92 ± 4.77	<0.05

Conclusions:

- Micorencapsulation process did not substantially modify sunscreen accumulation in the SC as demonstrated by *in vivo* tape stripping method.

Parenteral excretion control: None

TABLE 32.7

Plasma and Urine Concentrations of Oxybenzone and Octinoxate in 32 Volunteers

Urine and blood were collected for 96 hours. The dose was 2 mg/cm^2—twice the typical consumer dose. Sunscreen
formulation concentration was 10% for both. The analytic method was high-performance liquid chromatography (HPLC)

Maximum median plasma concentrations in women were 187 ng/mL oxybenzone and 7 ng/mL octinoxate, where the
median concentration in males was 238 ng/mL oxybenzone and 16 ng/mL octinoxate.

Maximum median urine concentrations in women were 44 ng/mL oxybenzone and 6 ng/mL octinoxate, where the median
concentration in males was 81 ng/mL oxybenzone and 4 ng/mL octinoxate.

Neither the area under the curve nor the percentage of dose of absorbed in urine were stated. There was no parenteral control.

These data permit the conclusion of these maximum urine and plasma concentrations, but cannot be compared directly to
the recent Matta data.

Objectives: Determine extent of oxybenzone (benzophenone-3 [BP3]) and octinoxate (octyl methoxycinnamate [OMC])
absorption.

Methods:

- Thirty-two healthy volunteers (n = 15 males aged 23–29, n = 17 postmenopausal women aged 54–86).
- Five-day study.
- Cream application and blood sampling conducted daily.
- Blood samples a: 0, 1, 2, 3, 4, 24, and 96 hours.
- Urine concentration measured at 0, 24, 48, 72, and 96 hours.
- Dose of 2 mg/cm^2 body surface area (BSA)—twice the typical consumer dosage.
- Sunscreen formulation concentration was 10% (w/w) for both sunscreens.
- Samples analyzed with HPLC.

Results:

- Prior to application, undetectable in plasma and urine.
- Maximum median plasma concentrations in females: 187 ng/ml BP3, 7 ng/ml OMC.
- Maximum median plasma concentrations in males: 238 ng/ml BP3, 16 ng/ml OMC.
- Maximum median urine concentrations in females: 44 ng/ml BP3, 6 ng/ml OMC.
- Maximum median urine concentrations in males: 81 ng/ml BP3, 4 ng/ml OMC.
- Absorbed quantity as a percent value unstated.

Parenteral excretion control: None

Penetration was directly quantifiable from blood and urine data (Tables 32.2, 32.3, 32.7, 32.8,
32.10, and 32.11). These data support the conclusions formulated by Matta (Table 32.9).

32.4 DISCUSSION

We strongly benefit from Matta's data and add similar data for other widely used sunscreens. In our
search of various online databases, percutaneous absorption data *in vivo* in man was not found for
cinoxate, trolamine salicylate, dioxybenzone, and meradimate.

Data provided by studies that utilized the stripping method (Tables 32.4, 32.5, and 32.6) were
unusable for quantification of sunscreen percutaneous concentrations. These studies were not conducted utilizing the Rougier method of tape stripping [6] where there was a skin wash at 30 minutes
post-application, which provides an estimate of systemic absorption.

We can more readily interpret blood level and urine concentration data provided by the studies
outlined in Tables 32.2, 32.3, 32.7, 32.8, 32.10, and 32.11. Some sunscreens such as PABA (Tables
32.2 and 32.3), as well as oxybenzone (Tables 32.7 and 32.9), demonstrate high levels of percutaneous absorption, while others, such as ecamsule (Tables 32.8 and 32.9), demonstrate much lower
levels. However, each supports the conclusion of Matta—that they penetrate the skin beyond FDA
systemic absorption thresholds.

TABLE 32.8
Data for Ecamsule Utilizing Carbon-14 Dosing

Five males received a dose of 2 mg/cm² on the forearm. This is twice the usual consumer exposure. The exposed site was protected with an aluminum device to decrease the likelihood of rub and wash loss. Test site was unspecified.

Urine was collected for 120 hours and blood for 168 hours with feces up to 120 hours.

This study cannot be directly compared to that of Matta and Feldmann. They observed $0.011 \pm 0.003\%$ in urine and had a total mass balance of $91.91 \pm 1.66\%$, which is within the range of current recovery standards. There was no parenteral control.

Objectives: Determine extent of absorption and excretion of radioactivity in humans after dermal application of ecamsule cream.

Methods:

- Five Caucasian males: age range 19–29, weight 62.2–74.3 kg, height 175.1–187.3 cm
- Dosing: 2 mg/cm² of formulation spread on forearm (5.95 cm × 16.90 cm). Exposure four hours (protected with perforated aluminum). Unspecified whether ventral or dorsal.
- Skin wash sample collected at four hours and excess formulation washed off by wiping area wet with 5% sodiumlaurylethersulfate.
- Urine samples collected at 0–4, 4–12, and 9–12 hour intervals up to 120 hours.
- Blood samples collected at 0, 1, 2, 3, 4, 6, 8, 10, 12, 14, 24, 34, 48, 72, 96, and 168 hours after application.
- Feces collected up to 120 hours post-application.
- Thirteen to sixteen skin strips, which covered 31% of test area, taken per subject. Strips taken on day 6, about 120 hours post-application.

Results:

- Radioactivity in the samples as a percentage of applied dose
- Skin wash: 91.52 ± 1.61
- Blood and feces: Nothing above background
- Urine: 0.011 ± 0.003
- Skin strips: 0.008 ± 0.005
- Perforated aluminum: 0.073 ± 0.075
- Total: 91.91 ± 1.66
- Approximately 0.02% of ecamsule was available for system absorption from urine, feces, and skin strip data

Parenteral excretion control: None

TABLE 32.9

Plasma Concentrations under Maximal Use Conditions of Avobenzone, Oxybenzone, Octocrylene, and Ecamsule

Twenty-four healthy volunteers received formulations, with six in each group. The dose was 2 mg/cm^2 over 75% of the body surface area for four times daily over four days. This is twice the typical consumer dosage.

Maximum plasma concentration for avobenzone was 4.0 ng/mL for spray 1, 3.4 ng/mL for spray 2, 4.3 ng/mL for the lotion, and 1.8 ng/mL for the cream. Maximum plasma concentration for oxybenzone was 209.6 ng/mL for spray 1, 194.9 ng/mL for spray 2, and 169.3 ng/mL for the lotion. Maximum plasma concentration for octocrylene was 2.9 ng/mL for spray 1, 7.8 ng/mL for spray 2, 5.7 ng/mL for the lotion, and 5.7 ng/mL for the cream. Mean maximum plasma concentration of ecamsule in the cream was 1.5 ng/mL. Spray 1, spray 2, and the lotion did not contain ecamsule. ecamsule.

All four sunscreens exceeded the FDA systemic threshold of 0.5 ng/mL under maximal use conditions.

Objectives: Determine systemic absorptions of avobenzone, oxybenzone, octocrylene, and ecamsule.

Methods

- Twenty-four healthy volunteers.
- Participants randomly assigned to one of four sunscreen formulations: spray 1 ($n = 6$), spray 2 ($n = 6$), lotion ($n = 6$), and cream ($n = 6$).
- Dosing regimen: 2 mg/cm^2 over 75% body surface area (BSA) four times daily for four days. This is twice the typical consumer dosage.
- Thirty blood samples over seven-day period from each volunteer.

Results

- Avobenzone: mean maximum plasma concentration in spray 1: 4.0 ng/mL, spray 2: 3.4 ng/mL, lotion: 4.3 ng/mL, cream: 1.8 ng/mL.
- Oxybenzone: mean maximum plasma concentration in spray 1: 209.6 ng/mL, spray 2: 194.9 ng/mL, lotion: 169.3 ng/mL, cream did not contain oxybenzone
- Octocrylene: mean maximum plasma concentration in spray 1: 2.9 ng/mL, spray 2: 7.8 ng/mL, lotion: 5.7 ng/mL, cream: 5.7 ng/mL.
- Ecamsule: mean maximum plasma concentration in cream: 1.5 ng/mL. Spray 1, spray 2, and lotion did not contain ecamsule.

Conclusion

- All four sunscreens exceeded the FDA-approved systemic absorption threshold of 0.5 ng/mL under maximal use conditions.

Parenteral excretion control: None

TABLE 32.10

Penetration Data of Ethylhexyl Dimethyl PABA in an Ethanol Formulation Utilizing ^{14}C-Labeled Material

The dose was spread on 100 cm^2 on the forearm at a level of 0.5 mg/cm^2 at a final sunscreen concentration of 8%. The forearms were protected with gauze for 24 hours After the ethanol evaporated, blood was collected for 72 hours and urine for 24 hours. Radioactivity was not detected in the blood, and male urine contained 2.45%, whereas females contained 1.18%. The surface wash recovered 95.7%, suggesting a reasonable amount of mass balance demonstration. There was no parenteral control.

Objectives: Determine the extent of percutaneous absorption of ethylhexyl dimethyl PABA (padimate-O).

Methods:

- ^{14}C-labeled ethylhexyl dimethyl PABA in an ethanol solution applied to the forearms of subjects.
- $n = 4$ male and female.
- Dose spread over 100 cm^2 on forearms at 0.5 mg/cm^2 at a concentration of 8%. This is half the typical consumer dose.
- Forearms protected with gauze for 24 hours after ethanol evaporated.
- Blood collected at 0, 2, 4, 8, 24, and 72 hours.
- Urine collected in 24-hour period.

Results:

- Radioactivity not present in blood samples.
- 2.45% radioactivity in male urine and 1.18% radioactivity in females.
- Application site skin wash: average recovered radioactivity 95.7%.
- Using limited data, it is assumed that when 8% padimate-O was applied to 1.8 m^2 of skin, the absorbed amount was 13 mg (0.2 mg/kg).

Parenteral excretion control: None

TABLE 32.11

Penetration Data for a Lipophilic Octocrylene and Avobenzone

The dose was 2 mg/cm^2, which is twice the typical consumer dosage. the filter concentration was 2.34% for avobenzone and 10.85% of octocrylene. Twenty-eight volunteers were dosed, and blood was drawn up to 72 hours. The urine was collected over the duration of the study.

Neither avobenzone nor octocrylene were detected in urine or blood before this sunscreen exposure. Maximum plasma avobenzone concentration was 11 µg/L, and maximum octocrylene concentration was 25 µg/L

Low levels of avobenzone and octocrylene were measured in urine. There was no parenteral excretion control nor mass balance data. These data are readily compared to that of Matta.

Objectives: Determine the extent of octocrylene and avobenzone percutaneously absorbed.

Methods:

- Dose of 2 mg/cm^2 body surface area. This is the typical consumer dosage.
- UV filter concentration: 2.34% avobenzone, 10.85% octocrylene.
- Twenty-eight volunteers (14 men and 14 women).
- Mean age: 24.5, mean weight: 70.5 kg, mean height: 1.73 m.
- Blood samples drawn at 1.75, 3.75, 5.75, 7.75, 24, 48, and 72 hours.
- Urine collected over the duration of study.

Results:

- No avobenzone or octocrylene detected in urine or blood before sunscreen exposure.
- Maximum plasma avobenzone concentration: 11 µg/L.
- Maximum plasma octocrylene concentration: 25 µg/L.
- Low levels of octocrylene and avobenzone measured in urine.

Parenteral excretion control: None

Currently sunscreens are available as cosmetics in several vehicles, including creams, lotions, gels, and sprays. We have inadequate information regarding the effect of the vehicle on levels of sunscreen penetration. Table 32.5 demonstrates that the UV filters in an oil/water emulsion gel had far greater dermal penetration than the petroleum jelly vehicle, thus suggesting a considerable vehicle effect. Dragicevic and Maibach [13] provide a comprehensive overview of individual penetration enhancers, some of which have been considered for sunscreen usage.

The only data that allow us to know that the sunscreens are not stored in other body compartments such as fat and extracutaneous organs are the parenteral controls provided by Wester. Previously Feldmann had performed the study (but not with a parenteral control) on the forearm at a dose of 4 $\mu g/cm^2$ in an acetone vehicle with an absorption of 28.37%. Utilizing the subsequent parenteral control provided by Wester, this would be 4.5 times greater for the face, calculated by the Guy formula [14], such as that widely used in antiaging cosmetics. Clearly, future studies should clarify this aspect. An early Marzulli [15] study showed that the percutaneous penetration of hexachlorophene was greatly harmful in children and in newborns, explaining death in some. This suggests that percutaneous penetration of topically applied agents could be damaging in large quantities and for long periods of time, prompting the further study of the effects of the absorption of topically applied sunscreens.

REFERENCES

1. Matta MK, Zusterzeel R, Pilli NR, et al. Effect of Sunscreen Application Under Maximal Use Conditions on Plasma Concentration of Sunscreen Active Ingredients: A Randomized Clinical Trial. JAMA. 2019;321(21):2082–2091.
2. Sunscreens. (2018). The Medical Letter, 60(1553), 129–133.
3. Wester, R. C., Melendres, J., Sedik, L., Maibach, H., & Riviere, J. E. (1998). Percutaneous Absorption of Salicylic Acid, Theophylline, 2,4-Dimethylamine, Diethyl Hexyl Phthalic Acid, and p-Aminobenzoic Acid in the Isolated Perfused Porcine Skin Flap Compared to Man in Vivo. Toxicology and Applied Pharmacology, 151(1), 159–165.
4. Feldmann, R. J., and Maibach, H. I. (1970). Absorption of some organic compounds through the skin in man. Journal of Investigative Dermatology. 54, 399–404.
5. Couteau, C., Cullel, N. P., Connan, A., & Coiffard, L. (2001). Stripping method to quantify absorption of two sunscreens in human. International Journal of Pharmaceutics, 222(1), 153–157.
6. Rougier, A., Dupuis, D., Lotte, C., Roguet, R., Wester, R. C., and Maibach, H. I. (1986). Regional variation in percutaneous absorption in man: Measurement by the stripping method. Archives of Dermatological Research. 278, 465–469.
7. Chatelain, E., Gabard, B., & Surber, C. (2003). Skin Penetration and Sun Protection Factor of Five UV Filters: Effect of the Vehicle. Skin Pharmacology and Physiology, 16(1), 28–35.
8. Iannuccelli, V., Coppi, G., Sergi, S., Mezzena, M., & Scalia, S. (2007). In Vivo and In Vitro Skin Permeation of Butyl Methoxydibenzoylmethane from Liposheres. Skin Pharmacology and Physiology, 21(1), 30–38.
9. Janjua, N., Kongshoj, B., Andersson, A.-M., & Wulf, H. (2008). Sunscreens in Human Plasma and Urine after Repeated Whole-Body Topical Application. Journal of the European Academy of Dermatology and Venereology, 22(4), 456–461.
10. U.S. Food and Drug Administration (FDA). Clinical Pharmacology Review: NDA Number 22-009 2008: 23–24. https://www.accessdata.fda.gov/drugsatfda_docs/nda/2008/022009s000_ClinPharmR. pdf. Accessed March 25, 2020.
11. Sung, C. R., Kim, K.-B., Lee, J. Y., Lee, B.-M., & Kwack, S. J. (2019). Risk Assessment of Ethylhexyl Dimethyl PABA in Cosmetics. Toxicological Research, 35(2), 131–136.
12. Hiller, J., Klotz, K., Meyer, S., Uter, W., Hof, K., Greiner, A., Drexler, H. (2019). Systemic Availability of Lipophilic Organic UV Filters through Dermal Sunscreen Exposure. Environment International, 132, 105068.

13. Dragicevic, N., & Maibach, H. I. (2016). Percutaneous Penetration Enhancers: Chemical Methods in Penetration Enhancement. Springer.

14. Guy, R. H., & Maibach, H. I. (1984). Correction Factors for Determining Body Exposure from Forearm Percutaneous Absorption Data. Journal of Applied Toxicology,4(1), 26–28.

15. Marzulli F, Maibach H (1975) Relevance of Animal Models: The Hexachlorophene Story. In: Maibach H (ed) Animal Models in Dermatology. Churchill Livingstone, pp. 156–167.

16. Matveev, N. V., & Maibach, H. I. (2002). Factors Influencing the Amount of Topical Preparations Applied. Exogenous Dermatology, 1(2), 64–67.

33 Cutaneous Metabolism of Xenobiotics

Howard I. Maibach
University of California, San Francisco, California

CONTENTS

33.1 INTRODUCTION

The human skin is exposed to many topical agents, either intentionally or by accident. The variety of these foreign agents (xenobiotics) reflects the variety of their intended uses: cosmetics are intended, in theory, to decorate the skin rather than penetrate it, while dermatological drugs such as corticosteroids are intended to act locally within the skin, with little or minimal systemic action. Some drugs, such as nitroglycerin, are not intended to act at the skin, but at distant target organs, in this case, the coronary arteries.

Therefore, it is clear that the application of substances to human skin is widespread. One must pause to consider the consequences of this behavior with respect to the skin and the body as a whole. Although many preparations are placed on the skin on the assumption that the skin is biologically inert, this chapter demonstrates that many exogenous compounds are metabolized in skin (xenobiotic metabolism). We review the existence of enzymes that are capable of metabolizing cutaneous xenobiotics and some of the factors regulating their activity. Recent work documenting the metabolism of commonly prescribed drugs and environmental agents on the skin is also reviewed.

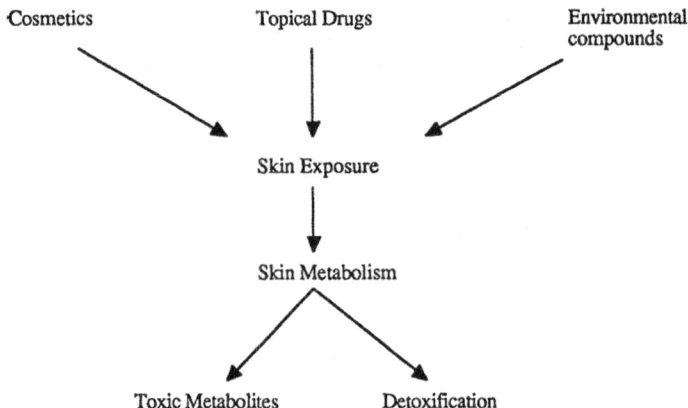

FIGURE 33.1   Metabolism of xenobiotics.

The role of cutaneous xenobiotic metabolism in the production of toxic metabolites, irritants, and allergens is discussed, in addition to the implication of cutaneous metabolism on transdermal drug delivery in healthy and damaged skin (Figure 33.1).

33.2   XENOBIOTIC-METABOLIZING ENZYMES

These are enzymes participating in the metabolism of foreign compounds. They metabolize substrates that are predominantly lipophilic (and thus penetrate the skin well) into substances that are hydrophilic and less active and can then be excreted in the urine via the kidney.

There are two distinct metabolic steps in their process. The first step is known as phase I reaction and introduces a polar reactive group into a molecule, which renders the molecule suitable for further metabolism as part of phase II reaction.

Phase I reactions include metabolism by cytochrome P450–dependent monooxygenases, which have been demonstrated in skin (1). These enzymes add a single oxygen atom from a molecule of O_2 to a carbon atom, resulting in the formation of an OH group on the substrate (hydroxylation) and one molecule of water, H_2O.

Subsequently, these metabolites formed by the phase I reaction by undergo further metabolism, known as phase II reactions. These are conjugation reactions, which render the substrate more hydrophilic, allowing renal excretion. Metabolites can be conjugated with substances such as glucuronic acid, sulfur, or glutathione, resulting in the production of easily excretable products.

33.3   PHASE I METABOLISM: CYTOCHROME P450 MONOOXYGENASES

The cytochrome P450 monooxygenase enzymes are microsomal enzymes demonstrated in the liver and other organs, including skin (2). They play an important role in the phase I metabolism of both exogenous and endogenous compounds such as fatty acids, prostaglandins, leukotrienes, and steroid hormones, and it has been suggested that many dermatological topical drugs are suitable substrates for their enzymes (3).

Cytochrome P450 enzymes are cofactor-dependent enzymes: They require energy from an external source such as NADPH to catalyze the reaction. This is in contrast to cofactor-independent reactions, which require only the enzyme to catalyze the reaction.

Cytochrome P450 exists in both prokaryotes and eukaryotes. In eukaryotes, the enzyme is mainly located in the membranes of the endoplasmic reticulum and the mitochondria. The structure of cytochrome P450 is a protoporphyrin ring that contains a centrally placed Fe^{3+} and a polypeptide chain of approximately 45,000 to 55,000 kDa (4).

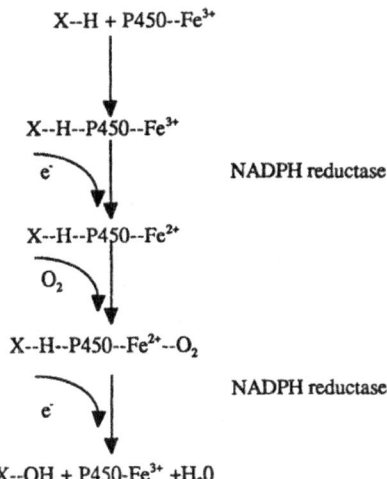

FIGURE 33.2   Mechanism of action of cytochrome P450. *Abbreviations*: X, Substrate; P450, cytochrome P450 enzyme.

The substrate to be metabolized binds to the protein moiety of the cytochrome P450, inducing a conformational change. This triggers the necessary cofactor NADPH–P450 reductase, which donates an electron to the cytochrome P450; the Fe^{3+} is reduced to Fe^{2+}.

This reduced cytochrome P450–substrate complex may now bind to a molecule of oxygen. Another electron is donated from NADPH–P450 reductase; the oxygen molecule is split into two oxygen atoms, with one binding to the substrate, which is then released from the enzyme as a hydroxylated product. The second oxygen atom is released as water (Figure 33.2) (4).

Evidence for the existence of cutaneous cytochrome P450 was initially obtained from the study of the carcinogenic effects of polycyclic aromatic hydrocarbons on the skin. The carcinogenic consequences of cutaneous metabolism are discussed later. Other more recent studies have demonstrated that cytochrome P450 metabolizes topically applied medications in a fashion similar to the metabolism of systemic medications by the liver.

For example, recent work has demonstrated the relevance of cytochrome P450 in the context of therapeutic agents. Ademola et al. (5) studied the diffusion and metabolism of theophylline using a flow-through *in vitro* system. Theophylline is metabolized in the liver by monooxygenases to the metabolites 1,3-dimethyluric acid, 3-methylxanthine, and 1-methyluric acid. In this study of *in vitro* human skin metabolism of theophylline, these metabolites were also found, suggesting that the cytochrome P450–dependent enzymes in the skin metabolized the xenobiotic.

33.3.1   ISOENZYMES OF CYTOCHROME P450

Many isoenzymes of cytochrome P450 exist (Table 33.1), and there are many genes that encode for them. No particular isoenzyme has unique substrate specificity; rather, there is an overlap of substrates. The isoenzymes are categorized by their amino acid similarities into families, named with the root CYP followed by the family number, a capital letter denoting the subfamily, and a number identifying the particular form.

The family CYP1 has been implicated in xenobiotic metabolism, and the families CYP2 and CYP3 in the metabolism of both xenobiotics and steroids. The CYP1A1 is a well-studied member of the cytochrome P450 family and is expressed in the skin (6). The CYPs, including CYP1A1, are normally expressed at a low level in the skin; however, their activity can be induced by a variety of agents, discussed later in this chapter.

TABLE 33.1

Cytochrome P450 Isomers Determined in Mammals and Their Functions

Isomer	Function
CYP 1	Metabolism of xenobiotics
CYP 2	Metabolism of xenobiotics and steroids
CYP 3	Metabolism of xenobiotics and steroids
CYP 4	Fatty acid ω and ω-1 hydroxylation
CYP 5	Thromboxane synthase
CYP 7	Cholesterol 7α-hydroxylase
CYP 11	Steroid 11 β-hydroxylase
CYP 17	Steroid 17 β-hydroxylase
CYP 19	Aromatase
CYP 21	Steroid 21-hydroxylase
CYP 24	Vitamin D-25 hydroxylase
CYP 27	Cholesterol 27-hydroxylase

33.4   PHASE II METABOLISM

Much of the literature on cutaneous metabolism of xenobiotics focuses on phase I reactions, especially on the role of cytochrome P450 enzymes. However, phase I reactions are only part of the metabolic process. Following the phase I reaction, the metabolite must be conjugated to facilitate its elimination.

33.4.1   TRANSFERASES

Transferase activities in the skin can be as high as 10% of that of the liver. In comparison, the relative activity of cytochrome P450 in skin may be only 1% to 5% of the liver's (7). Raza et al. (8) have demonstrated the presence of glutathione S-transferase in skin. Higo et al. (9) have shown that the cutaneous metabolism of nitroglycerin (GTN) to 1,2-GDN (glyceryl di-nitrate) and 1,3-GDN is heavily dependent on the presence of glutathione, which is a cofactor for the transferase enzyme. They exposed GTN to skin homogenates with and without the glutathione cofactor to determine its role in cutaneous metabolism. In the tissue with the cofactor, 30% of the GTN was metabolized within two hours, whereas only 5% of the GTN was metabolized in the tissue without glutathione.

Glycine conjugation is another mechanism of metabolism in the skin. Nasseri-Sina et al. (10) described glycine conjugation in both human and rat keratinocytes.

The metabolic pathway involves the activation of the carboxylic acid group with coenzyme A (CoA) in an adenosine triphosphate (ATP)–dependent reaction. This is followed by the reaction of the S-CoA derivative with the glycine molecule, catalyzed by a mitochondrial acyltransferase. The resulting glycine conjugation renders the metabolite more polar than the parent compound, and it can then be excreted renally (Figure. 33.3).

Nasseri-Sina et al. (10) investigated the metabolism of benzoic acid, used topically for the treatment of tinea infestations. Benzoic acid, when administered systemically, is excreted as hippuric acid in urine. This group found that cultured keratinocytes in both humans and rats also metabolized benzoic acid to hippuric acid, but to a much smaller extent than hepatocytes.

Both of the studies just described demonstrated that transferase activity may play a significant role in the metabolism of topically applied compounds.

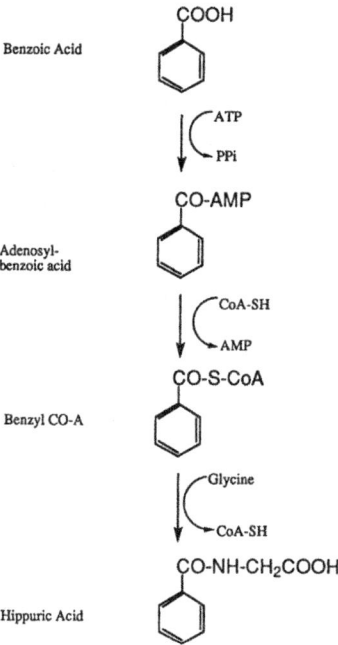

COOH

Benzoic Acid

ATP
PPi

CO-AMP

Adenosyl-
benzoic acid

CoA-SH
AMP

CO-S-CoA

Benzyl CO-A

Glycine
CoA-SH

CO-NH-CH₂COOH

Hippuric Acid

FIGURE 33.3 Metabolism of benzoic acid: An example of a conjugation reaction.

33.5 EXAMPLES OF XENOBIOTIC METABOLISM

33.5.1 CORTICOSTEROIDS

Topical corticosteroids are extensively prescribed for dermatological conditions. Kubota et al. (11) studied the metabolism of betamethasone 17-valerate (B-17) in the living skin equivalent (LSE) model. The betamethasone 17-valerate was initially isomerized to beta-methasone 21-valerate (B-21) before it was hydrolyzed to the more polar betamethasone. The rate of conversion of B-17 to B-21 was the same with or without skin homogenate, suggesting that the initial isomerization step was not enzyme dependent but possibly a passive chemical degradation.

Taking this study further, Kubota et al. (12) compared the rates of metabolism of the two isomers B-17 and B-21. When the B-17 isomer was applied to the LSE, half of the drug was left unchanged. In contrast, when B-21 was applied to the LSE, almost all of the drug was metabolized. Thus, the esterases that are responsible for this second, enzyme-dependent step demonstrate preference for the B-21 isomer.

Applying this knowledge in the human setting, Ademola and Maibach (13) demonstrated that the B-17 isomer is metabolized to form the B-21 isomer and betamethasone in both human skin *in vivo* and in the LSE model. This work showed that the B-17 isomer accumulated in the human skin. This was possibly because the B-21 isomer was metabolized faster than the B-17 isomer, which would be consistent with isomeric preference shown *in vitro*.

These studies have therefore shown that corticosteroids are metabolized in human skin. Further, this metabolism may involve a passive step of chemical degradation as well as active enzyme-dependent metabolism. Importantly, the isomeric structure of the topical agent may influence the rate of metabolism within the skin. Therefore, different isomers of the same compound may be more or less suitable than one another for topical application. This must be considered in the study of any agent to which the skin is exposed.

33.5.2 BETA-ADRENOCEPTOR ANTAGONISTS

Propranolol is a widely prescribed, highly lipophilic beta-adrenoceptor antagonist. As it is lipophilic, having a partition coefficient of 5.39 at pH 7.0, the topical route of administration may theoretically achieve a steady drug release and plasma concentration. Oral propranolol is subject to first-pass metabolism, leading to variable adsorption and low systemic bioavailability.

Ademola et al. (14), studying percutaneous absorption and metabolism of propranolol *in vitro* using intact human skin and microsomal preparations, found that between 10.4% and 36.6% of the drug was absorbed, but only 4.1% to 16.1% of the drug penetrated the skin. Some propranolol was retained in the skin, and metabolites of propranolol were found. Naphthoxyacetic acid, 4-hydroxypropanolol, and N-desisopropyl propranolol were formed by intact human skin. The concentration of these metabolites was lower compared with hepatic metabolism, suggesting less enzymatic activity in the skin compared to the liver. These metabolites were also formed by the skin microsomes in a greater concentration than in intact skin. This may be the result of the greater surface area that the microsomes (everted endoplasmic reticulum) had to react with the drug. Additionally, the microsomes biotransformed propranolol to norpropranolol, which the intact skin did not form.

Ademola and Maibach (13) took this study further, using human, LSE, and keratinocyte models. Propranolol does indeed accumulate in human skin, which may be responsible for its irritant or toxic effects. They suggest that the differences between the metabolism of propranolol in skin and liver may explain the accumulation of the drug in the skin. This difference could not be attributed to the degree of enzyme activity, as the enzyme saturation points in the metabolism of propranolol in liver and skin were similarly high.

Ademola and Maibach postulated that the difference in metabolism may lie in the stereoisomeric structure. Using racemic propranolol, they demonstrated that the S-enantiomer was eliminated more efficiently by the skin than the R-enantiomer. This is in contrast to hepatocytes, which are more efficient at removing the R-enantiomer (15). Therefore, the irritation caused by the topical application of propranolol may be the result of accumulation of the R-enantiomer (16).

These studies therefore suggest that propranolol is metabolized by human skin and that its metabolism may be stereoselective. This metabolism and the retention of propranolol in the skin may explain both the low plasma concentration and irritant dermatitis after topical application.

33.5.3 TOPICAL NITRATES

Higo et al. (9) used intact skin and homogenates from hairless mice to study the metabolism of nitroglycerin. In the homogenate study, GTN was incubated with homogenized tissue. After two hours of incubation, 30% of the GTN had been metabolized to the breakdown products 1,2- and 1,3-GDN. This metabolism was shown to be heavily dependent on the presence of glutathione (see earlier). Using the intact skin model, the investigators compared the extent of metabolism using different formulations of the GTN: a 1-mg/mL aqueous solution, a 2% ointment, and a transdermal delivery system. The percentage of metabolites formed was greatest with the aqueous solution (61%), followed by the patch (49%), and least of all with the ointment (35%). This difference is thought to be explained by the greater transdermal flux with the patch and ointment compared to the solution: The smaller the flux, the greater the relative level of skin metabolism.

33.5.4 THEOPHYLLINE

Theophylline is a xanthine derivative that is used as a bronchodilator. Ademola et al. (5) studied the effect of cutaneous metabolism on its topical administration. This drug has a narrow therapeutic index at which optimal bronchodilation is maintained with minimal adverse effects occurring. Considering this, topical administration may give theoretical advantage over the oral route, as the latter results in variable plasma concentrations and is subject to altered absorption with the presence

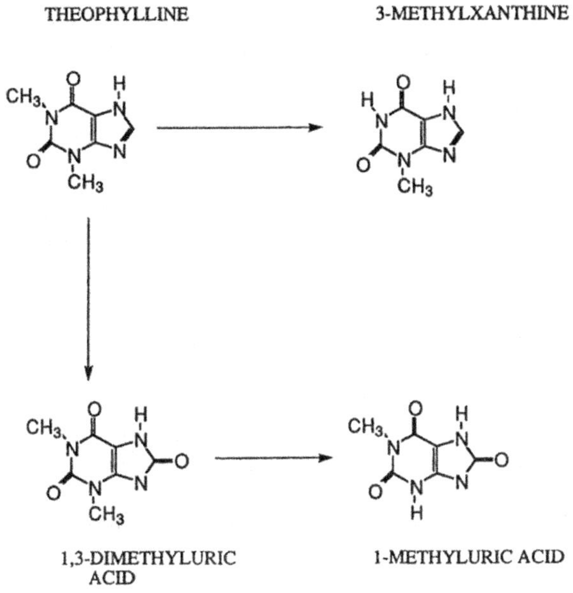

FIGURE 33.4 Pathways of theophylline metabolism.

or absence of food in the gastrointestinal tract. Using both human skin samples and its microsomes, Ademola et al. determined that theophylline was metabolized with the production of 1,3-dimethyl uric acid, 3-methyl uric acid, and 3-methylxanthine from the skin samples. These metabolites of theophylline are produced via cytochrome P450–dependent metabolism in the liver, and the authors proposed that a similar mechanism may occur in skin (Figure 33.4).

33.6 METABOLISM OF ENVIRONMENTAL XENOBIOTICS

An important consideration in this subject is the metabolism by the skin of compounds it is exposed to in the environment. The skin forms a barrier against our environment and is constantly exposed to compounds both natural and manmade. In this section, we address the effects of their metabolism.

33.6.1 POLYCYCLIC AROMATIC HYDROCARBONS

Polycyclic aromatic hydrocarbons (PAHs) are produced by the incomplete combustion of fossil fuels and other organic matter. Their potential role in human carcinogenesis is suggested by their presence in the environment and the carcinogenicity of their metabolites.

Cutaneous metabolism of PAH is capable of forming carcinogenic metabolites (see Ref. 17 for review). Studies with model compounds such as benzo[a]pyrene have demonstrated that cutaneous metabolism of PAHs can lead to the formation of phenols, quinones, dihydrodiols, and reactive diol epoxides. The diol epoxides are thought to be responsible for the carcinogenic effect, binding covalently to macromolecules. Covalent binding with DNA correlates well with the tumorigenicity of the metabolites of benzo[a]pyrone (18).

The PAHs are present in crude coal tar, which is extensively used in dermatological practice. Merk et al. (19) demonstrated that exposure of crude coal tar to the human hair follicle results in the induction of aromatic hydrocarbon hydroxylase (AHH), which is a cytochrome P450–dependent enzyme. This resulted in the production of benzo[a]pyrene derivatives that were shown to bind to DNA.

These studies of PAHs therefore exemplify the potentially hazardous nature of the cutaneous metabolism of environmental xenobiotics. We discuss the metabolism of other environmental agents and their potential for toxicity next.

33.6.2 PESTICIDES

Ademola et al. (20) studied the cutaneous metabolism of an environmental pesticide, 2-chloro-2,6-diethyl-*N*-(butoxymethyl) acetanilide (butachlor), on human skin *in vitro*. This study is significant in our discussion of the role of cutaneous metabolism in our everyday lives and its potential consequences. Skin is the most important route of exposure to such agents; topical exposure could result in systemic absorption, which may be toxic, and also could result in cutaneous or systemic metabolism, either of which could toxify or detoxify the compound. In this study, the butachlor was metabolized to 4-hydroxybutachlor and was NADPH dependent, implying that the metabolism may be dependent on monooxygenases in the skin. The 4-hydroxy-butachlor metabolite was noted to accumulate in skin.

Cysteine- and glutathione-conjugated metabolites were also found. The formation of glutathione conjugates is consistent with the known presence of glutathione in human skin (8). Although the significance of these metabolites is not yet known, their formation and accumulation in the skin may be potentially hazardous.

Ademola et al. (21) also investigated the metabolism of a widely used herbicide, atrazine, within the skin. The metabolites 2-chloro-4-ethyl-amino-6-amino-*s*-triazine (desisopropylatrazine) and 2-chloro-4,6-diamino-s-triazine were found in the receptor fluid and the skin supernates. An additional metabolite (2-chloro-4-amino-6-iso-propylamino-s-triazine) was found in the skin supernates. This study again showed that metabolites of an environmental agent can be produced in the skin, further reinforcing the need for the detailed study of skin metabolism as a possible source of pathology (Table 33.2).

TABLE 33.2
Examples of Some Xenobiotics and Their Metabolites

Compound	Major Metabolites	Comment
Betamethasone 17-valerate	Betamethasone 21-valerate	Chemical degradation
Propranolol	Betamethasone	Active metabolism
	Naphthoxyacetic acid	Produced by intact skin
	4-Hydroxypropanolol	Produced by intact skin
	N-Desisopropyl propranolol	Produced by intact skin
	Norpropranolol	Only produced by microsomes
Nitroglycerin	1,2-GDN	
Theophylline	1,3-GDN	
	1,3-Dimethyl uric acid	
	3-Methyl uric acid	
	3-Methyl xanthene	
Polycyclic aromatic hydrocarbons	Phenols	
	Quinones	
	Dihydrodiols	
	Diol epoxides	Carcinogenic
Butachlor	4-Hydroxybutachlor cysteine conjugates	
	Glutathione conjugates	
Atrazine	Desisopropylatrazine	
	2-Chloro-4,6-diamino-*s*-triazine	

33.7 FACTORS AFFECTING CUTANEOUS METABOLISM

The factors that influence the metabolism of cutaneous xenobiotics can be dynamic or static. Dynamic metabolism may vary according to the physiological and pathological condition of the skin. In contrast, static factors may be related to the structure of the skin at a particular site.

33.7.1 DYNAMIC FACTORS

The dynamic response of enzymes to inductive and inhibitory stimuli could be an important factor in determining the extent of metabolism within the skin. Also, in the case of isoenzymes, such as the cytochrome P450 family, which particular isoenzymes are induced and in what proportions must be considered.

33.7.1.1 Enzyme Induction

The induction of enzymes that metabolize xenobiotics may increase the rate and/or amount of metabolites produced. Some xenobiotics may induce enzymes for which they themselves are substrates or may induce enzymes that act on other exogenous or endogenous substrates.

Schlede and Connely (22) demonstrated a tenfold increase in AHH activity in skin homogenates from rats pretreated with 3-methychloranthene. The AHH is a cytochrome P450–dependent enzyme associated with the expression of CYP1A1 (3). Further studies have shown that topically applied polycyclic hydrocarbons, coal tar, and petroleum derivatives are also effective in the induction of AHH in human skin (17).

Jugert et al. (23) studied the effect of topically applied dexamethasone on the induction of cutaneous cytochrome P450 isoenzymes in murine skin. The induction of cytochromes 1A1, 2B1, 2E, and 3A was seen, in addition to induction of the monooxygenase enzymes catalyzed by these CYPs. The group further employed immunohistochemistry to localize the expression of the CYP2B1 isoenzyme within the epidermis. This particular isoenzyme was investigated, as it was involved in the greatest enzyme induction. The isoenzyme was localized to the suprabasal layer of the epidermis and the cells of the hair follicle.

That dexamethasone can induce several isoenzymes of cytochrome P450 is a significant finding because the cytochrome P450 monooxygenases are not substrate specific. Therefore, if one substrate induces a series of enzymes, other xenobiotics that are applied to the skin, either intentionally or unintentionally, may be metabolized at an increased rate. For example, if one comes in contact with benzo[a]pyrone while using topical corticosteroids for atopic dermatitis, the metabolism of carcinogenic metabolites could be increased.

33.7.1.2 Enzyme Activity Inhibition

In contrast to induction, the inhibition of enzymes must also be considered. Inhibition of the cutaneous metabolism of xenobiotics has several theoretical advantages. For example, selectively inhibiting an enzyme may increase the overall percutaneous absorption of a particular medication. Kao and Carver (17) reviewed work in this field. The imidazole antifungal agents, widely prescribed in dermatological practice, are potent inhibitors of the microsomal P450–dependent monooxygenases. In skin, they inhibit the activity of AHH and epoxide hydrolase activity (EPOH). Also, imidazoles induce glutathione-s-transferase activity and inhibit the cutaneous metabolism, macromolecular binding, and carcinogenicity of topically applied benzopyrene in cultured mouse keratinocytes (24). Plant phenols also inhibit the monooxygenase metabolism of benzo[a]pyrene *in vitro* (25). The studies suggest that inhibitors of xenometabolizing enzymes may be useful in the prevention of polycyclic hydrocarbon skin malignancies.

33.7.2 BARRIER DISRUPTIONS AND CUTANEOUS XENOMETABOLISM

Several studies have attempted to study the metabolism of xenobiotics following disruption of the skin barrier. Higo et al. (26) studied the effect of skin condition *in vitro* on the cutaneous metabolism of nitroglycerin. Full-thickness excised skin from hairless mice was placed in a plastic bag prior to immersion in boiling water for 10 minutes. Heating the skin disrupted its barrier function, a fact that can be inferred from the increased total nitrate flux across the heated skin compared to controls. The skin did continue to metabolize the GTN; however, compared to control skin, the heated skin showed a preference for the formation of 1,3-GDN rather than 1,2-GTN. The heated tissue continued to metabolize the nitroglycerin at a steady rate during the 10-hour experiment, whereas the control specimen's metabolism decreased with time. This suggests that the altered metabolism may be the result of nonenzymatic metabolism of the drug. In the same study, the authors also damaged the skin barrier using tape stripping. The greater the number of strippings, the more damaged the skin was, with greater flux of nitrates and less metabolic activity.

However, Shaikh et al. (27) demonstrated that freezing human skin did not alter its metabolic capacity. Investigating the metabolism of 8-methoxypsoralen (8-MOP) on human skin *in vitro*, it was demonstrated that the skin barrier had been perturbed, as there was a greater flux of 8-MOP in the frozen specimen compared to the control. However, the metabolic capacity of the skin remained constant.

Different insults to the human skin barrier may alter the metabolism of xenobiotics in different ways. These studies demonstrate that further investigation of skin barrier function in cutaneous metabolism is necessary. As products for topical use become increasingly popular, their use on damaged skin must be investigated.

33.8   CONSEQUENCES OF CUTANEOUS XENOBIOTIC METABOLISM

For any drug metabolized in the skin, the potentially toxic nature of any metabolite must be considered. For example, a metabolite may be irritant, allergenic, or even carcinogenic, either locally or systemically. The precarcinogen benzo[a]pyrene was described earlier as an example of this, as was the metabolism of propranolol.

The ability of the enzymes responsible for xenometabolism to be induced or inhibited may affect the rate and extent of metabolism of any compound on the skin. This may affect the efficacy of drugs applied topically either for local or systemic administration. Indeed, there is potential for topical formulations to include inhibitors of enzymes to enhance drug delivery.

Metabolism of the drug at the cutaneous level constitutes "first-pass metabolism," which may result in subtherapeutic doses reaching the systemic circulation. Indeed, the metabolic activity of the enzymes may be dynamic rather than static; this implies that under different physiological and pathological conditions, variable doses of the drug may be delivered through the skin, perhaps resulting in toxicity or decreased effectiveness. Particular regard must therefore be paid to drugs of narrow therapeutic index.

33.9   CONCLUSION

This chapter has demonstrated that cutaneous metabolism is relevant in the application of any topical agent to the skin, whether for superficial use or end-organ effect.

REFERENCES

1. Goerz G. Animal models for cutaneous drug metabolising enzymes. In: Maibach HI, Lowe NJ, eds. Models in Dermatology. Vol. III. Basel: Karger, 1989:93–105.
2. Gonzalez FJ. The molecular biology of cytochrome P450s. Pharmacol Rev 1989; 40:243–388.
3. Ahmad N, Agarwal R, Mukhtar H. Cytochrome P450-dependent drug metabolism in skin. Clin Dermatol 1996; 14:407–415.
4. Goeptar AR, Scheerens H, Vermeulen NP. Oxygen and xenobiotic reductase activities of cytochrome P450. Crit Rev Toxicol 1995; 25(1):25–65.
5. Ademola JI, Wester RC, Maibach HH. Cutaneous metabolism of theophylline by human skin. J Invest Dermatol 1992; 98(3):310–314.

6. Bickers DR, Dutta-Chaudhury T, Mukhtar H. Epidermis: A site of drug metabolism in rat skin. Studies on cytochrome P450 content and mixed function oxidase and epoxide hydrolase activity. Mol Pharmacol 1982; 21:239–247.
7. Merk HF, Jergert FK, Frankenberg S. Biotransformations in the skin. In: Marzulli FN, Maibach HI, eds. Dermatoxicology. 5th ed. Ch. 6. Washington, DC: Taylor & Francis, 1996:61–76.
8. Raza H, Awasthi YC, Zaim MT, Eckert RL, Mukhtar H. Glutathione-S transferase in human and rodent skin; Multiple forms and species specific expression. J Invest Dermatol 1991; 96:463–467.
9. Higo N, Hinz RS, Lau DTW, Benet LZ, Guy RH. Cutaneous metabolism of nitroglycerin in vitro. Pharm Res 1992a; 9(2):187–191.
10. Nasseri-Sina P, Hotchkiss SA, Caldwell J. Cutaneous xenobiotic metabolism glycine conjugation in human and rat keratinocytes. Food and Chemical Toxicology 1997; 35(3–4):409–416.
11. Kubota K, Ademola JI, Maibach HI. Metabolism of topical drugs within the skin, in particular glucocorticoids. In: Korting HC, Maibach HI, eds. Topical Glucocorticoids with Increased Benefit/Risk Ratio. Current Problems in Dermatology. Vol. 21. Basel: Karger, 1993:61–66.
12. Kubota K, Ademola JI, Maibach HI. Simultaneous diffusion and metabolism of betamethasone 17-valerate in the living skin equivalent. J Pharm Sci 1995; 84(12):1478–1481.
13. Ademola JI, Maibach HI. Cutaneous metabolism and penetration of methoxypsoralen, betamethasone 17-valerate, retinoic acid, nitroglycerin and theophylline. Curr Problems Dermatol 1995; 22:201–213.
14. Ademola JI, Chow CA, Wester RC, Maibach HI. Metabolism of propanolol during percutaneous absorption in human skin. J Pharm Sci 1991; 82(8):767–770.
15. Ward S, Walle T, Walle K, Wilkinson GR, Branch RA. Propanolol's metabolism is determined by both mephenytoin and debrisoquin hydroxylase. Clin Pharm Ther 1989; 45:72–78.
16. Melendres JL, Nangia A, Sedik L, Mitsuhiko H, Maibach HI. Nonane enhances propanolol hydrochloride penetration in human skin. Int J Pharm 1992; 92:243–248.
17. Kao J, Carver MP. Skin metabolism. In: Marzulli N, Maibach HI, eds. Dermatotoxicology. 4th ed. Washington, DC: Hemisphere, 1991:143–200.
18. Mukhtar H, Agarwal R, Bickers DR. Cutaneous metabolism of xenobiotics and steroid hormones. In: Mukhtar H, ed. Pharmacology of the Skin. Boca Raton, FL: CRC Press, 1992:89–110.
19. Merk HF, Mukhtar H, Kaufmann I, Das M, Bickers DR. Human hair follicle benzo(a)-pyrene and benzo(a)pyrene 7,8-diol metabolism; Effect of exposure to a crude coal tar containing shampoo. J Invest Dermatol 1987; 88:71–76.
20. Ademola JI, Wester RC, Maibach HI. Absorption and metabolism of 2-chloro-2,6-diethyl-N-(butoxymethyl)acetanilide (butachlor) in human skin in vitro. Toxicol Appl Pharmacol 1993a; 121(1):78–86.
21. Ademola JI, Sedik LE, Wester RC, Maibach HI. In vitro percutaneous absorption and metabolism in man of 2-chloro-4-ethyl amino-6-isopropylamine-s-triazine (atrazine). Arch Toxicol 1993b; 67(2):85–91.
22. Schlede E, Connely AH. Induction of benzo(a)pyrene hydroxylase activity in rat skin. Life Sci 1970; 9(II):1305–1303.
23. Jugert FK, Agarwal R, Kuhn A, Bickers DR, Merk HF, Mukhtar H. Multiple cytochrome P450 isozymes in murine skin: induction of P450 1A, 2B, 2E, and 3A by dexamethasone. J Invest Dermatol 1994; 102(6):970–975.
24. Das M, Mukhtar H, Del Tito BJ Jr, Marcelo CL, Bickers DR. Clotrimaozole, an inhibitor of benzo(a) pyrene metabolism and its subsequent glucuronidation, Sulfation, and macromolecular binding in BALB/c mouse culured keratinocytes. J Invest Dermatol 1986; 87:4–10.
25. Das M, Mukhtar H, Bik DP, Bickers DR. Inhibition of epidermal xenobiotic metabolism in SENCAR mice by naturally occurring phenols. Cancer Res 1987; 47:760–766.
26. Higo N, Hinz RS, Lau DTW, Benet LZ, Guy RH. Cutaneous metabolism of nitroglycerin in vitro. II. Effects of skin condition and penetration enhancement. Pharm Res 1992a; 9(3):303–306.
27. Shaikh NA, Ademola JI, Maibach HI. Effects of freezing and azide treatment of in vitro human skin on the flux and metabolism of 8-methoxypsoralen. Skin Pharmacol 1996; 9:274–280.

34 Chemical Modification

An Important and Feasible Method for Improving Peptide and Protein Dermal and Transdermal Delivery

Seyedeh Maryam Mortazavi and Hamid R. Moghimi
Shahid Beheshti University of Medical Sciences,
Tehran, Iran

Howard I. Maibach
University of California, San Francisco, California

CONTENTS

34.1 INTRODUCTION

While peptides and proteins have attracted much attention as therapeutic agents (Bruno et al. 2013), their delivery through almost all administration routes encounters considerable challenges. Routes of administration for peptides and proteins include parenteral, oral, nasal, buccal, ocular, rectal, vaginal, pulmonary, and topical/transdermal pathways (Sanders 1990). Each administration route has advantages and limitations over other routes. Among these routes, paying attention to the skin for the delivery of peptides and proteins is remarkable for the following reasons: avoidance of gastrointestinal degradation and hepatic first-pass effect (some limitations of the oral route) (Bodde et al. 1989; Bruno et al. 2013); increasing patient compliance (Brown et al. 2006; Prausnitz & Langer 2008) (one of the most important limitations of the parenteral route and, to some extent, the rectal route); longer residence time in the case of controlled drug delivery, especially by adhesive systems compared to nasal and pulmonary routes (due to lack of mucociliary clearance) and also buccal, rectal and vaginal routes (because of lower membrane turnover and possibility of detachment); lower proteolytic activity compared to the mucosal routes (Foldvari et al. 1998); and finally the possibility of abrupt termination of drug delivery (Brown et al. 2006). However, in spite of their advantages, it has not been possible to deliver most peptides and proteins through the skin in therapeutic amounts due to the hydrophilic nature and high molecular weight (Benson & Namjoshi 2008; Gorouhi & Maibach 2009; Zhou et al. 2017). To overcome these problems, various approaches have been applied from penetration enhancers to physical methods (Amsden & Goosen 1995; Benson & Namjoshi 2008; Kalluri & Banga 2011).

Here, the possibility of skin permeation of peptides and proteins and chemical modification approaches for the enhancement of transdermal and topical delivery of these difficult molecules are reviewed.

34.2 SKIN PERMEATION OF PEPTIDES AND PROTEINS

Given the nature of the intercellular space, hydrophobic compounds are more appropriate to permeate across the intact stratum corneum than hydrophilic compounds, but considering the permeation process, a balance between hydrophilicity and hydrophobicity is essential to cross the skin (Subedi et al. 2010). Hence, there is an optimum value for hydrophobicity so that the desired log partition coefficient (1-octanol/water) is in the range of 1 to 3. In addition to hydrophobicity, another important limitation is to have a molecular weight of approximately less than 500 Da (Gujjar et al. 2016; Subedi et al. 2010). As a result, peptides and proteins are not good candidates for topical/transdermal delivery due to their high molecular size and hydrophilic nature (Falconer & Toth 2007). Apart from these, the peptides and proteins are mainly charged molecules at physiological pH (Benson & Namjoshi 2008) and in this respect also they are not suitable for crossing the skin (Wang et al. 2005).

Different approaches have been applied to increase skin permeation of peptides and proteins. These approaches include application of chemical penetration enhancers, encapsulation into hydrophobic carriers, physical enhancement methods, and chemical modification. The first three strategies have been extensively reviewed (Alexander et al. 2012; Naik et al. 2000; Singh et al. 2012), but there is a considerable absence of information about research performed in the field of chemical modification of peptides and proteins. However, chemical modification could increase the metabolic and chemical stability (Bundgaard & Møss 1999; Toth et al. 1994), as well as skin absorption of peptides and proteins (Foldvari et al. 1998; Møss & Bundgaard 1990). Thus, the investigations on the influences of chemical modification on biological activity, enzymatic stability, and skin permeation are comprehensively reviewed here.

34.3 CHEMICAL MODIFICATION OF PEPTIDES AND PROTEINS

Chemical modification can be defined as a process in which a chemical moiety is incorporated into the native structure of peptides or proteins (Buckley et al. 2016). Such modifications can be used to increase the permeability of molecules across biological barriers, as well as to increase the metabolic or enzymatic stability. The two main categories of chemical moieties that have been employed to date for the improvement of topical and transdermal delivery of peptides and proteins include hydrophobic moieties and cell-penetrating peptides (CPPs). Thus, two approaches are discussed here.

From a mechanistic view, hydrophobic moieties increase the tendency of peptides and proteins to the intercellular lipid matrix by enhancing the partition coefficient of these macromolecules. In fact, they change the physicochemical properties of peptides and proteins. CPPs act in a different manner; they decrease the resistance of the diffusional barrier (intercellular lipid matrix and keratins) and consequently increase the diffusion coefficient of peptides and proteins.

34.3.1 Peptide or Protein Conjugation with Hydrophobic Moieties

Various hydrophobic moieties (e.g., simple lipoamino acids [LAA], fatty acids, etc.) have been applied to improve skin delivery of peptides and proteins. Simple LAA is a single amino acid that is combined with a fatty acid (Xia 2001), but fatty acids are straight hydrocarbon chains with a functional group of carboxylic acid. Butyric acid (C4), caproic acid (C6), octanoic acid (C8), lauric acid (C12), myristic acid (C14), palmitic acid (C16), stearic acid (C18), oleic acid (C18), C6 LAA, C8 LAA, and C10 LAA are some hydrophobic moieties that have been used to increase skin permeation of peptides and proteins (see Table 34.1) (Caccetta et al. 2006; Choi et al. 2014; Foldvari et al. 1998, 1999; Gozes et al. 1994; Namjoshi et al. 2014; Setoh et al. 1995; Toth et al. 1995; Yamamoto et al. 2003). The chemical structures of some parent peptides that have undergone chemical modification are presented in Figure 34.1.

LAAs, which possess the structural characteristics of lipids and α-amino acids, can increase percutaneous drug absorption (Ziora et al. 2012). Namjoshi et al. (2014) applied a racemic mixture of LAAs (carbon chain length C6, C8, and C10) for conjugation to the tetrapeptide AAPV (Ala-Ala-Pro-Val), a human neutrophil elastase inhibitor. Human epidermal permeation of all conjugates exceeded that of AAPV. The ability for epidermal permeation of AAPV and its derivatives was in the following order: C8 (D,L)-LAA-AAPV > C10 (D,L)-LAA-AAPV > C6 (D,L)-LAA-AAPV > AAPV. The authors concluded that there is an optimal carbon chain length for skin permeation. The stereoselective epidermal permeation was also reported so that the D-diastereomers were

TABLE 34.1
Examples of Chemically Modified Peptides and Proteins by Hydrophobic Moieties

Peptide or Protein Name	MW (Da)	Length (aa)	Conjugated Moiety (Carbon Atoms Number)	Permeation Study Type	Formulation Vehicle	Reference
Phe-Gly	222.2	2	Short-chain fatty acids (C4,C6,C8)	Franz-diffusion cells (statistic)	Not mentioned	(Yamamoto et al. 2003)
AAPV	356.4	4	Short-chain LAAs (C6, C8, and C10) and short-chain fatty acids (C7)	Franz-diffusion cells (statistic)	Propylene glycol	(Caccetta et al. 2006; Namjoshi et al. 2014; Rocco et al. 2016)
TRH	362.4	3	Chloroformate (C5, C9)	Franz-diffusion cells (statistic)	Phosphate buffer or propylene glycol	(Møss & Bundgaard 1990)
KTTKS	563.6	5	Long-chain fatty acid (C16)	Franz-diffusion cells (statistic)	15% ethanol	(Choi et al. 2014)
Tetragastrin	596.7	4	Short-chain fatty acids (C2,C4,C6)	Franz-diffusion cells (statistic)	Not mentioned	(Setoh et al. 1995)
[D-Lys][6] GnRH	1253.4	10	Short- and long-chain fatty acids (C2, C6, C12, C18)	Measurement of LH level in the blood	DMSO	(Yahalom et al. 1999)
VIP	3326.8	28	Long-chain fatty acid (C18)	Distribution measurement of radioactively labeled compounds in the various organs	I-Monocapryloyl-rac-glycerol and DMSO	(Gozes et al. 1994)
IFN-α2b	19271	165	Long-chain fatty acid (C16)	Franz-diffusion cells (flow-through)	Phosphate buffer or methylcellulose gel hydrated with phosphate buffer	(Foldvari et al. 1998)

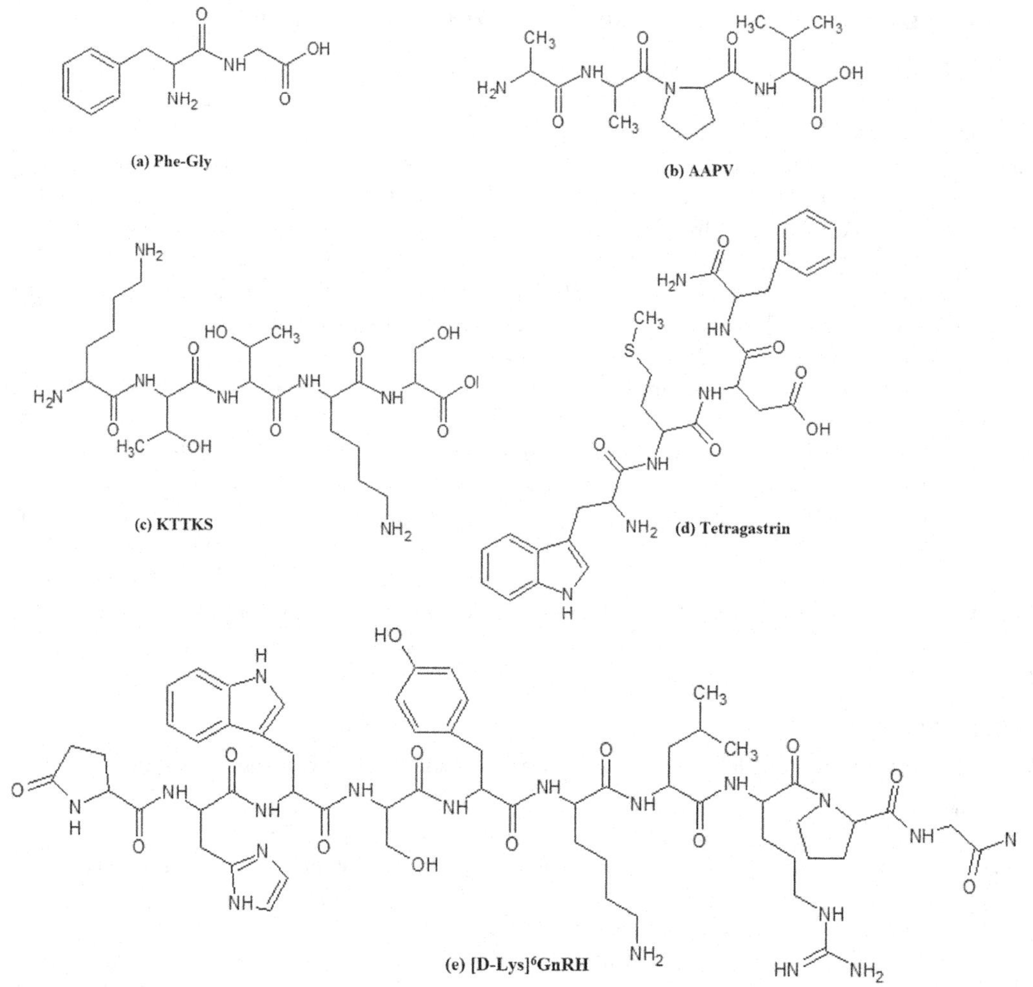

FIGURE 34.1 Chemical structures of some parent peptides that have undergone chemical modification.

more permeable than L-diastereomers. This stereoselectivity in skin permeation was attributed to the presence of chiral ceramide molecules in the intercellular lipid domain of the stratum corneum, which led to stereospecific interactions with the conjugates. In addition, conjugation caused enhanced peptide stability against enzymatic attack in the skin without causing much reduction in the biological activity of AAPV.

Chemical modification of a peptide using a racemic mixture of LAA leads to generation of a mixture of D and L stereoisomers, which interact with the skin lipids differently (Caccetta et al. 2006; Namjoshi et al. 2014; Rocco et al. 2016). However, production of the single stereoisomer is expensive and time-consuming (Rocco et al. 2016).

In addition to LAA lipidation of AAPV (Caccetta et al. 2006; Namjoshi et al. 2014; Toth et al. 1995), acyl lipidation was reported (Rocco et al. 2016). Transepidermal permeation of L-C7-AAPV and L-AAPV-C7 analogs of AAPV through human abdominal skin was evaluated with Franz-type diffusion cells. Based on the result, acyl lipidation was an efficient approach to enhance permeation of AAPV so that both analogs were more permeable than the parent peptide. Permeability of both analogs was the same. Importantly, both analogs exhibited greater inhibitory activity than AAPV. This finding agrees with the study conducted by Toth et al. (1995), who reported that peptide lipidation could increase human neutrophil elastase inhibitory activity of AAPV. Note that the results of the Namjoshi et al. (2014) study showed that LAA lipidation reduced the elastase inhibition activity of AAPV slightly. Due to the fact that there is a hydrophobic pocket near the active center of human neutrophil elastase (Toth et al. 1995), it seems reasonable to increment the inhibitory activity of lipophilic analogs of AAPV.

Successful transdermal delivery of tetragastrin as a model peptide was also reported after conjugation to fatty acids (Setoh et al. 1995). Tetragastrin is the smallest fragment of the gastrin hormone, and its physiological effect is similar to gastrin (Tenma et al. 1993). *In vitro* skin permeation of the acyl derivatives of tetragastrin (acetyl, butyryl, and caproyl) was evaluated by Franz-type diffusion cells using full-thickness and tape-stripped abdominal skin of the rat. Acetic acid and butyric acid improved the skin permeation of tetragastrin across the full-thickness skin, but caproyl-tetragastrin, like tetragastrin, could not permeate across the intact skin. All three derivatives permeated tape-stripped skin. Due to hydrophilic nature of viable epidermis, acetyl-tetragastrin and caproyl-tetragastrin had the most and the least permeation ability, respectively. This difference between the obtained results was attributed to the contribution of stratum corneum, so that caproyl-tetragastrin (a more lipophilic derivative) because of binding to the intercellular lipids of stratum corneum was not detected in the receptor phase, but after removing the stratum corneum it became detectable. The parent tetragastrin did not permeate across intact and tape-stripped skin. This observation was attributed to the rapid degradation of parent peptide in the skin. The results indicated that all derivatives were more stable than tetragastrin. Furthermore, in another research conducted by the same group, the pharmacological activities of the derivatives were similar to the parent tetragastrin (Setoh et al. 1995; Tenma et al. 1993). In conclusion, chemical modification enhanced the skin permeation and stability of tetragastrin without affecting the pharmacological activity.

Yamamoto et al. (2003) also found that transdermal delivery of peptide could be increased by chemical modification by fatty acids. Using full-thickness abdominal skin of the rat, three acyl derivatives (butyryl, caproyl, and octanoyl) of phenylalanine-glycine (Phe-Gly) were evaluated in terms of skin permeability, stability, and accumulation in the skin layers. Accordingly to results, caproyl-Phe-Gly was the most permeable analog. All three derivatives were more stable against enzymatic degradation than Phe-Gly, and there were no differences between analogs in this respect. The accumulation of octanoyl–Phe-Gly in the skin was more than that of other analogs.

Besides short-chain fatty acids, as discussed earlier, long-chain fatty acids, for example, palmitic acid, have also been used to increase permeation of peptides across the skin. Topical delivery of KTTKS, Lys-Thr-Thr-Lys-Ser, and its palmitoyl derivative, Pal-KTTKS, across full-thickness mouse skin was evaluated by Choi et al. (2014). The results of the full-thickness skin permeation test revealed that neither the parent peptide nor its derivative was detected in the receptor phase of Franz-type diffusion cells. Nevertheless, contrary to the parent peptide, Pal-KTTKS was detected in all skin layers from 8.3% of the applied dose in the stratum corneum to 0.6% of the applied dose in the dermis. KTTKS is a signaling peptide that acts in the dermis layer and leads to promotion in type I collagen production. Thus, it is necessary that the adequate amount of KTTKS enters the dermis layer. Pal-KTTKS conjugate with 16 carbon atoms in the acyl chain is considered a high hydrophobic compound with a clogP of 3.72 (Palladino et al. 2012). Given the results of the studies described earlier, it seems that an optimal hydrophobicity can be obtained by reducing the carbon chain length of the hydrophobic moiety, and therefore the likelihood of retention in the lipid bilayer of the stratum corneum is reduced. Note that palmitic acid is one component of stratum corneum lipid composition and has a linear structure. On the other hand, KTTKS also possesses a linear structure, and contrary to all mentioned peptides, has no cyclic amino acid in its sequence. Therefore, it might be possible to accommodate Pal-KTTKS with a lipid bilayer instead of permeation across it, as was suggested by Moghimi et al. for the permeation of fluorouracil straight-chain terpene alcohol complexes across human skin (Moghimi et al. 1998). Both KTTKS and Pal-KTTKS were degraded in the skin homogenate rapidly. However, the stability of Pal-KTTKS was more than that of KTTKS.

In general, all of the studies mentioned have demonstrated that chemical modification is a suitable technique for increasing the stability and topical delivery of peptides. Note that the correlation between hydrophobicity and permeability is not linear, and there is an optimal value for hydrophobicity so that excessive increase in hydrophobicity results in the accumulation of compound in the intercellular lipid domain. Although chemical modification can improve the lipophilicity of compounds, it can affect both structure and molecular weight of the peptides and therefore their permeability.

All mentioned peptides have fewer than six amino acids and relatively low molecular weight. The molecular weights of AAPV (a tetrapeptide), tetragastrin (a tetrapeptide), Phe-Gly (a dipeptide), and KTTKS (a pentapeptide) are 356.4, 596.7, 222.2, and 563.6 Da, respectively. The question that arises is whether the results obtained for such peptides are generalizable to longer peptides as well as proteins. The following attempts to answer this question.

Gozes et al. (1994) introduced two novel analogs of vasoactive intestinal peptide (VIP): stearyl VIP (St-VIP) and stearyl- norleucine[17]-VIP (St-Nle[17]-VIP). VIP is employed for the treatment of male impotence. In order to prepare St-VIP, stearic acid as a hydrophobic moiety was conjugated to VIP, and in the case of St-Nle[17]-VIP, the methionine in position 17 was replaced with norleucine (a more hydrophobic amino acid) and then stearic acid was conjugated to Nle[17]-VIP. The norleucine replacement enhances the biological activity of VIP (Gozes et al. 1994; White et al. 2010). The sexual activity in rats after topical application of the ointment containing any of these derivatives on the sex organ was compared to the control (the ointment without peptide). The results demonstrated that the most effectiveness belonged to St-Nle[17]-VIP and then St-VIP. In addition, the results of *in vivo* skin permeation measurement using ^{125}I derivatives of peptide and its analogs showed that the derivatives had greater skin permeation ability than VIP. St-Nle[17]-VIP was also more permeable than St-VIP. According to these results, conjugation increases skin permeation and, as a result, increases efficiency of the peptide after topical application.

Yahalom et al. (1999) reported that chemical modification of [D-Lys][6]GnRH (a superactive GnRH agonist) by conjugation to fatty acids (acetic acid, caproic acid, lauric acid, and stearic acid) decreased the binding affinity to the GnRH receptor as a function of hydrophobicity increment. Nevertheless, the results of evaluation of *in vitro* and *in vivo* luteinizing hormone (LH) release capability indicated that the capability of [D-Lys-acetyl], [D-Lys-caproyl], and [D-Lys-lauryl][6]GnRH derivatives were rather similar to the parent peptide, but the capability of [D-Lys-stearyl][6]GnRH was less than other analogs. The aqueous solution of [D-Lys][6]GnRH or its analogs could not induce the release of LH after application to the skin surface of the proestrus rat, but LH release was induced by using dimethyl sulfoxide (DMSO) as a solvent to dissolve [D-Lys][6]GnRH, as well as its analogs. The potency of derivatives after skin application decreased with increasing acyl chain length so that the capability of [D-Lys-acetyl][6]GnRH for LH release was more than the other two analogs ([D-Lys-caproyl] and [D-Lys-lauryl][6]GnRH) and rather similar to [D-Lys][6]GnRH. The researchers explained that, apart from hydrophobicity, other parameters such as molecular weight and molecular conformation of analogs could affect skin penetration.

Structural modification alone is sometimes not enough for effective permeation enhancement of peptides, and therefore other strategies, such as application of chemical permeation enhancers, are required for a good permeation, such as application of DMSO for VIP, as described earlier. In the study about [D-Lys][6]GnRH, application of DMSO was also necessary for skin permeation, and chemical modification could not increase the tendency of molecules to the intercellular lipid domain of the stratum corneum. Molecular weights of VIP (28 amino acid residues in length) and [D-Lys][6]GnRH (10 amino acid residues in length) are 3326.8 and 1253.4 Da, respectively. Given the optimum molecular weight of about 500 Da to cross the skin, it could be concluded that the sizes of both peptides are too large for good permeation, and attachment of hydrophobic moieties decreases the permeation possibility. Accordingly, it is expected that chemical modification acts more efficiently about [D-Lys][6]GnRH, which has lower molecular weight as well as higher logP, but that did not happen. Yahalom et al. believed that molecular conformation of a short peptide (like [D-Lys]⁶GnRH) was more affected by the chemical modification. Note that DMSO, which is a dipolar aprotic solvent, was used as a vehicle by Yahalom et al.; therefore, the barrier function of the skin might be decreased so that the increase in hydrophobicity did not affect the permeability of molecules.

Opposite to peptides, unfortunately, few studies have been conducted on chemical modification of proteins for skin delivery, especially by attachment of hydrophobic moieties. Protein lipidation is a natural process that occurs in the body either in the cytoplasm of cells or in the lumen of the secretory pathway. This process is important for the protein functionality. Fatty acids, isoprenoids, and cholesterol are some lipids that are used in lipid modification of proteins. Palmitoylation is a reversible process in which long-chain fatty acids like palmitic acid are covalently added to proteins. Palmitoylation promotes the association of soluble proteins with plasma membranes (Nadolski & Linder 2007).

Covalent attachment of palmitic acid to the lysine residues in interferon α2b (IFNα2b) was conducted by Foldvari et al. (1998). This process led to the production of different palmitoyl derivatives of IFNα2b with 10, 11, and 12 palmitoyl substitutions. Using full-thickness human breast skin in permeation studies, Foldvari et al. reported that cutaneous absorption of palmitoyl IFNα2b (p-IFNα2b) was five to six times higher than that of IFNα2b. The antiviral activity of IFNα2b decreased by 50% due to chemical modification. Interferon α2b, a hydrophilic protein, has a molecular weight of 19.3 kDa and 165 amino acids. The attachment of 10 to 12 palmitic acids to IFNα2b, which is already a large molecule, increases its molecular weight. Therefore, the increased partitioning of the protein due to lipidation is apparently able to compensate for molecular weight increments and therefore reduction of the diffusion coefficient.

This study was conducted in 1998, and so far, about 20 years later, no studies have been reported for the application of lipidation in skin absorption enhancement of proteins.

34.3.2 Peptide or Protein Conjugation with Cell-Penetrating Peptides

CPPs or protein transduction domains (PTDs) are short peptides (generally less than 30 residues in length) that are inherently able to cross cellular membranes without causing serious membrane damage (Bechara & Sagan 2013; Buckley et al. 2016; Guo et al. 2016). These types of peptides are usually highly cationic or/and amphipathic molecules that are capable of transporting biomolecules (e.g., protein, peptide, plasmid DNA, oligonucleotide, siRNA) across biological barriers (Brasseur & Davita 2010; Munyendo et al. 2012). CPPs can internalize into the cell by two main mechanisms: energy-dependent, endocytotic pathways and non-energy-dependent, nonendocytotic pathways (Zhang et al. 2016).

The mechanisms of CCPs for increasing skin penetration are not fully understood. The stratum corneum consists of keratin-containing dead cells embedded in a lipid matrix (Menegatti et al. 2016). The molecular weights of CCPs are mostly more than 1000 Da, and it has been argued that these molecules do not interact with the intercellular lamellar structure of the SC (Gennari et al. 2016). Using coadministration of five different CCPs with cyclosporine A (CsA) individually, Kumar et al. (2015) found that CCPs interacted with the skin proteins and led to changes in their secondary structure; as a result, they increased partitioning of CsA into the corneocytes. However, Gennari et al. (2016) reported that both the fluidity of intercellular lipids and extension of keratins were induced by the skin penetration enhancer heptapeptide.

CPPs are added to peptides and proteins through either physical complexation or covalent conjugation (Brasseur & Davita 2010; Kristensen et al. 2016). Most studies are about coadministration of CPPs with peptides and proteins, but since this chapter is about chemical modification, it continues to focus only on conjugation.

The successful topical delivery of CsA because of conjugation to short oligomers of arginine was reported by Rothbard et al. (2000). CsA, a cyclic peptide with 11 amino acids and molecular weight of 1202.6 Da, has poor skin penetration. CsA was conjugated to a heptamer of arginine through a pH-dependent linkage, thus allowing CsA to be released at physiological pH. The conjugate efficiently penetrated into the skin so that it was detected not only in epidermis and dermis but also in T lymphocytes in the dermis, although the water solubility, as well as polarity of the conjugate, was substantially more than that of CsA alone.

Gautam et al. (2016) reported that IMT-P8 (15 amino acid residues in length) as a CCP mediated delivery of KLA (a proapoptotic peptide) and GFP (green fluorescent protein) into the human tumor cells, as well as epidermis layer and hair follicles. KLA is a cationic amphipathic peptide with 14 amino acid residues, which could disturb the mitochondrial membrane, but it does not alone enter the cell and also the skin in the intact form. Recombinant protein GFP is a 27-kDa macromolecule and similar to KLA could not permeate across the cell membrane or skin barrier on its own. However, conjugation with IMT-P8 increased permeation of KLA and GFP across mouse skin. Similar to this report, the successful topical delivery of GFP by conjugation to the POD peptide and accumulation of conjugate into the epidermis and hair follicles were reported by Johnson et al (2010). It is suggested that some CPPs enter the skin layers through a transfollicular route (Gautam et al. 2016).

According to these studies, it can be said that CPPs exert their actions through different mechanisms, and depending on the molecular size, hydrophobicity, electrical charge, secondary structures, and so on, different mechanisms could be proposed for their permeation. Finally, it seems that CPPs are an attractive, powerful, and promising tool to overcome the skin barrier.

34.4   CONCLUSION

As therapeutic and cosmetic peptides and proteins are developing, appropriate and noninvasive delivery strategies should also be developed. Transdermal delivery of peptides and proteins could be a convenient alternative to the parenteral route. As highlighted here, attaining efficacious skin delivery of peptides and proteins (either topical or transdermal) is a laborious task. Chemical modification is one of the effective approaches to overcome the barrier properties of skin. The results of studies performed so far suggest that covalent conjugation of a hydrophobic moiety or CPP to macromolecules could mostly enhance the skin permeation of peptides and proteins. CPPs seem to be more potent in increasing skin permeation, at least about proteins in comparison to hydrophobic moieties. However, skin side effects of both moieties should also be evaluated. Chemical modifications not only increase skin permeation ability but also increase the metabolic stability of peptides and proteins in the skin. However, it might be possible that covalent conjugation leads to a decrease of biological activity, but not so much that the peptide or protein activity is completely eliminated. Of course, it's presumed that reducing activity will be neutralized by increased penetration and stability. Given these findings, it seems that chemical modification will have a major impact on the topical and transdermal delivery of peptides and proteins.

REFERENCES

Alexander, A., Dwivedi, S., Ajazuddin, et al. 2012. Approaches for breaking the barriers of drug permeation through transdermal drug delivery. J Control Release. 164 (1):26–40.

Amsden, B., and Goosen, M. 1995. Transdermal delivery of peptide and protein drugs: An overview. Vol. 41.

Bechara, C., and Sagan, S. 2013. Cell-penetrating peptides: 20 years later, where do we stand? FEBS Letters. 587 (12):1693–1702.

Benson, H. A., and Namjoshi, S. 2008. Proteins and peptides: strategies for delivery to and across the skin. J Pharm Sci. 97 (9):3591–610.

Bodde, H. E., Verhoef, J., and Ponec, M. 1989. Transdermal peptide delivery. Biochem Soc Trans. 17 (5):943–945.

Brasseur, R., and Divita, G. 2010. Happy birthday cell penetrating peptides: Already 20 years. Biochimica et Biophysica Acta (BBA) - Biomembranes. 1798 (12):2177–2181.

Brown, M. B., Martin, G. P., Jones, S. A., et al. 2006. Dermal and transdermal drug delivery systems: current and future prospects. Drug Deliv. 13 (3):175–87.

Bruno, B. J., Miller, G. D., and Lim, C. S. 2013. Basics and recent advances in peptide and protein drug delivery. Ther Deliv. 4 (11):1443–1467.

Buckley, S.T., Hubálek, F., and Rahbek, U.L. 2016. Chemically modified peptides and proteins - critical considerations for oral delivery. Tissue Barriers. 4 (2):e1156805.

Bundgaard, H., and Møss, J. 1999. Prodrugs of peptides. 6. Bioreversible derivatives of thyrotropin-releasing hormone (trh) with increased lipophilicity and resistance to cleavage by the trh-specific serum enzyme. Pharm Res. 7 (9):885–892.

Caccetta, R., Blanchfield, J. T., Harrison, J., et al. 2006. Epidermal penetration of a therapeutic peptide by lipid conjugation; stereo-selective peptide availability of a topical diastereomeric lipopeptide. Int J Pept Res Ther. 12 (3):327–333.

Choi, Y. L., Park, E. J., Kim, E., et al. 2014. Dermal Stability and In Vitro Skin Permeation of Collagen Pentapeptides (KTTKS and palmitoyl-KTTKS). Biomol Ther. 22 (4):321–327.

Falconer, R. A., and Toth, I. 2007. Design, synthesis and biological evaluation of novel lipoamino acid-based glycolipids for oral drug delivery. Bioorg Med Chem. 15 (22):7012–7020.

Foldvari, M., Attah-Poku, S, Hu, J, et al. 1998. Palmitoyl derivatives of interferon alpha: potential for cutaneous delivery. J Pharm Sci. 87 (10):1203–8.

Foldvari, M., Baca-Estrada, M. E., He, Z., et al. 1999. Dermal and transdermal delivery of protein pharmaceuticals: lipid-based delivery systems for interferon alpha. *Biotechnol Appl Biochem*. 30 (Pt 2):129–37.

Gautam, A., Nanda, J. S., Samuel, J. S., et al. 2016. Topical delivery of protein and peptide using novel cell penetrating peptide IMT-p8. Sci Rep. 6

Gennari, C. G. M., Franzè, S., Pellegrino, S., et al. 2016. Skin penetrating peptide as a tool to enhance the permeation of heparin through human epidermis. Biomacromolecules. 17 (1):46–55.

Gorouhi, F., and Maibach, H. I. 2009. Role of topical peptides in preventing or treating aged skin. *Int J Cosmet Sci*. 31 (5):327–45.

Gozes, I., Reshef, A., Salah, D., et al. 1994. Stearyl-norleucine-vasoactive intestinal peptide (VIP): a novel VIP analog for noninvasive impotence treatment. Endocrinology. 134 (5):2121–5.

Gujjar, M., Arbiser, J., Coulon, R., et al. 2016. Localized delivery of a lipophilic proteasome inhibitor into human skin for treatment of psoriasis. J Drug Target. 24 (6):503–507.

Guo, Z., Peng, H., Kang, J., et al. 2016. Cell-penetrating peptides: Possible transduction mechanisms and therapeutic applications. Biomed Rep. 4 (5):528–34.

Johnson, L. N., Cashman, S. M., Read, S. P., et al. 2010. Cell penetrating peptide POD mediates delivery of recombinant proteins to retina, cornea and skin. Vision Res. 50 (7):686–97.

Kalluri, H., and Banga, A.K. 2011. Transdermal delivery of proteins. AAPS PharmSciTech. 12 (1):431–441.

Kristensen, M., Ditlev, B., and Nielsen, H. M. 2016. Applications and challenges for use of cell-penetrating peptides as delivery vectors for peptide and protein cargos. Int J Mol Sci. 17 (2):185.

Kumar, S., Zakrewsky, M., Chen, M., et al. 2015. Peptides as skin penetration enhancers: mechanisms of action. J Control Release. 199:168–78.

Menegatti, S., Zakrewsky, M., Kumar, S., et al. 2016. De novo design of skin-penetrating peptides for enhanced transdermal delivery of peptide drugs. Adv Healthc Mater. 5 (5):602–9.

Moghimi, H. R., Williams, A. C., and Barry, B. W. 1998. Enhancement by terpenes of 5-fluorouracil permeation through the stratum corneum: model solvent approach. J Pharm Pharmacol. 50 (9):955–64.

Møss, J., and Bundgaard, H. 1990. Prodrugs of peptides. 7. Transdermal delivery of thyrotropin-releasing hormone (TRH) via prodrugs. Int J Pharm. 66 (1):39–45.

Munyendo, W. L. L., Lv, H., Benza-Ingoula, H., et al. 2012. Cell penetrating peptides in the delivery of biopharmaceuticals. Biomolecules. 2 (2):187–202.

Nadolski, M. J., and Linder, M. E. 2007. Protein lipidation. FEBS J. 274 (20):5202–5210.

Naik, A., Kalia, Y. N., and Guy, R. H. 2000. Transdermal drug delivery: overcoming the skin's barrier function. Pharm Sci Technolo Today. 3 (9):318–326.

Namjoshi, S., Toth, I., Blanchfield, J.T., et al. 2014. Enhanced transdermal peptide delivery and stability by lipid conjugation: Epidermal permeation, stereoselectivity and mechanistic insights. Pharm Res. 31 (12):3304–3312.

Palladino, P., Castelletto, V., Dehsorkhi, A., et al. 2012. Conformation and Self-Association of Peptide Amphiphiles Based on the KTTKS Collagen Sequence Langmuir. 28 (33):12209–12215.

Prausnitz, M. R., and Langer, R. 2008. Transdermal drug delivery. Nat Biotechnol. 26 (11):1261–1268.

Rocco, D., Ross, J., Murray, P. E., et al. 2016. Acyl lipidation of a peptide: effects on activity and epidermal permeability in vitro. Drug Des Devel Ther. 10:2203–9.

Rothbard, J. B., Garlington, S., Lin, Q., et al. 2000. Conjugation of arginine oligomers to cyclosporin A facilitates topical delivery and inhibition of inflammation. Nat Med. 6:1253.

Sanders, L. M. 1990. Drug delivery systems and routes of administration of peptide and protein drugs. Eur J Drug Metab Pharmacokinet. 15 (2):95–102.

Setoh, K., Murakami, M., Araki, N., et al. 1995. Improvement of transdermal delivery of tetragastrin by lipophilic modification with fatty acids. J Pharm Pharmacol. 47 (10):808–11.

Singh, N., Kalluri, H., Herwadkar, A., et al. 2012. Transcending the skin barrier to deliver peptides and proteins using active technologies. Crit Rev Ther Drug Carrier Syst. 29 (4):265–98.

Subedi, R. K., Oh, S. Y., Chun, M. K., et al. 2010. Recent advances in transdermal drug delivery. Arch Pharm Res. 33 (3):339–51.

Tenma, T., Yodoya, E., Tashima, S., et al. 1993. Development of new lipophilic derivatives of tetragastrin: physicochemical characteristics and intestinal absorption of acyl-tetragastrin derivatives in rats. Pharm Res. 10 (10):1488–92.

Toth, I., Christodoulou, M., Bankowsky, K., et al. 1995. Design of potent lipophilic-peptide inhibitors of human neutrophil elastase: In vitro and in vivo studies. Int J Pharm. 125 (1):117–122.

Toth, I., Flinn, N., Hillery, A., et al. 1994. Lipidic conjugates of luteinizing hormone releasing hormone (LHRH)+ and thyrotropin releasing hormone (TRH)+ that release and protect the native hormones in homogenates of human intestinal epithelial (Caco-2) cells. Int J Pharm. 105 (3):241–247.

Wang, Y., Thakur, R., Fan, Q., et al. 2005. Transdermal iontophoresis: combination strategies to improve transdermal iontophoretic drug delivery. Eur J Pharm Biopharm. 60 (2):179–91.

White, C. M., Ji, S., Cai, H., et al. 2010. Therapeutic potential of vasoactive intestinal peptide and its receptors in neurological disorders. CNS Neurol Disord Drug Targets. 9 (5):661–6.

Xia, J. 2001. Protein-based surfactants: synthesis: physicochemical properties, and applications. 101 vols. New York: Taylor & Francis.

Yahalom, D., Koch, Y., Ben-Aroya, N., et al. 1999. Synthesis and bioactivity of fatty acid-conjugated GnRH derivatives. Life Sci. 64 (17):1543–52.

Yamamoto, A., Setoh, K., Murakami, M., et al. 2003. Enhanced transdermal delivery of phenylalanyl-glycine by chemical modification with various fatty acids. Int J Pharm. 250 (1):119–28.

Zhang, D., Wang, J., and Xu, D. 2016. Cell-penetrating peptides as noninvasive transmembrane vectors for the development of novel multifunctional drug-delivery systems. J Control Release. 229:130–139.

Zhou, Y., Kumar, V., Herwadkar, A., et al. 2017. Transdermal delivery of peptides and proteins by physical methods. In *Percutaneous penetration enhancers physical methods in penetration enhancement*, edited by Dragicevic, N. and Maibach, H. I., 423–437. Berlin, Heidelberg: Springer Berlin Heidelberg.

Ziora, Z. M., Blaskovich, M. A., Toth, I., et al. 2012. Lipoamino acids as major components of absorption promoters in drug delivery. Curr Top Med Chem. 12 (14):1562–1580.

35 Percutaneous Penetration of Oligonucleotide Drugs

Howard I. Maibach
University of California, San Francisco, California

Myeong Jun Choi
Charmzone Research and Development
Center, Wonju, Kangwon-do, Korea

CONTENTS

35.1   INTRODUCTION

Antisense oligonucleotides (ONs) technology uses single-stranded DNA to modulate gene expression. Antisense ONs with base sequences complementary to a specific messenger RNA (mRNA) can selectively modulate gene expression (1). Thus, antisense ONs may have potential as therapeutic agents against systemic and local diseases (2). Carcinoma, melanoma, psoriasis, xeroderma pigmentation, and viral diseases are potential candidates.

Despite major research and development efforts in topical systems and the advantages of the topical route, low stratum corneum (SC) permeability remains a major problem limiting the usefulness of the topical approach (3–5). To increase permeability, chemical and physical approaches have been examined to lower SC barrier properties.

Physical approaches for skin penetration enhancement, such as tape stripping (6–8), intradermal injection (8, 9), iontophoresis (7, 10), and electroporation (7, 11, 12) have been evaluated. In addition, vehicle systems have been used to enhance permeability (13, 14).

Topical antisense therapy may offer advantages over systemic therapy: ready access to targeted tissue, intervention in the case of toxicity, and the use of powerful and convenient animal models such as grafted skin on severe combined immunodeficiency (SCID) and nude mice (8, 15). This method should decrease cost, enhance patient compliance, and, in some cases, improve pharmacokinetics. In addition, the method provides a simple and convenient delivery system (13, 16).

Clinical applications of antisense ONs depend on the development of new approaches to delivery. Improvement of ONs administration can be achieved either by chemical modifications of ONs or by utilizing carrier systems. This chapter reviews percutaneous delivery methods of antisense ONs and summarizes recent data.

35.2   SKIN BARRIER AND FUNCTIONS

The SC is a permeability barrier that depends upon the presence of a unique mixture of lipids in the SC's intercellular domains. The SC comprises nonviable cornified cells (corneocytes) embedded in lipid-rich intercellular domains (intercorneocyte spaces). Intercellular domains comprise ceramides (CER), cholesterol (CHOL), and free fatty acid (FFA), with smaller amounts of cholesteryl sulfate, sterol, triglycerides, squalene, n-alkanes, and phospholipids. The composition of the SC intercellular lipids is unique in biological systems. These lipids exist as a continuous lipid phase, occupying about 20% of the SC volume, and arranged in multiple lamellar structures. All CER and fatty acids found in the SC are rod and cylindrical in shape; this physical attribute makes them suitable for the formation of highly ordered gel-phase membrane domains. The CHOL is capable of either fluidizing membrane domains or of enhancing rigidity, depending on the physical properties of the other lipids and the proportion of CHOH relative to the other components (17). Intracellular lipids that form the only continuous domain in the SC are required for a competent skin barrier. Based on electron microscopic and x-ray diffraction studies, the lipids appear arranged as lamellar structures, the organization of which is strongly dependent on lipid composition (18).

Skin barrier functions vary in skin conditions such as atopic dermatitis, psoriasis, and Gaucher disease (5, 19). Some skin barrier functions are reduced in atopic dermatitis and psoriasis. Hence, larger and charged molecules can penetrate into the SC of some diseased skin. White et al. (5) observed that ON penetrated into psoriatic but not normal skin. When ONs are applied to skin, these lamellar structures prevent ONs from penetrating. Methods to overcome this barrier are required to develop ON drugs against systemic and local skin diseases.

35.3   SKIN INTERACTION OF OLIGONUCLEOTIDES

When ONs are applied, they can interact with skin components and be destroyed by skin enzymes. Regnier et al. (3) reported the affinity of various ONs with SC components. Passive accumulation of the phosphorothioate (PS) ON in the SC was much higher than 3'-end modified phosphodiester (3'-PO) ON accumulation (Table 35.1). Immediately after pulsing (electroporation), the accumulation of PS on the SC was significantly higher than the accumulation of 3'-PO, and the quantity of PS was almost unchanged in the SC during four hours incubation after pulsing, one- third of the quantity of 3'PO was found in the SC. In the viable skin, the transport of 3'-PO was more efficient than that of PS immediately after pulsing (Table 35.1). These results indicate a stronger interaction of the PS with the SC components. The PS and 3'-PO were stable in the skin, while the nonprotected PO exhibited significant degradation within the viable skin. Hence, 3'-PO with high stability and low SC retention may be a good candidate for antisense ON therapy.

White et al. (8) found that ON in aqueous solution and gel does not significantly penetrate normal human skin grafts on athymic mice. The lack of penetration of ON across normal SC was consistent with the finding of Butler et al. (20), but in contrast to those of others (13, 14). Mehta et al. (13) and Valssov et al. (14) found that ON crossed the SC of human skin grafts and mouse skin after application in a cosmetic cream and lotion. Because the cosmetic cream and lotion contained penetration enhancers, ON had different penetration properties. Others reported that ONs/DNA penetrated the skin through follicular ducts (21, 22).

TABLE 35.1

Effect of Oligonucleotide Types on the Affinity for the Stratum Corneum of Intact Skin and on the Ability of the Oligonucleotide to Penetrate into Intact Skin after Pulsing

Type of ONs	Passive Diffusion ON Concentration in the SC (µM)[a]	Accumulation after Pulsing (pmol/cm²)[b]			
		Stratum Corneum		Viable Tissue	
		5 min	4 hr	5 min	4 hr
PS[c]	100 µM ± 10	225 ± 12.5	180 ± 10	23	33±2
3'-PO[d]	25 µM ± 3	200 ± 10	75 ± 3	71 ± 4	39 ± 2

[a] Effect of the ON types on the ON affinity for the stratum corneum of intact skin after four hours passive diffusion. Donor solution: ON 3.2 µM, EDTA 1mM, sucrose 8% in 0.04M HEPES buffer, pH 7.

[b] Mean quantity of PS or 3'-end modified PO oligonucleotide (pmol/cm²) recovered from the SC and viable skin of hairless rat skin immediately or four hours after pulsing. Donor solution: ON 3.2 µM, EDTA 1 mM, sucrose 8% in 0.04 M HEPES buffer, pH 7.

[c] Sequence of ON is 5'-ACC AAT CAG ACA CCA-3' and molecular weight and net electric charge are 4727 and –14, respectively. Nonbridging oxygen of the phosphodiester backbone is replaced by sulfur.

[d] Sequence of ON is 5'-ACC AAT CAG ACA C*C*A*-3' and molecular weight and net electric charge are 4593 and –14, respectively. Hydrogen at the deoxyribose 2' position is replaced by hydroxymethyl group at three bases (C*C*A*) of the 3'-end.

Abbreviations: PO, phosphodiester; PS, phosphorothioate.

35.4 OLIGONUCLEOTIDE MODIFICATION

Antisense ONs are short synthetic fragments of genes that inhibit gene expression. Antisense ONs consist in natural PO compounds. These compounds have poor stability in nuclease enzyme *in vitro* and *in vivo* and minimal skin-penetrating properties. To improve stability, chemical modifications have focused on the PO backbone and/or the sugar moiety (23).

Replacement of the nonbridging oxygen of the PO backbone by sulfur results in a PS with enhanced stability to enzymatic degradation. Replacement of the nonbridging oxygen by a methyl group results in increased hydrophobicity due to the loss of the negative charge. Replacement of hydrogen at the deoxyribose 2' position with a hydroxymethyl group converts the sugar to a modified ribose. One modification replaces the deoxyribose phosphate backbone, as in peptide nucleic acids (24).

Although chemical modifications provide improved stability and penetration, they have also resulted in non-antisense activities, such as an aptameric effect (25, 26), clotting and complement system (27), and immunomodulation property (28). Thus, an alternative strategy to the use of chemically modified ONs would be the association of natural PO molecules (including 3'-end modification) with a drug carrier such as liposomes that might provide increased stability and transport.

35.5 TAPE STRIPPING

A topically applied ON does not penetrate normal human SC. But removal by tape stripping leads to extensive penetration of ONs throughout the epidermis. Stripping increased the penetration of ONs in the viable skin. Regnier et al. (3) compared penetration through intact and stripped skin. After four-hour passive diffusion, between 15 and 25 pmol/cm² of ONs were found in the SC and

TABLE 35.2

Influence of Stripping and Electroporation on Oligonucleotides Topical Delivery

| | | ON Concentration in the Skin (after 4 hr) | |
		Passive Diffusion (μM)	Electroporation (μM)
Intact skin	Stratum corneum	9–25[a]	30–70
	Viable tissues	0.003–0.05[b]	0.5–0.6
Stripped skin	Viable tissues	0.5–1.2	2.5–3.5

[a] Average ON concentration in the stratum corneum (SC) was calculated based on a stratum thickness of 14 μm. Mean quantities of ON recovered from the SC of intact skin after four hours passive diffusion. Donor solution: ON 3.2 μM, EDTA 1 mM, sucrose 8% in 0.04 M HEPES buffer, pH 7.

[b] Average ON concentration in the viable skin was calculated based on a tissue thickness of 0.65 mm. Mean quantities of ON recovered from the viable skin four hours after passive diffusion. Donor solution: ON 3.2 μM, EDTA 1 mM, sucrose 8% in 0.04M HEPES buffer, pH 7.

0.5 and 3 pmol/cm² found in viable skin. In contrast, stripping increased ON concentration in the viable skin by one or two orders of magnitude. Table 35.2 shows the effect of tape stripping on ON penetration. In addition, topical application of a high concentration of ON (500 nmol) to human skin grafts over 24 hours resulted in localization of the ON in the SC, with no penetration into viable epidermis. In contrast, when 5 nmol of ON was topically applied after tape stripping (10 times with Scotch Crystal), ON could be detected in all epidermal layers. Stripping of the human skin or skin grafts resulted in a significant change in penetration of ON into the lower epidermis and ultimately keratinocyte ON uptake. In addition to ON, tape stripping increased the penetration of peptide and DNA antigens into viable skin. Hence, tape stripping has been used to disrupt the skin barrier before percutaneous peptide and DNA vaccines (29–31).

35.6   ELECTROPORATION AND IONTOPHORESIS

Electroporation is a phenomenon in which lipid bilayers exposed to high-intensity electric field pulses are temporarily destabilized and permeated (12, 32). The most common use of high-voltage pulsing is the introduction of DNA into isolated cells and for introducing ONs into cells. In addition, this technique enhances topical ON delivery and facilitates ON uptake by skin cells (33–35).

Iontophoresis enhances ON across hairless skin *in vitro* (36). In contrast to electroporation, iontophoresis is not believed to permeate the cells of the treated tissue. Oldenburg et al. (10) investigated the effect of pH, salt concentration, current density, and ON structure by iontophoretic delivery across hairless mouse skin. Brand et al. (37) evaluated 16 biologically relevant PS ONs with lengths from 6 to 40 bases for their iontophoretic transport across hairless mouse skin. The base located at the 3′-end affected the ability of an ON to be iontophoretically transported.

Electroporation and iontophoresis for the transdermal delivery of drugs were compared by Banga et al. (38). Electroporation applies a high voltage pulse of short duration to permeate the skin barrier, while iontophoresis applies a small low voltage with constant current to push charged drug into the skin. The ON transport across the SC was primarily transcellular during electroporation and paracellular during iontophoresis. In addition, electroosmosis is important in delivering ON in iontophoresis, but electroporation is not. Compared with the passive diffusion, electroporation and iontophoresis increased the topical delivery of the macromolecule greater than one order of magnitude. Table 35.2 shows the effect of electroporation on ON delivery. Regnier et al. (11)

also compared electroporation with that of iontophoresis for ON delivery; ON was delivered to the viable skin tissue equally by both. This result was inconsistent with Regnier and Preat (7), who reported electroporation less efficient than iontophoresis to deliver ON in the viable tissues of intact skin.

The most important advantage of topical delivery of antisense ON by skin electroporation is the rapid cellular and nuclear uptake of antisense compounds by the keratinocytes. Advantages of skin electroporation are (1) reducing ON exposure to the nuclease present in both extracellular fluids and endocytic compartments, (2) shortening the time of onset of the antisense effect, and (3) lowering the threshold ON concentration necessary to achieve such an effect. Iontophoresis facilitates the transport of charged and high molecular compounds, which cannot be normally delivered by passive delivery. Iontophoresis provides a rapid onset of action, since the lag time is on the order of minutes, as compared to hours in passive transport. Disadvantages of iontophoresis are a slight feeling of tingling or itch. Transient erythema and local vasodilatation are two common side effects associated with iontophoresis (39, 40). However, with rapid and significant advances in the area of biotechnology resulting in increased number of peptide, protein, ON, and DNA drugs, iontophoresis and electroporation provide unique opportunities for noninvasive, safe, convenient, effective, and patient-controlled delivery of such drugs.

McAllister et al. (41) developed micro-scale projections that penetrate only the outermost layers of the skin using microelectrical mechanical system (MEMS)–based fabrication. With this device, Mikszta et al. (42) improved genetic immunization via microfabricated silicon projections, termed microenhancer arrays (MEAs), to mechanically disrupt the skin barrier and targeted epidermal delivery of genetic vaccines. The MEA-based delivery enabled topical gene transfer resulting in reporter gene activity up to 2800-fold above topical controls in a mouse model. This technology may be applicable to targeted therapy of epidermal disorders and skin cancer. The skin is a privileged target for antisense ON given its accessibility; many have thought that electroporation, iontophoresis, and MEA technology, which enhance SC and keratinocyte permeability, might be a useful method for their topical delivery.

35.7 ANTISENSE OLIGONUCLEOTIDES SEMISOLID FORMULATIONS

Vlassov et al. (14) first reported ON penetration through skin. They applied ON lotion on mouse ear and recovered intact ON from the blood and pancreas. Subsequently, several methods were developed to deliver ON into skin. C-5 propyne–modified antisense ON in aqueous solution penetrated psoriatic SC, but not normal skin. This result suggests that ONs can be topically applied to psoriatic skin in simple topical formulations and efficiently reach the basal epidermis fully intact. Thus, simple formulations, including cream and lotion, might be used to treat psoriasis. In contrast to systemic ON injection, there was no apparent degradation of the ON after topical application for either normal or psoriatic skin in spite of extensive enzymatic activity in the skin (3, 5). Hence, psoriasis is a reasonable target for antisense ON therapy.

Mehta et al. (13) topically applied 20-nucleotide PS intercellular adhesion molecule-1 (ICAM-1) antisense ON (ISIS-2302) in a cream formulation. ISIS-2302 topical cream is being developed as a potential therapeutic agent for plaque psoriasis. The vehicle contained glyceryl monostearate (10%), hydroxypropyl methylcellulose (0.5%), isopropyl myristate (10%), methylparaben (0.5%), propylparaben (0.5%), polyoxy-40-stearate (15%), and water. Antisense ON effects were concentration dependent, sequence specific, and resulted from reduction of ICAM-1 mRNA levels in the skin. Compared with intravenous ON administration that had no pharmacological effects, topical delivery produced a rapid and a significantly higher accumulation of ON in the epidermis and dermis. ISIS-2302 (ALICAFORSEN) is in phase 2a human clinical trials. In preclinical studies, topical ISIS-2302 formulation showed suppression of upregulated ICAM-1 by the epidermal and dermal skin layers implicated in the pathogenesis of psoriasis. Topical formulations were well tolerated, with more than 4000-fold greater accumulation of the intact drug observed in the epidermis and

150-fold more in dermal layers of the skin than with the intravenous injection (13). From these results, topically applied antisense ON in a cream-type formulation can be delivered to target sites in the skin and may be of value in the treatment of psoriasis and other inflammatory skin disorders.

35.8 LIPOSOMAL FORMULATIONS

Although the SC is considered a major barrier to percutaneous absorption, it is also regarded as the main pathway for penetration. Compounds and vehicle systems that loosen or fluidize the lipid matrix of the SC may enhance permeation. Among these delivery systems, liposome formulations offer several advantages over more conventional formulations (43). Liposomes are of great interest for the delivery of ONs, and their application in medicine has been extensively studied.

Topical delivery of ON and/or DNA using liposome formulations included conventional liposomes; stealth liposomes coated with polyethylene glycol; targeted liposomes containing antibodies, ligands, and polysaccharides; and cationic and nonionic liposomes. Raghavachari and Fahl (22) reported that nonionic liposomes were their most efficient vehicles for transdermal systems. Rat pups treated with nonionic liposomes formulations showed the highest reporter gene expression 24 hours following liposome application, followed by nonionic/cationic liposomes and phospholipid formulations (Table 35.3). Surprisingly, the traditional phospholipid-based liposome carriers were not effective as delivery vehicles for luciferase or galactosidase DNA when compared to nonionic liposomes. Jayaraman et al. (44) explained the high efficiency of nonionic liposomes as a facilitator of drug delivery to the unique lipid composition. They suggest that polyoxyethylene and glyceryl dilaurate act as penetration enhancers. Raghavachari and Fahl (22) also showed kinetic studies to assess the longevity of expression of the delivered luciferase and galactosidase genes. The maximum expression was 24 hours postdelivery, and expression level returned to near-basal levels at 72 hours. This indicated that the process of topical delivery of DNA facilitates a transient, high-level expression of the exogenous gene delivered into the skin cells. This result is important in treating skin diseases and immunization.

TABLE 35.3
Luciferase and Galactosidase Activity in Rat Pup Skin Following Treatment with Liposome–DNA Formulations

Liposome Composition	Relative Luciferase Activity (RLU/mg protein)[d]	Relative Galactosidase Activity (m units/mg Protein)[e]
Nonionic[a]	57,000	6.0
Nonionic/cationic[b]	32,000	5.4
Phospholipid[c]	8900	3.3

[a] Composition: glyceryldilaurate (GDL)/cholesterol (CHOL)/polyoxyethylene-10 stearyl ether (POE-10) (58:15:27, w/w ratio)

[b] Composition: GDL:CHOH:POE-10:DOTAP (50:15:23:12 w/w ratio)

[c] Composition: dioleoylphosphatidylethanolamine-2000 (PEGylated):CHOH:DSPC (1:5:0.1, molar ratio)

[d] Treated skin was dissected out and homogenized. To 100 μL of the tissue homogenate was added, with 100 μL of the luciferase assay buffer containing substrate, and the emitted light was measured in a Monolight 2010 luminometer.

[e] Galactosidase activity was measured by adding 100 μL of the tissue homogenate to an equal volume of assay buffer. The reaction mixture was incubated for 30 minutes at 37°C and terminated by the addition of 100 μL 1 M sodium carbonate, and the absorbance at 420 nm was measured.

Liposomes are widely used in the topical ocular delivery of ON. Among these applications, the treatment of viral diseases has been approached using liposome-encapsulated ONs. Bochot et al. (45) reported on an ophthalmic delivery system for ON based on a liposomal dispersion within a thermosensitive gel. Ocular distribution and clearance from the vitreous humor of a model antisense ON were investigated after intravitreal injection to rabbits of the ON either free or encapsulated into liposomes. Liposomes provided higher drug levels than the control solution one day postinjection. After 14 days, the residual concentration of ON using liposomal suspension was 9.3-fold higher than that obtained with the ON control solution. The intravitreal injection ON containing liposomes led to a controlled release, thus offering an interesting prospective in the ocular delivery of ONs effective for the treatment of some retinal infections.

Enhancers can be also used with liposome formulations. Dimethyl sulfoxide increased ON skin delivery with a liposome formulation (46). Brand and Iversen (16) reported the combined effect of skin enhancers: a mixture of polyethylene glycol and linoleic acid reduced the SC barrier function. The ON flux was near 20 times greater than iontophoretic delivery of the same sequence containing a PS backbone. Recently, we have tested the percutaneous delivery of an NF-kB decoy with various formulation systems. Among these formulation systems, liposomes containing 10% urea were an efficient composition to transfer into skin (personal communication). Hence, liposomal creams containing these enhancers may be suited to use in the delivery of therapeutic ON.

35.9   FIRST OLIGONUCLEOTIDE DRUG: ISIS 2922

The ONs have potential for the treatment of ocular severe viral infections due to herpes simplex virus or to cytomegalovirus (CMV). The use of ONs to inhibit CMV was evaluated by two groups. A series of ONs complementary to the translation start sites, coding regions, intron/exon region, and 5'caps in RNAs, including the DNA polymerase, and immediate early genes IE 1 and IE 2 was evaluated by Azad et al. (47, 48). The most potent was a 21-mer (ISIS 2922) against the coding regions of IE 2, with an IC_{50} of about 0.1 µM. Recently, the first ON drug was marketed: Vitravene (ISIS 2922) is delivered to the eye by intravitreal administration for the treatment of CMV infections in patients with AIDS.

Marketed ONs require repeated administrations. In order to more effectively target these ONs and to obtain a slow-release pattern of the compounds, the use of liposomes would be a good alternative. The use of liposomes for intravitreal administration can be promising, since these lipid vehicles are stable and protect ONs against degradation by nuclease, and they allow increased retention time in the vitreous.

35.10   CONCLUSION

The technology of ON antisense for the manipulation of specific gene expression has therapeutic potential. Topical delivery of ONs is highly feasible and offers the advantages for local treatment of skin diseases. ISIS-2922 as an antisense ON drug for viral therapy is commercially available, and many other ON drugs are in clinical trials. Liposomal creams containing enhancers are well suited to use in the delivery of therapeutic ON in terms of cost, efficacy, compliance, and comfort. These systems provide a likely direction for future studies.

REFERENCES

1. Zon G. Oligonucleotide analogues as potential chemotherapeutic agents. Pharm Res 1988; 5:539–549.
2. Stein CA, Cheng YC. Antisense oligonucleotides as therapeutic agents – Is the bullet really magical? Science 1993; 261:1004–1012.
3. Regnier V, Tahiri A, Andre N, Lemaitre M, Le Doan T, Preat V. Electroporation- mediated delivery of 3'-protected phosphodiester oligonucleotides to the skin. J Control Rel 2000; 67:337–346.

4. Rojanasakul Y. Antisense oligonucleotide therapeutics: drug delivery and targeting. Adv Drug Deliv Rev 1996; 18:115–131.

5. White PJ, Gray AC, Fogarty RD, Sinclair RD, Thuminger SP, Werther GA, Wraight CJ. C-5 propyne-modified oligonucleotides penetrate the epidermis in psoriatic and not normal human skin after topical application. J Invest Dermatol 2002; 118:1003–1007.

6. Choi MJ, Zhai H, Maibach HI. Effect of tape stripping on percutaneous penetration and topical vaccination. Exogenous Dermatol 2003; 2:262–269.

7. Regnier V, Preat V. Localization of a FITC-labeled phosphorothioate oligonucleotide in the skin after topical delivery by iontophoresis and electroporation. Pharm Res 1998; 15: 1596–1602.

8. White PJ, Fogarty RD, Liepe IJ, Delaney PM, Werther GA, Wraight CJ. Live confocal microscopy of oligonucleotide uptake by keratinocytes in human skin grafts on nude mice. J Invest Dermatol 1999; 112:887–892.

9. Wraight CJ, White PJ, Mckean SC, Fogarty RD, Venables DJ, Liepe IJ, Edmondson SR, Werther GA. Reversal of epidermal hyperproliferation in psoriasis by insulin-like growth factor I receptor antisense oligonucleotides. Nat Biotechnol 2000; 18:521–526.

10. Oldenburg KR, Vo KT, Smith GA, Selick HE. Iontophoretic delivery of oligonucleotides across full thickness hairless mouse skin. J Pharm Sci 1995; 84:915–921.

11. Regnier V, De Morre N, Jadoul A, Preat V. Mechanism of a phosphorothioate oligonucleotide delivery by skin electroporation. Int J Pharm 1999; 184:147–156.

12. Weaver J. Electroporation theory. Concepts and mechanism. Methods Mol Biol 1995; 47:1–26.

13. Mehta RC, Stecker KK, Cooper SR, Templin MV, Tsai YJ, Condon TP, Bennett CK, Hardee GE. Intercellular adhesion molecule-1 suppression in skin by topical delivery of anti-sense oligonucleotides. J Invest Dermatol 2000; 115:805–812.

14. Vlassov VV, Karamyshev VN, Yakubov LA. Penetration of oligonucleotides into mouse organism through mucosa and skin. FEBS Lett 1993; 327:271–274.

15. Raychaudhuri SP, Sanyal M, Raychaudhuri SK, Duff S, Farber EM. Severe combined immunodeficiency mouse-human skin chimeras: a unique animal model for the study of psoriasis and cutaneous inflammation. Br J Dermatol 2001; 144:931–939.

16. Brand RM, Iversen PL. Transdermal delivery of antisense compounds. Adv Drug Deliv Rev 2000; 40:51–57.

17. Wertz PW. Lipids and barrier function of the skin. Acta Derm Venereol 2000; 208:7–11.

18. Weerheim A, Ponec M. Determination of stratum corneum lipid profile by tape stripping in combination with high-performance thin-layer chromatography. Arch Dermatol Res 2001; 293:191–199.

19. Hollern WM, Ginns EI, Menon GK, Ginndmann J-U, Fartasch M, Mckinney CE, Elias PM, Sidransky E. Consequences of beta-glucocerebrosidase in epidermis. J Clin Invest 1994; 93:1756–1764.

20. Butler M, Stecker K, Bennett CF. Cellular distribution of phosphorothioate oligodeoxynucleotides in normal rodent tissues. Lab Invest 1997; 77:379–388.

21. Fan H, Lin Q, Morrissey GM, Khavari PA. Immunization via hair follicles by topical application of naked DNA to normal skin. Nat Biotechnol 1999; 17:870–872.

22. Raghavachari N, Fahl WE. Targeted gene delivery to skin cells in vivo: a comparative study of liposomes and polymers as delivery vehicles. J Pharm Sci 2002; 91:615–622.

23. Bochot A, Couvreur P, Fattal E. Intravitreal administration of antisense oligonucleotides: potential of liposomes delivery. Prog Retin Eye Res 2000; 19:131–147.

24. Hanvey JC, Peffer NJ, Bisi JE, Thomson SA, Cadilla R, Josey JA, Ricca DJ, Hassman CF, Bonham MA, Au KG, Carter SG, Bruckenstein DA, Boyd AL, Noble SA, Babiss LE. Antisense antigene properties of peptide nucleic acids. Science 1992; 258:1481–1485.

25. Castier Y, Chemla E, Nierat J, Heudes D, Vasseur MA, Rajnoch C, Bruneval P, Carpentier A, Fabbiani JN. The activity of c-myb antisense oligonucleotide to prevent intimal hyperplasia is non-specific. J Cardiovasc Surg 1998; 38:1–7.

26. Ellington AD, Szostak JW. Selection in vitro of single strand DNA molecules that fold into specific ligand-binding structures. Nature 1992; 355:850–852.

27. Galbraith WM, Hobson WC, Giclas PC, Schechter PJ, Agrawal S. Complement activation and homodynamic changes following intravenous administration of phosphor-othioate oligonucleotides in the monkey. Antisense Res Dev 1994; 4:201–206.

28. Krieg AM. CpG DNA: a novel immunomodulator. Trends Microbiol 1999; 7:64–65.

29. Seo N, Tokura Y, Nishijima T, Hashizume H, Furukawa F, Takigawa M. Percutaneous peptide immunization via corneum barrier-disrupted murine for experimental tumor immunoprophylaxis. Proc Natl Acad Sci USA 2000; 97:371–376.

30. Takigawa M, Tokura Y, Hashizume H, Yagi H, Seo N. Percutaneous peptide immunization via corneum barrier-disrupted murine for experimental tumor immunoprophylaxis. Ann NY Acad Sci 2001; 941:139–146.
31. Watabe S, Xin K-Q, Ihata A, Liu L-J, Honsho A, Aoki I, Hamajima K, Wahren B, Okuda K. Protection against influenza virus challenge by topical application of influenza DNA vaccine. Vaccine 2001; 19:4434–4444.
32. Zhang L, Li L, Hoffmann GA, Hoffmann RM. Depth-targeted efficient gene delivery and expression in the skin by pulsed electric fields: an approach to gene therapy of skin aging and other diseases. Biochem Biophys Res Commun 1996; 220:633–636.
33. Prausnitz MR, Edelman ER, Gimm JA, Langer R, Weaver JC. Transdermal delivery of heparin by skin electroporation. Biotechnol 1995; 13:1205–1209.
34. Vanbever R, LeBoulange E, Preat V. Transdermal drug delivery of fentanyl by electroporation. I. Influence of electrical factors. Pharm Res 1996; 13:557–563.
35. Zewert TE, Pilquett UF, Langer R, Weaver JC. Transdermal transport of DNA antisense oligonucleotide by electroporation. Biochim Biophys Res Commun 1995; 212: 286–292.
36. Brand RM, Iversen PL. Iontophoretic delivery of a telomeric oligonucleotides. Pharm Res 1996; 13:851–854.
37. Brand RM, Wahl A, Iversen PL. Effects of size and sequence on the iontophoretic delivery of oligonucleotides. J Pharm Sci 1998; 87:49–52.
38. Banga AK, Bose S, Ghosh TK. Iontophoresis and electroporation: comparisons and contrasts. Int J Pharm 1999; 179:1–19.
39. Ledger PW. Skin biological issues in electrically enhanced transdermal delivery. Adv Drug Deliv Rev 1992; 9:289–307.
40. Branda RM, Singh P, Aspe-Carranza E, Maibach HI, Guy RH. Acute effects of iontophoresis on human skin in vivo: cutaneous blood flow and transepidermal water loss measurements. Eur J Pharm Biopharm 1997; 43:133–138.
41. McAllister DV, Allen MG, Prauznitz MR. Microfabricated microneedles for gene and drug delivery. Ann Rev Biomed Eng 2000; 2:289–313.
42. Mikszta JA, Alarcon JB, Brittingham JM, Dutter DE, Pettis RJ, Harvey NG. Improved genetic immunization via micromechanical disruption of skin-barrier function and targeted epidermal delivery. Nat Med 2002; 8:415–419.
43. Egbaria K, Weiner N. Liposomes as a topical drug delivery system. Adv Drug Deliv Rev 1990; 5:287–300.
44. Jayaraman SC, Ramachandran C, Weiner N. Topical delivery of erythromycin from various formulation: an in vivo hairless mouse study. J Pharm Sci 1996; 85:1082–1084.
45. Bochot A, Fattal E, Couvreur P. Design of a new eye delivery system for oligonucleotide based on a liposomal dispersion within a thermosensitive gel. In: Proceeding of the 2nd World APGI/APV Meeting on Pharmaceutics, Biopharmaceutics and Pharmaceutical Technology, Paris, 1998:1089–1090.
46. Heckert RA, Elankumaran S, Oshop GL, Vakharia VN. A novel transcutaneous plasmid-dimethyl-sulfoxide delivery technique for avian nucleic acid immunization. Vet Immunol Immunopathol 2002; 89:67–81.
47. Azad RF, Driver VB, Tanaka K. Antiviral activity of a phosphorothioate oligonucleotide complementary to RNA of the human cytomegalovirus major immediate-early region. Antimicrob Agents Chemother 1993; 37:1945–1954.
48. Azad RF, Brown-Driver VB, Buckheit RW, Anderson KP. Antiviral activity of a phosphorothioate oligonucleotide complementary to human cytomegalovirus RNA when used in combination with antiviral nucleoside analogs. Antiviral Res 1995; 28:101–111.

36 Use of Microemulsions for Topical Drug Delivery

Efrem N. Tessema, Sandra Heuschkel, Anuj Shukla, and Reinhard H. H. Neubert
Martin-Luther-University Halle-Wittenberg, Halle (Saale), Germany

CONTENTS

36.1 INTRODUCTION

Over the past several years great efforts have been made in the dermatopharmaceutical area for the development of new colloidal drug delivery systems, including micelles, mixed micelles, nanoparticles, liposomes, and microemulsions (MEs). Among these carriers, MEs play the most important role and represent a promising alternative to conventional formulations. MEs are optically isotropic, transparent, or slightly opalescent, one-phase colloidal systems with low viscosity. The size of the colloidal phase is typically in the range of 10 to 100 nm. MEs are thermodynamically stable systems, formed without (or with minimal) energy input. The thermodynamic stability of MEs can be characterized by Gibbs-Helmholtz (Equation [36.1]).

$$\Delta G = \gamma \Delta A - T \Delta S \qquad (36.1)$$

where ΔG is the free energy of formation, γ is the oil–water interfacial tension, ΔA is the change in the interfacial area upon emulsification, ΔS is the change in entropy, and T is the absolute temperature. The enormous surface area resulting from the formation of MEs tends to increase the surface free energy of the system. The thermodynamic stability and spontaneity of formation of MEs can be explained by a negative free energy of formation due to a remarkable reduction of interfacial tension accompanied by a dramatic change in the entropy of the system [1].

MEs consist of hydrophilic and lipophilic phases as well as surfactants (SAAs). Besides, in most of the cases, cosurfactants (co-SAAs) are needed. Depending on the oil-to-water ratio and the type of the SAA, a characteristic microstructure of either small oil droplets in an aqueous surrounding (o/w) or water droplets in an oil continuous matrix (w/o) exists. However, bicontinuous structures (in which the aqueous and oil phases are intertwined) are also possible. In bicontinuous MEs, both water and oil form continuous domains separated by SAA-rich interfaces. All microstructures are highly dynamic, undergoing continuous and spontaneous fluctuations.

Pharmaceutical MEs offer several advantages, including ease of preparation (spontaneous formation), long-term stability, high solubilization capacity for hydrophilic and lipophilic drugs, and improved drug delivery. The latter provides a wide range of pharmaceutical applications that ensure improved topical and systemic drug availability via dermal, oral, parenteral, and ophthalmic administrations [2–5]. In this chapter an overview is given of the formulation components of MEs, selected methods for the physicochemical characterization of MEs, and current developments in the field of cutaneous application.

36.2 FORMULATION COMPONENTS

MEs are prepared by simple mixing of the oil phase, aqueous phase, SAA, and co-SAA in appropriate compositions and concentrations. In some cases a rapid microemulsification process requires a very low energy input (heat or mechanical agitation) to overcome the kinetic barriers to the formation of MEs [1]. As the emulsification process is mainly governed by the amount and nature of the formulation components (and the physicochemical properties of the drug) [6], careful selection of oil phase, SAA, co-SAA, and/or cosolvents is needed [7].

36.2.1 SURFACTANTS

Previously, various SAAs and SAA blends have been used for the stabilization of MEs. Zwitterionic and nonionic SAAs are generally less toxic and less irritating to the skin than ionic SAAs for the formulations of topical MEs [4, 7]. Zwitterionic SAAs are represented by one of the most promising natural, biodegradable, and biocompatible SAAs: lecithins [8]. Lecithins showed no skin irritancy even at high concentrations in topical formulations [9–12]. An alternative to lecithins, nonionic SAAs such as polyethylene glycol alkyl ethers (Brij, e.g. Brij 97) [13], sorbitan esters (Spans; e.g. Span 20 and 80), and ethoxylated sorbitan esters (polysorbates, Tweens; e.g. Tween 20, 40, 80) [1, 13–16] have been used for oral, parenteral, and topical MEs. The other nonionic SAAs include polyglycerol esters such as HYDRIOL PGCH.4 (polyglyceryl-4-caprate) and TEGO CARE PL 4 (polyglycerol-4-laurate) [17, 18], block copolymers of polyethylene glycol and polypropylene glycol (Poloxamers e.g. Pluronics, Synperonics) [19], polyoxyethylene glycerol fatty acid esters (e.g. TagatO2) [19, 20], and sugar-based SAAs (such as Plantacare 1200 UP) [21, 22]. Cationic SAAs such as quaternary ammonium alkyl salts (e.g. hexadecyltrimethyl-ammonium bromide [CTAB] and didodcecylammonium bromide [DDAB]) have also been used in the stabilization of MEs [23]. The most widely studied anionic SAA that forms stable MEs without the addition of co-SAAs is sodium bis(2-ethyl hexyl) sulfosuccinate (AOT).

In the past, the crucial point in topical MEs was the high SAA content needed to stabilize the colloidal phase of MEs. Hence, a lot of research work was focused on both diminishing their concentration and searching for well-tolerated SAAs. Taking into account the fact that MEs can be applied in the treatment of skin diseases, an amount of 20% to 30% of SAAs appears to be the threshold of acceptance in dermal use.

36.2.2 COSURFACTANTS

Mostly MEs contain co-SAAs to sufficiently lower the oil–water interfacial tension and to fluidize the interfacial film [6]. They are amphiphilic molecules accumulating at the interfacial layer, with the SAA thereby affecting the interfacial structure, disrupting the liquid crystalline phases, promoting drug solubility, and expanding the one-phase region in the phase diagram [6, 24]. They also modify the chemical composition and relative polarities of the phases by partitioning themselves between lipophilic and hydrophilic phases [6]. Different alcohols (such as ethanol, butanol, propylene glycol, pentylene glycol [1,2-pentanediol], and glycerol) [12, 25, 26], polyethylene glycols (PEGs) (such as PEG 400) [1], and nonionic SAAs (such as diethylene glycol monoethyl ether [Transcutol P]) [14, 27] have been used as co-SAAs in the formulation of MEs. Unlike the medium-chain alcohols, which are potentially toxic/irritating to the skin, alkanediols and alkanetriols are nontoxic co-SAAs but, due to their extreme hydrophilic nature, they are used at high amounts to produce MEs. Generally, however, nonalcohol co-SAAs are promoted for the formulation of MEs [6, 28, 29]. As a result of the low toxicity and irritancy and biodegradability of the nonionic SAAs, the interest in using them both as a SAA and as a co-SAA is increasing [30]. On the other hand, some twin-tailed SAAs such as AOT are capable of forming MEs by themselves and they don't need the addition of co-SAAs [1].

36.2.3 OIL PHASES

Several lipophilic compounds such as fatty acids (e.g. oleic acid) [14], fatty acid esters (e.g. isopropyl myristate [IPM], isopropyl palmitate, ethyl oleate, and decyl oleate) [22, 30, 31], alcohols, medium-chain triglycerides (e.g. Miglyol 812) [10, 32], terpenes (e.g. menthol and limonene) [15], and vegetable oils (e.g. jojoba oil) [33] have been used in the formulation of MEs. A lipophilic component is mostly selected based on its drug solubilization capacity and penetration-enhancing properties [22]. The ability of the oil to produce a broader ME region is also important, though fulfilling both requirements (high drug loading capacity and producing a broader ME region) by a single oil component is difficult. Sometimes a mixture of lipophilic components is used to meet these requirements [6]. It has been shown that, compared to high molecular volume, oils with low molecular volume such as fatty acid esters and medium-chain triglycerides improve the solubilization efficiency of SAAs possibly by penetrating the interfacial monolayer and providing optimal film curvature [30]. As a result they are easily microemulsified and give a wider homogeneity, unlike oils with long hydrocarbon chains such as soybean oil [6].

36.2.4 PENETRATION MODIFIERS AND SOLUBILIZERS

MEs often contain cosolvents to increase the solubility of the drug and to stabilize the dispersed phase [24]. Besides, chemical penetration enhancers such as oleic acid (also used as a lipophilic phase) [12, 34], N-methyl-pyrrolidone [35], terpenes [36], dimethyl sulfoxide (DMSO) [37], and propylene glycol may be incorporated in the ME formulations. Nevertheless, the necessity of these ingredients is still contentious because of the superior penetration properties of the vehicle ME itself. Solubilizers such as β-cyclodextrin have also been used in MEs.

36.3 CHARACTERIZATION

Combinations of various complementary techniques have been used to fully characterize MEs. The physicochemical characterization of MEs include phase stability and phase behavior, microstructure, dimension (size and distribution), shape (or conformation), surface features (specific area, charge and distribution), local molecular arrangements, interactions, and dynamics. Among these properties, particle size, interactions, and dynamics are of fundamental importance, since they control many of the general properties of MEs. In particular, the size distribution of MEs gives essential information for a reasonable understanding of the mechanism governing both the stability and the penetration into the skin [38, 39]. Many technologies such as scattering techniques (static light scattering, dynamic light scattering, small-angle neutron scattering, and small-angle x-ray scattering) and transmission electron microscopy and nuclear magnetic resonance have been used for particle characterization. Other methods such as electrokinetic chromatography, conductance, viscosity, electrical birefringence, infrared spectroscopy, and calorimetry have also been employed for investigating the internal physicochemical states of MEs [40–44]. Furthermore, the electron paramagnetic resonance method was also used to reveal the nanostructure, as well as to measure the micropolarity and microviscosity of MEs [10, 17]. Among these techniques, in this section, the applications of the most practically relevant techniques i.e., microscopy, viscosity, and scattering experiments are discussed in detail.

36.3.1 MICROSCOPY

Optical isotropy is one important feature of MEs. Unlike lamellar or hexagonal liquid crystals, isotropic structures do not cause birefringence between crossed polarizers. Therefore, polarized light microscopy is used to detect this ME behavior.

Freeze fracture electron microscopy (FFEM) is a method to visualize the microstructure of colloidal systems, mainly the size and shape of the ME droplets. The sample is rapidly frozen, applying cooling rates of about 10^4 K/sec, and subsequently fractured. It is possible to etch the frozen and fractured sample, which yields an amplification of the characteristic relief by lyophilization of the frozen water along the fractured surface. In either case the surface is shadowed in a 45-degree angle with a thin layer of platinum and then immediately in a vertical angle, with carbon providing a mechanical stabilization. After a washing procedure, the resulting replica can be observed in a transmission electron microscope (TEM). Due to shadowing in the transversal angle, the platinum-layer thickness depends on the surface structure, which causes light-dark contrasts in the micrographs [45]. Instead of platinum, gold or tantalum-wolfram can be used as shadow materials, showing the advantage of decoration effects only on the oil fracture face. Therefore, it is possible to differentiate between water and oil fractions within the specimen [46].

A negative aspect of this method is that only replicas can be observed, never the sample itself. Furthermore, the formation of artifacts by cryofixation cannot always be excluded. For example, ice decoration is a frequently occurring artifact in FFTEM [47]. According to Jahn and Strey, high cooling rates, a limited number of components, large and slowly reorganizing structures, and detailed structural knowledge from other experimental techniques are essential to minimize these effects [46].

Schulman et al. applied electron microscopy to get the structural information of MEs. In this case, visualization was attained by staining the double bonds in the oil phase with osmium tetroxide [48]. Alany et al. used electron microscopy to characterize the colloidal structures of two pseudo-ternary phase diagrams and to identify phase transitions between the colloidal phases formed [47]. The studied systems were composed of a lipophilic phase, water, and a SAA blend either with or without a co-SAA, 1-butanol. In the co-SAA–free phase diagram, an ME region and a phase of lamellar liquid crystals were identified, whereas the 1-butanol–containing system showed only an increased ME area without any other structures. Electron micrographs enabled the visualization of the structural differences between droplet and bicontinuous MEs, as well as lamellar phases.

36.3.2 VISCOSIMETRY

Determination of rheological behavior and viscosity of MEs can be used to obtain different kinds of information. In many cases, shear rate and shear stress are proportional i.e. MEs exhibit Newtonian flow. The results of such measurements can carry structural information [49].

Ktistis investigated the viscosity of o/w MEs containing IPM, polysorbate 80, sorbitol, and water, varying oil–volume fraction ϕ, total SAA concentration, and SAA/co-SAA mass ratio in order to determine their effect on the hydration of the dispersed droplets [50]. The increase of the relative viscosity η_{rel} with increasing ϕ could be described by the following equation:

$$\eta_{rel} = \exp\left[\frac{a\phi}{1 - K\phi}\right] \tag{36.2}$$

where a is the constant with a theoretical value of 2.5 for solid spheres and K is the hydrodynamic interaction coefficient [51]. A decrease in the polysorbate/sorbitol mass ratio, as well as increasing total SAA concentration, yielded an increase of a and a decrease of K. The deviation of the obtained a values from the theoretical value for spheres was attributed to the hydration of the droplets. The ratio of bound solvent layer to droplet core radius was calculated, resulting in an increase of this parameter with increasing total SAA concentration due to a greater hydrodynamic volume of the droplets.

Primorac et al. studied the rheological behavior of o/w MEs with different emulsifying agents and observed an increase in viscosity with decreasing hydrophilic lipophilic balance (HLB) of coemulsifiers [52]. All systems studied behaved as Newtonian fluids, indicating the existence of spherical particles, but it is also reported about non-Newtonian properties of MEs, e.g., pseudoplastic and thixotropic flow [53].

The aforementioned studies of Alany et al. demonstrated that rheological behavior could be used to differentiate between MEs that change from droplet to bicontinuous systems [47]. Although both exhibit Newtonian flow, only the viscosity of the latter was independent of the water volume fraction. Additionally, it was possible to distinguish between MEs and lamellar liquid crystals. Because of their geometrically ordered and rigid structure, lamellar phases show a higher viscosity and pseudoplastic flow.

Rheological characteristics are important features for the development of innovative dosage forms, particularly for the special route of administrations. The effects of formulation components (oil phase content, total SAA concentration, and polysorbate 80/lecithin weight ratio K_m) on rheological properties of lecithin-based o/w MEs for parenteral use were studied [54]. It was shown that an increase in the amount of SAA and oil, respectively, resulted in a change of the rheological behavior from non-Newtonian into Newtonian flow and rising viscosity values, whereas K_m influenced these properties only marginally. The results of this method in combination with particle size analysis led to the selection of a Newtonian ME system containing 10% oil (IPM), 30% SAA blend, and 60% water, which was further tested in terms of stability and acute toxicity. From the results, the authors concluded that lecithin-based o/w MEs are valuable technological alternatives for intravenous administration of low-water-soluble drugs.

36.3.3 LIGHT AND NEUTRON SCATTERING

Elucidation of ME microstructure, an important feature for the development of these drug delivery systems, can be very complex. Here, the application of three scattering techniques has been described. These methods involve only weak perturbation and hence are readily used to monitor particle size and size distribution of MEs nondestructively. The aspects are discussed by recalling the theoretical background and illustrating the potential of the techniques with experimental results.

36.3.3.1 Light Scattering from Microemulsion Droplets

Interaction of light with matter can be used to obtain important information about the structure and dynamics of matter. Investigation of this interaction is possible by light scattering experiments, which offer two ways of gleaning information. The first method, called dynamic light scattering (DLS), monitors fluctuations in scattered light as a function of time $I(t)$. The second method, called static light scattering (SLS), observes interparticle interference patterns of scattered light by measuring the time average intensity as a function of angle $\langle I(\theta)\rangle$.

36.3.3.1.1 SLS from Microemulsion Droplets

For MEs, time-average (or "total") intensity of the scattered light arises from concentration fluctuation of the droplets of the dispersed phase. The scattering intensity $\langle I \rangle$ at a selected scattering angle θ can be written as [55]:

$$\langle I(q)\rangle = kV\phi P(q)S(q) \tag{36.3}$$

where q is the scattering wave vector with $q = \left(\frac{4\pi n}{\lambda}\right)sin\frac{\theta}{2}$, depending on the wavelength λ of the incident light, the refractive index n of the ME, and the scattering angle θ. K is a constant characteristic of the instrument, V the ME droplet volume, ϕ the droplet volume fraction, P the form factor of an isolated colloidal particle, and S the structure factor that carries all the information about correlations among colloidal particles. Often, ME droplets have a small radius R compared to the wavelength of the light λ, and $qR \ll 1$. In this case, scattering intensity is independent of the scattering angle, and for spherical droplets Equation (36.3) can be rewritten as [56]:

$$\frac{\phi}{\langle I \rangle} \approx G \frac{1}{R^3}\left(\frac{\partial n}{\partial \phi}\right)^{-2}(1 + K_I \phi) \tag{36.4}$$

where G is the constant for all samples, and K_I describes perturbation due to thermodynamic effects and is therefore related to the interaction potential. For hard sphere potential $K_I = 8$. The coefficient K_I becomes smaller if there are supplementary attractive interactions and larger in the case of additional repulsive interaction.

If the studied systems are ideal mixtures, $(\partial n/\partial \phi)$ is constant and $(\phi/\langle I \rangle)$ should be a linear function of ϕ provided that droplet size does not vary significantly over the concentration range. By extrapolating the linear plot of $(\phi/\langle I \rangle)$ to $\phi = 0$, the radius of ME droplets R can be obtained if a calibration has been made by applying samples of known size [57]. By the slope of the linear plot of $(\phi/\langle I \rangle)$ versus ϕ, determination of interdroplet interaction is possible. From this interaction potential, parameters describing stability, i.e., coagulation time of systems can be estimated [58].

36.3.3.1.2 DLS from Microemulsion Droplets

The Brownian motion of ME droplets within the continuous phase causes time-dependent fluctuations of the scattered light intensity dependent on the hydrodynamic properties of the system. In DLS, the autocorrelation function of the scattered light $g_2(\tau) = \langle I(t)I(t+\tau)\rangle_t$ is detected. Since the normalized field autocorrelation function $g_1(\tau)$ is a quantity of basic interest in DLS and carries the information about droplet motions in a system, it has been derived from the measured scattered intensity autocorrelation function $g_2(\tau)$ via the Siegert relation [59]:

$$g_1(\tau) = C\sqrt{1 - g_2(\tau)} \tag{36.5}$$

where the constant C is in the order of unity, dependent on instrumental conditions and the amount of background scattering from solvent, etc.

For dense polydisperse interacting systems of ME droplets, $g_1(\tau)$ can be represented as the sum of two exponentials, provided that the extent of polydispersity is not too large [60]:

$$g_1(\tau) = \frac{A_1}{A_1 + A_2}\exp(-D_c q^2 \tau) + \frac{A_2}{A_1 + A_2}exp(-D_s q^2 \tau) \tag{36.6}$$

The two exponentials in Equation (36.6) are attributed to the existence of two relaxation modes: fast mode is due to collective diffusion D_c (i.e., total number of density fluctuations), whereas slow mode is due to self-diffusion D_s (i.e., concentration fluctuations that decay by the exchange of species by single droplet diffusion). $A_1/(A_1 + A_2)$ and $A_2/(A_1 + A_2)$ are the intensities of their exponentials. Relative amplitude of slower decaying mode, $A_2/(A_1 + A_2)$, can be used as measure of the size polydispersity index $\sigma_s = \sqrt{\frac{\langle R^2 \rangle}{\langle R \rangle^2} - 1}$ [60–62].

The average hydrodynamic radius of scattering droplets R_h can be determined from the free particle diffusion coefficient D_0 using the Stokes-Einstein equation:

$$R_h = \frac{k_B T}{6\pi\eta D_0}$$

(36.7)

where K_B is the Boltzmann's constant, T is the absolute temperature, and η is the coefficient of the continuous-phase viscosity. For spherical particles, interacting through essentially a hard sphere or excluded-volume forces, D_0 can be deduced from the collective diffusion coefficient D_c by means of the droplet volume fraction ϕ following (25):

$$D_c = D_0 \left(1 + 1.56\phi + 0.91\phi^2 + ...\right)$$

(36.8)

The results of this kind of double exponential fit for o/w MEs consisting of Poloxamer 331/Tagat O2 as SAAs, water/propylene glycol as continuous phase, and two different pharmaceutical oils (Eutanol G and isopropyl palmitate IPP]) studied by Shukla et al. are summarized in Table 36.1. The obtained values are close to the results deduced by approximate analysis of small-angle neutron scattering and indicate that the kind of oil (comparable molecular size provided) only marginally influences the droplet size of an ME [20].

In diluted regions, the difference between D_c and D_s is expected to be small. Therefore, resolution of the measured autocorrelation function by a sum of two exponentials will be difficult. In this case, analyzing the obtained normalized field autocorrelation function $g_1(\tau)$ by a single exponent [63] (for monodispersed systems) or cumulants [64] (for polydispersed systems) gives an apparent diffusion coefficient D_{app}. D_0 can be identified with D_{app} when $\phi \to 0$ and is used for the calculation of R_h.

Shukla et al. investigated o/w MEs by means of DLS using a dilution procedure in the region of the phase diagram where SAA-covered oil droplets were formed [65]. The aim of the studies was to determine information about the diffusion coefficient, droplet size, interparticle interaction, and polydispersities from experimental data applying cumulant fitting. With a suitable model, scattering data were corrected for interparticle interactions that occur in concentrated nonideal systems. The results indicate a considerable increase in coagulation time due to the observed particle–particle interaction compared with rapid coagulation that happens when there is no interaction between

TABLE 36.1
Particle Size Parameters of MEs

ME	DLS		SANS		
	R_h (nm)	σ_s	R_{core} (nm)	R_{shell} (nm)	σ_s
IPP	9.58	0.156	7.75	11.49	0.174
Eutanol	9.01	0.180	7.98	10.81	0.209

Source: From Reference [20].
Note: Errors are smaller than ±2% for the radii and ±10% for the size polydispersity index σ_s

particles except a sharp attraction by touching each other. These stability results were consistent with the observed long-term stability of the studied MEs.

The DLS results have also been used as a means of identifying the microstructure of MEs [10, 17, 66]. In droplet MEs, the apparent diffusion coefficients (from which the droplet size of the ME was determined using the Stokes-Einstein equation) obtained at various scattering angles showed no significant difference. Besides, the angular independence of diffusion coefficients suggests that ME droplets are spherical in shape. On the other hand, bicontinuous MEs were shown to have a very high pseudo-droplet diameter and relative standard deviation, which was attributed to the dynamics and structural alterations of the bicontinuous channels. Furthermore, the apparent diffusion coefficients of bicontinuous MEs vary with the scattering angles.

36.3.3.2 Neutron Scattering from Microemulsion Droplets

The principle of neutron scattering is similar to that of light scattering. The scattering intensity of thermal neutrons from soft matter can also be expressed by Equation 36.3 [67]. In the case of light, the interaction is between the electric field of the radiation and the electronic charges. Neutrons, having no electrical charge, interact in almost all situations via their scattering length with the nuclei exclusively. Their penetration is very large and allows the study of materials containing heavy elements. The typical wavelength associated with thermal neutrons is in the order of 1 to 10 Å, which means an increased resolution. Considering the droplet sizes present in colloidal systems, it can be deduced that neutrons are very often the more appropriate way of studying their structure. Mostly small scattering angles are applied. This constitutes the technique of small-angle neutron scattering (SANS).

Shukla et al. used a core shell sphere form factor with an internal core of radius R_{core} and a scattering length density ρ_{core} surrounded by a shell with an outer radius R_{shell} and a scattering length density ρ_{shell} [67] for fitting their data. A useful expression of the structure factor $S(q)$ for hard spheres is obtained from the Percus-Yevick approximation [69].

Applying the aforementioned procedure, the authors obtained the size and polydispersity index of the two o/w MEs already investigated by DLS (Table 36.1) [20]. In their computation, a Schultz size distribution function was used, and the fits were generated by allowing R_{core}, ρ_{shell}, and σ_s to vary. As shown in Figure 36.1, the R_{core} radius corresponds to the size of the oil droplet (dark black

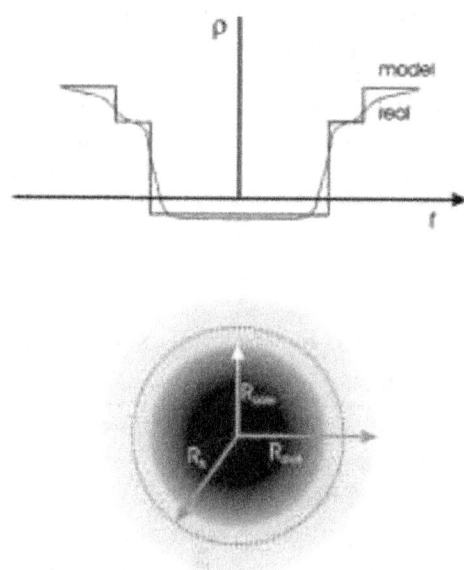

FIGURE 36.1   Model of an o/w ME droplet as a core shell sphere. (From Reference [20].)

part:pure oil and residue:penetration of SAA tails into the oil), whereas R_{shell} describes the distance between the center of the particle and a position in the surface film, where the difference in scattering length density has its maximum. As expected, the outer radius incorporates looser-bounded SAA molecules and is substantially bigger than the hydrodynamic radius R_h, obtained by DLS. The latter is supposed to consist of the oil core and a stronger bounded SAA film, perhaps containing some solvent molecules too.

Although ME structure elucidation by SANS has been advanced by several workers (e.g., [70–73]) there are still many complications. First, the scattering length density of the attached SAA layer is usually of the value between those of adsorbed molecules comprising the layer and solvent molecules as a consequence of penetration or adsorption of solvent into the attached layer. Second, for other than hard sphere potentials, SANS data analysis, incorporating polydispersity, may not be straightforward due to complexity in the structure factor. Nevertheless, scattering techniques are valuable tools for determining the structure of colloidal systems.

36.4 DERMAL AND TRANSDERMAL DRUG DELIVERY USING MICROEMULSIONS

The barrier nature of the skin, resulting in poor permeability of drugs, has limited the dermal and transdermal delivery of several drugs [15, 16]. Several chemical and physical methods such as chemical penetration enhancers, iontophoresis, electroporation, and sonophoresis have been employed to overcome this barrier and improve the skin drug permeation [16]. However, these approaches have their own limitations such as skin irritation and sensitization by the chemical enhancers and the physical disruption by the other methods [74, 75].

In dermatopharmacy MEs are promising colloidal carriers for dermal and transdermal delivery of drugs due to their high drug-loading capacity and drug-permeation-enhancing effects. The high drug solubilization capacity of MEs is attributed to the enormous interfacial area and existence of microenvironments of different polarity within the same single-phase system [1].

Confocal laser scanning microscopy investigations revealed the involvement of paracellular, transcellular, and transfollicular pathways [76, 77] during ME-mediated percutaneous absorption of topically applied drugs. Mostly, the transepidermal routes (paracellular as well as transcellular) are the dominant skin permeation pathways for several drugs. The very low interfacial tension between the formulation and skin ensures an excellent contact to the skin surface, where the good spreading is additionally supported by the low viscosity. Hence, the formulation is capable of entering the skin easily. Due to their hydrophilic and lipophilic domains, it can be suggested that MEs are able to interact with both the lipid and the polar pathways by entering the stratum corneum (SC) via the intercellular route.

MEs are valuable vehicles for the localization (retention) of drugs within skin layers (local effects), as well as for systemic delivery [7]. The localization of drugs in the skin layer can be used for both cosmetic and therapeutic purposes. Site-specific treatment of dermatological diseases is a classical field of topical administration. A wide range of hydrophilic and lipophilic actives can be solubilized in MEs, as there are plenty of combinations of ME constituents which principally can form MEs [4]. In the case of lipophilic substances, application of conventional vehicles such as ointments often causes formation of a drug depot in SC. This phenomenon is attributed to the high affinity of these drugs to the lipophilic structure of the outermost skin layer. MEs are capable of increasing their permeation extent.

During the past several years, improving the effect of MEs on dermal drug delivery has been demonstrated in several *in vitro*, *ex vivo*, and *in vivo* studies, showing the influence of different factors on the enhancing activity. Some of the selected investigations in delivering various classes of actives, including highly lipophilic molecules such as ceramides (CERs) and highly hydrophilic molecules such as peptides, are discussed next.

36.4.1 Epidermal Lipids

The lipid regions in the SC, consisting of mainly CERs, cholesterol, and fatty acids, are essential for the barrier function of the skin, as they are the only continuous structure in the SC. Studies have shown that some skin diseases such as psoriasis and atopic dermatitis and aging are associated with reduced levels of SC lipids and/or altered lipid compositions [78–80]. Therefore, these lipids have been used in some skin care products to replenish the depleted lipids.

CERs play a crucial role in the skin barrier function and skin hydration. The depleted CERs (in some skin conditions) can be replenished with exogenous skin-identical CERs. By virtue of their head groups, CERs are substantially important in forming super-stable lipid lamellae. The CERs, however, need to be delivered deep into the stratum granulosum–SC interface where the SC lipid organization into lipid bilayers takes place [81–83]. Since the penetration of CERs across the skin from conventional formulations such as ointment and cream is poor (which is attributed to their extreme lipophilicity) [66, 84], MEs have been investigated to improve the poor solubility, facilitate the permeation, and target the delivery of CERs into the SC [10, 17, 22, 66]. Sahle et al. developed and characterized stable lecithin- and polyglycerol fatty acid ester SAA–based MEs for controlled delivery of CER [AP] into the SC [10, 17]. The release and penetration from the MEs were assessed *in vitro* by using a multilayer membrane model. The *in vitro* investigations showed that the MEs exhibited excellent rate and extent of release and penetration as compared to hydrophilic cream. The lecithin-based MEs were also shown to have better properties (smaller globule size, spherical shape, better stability, and lipid loading capacity) than polyglycerol fatty acid SAA–based MEs.

Sahle et al. also investigated the penetration of CER [NP] from various ME formulations (using lecithin or TEGO CARE PL 4 as base SAAs) *ex vivo* using excised human skin mounted on Franz diffusion cells [66]. Unlike the conventional hydrophilic cream, CER [NP] loaded in the MEs permeated into the deeper layers of the SC. It was also shown that type, microstructure, and viscosity of MEs influence the extent of permeation. Compared to TEGO CARE PL 4 containing MEs, lecithin-based MEs permeated into the deeper skin layers and smaller and/or o/w MEs permeated more into the deeper skin layers than bigger and/or bicontinuous MEs, respectively. As the penetration from ME gels was minimal and shallow, they can be used as a means of localizing the MEs into the desired site.

In another study by Tessema et al. [85], plant-derived CERs (phytoceramides) were incorporated into lecithin-based MEs and ME gel (using Carbopol 980 as a gelling agent). Both *in vitro* (using an artificial four-layer membrane system) and *ex vivo* (using excised human skin) studies revealed the penetration-enhancing effect of ME compared to the standard amphiphilic cream formulation. Compared to the ME, the ME gel exhibited reduced depth and extent of phytoceramides permeation and was effective in concentrating phytoceramides in the SC where they need to be.

On the other hand, development of well-tolerated MEs containing fatty acids, particularly linoleic acid, as the active ingredient has been described Goebel et al. [21]. Penetration studies showed higher amounts of linoleic acids were penetrated after ME application (up to 23% of the applied dose) compared to the reference standard cream formulation (at most 8%) at all the investigated incubation times. Linoleic acids were also found to accumulate in the epidermis at longer incubation times. The penetration-enhancing effect of MEs suggests that these colloidal systems might be an interesting vehicle for the delivery of linoleic acids into the epidermis for barrier-enhancing and possibly for antiinflammatory effects.

36.4.2 Peptides

Most peptide drugs and cosmetic actives have poor oral bioavailability due to extensive proteolytic degradation by enzymes in the gastrointestinal tract and their poor permeability into the intestinal mucosa (high hydrophilicity and high molecular weight). As an alternative route of administration, dermal/transdermal delivery has received attention in recent years as a promising means of enhancing the delivery of peptides across the skin. The SC, however, hampers the transport of the hydrophilic peptides into skin. Incorporation of peptides into MEs helps overcome SC barrier.

A series of studies aiming at delivering various peptides into the skin using colloidal carrier systems have been made to show the beneficial effects of MEs in enhancing skin penetration of peptides. To show the potential application of MEs in the dermal and transdermal delivery of peptides, the skin penetration profiles of desmopressin acetate from w/o ME and amphiphilic cream, a standard formulation, were determined using Franz diffusion cells [86]. A higher amount of desmopressin acetate was found in the deeper skin layers and in the acceptor compartment from the ME compared to the standard cream.

Goebel et al. investigated the topical bioavailability of hydrophilic dipeptides, L-carnosine, and its related compound, N-acetyl-L-carnosine, from standard formulations containing enhancer molecules and MEs [87]. In *ex vivo* penetration studies, an enhancer (1,2-pentylene glycol) containing a standard formulation resulted in higher dipeptide concentrations in the SC and viable skin layers at all experimental periods compared to enhancer-free formulations and MEs. The relatively lower penetration of dipeptide from MEs was attributed to the inappropriateness of the microstructure of the MEs prepared for the delivery of such a hydrophilic molecule, suggesting the need to undertake further investigations to enhance and optimize the penetration of the dipeptide from MEs.

In attempt to improve the topical bioavailability of the polar tetrapeptide PKEK (amino acid sequence in one-letter notation), an ME was developed by Neubert et al. [88], and the *ex vivo* human skin penetration of PKEK from the ME was compared to a standard formulation. The penetration study showed that relatively high amounts (40% to 58%) of the PKEK penetrated into the skin from the standard cream and mainly remained in the SC. The PKEK did not reach the target layer of the skin. On the other hand, very high amounts of PKEK loaded in MEs penetrated into the human skin after 100 minutes (94%) and 300 minutes (88%) incubation times. The largest proportion of PKEK did not remain in the skin, but rather permeated into the acceptor compartment. The relative peptide content in the viable skin layers, however, was predominantly comparable for the cream and the ME.

In another study, the authors developed w/o ME to enhance the penetration of another tetrapeptide, GEKG [89]. The *ex vivo* studies were performed to investigate the dermal penetration, as well as localization and distribution of the tetrapeptide in the skin layer. The results showed that the nano-sized carrier system significantly enhanced the transport of GEKG into upper and deeper vital skin layers, as well as through the skin, compared to the standard cream. Therefore, liquid nano-sized systems such as MEs are more effective as carriers for extremely hydrophilic peptides used in cosmetics and in therapeutics than the classical cosmetic emulsions or enhancer-containing emulsions.

36.4.3 LOCAL ANESTHETICS

MEs have been investigated for the topical administration of some local anesthetics. Kreilgaard et al. studied the potential use of MEs in improving dermal delivery of hydrophilic (prilocaine HCl) and lipophilic (lidocaine) model drugs *in vitro* (using excised rat skin mounted on Franz-type diffusion cells) [90] as well as *in vivo* (microdialysis in rats) [91]. The ME increased the flux and *in vivo* penetration rate of both drugs compared to the commercial products. This was attributed to the high drug solubilization capacity of MEs causing a larger concentration gradient towards the skin. The transdermal flux was found to be dependent on the drug mobility in the individual vehicle. A pharmacokinetic model, reliably estimating cutaneous absorption coefficient and lag time from microdialysis data, revealed a good *in vitro–in vivo* correlation. The MEs also showed low skin irritancy.

Further studies were also carried out to investigate the cutaneous bioequivalence of lidocaine from MEs and an o/w emulsion–based cream in volunteers using a minimal invasive microdialysis technique and determining the pharmacodynamic effect [92]. Applying the ME, the mean absorption coefficient of the local anesthetic drug was shown to increase about threefold, and the lag time entering the dermis was reduced considerably compared to the conventional vehicle. However, the anesthetic effect did not diverge significantly between the two formulations.

Junyaprasert et al. developed Brij 97– and Aerosol OT–based MEs for transdermal delivery of hydrophobic (lidocaine, tetracaine, and dibucaine) and hydrophilic (their respective HCl salts) local anesthetics and investigated the effect of ME microstructures on skin permeability using heat-separated human epidermis mounted on modified Franz diffusion cells [93, 94]. The results from *in vitro* skin permeation studies showed that the type of MEs, drug intrinsic properties, and drug–SAA interactions have effects on the skin permeation of the drugs from the ME formulations.

Transdermal transport of hydrophilic (diltiazem HCl, lidocaine HCl) and lipophilic (lidocaine-free base, estradiol) drugs from w/o and o/w MEs containing IPM, polysorbate 80, water, ethanol, N-methyl-pyrrolidone (NMP), and oleyl alcohol as an enhancer was studied by Lee et al. [36]. For all the drugs MEs considerably improved the drug transport compared to solution in either water or IPM, with a significantly better flux from the o/w system than from w/o. The results suggest that transport from the aqueous phase is the most important factor for both kinds of drugs, whereas the oil phase serves as a drug depot. This could be confirmed by removing the SAA and oil from the system. The flux from the remaining water-phase components was comparable to that from the o/w ME. It was concluded that the presence of NMP increases the partition of the lipophilic drugs into the water phase, hence making them available for transport across the skin.

Changez and Varshney developed w/o MEs made of AOT (sodium bis[2-ethyl hexyl] sulfosuc-cinate), IPM, and water for topical application of tetracaine HCl and studied the local analgesic response on rats [95]. The optimal formulation exhibited an eightfold enhancement of this param-eter compared to an aqueous solution of the drug. It was assumed that AOT as an anionic SAA is able to soften the SC. The safety of MEs as a transdermal carrier has also been confirmed by histo-pathological, irritation, and oxidative stress investigations on mice.

36.4.4 ANALGESICS AND ANTIINFLAMMATORY DRUGS

Previously, ME formulations have been developed for transdermal delivery of nonsteroidal antiin-flammatory drugs, as these drugs are mostly sparingly soluble, induce gastrointestinal side effects, and are liable to first-pass metabolism.

Kriwet and Mueller-Goymann obtained different colloidal structures (liposomes, MEs, and lamellar liquid crystals) by varying the mass ratio of the components of a ternary system contain-ing phospholipids, diclofenac diethylamine, and water [96]. In this case, the amphiphilic drug takes part essentially in forming the microstructure. *In vitro* drug release studies, as well as permeation studies through excised human SC, exhibited a dependence of diffusion behavior on the colloidal structure. Whereas in liposomes and lamellar phases strongly bound drug and phospholipids ham-per the interaction with the horny layer, incorporation into MEs leads to enhanced SC permeability.

Fouad et al. developed and optimized ME- and poloxamer ME–based gel formulations for sus-tained transdermal delivery of diclofenac epolamine [97]. Unlike the gel formulations, the opti-mized ME showed high drug permeability in *ex vivo* newly born rat skin. In addition, an *in vivo* antiinflammatory efficacy study in rat paw edema demonstrated sustained effect (for 12 hours) after removal of ME applied to the skin. According to the authors, this result shows the formation of in-skin drug depot.

Cationic MEs containing piroxicam and a piroxicam-ß-cyclodextrin inclusion complex were developed by Dalmora et al. [98, 99]. The drug solubility was remarkably increased in MEs compared to simple solutions. *In vitro* piroxicam release studies demonstrated a reservoir effect. Furthermore, *in vivo* assessment of antiinflammatory activity on rats resulted in significantly inhib-ited inflammatory reactions after topical application relative to control and an improved effect of the MEs after subcutaneous administration compared to a buffered solution of the drug. The prolonged pharmacological activity after subcutaneous application confirmed the potential of modifying der-mal drug delivery by ME systems.

Yuan et al. developed an o/w ME for transdermal delivery of meloxicam and evaluated various formulation factors to obtain high skin permeation of the drug [27]. Among the various SAAs and co-SAAs studied, polyoxyethylene sorbitan trioleate (Tween 85) and ethanol showed excellent solubility and skin drug permeation–enhancing effects, respectively. The optimum ME with the highest skin permeation rate consisted of 5% IPM, 50% Tween 85/ethanol (1:1), and water.

The potential application of lecithin-based o/w ME as a carrier system for percutaneous delivery of ketoprofen was investigated by Paolino et al. [12]. Ketoprofen-loaded MEs showed an enhanced permeation through human skin compared to conventional formulations (o/w and w/o cream and gel). A good human skin tolerability (evaluated on human volunteers) of ME was observed compared to the conventional vehicles. In another study, Rhee et al. developed o/w MEs containing Labrasol/Cremophor RH 40 and oleic acid for topical application of ketoprofen [36]. They carried out permeation experiments on excised rat skin in order to investigate the influence of oil and SAA content on transdermal transport. With increasing SAA content a twelvefold to twenty-threefold decrease in permeation rate was detected, which was probably caused by a lower thermodynamic activity at higher SAA amounts. At SAA concentrations of 30% and 55%, respectively, an optimum oil content of 6% was found. Incorporating several terpenes as an enhancer, only limonene exhibited improved permeation properties.

Subramanian et al. developed an ME system containing IPM, medium-chain glyceride, polysorbate 80, and water for topical delivery of celecoxib, a selective cyclooxygenase inhibitor [100]. The *in vitro* percutaneous absorption and *in vivo* antiinflammatory effect of celecoxib were found to be enhanced by using MEs. The MEs were found to increase the permeation rate of celecoxib up to 5 and 11 times compared with those of ME gel and cream, respectively. The study suggested that the developed ME formulations might serve as a potential drug vehicle for the prevention of UVB-induced skin cancer.

Recently ME-based gel formulations have been prepared and characterized for transdermal delivery of celecoxib [101, 102]. The ME gels improved the transdermal permeation of celecoxib compared to the conventional gel. *In vivo* pharmacokinetic study in rabbits revealed better bioavailability of celecoxib compared to the commercial product, Celebrex [101]. Incorporation of a gelling agent in the MEs also made the formulation suitable for topical application and controlled the drug release, suggesting improved therapeutic effects of celecoxib for arthritis [102]. Therefore, ME-based gels could be promising formulations over the conventional dosage forms.

Niflumic acid was incorporated into sucrose fatty acid ester–stabilized bicontinuous MEs by Bolzinger-Thevenin et al. [103]. The antiinflammatory effect of an ME system that was saturated with the drug (1%) was comparable to that from a commercially available 3% o/w emulsion. Occurring lag time was attributed to the accumulation of niflumic acid in the interfacial film of the ME, which could control the drug release.

Heuschkel et al. developed MEs containing dihydroavenanthramide D, a synthetic analogue to naturally occurring avenanthramides, to investigate the effects of various enhancer molecules on drug release and skin penetration from conventional cream [104]. Later, they developed MEs based on a vegetable protein SAA and 1,2-alkanediols as co-SAAs [105]. Compared to the previously investigated glycol-containing cream, a smaller fraction of the drug loaded in ME was found within viable epidermis and dermis, but the amount in the acceptor fluid increased significantly.

36.4.5 STEROIDS

Steroids such as hydrocortisone (HC), estradiol, and testosterone have been formulated as topical MEs. An *in vitro* release study (using a multilayer membrane system) of HC loaded in ME, as well as commercially available vehicles, showed good release properties, suggesting that the drug release is not the rate-limiting factor in the penetration process [106]. Using Franz-type diffusion cells, the penetration of HC from the innovative ME was subsequently compared to that of an o/w cream (Nubral 4HC, proven to be effective in treatment of dermatologic conditions). Drug content in different layers of human breast skin, as well as in the acceptor solution, was analyzed after 30 and 300 minutes, respectively. Application of the conventional vehicle yielded a considerable accumulation of HC in the SC, and only small amounts of the drug were detected in lower skin layers and the acceptor. On the other hand, the ME caused inferior drug depot in the horny layer and the amount of HC permeated into the acceptor increased significantly, confirming the ability of MEs in transporting drugs in a greater extent through the main permeability barrier, the SC.

Lehmann et al. tested an o/w and a w/o ME for their suitability in dermatological use [107]. In a hen's egg test on chorioallantoic membrane (HET-CAM), both formulations, containing either sucrose esters or Tagat S/Plurololeat WL1173 as nonionic SAAs and IPM as the lipophilic phase, were classified as a nonirritant. But an *in vivo* test on human subjects demonstrated a significant increase in transepidermal water loss (TEWL) by the MEs compared to untreated control sites. The water-continuous system caused dehydration of SC as well. Furthermore, the influence of the MEs on HC penetration was evaluated in terms of a skin-blanching test. Despite the observed enhanced drug penetration from the colloidal systems as compared to an amphiphilic cream, neither ME confers benefit in HC therapy because irritant effects of the formulations outbalance the improved penetration of the antiirritant drug. The authors concluded that use of MEs as drug delivery systems is more valuable when irritant effects are negligible.

Fini et al. evaluated the release and transdermal permeation of HC acetate from MEs and conventional formulations [108]. The MEs enhanced the permeation of HC acetate across an *ex vivo* membrane compared to gel and ointment formulations, and hence, the later formulations were shown to be suitable in minimizing the absorption of topically applied HC acetate and preventing systemic side effects.

Transdermal application of estradiol is a frequently used way for increasing systemic bioavailability by avoiding the first-pass metabolism that occurs after oral treatment. *In vitro* permeation experiments through human cadaver skin demonstrated that MEs are appropriate vehicles for this purpose [109]. The observed 200- to 700-fold increase in steady-state flux compared to a saturated solution in phosphate buffered saline was assumed to be due to the improved solubility in the MEs and the resulting increased concentration gradient towards the skin. Considering therapeutic plasma concentration and estradiol clearance, pharmacological effects can be expected by topical application of the systems.

Hathout et al. developed an ME formulation for the transdermal delivery of testosterone using oleic acid as the oil phase, Tween 20 as an SAA, and Transcutol as the co-SAA [14]. The study demonstrated that the drug mainly located in the oily domains of the MEs and the ME-mediated transdermal delivery was successful.

36.4.6 IMMUNOSUPPRESSANTS

Immunosuppressants such as cyclosporine A (CsA) and methotrexate (MTX) are among the standard treatments for psoriasis vulgaris and are mostly applied orally or parenterally. Systemic administration of these drugs has severe side effects such as nephrotoxicity and hepatotoxicity. In the past, several conventional topical formulations were ineffective in treating psoriasis compared to systemic or intradermal application. Due to high lipophilicity and molecular weight, CsA poorly penetrates the skin and mainly accumulates in the SC. The T cell as a target structure, however, is localized in the dermoepidermal junction region and in the upper dermis layer. Likewise, the topical application of MTX is problematic because of its hydrophilic character, the high molecular weight, and the high dissociation degree at physiological pH. A number of *in vitro* and *in vivo* studies have shown enhanced dermal delivery of these drugs using MEs [37, 110–112].

Jahn succeeded in developing CsA containing o/w MEs of therapeutic importance [37]. In *ex vivo* penetration studies on human breast skin using Franz-type diffusion cells, higher concentrations of CsA were detected in viable epidermis and dermis layers following the application of an o/w cream than MEs. But the conventional vehicle was not able to transport the drug through all the skin

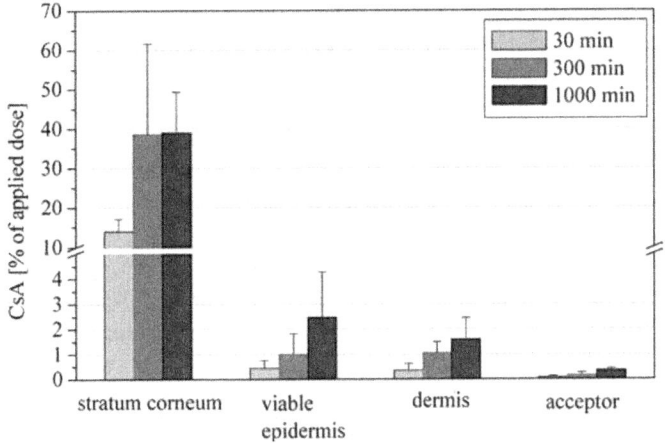

FIGURE 36.2 Penetration of cyclosporine A (CsA) from an o/w cream into human skin *ex vivo* after 30, 300, and 1000 minutes (mean ± SD, $n = 3$). (From Reference [37].)

layers, whereas 20% to 30% of the applied dose from the ME reached the acceptor (Figures 36.2 and 36.3), which is assumed to be responsible for a pharmacological effect.

An *in vivo* study involving 10 patients with chronic plaque-type psoriasis demonstrated CsA containing ME to be comparable to commercially available creams containing calcipotriol and betamethasone-17-valerate (a common therapy for psoriasis). The slight advantage of a system with DMSO as an enhancer in addition to oleic acid as the lipophilic phase in preceding penetration studies could not be established *in vivo*. Application of this ME on chronically inflamed skin caused irritant effects and is therefore concluded not to be suited for the treatment of damaged skin.

Alvarez-Figueroa and Blanco-Méndez carried out *in vitro* studies on pig skin for transdermal delivery of MTX [110]. MEs were found to be more effective compared to simple solutions. However, iontophoretic delivery from solutions exceeded the ME results, probably due to the lower solubility of MTX in MEs than in aqueous solutions.

Goebel et al. developed MEs containing tacrolimus and investigated the skin penetration *ex vivo* [113]. The penetration studies demonstrated that ME formulations resulted in higher concentrations of tacrolimus in the deeper skin layers independent of the time of incubation compared to

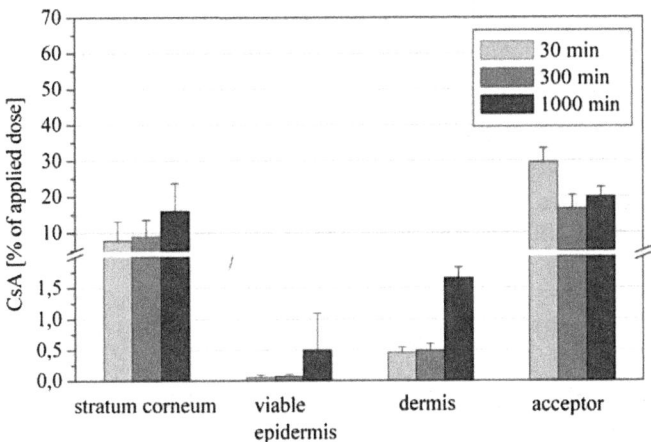

FIGURE 36.3 Penetration of cyclosporine A (CsA) from an o/w ME into human skin *ex vivo* after 30, 300, and 1000 minutes (mean ± SD, $n = 3$). (From Reference [37].)

the standard vehicle ointment. The colloidal carrier systems significantly enhanced the penetration profile of tacrolimus ($p < 0.01$). High amounts of drug loaded in the MEs penetrated the target site in a short period of time.

36.4.7 OTHER DRUGS

Several antiacne drugs including antimicrobial agents like basil oil [114], tea tree oil [115], retinoic acid [25], and azelaic acid [116, 117], as well as some antibiotics, have been incorporated into MEs. Bhatia et al. developed an ME formulation for the transfollicular delivery of adapalene, a synthetic analog of retinol used for the treatment of acne [76]. Confocal laser scanning microscopy images suggested the transfollicular permeation of the ME. The microstructure was also shown to affect drug penetration into hair follicles (bicontinuous ME enhanced the drug penetration compared to o/w ME). The proposed transfollicular pathway of MEs might be advantageous for acne treatment.

Dermal delivery of antioxidants plays a role in prophylaxis and treatment of ultraviolet-induced damage of the skin such as photoaging and photocarcinogenesis, which are related to increased levels of free radicals. An effective skin protection by ascorbyl palmitate, incorporated into an ME, has been demonstrated [117], but also α-tocopherol is in use [119].

8-Methoxsalen (8-MOP), a photoactive furocoumarin, has been widely used for the treatment of hyperproliferative skin diseases such as psoriasis. The cutaneous accumulation and *in vitro* penetration on newborn pig skin of 8-MOP–loaded MEs containing varying amounts of SAA, IPM, and water were investigated [120]. All MEs exhibited an increase in both parameters compared to a saturated IPM solution and a clinically used aqueous solution. Since 8-MOP is effective in psoriasis therapy, retaining of the drug in the skin is required and can be realized by varying the composition of the MEs.

ME-based transdermal delivery has also been investigated for the administration of a number of other classes of drugs, including beta-blockers, antihypertensives, antiparkinsonian agents, antivirals, and others. Kemken et al. studied the pharmacodynamic effects of several beta-blockers incorporated into water-free ME preformulations [121]. The vehicles were saturated with the drugs and, after application under occlusion, water uptake from the skin leads to *in situ* formation of water containing MEs, decreasing the solubility of the lipophilic drugs (therefore supersaturated). The observed high pharmacodynamic effects were assumed to be due to rising thermodynamic activity as the driving force for enhanced dermal drug uptake. Trotta et al. studied the *in vitro* skin permeation of felodipine loaded in o/w MEs [122]. Keeping the amount of the other phases nearly constant, it was shown that drug flux depends on the composition of the lipophilic phase. The ME system with the highest drug solubility could favor permeability, probably due to the droplets of the internal phase acting as an effective drug reservoir.

In vitro (using hairless mouse skin) as well as clinical studies have shown the use of MEs for the transdermal delivery of apomorphine in the treatment of Parkinson disease [26, 123]. In the former study, lipophilic apomorphine–octanoate ion pairs were formed to improve drug permeability [26]. The *in vivo* steady-state plasma concentration was estimated from the *in vitro* steady-state flux, suggesting the future *in vivo* application. The *in vivo* studies on Parkinson disease patients also demonstrated the clinical efficacy and long action of ME-mediated transdermal delivery of apomorphine [123].

ME has been investigated as a possible carrier for transdermal delivery of theophylline using oleic acid and Cremophor RH40/Labrasol (1:2) as the oil phase and SAA/co-SAA, respectively [124]. The *in vivo* pharmacokinetic study using rabbits indicated that $AUC_{0\to\infty}$ of transdermal administration was 1.65-fold higher than that of oral solution administration. In another study, the potential application of ME containing oleic acid, Cremophor EL, and ethanol was investigated for the dermal delivery of penciclovir [125]. The optimized ME formulation significantly increased the permeation of penciclovir through excised mouse skins compared to the commercial cream.

Schmalfuß et al. studied the amount of a hydrophilic model drug, diphenhydramine HCl (DPH), in different skin layers using *ex vivo* human skin [34]. A standard w/o ME resulted in an accumulation of the drug in the dermis. Addition of cholesterol as a penetration enhancer caused a generally higher penetration rate and a shift of the drug towards the epidermis. Cholesterol was assumed to loosen the SC lipid bilayers, enabling an increased hydration of the polar head groups and therefore facilitating penetration of DPH along the polar route. This mechanism is proposed for hydrophilic substances. This incorporation of oleic acid as an enhancer did not change the penetration rate or concentration profile, probably because it influences only the lipophilic pathway by altering the CER chain's mobility.

36.5 FACTORS AFFECTING THE SKIN PENETRATION OF MICROEMULSIONS

As has been shown, numerous studies confirm MEs as potential vehicles for dermal and transdermal drug delivery. The exact mechanism by which MEs enhance the cutaneous drug permeation is not yet fully elucidated. The superior transport of bioactive agents into and across the skin could be attributed to several factors. The small droplet size and large surface area/volume ratio, the high concentration gradient across the skin due to high drug-loading capacity, the prolonged absorption due to a continuous supply of drug from the internal phase (acting as a reservoir) to the external phase, and/or the permeation-enhancing effects of the formulation components such as SAAs, co-SAAs, and oils (either by disrupting the SC lipid organization or increasing drug partitioning into the skin) might contribute to the improved dermal and transdermal drug delivery [9]. The high solubilization capacity of MEs for hydrophilic and lipophilic drugs, which leads to a large concentration gradient towards the skin, is an important feature. If high thermodynamic activity is achieved by incorporating drugs at a saturation or even supersaturation level, it results in a large concentration gradient towards the skin, which is a driving force for drug transport [109, 121, 122]. The type and internal structure of the ME also affect the penetration of drugs from MEs. The MEs can also increase the skin hydration [7]. The combination of these mechanisms might result in the penetration-enhancing effect of MEs.

Most MEs require a relatively large amount of SAAs that might be able to alter the structure of the SC and facilitate drug diffusion or increase the drug's partitioning into the skin. Several studies, however, have shown that increasing the levels of SAAs in the MEs have a detrimental effect on the drug flux across the skin [27, 90, 126, 127]. Some authors explained this by the decrease in the thermodynamic activity of the drugs due to increasing SAA amounts [27, 128]. Furthermore, an optimum SAA/co-SAA mass ratio exists. In the case of nonionic SAAs combined with glycols or Transcutol as a co-SAA, broader ME area in the phase diagram were obtained at higher SAA/co-SAA ratios, though higher drug fluxes were obtained at lower SAA/co-SAA ratios [127, 129].

Another important factor is the amount of water in an ME. Osborne et al. investigated the transdermal permeation of glucose as a hydrophilic model drug from MEs and found a correlation between glucose flux and water content in the ME. The presence of free water was shown to be essential for glucose transport into skin. At lower water contents, all molecules are used for hydrating the SAA head groups and thus are not available for partitioning into the skin [129]. Other studies by Sintov and Shapiro using lidocaine ME [127] and Changez et al. using lecithin-based MEs containing tetracaine HCl [31] also reported similar effects. It was also shown that the drug release is a function of water content. Djordjevic et al. found that the drug flux proportionally increases with the amount of water in the MEs [131].

The penetration-enhancing effect of MEs could also be attributed to the fact that the continuous and spontaneous fluctuations of the domains within the MEs allow a high drug mobility, thereby improving the diffusion process [22]. NMR studies by Kreilgaard et al. [90] and Hua et al. [129] on dynamics within the colloidal formulations have shown a correlation between drug mobility in the vehicle resulting from a certain microstructure and drug flux. An optimum extent of hydration of the SAA head groups seems to be essential where enough free water is additionally present to enable fast drug diffusion. The necessary amount of water is specific for each quaternary system and probably depends on the kind of SAA and co-SAA, mainly size and water binding capacity of the polar moiety. The permeability of lipophilic drugs is also correlated to water diffusivity [129]. In this context it was suggested that the hydration of the SC by the vehicle plays a role.

The full drug diffusivity potential of MEs can also be hampered by their composition and microstructure, e.g., due to adsorption of drug molecules to the SAA film, encapsulation, or unfavorable partitioning of the drug between formulation and skin [4, 90]. The probability is obviously higher in the case of amphiphilic drugs and when high amounts of SAAs are employed.

Skin pretreatment with MEs and/or ME components could affect the percutaneous absorption of drugs. Osborne et al. pretreated skin with either SAA (dioctyl sodium sulphosuccinate), co-SAA (octanol), or a mixture and compared the transdermal water flux with the one obtained by applying an ME containing these ingredients [132]. Whereas pretreatment with the single substance had marginal influence, the combination was as effective in increasing the water flux as the ME itself. Therefore, it was concluded that the enhancing activity of the ME is a result of the synergism between SAA and co-SAA, independent of the formulation's microstructure. Along those lines, pretreatment with a w/o ME increased the percutaneous absorption of the subsequently applied cetyl alcohol included in a cream and a lotion, respectively [133].

The physicochemical properties of a penetrating molecule such as molecular weight, partition coefficient, and solubility also affect the rate and extent of skin penetration from colloidal systems. In summary, there are a number of factors influencing the penetration of MEs loaded with biologically active agents. A strong relationship between microstructure and drug delivery potential exists. Nevertheless, more systematic study is required for a detailed clarification of the penetration mechanism.

36.6   CONCLUSION

Plenty of studies confirmed the benefit of MEs as drug delivery systems, in particular in the field of dermatopharmacy. In addition to the ease of preparation and long-term stability as practical advantages, the high skin penetration power and the high solubilization capacity (hence high drug loading capacity) for hydrophilic as well as lipophilic drugs make MEs superior nano-sized carriers for dermal and transdermal delivery of drugs from various categories. Those actives, causing several problems in dermal and transdermal administration due to their physicochemical properties, were shown to be effectively transported to their target region in the skin or blood circulation, respectively. Topical application of MEs might not be convenient for all patients because of their low viscosity. Therefore, thickening agents are added to obtain the desired semisolid consistency for cutaneous application.

Moreover, the growing use of nonirritating ingredients, mainly SAAs, leads to the creation of ME systems that are suitable for dermal application. Tolerability studies are basically required for future clinical use. Since they are often missing or have been performed applying animal models, such tests have to be carried out on human skin *in vivo*. These investigations, in conjunction with the variety of available characterization methods, offer the opportunity for the development of optimized colloidal formulations and a better understanding of the drug delivery mechanism from MEs. In summary, all the foregoing studies have shown that MEs are promising carriers to overcome the SC barrier and deliver biologically active substances into and across the skin.

REFERENCES

1. Lawrence MJ, Rees GD. Microemulsion-based media as novel drug delivery systems. Adv Drug Del Rev 2000; 45:89–121.
2. Tenjarla S. Microemulsions: an overview and pharmaceutical applications. Crit Rev Ther Drug Carrier Syst 1999;16:461–521.
3. Jahn K, Krause A, Janich M, Neubert RHH. Colloidal drug carrier systems. In: Bronaugh RL, Maibach HI, editor. Topical Absorption of Dermatological Products. New York: Marcel Dekker; 2002. p. 483–493.

4. Kreilgaard M. Influence of microemulsions on cutaneous drug delivery. Adv Drug Del Rev 2002; 54:S77–S98.
5. Vandamme TF. Microemulsions as ocular drug delivery systems: recent developments and future challenges. Prog Retin Eye Res 2002; 21:15–34.
6. Date AA, Nagarsenker MS. Parenteral microemulsions: An overview. Int J Pharm 2008; 355:19–30.
7. Lopes LB. Overcoming the cutaneous barrier with microemulsions. Pharmaceutics. 2014; 6:52–77.
8. Nguyen TTL, Edelen A, Neighbors B, et al. Biocompatible lecithin-based microemulsions with rhamnolipid and sophorolipid biosurfactants: Formulation and potential applications. J Colloid Interface Sci 2010; 348:498–504.
9. Santos P, Watkinson AC, Hadgraft J, et al. Application of microemulsions in dermal and transdermal drug delivery. Skin Pharmacol Phys 2008; 21:246–259.
10. Sahle FF, Metz H, Wohlrab J, et al. Lecithin-based microemulsions for targeted delivery of ceramide AP into the stratum corneum: formulation, characterizations, and in vitro release and penetration studies. Pharm Res 2013; 30:538–51.
11. Dreher F, Walde P, Luisi PL, et al. Human skin irritation studies of a lecithin microemulsion gel and of lecithin liposomes. Skin Pharmacol 1996; 9:124–129.
12. Paolino D, Ventura CA, Nisticon S, et al. Lecithin microemulsions for the topical administration of ketoprofen: percutaneous adsorption through human skin and in vivo human skin tolerability. Int J Pharm 2002; 244:21–31.
13. Chaiyana W, Saeio K, Hennink WE, et al. Characterization of potent anticholinesterase plant oil based microemulsion (vol 401, pg 32, 2010). Int J Pharm 2011; 414:333–334.
14. Hathout RM, Woodman TJ, Mansour S, et al. Microemulsion formulations for the transdermal delivery of testosterone. Eur J Pharm Sci 2010; 40:188–196.
15. Liu C-H, Chang F-Y, Hung D-K. Terpene microemulsions for transdermal curcumin delivery: Effects of terpenes and cosurfactants. Colloids Surf B Biointerfaces 2011; 82:63–70.
16. El Maghraby GM. Self-microemulsifying and microemulsion systems for transdermal delivery of indomethacin: Effect of phase transition. Colloids Surf B Biointerfaces. 2010; 75:595–600.
17. Sahle FF, Metz H, Wohlrab J, et al. Polyglycerol fatty acid ester surfactant-based microemulsions for targeted delivery of ceramide AP into the stratum corneum: formulation, characterisation, in vitro release and penetration investigation. Eur J Pharm Biopharm 2012; 82:139–50.
18. Ho HO, Hsiao CC, Sheu MT. Preparation of microemulsions using polyglycerol fatty acid esters as surfactant for the delivery of protein drugs. J Pharm Sci 1996; 85:138–143.
19. Teichmann A, Heuschkel S, Jacobi U, et al. Comparison of stratum corneum penetration and localization of a lipophilic model drug applied in an o/w microemulsion and an amphiphilic cream. Eur J Pharm Biopharm 2007; 67:699–706.
20. Shukla A, Janich M, Jahn K, et al. Investigation of pharmaceutical oil/water microemulsions by small-angle scattering. Pharm Res 2002; 19:881–886.
21. Goebel ASB, Knie U, Abels C, et al. Dermal targeting using colloidal carrier systems with linoleic acid. Eur J Pharm Biopharm 2010; 75:162–172.
22. Heuschkel S, Goebel A, Neubert RH. Microemulsions—modern colloidal carrier for dermal and transdermal drug delivery. J Pharm Sci 2008; 97:603–31.
23. Sathishkumar M, Jayabalan R, Mun SP, et al. Role of bicontinuous microemulsion in the rapid enzymatic hydrolysis of (R,S)-ketoprofen ethyl ester in a micro-reactor. Bioresour Technol 2010; 101:7834–7840.
24. Narang AS, Delmarre D, Gao D. Stable drug encapsulation in micelles and microemulsions. Int J Pharm 2007; 345:9–25.
25. Trotta M, Ugazio E, Peira E, et al. Influence of ion pairing on topical delivery of retinoic acid from microemulsions. J Control Release 2003; 86:315–321.
26. Peira E, Scolari P, Gasco MR. Transdermal permeation of apomorphine through hairless mouse skin from microemulsions. Int J Pharm 2001; 226:47–51.
27. Yuan Y, Li SM, Mo FK, et al. Investigation of microemulsion system for transdermal delivery of meloxicam. Int J Pharm 2006; 321:117–123.
28. Yuan JS, Yip A, Nguyen N, et al. Effect of surfactant concentration on transdermal lidocaine delivery with linker microemulsions. Int J Pharm 2010; 392:274–284.
29. Lin C-C, Lin H-Y, Chen H-C, et al. Stability and characterisation of phospholipid-based curcumin-encapsulated microemulsions. Food Chem 2009; 116:923–928.
30. Djekic L, Primorac M. The influence of cosurfactants and oils on the formation of pharmaceutical microemulsions based on PEG-8 caprylic/capric glycerides. Int J Pharm 2008; 352:231–239.

31. Changez M, Varshney M, Chander J, et al. Effect of the composition of lecithin/n-propanol/isopropyl myristate/water microemulsions on barrier properties of mice skin for transdermal permeation of tetracaine hydrochloride: In vitro. Colloid Surface B. 2006; 50:18–25.

32. Warisnoicharoen W, Lansley AB, Lawrence MJ. Nonionic oil-in-water microemulsions: the effect of oil type on phase behaviour. Int J Pharm 2000; 198:7–27.

33. Shevachman M, Garti N, Shani A, et al. Enhanced percutaneous permeability of diclofenac using a new U-Type dilutable microemulsion. Drug Dev Ind Pharm. 2008; 34:403–412.

34. Schmalfuß U, Neubert R, Wohlrab W. Modification of drug penetration into human skin using microemulsions. J Control Release 1997; 46:279–285.

35. Lee PJ, Langer R, Shastri VP. Novel microemulsion enhancer formulation for simultaneous transdermal delivery of hydrophilic and hydrophobic drugs. Pharm Res 2003; 20:264–9.

36. Rhee YS, Choi JG, Park ES, et al. Transdermal delivery of ketoprofen using microemulsions. Int J Pharm 2001; 228:161–70.

37. Jahn K. Moderne galenische Zubereitungen zur dermalen Anwendung von Ciclosporin A und Mycophenolatmofetil. [PhD Dissertation]: Martin-Luther-University, Halle-Wittenberg, Germany; 2002.

38. Constantinides PP, Yiv SH. Particle size determination of phase-inverted water-in-oil microemulsions under different dilution and storage conditions. Int J Pharm 1995; 115:225–234.

39. Müller BW, Müller RH. Particle Size Distributions and Particle Size Alterations in Microemulsions. J Pharm Sci 1984; 73:919–922.

40. Mrestani Y, El-Mokdad N, Rüttinger HH, et al. Characterization of partitioning behavior of cephalosporins using microemulsion and micellar electrokinetic chromatography. Electrophoresis. 1998; 19:2895–2899.

41. Mrestani Y, Neubert RH, Krause A. Partition behaviour of drugs in microemulsions measured by electrokinetic chromatography. Pharm Res 1998; 15:799–801.

42. Moulik SP, Paul BK. Structure, dynamics and transport properties of microemulsions. Adv Colloid Interface Sci 1998; 78:99–195.

43. Kumar PM, K.L. Handbook of Microemulsion Science and Technology. New York: Marcel Dekker; 1999.

44. Attwood D. Microemulsions. In: Kreuter J, editor. Colloidal Drug Delivery Systems. New York: Marcel Dekker; 1994. p. 31–71.

45. Junginger HE, Heering W. Darstellung kolloider Strukturen von Salben, Cremes, Emulsionen und Mikroemulsionen mittels Gefrierbruch-Ätztechnik und TEM. Acta Pharm Technol 1983; 29:85–96.

46. Jahn W, Strey R. Microstructure of microemulsions by freeze fracture electron microscopy. J Phys Chem 1988; 92:2294–2301.

47. Alany RG, Tucker IG, Davies NM, et al. Characterizing colloidal structures of pseudoternary phase diagrams formed by oil/water/amphiphile systems. Drug Dev Ind Pharm 2001; 27:31–38.

48. Schulman JH, Stoeckenius W, Prince LM. Mechanism of Formation and Structure of Micro Emulsions by Electron Microscopy. J Phys Chem 1959; 63:1677–1680.

49. Gradzielski M, Hoffmann H. Rheological properties of microemulsions. In: Kumar P MK, editor. Handbook of Microemulsion Science and Technology. New York: Marcel Dekker; 1999.

50. Ktistis G. A viscosity study on oil-in-water microemulsions. Int J Pharm 1990; 61:213–218.

51. Saunders FL. Rheological properties of monodisperse latex systems I. Concentration dependence of relative viscosity. J Colloid Sci1961; 16:13-22.

52. Primorac M, Stupar, M., Vuleta, G., Vasiljevic´, D. Rheological properties of oil/water microemulsions. Die Pharmazie. 1992; 47:645–646.

53. Primorac M, Dakovic´, L.J., Stupar, M., Vasiljevic´ D. The influence of temperature on the rheological behaviour of microemulsions. Die Pharmazie. 1994; 49:780–781.

54. Moreno MA, Ballesteros MP, Frutos P. Lecithin-based oil-in-water microemulsions for parenteral use: Pseudoternary phase diagrams, characterization and toxicity studies. J Pharm Sci 2003; 92:1428–1437.

55. Langevin D, Rouch, J. Light scattering of microemulsion systems. In: Kumar P MK, editor. Handbook of Microemulsion Science and Technology. New York: Marcel Dekker; 1999. p. 387–410.

56. Cazabat AM, Langevin D. Diffusion of interacting particles: Light scattering study of microemulsions. J Chem Phys. 1981; 74:3148–3158.

57. Gan LM, Ng SC, Ong SP, et al. A light scattering study of the influence of poly(ethylene glycol) on the droplet size and the interdroplet interaction in a water-in-oil-microemulsion. Colloid Polym Sci 1989; 267(12):1087–1095.

58. Verwey EJW, Overbeek JTG. Theory of the stability of lyophobic colloids. New York: Elsevier Publishing; 1948.

59. Pusey PN. Diffusion of spherical particles in concentrated dispersion. In: Degiorgio V, Corti, M., editor. Physics of Amphiphiles: Micelles, Vesicles and Microemulsions. Amsterdam: Elsevier; 1995. p. 152–159.

60. Yan YD, Clarke JHR. Dynamic light scattering from concentrated water-in-oil microemulsions: The coupling of optical and size polydispersity. J Chem Phys 1990; 93:4501–4509.

61. Shukla A. Characterization of Microemulsions Using Small Angle Scattering Techniques [PhD Dissertation]: Martin-Luther-University, Halle-Wittenberg, Germany; 2003.

62. Kops-Werkhoven MM, Fijnaut HM. Dynamic behavior of silica dispersions studied near the optical matching point. J Chem Phys 1982; 77:2242–2253.

63. Pusey P N, Tough, R.J.A. Particle interaction. In: R P, editor. Dynamic Light Scattering. New York: Plenum Press; 1985. p. 85–179.

64. Koppel DE. Analysis of Macromolecular Polydispersity in Intensity Correlation Spectroscopy: The Method of Cumulants. J Chem Phys 1972; 57:4814–4820.

65. Shukla A, Janich M, Jahn K, et al. Microemulsions for dermal drug delivery studied by dynamic light scattering: effect of interparticle interactions in oil-in-water microemulsions. J Pharm Sci 2003; 92:730–8.

66. Sahle FF, Wohlrab J, Neubert RH. Controlled penetration of ceramides into and across the stratum corneum using various types of microemulsions and formulation associated toxicity studies. Eur J Pharm Biopharm 2014; 86:244–50.

67. Kotlarchyk M, Chen SH. Analysis of small angle neutron scattering spectra from polydisperse interacting colloids. J Chem Phys 1983; 79:2461–2469.

68. Chen SH. Small Angle Neutron Scattering Studies of the Structure and Interaction in Micellar and Microemulsion Systems. Annu Rev Phys Chem 1986; 37:351–399.

69. Percus JK, Yevick GJ. Analysis of Classical Statistical Mechanics by Means of Collective Coordinates. Phys Rev 1958; 110:1–13.

70. Kotlarchyk M, Chen S-H, Huang JS, et al. Structure of three-component microemulsions in the critical region determined by small-angle neutron scattering. Phys Rev A. 1984; 29:2054–2069.

71. Kotlarchyk M, Chen SH, Huang JS. Temperature dependence of size and polydispersity in a three-component microemulsion by small-angle neutron scattering. J Phys Chem 1982; 86:3273–3276.

72. Huang JS, Safran SA, Kim MW, et al. Attractive Interactions in Micelles and Microemulsions. Phys Rev Lett 1984; 53:592–595.

73. Lisy V, Brutovsky B. Interpretation of static and dynamic neutron and light scattering from microemulsion droplets: Effects of shape fluctuations. Phys Rev E 2000; 61:4045–4053.

74. Yuan JS, Ansari M, Samaan M, et al. Linker-based lecithin microemulsions for transdermal delivery of lidocaine. Int J Pharm 2008; 349:130–143.

75. Banga AK, Bose S, Ghosh TK. Iontophoresis and electroporation: comparisons and contrasts. Int J Pharm 1999; 179:1–19.

76. Bhatia G, Zhou Y, Banga AK. Adapalene Microemulsion for Transfollicular Drug Delivery. J Pharm Sci 2013; 102:2622–2631.

77. Hathout RM, Nasr M. Transdermal delivery of betahistine hydrochloride using microemulsions: Physical characterization, biophysical assessment, confocal imaging and permeation studies. Colloids Surf B Biointerfaces 2013; 110:254–260.

78. Imokawa G, Abe A, Jin K, et al. Decreased Level of Ceramides in Stratum-Corneum of Atopic-Dermatitis - an Etiologic Factor in Atopic Dry Skin. J Invest Dermatol 1991; 96:523–526.

79. Motta S, Monti M, Sesana S, et al. Abnormality of Water Barrier Function in Psoriasis – Role of Ceramide Fractions. Arch Dermatol 1994; 130:452–456.

80. Rogers J, Harding C, Mayo A, et al. Stratum corneum lipids: The effect of ageing and the seasons. Arch Dermatol Res 1996; 288:765–770.

81. Bouwstra JA, Ponec M. The skin barrier in healthy and diseased state. Biochim Biophys Acta 2006; 1758:2080–95.

82. Loden M. The skin barrier and use of moisturizers in atopic dermatitis. Clin Dermatol 2003; 21:145–57.

83. Sahle FF, Gebre-Mariam T, Dobner B, et al. Skin Diseases Associated with the Depletion of Stratum Corneum Lipids and Stratum Corneum Lipid Substitution Therapy. Skin Pharmacol Phys 2015; 28:42–55.

84. Zhang Q, Flach CR, Mendelsohn R, et al. Topically applied ceramide accumulates in skin glyphs. Clin Cosmet Investig Dermatol 2015; 8:329–37.

85. Tessema EN, Gebre-Mariam T, Paulos G, et al. Delivery of Oat-derived Phytoceramides into the Stratum Corneum of the Skin using Nanocarriers: Formulation, Characterization and in vitro and ex-vivo Penetration Studies. Eur J Pharm Biopharm 2018; 127:260–269.

86. Getie M, Wohlrab J, Neubert RHH. Dermal delivery of desmopressin acetate using colloidal carrier systems. J Pharm Pharmacol 2005; 57:423–427.

87. Goebel AS, Schmaus G, Neubert RH, et al. Dermal peptide delivery using enhancer molecules and colloidal carrier systems–part I: carnosine. Skin Pharmacol Physiol 2012; 25:281–7.

88. Neubert RHH, Sommer E, Scholzel M, et al. Dermal peptide delivery using enhancer moleculs and colloidal carrier systems. Part II: Tetrapeptide PKEK. Eur J Pharm Biopharm 2018; 124:28–33.

89. Sommer E, Neubert RHH, Mentel M, et al. Dermal peptide delivery using enhancer molecules and colloidal carrier systems. Part III: Tetrapeptide GEKG. Eur J Pharm Biopharm 2018; 124:137–144.

90. Kreilgaard M, Pedersen EJ, Jaroszewski JW. NMR characterisation and transdermal drug delivery potential of microemulsion systems. J Control Release 2000; 69:421–33.

91. Kreilgaard M. Dermal pharmacokinetics of microemulsion formulations determined by in vivo microdialysis. Pharm Res 2001; 18:367–73.

92. Kreilgaard M, Kemme MJ, Burggraaf J, et al. Influence of a microemulsion vehicle on cutaneous bioequivalence of a lipophilic model drug assessed by microdialysis and pharmacodynamics. Pharm Res 2001; 18:593–9.

93. Junyaprasert VB, Boonme P, Songkro S, et al. Transdermal delivery of hydrophobic and hydrophilic local anesthetics from o/w and w/o Brij 97-based microemulsions. J Pharm Pharm Sci 2007; 10:288–98.

94. Junyaprasert VB, Boonme P, Wurster DE, et al. Aerosol OT microemulsions as carriers for transdermal delivery of hydrophobic and hydrophilic local anesthetics. Drug Deliv 2008; 15:323–30.

95. Changez M, Varshney M. Aerosol-OT microemulsions as transdermal carriers of tetracaine hydrochloride. Drug Dev Ind Pharm 2000; 26:507–12.

96. Kriwet K, Müller-Goymann CC. Diclofenac release from phospholipid drug systems and permeation through excised human stratum corneum. Int J Pharm 1995; 125:231–242.

97. Fouad SA, Basalious EB, El-Nabarawi MA, et al. Microemulsion and poloxamer microemulsion-based gel for sustained transdermal delivery of diclofenac epolamine using in-skin drug depot: in vitro/in vivo evaluation. Int J Pharm 2013; 453:569–578.

98. Dalmora ME, Oliveira AG. Inclusion complex of piroxicam with beta-cyclodextrin and incorporation in hexadecyltrimethylammonium bromide based microemulsion. Int J Pharm 1999; 184:157–164.

99. Dalmora ME, Dalmora SL, Oliveira AG. Inclusion complex of piroxicam with beta-cyclodextrin and incorporation in cationic microemulsion. In vitro drug release and in vivo topical anti-inflammatory effect. Int J Pharm 2001; 222:45–55.

100. Subramanian N, Ghosal SK, Moulik SP. Enhanced in vitro percutaneous absorption and in vivo anti-inflammatory effect of a selective cyclooxygenase inhibitor using microemulsion. Drug Dev Ind Pharm 2005; 31:405–416.

101. Cao M, Ren L, Chen G. Formulation optimization and ex vivo and in vivo evaluation of celecoxib microemulsion-based gel for transdermal delivery. AAPS PharmSciTech 2017; 18:1960–1971.

102. Seok SH, Lee S-A, Park E-S. Formulation of a microemulsion-based hydrogel containing celecoxib. J Drug Deliv Sci Tec 2018; 43:409–414.

103. Bolzinger MA, Carduner TC, Poelman MC. Bicontinuous sucrose ester microemulsion: a new vehicle for topical delivery of niflumic acid. Int J Pharm 1998; 176:39–45.

104. Heuschkel S, Wohlrab J, Schmaus G, et al. Modulation of dihydroavenanthramide D release and skin penetration by 1,2-alkanediols. Eur J Pharm Biopharm 2008; 70:239–247.

105. Heuschkel S, Wohlrab J, Neubert RH. Dermal and transdermal targeting of dihydroavenanthramide D using enhancer molecules and novel microemulsions. Eur J Pharm Biopharm 2009; 72:552–560.

106. Krause SA. Entwicklung und Charakterisierung von Mikroemulsionen zur dermalen Applikation von Arzneistoffen. [PhD Dissertation]: Martin-Luther-University, Halle-Wittenberg, Germany; 2001.

107. Lehmann L, Keipert S, Gloor M. Effects of microemulsions on the stratum corneum and hydrocortisone penetration. Eur J Pharm Biopharm 2001; 52:129–136.

108. Fini A, Bergamante V, Ceschel GC, et al. Control of transdermal permeation of hydrocortisone acetate from hydrophilic and lipophilic formulations. AAPS PharmSciTech 2008; 9:762–768.

109. Peltola S, Saarinen-Savolainen P, Kiesvaara J, et al. Microemulsions for topical delivery of estradiol. Int J Pharm 2003; 254:99–107.

110. Alvarez-Figueroa MJ, Blanco-Mendez J. Transdermal delivery of methotrexate: iontophoretic delivery from hydrogels and passive delivery from microemulsions. Int J Pharm 2001; 215:57–65.

111. Trotta M, Pattarino F, Gasco MR. Influence of counter ions on the skin permeation of methotrexate from water-oil microemulsions. Pharm Acta Helv 1996; 71:135–140.

112. Liu H, Li S, Wang Y, et al. Bicontinuous water-AOT/Tween85-isopropyl myristate microemulsion: a new vehicle for transdermal delivery of cyclosporin A. Drug Dev Ind Pharm 2006; 32:549–557.

113. Goebel AS, Neubert RH, Wohlrab J. Dermal targeting of tacrolimus using colloidal carrier systems. Int J Pharm 2011; 404:159–68.

114. Viyoch J, Pisutthanan N, Faikreua A, et al. Evaluation of in vitro antimicrobial activity of Thai basil oils and their micro-emulsion formulas against Propionibacterium acnes. Int J Cosmet Sci 2006; 28:125–133.

115. Biju SS, Ahuja A, Khar RK. Tea tree oil concentration in follicular casts after topical delivery: determination by high-performance thin layer chromatography using a perfused bovine udder model. J Pharm Sci 2005; 94:240–245.

116. Gasco MR, Gallarate M, Pattarino F. In vitro permeation of azelaic acid from viscosized microemulsions. Int J Pharm 1991; 69:193–196.

117. Pattarino F, Carlotti ME, Gasco MR. Topical delivery systems for azelaic acid: effect of the suspended drug in microemulsion. Die Pharmazie 1994; 49:72–73.

118. Jurkovic P, Sentjurc M, Gasperlin M, et al. Skin protection against ultraviolet induced free radicals with ascorbyl palmitate in microemulsions. Eur J Pharm Biopharm 2003; 56:59–66.

119. Rangarajan M, Zatz JL. Effect of formulation on the topical delivery of alpha-tocopherol. J Cosmet Sci 2003; 54:161–174.

120. Baroli B, Lopez-Quintela MA, Delgado-Charro MB, et al. Microemulsions for topical delivery of 8-methoxsalen. J Control Release 2000; 69:209–218.

121. Kemken J, Ziegler A, Muller BW. Investigations into the pharmacodynamic effects of dermally administered microemulsions containing beta-blockers. J Pharm Pharmacol 1991; 43:679–684.

122. Trotta M, Morel S, Gasco MR. Effect of oil phase composition on the skin permeation of felodipine from o/w microemulsions. Die Pharmazie 1997; 52:50–3.

123. Priano L, Albani G, Brioschi A, et al. Transdermal apomorphine permeation from microemulsions: a new treatment in Parkinson's disease. Mov Disord 2004; 19:937–942.

124. Zhao X, Liu JP, Zhang X, et al. Enhancement of transdermal delivery of theophylline using microemulsion vehicle. Int J Pharm 2006; 327:58–64.

125. Zhu W, Yu A, Wang W, et al. Formulation design of microemulsion for dermal delivery of penciclovir. Int J Pharm 2008; 360:184–190.

126. Delgado-Charro MB, Iglesias-Vilas G, Blanco-Méndez J, et al. Delivery of a hydrophilic solute through the skin from novel microemulsion systems. Eur J Pharm Biopharm 1997; 43:37–42.

127. Sintov AC, Shapiro L. New microemulsion vehicle facilitates percutaneous penetration in vitro and cutaneous drug bioavailability in vivo. J Control Release 2004; 95:173–183.

128. Chen H, Chang X, Weng T, et al. A study of microemulsion systems for transdermal delivery of triptolide. J Control Release 2004; 98:427–436.

129. Hua L, Weisan P, Jiayu L, et al. Preparation, evaluation, and NMR characterization of vinpocetine microemulsion for transdermal delivery. Drug Dev Ind Pharm 2004; 30:657–666.

130. Osborne DW, Ward AJI, O'neill KJ. Microemulsions as topical drug delivery vehicles: in-vitro transdermal studies of a model hydrophilic drug. J Pharm Pharmacol 1991;43:451–454.

131. Djordjevic L, Primorac M, Stupar M. In vitro release of diclofenac diethylamine from caprylocaproyl macrogolglycerides based microemulsions. Int J Pharm 2005; 296:73–79.

132. Osborne DU, Ward AJI, O'Neill KJ. Microemulsions as topical drug delivery vehicles. I. Characterization of a model system. Drug Dev Ind Pharm 1988; 14:1203–1219.

133. Linn EE, Pohland RC, Byrd TK. Microemulsion for intradermal delivery of cetyl alcohol and octyl dimethyl PABA. Drug Dev Ind Pharm 1990; 16:899–920.

37 Transdermal Delivery of Vesicular Nanocarriers under Electrical Potential

Ebtessam A. Essa and Gamal M. El Maghraby
Tanta University, Tanta, Egypt

Michael C. Bonner and Brian W. Barry
University of Bradford, Bradford, United Kingdom

CONTENTS

37.1 INTRODUCTION

Human skin is the most accessible organ for pharmaceutical formulators. It constitutes approximately 16% of body weight and has a very large surface area. It is a complex, multilayered structure, providing a barrier that preserves the components of the body and protects the body from being invaded by exogenous xenobiotics and microorganisms. There is an increasing interest in using the skin as a port for delivering therapeutic agents into the systemic circulation. This drug delivery route offers several advantages over other pathways. The advantages include bypassing the presystemic disposition, providing a chance for continuous drug input with direct control of drug delivery rate, and upgraded patient compliance due to the noninvasive and painlessness nature of transdermal delivery. However, the defensive nature of the skin hinders the partitioning and diffusion of most drugs into and through the successive skin strata. The hindrance of transdermal delivery relies mainly on the stratum corneum (SC), which is made of corneocytes (dead keratinocytes). These keratinocytes are assembled by a well-organized matrix coated with a layer of lipids (ceramides, cholesterol, and other free fatty acids) [1]. This lipid matrix of the SC has been subjected to extensive characterization over the last few decades. Freeze fracture electron microscopic studies reflected the existence of lipid lamellae in the intercellular regions. The lipid can be crystalline, gel, liquid crystalline, or liquid. The predominantly semisolid nature of the lipid matrix contributes to its strength and resistance to drug permeation. The SC with its lipophilic matrix prevents the passive permeation of drug molecules over 500 kDa [2–3]. For this reason, the SC, which has a thickness between 15 and 20 μm, is the rate limiting barrier during transdermal drug diffusion.

Authors are trying to widen the spectrum of drugs that can be delivered into and through the skin, with the goal of increasing systemic availability of the drug after topical application. This requires modulation of the skin barrier properties in order to increase permeability. Many strategies have been adopted to overcome this barrier, which include disrupting and/or fluidizing the intercellular lipid structure of the SC, altering cellular proteins, and in some cases, extracting intercellular lipids. However, these enhancers do not add much, especially for large molecules and hydrophilic drugs. Physical approaches such as iontophoresis, electroporation, sonophoresis, and the use of microneedles are thus introduced and are being extensively studied to improve the permeation of both hydrophilic and lipophilic drugs [4].

This chapter summarizes our present knowledge of the means by which colloidal particles under iontophoresis, electroporation, and combinations of these electrical methods can alter drug transport through skin.

37.1.1 LIPID NANOVESICULAR SYSTEMS

Liposomes are the most extensively studied nanostructure for dermal and transdermal drug delivery, and their history began in 1980 by Mezei and Gulasekharam who were the first to employ liposomes in skin drug delivery [5]. Liposomes are colloidal carriers made of lipid bilayer(s) enclosing an aqueous volume. Vesicles of a single lipid bilayer and one aqueous core are classified as unilamellar vesicles (ULVs), with those containing alternating aqueous compartments and lipid bilayers being categorized as multilamellar vesicles (MLVs). The basic component of bilayer structures is amphiphilic substances, which comprise phospholipids as the integral component, with surfactants, cholesterol (CH), or charging agents being included to modulate the specifications of the vesicular system. The secondary material may control the charge of the vesicles and/or the fluidity of the vesicular membrane [6, 7]. The vesicular systems can be formulated by hydrating a thin film of the amphiphilic and lipophilic components with the aqueous phase to produce crude vesicles. The vesicular size and lamellarity can be controlled by bath sonication or membrane extrusion. Details of the preparation techniques of vesicular nanostructures can found in the practical approach, which provides a step-by-step guide for the preparation of ULVs and MLVs [8].

Early investigations recorded a localizing effect in which the amount of drug deposited into the skin strata was increased after the application of liposomes [8]. Many researchers suggested that phospholipid vesicles administered on the skin first disintegrate with subsequent diffusion of lipid molecules through the SC. This may disrupt the skin lipid with subsequent permeation enhancement [9]. Another mechanism depends on the adsorption and fusion of liposomes with the skin surface, with their constituents changing the ultrastructure of the intercellular regions in the deeper layers of the skin barrier [10]. Although it has been generally accepted that vesicles normally increase drug transport across the skin, the mechanism of action of these formulations are still debated.

The research in this area was intensified to develop new vesicular systems (Transfersomes), which were claimed to penetrate the intact skin, delivering measurable concentrations of drugs to the systemic circulation [11]. Transfersomes are a new generation of traditional liposomes with highly deformable properties (also designated as ultra-deformable, flexible, or elastic). Cevc and Blume [11] were the first to use the term Transfersomes to describe lipid vesicles comprising a PC with sodium cholate, which was described as an edge activator. The inventors of these vesicles claimed that such vesicles squeeze themselves through pores in the SC that are less than one-tenth the liposome's diameter after open application to the skin. Thus, sizes up to 200 to 300 nm could potentially penetrate intact to the deep layers of the skin and may progress far enough to reach the systemic circulation [11, 12]. The exceptional features of these vesicular nanostructures include xerophobia and high deformation. These characteristics are responsible for vesicle infiltration into the skin interior towards the more hydrated layers. It was thus believed that the transdermal water gradient plays a major role in Transfersomal skin invasion. To verify vesicular skin infiltration, the fate of radiolabeled Transfersomes was monitored in comparison to standard vesicles. This research was conducted after occlusive and open application to skin. Transfersomes showed superior ability to invade the intact skin, traveling far enough to reach the subdermis and even the blood after open application. Occlusion inhibited such effect, and traditional vesicles accumulated in the SC. This was considered an indication for the success of the ultra-deformable vesicles, but this required open application [11]. In contrast to this hypothesis, Transfersomes enhanced the local anesthetic effect after occlusive application compared with standard liposomes [13]. The striking report revealed the ability of the highly deformable vesicular nanostructures to deliver large proteins through the skin to provide transdermal immunization [14].

37.1.2 ELECTRICAL METHODS FOR ENHANCING SKIN DELIVERY

Electrotransport (iontophoresis and electroporation) is a technique originally designed to deliver challenging molecules into and through the skin. Challenging candidates include ionized drugs and hydrophilic macromolecules. This strategy has now been extended to particulate delivery systems, including vesicular carriers.

37.1.2.1 Iontophoresis

The highly lipophilic nature of the skin hinders the permeation of hydrophilic, large-molecular-weight, and charged compounds into and through the SC. This is a major challenge, as many of the therapeutically valuable molecules are of a hydrophilic nature with high molecular weights, such as peptides. The introduction of iontophoresis provided a possible solution for this problem. Iontophoresis in the present context can be defined as the enhanced movement of molecules through the tissue using a low, physiologically acceptable electric current. It hastens the delivery of ionized hydrophilic moieties, though delivery of un-ionized species can be facilitated. This procedure extended the range of drug molecules that can be driven via the transdermal route. Iontophoresis utilizes the electropotential energy and the charge present on a drug molecule or the surface of colloidal particles to facilitate skin permeability. In transdermal iontophoretic delivery, and electrical field is created by mounting suitable electrodes (anode and cathode) close to the skin. The two electrodes are connected via a battery. The electrode containing the drug or colloidal system is termed the active electrode, whereas the return electrode (located nearby the active electrode on the skin) completes the circuit and is termed the return electrode [15–17].

The method is based on the general principle that like charges repel each other and opposite charges attract. Accordingly, to drive a negatively charged molecule across the skin, it is placed under the negative electrode (cathode), where it is repelled towards a positive electrode (anode), which can be located elsewhere on the body, and vice versa for a drug cation. Thus ions on either side of the skin will migrate in the direction dictated by their charges. The speed of migration depends on the physicochemical properties of the migrating species and the properties of the diffusion media [18, 19]. The sum of individual ion fluxes must equal the current supplied by the power source; thus all ions compete to carry the charge. Iontophoresis has been clinically employed to deliver medication to surface tissue for several decades. Its potential has been advanced to cover transdermal delivery of ionic drugs, including peptides and oligonucleotides that are normally difficult to administer except by the parenteral route [16].

In addition to electrorepulsion, the driving force for iontophoretic drug delivery can depend on electro-osmosis—a bulk solvent flow across a membrane under an electric potential gradient. At normal pH, skin is negatively charged and fluid flows in the direction of cation flux. Such flow either enhances the transport of cations or retards anion movement. The contribution of electro-osmotic flux to the overall transport of charged compounds is likely to be small, as fluid flow is estimated at mL/hr [20]. An additional transport mechanism relies on the possible disorganization of an intercellular lipid matrix under the influence of the weak electric current, which can subsequently produce more permeable SC [21].

The pathways of iontophoretic transdermal delivery are believed to primarily employ preexisting routes such as skin appendages [22, 23] and intercellular routes [24]. The development of new aqueous pores can play a measurable role as well [25]. The dominant iontophoretic pathway depends on the physicochemical properties of the permeant and its affinity to the existing environment, where lipophilic permeants favor the intercellular route and hydrophilic compounds mainly penetrate through the appendageal pathway [26].

37.1.2.2   Electroporation

Electroporation is an electrical enhancement technique that could work alone or in combination with iontophoresis. Electroporation (or electropermeabilization) is a long-established technique for permeabilizing biological membranes and is widely employed to input genetic material into bacterial cells. It is a noninvasive transdermal delivery technique for macromolecules (up to least 40 kDa). It involves application of high-voltage pulse(s) (usually from 100 to 1000 V) to skin for a very short duration (from microseconds to milliseconds). This will create transient aqueous pores in lipid bilayers of the SC. These electropores provide routes for drug permeation via the horny layer of the skin [27–30]. Localized heating of lipids, causing a phase transition, forms the pores [31]. Drug transport through these transient pores can also be facilitated by electrophoresis during the pulse "on" time, or by simple diffusion through these aqueous domains that remain open for some time after pulsing. Unlike iontophoresis, electroosmotic solvent flow is much less significant [32–34]. In spite of the marked enhancement in transdermal drug permeation under the applied electromotive force (EMF), safety issues are challenging, although many authors suggested that skin damage is usually mild and reversible [34, 35].

37.2   LIPID VESICLES UNDER ELECTRICAL POTENTIAL

Topical application of liposomes under the influence of a weak electric current can get the benefits of enhancing transdermal drug delivery by combined mechanisms. This approach has gained interest [36]. Nanostructures have been extensively investigated for skin dermal/transdermal drug delivery. However, their effect is mainly confined to achieving localized skin delivery of drugs, while transdermal drug delivery is less likely to be achieved. Therefore, there was a need for combining between nanocarriers and other penetration enhancement techniques to enhance both dermal and transdermal drug delivery. For a comprehensive review on the combination of different nanocarriers with other physical means to enhance the drug penetration into/through the skin, the reader should refer to Dragicevic and Maibach [37]. In the proceeding section we will focus on the combined use of liposomes and electric current (iontophoresis or electroporation).

37.2.1   Iontophoresis and Ultra-Deformable Liposomes

Combining lipid vesicles with the iontophoresis strategy is a relatively recent approach, and few reports have been published on this mode of transdermal drug delivery. Here, we briefly review their conjoined use.

37.2.1.1   Electrical Enhancement of Liposome Delivery

While there are numerous reports on the use of liposomes for penetration enhancement, the combination of liposomes and iontophoresis has received little attention, though it could offer some additional benefits. A charge can effectively be imparted to neutral drugs by encapsulating them in charged liposomes, thus enhancing their iontophoretic delivery. Charging the vesicles can be achieved using stearylamine which is commonly used to induce positive charges, with dicetyl phosphate to create negatively charged vesicles [16]. An early report of the combined use of iontophoresis and traditional liposomes in skin delivery was for enkephalin entrapped in positive or negative vesicles [38]. Iontophoresis increased liposomal enkephalin penetration compared to the control solution. During transport, the enkephalin solution underwent degradation, with a minimal amount being degraded after liposomal encapsulation. This reflects the potential protective effect of the vesicles for the encapsulated drug.

Iontophoretic delivery of neutral colchicine encapsulated in positively charged liposomes was able to augment the drug flux by four to five times compared to free colchicine [39]. The effect of different liposomal formulations on the iontophoretic transport of enoxacin through rat skin has been investigated *in vitro* [40]. The iontophoretic penetration of enoxacin depended on vesicular composition, with better flux being recorded by decreasing the fatty acid chain length of the phospholipid. This was attributed to the decrease in the phase transition temperature of the lipid.

The effects of zwitterionic lipids (phosphatidylcholine [PC] and distearoyl phosphatidylcholine DSPC]), cationic lipid (stearylamine), and the penetration enhancer Azone on the iontophoretic transdermal flux of neutral mannitol through human skin were examined [41]. The skin was pretreated with the placebo lipid suspensions or Azone solution, all containing 32% ethanol, prior to iontophoresis.

For the lipid suspensions, only PC increased mannitol flux compared to control (without pretreatment). Interestingly, the authors recorded an increase in mannitol flux after the combination of PC with electric current, with the recorded increase being comparable to Azone, suggesting a synergistic effect between PC and the electric current.

The combined use of iontophoresis and ultra-deformable (ultra-flexible or elastic) liposomes has been studied. Offering the potential to stabilize therapeutic agents undergoing iontophoresis, surfactant-based elastic vesicles (composed of octaoxyethylene laurate ester, sucrose laurate ester, and cholesterol sulfate) were used to deliver apomorphine through human skin *in vitro* [42].

Negatively charged Transfersomes were prepared using sodium cholate as the edge activator (PC: sodium cholate; 86:14% w/w). Using human epidermal membranes, cathodic iontophoresis (0.2 to 0.8 mA/cm^2 constant current) increased the delivery of estradiol compared to the control (saturated estradiol aqueous solution), even though the vesicles were delivered against electro-osmotic flow [43]. The steroid flux increased linearly with the applied current, confirming the ability of iontophoresis to provide programmed drug delivery. The fifteenfold enhancement in estradiol flux from liposomes under iontophoresis (0.8 mA/cm^2) was attributed to the synergistic effect of both electric current and phospholipid monomers released from the lipid vesicles under electric field. Both processes modulated the intercellular lipid lamellae of the SC, increasing membrane permeability. It was also suggested that under such conditions of a permeabilized skin structure, intact vesicles might penetrate someway down the SC because of their flexibility. Importantly, iontophoresis induced tritium exchange of the ^{3}H-labeled estradiol with water and had to be allowed for so as not to falsely elevate the flux data. Tritium exchange increased with increasing current density and time of application. Interestingly, the liposomal structure shielded the drug against the effect, producing a protective action [43].

To estimate the role of vesicle deformability on the enhanced drug penetration from ultra-deformable vesicles, iontophoresis (six hours of 0.8 mA/cm^2) of estradiol from the same ultra-deformable vesicles (containing sodium cholate as the edge activator) was compared with that from traditional liposomes (i.e., without edge activator).

The prototype nonrigid pure PC and membrane-stabilized (PC: cholesterol; 1:1 molar ratio) formulations were used. All preparations improved skin delivery of estradiol in terms of flux and skin deposition compared with the control solution, with ultra-deformable liposomes being the most effective. Nevertheless, there was no strong evidence that such higher results were due to any special capability of Transfersomes to deform. Moreover, by comparing the zeta potentials of the three liposomal formulations with their flux values, it was concluded that the highest result obtained from Transfersomes was because of the greater electrophoretic repulsion force imposed by the current acting on the more charged vesicles [44]. Despite the encouraging data in these studies, the question arises whether or not the relatively high current density of 0.8 mA/cm² is suitable for practical application, knowing that most reports recommend a maximum of 0.5 mA/cm², for clinical relevance [35]. To probe the safety of iontophoresis using such a relatively high current, an *in vitro* experimental protocol was designed to examine skin barrier integrity before and after current application. The same Transfersome formulations and saturated drug solution were used [43]. This protocol involved three consecutive four-hour stages: a first passive diffusion stage, then iontophoresis (0.8 mA/cm²), and finally a second passive regimen applied to the same piece of the skin. This sequence of drug delivery thus assessed the effect of current on the skin barrier properties. Theoretically, if skin barrier modulation due to iontophoresis is a reversible process, estradiol passive penetration following current termination would be similar to that of the first passive stage. The transepidermal estradiol fluxes from ultra-deformable liposomes and control at different stages, as shown in Figure 37.1, indicated that iontophoresis reversibly changed the skin barrier. The passive flux after iontophoresis was similar to that before current application for both solution and liposomes, suggesting the suitability of such current density for *in vitro* application. For clinical usage, of course, we would also need to do *in vivo* studies.

There is considerable debate about the pathways taken by ions traversing the skin during iontophoresis. However, there is general agreement that a low-resistance route is involved. The current flows via domains of low resistance, and these are clearly provided by the shunt route (comprising hair follicles and sweat glands).

Assessment of the contribution of different transport pathways during iontophoresis is difficult to extract from the literature due to the diversity of the experimental protocols used. With ultra-deformable liposomes, the shunt route was shown to contribute minimally to passive delivery, and

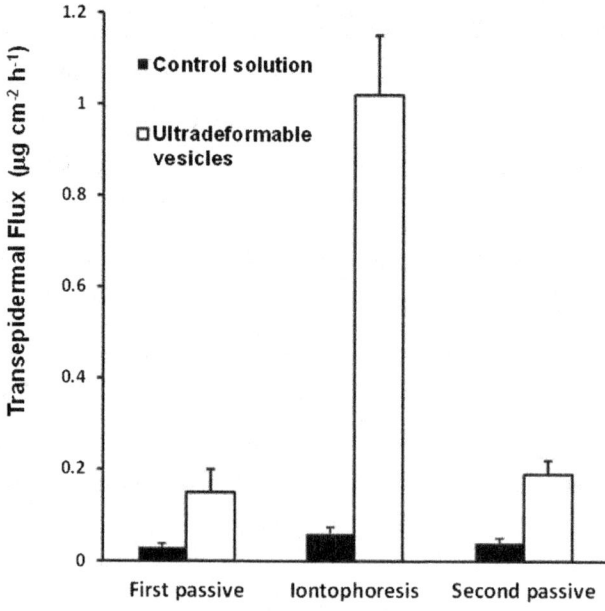

FIGURE 37.1   *In vitro* iontophoretic estradiol flux values through human epidermis from saturated aqueous control and ultra-deformable liposomes using the three 4-hour stages protocol: passive, iontophoresis (0.8 mA/cm²), then passive (*n* = 5–6).

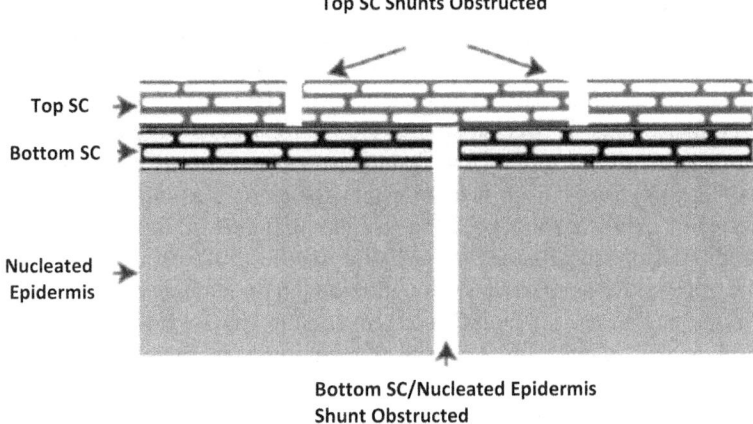

FIGURE 37.2 Diagrammatic representation of the stratum corneum epidermal sandwich (not to scale). (Modified from El Maghraby et al. [46].)

the intercellular lipid domain was suggested to be the main pathway [45, 46]. Therefore, the role of the shunt route in the skin penetration of estradiol during occluded passive and iontophoretic (0.5 mA/cm^2) delivery of the drug from saturated solution and negatively charged Transfersomes was investigated [47]. The technique of using a stratum corneum/epidermis (SC/Ep) sandwich designed by El Maghraby et al. [46] was utilized (Figure. 37.2). The study monitored the delivery of estradiol through human epidermal membrane compared to that through a sandwich of SC/Ep. In the SC/Ep sandwich, the additional SC formed the top layer. Because skin shunts occupy only about 0.1% of skin surface area, it was assumed that the top layer of the SC would essentially block all shunts available in the bottom membrane. The presence of the top layer of the SC effectively doubles the thickness of the skin barrier. This doubling should reduce the transepidermal flux by half compared to that through the epidermal membrane alone if the shunt route was unimportant for drug penetration [48]. A much greater reduction in flux would indicate a major shunt contribution to estradiol penetration. The reduction in the iontophoretic flux of the steroid indicated an important role for the shunt route, which was estimated to represent up to about 50% of the total iontophoretic pathway. In spite of their lipophilic nature and relatively large size (126 ± 4.2 [SD] nm), ultra-deformable liposomes were capable of penetrating at least some way down the shunts under the effect of iontophoresis. The data also suggested that anatomical shunts were not the only possible iontophoretic pathway, as due to disorganization of the intercellular lipid lamella under electrical treatment, some additional pores formed.

Lee and coworkers [49] encapsulated ascorbyl palmitate (AsP) in liposomes. Neutral liposomes were prepared using dimyristoylphosphatydilcholine (DMPC), and negatively charged liposomes were prepared with DMPC and dicetylphosphate at 10% and 20% concentration. Liposomal gel (LipoGel) was prepared by dispersing each liposome system into a hydrogel matrix (poloxamer 25%). They investigated passive and electrically assisted (0.4 mA/cm^2) delivery of AsP from different LipoGels, using dorsal rat skin. In the passive transport study, the permeated amounts of AsP from all the LipoGels tested were higher than that of control hydrogel which contains AsP. In the cathodal delivery, the skin permeation of AsP from the negative LipoGels (containing negative liposomes) were superior to that obtained with the neutral one. Increasing surface negativity of liposomes increased drug permeation. Combined use of negative LipoGel with cathodal electric current was found to be promising in enhancing the skin delivery of AsP [49].

Chen et al. [50] provided a new strategy for noninvasive delivery of insulin using a combination of physical means and nanovesicles. This involved the use of a microneedle together with iontophoresis for skin delivery of insulin containing liposomes. Insulin-loaded nanovesicles were driven by iontophoresis through skin containing microchannels created by microneedles both *in vitro* and *in vivo*. Liposomes were devised from soybean lecithin. Positively or negatively charged vesicles were prepared by the addition of 0.4 cetyltrimethyl ammonium bromide or sodium dodecyl sulfate (0.4%, 0.03%), respectively. Both passive and iontophoretic (0.2 mA/cm^2) delivery were assessed in both intact and microneedle-pretreated skin. Under iontophoresis, all liposomes showed higher skin permeation rates compared to the control solution, with the positive vesicles being superior. The permeation rates of insulin from positive nanovesicles driven under iontophoresis through microneedle-pretreated skin were about 713 times higher than that of its passive diffusion.

The *in vivo* studies, using rats, showed that the blood glucose levels of diabetic rats induced by iontophoretic delivery of positive nanovesicles through skin with microchannels were 33.3% and 28.3% of the initial levels after four and six hours. Such reduction in glucose level was comparable to that produced after subcutaneous injection of insulin. The fluorescence imaging study of nanovesicles containing FITC-labeled insulin confirmed the penetration of insulin from the nanovesicles driven by iontophoresis through skin following microchannel formation [50]. The results of this study introduced an efficient noninvasive delivery method of peptides and other macromolecules employing a combined triple means acting synergistically to temporarily modify skin barrier properties. In a more recent investigation, Bernardi et al. [51] investigated the potential use of iontophoresis and liposomes for transcutaneous immunization. Ovalbumin (OVA) was used as a model antigen. The goal was to enhance penetration of OVA down to the viable epidermis, where antigen-presenting cells are found. Cathodal iontophoresis of the liposomes encapsulating OVA together with silver nanoparticles increased OVA permeation to the viable epidermis by ninety-twofold compared to passive delivery *in vitro*. For *in vivo* study using rats, the increase in OVA skin penetration resulted in a humoral immune response similar to that obtained following a subcutaneous injection of the same agent [51].

37.2.1.2 Combined Iontophoresis and Ethosomes

The advancement in skin delivery by the introduction of ultra-deformable vesicles encouraged researchers in the field to modulate the vesicular compositions to enhance their stability and/or to improve their transdermal drug delivery potential. Ethosomes are such a new modified vesicular system. These are phospholipid vesicles incorporating a high concentration of ethanol. Ethosomes can be prepared at low temperature, producing nanostructures with the size decreasing at a higher concentration of ethanol. These vesicles are elastic and can deliver the drug deep into and through the skin [52]. Touitou and coworkers were the first to employ a high concentration of ethanol (up to 45%) in the vesicular nanoarchitectures to develop ethosomes for transdermal delivery of drugs [52, 53].

Being used as a skin penetration enhancer, ethanol was believed to destroy the vesicular structure. The proponents of ethosomes challenged this hypothesis by employing phosphorus nuclear magnetic resonance to prove the preservation of the vesicular structure in the presence of high ethanol content. They adopted differential scanning calorimetry to indicate the fluidizing effect of ethanol on the vesicular membrane. This effect is believed to provide ethosome elasticity, which is one of the driving forces for enhanced ethosomal transdermal delivery of drugs [54–56].

Combined delivery of ethosomes and iontophoresis was recently investigated for the skin delivery of vancomycin hydrochloride. The target goal was to augment the pharmacodynamic and pharmacokinetic characteristics and reduce the toxicity of vancomycin hydrochloride [57]. The ethosomal dispersion of vancomycin hydrochloride was composed of 1% w/v soya phospholipids, 45% v/v of ethanol, 10% v/v propylene glycol, and water up to 100% v/v. Stearylamine was included in the composition of ethosomes to impart a positive charge. Cathodal iontophoresis was employed for negatively charged ethosomes and anodal iontophoresis for positively charged vesicles and the free drug solution. Cathodal iontophoresis of negatively charged vesicles showed significant increase in transdermal flux compared to other ethosomal formulations and free drug solution. Continuous current was better than alternating ON/OFF mode. In the *in vivo* study, using rats with induced mediastinitis revealed similar results obtained after intramuscular vancomycin administration and treatment by combined iontophoretic skin delivery of vancomycin encapsulated in ethosomes.

Another study tested a system combining iontophoresis and drug-loaded lipid vesicles for the controlled transdermal delivery of diclofenac sodium [58]. Four different types of lipid vesicles were prepared. The conventional vesicles comprised phophatidylecholine (PC) and cholesterol (Chol) (3:1). The pegylated liposomes contained PC and Chol (3:1) with 2.5% (mol/mol%) of DSPE-PEG2000. Transfersomes were made of PC with Tween 80 as the edge activator, and ethosomes were fabricated from PC and Chol in the presence of 20% ethanol. The pegylated liposomes were prepared to reduce the electro-negativity of the conventional one by shielding the negative charge of the vesicle so as to study the effect of the surface charge of the lipid nanocarriers on the diclofenac sodium transport under iontophoretic current. Using full-thickness porcine skin, passive and iontophoretic (direct current or pulsed current 0.5 mA/cm^2 for eight hours) models were tested. The results indicated that the use of drug-loaded vesicles led to decreased flux values with increased lag times compared to that from the aqueous solution, both under passive delivery. This was explained by the hydrophilic nature of the drug. Iontophoretic drug transport from the liposomes was significantly affected by the composition and the charge of the lipid bilayer of the vesicles and the current mode used. Ethosomes resulted in the highest iontophoretic flux under direct constant current. Conventional liposomes with the highest negative surface charge led to better transport efficiencies of the model drug due to the higher mobility of the drug carriers under iontophoretic current. Based on their findings, pulsed current treatment has no clear advantage over constant current treatment in combination with any type of lipid vesicles, opposite to what has been described earlier with polymeric nanocarriers by Malinovskaja-Gomez [59, 60].

37.2.2 ELECTROPORATION AND ULTRA-DEFORMABLE LIPOSOMES

Enhanced transdermal penetration by electroporation is believed to depend on many mechanisms. These include increased permeability of the skin due to electrical breakdown, electrophoresis (repulsion force between the applied current and the entity of the same polarity), and/or—but less likely—from electro-osmosis. The mechanism of pore formation was reported to be due to a temperature rise within the SC intercellular lipids to above their phase transition temperature. The temperature rises in localized regions known as local transport regions (LTRs) [31, 61]. Additionally, the bulk of the SC is not homogenous, but exhibits defects, so it is likely that at least temporary aqueous pathways exist, e.g., in desmosomes or protein structures between adjacent corneocytes. The electric field can force electrolytes into such areas, expanding them so that SC resistance reduces markedly [62].

Few investigations are available on the combined use of liposomes and electroporation. For example, electroporation was achieved by application of electrical pulses (250 V, 20 ms, 10 pulses/min for five minutes), and its effect on the epidermal delivery of colchicine encapsulated in positively charged standard liposomes (DSPC: cholesterol;1:0.5 molar ratio) was investigated [63]. The total charge and cumulative amount of colchicine delivered over 24 hours were less than that after iontophoresis (0.5 mA/cm^2) for six hours. Interestingly, the authors proposed that intact vesicles could penetrate through such a potentially modified skin structure.

The investigation of vesicular transdermal delivery under electroporation has been extended to the highly deformable liposomes, which comprised PC with sodium cholate (86:14 w/w) [64]. The study employed human epidermal membrane and applied five pulses (100 V, 100 ms, and one-minute spacing) to negatively charged vesicles containing estradiol. Saturated aqueous solution of estradiol was used as the control. Electroporation resulted in significant increase in skin permeation and deposition of estradiol over eight hours from control solution (about sixteenfold relative to passive diffusion). Contrary to this, the permeation parameters were not enhanced after delivering the ultra-deformable liposomes under electroporation compared to simple occluded passive delivery from the same vesicles. Such low penetration was unexpected for ultra-deformable liposomes, as it would be reasonable to assume that the combination of the two accelerant strategies (released phospholipids acting as chemical enhancer and electroporation as a physical force) would augment each other, increasing penetration. This surprising result was attributed in part to the possible attenuated effect of the electrical pulses on the skin due to voltage/liposomes interaction. Nevertheless, as liposomes were suspended in a saturated (nonentrapped) estradiol solution, it would be logical to expect a result at least similar to that of the control, or even higher, due to the well-accepted enhancing effect of liposomes. Therefore, a possible role of PC (present in liposomes but not in solution) in restoring some of the skin's barrier properties was suggested.

To delineate this effect of PC on the skin barrier after electroporation, a two-stage protocol was designed so as to introduce the same number of pores within the skin using the same pulsing regimen detailed earlier. Membranes were dosed with empty liposome suspension (i.e., without estradiol) with or without edge activator for 30 minutes, with control membranes being treated with water. After washing the donor chambers, penetration from estradiol solution through control and treated skin was followed for 2.5 hours (Stage I). To examine the skin integrity further, another set of pulses was applied while estradiol solution remained in the donor (Stage II), and penetration was followed for a further two hours [64]. The results of this investigation are displayed as cumulative amount penetrated versus time plot in Figure 37.3. The graph displays a steady increase in estradiol penetrated during Stage I, with control (water-treated) showing the highest penetration rate. After the second pulsing (Stage II), drug penetration was once again increased, with the control showing a marked rise compared to that through skin treated with the two types of empty vesicles. It was therefore suggested that during skin electroporation using liposomes, PC molecules released from liposomes at the highly altered skin sites could improve skin repair. The PC monomers reaching the site of high skin perturbation (LTRs) would replace some of the water molecules at these particular regions. Although in a liquid-crystalline state, PC microdomains would be more resistant to molecular penetration than are water molecules. Thus, such new liquid crystalline microdomains acted in

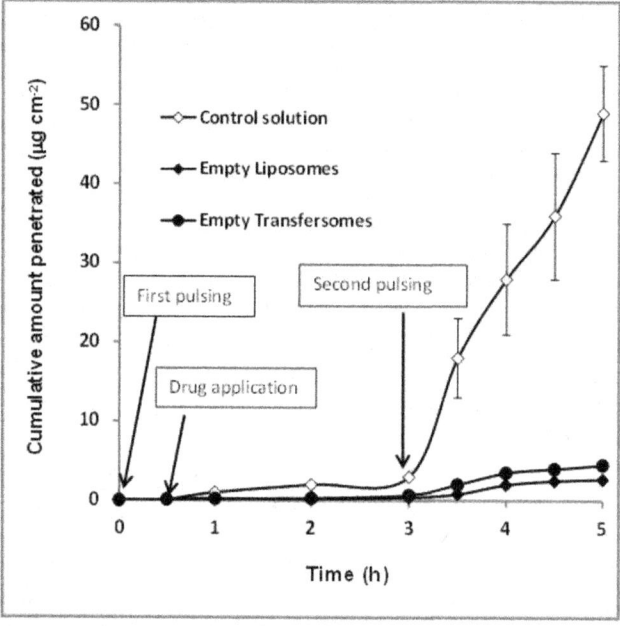

FIGURE 37.3 Two-stage *in vitro* human epidermal penetration of estradiol from saturated aqueous solution after two sets of pulses (five pulses, 100 V, 100 ms, and one-minute spacing) through control (water-treated) and empty liposome (with or without cholate)–treated skin (*n* = 6–10). (Modified from Essa et al. [64].)

opposition to the more usual penetration-enhancing effect of phospholipids operating particularly at gel regions of the intercellular lipid.

Accordingly, under such conditions, phospholipids would act as penetration retardants, in reasonable agreement with Fang et al. [65], who also reported a retardation of flurbiprofen permeation through mice skin *in vitro* when phospholipids were mixed with cellulose hydrogel.

37.2.3 COMBINED PHYSICAL MEANS AND ULTRA-DEFORMABLE LIPOSOMES

The combined use of electroporation and iontophoresis in improving transepidermal drug delivery was first investigated in the early nineties [66]. Transport of luteinizing hormone–releasing hormone in solution through human skin *in vitro* was enhanced by this combination by 5 to 10 times compared to the corresponding iontophoretic flux [66]. However, later on many reports gave outcomes where the combined techniques were less encouraging [67, 68]. After that, a study investigated the delivery of liposomally encapsulated estradiol under the two physical enhancers [44]. Transdermal fluxes and skin deposition from solution and ultra-deformable vesicles under iontophoresis, electroporation, and the combined two electric methods are shown in Figure 37.4.

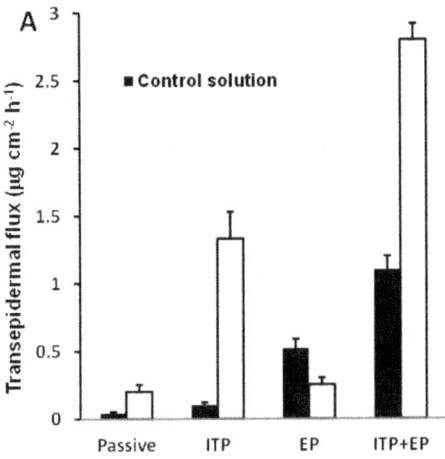

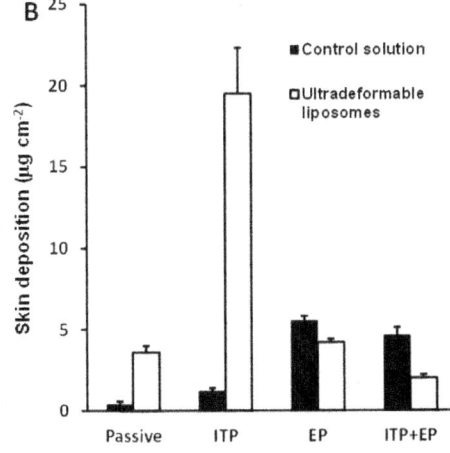

FIGURE 37.4 Transepidermal estradiol fluxes (A) and skin deposition (B) after iontophoresis (ITP), electroporation (EP), and combined electroporation and iontophoresis (EP + ITP) delivery from saturated aqueous solution and ultra-deformable liposomes, through human epidermal membranes *in vitro* (n = 6–12).

The histograms reveal that ultra-deformable liposomes improved drug penetration and deposition under passive and iontophoretic deliveries compared to the control saturated solution. Under electroporation, only the solution improved drug skin penetration compared to the passive one and liposomes under electroporation. This was attributed to the possible retarding effect of the phospholipid. While electroporation alone did not improve estradiol parameters from ultra-deformable liposomes over its passive delivery, iontophoresis (0.8 mA/cm^2) after skin pulsing (five pulses, 100V, 100 ms, and one-minute spacing) increased drug flux by seventeenfold compared to passive delivery.

Together, the barrier-distorting factors (electroporation, iontophoresis, and phospholipids) may have disturbed more of the stratum corneal lipid domain. However, the penetration data were still low. While iontophoretic delivery enhanced estradiol flux from ultra-deformable vesicles by up to about 15-fold compared to control, combined electroporation and iontophoresis raised the flux by only 2.5-fold. This low ratio suggested an increased skin barrier towards estradiol penetration, a result that supports the earlier finding of the penetration-retarding effect of PC monomers when present during skin electroporation. Thus, the overall results supported the concept that phospholipid protects the skin after high-voltage pulses. The dramatic fall in skin deposition value to 0.46-fold compared to control solution further emphasizes the protective effect of phospholipid monomers against estradiol diffusion into, and through, the skin.

Recently, Zorec et al. [69] investigated the combined use of lipid nanovesicles (ethosomes, liposomes) with electroporation or sonoporation or a combination of the two physical means for the skin delivery of calcein (model hydrophilic drug). Passive diffusion of ethosomes (2% phospholipon 90G and 30% ethanol) greatly enhanced calcein delivery compared to liposomes (phospholipon 90G and cholesterol) and control aqueous drug solution when investigated *in vitro* using porcine skin. When lipid vesicles were driven under electroporation (200/100/100 pulse voltage [V]/duration [μs]/spacing [μs] applied for 5 or 15 seconds), molecular delivery was significantly improved, with ethosomes producing a pronounced effect compared to traditional liposomes. Surprisingly, when electroporation was combined with sonophoresis (30/100/166 kHz, duty cycle [%], kPa applied for 2.5 or 5 minutes), this did not result in a synergistic or additive effect over electroporation alone. The experimental setups and treatment protocols they used were close to *in vivo* and potential clinical conditions. This would increase the relevance of the obtained data and make this translation easier and quicker.

37.3   CONCLUSION

Development of electrically assisted transdermal delivery broadened the spectrum of transdermal drug delivery. Using these strategies allowed the delivery of large-molecular-weight hydrophilic compounds that had been waiting for years to get the benefits of the advantages of controlled transdermal transport. A combination of particulate drug delivery systems with the electrical driving has increased the chance of the delivery of noncharged drug candidates. In this case, the neutral drug can be loaded in charged particulate carriers such as liposomes. Studies have indicated that iontophoresis of such vesicles can indeed augment the penetration of entrapped drugs, irrespective of the flexibility of the liposomal membrane. Despite the encouraging data, much work is required, and authors have to investigate liposome substitutes such as niosomes to reduce the cost of the process.

REFERENCES

1. Smeden JV, Janssens M, Gooris GS, Bouwstra JA. The important role of stratum corneum lipids for the cutaneous barrier function. Biochim Biophys Acta (BBA) – Mol. Cell Biol. Lipids 2014; 1841:295–313.
2. Bos JD, Meinardi MM. The 500 Dalton rule for the skin penetration of chemical compounds and drugs. Exp Dermatol 2000; 9:165–169.
3. Bouwstra JA, Gooris GS, van der Spek JA, Lavrijsen S, Bras W. The lipid and protein structure of mouse stratum corneum: a wide and small angle diffraction study. Biochim Biophys Acta 1994; 1212:183–192.
4. Wang Y, Thakur R, Fan Q, Michniak B. Transdermal iontophoresis: combination strategies to improve transdermal iontophoretic drug delivery. Eur J Pharm Biopharm 2005; 60:179–191.

5. Mezei M, Gulasekharam V. Liposomes: a selective drug delivery system for the topical route of administration I: lotion dosage form. Life Sci 1980; 26:1473–1477.

6. El Maghraby GM, Williams AC. Vesicular systems for delivering conventional small organic molecules and larger macromolecules to and through human skin. Expert Opin Drug Deliv 2009; 6:149–163.

7. El Maghraby GMM. Ultra-deformable vesicles as skin drug delivery systems: mechanisms of action, in: N. Dragicevic, H.I. Maibach (Eds.), Percutaneous Penetration Enhancers, Chemical Methods in Penetration Enhancement: Nanocarriers, Springer-Verlag Berlin Heidelberg, 2016:137–145.

8. New RRC. Liposomes: A Practical Approach, Oxford University Press, Oxford, 1990.

9. Schreier H, Bouwstra JA. Liposomes and niosomes as topical drug carriers: dermal and transdermal drug delivery. J Control Rel 1994; 30:1–15.

10. Hofland HEJ, Bouwstra JA, Bodde′ HE, Spies F, Junginger HE. Interactions between liposomes and human stratum corneum in-vitro: freeze fracture electron microscopical visualization and small angle X-ray scattering studies. Br J Dermatol 1995; 132:853–856.

11. Cevc G, Blume G. Lipid vesicles penetrate into intact skin owing to the transdermal osmotic gradient and hydration force. Biochim Biophys Acta 1992; 1104:226–232.

12. Nounou MM, El-Khordagui LK, Khalafallah NA, Khalil SA. Liposomal formulation for dermal and transdermal drug delivery: past, present and future. Recent Pat. Drug Deliv Formul. 2008; 2: 9–18.

13. Planas ME, Gonzalez P, Rodriguez L, Sanchez S, Cevc G. Noninvasive percutaneous induction of topical analgesia by a new type of drug carrier, and prolongation of local pain insensitivity by anesthetic liposomes. Aneth Analg 1992; 75:615–621.

14. Paul A, Cevc G, Bachhawat BK. Transdermal immunization with large proteins by means of ultra-deformable drug carriers, Eur J Immunol. 1995; 25:3521–3524.

15. Green PG, Flanagan M, Shroot B, Guy RH. Iontophoretic drug delivery, In: Walters KA, Hadgraft J, eds. Pharmaceutical Skin Penetration Enhancement. New York: Marcel Dekker Inc., 1993:311–333.

16. Banga AK. In: Electrically Assisted Transdermal and Topical Drug Delivery. London: Taylor and Francis, 1998.

17. Guy RH. Iontophoresis-recent developments. J Pharm Pharmacol 1998; 50:371–374.

18. Sage BH, Riviere JE. Model system in iontophoresis transport efficacy. Adv Drug Deliv Rev 1992; 9:265–237.

19. Phipps JB, Padmanabhan RV, Lattin GA. Iontophoretic delivery of model inorganic and drug ions. J Pharm Sci 1989; 78:365–369.

20. Pikal MJ, Shah S. Transport mechanisms in iontophoresis. III. An experimental study of the contributions of electroosmotic flow and permeability change in transport of low and high molecular weight solutes. Pharm Res 1990; 7:222–229.

21. Jadoul A, Bouwstra J, Pre′at V. Effect of iontophoresis and electroporation on the stratum corneum. Adv Drug Deliv Rev 1999; 35:89–105.

22. Cullander C, Guy RH. Sites of iontophoretic current flow into the skin: identification andcharacterisation with the vibrating probe electrode. J Invest Derm 1991; 97:55–64.

23. Cullander C. What are the pathways of iontophoretic current flow through mammalian skin? Adv Drug Deliv Rev 1992; 9:119–135.

24. Monteiro-Riviere NA, Inman AO, Riviere JE. Identification of the pathway of iontophoretic drug delivery: light and ultrastructural studies using mercuric chloride in pigs. Pharm Res 1994; 11:251–256.

25. Graaff AM, Li GL, Van Aelst AC, Bouwstra JA. Combined chemical and electrical enhancement modulates stratum corneum structure. J Control Rel 2003; 90:49–58.

26. Turner NG, Guy RH. Iontophoretic transdermal pathways: dependence on penetrant physicochemical properties. J Pharm Sci 1997; 86:1385–1389.

27. Pliquett UF, Zewert TE, Chen T, Langer R, Weaver JC. Imaging of fluorescent molecules and small ion transport through human stratum corneum during high voltage pulsing: localised transport regions are involved. J Biophys Chem 1996; 58:185–204.

28. Prausnitz MR, Lee CS, Liu CH, Pang JC, Singh TP, Langer R, Weaver JC. Transdermal transport efficiency during skin electroporation and iontophoresis. J Control Rel 1996; 38:205–217.

29. Higuchi WI, Li SK, Ghanem AH, Zhu HG, Song Y. Mechanistic aspects of iontophoresis in human epidermal membrane. J Control Rel 1999; 62:13–23.

30. Prausnitz MR. A practical assessment of transdermal drug delivery by skin electroporation. Adv Drug Del Rev 1999; 35:61–76.

31. Pliquet UF, Gusbeth CA. Perturbation of human skin due to application of high voltage. J Bioelectrochem 2000; 51:41–51.

32. Pliquett U, Weaver JC. Electroporation of human skin: simulation measurement of changes in transport of two fluorescent molecules and in the passive electrical properties. Bioelectrochem Bioenerget 1996; 39:1–12.

33. Vanbever R, Morre ND, Pre´at V. Transdermal delivery of fentanyl by electroporation. II Mechanisms involved in drug transport. Pharm Res 1996; 13:1359–1365.

34. Vanbever R, Leroy MA, Pre´at V. Transdermal penetration of neutral molecules by skin electroporation. J Control Rel 1998; 54:243–250.

35. Curdy C, Kalia YN, Guy RH. Non-invasive assessment of the effects of iontophoresis on human skin in vivo. J Pharm Pharmacol 2001; 53:769–777.

36. Williams AC. Transdermal and Topical Drug Delivery. London and Chicago: Pharmaceutical Press, 2003.

37. Dragicevic N, Maibach H. Combined use of nanocarriers and physical methods for percutaneous penetration enhancement. Advanced Drug Delivery Reviews 2018; 127:58–84.

38. Vutla NB, Betageri GV, Banga AK. Transdermal iontophoretic delivery of encephalin formulated in liposomes. J Pharm Sci 1996; 85:5–8.

39. Kulkarni SB, Banga AK, Betageri GV. Transdermal iontophoretic delivery of colchicine encapsulated in liposomes. Drug Del 1996; 3:245–250.

40. Fang J, Sung KC, Lin H, Fang C. Transdermal iontophoretic delivery of enoxacin from various liposome-encapsulated formulations. J Control Rel 1999; 60:1–10.

41. Kirjavainen M, Urtti A, Monkkonen J, Hirvonen J. Influence of lipid on the mannitol flux during transdermal iontophoresis in vitro. Eur J Pharm Sci 2000; 10:97–102.

42. Li GL, Danhof M, Bouwstra JA. Effect of elastic liquid state vesicle on apomorphine iontophoresis transport through human skin in vitro. Pharm Res 2001; 11:1627–1630.

43. Essa EA, Bonner MC, Barry BW. Iontophoretic estradiol skin delivery and tritium exchange in ultradeformable liposomes. Int J Pharm 2002; 240:55–66.

44. Essa EA, Bonner MC, Barry BW. Electrically assisted skin delivery of liposomal estradiol; phospholipid as damage retardant. J Control Rel 2004; 95:535–546.

45. Cevc G, Gebauer D, Stieber J, Schätzlein A, Blume G. Ultraflexible vesicles, Transfersomes, have an extremely low pore penetration resistance and transport therapeutic amounts of insulin across the intact mammalian skin. Biochim Biophys Acta 1998; 1368:201–215.

46. El Maghraby GMM, Williams AC, Barry BW. Skin hydration and possible shunt route penetration in controlled estradiol delivery from ultra-deformable and standard liposomes. J Pharm Pharmacol 2001; 53:1311–1322.

47. Essa EA, Bonner MC, Barry BW. Human skin sandwich for assessing shunt route penetration during passive and iontophoretic drug and liposome delivery. J Pharm Pharmacol 2002; 54:1481–1490.

48. Barry BW. Drug delivery routes in skin: a novel approach. Adv Drug Deliv Rev 2002; 54:31–40.

49. Lee S, Lee J, Choi YW. Skin permeation enhancement of ascorbyl palmitate by liposomal hydrogel (LipoGel) formulation and electrical assistance. Biol Pharm Bull 2007; 30:393–396.

50. Chen H, Zhu H, Zheng J, Mou D, Wan J, Zhang J, Shi T, Zhao Y, Xu H, Yang X. Iontophoresis-driven penetration of nanovesicles through microneedle-induced skin microchannels for enhancing transdermal delivery of insulin. J Control Release 2009; 139:63–72.

51. Bernardi DS, Bitencourt C, Silveira DS, Cruz EL, Pereira-da-Silva MA, Faccioli LH, Lopez RF. Effective transcutaneous immunization using a combination of iontophoresis and nanoparticles, Nanomed 2016; 12:2439–2448.

52. Touitou E, Alkabes M, Dayan N, Eliaz M. Ethosomes: the novel vesicular carriers for enhanced skin delivery. Pharm Res 1997; 14:S305.

53. Touitou E. Composition for applying active substances to or through the skin. U.S. Patent 1998.

54. Dayan N, Touitou E. Carriers for skin delivery of trihexyphenidyl HCl: ethosomes vs. liposomes. Biomaterials 2000; 21:1879–1885.

55. Godin B, Touitou E. Intracellular and dermal delivery of polypeptide antibiotic bacitracin. Proceedings of the Drug Research Between Information and Life Sciences, ICCF, 3rd Symposium, Bucharest, Romania 2002.

56. Touitou E, Dayan N, Bergelson L, Godin B, Eliaz M. Ethosomes -novel vesicular carriers for enhanced delivery; characterization and skin penetration properties, J Control Rel 2000; 65:403–418.

57. Mohammed MI, Makky AMA, Teaima MHM, Abdellatif MM, Hamzawy MA, Khalil MAF. Transdermal delivery of vancomycin hydrochloride using combination of nano-ethosomes and iontophoresis: in vitro and in vivo study. Drug Deliv 2016; 23:1558–1564.

58. Malinovskaja-Gomez K, Espuelas S, Garrido MJ, Hirvonen J, Laaksonen T. Comparison of liposomal drug formulations for transdermal iontophoretic drug delivery. Eur J Pharm Sci 2017; 106: 294–301.

59. Malinovskaja-Gomez K, Labouta H, Schneider M, Hirvonen J, Laaksonen T. Transdermal iontophoresis of flufenamic acid loaded PLGA nanoparticles. Eur J Pharm Sci 2016; 89:154–162.

60. Malinovskaja K, Laaksonen T, Hirvonen J. Controlled transdermal delivery of leuprorelin by pulsed iontophoresis and ion-exchange fiber. Eur J Pharm Biopharm 2014; 88: 594–601.

61. Pliquett UF, Martin GT, Weaver JC. Kinetics of the temperature rise within human stratum corneum during electroporation and pulsed high voltage iontophoresis. Bioelectrochem 2002; 57:65–72.

62. Bodde´ HE, van den Brink I, Koerten HK, de Haan FHN. Visualization of in vitro percutaneous penetration of mercuric chloride transport through intercellular space versus cellular uptake through desmosomes. J Control Rel 1991; 15:227–236.

63. Badkar AV, Betageri GV, Hofmann GA, Banga AK. Enhancement of transdermal iontophoretic delivery of a liposomal formulation of colchicine by electroporation. Drug Deliv 1999; 6:111–115.

64. Essa EA, Bonner MC, Barry BW. Electroporation and ultra-deformable liposomes; human skin repair by phospholipid. J Control Rel 2003; 92:163–172.

65. Fang JY, Hwang TL, Leu YL. Effect of enhancers and retarders on percutaneous absorption of furbiprofen from hydrogels. Int J Pharm 2003; 250:313–325.

66. Bommannan D, Tamada J, Leung L, Potts RO. Effect of electroporation on transdermal iontophoretic delivery of luteinizing hormone releasing hormone (LHRH) in vitro. Pharm Res 1994; 11:1809–1814.

67. Badkar AV, Banga AK. Electrically enhanced transepidermal delivery of a macromolecule. J Pharm Pharmacol 2002; 54:907–912.

68. Fang JY, Hwang TL, Huang YB, Tsai YH. Transepidermal iontophoresis of sodium nonivamide acetate V. Combined effect of physical enhancement methods. Int J Pharm 2002; 235:95–105.

69. Zorec B, Zupančič S, Kristl J, Pavše N. Combinations of nanovesicles and physical methods for enhanced transdermal delivery of a model hydrophilic drug. Euro J Pharm Biopharm 2018; 127: 387–397.

38 Lipid-Based Vesicles (Liposomes) and Their Combination with Physical Methods for Dermal and Transdermal Drug Delivery

Nina Dragićević
Singidunum University, Danijelova 32, Belgrade, Serbia

Howard I. Maibach
University of California, San Francisco, California

CONTENTS

38.1 INTRODUCTION

The skin has been recognized as an important drug delivery route in topical pharmacotherapy treatments of various skin diseases, as well as for systemic drug administration. Thus, the skin represents a site of drug application both for local (topical/dermal) and systemic (transdermal) effects. Topical and transdermal drug delivery systems are of great interest, since they offer a number of advantages compared to other conventional routes (Predic Atkinson et al., 2015).

Unlike most other organs in the body, the skin can be reached directly, and so drug delivery to this tissue is assumed to be relatively easy. However, dermal/transdermal drug delivery is far away of being easy to achieve, especially if the goal is systemic drug delivery. When a drug possesses ideal physicochemical properties (as in the case of nicotine and nitroglycerin), transdermal delivery is feasible.

According to Benson and Watkinson (2012) ideal properties for a molecule in order to penetrate the stratum corneum (SC) well, being the uppermost skin layer, would be the following: low molecular mass (preferably less than 600 Da, when the diffusion coefficient D tends to be high), adequate solubility in oil and water (in order to achieve a high membrane concentration gradient), a high but balanced (log K octanol/water of 1 to 3) partition coefficient K (a too high coefficient may inhibit clearance from viable tissues), and low melting point (which correlates with good solubility).

If the drug does not match these ideal characteristics, its penetration into or permeation through the skin will be insufficient to achieve the desired drug effects. The major problem in topical/transdermal drug delivery is the low permeability of the most apical layer of the skin, the SC. Since percutaneous absorption is pivotal to the effectiveness of both topical and transdermal systems, significant efforts have been devoted to developing strategies to overcome the impermeability of intact human skin. There are many strategies for circumventing the SC providing the main barrier for drug penetration. Methods to enhance percutaneous drug penetration are based, on one hand, on the manipulation of the drug or vehicle to enhance drug diffusion, such as the use of a special drug form or pro-drug, ion pairs or coacervates, eutectic systems, saturated or supersaturated solutions, complexes, different nanocarriers (vesicles, nanoparticles, dendrimers, etc.), etc. (Dragicevic and Maibach, 2015, 2016). On the other hand, to enhance percutaneous penetration, SC modification is achieved through physical enhancement techniques, such as bypass/removal of SC (ablation, microneedles) and electrical methods (ultrasound, iontophoresis, electroporation, etc.), as well as by chemical penetration enhancers. For a comprehensive review of different physical penetration enhancement methods being used to enhance drug penetration into/through the skin, the reader should refer to Dragicevic and Maibach (2017).

Among formulation methods nanocarriers are often used, especially vesicles. Vesicles comprise a wide range of lipid-based vesicles (e.g., liposomes), which can be conventional phospholipid vesicles or elastic/deformable phospholipid vesicles (containing different penetration enhancers) and will be discussed in this chapter, as well as surfactant-based vesicles (e.g., niosomes), penetration enhancer-containing vesicles (Ainbinder et al., 2016; Cevc and Chopra, 2016; Dragicevic et al., 2016; Manconi et al., 2016, n.d.; Muzzalupo, 2016; Siler-Marinkovic, 2016) The use of vesicles and other nanocarriers for drug delivery has gained growing interest as a noninvasive means for improving dermal and transdermal delivery of drugs possessing unfavorable penetration properties.

As to physical methods, ultrasound (Azagury et al., 2015; Daftardar et al., 2019; Oberli et al., 2014; Seah and Teo, 2018), electroporation (Bernelin-Cottet et al., 2019; Escobar-Chávez et al., 2009; Feng et al., 2017; Ita, 2016), iontophoresis (Mohammed et al., 2016; Park et al., 2019; Takeuchi et al., 2016), microneedles (Ahmed et al., 2019; Moffatt et al., 2017; Nguyen and Banga, 2017; Nguyen et al., 2018; Sabri et al., 2020), radiofrequency ablation (Banga, 2009; Birchall et al., 2006; Kalluri and Banga, 2011), and others are being used. For details on different physical methods, the reader should refer to Dragicevic and Maibach (2017).

The use of nanocarriers is mainly confined to achieving skin delivery of drugs, while transdermal drug delivery is infrequently achieved. On the other hand, the combination of nanocarriers with another penetration enhancement methods with the aim to enhance dermal, as well as transdermal, drug delivery has been the subject of numerous investigations. Therefore, nanocarriers are often used together with physical methods. These two approaches applied to enhance drug penetration act via different enhancement mechanisms. Thus, it is assumed that these methods will act synergistically to overcome the low permeability of the most apical layer of the skin, the SC, leading to enhanced drug penetration. Among physical enhancement methods, especially microneedles (MNs), iontophoresis, ultrasound, and electroporation can be used together with nanocarriers to induce a synergistic penetration enhancement of drugs into/through the skin (Balázs et al., 2016; Charoenputtakun et al., 2015; Elsabahy and Foldvari, 2013; Park et al., 2010; Rastogi et al., 2010).

Conventional liposomes and especially the new generation of elastic/deformable vesicles, such as Transfersomes (Idea AG, Germany), ethosomes, invasomes, etc., have been widely studied as drug carriers for dermal and transdermal delivery of different drugs (analgesics, anticancers, proteins and peptides, immunomodulators, steroidal hormones, etc.) when used alone or in combination with other penetration enhancement methods (Abd El-Alim et al., 2019; Ascenso et al., 2015; Avadhani et al., 2017; Caddeo et al., 2018; Elsabahy and Foldvari, 2013; Hussain et al., 2020; Priyanka and Singh, 2014; Zhang et al., 2014).

38.2 LIPID-BASED VESICLES (LIPOSOMES)

38.2.1 CONVENTIONAL LIPID-BASED VESICLES

Lipid-based vesicles i.e., liposomes are colloidal spherical particles typically consisting of phospholipids, cholesterol, and other possible ingredients. These lipid molecules tend to self-aggregate, forming one or more concentric bimolecular layers enclosing an equal number of aqueous compartments. Thus, liposomes can be unilamellar or multilamellar. Liposomes containing only phospholipids and cholesterol are usually termed *conventional liposomes*. Further, liposomes can encapsulate hydrophilic drugs within the aqueous regions and lipophilic molecules within the lipid bilayers. They were discovered in the 1960s by Bangham and represent, among a variety of nanocarriers, the first ones studied for skin delivery of drugs (Siler-Marinkovic, 2016). The first approved and clinically available liposomal dermatic, Pevaryl Lipogel, containing 1% econazole, was marketed by Cilag AG, in Switzerland in 1988. This liposomal gel formulation revealed a quicker onset of drug action and shorter treatment duration due to increased drug levels in the stratum corneum (Kriftner, 1992). Conventional liposomes have been used since the 1980s as drug carrier systems for topical/dermal delivery, as they indeed have the potential to enhance drug penetration into/through the skin (Belhaj et al., 2017; Betz et al., 2005; El Maghraby et al., 2000; Joseph et al., 2018; Mostafa et al., 2018), improve therapeutic effectiveness (Jeong et al., 2017; Manca et al., 2016; Mura et al., 2007; Oh et al., 2011) and decrease side effects (Seth et al., 2004). Liposomes have also been used to deliver drugs to hair follicles, i.e., to the pilosebaceous unit, which is the desired target site in treating acne vulgaris. Adapalene encapsulated in liposomes showed enhanced drug delivery into the skin and hair follicles (Ingebrigtsen et al., 2017; Kumar and Banga, 2016), as well as retinoids (Latter et al., 2019). The application of argan oil–enriched liposomes containing allantoin seemed to provide a softening and relaxing effect on the skin, thus facilitating the drug penetration into and through the skin (Manca et al., 2016). Further, liposomes are used in cosmetology, noncoated as well as polysaccharide-coated (Ionosomes), and both types have shown to significantly improve penetration of hydrophilic-active molecules (caffeine, hexapeptide) into the skin (Belhaj et al., 2017). An interesting approach is the preparation of lipase-sensitive liposomes by coating of lipase-sensitive moieties onto conventional erythromycin liposomes for achieving an enhanced antimicrobial effect in treating acne vulgaris (Jeong et al., 2017). A further approach is the encapsulation of azithromycin into different liposomes, including conventional liposomes, to locally treat skin infections caused by methicillin-resistant *Staphylococcus aureus* (MRSA) strains. All liposomes delivered azithromycin into the skin more efficiently than the control and were shown to be biocompatible with keratinocytes and fibroblasts (Rukavina et al., 2018). Liposomes encapsulating active compounds have been used with high therapeutic effectiveness in wound healing and skin regeneration (Wang et al., 2017, 2019). Moreover, liposomes with co-incorporated quercetin and resveratrol led to a remarkable amelioration of the tissue damage in skin lesions, with a significant reduction of edema and leukocyte infiltration (Caddeo et al., 2016), which caused further investigation of resveratrol liposomes for the treatment of skin disorders such as chloasma, acne vulgaris, and skin aging, as well as wound and facial redness (Soleymani et al., 2019). Liposomes and other nanocarriers have been formulated to enhance the bioavailability and stability, as well as the therapeutic efficacy, of different polyphenols used for prevention and treatment of melanoma (Heenatigala Palliyage et al., 2019). Conventional liposomes are the most commonly and extensively studied vesicle carrier systems for the skin/dermal delivery of drugs.

38.2.2 NOVEL DEFORMABLE LIPID-BASED VESICLES

As conventional liposomes are used for dermal drug delivery, i.e., they are not successful in achieving transdermal drug delivery, there was a need to develop a new generation of lipid-based vesicles. Different approaches were used to obtain these vesicles. At the end, vesicles were obtained that contain besides phospholipids in their membranes, i.e., bilayers, small amounts of edge activators, such as surfactants (e.g., polysorbate 80 or polysorbate 20), ethanol, terpenes, etc., to enhance their membrane fluidity and deformability, i.e., elasticity, and hence their penetration-enhancing ability. Therefore these vesicles are called *elastic* or *deformable or flexible vesicles*. These elastic liposomes, such as Transfersomes (Ahmed, 2015; Al Shuwaili et al., 2016; Cevc and Chopra, 2016; Khan et al., 2015), ethosomes (Abdulbaqi et al., 2016; Ainbinder et al., 2010, 2016; Garg et al., 2016; Zhai et al., 2015), transethosomes (Ascenso et al., 2015), invasomes (Dragicevic et al., 2016; Dragicevic-Curic et al., 2008, 2009, 2010), are being investigated for dermal as well as transdermal drug delivery. They have been studied as drug carriers for a range of small molecules—peptides, proteins, and vaccines—both *in vitro* and *in vivo* (Benson, 2017). For a comprehensive review of different vesicles, the reader should refer to Dragicevic and Maibach (2016).

Transfersomes (termed by the inventors) present one of the first deformable vesicles, which were introduced by Cevc and his group (Cevc et al., 1995). These vesicles contain phosphatidylcholine (PC) and edge activators (sodium cholate, polysorbate 80, or polysorbate 20), which can impart deformability to the carrier, being responsible for improved transdermal drug delivery (Cevc, 2003; Cevc and Blume, 1992, 2001, 2004; Cevc et al., 2002, 2008; Fesq et al., 2003; Schätzlein and Cevc, 1998). The main benefit of using Transfersomes as a carrier is the delivery of macromolecules through the skin by a noninvasive route, therefore increasing the patient's compliance. It is used for the delivery of growth hormones, anesthetics, insulin, proteins, vaccines, and herbal drugs (Gupta and Kumar, 2020). Transfersomes encapsulating lidocaine and tetracaine provided a higher local analgesic effect than liposomes and the drug solution (Cevc, 1996). Further, it was shown that these ultra-deformable vesicles improved the regio-specificity and the biological activity of the corticosteroids *in vivo* (Cevc et al., 1997). Studies with Transfersomes entrapping TRMA (Cevc and Blume, 2003), hydrocortisone, and dexamethasone (Cevc and Blume, 2004) reported that the use of Transfersomes significantly reduced the required drug doses and enabled a sustained release in comparison to commercial preparations. Jain et al. (2003) also showed that Transfersomes entrapping dexamethasone induced better antiedema activity in comparison to liposomes and ointment. The authors concluded that Transfersomes can increase the transdermal flux, prolong the release, and improve the site specificity of bioactive molecules. The use of Transfersomes containing diclofenac resulted in tenfold higher drug concentration in the subcutaneous tissue compared to a commercial diclofenac gel, thus forming a drug reservoir with sustained drug release (Cevc and Blume, 2001). It has been reported that Diractin, a new formulation containing ketoprofen encapsulated in Transfersomes, can deposit ketoprofen in deep subcutaneous tissues, which the drug from conventional gels (Gabrilen gel, Togal Mobil Gel, Fastum gel) reaches mainly via systemic circulation (Cevc et al., 2008). Further, *in vivo* studies in mice and humans revealed that Transfersomes enabled a systemic delivery of insulin and that the efficiency of the formulation was comparable to that obtained after a subcutaneous (s.c.) injection of the same preparation, but with a longer lag time (Cevc et al., 1995, 1998). It has also been reported that systemic normoglycemia that lasting at least 16 hours has been achieved using a single noninvasive, epicutaneous administration of insulin in Transfersomes (Cevc, 2003). Transfersomes can also be used as a transdermal delivery system for the poorly soluble drug sertraline in order to overcome the troubles associated with its oral delivery (Gupta et al., 2012). Different transfemoral formulations were prepared with nonionic surfactant (Span 80), soya lecithin, and carbomer. The transfersomal gel showed a significantly higher cumulative amount of drug permeation and flux along with lower lag time than the drug solution and drug gel, indicating the possibility of its application for transdermal delivery of sertraline. Transfersomes can also be used for topical immunization (Mahor, Gupta, et al., 2007). An *in vivo* study in rats revealed that the topically applied tetanus toxoid (TT) entrapped in Transfersomes, after secondary immunization, could elicit an immune response (anti-TT-IgG) equivalent to one that was produced following intramuscularly alum-adsorbed TT-based immunization (Gupta et al., 2005). In addition, cationic Transfersomes loaded with DNA encoding the hepatitis B surface antigen (HBsAg) elicited *in vivo* in mice a significantly higher anti-HBsAg antibody titer and cytokines level as compared to unentrapped DNA, and they were comparable to levels achieved after intramuscular recombinant HBsAg administration (Mahor, Rawat, et al., 2007). It has been shown that transferosomes incorporated in a gel can be used as a carrier of papaverine hydrochloride for both diagnosis and treatment of erectile dysfunction (Ali et al., 2015). Topically applied lyophilized gel containing felodipine-loaded transferosomes has been reported to be a promising transdermal delivery system to enhance its bioavailability compared to Plendil (Kassem et al., 2018). An optimized protransfersomal system encapsulating the antihypertensive drug timolol maleate, topically applied, has been compared to its oral administration, and it revealed excellent permeation rate through shaved rat skin (780.69 $\mu g/cm^2/h$) and showed a sixfold increase in relative bioavailability with prolonged plasma profile up to 72 hours (Morsi et al., 2018). D-α-tocopherol polyethylene glycol 1000 succinate–based Transfersomes enhanced the permeation of raloxifene (used for breast cancer protection) through rat skin, indicating its potential for transdermal drug delivery (Alhakamy et al., 2019). Transfersomes containing different edge activators (sodium deoxycholate, sodium cholate, and sodium taurocholate) and ethosomes with variable ethanol contents (10%, 30%, and 50%) were prepared, and after their characterization ethosomes with 30% ethanol and sodium deoxycholate–containing Transfersomes were incorporated into hydrogels. Hydrogels containing deformable vesicles exhibited a more sustained release of diflunisal than the corresponding dispersions. Compared to the liposomal hydrogel, both hydrogels containing deformable vesicles were superior regarding diflunisal permeation and flux across the skin. Further, they exhibited remarkable antinociceptive and antiinflammatory effects, which was manifested by significant reduction in the number of writhings and significantly higher inhibition of paw edema, indicating their use for pain and inflammation management (Abd El-Alim et al., 2019).

Peptide-modified, vemurafenib-loaded, deformable liposomes (containing sodium cholate) were successfully used for the targeted inhibition of subcutaneous melanoma after their application to the skin (Zou et al., 2018). Transfersomes as well as ethosomes were shown to be able to effectively deliver cyclosporine A *in vitro* into the skin (Carreras et al., 2020). Tocopherol-loaded Transfersomes (containing Tween 20, 40, 60, and 80) have shown to bear potential as a topical delivery system with antioxidant activity and wound healing properties (Caddeo et al., 2018). Further, the encapsulation of the 19–amino acid synthetic peptide PnPP-19 in cationic Transfersomes protected the peptide from degradation and enabled its topical administration (De Marco Almeida et al., 2018). Baicalin was incorporated into new self-assembling core-shell gellan-Transfersomes, and their ability to improve baicalin efficacy in antiinflammatory and skin repair tests was confirmed *in vivo* in mice, providing complete skin restoration and inhibiting all the studied inflammatory markers (Manconi et al., 2018). Transfersomes have also been investigated as a transdermal delivery system to encapsulate the growth hormone as an antiaging strategy (Azimi et al., 2019).

Ethosomes (as termed by the inventors) present vesicles composed of phospholipids, ethanol, and water. The incorporation of ethanol into lipid vesicles is an alternative approach to fluidize the lipid membrane and thus enhance drug penetration into deep skin layers and/or the systemic circulation (Ainbinder et al., 2016; Touitou et al., 2000). The ethosomal system enhanced *in vitro* the amount of minoxidil permeated through and the amount deposited in nude mice skin (Touitou et al., 2000). The transdermal delivery of testosterone from the ethosomal patch Testosome was greater both *in vitro* and *in vivo* than from the commercially available Testoderm patch (Alza, USA) (Touitou et al., 2000). Ethosomes improved the transdermal delivery of melatonin (Dubey et al., 2007) and testosterone (Ainbinder and Touitou, 2005) across human skin *in vitro* and enabled systemic absorption of testosterone in rats (Ainbinder and Touitou, 2005), i.e. ethosomal testosterone was superior compared to the commercial preparation Androgel (Unimed, USA). The ethosomal buspirone transdermal system for the potential treatment of menopausal syndromes enhanced *in vitro* drug permeation into porcine ear skin and provided good bioavailability and efficient pharmacodynamic responses in rats (Shumilov and Touitou, 2010). A binary combination of the lipophilic pro-drug acyclovir palmitate and ethosomes synergistically enhanced acyclovir absorption into the mice skin *in vitro* (Zhou et al., 2010). For more details on ethosomes, refer to Ainbinder et al. (2016). Further, the blood profile of cytarabine after its transdermal administration in ethosomes indicated a lower lag time with the high amount of drug within 3 to 12 hours, demonstrating the enhanced percutaneous penetration of cytarabine (Raj et al., 2018). Ethosomes have been shown to be a promising vehicle for transdermal delivery of paeonol, which shows antiinflammatory, antidiabetic, and pain-relieving activities (Ma et al., 2018). Further, ethosomal hydrogel was able to significantly enhance the skin permeation parameters and skin deposition of encapsulated resveratrol in comparison to the conventional cream (Arora and Nanda, 2019).

Besides ethosomes and Transfersomes, there is an additional type of deformable vesicle i.e., transethosomes, which contain surfactants as well as ethanol. Transethosomes enhanced both *in vitro* and *in vivo* skin deposition of voriconazole in the dermis/epidermis region compared to conventional and deformable liposomes and control (Song et al., 2012). Ascenso et al. (2015) studied Transfersomes, ethosomes, and transethosomes for the incorporation of actives of different polarities, i.e., vitamin E and caffeine, in order to evaluate the effect of the carrier on skin permeation and penetration of actives. Transethosomes were shown to be more deformable than ethosomes and Transfersomes due to the presence of both ethanol and surfactant in their composition. However, all these vesicles, especially transethosomes, were shown to be suitable as skin delivery systems, being capable of delivering active molecules into different skin layers under certain conditions. Moreover, transethosomes have been shown to enhance the transdermal delivery of the antihypertensive drug olmesartan medoxomil (Albash et al., 2019). Transethosomes have also been shown to be a promising transdermal drug delivery system for sinomenine hydrochloride in the treatment of rheumatoid arthritis (Song et al., 2019).

Elastic liposomes showed higher efficiency in the transdermal delivery of gabapentin through porcine skin than the compounded pluronic lecithin organogel (Le et al., 2018).

A new interesting approach is the combination of flexible liposomes (FL) and sponge *Haliclona* sp. spicules (SHS), referred to as SFLS (SHS-Flexible Liposomes Combined System), for topical drug delivery, which has been shown to result in improved skin absorption and deposition of hyaluronic acid, especially in deep skin layers, due to the synergistic effect of liposomes and sponge spicules (Zhang et al., 2019).

Invasomes have been invented by the group of Prof. Alfred Fahr (Verma, 2002). These vesicles for enhanced skin delivery of drugs are composed of phosphatidylcholine, ethanol, and a mixture of terpenes as penetration enhancers, which increase the fluidity of the vesicles' bilayers. Invasomes provided *in vitro* a significantly higher amount of incorporated cyclosporine A and temoporfin in the deeper layers of human skin (viable epidermis and dermis) as compared to conventional liquid-state liposomes and aqueous/ethanolic drug solution (Dragicevic-Curic et al., 2008, 2009; Verma, 2002). Invasomes loaded with cyclosporine A induced a faster visible hair regrowth in alopecia areata in the Dundee Experimental Bald Rat (DEBR) model than conventional liposomes (Verma et al., 2004). Dapsone-loaded invasomes enhanced *in vivo* in Wistar rats skin delivery of dapsone, which is used to treat mild to moderate acne, showing about 2.5-fold higher deposited drug amount in the skin compared to the drug solution (El-Nabarawi et al., 2018). Invasomes and Transfersomes have been shown to efficiently deliver the skin lightening agent phenylethyl resorcinol into the deep skin layers in high amounts and provided anti-tyrosinase activity up to 80%, being better than conventional liposomes (Amnuaikit et al., 2018). Invasomes loaded with azelaic acid exhibited the best antiacne efficacy in rats, followed by liposomes and LeciPlex (Shah et al., 2015). Isotretinoin-loaded invasomal gel targeted and delivered the drug to the pilosebaceous follicular unit in the treatment of eosinophilic pustular folliculitis (Dwivedi et al., 2017). Further, they have been shown to be more effective in *in vitro* delivery of hydrophilic compounds (carboxyfluorescein and radiolabeled mannitol) into and through human skin compared to aqueous drug solutions (Badran et al., 2009). As to the transdermal delivery by invasomes, isradipine-loaded invasomes enhanced the transdermal flux of the antihypertensive drug isradipine and showed a substantial and constant decrease in blood pressure for up to 24 hours, indicating their potential to be used for the management of hypertension (Qadri et al., 2017). Invasomes provided a 1.15 times improved bioavailability of the antihypertensive olmesartan with respect to the control formulation in Wistar rats (Kamran et al., 2016).

Invasomes loaded with avanafil (used for the oral treatment of erectile dysfunction) and incorporated into the hydroxypropyl methyl cellulose–based transdermal film showed *ex vivo* in rats avanafil enhanced permeation with an enhancement factor of 2.5 and a more than fourfold increase in the relative bioavailability compared to the conventional avanafil film (Ahmed and Badr-Eldin, 2019).

38.2.3   MECHANISM OF ACTION OF LIPOSOMES

As to the penetration of intact liposomes, one of the first theories was that intact conventional liposomes could penetrate into and even through the SC under the influence of a transepidermal osmotic gradient, acting as drug carrier systems (Cevc and Blume, 1992). This theory has been rejected by authors, who did not find evidence of intact vesicle penetration into the deeper skin layers (Lasch et al., 1992; Van Kuijk-Meuwissen et al., 1998; Zellmer et al., 1995, 1998).

As to the deformable vesicles (Transfersomes), it has been reported that these vesicles, being ultra-deformable (up to 10^5 times that of unmodified liposomes), squeeze through pores in the SC, being less than one-tenth the vesicles' size, under the influence of transepidermal osmotic gradient, and go into deep subcutaneous tissue and even into systemic circulation (Cevc and Gebauer, 2003; Cevc et al., 1998, 2002, 2008;).

However, recently other authors who used conventional liposomes and more flexible liposomes containing the surfactant sodium cholate and the combination of super resolution optical microscopy and raster image correlation spectroscopy, suggested that liposomes do not act as carriers that transport their cargo directly through the skin barrier, but mainly burst and fuse with the outer lipid layers of the SC (Dreier et al., 2016). Further, these authors found that flexible liposomes delivered higher amounts of the fluorophore into the SC, indicating that they functioned as chemical penetration enhancers.

In contrast, another study with flexible/deformable liposomes showed that these intact liposomes were indeed observed in the epidermis layers and that a direct relationship between the depth of penetration and the liposome flexibility was found, supporting the hypothesis of the whole vesicle penetration mechanism (Franzé et al., 2017).

As to ethosomes, their inventors proposed a mechanism of skin permeation enhancement which is based on the dual effect of ethanol, i.e., it fluidizes lipid bilayers in the vesicles and the lipids in the SC, causing changes in the arrangement of lipids. As a consequence, ethosomes penetrate the altered SC barrier releasing the active ingredient in the deeper skin layers. They suggest that vesicles penetrate into deep skin layers (Ainbinder et al., 2016). Other authors who investigated ethosomes proposed also that ethosomes could penetrate the skin through open hair follicles and SC pathways, while during the process of penetration, the vesicles were broken and the phospholipids were retained in the upper epidermis, with the test compounds penetrating gradually (Yang et al., 2017). Further, other authors showed that ethosomes could penetrate the skin via the SC mainly through the intercellular route, while during the process of penetration, phospholipids were retained in the upper epidermis, and cell experiments confirmed that ethosomes were distributed mainly on the cell membrane (Niu et al., 2019).

In conclusion, the possibility that intact conventional liposomes penetrate the skin is generally rejected, while for deformable vesicles and their penetration as intact vesicles through the skin having a highly organized multilamellar structure, there are still doubts and their penetration is under investigation. For a comprehensive review on liposomes and other vesicles, their mechanism of action, and penetration ability, the reader should refer to the Dragicevic and Maibach (2016).

38.2.4   COMBINED USE OF DIFFERENT LIPOSOMES AND MICRONEEDLES

In order to further enhance the drug penetration/permeation through the skin, liposomes are often used in combination with microneedles (MNs).

MNs are micron-sized needles with a height of 10 to 2000 μm and a width of 10 to 50 μm, which can penetrate through the epidermis layer to the dermal tissue directly without pain

(Hao et al., 2017). MNs have been used frequently, as they facilitate intra/transdermal delivery of drugs in a minimally invasive fashion (Arya et al., 2017; Baek et al., 2017; Dul et al., 2017; Jamaledin et al., 2020; Ripolin et al., 2017; Singh et al., 2019; Ye et al., 2018). Recently, they have been started to be extensively investigated for their use in dermatology (Sabri et al., 2019).

In brief, the mechanism of action of MNs is based on creating transient microconduits, which penetrate through the SC, extend into the viable epidermis, and hence facilitate drug permeation, as well as the penetration of drug carriers. It represents a powerful enhancement method when used alone, e.g., for intradermal vaccination and gene delivery (Dul et al., 2017; Sabri et al., 2020; Sala et al., 2018), intradermal delivery of cosmetic actives (Puri et al., 2016), transdermal delivery of insulin and other drugs (Kearney et al., 2016; Sabri et al., 2020), and combined with other physical methods, such as with iontophoresis (Ronnander et al., 2019), electroporation (Fang et al., 2001), and with sonophoresis (Chen et al., 2009a). Also the combination between ultrasonic waves and iontophoresis for improving the efficiency of MNs has been reported (Bok et al., 2020).

As to the safety of MNs, it has been shown recently in an *in vivo* study that insertions on multiple occasions of dissolving polymeric MN patches induced no significant changes to skin appearance or skin barrier function, regardless of the MN formulation applied, needle density, or number of insertions, as well as that serum biomarkers of irritation/inflammation, infection, and immunity were not significantly disturbed by the end of the study periods. These findings were encouraging, suggesting that their repeated use by patients will not cause undesirable side effects (Vicente-Perez et al., 2017).

Badran et al. (2009) have shown that invasomes containing 1% w/v of the terpene mixture (cineole:citral:d-limonene = 0.45:0.45:0.10 v/v) and 3.3% w/v ethanol were more effective in delivering hydrophilic radiolabeled mannitol into and through human skin *in vitro* compared to the aqueous drug solutions. The amount of radiolabeled mannitol in the SC and in the stripped skin was 3.8- and 5.7-fold higher for invasomes compared to the buffer solution. The authors additionally applied the Dermaroller in order to induce skin perforation and, hence, further enhancement of drug penetration and permeation into/through the skin. The Dermaroller with 150-μm-long needles used together with invasomes provided the highest drug amount in the SC (1.4-fold higher) and an increased drug amount in the stripped skin (3.1-fold higher) as well as in the receptor fluid (13.6-fold higher) compared to invasomes applied alone. Increasing the needle length to 500 and 1500 μm led to an increase of mannitol deposition into deeper skin layers and the receptor fluid, while mannitol amounts in the SC were reduced, i.e., the amounts of mannitol were 8.7- and 6.5-fold higher in the stripped skin (deeper skin) and 30.3- and 49.2-fold higher in the receptor fluid (for 500 and 1500 μm needle lengths, respectively) compared to the application of invasomes. According to the authors, the Dermaroller with a needle length of 500 μm appeared most promising for the delivery of hydrophilic compounds into deeper skin layers or through the skin (Badran et al., 2009).

Ding et al. (2011) investigated the combined use of two diphtheria toxoid–loaded vesicle formulations, i.e., cationic SPC liposomes (composed of soybean-phosphatidylcholine, Span80 and DOTAP) and anionic surfactant–based L595 vesicles/niosomes (composed of sucrose-laurate ester, octaoxyethylene-laurate ester, and sodium bistridecyl sulfo succinate as a stabilizer) and MN to induce transcutaneous immunization in mice. Substantial antibody titers were achieved only if MN pretreatment was applied. The co-administration of cholera toxin further augmented the immune responses of transcutaneous immunization. However, the authors reported that vesicle formulations did not enhance the immunogenicity of diphtheria toxoid, regardless if intact or MN-treated skin was used. They induced low stimulation of dendritic cells as well. The authors found that antigen association to vesicles (regardless if rigid or elastic, anionic or cationic) does not enhance the immunogenicity of topically applied diphtheria toxoid, but only MN pretreatment and cholera toxin do (Ding et al., 2011).

Hirschberg et al. (2012) investigated transcutaneous immunization of HBsAg *in vitro* and *in vivo* in mice using two vesicle formulations: cationic SPC liposomes (composed of soybean-phosphatidylcholine, Span 80 and DOTAP) and anionic surfactant–based L595 vesicles/niosomes with HBsAg associated with the vesicles. Both vesicle formulations induced an antibody response in mice, but only when the skin was pretreated with MNs. Co-administration of cholera toxin further augmented the immune responses. The highest transcutaneous immunization was achieved by the use of SPC-HBsAg vesicles, being superior to L595-HBsAg vesicles due to the higher degree of HBsAg association, adjuvanted with cholera toxin, on MN-pretreated skin. This transcutaneous immunization achieved in mice was comparable to immunization by conventional intramuscular (i.m.) vaccination.

DeMuth et al. (2012) coated poly(lactide-co-glycolide) MN arrays with multilayer films via layer-by-layer (LbL) assembly of a biodegradable cationic poly(β-amino ester) (PBAE) and negatively charged interbilayer-cross-linked multilamellar lipid vesicles (ICMVs) as a potential device for vaccine delivery. This approach enhances the stability of lipid vesicles, as covalent crosslinks are introduced between adjacent phospholipid bilayers in the walls of multilamellar vesicles to create a robust lipid nanocapsule. Without such stabilizing measures, LbL deposition would result in spontaneous vesicle disruption into lipid bilayers on the target substrate. Obtained ICMVs were loaded with a protein antigen and the molecular adjuvant monophosphoryl lipid A. The study revealed that MNs with ICMV-carrying multilayers promoted in mice robust antigen-specific humoral immune responses, while bolus delivery of soluble or vesicle-loaded antigen via intradermal injection or transcutaneous vaccination with MNs encapsulating soluble protein elicited a weak humoral immune response, indicating the potential of nanocarriers delivered by MNs as a promising approach for noninvasive vaccine delivery applications (DeMuth et al., 2012).

Guo et al. (2013) used dissolving microneedle arrays (DMAs) for achieving transcutaneous immunization polyvinylpyrrolidone (PVP), where the tips were loaded with an antigen and adjuvant encapsulated in cationic phospholipid liposomes. Ovalbumin (OVA) was used as a model antigen, CpG oligodeoxynucleotide (CpG OND) as an adjuvant, and cationic liposomes to deliver the antigen and adjuvant. It was shown that mice were indeed transcutaneously immunized with DMAs containing OVA, OVA-CpG OND, OVA encapsulated in liposomes, OVA-CpG OND encapsulated in liposomes, and conventional i.m. injection with OVA solution. The anti-OVA IgG antibody level was highest in the group immunized with the DMAs containing OVA-CpG OND encapsulated in liposomes. Thus, the described device could effectively deliver the liposomes encapsulating CpG OND-OVA into the skin, enhancing the immune response and changing the immune type.

Chen et al. (2015) investigated in a rat model of rheumatoid arthritis a triptolide-loaded trans-dermal delivery system, termed the triptolide-loaded liposome hydrogel patch (TP-LHP), applying it together with a microneedle array. The pharmacokinetic results showed that MNs together with TP-LHP yielded plasma drug levels which fit a one-compartment open model. Further, TP-LHP treatment mitigated the degree of joint swelling and suppressed the expressions of fetal liver kinase-1, fetal liver tyrosine kinase-4, and hypoxia-inducible factor-1α in synovium. Hyperfunction of the immune system was also observed. The authors proposed that the therapeutic mechanism of TP-LHP might rely on the regulation of the balance between Th1 and Th2, as well as inhibition of the expression and biological effects of vascular endothelial growth factor (Chen et al., 2015).

Qiu et al. (2016) developed dissolving microneedle arrays (DMAs) loaded with cationic phospholipid liposomes encapsulating hepatitis B DNA vaccine and adjuvant CpG ODN and applied them *in vivo* in mice to investigate their capability to induce an immune response after DNA delivery. The results showed that pGFP could be delivered into skin by DMAs and expressed in skin, and the amount of expressed GFP was likely to peak at day 4. DMAs-based DNA vaccination could induce an effective immune response, while CpG ODN significantly improved the immune response and achieved the shift of immune type from predominate Th2 type to a balance Th1/Th2 type, while cationic liposomes further improved the immunogenicity of the DNA vaccine. In conclusion, the authors showed that this novel system based on microneedles and liposomes can effectively deliver hepatitis B DNA vaccine into skin, inducing an effective immune response and changing the immune type by adjuvant CpG ODN.

Zhao et al. (2017) combined the model subunit vaccine ovalbumin (OVA) with platycodin (PD), a saponin adjuvant, in order to enhance its immunogenicity and loaded them together into liposomes. Afterwards liposomes were incorporated into a dissolving microneedle array. The authors showed in mice that the uptake of OVA by dendritic cells was greatly enhanced when OVA was applied in the aforementioned liposomes. Further, it was shown that mice treated with OVA-PD–loaded liposomes incorporated in MNs showed a significantly enhanced immune response. Liposomes with PD and OVA elicited a balanced Th1 and Th2 humoral immune response in mice and caused minimal irritation in rabbit skin (Zhao et al., 2017).

Van der Maaden et al. (2018) developed a digitally DMAs-based system for transcutaneous immunization that can effectively deliver hepatitis B DNA vaccine in a controlled hollow MN injection system (DC-hMN-iSystem) with an ultra-low dead volume to perform microinjections into skin in an automated manner. They used this system for the application of a synthetic long peptide $E7_{43\text{-}63}$ derived from human papillomavirus (HPV E743–63 SLP) formulated in cationic liposomes onto the skin. Intradermal administration of the therapeutic cancer vaccine by these MNs induced strong functional cytotoxic and T-helper responses in mice and required much lower volumes as compared to classical intradermal immunization. The authors demonstrated that the DC-hMN-iSystem allowed very low vaccine volumes to be precisely injected into the skin in an automated manner, showing potential for minimally invasive and potentially pain-free therapeutic cancer vaccination (van der Maaden et al., 2018).

Du et al. (2018) studied the immunogenicity of different cationic liposomes loaded with diphtheria toxoid and poly(I:C) (i.e., DT-loaded liposomes, a mixture of free DT and poly[I:C]-loaded liposomes, a mixture of DT-loaded liposomes and free poly[I:C], and liposomes with DT and poly[I:C] either individually or co-encapsulated in the liposomes) after hollow microneedle-mediated intradermal vaccination in mice. All liposomes induced similar total IgG and IgG1 titers. All liposomes containing both DT and poly(I:C) showed similar enhanced IgG2a titers compared to DT/poly(I:C) solution. The authors concluded that a mixture of diphtheria toxoid–loaded liposomes and poly(I:C)-loaded liposomes has a similar effect on the antibody responses as DT and poly(I:C) co-encapsulated liposomes, being an important finding for the formulation of liposomal vaccine delivery systems (Du et al., 2018).

Transfersomes were loaded with eprosartan mesylate, incorporated into the Carbopol gel, and applied to rat skin pretreated with microneedles (Dermaroller) (Ahad et al., 2017). A pharmacodynamic study in rats with experimentally induced hypertension showed prolonged and better management of hypertension after the application of transfersomal gel compared to oral control formulation. The authors showed that the *in vivo* angiotensin II type-1 blocking efficacy of the investigated transfersomal gel and control formulation was also supported with RT-PCR and Western blot analysis of AT_1R mRNA and protein expressions on smooth vascular muscles of aorta (Ahad et al., 2017). Regarding skin irritation, the transfersomal gel has been shown to be safe. The authors concluded that Transfersomes together with MNs appeared to be a suitable transdermal drug delivery system for eprosartan mesylate in the management of hypertension in Wistar rats (Ahad et al., 2017).

Yang et al. (2019) developed dissolving MNs made from hyaluronic acid, which they integrated with doxorubicin-loaded Transfersomes. This Transfersomes/microneedles complex was expected to enhance lymphatic delivery of doxorubicin. It has been shown that indeed MNs were able, due to efficient insertion into rat skin and their dissolution, to release doxorubicin-loaded Transfersomes in the dermis. This approach provided a significantly enhanced accumulation of doxorubicin in lymph nodes compared to drug diffusion through the skin and increased its bioavailability in plasma, being promising for chemotherapy of tumors through lymphatic drug delivery, as it kills metastasized tumor cells present in lymph nodes (Yang et al., 2019). Thus, according to obtained results, this Transfersomes/microneedles complex could be used as a transdermal drug delivery system for tumor therapy.

Wu et al. (2019) used a similar approach, i.e., they integrated dissolving MNs with antigen-loaded Transfersomes. They used Transfersomes with opposite surface charges for antigen encapsulation and investigated the effect of surface charge on immune responses via transdermal immunization. As mentioned, MNs dissolved in mouse skin during insertion and released Transfersomes into the dermis. Cationic Transfersomes significantly increased the IgG2a/IgG1 ratio and enhanced cytokine secretion from Th1 cells, while not enhancing the Th2 response and, thus, they more efficiently activated maturation of dendritic cells and induced Th1 immunity, compared to anionic

Transfersomes. This enhanced Th1 antigen-specific immune response in lymph nodes is promising for potential immunotherapy (Wu et al., 2019).

Ethosomes were also used in combination with MNs. Raloxifene hydrochloride, a selective estrogen receptor modulator, was encapsulated into ethosomes, which were incorporated into a hydrogel. This hydrogel was applied together with MNs in order to achieve transdermal delivery of raloxifene hydrochloride. The *ex vivo* skin permeation study revealed a transdermal flux of 4.621 $\mu g/cm^2/h$ through the intact pig ear skin, which was further enhanced through the microporated skin (transdermal flux, 6.194 $\mu g/cm^2/h$) with a 3.87-fold rise when compared to drug permeation from plain solution applied over intact skin (transdermal flux, 1.6 $\mu g/cm^2/h$) (Thakkar et al., 2016).

Paeoniflorin-loaded ethosomes were developed and applied together with MNs (Cui et al., 2018). The optimal MN-assisted conditions were obtained at a microneedle length of 500 μm, a pressure of 3 N, and an action time of 3 minutes. The cumulative penetrated amounts of paeoniflorin from solution and MN-assisted solution were 24.42 ± 8.35 $\mu g/cm^2$ and 548.11 ± 10.49 $\mu g/cm^2$, respectively, indicating that MNs significantly enhanced the drug permeation. The encapsulation of the drug into ethosomes enhanced the cumulative penetrated drug amount, as it was 54.97 ± 4.72 $\mu g/cm^2$, while the additional use of MNs enhanced it further to the amount of 307.17 ± 26.36 $\mu g/cm^2$. Thus, results indicated that the use of ethosomes and MNs both enhanced the penetration of the water-soluble drug paeoniflorin, but there was no synergism in skin penetration enhancement between the nanocarrier/ethosomes and MNs (Cui et al., 2018).

In another comprehensive study, in order to find an efficient delivery system able to transport macromolecules such as genes into the skin, in *in vitro* and *ex vivo* experiments, the influence of various vesicle parameters (surface charge—using cationic [DOTAP], anionic [DOPG], or neutral [DOPC] lipid deformability—addition of ethanol and/or edge activators, such as sodium cholate, Tween 80, and Span 80 to enhance the vesicle deformability) on the vesicle penetration were studied, as well as the influence of physical enhancement methods, such as the tape stripping of the SC and MNs (Bellefroid et al., 2019). The authors showed that all formulations were not able to cross the SC (including deformable formulations) when the SC was intact. Regarding the tape-stripped skin, the addition of ethanol significantly enhanced vesicle penetration into the skin compared to liposomes without ethanol. Furthermore, it was obvious that edge activators favor a deeper penetration compared to formulations without them. The kind of edge activator was also important. Whereas liposomes containing Tween 80 remained in the first cell layers of viable epidermis, liposomes containing sodium cholate were able to penetrate more profoundly. Liposomes containing ethanol and sodium cholate allowed the deepest penetration, since fluorescence was localized across the viable epidermis until the upper dermis was reached. As to the surface charge, cationic nanocarrier penetration increased when ethanol was added to the formulation. Cationic vesicles containing edge activators (sodium cholate) and ethanol improved further the skin penetration of vesicles. As to the use of MNs together with liposomes, it has been shown that sodium cholate and ethanol were necessary to ensure an appropriate diffusion of liposomes into the dermis. The authors concluded that combined use of these liposomes and MNs could be a promising approach to efficiently deliver macromolecules into the skin (Bellefroid et al., 2019).

38.2.5 Combined use of Liposomes and Iontophoresis

Iontophoresis represents an electrical physical penetration enhancement method. It is noninvasive and involves the application of a small electric current to drive ionic and polar drugs such as peptides across the skin, which usually exhibit poor skin permeation. Hydrophilic molecules with good aqueous solubility and little affinity for lipids are excellent candidates for this method. The drug transport is determined by the duration, intensity, and profile of the applied current and on the area of current application. Thus, modulation of the current profile provides a simple and convenient method to control drug delivery kinetics (Gratieri and Kalia, 2017a, b). In brief, an iontophoretic device consists of a power source and two electrodes, i.e., the "active" electrode is placed in the compartment containing the drug formulation, and the circuit is completed by the "return" electrode placed at an adjacent area on the skin. Due to the electric field, ordered movement of ions to and from the active and return electrode compartments occurs and is called electromigration, being the principal electrotransport mechanism (Gratieri and Kalia, 2017a). Transdermal drug transport enhancement by iontophoresis is promoted by three main mechanisms: electrorepulsion of charged solutes by the electrode; electro-osmotic effects on unionized, polar species; and permeabilization of the skin by the electric current (Gratieri and Kalia, 2017b; Guy et al., 2000). Iontophoresis has been used for topical and transdermal drug delivery and for noninvasive skin sampling applications (Kalia et al., 2004; Merino et al., 2017). The most widespread therapeutic applications of iontophoresis are the treatment of palmoplantar hyperhidrosis and the diagnosis of cystic fibrosis. Other popular applications of iontophoresis are the delivery of lidocaine, acyclovir, and dexamethasone phosphate (Merino et al., 2017). For more detail on iontophoresis, the reader should refer to Gratieri and Kalia (2017a,b) and Merino et al. (2017). Iontophoresis has also been used in combination with nanocarriers as described in the following studies.

Essa et al. (2004) investigated *in vitro* in human epidermal membranes the influence of cathodic iontophoresis on the skin delivery of estradiol from different liposomes, sodium cholate (as an edge activator) containing ultra-deformable (Transfersomes), nonrigid conventional (pure phosphatidylcholine), and membrane-stabilized conventional (cholesterol-containing) liposomes. First, they found during passive delivery that traditional liposomes increased estradiol penetration, indicated by the fourfold and threefold enhancement in flux from nonrigid and membrane-stabilized liposomes, respectively, relative to control (aqueous solution) ($P < 0.05$), while the ultra-deformable vesicles induced a sixfold enhancement in flux compared to the control ($P < 0.05$). The drug deposited in the skin at the end of the permeation time was similarly improved. Iontophoresis improved drug penetration by about 4- and 3.5-fold for nonrigid and membrane-stabilized liposomes, respectively, and skin deposition was similarly improved. With ultra-deformable liposomes and iontophoresis, estradiol penetration was markedly improved, indicated by a fourteenfold enhancement in flux (1.23 ± 0.131 μg/cm^2/h, $P < 0.05$) and a twenty-twofold enhancement in skin deposition (19 ± 2.7 μg/cm^2), relative to control. Iontophoresis improved drug penetration over passive delivery for all systems, and ultra-deformable liposomes were the most efficient. A combination of electroporation and iontophoresis did not markedly improve estradiol penetration from ultra-deformable liposomes compared to the application of only iontophoresis.

Boinpally et al. (2004) succeeded in delivering the peptide drug cyclosporin A (CsA) with low skin penetration ability across human cadaver epidermis *in vitro* using negatively charged colloidal systems (microemulsion and lecithin liposomes) and anodal iontophoresis in contrast to passive diffusion. Liposomes were superior compared to the microemulsion (anodal iontophoresis was used), as they provided a mean cumulative CsA amount permeated across cadaver epidermis of approximately 230 μg after 22.5 hours compared to less than 50 μg provided by the microemulsion, and they appeared to have a potential in site-specific immunosuppression. In addition, the CsA flux from lecithin liposomes due to anodal iontophoresis was significantly higher than that from microemulsion. Further, according to the authors, electro-osmosis and compromised epidermis might have contributed to the higher skin flux of CsA. This finding, which demonstrates the ability of liposomes combined with anodal iontophoresis to deliver CsA across the skin, was very promising as a clinical potential of site-specific immunosuppression with topical CsA.

The dermal/transdermal delivery of high-molecular-weight drugs (such as insulin) is challenging. These drugs could be incorporated into liposomes, but in order to provide efficient transdermal drug delivery, another additional enhancement method is required, such as a physical enhancement method. Iontophoresis is a promising technique for enhancing transdermal administration of charged drugs, but it is not sufficient for an effective delivery of large, hydrophilic, or electrically neutral molecules. Hence, neutral drug molecules can be encapsulated into charged liposomes as carriers that can be applied with iontophoresis (Kajimoto et al., 2011). The application of iontophoresis and liposomes (1,2-dioleoyl-3-[trimethylammonium] propane [DOTAP]/egg phosphatidylcholine [EPC]/ Cholesterol [Chol] = 2:2:1) encapsulating insulin onto diabetic rat skin resulted in a gradual decrease in blood glucose levels, with levels reaching 20% of initial values at 18 hours after administration and the levels were maintained for up to 24 hours. Hence, the authors developed an efficient, noninvasive, and persistent transfollicular (as the transfollicular route was the main penetration route for liposomes) delivery system for insulin that used a combination of liposomes and iontophoresis.

In addition to dual penetration enhancement strategies, triple enhancement strategies can be used, i.e., nanocarriers can be used with two physical enhancement methods, and this approach was used to enhance the transdermal delivery of insulin. Chen et al. (2009b) showed *in vitro* in guinea pig skin that positively charged unilamellar insulin-loaded liposomes driven by iontophoresis through MNs-treated skin provided permeation rates of insulin 713.3 times higher than that during its passive diffusion. The positive surface charge and small diameters of liposomes were advantageous to the penetration of the insulin-loaded liposomes when combined with iontophoresis and MNs. *In vivo* studies in diabetic rats showed that the blood glucose levels in rats topically treated with insulin, as mentioned, were 33.3% and 28.3% of the initial levels at four and six hours after the application of insulin, which is comparable to those induced by subcutaneous injection of insulin. These results were encouraging, as they introduced a new, very efficient strategy for noninvasive delivery of peptides of large molecular weight using liposomes, which have been to date efficiently used mostly for intradermal delivery of drugs with low molecular weight.

By using the combination of DOTAP–EPC–Chol (2: 2: 1 molar ratio) cationic liposomes and iontophoresis, superoxide dismutase (SOD), representing a potent antioxidant agent protecting against UV-induced skin damage, can be delivered into the skin, besides its high molecular weight which normally prevents its efficient delivery into the skin (Kigasawa et al., 2012). Iontophoretic delivery of liposomes encapsulating SOD caused in rats *in vivo* a marked decrease in the production of oxidative products, such as malondialdehyde, hexanoyl lysine, and 8-hydroxi-2-deoxyguanosine, in UV-irradiated skin. Hence, SOD encapsulated in cationic liposomes and subjected to anodal iontophoresis represents an efficient intradermal SOD delivery approach, which could also be useful for delivering other macromolecules.

Mohammed et al. (2016) have investigated the transdermal delivery of vancomycin hydrochloride using the combination of ethosomes and iontophoresis *in vitro* and *in vivo*. They used cathodal iontophoresis for negatively charged ethosomes and anodal iontophoresis for the free drug solution and positively charged vesicles. The maximal transdermal flux was obtained with cathodal iontophoresis of negatively charged ethosomes (550 μg/cm^2/h) compared to the free drug solution and other ethosomes. The parameters of iontophoresis were varied, and the transdermal flux was reduced by altering the current mode from continuous to ON/OFF mode, reducing current density and by using normal saline as drug solvent, while the flux was increased by increasing the drug concentration. The performed *in vivo* study in rats revealed that there was no significant difference between the i.m. application of vancomycin and the iontophoretic delivery of vancomycin-loaded ethosomes, indicating a successful transdermal delivery of vancomycin by ethosomes and iontophoresis.

Bernardi et al. (2016) investigated the potential of employing iontophoresis for transcutaneous immunization using a formulation composed of OVA-loaded liposomes and silver nanoparticles (AgNPs). The *in vitro* cathodal iontophoresis of the OVA-liposomes associated with AgNPs increased OVA penetration into the viable epidermis by ninety-two-fold in comparison to passive delivery. *In vivo*, transcutaneous immunization with a suitable combination of liposomes and iontophoresis induced the production of antibodies, differentiation of immune-competent cells, and appeared to present an alternative strategy for needle-free vaccination.

Jose et al. (2017) investigated the liposomal delivery of curcumin and STAT3 siRNA when combined with iontophoresis in order to treat skin cancer. Curcumin was encapsulated in cationic liposomes and then complexed with STAT3 siRNA. Results showed that the co-delivery of curcumin and STAT3 siRNA using liposomes resulted in significantly greater ($P < 0.05$) cancer cell growth inhibition and apoptosis compared with neat curcumin and free STAT3 siRNA treatment. Penetration data obtained in excised porcine skin showed that iontophoresis enhanced skin penetration of the nanocomplex penetrating the viable epidermis (Jose et al., 2017). Hence, the authors concluded that cationic liposomes can be used with iontophoresis to deliver curcumin and siRNA to the skin to treat skin cancer.

A recent study *in vivo* in ovariectomized rats revealed that propranolol encapsulated at low doses in liposomes applied together with iontophoresis onto the skin enhanced the bone microarchitecture volumes and hence exhibited optimal effects against bone loss to a higher extent compared to propranolol used at higher doses in liposomes and applied by s.c. injection (Teong et al., 2017). Namely, liposomes with propranolol at low doses (0.05 mg/kg) elevated via iontophoresis over twofold the ratio between bone volume and total tissue volume (BV/TV) in proximal tibia to 9.0%, whereas treatment with liposomes containing propranolol at low and high (0.5 mg/kg) doses via s.c. injection resulted in smaller increases in BV/TV. The authors also reported a significant improvement of BV/TV and bone mineral density (BMD) in the fourth lumbar spine when low-dose liposomal propranolol was iontophoretically administered. In addition, iontophoretic low-dose liposomal propranolol also elevated trabecular numbers in tibia and trabecular thickness in spine (Teong et al., 2017).

38.2.5.1   Combined Use of Liposomes and Ultrasound

Liposomes may be used together with ultrasound. Percutaneous penetration enhancement induced by ultrasound is termed sonophoresis, indicating that the enhanced transport of molecules is under the influence of ultrasound. Various frequencies of ultrasound (in the range of 20 kHz to 16 MHz) have been used to enhance skin permeability. However, transdermal drug delivery induced by low-frequency ultrasound (f <100 kHz) has been found to be more efficient than that induced by high-frequency ultrasound. This method has been used to enhance transdermal transport of various drugs, including macromolecules (Mitragotri, 2017). For more information on ultrasound, the reader should refer to Escobar-Chávez et al. (2009), Lee et al. (2017), and Mitragotri (2017).

Elastic liposomes containing hydrogenated phosphatidylcholine and cholesterol as well as Tween 80 were used together with low-frequency ultrasound in order to enhance the transepidermal delivery of the hydrophilic and high-molecular-weight hyaluronic acid (Kasetvatin et al., 2015). The *in vitro* permeation studies demonstrated that hyaluronic acid in solution cannot permeate through the porcine epidermis. However, when elastic liposomes were applied with ultrasound, the skin permeation of hyaluronic acid was higher than those obtained with passive delivery of elastic liposomes and ultrasound-mediated delivery from the hyaluronic solution, 2.1 times and 6.4 times, respectively. In addition, no skin damage was observed at the optimized one-minute exposure time. Thus, the study demonstrated *in vitro* that the combination of elastic liposomes and ultrasound provided an efficacious transcutaneous delivery of hyaluronic acid.

Limonene-containing PEGylated liposomes (PL) and low-frequency sonophoresis were used to achieve transdermal delivery of galantamine HBr (GLT). It was shown that sonophoresis might improve drug permeation through the intracellular pathway, while limonene-containing liposomes play an important role in delivering GLT through an intercellular pathway by increasing the fluidity of intercellular lipids in the SC (Rangsimawong et al., 2018). As the authors showed that liposomes with the highest limonene content (2%) were superior to other liposomes, they concluded that small vesicle size and high membrane fluidity due to high limonene content might enhance the transportation of intact vesicles through the skin.

38.2.5.2   Combined Use of Liposomes and Electroporation

Electroporation is a physical technique that involves the application of very short duration (microsecond to millisecond) high-voltage electric pulses to reversibly enhance cell or tissue permeability for bioactive molecules such as drugs, dyes, vitamins, peptides, proteins, DNA, RNA, etc. (Medi et al., 2017). In comparison to other percutaneous penetration enhancement methods, it may not show significant difference in the penetration enhancement of small ions/molecules; however, compared to them it induces significantly higher fluxes of macromolecules. The major advantage of this technique is that the macromolecules, such as peptide and gene-based drugs, could be used for transdermal delivery, while for more detail on electroporation, the reader should refer to Angamuthu and Murthy (2017) and Medi et al. (2017).

Essa et al. (2003) investigated the influence of electroporation on the skin delivery of estradiol from ultra-deformable liposomes containing sodium cholate as an edge activator. They found that skin pulsing significantly increased estradiol penetration and skin deposition from the control solution, relative to passive delivery, while with liposomes, electroporation did not markedly affect estradiol skin penetration. It was also shown that liposomal phosphatidylcholine applied during or after pulsing accelerated skin barrier repair, i.e. provided an anti-enhancer or retardant effect.

Ethosomes and liposomes were combined with electroporation and sonoporation to enhance transdermal delivery of the hydrophilic model molecule calcein. Ethosomes significantly enhanced calcein permeation by passive diffusion compared to liposomes, which seem to remain confined to the outer layers of the skin, being better suited for topical dermal delivery than transdermal delivery. Sonication (five minutes) showed improvement over passive diffusion, but only for the ethosomes. Almost the same trend was seen for electroporation, which significantly enhanced the delivery of calcein, being more pronounced for ethosomes than liposomes and calcein in buffer. Ethosomes were also used with both electroporation and sonoporation. This combination did not achieve synergistic effects or additive effects. However, the combination of ethosomes with either electroporation or sonoporation achieved significant enhancement of the transdermal molecular delivery of calcein, being safe for its potential clinical use (Zorec et al., 2018).

38.3 CONCLUSION

Liposomes have been successfully applied for dermal and transdermal drug delivery, depending on their composition. Conventional phospholipid-based liposomes are only used for dermal drug delivery, i.e., in dermatology to treat cutaneous disorders or the cutaneous manifestations of general diseases. In contrast, deformable phospholipid-based vesicles can be used for both for dermal and transdermal drug delivery. However, when applied alone, even deformable vesicles are mostly used to provide drugs in the deeper skin layers. If the goal is to achieve systemic absorption of drugs i.e., transdermal drug delivery, the most promising results are obtained when vesicles are applied together with physical penetration-enhancing methods (microneedles, iontophoresis, ultrasound, and electroporation). This combination of enhancement methods has been shown to offer superiority to their single use. Due to their synergistic effect, these methods could possibly enable the use of drugs at a lower dose, reducing unwanted side effects.

In conclusion, deformable vesicles combined with physical enhancement methods enable even transdermal drug delivery, i.e., obtaining systemic drug effects by noninvasive drug administration, thus exhibiting numerous advantages compared to conventional drug administration, such as the avoidance of the first-pass metabolism, controlling the rate of drug input over a prolonged time, and ensuring constant plasma levels even for drugs with short half-times, better patient compliance, etc. Therefore, one of the most promising applications of vesicles and physical methods is their combined use for transcutaneous immunization (needle-free vaccination), which would circumvent drawbacks of the use of conventional syringes and needles (fear, pain, while in developing countries they may cause the spread of diseases due to the reuse of the needles). In addition, this strategy is important for the penetration enhancement of high-molecular-weight peptide/protein drugs, such as insulin, CsA, etc.

REFERENCES

Abd El-Alim, S. H. et al. (2019) 'Comparative study of liposomes, ethosomes and transfersomes as carriers for enhancing the transdermal delivery of diflunisal: *In vitro* and *in vivo* evaluation', International Journal of Pharmaceutics. 563, pp. 293–303.

Abdulbaqi, I. M. et al. (2016) 'Ethosomal nanocarriers: The impact of constituents and formulation techniques on ethosomal properties, *in vivo* studies, and clinical trials', International Journal of Nanomedicine. 11, pp. 2279–2304.

Ahad, A. et al. (2017) 'Pharmacodynamic study of eprosartan mesylate-loaded transfersomes Carbopol(®) gel under Dermaroller(®) on rats with methyl prednisolone acetate-induced hypertension.', Biomedicine & Pharmacotherapy = Biomedecine & Pharmacotherapie. 89, pp. 177–184.

Ahmed, K. S. et al. (2019) 'Derma roller® microneedles-mediated transdermal delivery of doxorubicin and celecoxib co-loaded liposomes for enhancing the anticancer effect', Materials Science and Engineering C. 99, pp. 1448–1458.

Ahmed, O. A. A. and Badr-Eldin, S. M. (2019) 'Development of an optimized avanafil-loaded invasomal transdermal film: *Ex vivo* skin permeation and *in vivo* evaluation', International Journal of Pharmaceutics. 570, p. 118657.

Ahmed, T. A. (2015) 'Preparation of transfersomes encapsulating sildenafil aimed for transdermal drug delivery: Plackett-Burman design and characterization', Journal of Liposome Research. 25(1), pp. 1–10.

Ainbinder, D. et al. (2010) 'Drug delivery applications with ethosomes', Journal of Biomedical Nanotechnology, 6, pp. 558–568.

Ainbinder, D., Godin, B. and Touitou, E. (2016) 'Ethosomes: Enhanced delivery of drugs to and across the skin', in: Dragicevic, N., Maibach, H.I. (eds.), Percutaneous penetration enhancers - Chemical methods in penetration enhancement: Nanocarriers, Springer Berlin Heidelberg New York, Dordrecht London, 77–92. ISBN 978-3-662-47861-5.

Ainbinder, D. and Touitou, E. (2005) 'Testosterone ethosomes for enhanced transdermal delivery', Drug Delivery: Journal of Delivery and Targeting of Therapeutic Agents, 12(5), pp. 297–303.

Albash, R. et al. (2019) 'Use of transethosomes for enhancing the transdermal delivery of olmesartan medoxomil: *In vitro*, *ex vivo*, and *in vivo* evaluation', International Journal of Nanomedicine. 14, pp. 1953–1968.

Alhakamy, N. A., Fahmy, U. A. and Ahmed, O. A. A. (2019) 'Vitamin E TPGS based transferosomes augmented TAT as a promising delivery system for improved transdermal delivery of raloxifene', PLoS ONE. 14(12):e0226639. doi: 10.1371/journal.pone.0226639.

Ali, M. F. M. et al. (2015) 'Preparation and clinical evaluation of nano-transferosomes for treatment of erectile dysfunction', Drug Design, Development and Therapy. 9, pp. 2431–2447.

Amnuaikit, T. et al. (2018) 'Vesicular carriers containing phenylethyl resorcinol for topical delivery system; liposomes, transfersomes and invasomes', Asian Journal of Pharmaceutical Sciences. 13(5), pp. 472–484.

Angamuthu, M. and Murthy, S. N. (2017) 'Therapeutic applications of electroporation', in: Dragicevic, N., Maibach, H.I. (eds.), Percutaneous penetration enhancers - Physical methods in penetration enhancement, Springer Berlin Heidelberg New York, Dordrecht London. ISBN 978-3-662-53271-3.

Arora, D. and Nanda, S. (2019) 'Quality by design driven development of resveratrol loaded ethosomal hydrogel for improved dermatological benefits via enhanced skin permeation and retention', International Journal of Pharmaceutics. 567:118448.

Arya, J. *et al.* (2017) 'Tolerability, usability and acceptability of dissolving microneedle patch administration in human subjects', Biomaterials. 128, pp. 1–7.

Ascenso, A. et al. (2015) 'Development, characterization, and skin delivery studies of related ultradeformable vesicles: transfersomes, ethosomes, and transethosomes.', International Journal of Nanomedicine. 10, pp. 5837–51.

Avadhani, K. S. et al. (2017) 'Skin delivery of epigallocatechin-3-gallate (EGCG) and hyaluronic acid loaded nano-transfersomes for antioxidant and anti-aging effects in UV radiation induced skin damage', Drug Delivery. 24(1), pp. 61–74.

Azagury, A. et al. (2015) 'The synergistic effect of ultrasound and chemical penetration enhancers on chorioamnion mass transport', Journal of Controlled Release. 200, pp. 35–41.

Azimi, M. et al. (2019) 'Impact of the Transfersome Delivered Human Growth Hormone on the Dermal Fibroblast Cells', Current Pharmaceutical Biotechnology. 20(14), pp. 1194–1202.

Badran, M. M., Kuntsche, J. and Fahr, A. (2009) 'Skin penetration enhancement by a microneedle device (Dermaroller®) *in vitro*: Dependency on needle size and applied formulation', European Journal of Pharmaceutical Sciences, 36(4–5), pp. 511–523.

Baek, S. H., Shin, J. H. and Kim, Y. C. (2017) 'Drug-coated microneedles for rapid and painless local anesthesia', Biomedical Microdevices. 19(1):2.

Balázs, B. et al. (2016) 'ATR-FTIR and Raman spectroscopic investigation of the electroporation-mediated transdermal delivery of a nanocarrier system containing an antitumour drug', Biomedical Optics Express. 7(1), p. 67.

Banga, A. K. (2009) 'Microporation applications for enhancing drug delivery', Expert Opinion on Drug Delivery. 6(4), pp. 343–354.

Belhaj, N. et al. (2017) 'Skin delivery of hydrophilic molecules from liposomes and polysaccharide-coated liposomes', International Journal of Cosmetic Science. 39(4), pp. 435–441.

Bellefroid, C. et al. (2019) '*In vitro* skin penetration enhancement techniques: A combined approach of ethosomes and microneedles'. Int J Pharm. 572:118793.

Benson, H. A. E. (2017) 'Elastic liposomes for topical and transdermal drug delivery', in Methods in Molecular Biology. 1522, pp. 107–117.

Benson, H. and Watkinson, A. (eds) (2012) Topical and Transdermal Drug Delivery: Principles and Practice. Wiley. Hoboken, New Jersey.

Bernelin-Cottet, C. et al. (2019) 'Electroporation of a nanoparticle-associated DNA vaccine induces higher inflammation and immunity compared to its delivery with microneedle patches in pigs', Journal of Controlled Release. 308, pp. 14–28.

Betz, G. et al. (2005) 'In vivo comparison of various liposome formulations for cosmetic application', International Journal of Pharmaceutics, 296(1–2), pp. 44–54.

Birchall, J. et al. (2006) 'Cutaneous gene expression of plasmid DNA in excised human skin following delivery via microchannels created by radio frequency ablation', International Journal of Pharmaceutics. 312(1–2), pp. 15–23.

Boinpally, R. R. et al. (2004) 'Iontophoresis of lecithin vesicles of cyclosporin A', International Journal of Pharmaceutics, 274(1–2), pp. 185–190.

Bok, M. et al. (2020) 'Ultrasonically and Iontophoretically Enhanced Drug-Delivery System Based on Dissolving Microneedle Patches', Scientific Reports. 10(1).

Caddeo, C. et al. (2016) 'Effect of quercetin and resveratrol co-incorporated in liposomes against inflammatory/oxidative response associated with skin cancer', International Journal of Pharmaceutics. 513(1–2), pp. 153–163.

Caddeo, C. et al. (2018) 'Tocopherol-loaded transfersomes: In vitro antioxidant activity and efficacy in skin regeneration', International Journal of Pharmaceutics. 551(1–2), pp. 34–41.

Carreras, J. J. et al. (2020) 'Ultraflexible lipid vesicles allow topical absorption of cyclosporin A', Drug Delivery and Translational Research. 10(2), pp. 486–497.

Cevc, G. (1996) 'Transfersomes, liposomes and other lipid suspensions on the skin: Permeation enhancement, vesicle penetration, and transdermal drug delivery', Critical Reviews in Therapeutic Drug Carrier Systems. 13(3–4), pp. 257–388.

Cevc, G. et al. (1998) 'Ultraflexible vesicles, transfersomes, have an extremely low pore penetration resistance and transport therapeutic amounts of insulin across the intact mammalian skin', Biochimica et Biophysica Acta - Biomembranes, 1368(2), pp. 201–215.

Cevc, G. (2003) 'Transdermal drug delivery of insulin with ultradeformable carriers', Clinical Pharmacokinetics, 42(5), pp. 461–474.

Cevc, G. et al. (2008) 'Occlusion effect on transcutaneous NSAID delivery from conventional and carrier-based formulations', International Journal of Pharmaceutics, 359(1–2), pp. 190–197.

Cevc, G. and Blume, G. (1992) 'Lipid vesicles penetrate into intact skin owing to the transdermal osmotic gradients and hydration force', BBA - Biomembranes, 1104(1), pp. 226–232.

Cevc, G. and Blume, G. (2001) 'New, highly efficient formulation of diclofenac for the topical, transdermal administration in ultradeformable drug carriers, Transfersomes', Biochimica et Biophysica Acta - Biomembranes, 1514(2), pp. 191–205.

Cevc, G. and Blume, G. (2003) 'Biological activity and characteristics of triamcinolone-acetonide formulated with the self-regulating drug carriers, Transfersomes®', Biochimica et Biophysica Acta - Biomembranes, 1614(2), pp. 156–164.

Cevc, G. and Blume, G. (2004) 'Hydrocortisone and dexamethasone in very deformable drug carriers have increased biological potency, prolonged effect, and reduced therapeutic dosage', Biochimica et Biophysica Acta - Biomembranes, 1663(1–2), pp. 61–73.

Cevc, G., Blume, G. and Schätzlein, A. (1997) 'Transfersomes-mediated transepidermal delivery improves the regiospecificity and biological activity of corticosteroids in vivo', Journal of Controlled Release, 45, pp. 211–226.

Cevc, G. and Chopra, A. (2016) 'Deformable (Transfersome®) vesicles for improved drug delivery into and through the skin', in: Dragicevic, N., Maibach, H.I. (eds), Percutaneous penetration enhancers - Chemical methods in penetration enhancement: Nanocarriers, Springer Berlin Heidelberg New York, Dordrecht London. ISBN 978-3-662-47861-5.

Cevc, G. and Gebauer, D. (2003) 'Hydration-driven transport of deformable lipid vesicles through fine pores and the skin barrier', Biophysical Journal, 84(2 I), pp. 1010–1024.

Cevc, G., Schätzlein, A. and Blume, G. (1995) 'Transdermal drug carriers: Basic properties, optimization and transfer efficiency in the case of epicutaneously applied peptides', Journal of Controlled Release, 36(1–2), pp. 3–16.

Cevc, G., Schätzlein, A. and Richardsen, H. (2002) 'Ultradeformable lipid vesicles can penetrate the skin and other semi-permeable barriers unfragmented. Evidence from double label CLSM experiments and direct size measurements', Biochimica et Biophysica Acta - Biomembranes, 1564(1), pp. 21–30.

Charoenputtakun, P., Li, S. K. and Ngawhirunpat, T. (2015) 'Iontophoretic delivery of lipophilic and hydrophilic drugs from lipid nanoparticles across human skin', International Journal of Pharmaceutics. 495(1), pp. 318–328.

Chen, G. et al. (2015) 'Pharmacokinetic and pharmacodynamic study of triptolide-loaded liposome hydrogel patch under microneedles on rats with collagen-induced arthritis', Acta Pharmaceutica Sinica B. 5(6), pp. 569–576.

Chen, H. et al. (2009a) 'Iontophoresis-driven penetration of nanovesicles through microneedle-induced skin microchannels for enhancing transdermal delivery of insulin', Journal of Controlled Release. 139(1), pp. 63–72.

Chen, H. et al. (2009b) 'Iontophoresis-driven penetration of nanovesicles through microneedle-induced skin microchannels for enhancing transdermal delivery of insulin', Journal of Controlled Release. 139(1), pp. 63–72.

Cui, Y. et al. (2018) 'Microneedle-assisted percutaneous delivery of paeoniflorin-loaded ethosomes', Molecules. 23(12):3371.

Daftardar, S. et al. (2019) 'Advances in ultrasound mediated transdermal drug delivery', Current Pharmaceutical Design. 25(4), pp. 413–423.

De Marco Almeida, F. et al. (2018) 'Physicochemical characterization and skin permeation of cationic transfersomes containing the synthetic peptide PnPP-19', Current Drug Delivery. 15(7), pp. 1064–1071.

DeMuth, P. C. et al. (2012) 'Releasable layer-by-layer assembly of stabilized lipid nanocapsules on microneedles for enhanced transcutaneous vaccine delivery', ACS Nano. 6(9), pp. 8041–8051.

Ding, Z. et al. (2011) 'Transcutaneous immunization studies in mice using diphtheria toxoid-loaded vesicle formulations and a microneedle array', Pharmaceutical Research. 28(1), pp. 145–158.

Dragicevic-Curic, N. et al. (2008) 'Temoporfin-loaded invasomes: Development, characterization and *in vitro* skin penetration studies', Journal of Controlled Release, 127(1), pp. 59–69.

Dragicevic-Curic, N. et al. (2009) 'Development of different temoporfin-loaded invasomes-novel nanocarriers of temoporfin: Characterization, stability and *in vitro* skin penetration studies', Colloids and Surfaces B: Biointerfaces, 70(2), pp. 198–206.

Dragicevic-Curic, N. et al. (2010) 'Efficacy of temoporfin-loaded invasomes in the photodynamic therapy in human epidermoid and colorectal tumour cell lines', Journal of Photochemistry and Photobiology B: Biology. 101(3), pp. 238–250.

Dragicevic, N., Maibach, H. I. (eds) (2015) *Percutaneous penetration enhancers - Chemical methods in penetration enhancement: Modification of the stratum corneum, Springer Berlin Heidelberg New York, Dordrecht London. ISBN: 978-3-662-47038-1.*

Dragicevic, N., and Maibach, H. I. (eds) (2016) *Percutaneous penetration enhancers - Chemical methods in penetration enhancement: Nanocarriers, Springer Berlin Heidelberg New York, Dordrecht London. ISBN 978-3-662-47861-5.*

Dragicevic, N., Maibach, H. I. (eds) (2017) *Percutaneous penetration enhancers - Physical methods in penetration enhancement, Springer Berlin Heidelberg New York, Dordrecht London. ISBN 978-3-662-53271-3;*

Dragicevic, N., Verma, D. D. and Fahr, A. (2016) 'Invasomes: Vesicles for enhanced skin delivery of drugs', in: Dragicevic, N., Maibach, H.I. (eds.), 2016. Percutaneous penetration enhancers - Chemical methods in penetration enhancement: Nanocarriers, Springer Berlin Heidelberg New York, Dordrecht London. ISBN 978-3-662-47861-5, pp. 77–92.

Dreier, J., Sørensen, J. A. and Brewer, J. R. (2016) 'Superresolution and fluorescence dynamics evidence reveal that intact liposomes do not cross the human skin barrier', PLoS ONE. 11(1).

Du, G. et al. (2018) 'Coated and hollow microneedle-mediated intradermal immunization in mice with diphtheria toxoid loaded mesoporous silica nanoparticles.', Pharmaceutical Research. 35(10), p. 189.

Dubey, V., Mishra, D. and Jain, N. K. (2007) 'Melatonin loaded ethanolic liposomes: Physicochemical characterization and enhanced transdermal delivery', European Journal of Pharmaceutics and Biopharmaceutics, 67(2), pp. 398–405.

Dul, M. et al. (2017) 'Hydrodynamic gene delivery in human skin using a hollow microneedle device', Journal of Controlled Release. 265, pp. 120–131.

Dwivedi, M., Sharma, V. and Pathak, K. (2017) 'Pilosebaceous targeting by isotretenoin-loaded invasomal gel for the treatment of eosinophilic pustular folliculitis: optimization, efficacy and cellular analysis', Drug Development and Industrial Pharmacy. 43(2), pp. 293–304.

El Maghraby, G. M. M., Williams, A. C. and Barry, B. W. (2000) 'Skin delivery of oestradiol from lipid vesicles: importance of liposome structure', International Journal of Pharmaceutics, 204(1–2), pp. 159–169.

El-Nabarawi, M. A. et al. (2018) 'Dapsone-loaded invasomes as a potential treatment of acne: preparation, characterization, and *in vivo* skin deposition assay', AAPS PharmSciTech. 19(5), pp. 2174–2184.

Elsabahy, M. and Foldvari, M. (2013) 'Needle-free gene delivery through the skin: an overview of recent strategies', Current Pharmaceutical Design. 19(41), pp. 7301–7315.

Escobar-Chávez, J. J. et al. (2009) 'Electroporation as an efficient physical enhancer for skin drug delivery.', Journal of Clinical Pharmacology, 49(11), pp. 1262–83.

Essa, E. A., Bonner, M. C. and Barry, B. W. (2003) 'Electroporation and ultradeformable liposomes; human skin barrier repair by phospholipid', Journal of Controlled Release, 92(1–2), pp. 163–172.

Essa, E. A., Bonner, M. C. and Barry, B. W. (2004) 'Electrically assisted skin delivery of liposomal estradiol; phospholipid as damage retardant', Journal of Controlled Release, 95(3), pp. 535–546.

Fang, J. Y. et al. (2001) 'In vitro skin permeation of estradiol from various proniosome formulations', International Journal of Pharmaceutics, 215(1–2), pp. 91–99.

Feng, S. et al. (2017) 'Controlled release of optimized electroporation enhances the transdermal efficiency of sinomenine hydrochloride for treating arthritis in vitro and in clinic', Drug Design, Development and Therapy. 11, pp. 1737–1752.

Fesq, H. et al. (2003) 'Improved risk-benefit ratio for topical triamcinolone acetonide in Transfersome® in comparison with equipotent cream and ointment: A randomized controlled trial', British Journal of Dermatology, 149(3), pp. 611–619.

Franzé, S. et al. (2017) 'Tuning the extent and depth of penetration of flexible liposomes in human skin', Molecular Pharmaceutics. 14(6), pp. 1998–2009.

Garg, B. J. et al. (2016) 'Nanosized ethosomes-based hydrogel formulations of methoxsalen for enhanced topical delivery against vitiligo: Formulation optimization, in vitro evaluation and preclinical assessment', Journal of Drug Targeting. 24(3), pp. 233–246.

Gratieri, T. and Kalia, Y. N. (2017a) 'Iontophoresis: basic principles', in Percutaneous Penetration Enhancers Physical Methods in Penetration Enhancement. Springer Berlin Heidelberg, pp. 61–65.

Gratieri, T. and Kalia, Y. N. (2017b) 'Iontophoretic transport mechanisms and factors affecting electrically assisted delivery', in Percutaneous Penetration Enhancers Physical Methods in Penetration Enhancement. Springer Berlin Heidelberg, pp. 67–76.

Guo, L. et al. (2013) 'Enhanced transcutaneous immunization via dissolving microneedle array loaded with liposome encapsulated antigen and adjuvant', International Journal of Pharmaceutics. 447(1–2), pp. 22–30.

Gupta, A. et al. (2012) 'Transfersomes: a novel vesicular carrier for enhanced transdermal delivery of sertraline: development, characterization, and performance evaluation', Scientia Pharmaceutica. 80(4), pp. 1061–1080.

Gupta, P. N. et al. (2005) 'Tetanus toxoid-loaded transfersomes for topical immunization', Journal of Pharmacy and Pharmacology. 57(3), pp. 295–301.

Gupta, R. and Kumar, A. (2020) 'Transfersomes: the ultra-deformable carrier system for non-invasive delivery of drug', Current Drug Delivery. doi: 10.2174/1567201817666200804105416.

Guy, R. H. et al. (2000) 'Iontophoresis: electrorepulsion and electroosmosis', Journal of Controlled Release. 64(1–3), pp. 129–132.

Hao, Y. et al. (2017) 'Microneedles-based transdermal drug delivery systems: a review', Journal of Biomedical Nanotechnology. 13(12), pp. 1581–1597.

Heenatigala Palliyage, G. et al. (2019) 'pharmaceutical topical delivery of poorly soluble polyphenols: potential role in prevention and treatment of melanoma', AAPS PharmSciTech. 20(6), p. 250.

Hirschberg, H. et al. (2012) 'A combined approach of vesicle formulations and microneedle arrays for transcutaneous immunization against hepatitis B virus', European Journal of Pharmaceutical Sciences. 46(1–2), pp. 1–7.

Hussain, A. et al. (2020) 'Vesicular elastic liposomes for transdermal delivery of rifampicin: In-vitro, in-vivo and in silico GastroPlus™ prediction studies', European Journal of Pharmaceutical Sciences. 151:105411.

Ingebrigtsen, S. G. et al. (2017) 'Successful co-encapsulation of benzoyl peroxide and chloramphenicol in liposomes by a novel manufacturing method - dual asymmetric centrifugation.', European Journal of Pharmaceutical Sciences. 97, pp. 192–199.

Ita, K. (2016) 'Perspectives on transdermal electroporation', Pharmaceutics. 8(1), p.9.

Jain, S. et al. (2003) 'Transfersomes – a novel vesicular carrier for enhanced transdermal delivery: development, characterization, and performance evaluation', Drug Development and Industrial Pharmacy, 29(9), pp. 1013–1026.

Jamaledin, R. et al. (2020) 'Progress in microneedle-mediated protein delivery', Journal of Clinical Medicine. 9(2), p. 542.

Jeong, S. et al. (2017) 'Combined photodynamic and antibiotic therapy for skin disorder via lipase-sensitive liposomes with enhanced antimicrobial performance', Biomaterials. 141, pp. 243–250.

Jose, A., Labala, S. and Venuganti, V. V. K. (2017) 'Co-delivery of curcumin and STAT3 siRNA using deformable cationic liposomes to treat skin cancer', Journal of Drug Targeting. 25(4), pp. 330–341.

Joseph, J., Vedha Hari, B. N. and Ramya Devi, D. (2018) 'Experimental optimization of Lornoxicam liposomes for sustained topical delivery', European Journal of Pharmaceutical Sciences. 112, pp. 38–51.

Kajimoto, K. et al. (2011) 'Noninvasive and persistent transfollicular drug delivery system using a combination of liposomes and iontophoresis', International Journal of Pharmaceutics. 403(1–2), pp. 57–65.

Kalia, Y. N. et al. (2004) 'Iontophoretic drug delivery', Advanced Drug Delivery Reviews. 56(5), pp. 619–658.

Kalluri, H. and Banga, A. K. (2011) 'Transdermal delivery of proteins', AAPS PharmSciTech. pp. 431–441.

Kamran, M. et al. (2016) 'Design, formulation and optimization of novel soft nano-carriers for transdermal olmesartan medoxomil delivery: *In vitro* characterization and *in vivo* pharmacokinetic assessment', International Journal of Pharmaceutics. 505(1–2), pp. 147–158.

Kasetvatin, C., Rujivipat, S. and Tiyaboonchai, W. (2015) 'Combination of elastic liposomes and low frequency ultrasound for skin permeation enhancement of hyaluronic acid', Colloids and Surfaces B: Biointerfaces. 135, pp. 458–464.

Kassem, M. A., Aboul-Einien, M. H. and El Taweel, M. M. (2018) 'Dry gel containing optimized felodipine-loaded transferosomes: a promising transdermal delivery system to enhance drug bioavailability', AAPS PharmSciTech. 19(5), pp. 2155–2173.

Kearney, M. C. et al. (2016) 'Microneedle-mediated delivery of donepezil: Potential for improved treatment options in Alzheimer's disease', European Journal of Pharmaceutics and Biopharmaceutics. 103, pp. 43–50.

Khan, M. A. et al. (2015) 'Novel carbopol-based transfersomal gel of 5-fluorouracil for skin cancer treatment: *in vitro* characterization and *in vivo* study', Drug Delivery. 22(6), pp. 795–802.

Kriftner, R. W. (1992) 'Liposome production: the ethanol injection technique and the development of the first approved liposome dermatic', in Liposome Dermatics. Springer Berlin Heidelberg, pp. 91–100.

Van Kuijk-Meuwissen, M. E. M. J., Junginger, H. E. and Bouwstra, J. A. (1998) 'Interactions between liposomes and human skin *in vitro*, a confocal laser scanning microscopy study', Biochimica et Biophysica Acta - Biomembranes, 1371(1), pp. 31–39.

Kumar, V. and Banga, A. K. (2016) 'Intradermal and follicular delivery of adapalene liposomes', Drug Development and Industrial Pharmacy. 42(6), pp. 871–879.

Lasch, J., Laub, R. and Wohlrab, W. (1992) 'How deep do intact liposomes penetrate into human skin?', Journal of Controlled Release. 18(1), pp. 55–58.

Latter, G. et al. (2019) 'Targeted topical delivery of retinoids in the management of acne vulgaris: Current formulations and novel delivery systems', Pharmaceutics. 11(10), p. 490.

Le, U. M., Baltzley, S. and AlGhananeem, A. (2018) 'Gabapentin in elastic liposomes: preparation, characterization, drug release, and penetration through porcine skin', International Journal of Pharmaceutical Compounding, 22(6), pp. 498–503.

Lee, S. E., Seo, J. and Lee, S. H. (2017) 'The mechanism of sonophoresis and the penetration pathways', in: Dragicevic, N., Maibach, H.I. (eds.), Percutaneous penetration enhancers - Physical methods in penetration enhancement, Springer Berlin Heidelberg New York, Dordrecht London. ISBN 978-3-662-53271-3, pp. 15–30.

Ma, H. et al. (2018) 'Paeonol-loaded ethosomes as transdermal delivery carriers: Design, preparation and evaluation', Molecules. 23(7), p. 1756.

Mahor, S., Gupta, P., et al. (2007) 'A Needle-Free Approach for Topical Immunization: Antigen Delivery via Vesicular Carrier System(s)', Current Medicinal Chemistry. 14(27), pp. 2898–2910.

Mahor, S., Rawat, A., et al. (2007) 'Cationic transfersomes based topical genetic vaccine against hepatitis B', International Journal of Pharmaceutics, 340(1–2), pp. 13–19.

Manca, M. L. et al. (2016) 'Combination of argan oil and phospholipids for the development of an effective liposome-like formulation able to improve skin hydration and allantoin dermal delivery', International Journal of Pharmaceutics. 505(1–2), pp. 204–211.

Manconi, M. et al. (2018) 'Nanodesign of new self-assembling core-shell gellan-transfersomes loading baicalin and *in vivo* evaluation of repair response in skin', Nanomedicine: Nanotechnology, Biology, and Medicine. 14(2), pp. 569–579.

Manconi, M., Sinico, C. and Fadda, A. M. (2016) 'Penetration enhancer-containing vesicles for cutaneous drug delivery', in: Dragicevic, N., Maibach, H.I. (eds.), Percutaneous penetration enhancers - Chemical methods in penetration enhancement: Nanocarriers, Springer Berlin Heidelberg New York, Dordrecht London. ISBN 978-3-662-47861-5, pp. 93–110.

Manconi, M., Sinico, C. and Fadda, A. M. (2016) 'Penetration enhancer-containing vesicles for cutaneous drug delivery', in: Dragicevic, N., Maibach, H.I. (eds.), Percutaneous penetration enhancers - Chemical methods in penetration enhancement: Nanocarriers, Springer Berlin Heidelberg New York, Dordrecht London. ISBN 978-3-662-47861-5, pp. 93–110.

Medi, B. M., Layek, B. and Singh, J. (2017) 'Electroporation for dermal and transdermal drug delivery', in: Dragicevic, N., Maibach, H.I. (eds.), Percutaneous penetration enhancers - Physical methods in penetration enhancement, Springer Berlin Heidelberg New York, Dordrecht London. ISBN 978-3-662-53271-3, pp. 105–122.

Merino, V., Castellano, A. L. and Delgado-Charro, M. B. (2017) 'Iontophoresis for therapeutic drug delivery and non-invasive sampling applications', in: Dragicevic, N., Maibach, H.I. (eds.), Percutaneous penetration enhancers - Physical methods in penetration enhancement, Springer Berlin Heidelberg New York, Dordrecht London. ISBN 978-3-662-53271-3, pp. 77–101.

Mitragotri, S. (2017) 'Sonophoresis: ultrasound-mediated transdermal drug delivery', in: Dragicevic, N., Maibach, H.I. (eds.), Percutaneous penetration enhancers - Physical methods in penetration enhancement, Springer Berlin Heidelberg New York, Dordrecht London. ISBN 978-3-662-53271-3, pp. 3–14.

Moffatt, K. et al. (2017) 'Microneedles for enhanced transdermal and intraocular drug delivery', Current Opinion in Pharmacology. 36, pp. 14–21.

Mohammed, M. I. et al. (2016) 'Transdermal delivery of vancomycin hydrochloride using combination of nano-ethosomes and iontophoresis: *in vitro* and *in vivo* study.', Drug Delivery. 23(5), pp. 1558–64.

Morsi, N. M., Aboelwafa, A. A. and Dawoud, M. H. S. (2018) 'Enhancement of the bioavailability of an anti-hypertensive drug by transdermal protransfersomal system: formulation and *in vivo* study', Journal of Liposome Research. 28(2), pp. 137–148.

Mostafa, M. et al. (2018) 'Optimization and characterization of thymoquinone-loaded liposomes with enhanced topical anti-inflammatory activity', AAPS PharmSciTech. 19(8), pp. 3490–3500.

Mura, S. et al. (2007) 'Liposomes and niosomes as potential cariers for dermal delivery of minoxidil', Journal of Drug Targeting, 15(2), pp. 101–108.

Muzzalupo, R. (2016) 'Niosomes and proniosomes for enhanced skin delivery', in: Dragicevic, N., Maibach, H.I. (eds.), Percutaneous penetration enhancers - Chemical methods in penetration enhancement: Nanocarriers, Springer Berlin Heidelberg New York, Dordrecht London. ISBN 978-3-662-47861-5, pp. 147–160.

Nguyen, H. X. et al. (2018) 'Poly (vinyl alcohol) microneedles: Fabrication, characterization, and application for transdermal drug delivery of doxorubicin', European Journal of Pharmaceutics and Biopharmaceutics. 129, pp. 88–103.

Nguyen, H. X. and Banga, A. K. (2017) 'Fabrication, characterization and application of sugar microneedles for transdermal drug delivery', Therapeutic Delivery. 8(5), pp. 249–264.

Niu, X. Q. et al. (2019) 'Mechanism investigation of ethosomes transdermal permeation', Int J Pharm X, 1:100027.

Oberli, M. A. et al. (2014) 'Ultrasound-enhanced transdermal delivery: recent advances and future challenges', Therapeutic Delivery. 5(7), pp. 843–857.

Oh, E. K. et al. (2011) 'Retained topical delivery of 5-aminolevulinic acid using cationic ultradeformable liposomes for photodynamic therapy', European Journal of Pharmaceutical Sciences. 44(1–2), pp. 149–157.

Park, J. *et al.* (2019) 'Enhanced transdermal drug delivery by sonophoresis and simultaneous application of sonophoresis and iontophoresis.', AAPS PharmSciTech. 20(3), p. 96.

Park, J. H. et al. (2010) 'A microneedle roller for transdermal drug delivery', European Journal of Pharmaceutics and Biopharmaceutics. 76(2), pp. 282–289.

Predic Atkinson, J., Maibach, H. and Dragicevic, N. (2015) 'Targets in dermal and transdermal delivery and classification of penetration enhancement methods', in Dragicevic, N. and Maibach, H. (eds) Percutaneous Penetration Enhancers - Chemical Methods in Penetration Enhancement: Drug Manipulation Strategies and Vehicle Effects. Springer Berlin Heidelberg New York Dordrecht London, pp. 93–108.

Priyanka, K. and Singh, S. (2014) 'A review on skin targeted delivery of bioactives as ultradeformable vesicles: overcoming the penetration problem', Current Drug Targets. 15(2), pp. 184–198.

Puri, A., Nguyen, H. X. and Banga, A. K. (2016) 'Microneedle-mediated intradermal delivery of epigallocatechin-3-gallate', International Journal of Cosmetic Science. 38(5), pp. 512–523.

Qadri, G. R. et al. (2017) 'Invasomes of isradipine for enhanced transdermal delivery against hypertension: formulation, characterization, and *in vivo* pharmacodynamic study', Artificial Cells, Nanomedicine and Biotechnology. 45(1), pp. 139–145.

Qiu, Y. et al. (2016) 'DNA-based vaccination against hepatitis B virus using dissolving microneedle arrays adjuvanted by cationic liposomes and CpG ODN', Drug Delivery. 23(7), pp. 2391–2398.

Raj, R., Raj, P. M. and Ram, A. (2018) 'Nanosized ethanol based malleable liposomes of cytarabine to accentuate transdermal delivery: formulation optimization, *in vitro* skin permeation and *in vivo* bioavailability', Artificial Cells, Nanomedicine and Biotechnology. 46(Suppl 2), pp. 951–963.

Rangsimawong, W. et al. (2018) 'Enhancement of galantamine hbr skin permeation using sonophoresis and limonene-containing PEGylated liposomes', AAPS PharmSciTech. 19(3), pp. 1093–1104.

Rastogi, R., Anand, S. and Koul, V. (2010) 'Electroporation of polymeric nanoparticles: An alternative technique for transdermal delivery of insulin', Drug Development and Industrial Pharmacy. 36(11), pp. 1303–1311.

Ripolin, A. et al. (2017) 'Successful application of large microneedle patches by human volunteers', International Journal of Pharmaceutics. 521(1–2), pp. 92–101.

Ronnander, J. P., Simon, L. and Koch, A. (2019) 'Transdermal delivery of sumatriptan succinate using iontophoresis and dissolving microneedles', Journal of Pharmaceutical Sciences. 108(11), pp. 3649–3656.

Rukavina, Z. et al. (2018) 'Azithromycin-loaded liposomes for enhanced topical treatment of methicillin-resistant Staphyloccocus aureus (MRSA) infections', International Journal of Pharmaceutics. 553(1–2), pp. 109–119.

Sabri, A. H. et al. (2019) 'Expanding the applications of microneedles in dermatology', European Journal of Pharmaceutics and Biopharmaceutics. 140, pp. 121–140.

Sabri, A. H. et al. (2020) 'Intradermal and transdermal drug delivery using microneedles – Fabrication, performance evaluation and application to lymphatic delivery', Advanced Drug Delivery Reviews. 153, pp. 195–215.

Sala, M. et al. (2018) 'Lipid nanocarriers as skin drug delivery systems: properties, mechanisms of skin interactions and medical applications', International Journal of Pharmaceutics. 535(1–2), pp. 1–17.

Schätzlein, A. and Cevc, G. (1998) 'Non-uniform cellular packing of the stratum corneum and permeability barrier function of intact skin: A high-resolution confocal laser scanning microscopy study using highly deformable vesicles (Transfersomes)', British Journal of Dermatology, 138(4), pp. 583–592.

Seah, B. C. Q. and Teo, B. M. (2018) 'Recent advances in ultrasound-based transdermal drug delivery', International Journal of Nanomedicine. 13, pp. 7749–7763.

Seth, A. K., Misra, A. and Umrigar, D. (2004) 'Topical liposomal gel of idoxuridine for the treatment of herpes simplex: Pharmaceutical and clinical implications', Pharmaceutical Development and Technology, 9(3), pp. 277–289.

Shah, S. M. et al. (2015) 'LeciPlex, invasomes, and liposomes: a skin penetration study', International Journal of Pharmaceutics. 490(1–2), pp. 391–403.

Shumilov, M. and Touitou, E. (2010) 'Buspirone transdermal administration for menopausal syndromes, in vitro and in animal model studies', International Journal of Pharmaceutics. 387(1–2), pp. 26–33.

Al Shuwaili, A. H., Rasool, B. K. A. and Abdulrasool, A. A. (2016) 'Optimization of elastic transfersomes formulations for transdermal delivery of pentoxifylline', European Journal of Pharmaceutics and Biopharmaceutics. 102, pp. 101–114.

Siler-Marinkovic, S. (2016) 'Liposomes as drug delivery systems in dermal and transdermal drug delivery', in Dragicevic, N. and Maibach, H. (eds) Percutaneous Penetration Enhancers Chemical Methods in Penetration Enhancement: Nanocarriers. Springer Berlin Heidelberg New York Dordrecht London, pp. 15–38.

Singh, P. et al. (2019) 'Polymeric microneedles for controlled transdermal drug delivery', Journal of Controlled Release. 315, pp. 97–113.

Soleymani, S. et al. (2019) 'Implications of grape extract and its nanoformulated bioactive agent resveratrol against skin disorders', Archives of Dermatological Research. 311(8), pp. 577–588.

Song, C. K. et al. (2012) 'A novel vesicular carrier, transethosome, for enhanced skin delivery of voriconazole: Characterization and in vitro/in vivo evaluation', Colloids and Surfaces B: Biointerfaces. 92, pp. 299–304.

Song, H. et al. (2019) 'Enhanced transdermal permeability and drug deposition of rheumatoid arthritis via sinomenine hydrochloride-loaded antioxidant surface transethosome', International Journal of Nanomedicine. 14, pp. 3177–3188.

Takeuchi, I. et al. (2016) 'Transdermal delivery of estradiol-loaded PLGA nanoparticles using iontophoresis for treatment of osteoporosis.', Bio-Medical Materials and Engineering. 27(5), pp. 475–483.

Teong, B. et al. (2017) 'Liposomal encapsulation for systemic delivery of propranolol via transdermal iontophoresis improves bone microarchitecture in ovariectomized rats', International Journal of Molecular Sciences. 18(4), p. 822.

Thakkar, P. H., Savsani, H. and Kumar, P. (2016) 'Ethosomal hydrogel of raloxifene hcl: statistical optimization & ex vivo permeability evaluation across microporated pig ear skin', Current Drug Delivery. 13(7), pp. 1111–1122..

Touitou, E. et al. (2000) 'Ethosomes - Novel vesicular carriers for enhanced delivery: Characterization and skin penetration properties', Journal of Controlled Release, 65(3), pp. 403–418.

van der Maaden, K. et al. (2018) 'Hollow microneedle-mediated micro-injections of a liposomal HPV E743–63 synthetic long peptide vaccine for efficient induction of cytotoxic and T-helper responses', Journal of Controlled Release. 269, pp. 347–354.

Verma, D. D. (2002) Invasomes: Novel Topical Carriers for Enhanced Topical Delivery: Characterization and Skin Penetration Properties. Philipps-University Marburg, Germany.

Verma, D. D. et al. (2004) 'Treatment of alopecia areata in the DEBR model using Cyclosporin A lipid vesicles', European Journal of Dermatology, 14(5), pp. 332–338.

Vicente-Perez, E. M. et al. (2017) 'Repeat application of microneedles does not alter skin appearance or barrier function and causes no measurable disturbance of serum biomarkers of infection, inflammation or immunity in mice *in vivo*', European Journal of Pharmaceutics and Biopharmaceutics. 117, pp. 400–407.

Wang, M., Hu, L. and Xu, C. (2017) 'Recent advances in the design of polymeric microneedles for transdermal drug delivery and biosensing', Lab Chip. 17(8), pp. 1373–1387.

Wang, W. et al. (2019) 'Nano-drug delivery systems in wound treatment and skin regeneration', Journal of Nanobiotechnology. 17(1), p. 82, doi: 10.1186/s12951-019-0514-y.

Wu, X. et al. (2019) 'A surface charge dependent enhanced Th1 antigen-specific immune response in lymph nodes by transfersome-based nanovaccine-loaded dissolving microneedle-assisted transdermal immunization', Journal of Materials Chemistry B. 7(31), pp. 4854–4866.

Yang, H. *et al.* (2019) 'Enhanced transdermal lymphatic delivery of doxorubicin via hyaluronic acid based transfersomes/microneedle complex for tumor metastasis therapy', International Journal of Biological Macromolecules. 125, pp. 9–16.

Yang, L. et al. (2017) 'Mechanism of transdermal permeation promotion of lipophilic drugs by ethosomes.', International Journal of Nanomedicine. 12, pp. 3357–3364.

Ye, Y. et al. (2018) 'Polymeric microneedles for transdermal protein delivery', Advanced Drug Delivery Reviews. 127, pp. 106–118.

Zellmer, S., Pfeil, W. and Lasch, J. (1995) 'Interaction of phosphatidylcholine liposomes with the human stratum corneum', BBA - Biomembranes, 1237(2), pp. 176–182.

Zellmer, S., Reissig, D. and Lasch, J. (1998) 'Reconstructed human skin as model for liposome-skin interaction', Journal of Controlled Release. 55(2–3), pp. 271–279.

Zhai, Y. et al. (2015) 'Ethosomes for skin delivery of ropivacaine: Preparation, characterization and *ex vivo* penetration properties', Journal of Liposome Research. 25(4), pp. 316–324.

Zhang, C. et al. (2019) 'Skin delivery of hyaluronic acid by the combined use of sponge spicules and flexible liposomes', Biomaterials Science. 7(4), pp. 1299–1310.

Zhang, Y.-T. et al. (2014) 'Evaluation of skin viability effect on ethosome and liposome-mediated psoralen delivery via cell uptake', J Pharm Sci, 103, pp. 3120–3126.

Zhao, J. H. et al. (2017) 'Enhanced immunization via dissolving microneedle array-based delivery system incorporating subunit vaccine and saponin adjuvant', International Journal of Nanomedicine. 12, pp. 4763–4772.

Zhou, Y. et al. (2010) 'Synergistic penetration of ethosomes and lipophilic prodrug on the transdermal delivery of acyclovir', Archives of Pharmacal Research, 33(4), pp. 567–574.

Zorec, B. et al. (2018) 'Combinations of nanovesicles and physical methods for enhanced transdermal delivery of a model hydrophilic drug', European Journal of Pharmaceutics and Biopharmaceutics. 127, pp. 387–397.

Zou, L. et al. (2018) 'Peptide-modified vemurafenib-loaded liposomes for targeted inhibition of melanoma via the skin', Biomaterials. 182, pp. 1–12.

39 Assessment of Microneedles for Transdermal Drug Delivery

Melissa Kirkby, Kurtis J. Moffatt, Aaron. R.J. Hutton, Inken K. Ramöeller, Peter E. McKenna, Marco T.A. Abbate, Sarah A. Stewart, and Ryan F. Donnelly
Queen's University Belfast, Belfast, United Kingdom

CONTENTS

39.1 INTRODUCTION

Microneedles (MNs) consist of multiple needlelike microprojections, ranging from 25 to 1000 μm in length, positioned on one side of a supporting baseplate [1, 2]. These microprojections pierce the epidermis, creating temporary microscopic aqueous channels through which drug molecules can diffuse into the microcirculation. However, they are not long enough to touch nerve endings and thus do not elicit a pain response [1]. The rationale behind the development of these minimally invasive devices was to offer pain-free drug administration and to increase the range of drugs that could be delivered transdermally via the production of temporary aqueous channels in a largely hydrophobic tissue [3].

MNs were first conceptualized in 1976 [4]; however, it was not until 1998 when advances in microelectronic technology and microfabrication allowed the fabrication of the first true MNs [5]. The first reported instance of MN-assisted drug delivery was in the late 1990s, where puncturing the skin using silicon MNs was shown to increase the skin's permeability to a model drug, calcein [5].

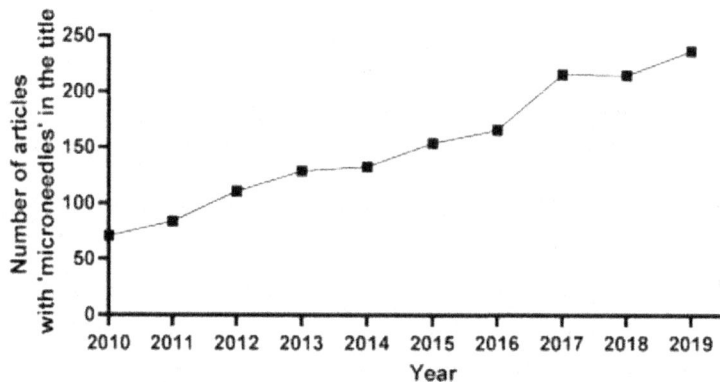

FIGURE 39.1 Number of journal articles published containing "microneedle" in the title each year since 2010. (Data acquired from PubMed (April 2020).)

Since then, there have been further advances in microengineering and polymer chemistry, leading to increasing numbers of publications (Figure 39.1), and significant progress has been made towards commercialization of this technology.

MNs combine the delivery capabilities of a hypodermic injection in the form of a patient-friendly transdermal patch. MNs minimize skin trauma and bleeding and are associated with significantly less microbial penetration than drug delivery by hypodermic injection [6]. Additionally, there are numerous reports documenting the reproducible insertion of MNs by patients (i.e., self-application) [7, 8]. Needle stick injuries are also a rare occurrence. Therefore, it can be assumed that medical personnel would not be required to administer or even supervise administration of MNs, as would be the case with a traditional hypodermic needle. There is reduced needle phobia in comparison to hypodermic needles, which should ultimately increase patient adherence to any MN device. The overriding benefit of MNs remains the promise of pain-free delivery of both small- and large-molecular-weight (MW) drugs [2].

Five types of MNs exist and are illustrated in Figure 39.2. They are solid, coated, hollow, dissolving, and hydrogel-forming MNs. Each type has advantages and disadvantages, and the most suitable type of MN for each purpose must be chosen after consideration of a number of factors, such as the drug properties and dose, among others.

Solid MNs (Figure 39.2A) typically employ a "poke and patch" technique, whereby the MNs are first applied to the skin, removed and subsequently a drug containing formulation (gel, ointment, cream, etc.) is applied to the site [10]. Drug delivery occurs via diffusion through the transient pores created in the skin by the MNs [11, 12]. The two-step process involved is the main drawback of this MN system.

Coated MNs (Figure 39.2B) are similar to solid MNs and are often referred to as the "coat and poke" approach [10]. These solid MNs are coated with a drug containing formulation prior to application to the skin. Once applied to the skin, the drug containing coating is deposited into the dermal tissue. This approach overcomes the problem of a two-step approach associated with solid MNs but is limited by the finite amount of drug that can be coated onto a MN.

Hollow MNs (Figure 39.2C) have a central bore or lumen through which drugs may pass through from a reservoir to the dermal microcirculation. Delivery of drugs via these devices may be driven by diffusion, electrical stimulation, or pressure [13]. This type of MN is capable of delivering higher amounts of drug than solid or coated MNs [14]; however, clogging of the bore/lumen or compression by the dense dermal tissue is a concern with this type of MN [15]. Furthermore, hollow MNs are often associated with bulky equipment, used to provide pressurized flow of the formulation into the skin, thus removing the advantage of convenience associated with MNs [16, 17].

Dissolving MNs (Figure 39.2D) are drug-containing MNs made of dissolving materials. As such, they may be applied to the skin in the solid state; once applied they are dissolved by the interstitial

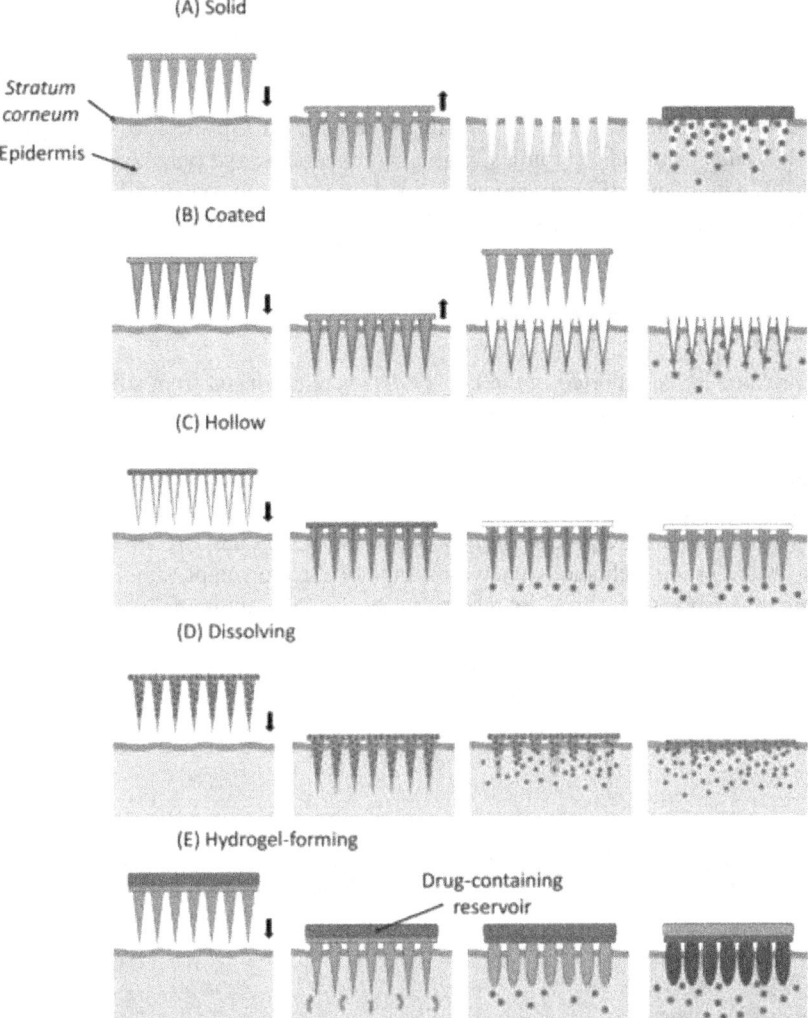

FIGURE 39.2 Schematic representation of the five types of MNs: (A) Solid; (B) coated; (C) hollow; (D) dissolving; and (E) hydrogel-forming. (Adapted from [9].)

fluid (ISF) and the drug load is thereby released. Similarly to coated MNs, this type is also associated with a low drug loading and is therefore only suitable for highly potent compounds. However, the dissolving nature of these types of MNs precludes them from being reinserted into the skin, thus reducing the risk of accidental reinsertion and the need for sharps disposal [18]. The long-term implications of polymer deposition in the skin need to be fully evaluated for this type of MN to allow for their repeated administration [19].

Hydrogel-forming MNs (Figure 39.2E) are a non-drug-containing MN system. Instead, the drug is contained within a reservoir (i.e., a compressed tablet or lyophilized wafer) which is placed on top of the MNs. The MN array is formed from materials, which when in contact with ISF, will swell. As such, when applied to the skin, the needles will imbibe ISF and will rapidly swell, thus forming continuous microconduits through which the drug contained within the reservoir may dissolve and be delivered [14]. This system has all the advantages of dissolving MNs, but polymer deposition in the skin is not an issue, and drug loading is not limited by what can be loaded into the MNs themselves [18].

39.2 MATERIAL TYPES AND FABRICATION TECHNIQUES IN MN MANUFACTURING

Over the last two decades, a wide range of materials and techniques have been employed for the manufacture of MNs. Starting with silicon in the late 1990s [5], the focus has since moved to other materials such as metals, ceramics, glass, carbohydrates, and polymers. The possibilities of designing MNs with many different geometries and properties to specifically modify transdermal release profiles of therapeutic agents has increased considerably with newly emerging fabrication techniques.

39.2.1 SILICON

The first fabricated MNs, reported in the late 1990s, were produced from silicon due to the recent developments in microfabrication technologies (i.e., microelectromechanical systems [MEMS]) [5]. The main advantage of silicon is its ability to be fabricated in a wide range of geometries using monocrystalline or polycrystalline silicon. Thus, it has been used to produce solid, hollow, and coated MNs that can successfully pierce the skin, facilitating transdermal drug delivery [9]. Existing manufacturing techniques are precise and can be easily scaled up [20], an attractive prospect for potential investors in the technology. However, high costs, the complex multistep manufacturing, and therefore long fabrication times are major drawbacks [20]. Additionally, concerns over the biocompatibility of silicon have been raised. After skin insertion, silicon fractures could remain in the skin, as it is a brittle material. Some pieces can be naturally discarded, but silicon-related granulomas have been reported in the past [21]. MEMS technology involves three basic sequential techniques. Briefly, the first fabrication step involves the coating of the substrate (in this case silicon)

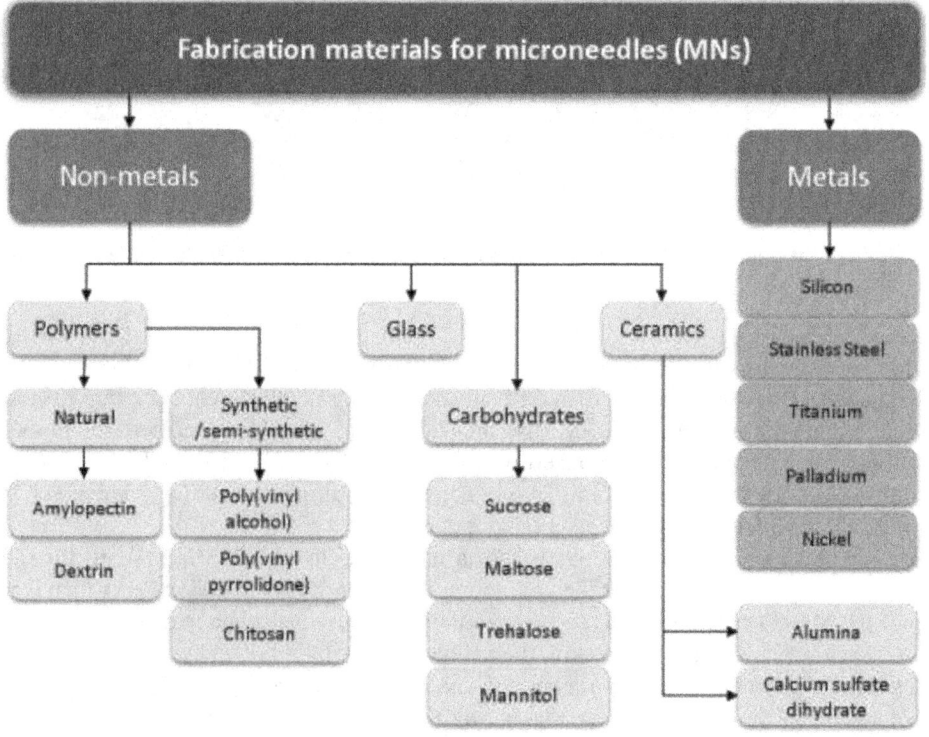

FIGURE 39.3 Materials used for the preparation of MNs.

with a photosensitive material. By photolithographic imaging, a master pattern is transferred to the substrate. A thin film is deposited on the substrate surface, and this film is then selectively etched (wet or dry etching) to achieve the desired three-dimensional structure [22].

39.2.2 METALS

Metals have been employed for the manufacture of medicinal products for many years. Stainless steel, which is the most common metal used for hypodermic needles, has been used successfully in MN production. Titanium, palladium, palladium-cobalt alloys, and nickel have also been reported [23]. These metals have not only been extensively characterized in terms of their biocompatibility, an important aspect for commercial and regulatory approval, but they also provide good mechanical properties (higher fracture toughness and similar yield strength compared to silicon) [24]. The simplest way of manufacturing metal MN arrays is to assemble an array of stainless-steel hypodermic needles of a desired length on supporting material [25]. Alternatively, metallic MNs can be fabricated by electroplating (e.g., palladium), photochemical etching (e.g., titanium) or laser cutting (e.g., stainless steel) [24].

39.2.3 CERAMICS

The main ceramic used for MNs is alumina (Al_2O_3), a porous material that can be coated with therapeutic agents for controlled release [26]. Despite its high resistance against corrosion and mechanical compression, alumina is brittle and has lower strength compared to metals [27]. Other ceramics for fabricating MNs are gypsum ($CaSO_4 \cdot 2\ H_2O$), brushite ($CaHPO_4 \cdot 2\ H_2O$) [28], and the organic-ceramic hybrid Ormocer (three-dimensional network of organically modified silicon alkoxides and organic monomers) [29]. The biocompatibility depends on the type of ceramic, but they have been used as replacement parts for the musculoskeletal system for years and are considered safe, especially in the short-term application that is needed for MNs [30]. Micromolding is the main technique for manufacturing ceramic MNs, a low-cost approach that is also used for e.g., polymeric MNs and can be easily scaled up. MNs of different designs can be fabricated by using different mold designs, and the process involves the casting of a ceramic slurry into a mold followed by a sintering process [26].

39.2.4 GLASS

Silica and borosilicate glass can be used for manufacture of MNs in various geometries. Brittleness and fracture toughness of glass are comparable to silicon. Its biocompatibility is not fully understood, as it is physiologically inert, but it might cause granulomas [21, 31]. Hollow glass MNs are manufactured by manually pulling glass pipettes using a micropipette puller and beveling the tips. Even though this can be done quickly in laboratory scale, scale-up to commercial use is not realistically feasible [9].

39.2.5 SIMPLE CARBOHYDRATES

Carbohydrate MNs are mainly prepared from maltose, but the use of trehalose, sucrose, mannitol, xylitol, and galactose has also been described [24]. The main advantages of carbohydrates are their low cost and the high biocompatibility. They are naturally present in food and have been used extensively in approved parenterals. However, mechanical properties have not been well studied, and they come with many limitations during their manufacture (thermal treatment), storage (disintegration), and use (sealing of created holes during dissolution). Carbohydrate MNs can be easily produced by micromolding of hot melts or solutions. The therapeutic agents are mixed with the carbohydrates before casting and are delivered upon in-skin dissolution of the prepared MNs [32].

39.2.6 POLYMERS

Polymers are commonly used for the manufacture of dissolving, biodegradable, or hydrogel-forming MNs, but solid, hollow, or coated polymeric MNs have also been reported. A wide range of synthetic polymers, proteins, and polysaccharides has been studied due to their excellent biocompatibility, degradability, and low cost [33]. Even though MNs prepared from polymers are not as strong as silicon, metal, ceramic, or glass MNs, they are able to penetrate the skin and show higher toughness than ceramic or glass MNs [9]. Dissolving MNs are mostly prepared from polysaccharides such as carboxymethyl cellulose (CMC), amylopectin, dextrin, hydroxypropyl cellulose (HPC), alginate, and hyaluronic acid or synthetic polymers such as poly(vinyl pyrrolidone) (PVP), poly(vinyl alcohol) (PVA), or poly(methyl vinyl ether/maleic anhydride (Gantrez AN-139). MNs manufactured from poly(lactic-co-glycolic acid) (PLGA), poly-L-lactic acid (PLLA), poly(glycolic acid) (PGA), and chitosan are biodegradable. Both types of polymeric MNs, dissolving and biodegradable, carry their payload inside the MNs and release it upon dissolution or biodegradation. In contrast, hydrogel-forming MNs consist of cross-linked polymers that absorb ISF upon skin insertion and form aqueous conduits through which the therapeutic agent, located in a separate reservoir, can permeate into the body (Figure 39.2E). The first hydrogel-forming MNs were made from poly (methyl vinyl ether/maleic anhydride) (Gantrez AN-139) or poly (methyl vinyl ether/maleic acid) (Gantrez S-97), crosslinked with polyethylene glycol. Sodium hydrogen carbonate was used as a pore-forming agent to modify the swelling properties. Other hydrogel-forming MNs were made from PVA in combination with either a mixture of polysaccharides or dextran and CMC or gelatin [24]. Most of these polymers have been previously used for other medical applications and are considered biocompatible. While some of them are biodegradable, others can be, if absorbed, eliminated in the kidney by glomerular filtration if their MW is below the glomerular threshold [34]. Most polymeric MNs are prepared by micromolding, with polydimethylsiloxane being the most commonly used mold material next to metals. Other techniques include hot embossing, droplet-borne air blowing, electro-drawing, injection molding, laser micromachining, drawing lithography, photolithography, investment molding, continuous liquid-phase interface production, dipping, solvent casting, and x-ray methods [35]. The long-term impact of repeated administration of polymers within the skin from repeated MN application is yet to be fully understood. The importance of the long-term safety of MNs, particularly when used for the treatment of chronic conditions, is discussed further in Section 39.7.2.

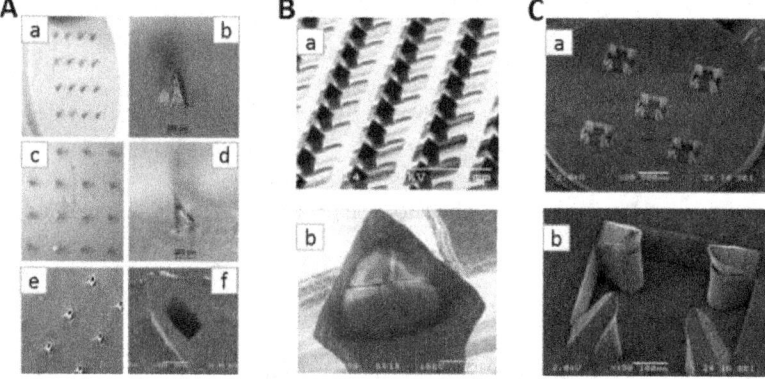

FIGURE 39.4 (A) Different types of stainless-steel MNs: (a) hollow stainless-steel 4 × 4 MN array, (b) higher magnification of a single hollow stainless-steel needle; (c) solid stainless-steel 4 × 4 MN array, (d) higher magnification of a single solid stainless-steel needle; (e) hollow silicon 4 × 4 MN array, (f) higher magnification of a single hollow silicon needle. (B) Scanning electron micrographs of titanium MNs coated with 80 µg of desmopressin per array: (a) general view, 1 mm scale, (b) front view of a single MN, 50 µm scale. (C) Scanning electron micrographs of ceramic MNs: (a) general view, 500 µm scale, (b) detailed view of a single MN, 100 µm scale. All images reproduced with permission [26, 36, 37].

To summarize, MNs exist in many forms and can be fabricated from a variety of materials to maximize efficiency for delivery of a specific compound. Each MN type in Figure 39.2 has been extensively investigated for drug delivery, examples of which will be described in detail in subsequent sections within this chapter, alongside any associated challenges with each particular method.

39.3 MICRONEEDLE-MEDIATED DRUG DELIVERY

39.3.1 Sustained/Long-Acting Delivery Using MNs

Controlled drug delivery systems, as the name suggests, deliver therapeutic agents to specific target cells, tissues, or organs in a controlled manner to achieve the desired therapeutic outcome [35]. With traditional transdermal delivery systems, such as patches, creams, ointments, gels, and lotions, achieving controlled delivery is difficult [35]. This is due to numerous factors that affect skin permeation, such as skin thickness, hydration, and age, in addition to the physiochemical properties of a therapeutic agent. MN-mediated delivery can address these issues by offering precise localization of the delivery cargo through the fabrication of needles of specific heights and geometries [9]. Furthermore, they can be used to maintain steady drug concentrations in blood, tissues, and specific target sites [38, 39]. Reducing the administration frequency improves patient compliance through enhanced convenience and by minimizing the chances of a missed dose [33, 40]. Therefore, employing MNs for sustained drug delivery can be perceived as one method of improving patient compliance.

Sustained transdermal drug delivery can be achieved through dissolving/biodegradable and hydrogel-forming MNs. As illustrated in Figure 39.2, dissolving/biodegradable polymeric MNs are designed to dissolve or degrade inside skin tissue, thus releasing their cargo. The numerous polymers available for dissolving MN fabrication can influence the time taken for the array to dissolve, hence influencing the release rate of the drug [9, 41–43]. Park et al. were the first to report sustained MN-mediated delivery by fabricating MNs out of PLGA loaded with microparticles (either PLGA or CMC), which encapsulated two model drugs: calcein and bovine serum albumin (BSA). This MN system achieved a sustained release profile ranging from hours to months, depending on the encapsulating method [44]. However, due to elevated temperatures during fabrication, 10% of the encapsulated BSA was irreversibly aggregated after a 10-minute exposure to the polymer melt. Addressing this issue, Chen et al. used chitosan MNs manufactured under aqueous conditions at ambient temperatures to highlight its ability to provide a sustained release of BSA. *In vitro* drug release showed that chitosan MNs provided a sustained release of BSA over a period of eight days [43]. Unfortunately, fabricating MNs from these polymers still remains a challenge, as good mechanical strength is difficult to achieve.

Regrettably, MNs have been rather narrowly viewed as vaccine delivery systems for the developing world. However, as MN technologies are becoming increasingly more advanced, two particular MN designs have recently demonstrated their potential for major enhancement in patient care outside of vaccine delivery. Li et al. have developed a reversible contraceptive MN patch that slowly releases levonorgestrel, a contraceptive hormone, for more than one month. In this unique design, an effervescent backing caused rapid separation of MNs from the patch upon skin penetration [45]. The detached MNs remained embedded under the skin's surface, where they slowly degraded, releasing the hormone for prolonged contraception. The second design, detailed by McCrudden et al., consisted of a two-layered dissolving MN system containing a long-acting rilpivirine nanosuspension for the treatment of human immunodeficiency virus (HIV). Currently, daily usage of oral antiretroviral drugs is the first-line treatment for HIV infection, however, many patients experience treatment fatigue, thus affecting regimen adherence [46]. Although there is an alternative in the form of a long-acting intramuscular (IM) injection, this requires access to health care facilities, dedicated sharps disposal, and the possibility of reduced compliance due to needle phobia. In this proof-of-concept study, following the application of the MN array, rilpivirine plasma concentration remained above the therapeutic level for seven days [46]. Furthermore, administration via IM produced comparable plasma results, thus indicating that MNs could potentially be used for the sustained release of antiretrovirals in humans [46].

With reference to hydrogel-forming MNs, as the MN itself is drug-free (Figure 39.2E), its key function is to act as a rate-controlling membrane, permitting sustained drug delivery from an attached drug-containing reservoir [47]. By adjusting the polymeric cross-linked density, which controls the rate of swelling, drug delivery across the skin is controlled by the formulator, rather than the stratum corneum. This was first demonstrated by Donnelly et al., in which MNs composed of poly(methyl vinyl ether/maleic acid) (PMVE/MA), cross-linked with poly(ethylene glycol) (PEG) delivered sustained doses of FITC-BSA, metronidazole, and insulin over 24 hours. To further exemplify the potential of this technology, Hardy et al. developed a stimulus responsive hydrogel-forming MN composed of 2-hydroxethly methacrylate and ethylene glycol dimethacrylate that enabled the delivery of ibuprofen upon application of light. *In vitro*, this light-responsive MN system delivered three doses of ibuprofen (50 mg) over a period of 160 hours [48]. Evidently, despite their infancy, hydrogel-forming MNs have the potential to further enhance the field of drug delivery; however, questions have been asked as to what applications this MN may have. Although in the early stages of development, hydrogel-forming MNs have successfully delivered clinically relevant drugs *in vivo*, including metformin, donepezil, and bevacizumab, in a sustained manner [49–51]. Therefore, with continued development, this minimally invasive form of administration offers a range of potential benefits for patients and health care providers alike.

39.3.2 IMMEDIATE TRANSDERMAL DRUG DELIVERY USING MICRONEEDLES

Given the difficulties associated with controlling drug delivery through traditional transdermal delivery systems, it is understandable why the controlled release of drugs using MNs has been explored extensively. Instant or rapid drug release from MNs has often been overlooked in MN-based controlled drug delivery, because it was considered a negative result when the aim was to develop long-term, controlled-release strategies. However, in some cases, instant or rapid delivery of a drug is desirable, for example, for analgesia and gene delivery for tissue repair [35].

Factors that affect drug release from MN formulations include polymer–drug interactions, polymer surface properties, and the porosity of the dry materials [52]. Drug release from dissolving MN formulations in particular therefore have been manipulated by the polymers used in fabrication. Often, water-soluble polysaccharides and similar compounds, e.g., sodium chondroitin sulfate (SCS), PVP, hyaluronic acid (HA), dextran, hydroxypropyl methylcellulose (HPMC), HPC, CMC, and amylopectin, are used in instant-release MN formulations [14, 53–55].

Thus, instant drug release from MNs may be considered beneficial for the treatment of various diseases, where the general advantages of MN treatment over other transdermal or intradermal devices will be of benefit. To overcome limitations of current dihydroergotamine mesylate (for acute migraine) formulations, such as pain, adverse side effects, and poor bioavailability, a dissolving MN system was utilized. The patches dissolved in two minutes within porcine skin and gave 97% bioavailability. Ito et al. developed a two-layered (dextran MN and hyaluronate MN) dissolving MN system for the delivery of sumatriptan in rats. The bioavailabilities of sumatriptan from the dissolving MNs were calculated as $100.7 \pm 18.8\%$ for hyaluronate MNs and $93.6 \pm 10.2\%$ for dextran MNs, with a release time of 30 minutes. Successful delivery of ibuprofen incorporated into dissolving MNs was demonstrated by McCrudden et al. [56]. C_{max} was achieved after four hours (339 µg/mL), approximately 26 times greater than the human therapeutic plasma level. Chen et al. formulated dissolving MNs for the delivery of meloxicam *in vitro*. Drug was rapidly released from the MNs (91.72% within 30 minutes) and gave a bioavailability of 122.3%.

Pain relief and reduced inflammation are not the only targets of instant-release MNs. For example, bleomycin, a potent wart treatment, is mostly delivered through intralesional injection. Lee et al. fabricated PVA MNs to make the treatment more patient friendly and found that >80% of the drug dissolved within 15 minutes [57]. Pamornapathomkul et al. fabricated acyclovir-containing dissolving MNs for the treatment of herpes labialis, as traditional therapy is limited by low skin permeability and poor efficacy. The MNs dissolved within 15 minutes when applied *in vivo* to mice, and the resulting skin permeation was approximately 45 times higher than a commercial cream formulation [58]. Qui et al. used artemether as a model drug to demonstrate drug delivery capabilities of dissolving MNs in mice. The maximum amount of artemether delivered into skin was 72.67 ± 2.69% of the initial dose loaded into the dissolving MNs, the same dose effect *in vivo* as IM injection. Peak plasma levels were achieved within five hours (600 µg loaded artemether MNs).

The treatment and management of diabetes has also been a target for MNs. While most studies have focused on delivery of insulin for extended periods in the hope that this will reduce the requirement for multiple daily subcutaneous (SC) injections, few studies have focused on rapid insulin release. Rapid insulin delivery may still be a requirement for certain insulin regimens, for example, short-acting insulins may be given before each meal when a glucose spike is anticipated [59]. Liu et al. encapsulated Exendin-4 into dissolvable MNs and found the majority of the drug (90%) was released from the dissolved MNs within five minutes. Insulin secretion was enhanced after application of exendin-4 tip-loaded MN arrays, and these effects were comparable to those after SC injection of exendin-4, with C_{max} achieved at 15 minutes [54]. Yang et al. [60] delivered insulin using hydrogel-forming MNs *in vitro* using porcine skin and found 30% of the total insulin load was released within the initial 30 minutes. This was followed by an additional 26% of the loaded cargo being released within four hours of patch application.

Rapid drug release has also been shown for recombinant human growth hormone (rhGH) and desmopressin [61], vitamin K for bleeding [62], and lidocaine for rapid analgesia [63].

39.3.3 DELIVERY OF PROTEIN- AND PEPTIDE-BASED THERAPIES USING MNs

Advances in biotechnology have led to the successful creation of numerous types of therapeutic proteins and peptides. Due to their high specificity and potency, these biotherapeutics are considered the most effective options for chronic diseases such as diabetes, cancer, dwarfism, hepatitis, and rheumatoid arthritis [64–67]. However, the rise of biotechnology as a tool to generate protein- and peptide-based therapeutics has far outpaced the development of delivery technologies. At present, these biomolecules are primarily administered via the parenteral route. This is due, in part, to their high MW, poor tissue permeability, and rapid degradation in the bloodstream [68]. However, it is well known that hypodermic injections induce pain, needle phobia, hypersensitivity, and lipohypertrophy [69]. This can result in reduced compliance and the need for medical supervision. Improper needle practices and disposal can also increase the risk of bloodborne pathogen transmission [70]. As a result, MN-mediated protein and peptide delivery has the potential to improve compliance, enhance safety, decrease costs, and reduce pain, as discussed next.

McAllister et al. fabricated solid silicon MNs to facilitate the delivery of insulin and BSA across human skin *in vitro*. Permeation of the two compounds was successful, with the concentration of insulin delivered across the skin from a 1 cm² patch containing 100 units/mL deemed sufficient to meet the basal needs of many diabetics. In a bid to improve the commercial viability of a solid MN device for the delivery of insulin, Li et al. used a thermal micromolding technique to create a biodegradable solid MN composed of PLA. Using the "poke and patch" technique in diabetic mice, blood glucose levels were reduced to 29% of the initial level at 5 hours, while for the SC injection, the blood glucose decreased rapidly to 19% after 1.5 hours, before gradually increasing to 100% after a further 1.5 hours.

By design, coated MNs have restricted drug loading, with approximately 1 mg available on the needle surface [71, 72]. For this reason, this MN design has been exploited for the transdermal delivery of potent macromolecules such as vaccines, proteins, peptides, and DNA [73–77]. Using Macroflux technology, Cormier et al. administered desmopressin, a potent synthetic peptide hormone indicated for enuresis in children and diabetes insipidus. In this proof-of-concept study, desmopressin was coated onto the tips of MNs in 2 cm² arrays and applied to the skin of hairless guinea pigs [36]. Pharmacologically relevant amounts of the peptide were delivered after five minutes [36]. In 2007, Macroflux Corporation changed their company name to Zosano Pharma, Inc. Since then, Zosano Pharma has been using a drug-coated titanium MN array and a handheld, reusable applicator on several different therapeutic candidates. The first clinical trial using this MN device was for the delivery of parathyroid hormone (PTH), indicated for the treatment of osteoporosis [78]. In phase 1 clinical studies, MN-mediated delivery demonstrated that irrespective of the application site, there was a rapid peak in plasma levels, with a T_{max} three times faster than FORTEO® the subcutaneously administered comparator. In phase 2, 20, 30, and 40 µg doses of PTH showed a proportional increase in plasma concentration in postmenopausal women with osteoporosis. Despite these promising results, Zosano halted the development of this PTH patch in 2015 due to regulatory issues in Japan.

In contrast to solid and coated MNs, hollow MNs are capable of delivering large quantities of pharmaceuticals either by diffusion or pressure-driven flow (Figure 39.2C) [79]. In some cases, hollow MNs can deliver their payload faster than SC injection, with the additional possibility of lymphatic targeting. Davis et al. used an array consisting of 16 hollow needles, 500 µm in length and a 75 µm tip diameter to deliver insulin as a model compound. Blood glucose levels dropped steadily over four hours to 47% of the initial level, which was then maintained for a further four hours [80].

Hollow MNs have also been tested as a means of targeting the lymphatic system. Using a delivery device consisting of three 1-mm 34G steel needles and a fluid disrupting hub, Harvey et al. examined the pharmacokinetics of etanercept (132 kDa) and somatropin (22 kDa). To control drug delivery rate and volume, these MN injections contained a syringe pump. The delivery of both proteins using MNs resulted in rapid lymphatic uptake and faster systemic availability compared to SC delivery. No lymphatic uptake was seen in the SC injection; instead, the dye was localized at the injection site. The authors concluded that these properties can provide an additional benefit in regimens such as hormone replacement or pain relief, where a rapid pharmacokinetic profile is required, or in cases where direct lymphatic targeting would be valuable, such as cancer therapy and diagnostic imaging [17].

Despite the commercial success of Soluvia and MicronJet600, there has been a conscious effort in recent years to move away from metals, silicon, and glass, instead focusing on biocompatible FDA-approved materials, discussed further in Section 39.7.1. This has resulted in the development of polymeric dissolving MNs, which encapsulate the drug within the needle formulation itself (Figure 39.2D). Importantly, polymeric materials are generally inexpensive and can be manipulated at ambient temperatures, thus facilitating the formulation of heat-labile drug compounds, such as peptides and proteins. In particular, dissolving MNs have been shown to enhance the transdermal delivery of insulin [81, 82], sulforhodamine B [83], low-MW heparin [84], ovalbumin [85–87], and a variety of vaccine antigens [88]. Despite this, previous studies have shown the difficulty in delivering large biomolecules from the entirety of the array, with delivery often limited to the drug loaded in the needles [85, 89]. This has resulted in two-step manufacturing processes in which the biomolecule is only housed within the needles themselves. Ling et al. developed a dissolving bilayer MN patch composed of starch and gelatin, which contained insulin-loaded needles and a drug-free baseplate. Importantly, insulin maintained its pharmacological activity after encapsulation and release from the MNs [90]. Pharmacokinetic and pharmacodynamic results showed a similar hypoglycaemic effect in rats receiving insulin-loaded MNs and a SC injection [90]. More recently, Chen et al. developed a dissolving MN for the intradermal delivery of interferon-α-2b (IFN). This fabrication process involved a two-solution system, with a PVP baseplate, upon which chondroitin sulfate and IFN MN tips were fixed [91]. *In vivo* pharmacokinetics in rats showed that MNs and an IM injection were bioequivalent. Furthermore, IFN remained stable at various temperatures and was applied safely [91]. This proves that dissolving MNs have the ability to deliver clinically relevant doses of biotherapeutics; however, their long-term stability in a polymeric formulation still requires further investigation.

To overcome the challenges of drug loading in other MN types, self-disabling hydrogel-forming MNs have been developed (Figure 39.2E). This particular MN type consists of drug-free micronscale needles situated in perpendicular orientation on a base plate to which a separate drug containing reservoir is attached. As a result, drug loading is no longer restricted, a considerable drawback with dissolving and coated MNs. For this reason, hydrogel-forming MNs have successfully delivered high doses of peptide- and protein-based molecules [47]. In particular, delivery of insulin from a 600 μm height, 19×19 MN resulted in blood glucose reduction to 90% of its original value in diabetic rats two hours after MN application [47]. Blood glucose levels fell further to 37% by the end of the 12-hour experimental period. In the same study, FITC-BSA plasma concentrations of 0.82 μg/mL and 8.86 μg/mL were registered after a MN application time of 2 and 12 hours, respectively, demonstrating the ability to achieve sustained delivery with this MN design.

With mAbs dominating the pharmaceutical market for several years now, the limited number of studies testing their MN-mediated delivery appears somewhat surprising. Addressing this perception, Courtenay et al. detailed, for the first time, the transdermal delivery of bevacizumab, an anticancer mAb, using both dissolving and hydrogel-forming MNs. It was observed that dissolving MNs produced a higher C_{max} at a faster rate (488.7 ng/mL at 6 hours) compared to hydrogel-forming MNs (81.2 ng/mL and 358.2 ng/mL at 48 hours for the hydrogel-forming MNs containing 5 mg and 10 mg of bevacizumab, respectively) [51]. In comparison to the IV control, the transdermal options did not provide equivalent circulating serum concentrations. One possibility is the drainage of bevacizumab into the lymphatic fluid, rather than permeating directly into the bloodstream [51]. Although further testing is required, MN-mediated delivery of bevacizumab could be used for the treatment of lymphoma carcinoma or secondary metastasis. In addition, as *in vivo* experiments were conducted using 0.5 cm² MN arrays, there is much scope for patch scale-up, as previous studies have shown that human patch sizes up to 30 cm² can be still be easily applied [51]. Although hydrogel-forming MNs are still in the early stages of development, with further optimization, it is still conceivable that this MN design can achieve clinically effective doses of high MW biotherapeutics, such as mAbs.

39.4 MN-MEDIATED VACCINE DELIVERY

The ability to vaccinate a population may be considered one of the most important, cost-effective, and successful public health interventions worldwide for the prevention of infectious diseases. A vaccine can be defined as "a biological preparation that improves immunity to a particular disease" [92] via imitation of the particular disease, instigating the production of T lymphocytes and antibodies but without the associated illness. The need for effective vaccination strategies is more apparent than ever before, given the increasing number of global pandemics, including severe acute respiratory syndrome (SARS) in 2003, the influenza H1N1 outbreak in 2009, and the coronavirus COVID-19 pandemic in 2020. Furthermore, an increasing fear of vaccinations has resulted in outbreaks of diseases that were once thought on the cusp of eradication, such as measles [93].

Traditionally, vaccines are delivered into the muscle or SC tissue via a hypodermic needle injection. Although universally successful in providing immunity against certain diseases, the injection is invasive and painful, and there is the potential for inappropriate reuse of equipment, particularly in developing countries. This may increase the risk of transmission of bloodborne pathogens. In addition, the use and disposal of needles are associated with the risk of needle stick injuries. An estimated 3 million health care workers worldwide are injured annually with a sharp object contaminated with the hepatitis C virus, hepatitis B virus, or HIV [94, 95].

An alternative to IM or SC injections is intradermal delivery of vaccines. The primary advantage of such a technique is the multiplicity of epidermal Langerhans cells and dermal dendritic cells [96, 97], which may allow for a greater immune response from a lower dose of vaccine [98]. Vaccination using MNs is particularly appealing because it offers the potential for painless, "needle-free" vaccination (via the use of dissolving or hydrogel-forming MNs, Figure 39.2E). Ideally, the production, transport, storage, and administration of vaccines should not be more costly than those that are currently available [92]. The use of inexpensive, widely available polymers in certain MN types allows MNs to be fabricated at a low cost on a large scale [9, 23, 99]. There has been a large amount of research pertaining to the removal of the "cold chain" through vaccine-MN manufacturing, which would result in huge cost savings if accomplished [100, 101]. These advantages are in addition to the expected advantages of MNs compared to other delivery routes previously discussed in Section 39.1.

Dissolving MNs are one of the most widely explored MN types for delivery of vaccines due to their inherent self-disabling nature. They have been explored as delivery devices for numerous vaccines against bacteria such as tetanus [88, 102] and viruses, such as influenza, polio, measles, HIV, and enterovirus [103–108]. In 2017, researchers from Emory University published results from a phase 1 clinical trial investigating the use of dissolving MNs to deliver the influenza vaccine [109]. Robust antibody responses were generated from the use of MNs containing the vaccine, and participants preferred MNs than the traditional IM injection, implying knock-on benefits in increasing acceptability of MN devices and concurrently increasing influenza vaccination rates. This is supported by a study that examined the use of a hyaluronic MN device in humans (MicroHyala) [110]. Volunteers showed no signs of severe local or systemic reactions.

Studies have demonstrated that a vaccine incorporated in MNs is able to retain its potency when stored at elevated temperatures [100, 101, 105, 111]. One of the more thorough studies [100] demonstrated that the influenza vaccine, incorporated into optimized dissolving MN arrays, remained stable after exposure to various conditions: 25°C, 24 months; 60°C, 4 months; five freeze–thaw cycles; or sterilization irradiation via electron beam. These studies clearly demonstrate the potential for MN-based vaccines to be used for seasonal and pandemic vaccination needs and for use in third world countries, where access to suitable storage facilities may be scarce.

To enable more controlled and efficient delivery, coated MNs have been extensively studied for vaccination purposes. Coating MNs has been a particularly popular method of vaccine delivery because the process of coating is not dissimilar to long-standing techniques such as spray coating [112, 113] and repeated dip coating [91, 114, 115]. Furthermore, only a small amount of vaccine is required to illicit an immune response; thus, the reported disadvantage of coated MNs (i.e., the small amount of drug able to be delivered) no longer applies. Influenza continues to be a popular target for vaccination using coated MNs [116–119]. Of upmost importance is ensuring the formulation used to coat the MNs does not reduce the activity of the vaccine [120]. For example, the presence of CMC in a coated MN formulation was found to contribute to the reduction of influenza vaccine activity to 2%. The addition of trehalose to the coating formulation was found to protect the antigen and retain 48% to 82% of antigen activity for all three major strains of seasonal influenza: H1N1, H3N2, and B [76]. Coated MN vaccine studies are not limited to the influenza [121–123], and numerous studies have utilized coated MNs to demonstrate equivalent antibody levels between the device and a traditional SC or IM injection [124–126]. Furthermore, delivery of vaccines using MNs is not limited to the skin, with several studies investigating vaccine delivery to the oral mucosa [127–130].

Vaccine delivery through a hollow MN could be seen to emulate the Mantoux technique (dermal needle technique based on shallow-angle needle insertion), which has produced inconsistent dermal cellular responses in some studies [131, 132]. Though hollow MNs have not induced the same wealth of published studies as their dissolving and coated counterparts, successful studies have been published [133–136], particularly those that have successfully demonstrated dose reduction. For example, hollow MN studies with anthrax vaccination in rabbit models showed the potential for an up to fiftyfold vaccine dose reduction [137, 138]. Hollow MNs were inserted perpendicularly to the skin surface of rats to control the dermal depth of needle penetration for influenza vaccine delivery. Intradermal delivery of the whole inactivated virus provided up to 100-fold dose-sparing compared with IM injection [139]. Similarly, a 2010 study effectively demonstrated that intradermal delivery of a rabies vaccine (combined with a Becton Dickinson skin abrader) at a quarter of the IM dose was enough to demonstrate adequate immune efficacy. The epidermal delivery route did not produce an immune response against the rabies vaccine [140].

The use of "poke and patch" techniques (Figure 39.2A) has mostly been replaced by more sophisticated MN devices. For example, it was demonstrated that antigen-coated, pH-sensitive MNs were superior to a poke and patch approach in terms of antigen-specific CD4+ and CD8+ T-cell responses [141]. Nonetheless, many studies using this technique have focused on delivery of diphtheria vaccine. In diphtheria toxoid intradermal immunization, MN array pretreatment of the skin was essential to achieve substantial IgG and toxin-neutralizing antibody titres [142]. Studies have also focused on adjuvants administered alongside the diphtheria toxoid vaccine and concluded that the potency and quality of the immune response can be modulated by the presence of adjuvants [143, 144].

MN-based systems, specifically dissolving MNs, appear to have huge potential for vaccine delivery. Many studies demonstrate dose-sparing effects compared to traditional vaccine administration routes, and the ability to formulate vaccines in the dry state could save huge amounts of money, as well as benefitting developing countries. Studies have demonstrated that studies are moving past "proof of concept" stages and into clinical trials [109, 145, 146]. If the maintenance of vaccine component stability can be assured, it is likely that a MN-based vaccine device will soon be available to use clinically as an alternative to traditional vaccine delivery methods.

39.5   MNs FOR COSMETIC APPLICATIONS

Skin health is affected by many factors such as lifestyle, genetics, hormones, nutrition, and aging [147]. Skin blemishes, be they wrinkling, stretching, or scarring, regardless of their causation, often resulting in reduced self-confidence. Considering the importance of the latter, it is unsurprising that, fueled by the rise of social media, the global cosmetic skincare market was valued at $135 billion USD in 2018 [148]. Successful use of cosmetic MN devices to rejuvenate and treat the skin was reported in 1995, and since then, growth has been exponential [149].

The earliest record of an MN-type therapy used solely for the treatment of skin blemishes was reported by Orentreich and Orentreich in 1995 [149]. Termed "SC incisionless surgery" or "subcision," this work described the successful treatment of acne scars through the promotion of substratum collagen production by needle application as deep as the dermis layer [149]. Based on the principle of subcision and in conjunction with subsequent advancements in the field of cosmetic MN therapy, Fernandes developed the first handheld device for cosmetic microneedling in 2002 [150]. This device comprised a handle with a rotating drum-shaped head that bore outwardly protruding fine needles and was designed to be rolled over skin blemishes such as scars or wrinkles to induce the aptly named process of percutaneous collagen induction (PCI) [150]. MN-mediated PCI (Figure 39.5) occurs in two distinct steps. The first step involves the disruption of preexisting collagen fibers that tether a scar or wrinkle to the underlying dermis by controlled incisions upon needle application [150, 151]. The second step aims to heal these microscopic wounds through angiogenesis and collagenesis as part of the skin's natural posttraumatic inflammatory cascade [150, 151]. The inflammatory cascade in this case is composed of three sequential phases: (1) initiation/inflammation, (2) proliferation, and (3) remodeling. Phase 1, i.e., after MN penetration, is characterized by the recruitment of platelets, neutrophils, and macrophages that stimulate the release of growth factors, including epidermal growth factor (EGF), transforming growth factor- alpha (TGF- α), TGF- beta (- β) and platelet-derived growth factor (PDGF) [152]. Growth factor release induces fibroblast proliferation and signals the commencement of phase 2 [151, 152]. In combination with keratinocytes and monocytes, which now increasingly replace neutrophils, these fibroblasts continue to produce growth factors [151, 152]. This sustained growth factor release results in angiogenesis leading to fibronectin matrix formation. Simultaneously, collagen III and other intercellular matrix proteins, including elastin, proteoglycans, and glycosaminoglycans (GAGs), are deposited at the wound site [152]. The final phase, remodeling, is the slowest phase and in some cases can take several months to complete [152]. This phase is characterized by the conversion of collagen III to collagen I through

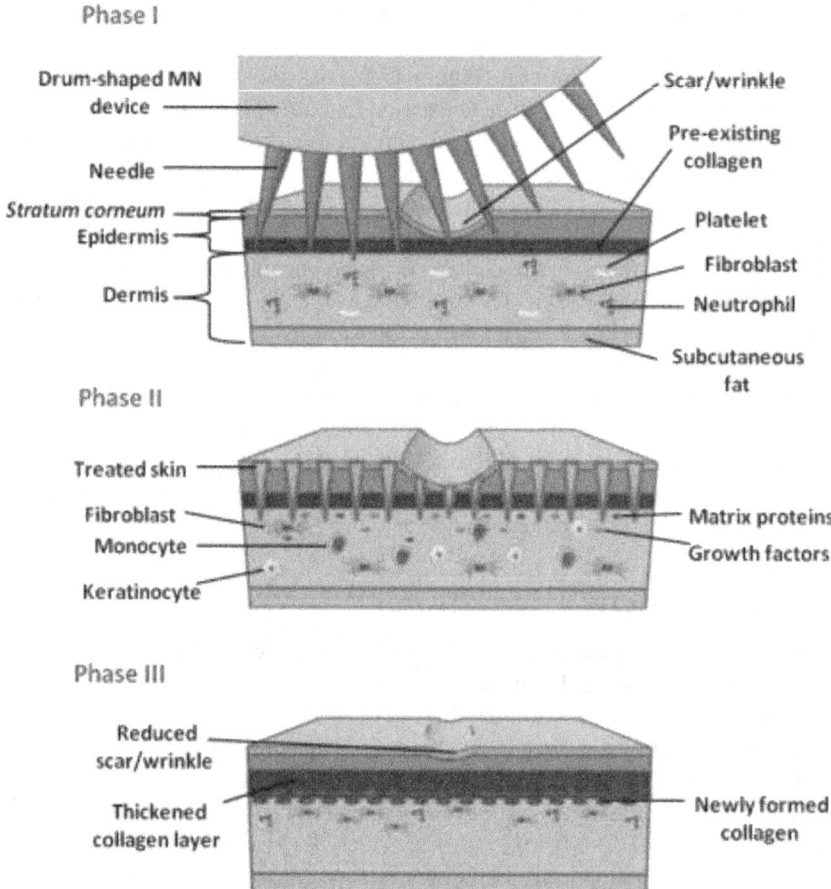

FIGURE 39.5 Schematic representation of PCI on a skin blemish using a handheld, drum-shaped device similar to that developed by Fernandes in 2002 [150–152].

tissue remodeling and vascular maturation, which results in the formation of a new, fully vascularized collagen layer and tightened skin with reduced blemish definition [152].

Microneedling in this fashion is associated with reduced disruption of skin architecture when compared to other cosmetic treatments that are highly ablative such as subcision, chemical peels, collagen injections, cortisone-like injections, cryosurgery, dermabrasion, and laser resurfacing [153]. The invasive nature of these methodologies can result in extended healing times and undesirable skin effects, including increased scarring and/or skin dyschromias (alteration in normal skin pigmentation) [154, 155]. In addition, nonablative microneedling has the advantage of being suited for delicate or hard-to-reach areas of the skin where ablative methods cannot be performed, for example, around the eyes. Currently, the most commonly used device used for cosmetic microneedling is an FDA-approved class I medical device known commercially as a Dermaroller. Based on the design first reported by Fernandes, the device is intended to be rolled across the skin, vertically, horizontally, and diagonally and, depending on the needle length used, is suitable for use in either a home or health care setting [41]. Treatment of skin aging is typically carried out using a device possessing true MNs i.e., needle height in the range of 100 to 1000 μm [156], whereas needles larger than 1000 μm, and therefore not strictly true MNs, are reserved for use by trained professionals for the treatment of scarring [156]. Subsequent modifications to the standard Dermaroller design in response to identified potential shortcomings have produced alternative forms of cosmetic microneedling devices. One such alternative is the Dermastamp (Figure 39.6), a miniaturized

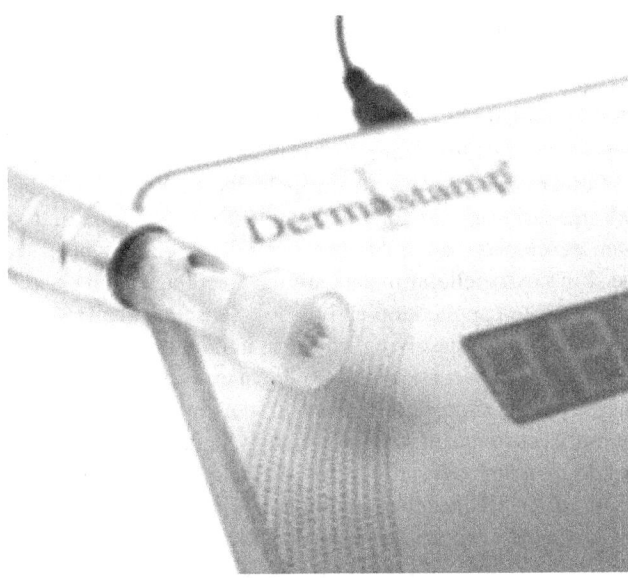

FIGURE 39.6   The Dermastamp, an example of the numerous MN devices marketed for cosmetic applications. (Reproduced with permission from [158].)

version of the Dermaroller technology. This device is designed to be applied in a vertical fashion by a trained clinician only and is highly suited for use on areas of the skin that are difficult for the conventional Dermaroller to reach [157]. Another is the Beauty Mouse, which is a computer mouse–shaped device with three separate Dermaroller heads situated on its underside. An approved medical device on the Australian Register of Therapeutic Goods (ARTG), the Beauty Mouse is designed to be used in a home care setting for the treatment of stretchmarks and cellulite over large areas of the body [157]. A further variation is the Dermapen, which is a spring-loaded oscillating MN device with the dimensions of a pen. This device is designed to overcome any issues associated with the variation in pressures applied by trained administrators, as well as being suited to use on areas of skin that are hard to reach [157]. Interestingly, a device similar in appearance to the Dermapen, known commercially as the INTRAcel, utilizes fractional radiofrequency emitted from MN tips to enhance tissue remodeling within the skin. Finally, a device comparable to the Dermaroller but with the addition of photodynamic therapy (PDT) (LED light emitted from MN tips) is commercially available for the treatment of skin aging.

In a similar fashion to the MN-mediated delivery of drugs not intended for cosmetic purposes, MN technology can be used to deliver many cosmeceutical agents. Leading on from the combination of MNs with PDT, the enhanced delivery of the photosensitizing agent 5-aminolevulinic acid (5-ALA) for the treatment of actinic keratosis caused by prolonged sun exposure was demonstrated in 2010 [159]. In this instance Clementoni et al. treated the skin with a rolling MN device like those described previously and then applied an ALA solution directly to the skin, which was washed off after one hour. Treated areas were then exposed to pulsed LED red light for a defined period of time [159]. At six months posttreatment, 90% of participants judged the improvement in skin condition to be greater than 50% compared to baseline photography [159]. Pretreatment of the skin with MNs followed by application of a topical preparation (without subsequent PDT) is an uncomplicated method of enhancing the permeation of a cosmeceutical. This methodology has been used to demonstrate improved delivery of multiple cosmeceutic agents, including eflornithine to treat hirsutism and minoxidil to treat androgenic alopecia [160, 161]. The delivery of a peptide-based cosmeceutical, melanostatin, was enhanced through a similar methodology by Mohammed et al. [162]. With the level of research into MN-mediated peptide delivery increasing, it is likely that advancements in this area of cosmetic microneedling are forthcoming. Similarly, the confirmation of skin rejuvenation through the MN-mediated delivery of endothelial precursor cells derived from human embryonic stem cells by Lee et al. has accelerated interest in cosmetic stem cell treatments using MNs [163]. Although pretreatment of skin with MNs followed by topical application of an active is a simple and effective use of MNs for cosmetic therapies (Figure 39.2A), there is an inherent need for the development of other types of MNs for this field. Thus, dissolving polymeric MNs containing transexamic acid and retinoic acid for the treatment of melesama and seborrheic keratosis, respectively, have been developed [164, 165]. The naturally occurring polysaccharide, HA, which is a component of the skin's extracellular matrix similar to collagen and elastin, has been shown to facilitate skin rejuvenation when applied topically [166]. Subsequently, HA has been highlighted as a promising candidate for use in a dissolving MN formulation both as a cosmeceutic agent and as a delivery enhancer for other cosmeceutics [167–169]. An example of the improved delivery of cosmeceutic agents using HA is the successful delivery of the antiwrinkle agent ascorbic acid via dissolving HA-MNs without occurrence of skin irritation by Kim et al. [170, 171]. The first HA-based cosmetic MN product, known commercially as MicroHyala, was introduced to Japan by CosMED Pharmaceutical Co. Ltd. in 2008. Since then, multiple HA-based cosmetic MN products have made it market, namely the Acute Care patch and the K-Wrinkle patch. However, due to the lack of international harmonization on the safety of cosmetics, the level of safety assurance surrounding these products is convoluted and unclear.

39.6 MNs FOR DIAGNOSTIC TESTS AND PATIENT MONITORING

Diagnostic tests and therapeutic monitoring play an essential role in modern medicine and refer to the detection and quantification of endogenous markers or drugs in the body, most commonly in the blood, plasma, or ISF. These tests can be used for diagnostic purposes in symptomatic patients, examples of which are in suspected iron-deficiency anaemia to assess serum ferritin levels or to screen for the presence of C-reactive protein in inflammatory bowel disorders, including Crohn's disease [172–174]. Diagnostic tests can also be carried out in asymptomatic cases, such as the detection of microRNAs in early stage breast cancer [175].

In cases involving chronic disease states, diagnostics can be used to measure biological markers to track disease progression, as seen with creatinine levels in chronic kidney disease, but can also be used to give direct or indirect indications of the patient's adherence to their medication regimens [176]. In those infected with HIV, patient adherence can be indirectly tracked by using their CD4 cell count as a measure of control, with low cell counts strongly indicating a lack of compliance [177]. Directly determining the patient's concordance with their medicines with drug plasma concentrations can be particularly useful in cases concerning those drugs with a narrow therapeutic index, including antiepileptics, immunosuppressants, and digoxin, particularly in vulnerable patient groups e.g., the elderly, neonates, pediatrics, and those with psychiatric disorders [178–183]. These results can be used to evaluate the efficacy of therapy and subsequently optimize drug treatment by monitoring plasma levels of the drug or outcomes post-dose change. In high-risk drugs these monitoring requirements are often essential, particularly involving cases with warfarin and determining the international normalized ratio associated with the treatment [184]. Not only is warfarin classed as high risk but it also exhibits variances in pharmacokinetic behavior between patient groups, further highlighting the requirement for regular blood tests. Monitoring can also be used to assess the undesirable effects of treatment. An example of this is liver toxicity associated with statin drugs, requiring liver function tests to be carried out at regular intervals [185].

Although diagnostic tests have been well established for many years and play an integral role in modern medicine, they are not without drawbacks. Most of the tests require a hypodermic needle to obtain a blood sample, with the issues associated mentioned previously. Additional problems are encountered when dealing with monitoring in neonates, as they have a decreased blood volume due to a decreased body weight, and so repeated blood sampling will have a marked effect, as well as bringing about the ethical dilemma surrounding the repeated use of needles and the pain this will cause [186, 187]. Diagnostic tests usually do not give a result at the point of care, with the test often having to be sent off-site for analysis. This process could take several hours or even days, which in many cases means the patient prognosis may change dramatically, such as in severe sepsis where the most common avoidable cause of death is failure to diagnose and provide appropriate antimicrobials in time [188]. With the increase in polypharmacy, particularly in the elderly, several blood samples may be required at repeated intervals, and this repeated assault on the aging blood vessels results in further problematic sampling [189].

Minimally invasive sampling methods may use ISF as a replacement for blood, as it has been shown in some cases that concentrations in ISF can be correlated to those in whole blood [190–195]. Pharmacologically the drug in the ISF will not be plasma protein bound, and therefore any detected drug can be classed as free and active [190, 191]. Confidence in using ISF has grown in recent years, and in 2014 the FreeStyle Libre was brought to market in Sweden and subsequently the rest of Europe, measuring glucose levels in ISF in those patients with type 1 diabetes [196]. The one barrier to accessing the ISF for monitoring is the stratum corneum. Two methods in the literature of bypassing this barrier for minimally invasive sampling are microdialysis and reverse iontophoresis, though both methods are complex to set up and may still need a blood sample to calibrate the analysis [190, 191, 197]. Another method of sampling the ISF is with the use of MNs.

MNs show their versatility with a number of different designs capable of sampling ISF. Hollow MNs can be used to extract both ISF and blood, depending on needle length. The hollowed centers enable the arrays to take up fluid via capillary action [187, 198–200]. These samples can then be analyzed conventionally at a testing center, or analysis can be completed at point of care with integrated microchip biosensors [200]. Hollow MNs coupled with paper-based sensors can be used to extract blood and rapidly measure cholesterol or glucose levels, simply requiring a one-touch activation under standard finger pressure to initiate the blood extraction, serum separation, and molecule detection, with results being available in real time [201]. Alternative arrays have been developed, where the inner lumen of the MN is functionalized to bind a specific target, resulting in an efficient system with no need for sample transfer [199, 202]. This analysis can be done with as little as 1 nanolitre of ISF, which would be of great benefit for use with neonates, who have a lower comparative volume of blood but a proportionally greater volume of ISF [187, 202].

Hydrogel-forming MNs can also be used for the uptake of ISF [192, 203]. They insert as a solid MN but when introduced to the ISF they swell, trapping fluid in the polymeric hydrogel matrix. Once removed from the skin, the array can be centrifuged to recover the sample for analysis, or alternatively the array can be incorporated into a system whereby the MN array forms the bottom of a microplate which enables *in situ* analysis [203]. A hydrogel-forming system using MNs formulated from PEG-cross-linked PMVE/MA has been shown to take up, detect, and quantify drugs such as theophylline and caffeine, and while the concentrations in the ISF did show trends indicative of blood levels, the levels could not be directly correlated [187]. The same group used a similar array to determine ISF glucose concentrations following oral administration of 75 g of glucose powder, which showed correlation when compared to finger-prick blood levels [187]. Hydrogel-forming MNs have been shown to be effective in monitoring lithium levels. This has the potential to be used in outpatient lithium clinics or for home monitoring of drug levels [192]. Methacrylated hyaluronic acid–based MNs have been shown to extract ISF rapidly and without any extra devices due to its affinity for water, and so can be used for rapid metabolic analysis [204].

With all MNs, sample analysis can be completed "on-chip" (within the MN system) or "off-chip" (i.e. extracted and analyzed externally), and while an on-chip analysis is preferred for economic reasons, integrated systems have the downside of needing up to microlitre samples for analysis, which also leads to prolonged collection times and the difficulty of transferring the fluid from the needle to the "analysis" part of the array [205].

Rapid, accurate diagnosis in secondary care is required to ensure optimum patient treatment, and MNs have a role to play in this area too. PLA MNs were coated with antibodies, which when inserted into the skin, could detect a specific antigen, or antigens, alongside result validation. An additional benefit is this test can produce results in less than five hours [206]. MNs have been used to detect nitric oxide levels in the body using a dual diagnostic system of an endomicroscope and MN biosensor, giving fast and accurate diagnoses of cancer [207]. Peptide aptamer–based MNs can also be used for detection of cancer by measuring vascular endothelial growth levels (VEGF) levels in the blood [208]. Point-of-care diagnostics using disposable MNs coupled with a wristwatch-type portable analyzer can measure blood oxygen levels, or other systems can measure potassium levels using an on-chip system, both giving rapid results, which lead to increased standards of patient care [209, 210]. Alternatively, MNs can be loaded with antigens and adjuvants, such that when inserted attract specific tissue-resident immune cells which can be sampled and analyzed. Changes in antibody levels can be tracked to assess immune responses over time [211].

MNs arrays were originally developed as a method of enhancing transdermal drug delivery, and the principle can be adapted to deliver diagnostic molecules across the skin. An example is with the Mantoux test, or tuberculin skin test (TST), for tuberculosis which involves intradermally injecting tuberculin purified protein derivative (PPD) from *Mycobacterium tuberculosis* [212]. Intradermal injections are painful for the patient and difficult to perform and require adequately trained health care workers. A MN array made from chitosan and coated with the PPD was subsequently developed, with the test being simplified to simply inserting the MN under thumb pressure [213]. This enables the PPD to be delivered to the correct depth consistently, with far greater ease, and with minimal training. The TST has also been carried out using the aforementioned MicronJet600 [214]. Comparing this device to traditional hypodermic needles used in the Mantoux test showed there was no significant difference in the TST reaction rates; however, the MN device exhibited significantly less pain and no additional adverse effects due to the device [214]. Allergen testing is often performed using skin patch tests, where traditionally different allergens would be injected into the patient's skin and the reaction to each allergen assessed for hypersensitivity. Along with the disadvantages mentioned previously (Section 39.1), the test also covers a substantial area of skin, which can be unsightly and uncomfortable. MNs have the potential to overcome this. Solid MNs could be coated with the allergen of choice, or the allergen could be incorporated into a dissolving MN array [215]. Both of these methods give quick responses, and when combined with an integrated sensor, give instantaneous results [216]. In an applicator device the numerous needle heights can be adjusted to deliver the allergen to various skin depths, or a different allergen could be combined with each needle to give multiple results at once.

MNs, and in particular hydrogel-forming arrays, are self-disabling and therefore can only be single use. Continuous monitoring is an area of great interest, with blood glucose monitoring alone worth an estimated $12 billion globally in 2020, and so it is no surprise that MNs have been explored for this purpose [197]. Arrays used for continuous glucose monitoring can be formulated from hollow MNs integrated with an enzyme-based flow-through sensor to give real-time data, which is essential for blood glucose control [217]. A different group has shown their hollow needles, which are coupled to an amperometric detector, to be clinically accurate at measuring glucose levels for up to 72 hours [218]. MNs coated in platinum and silver have been used to quantify glucose levels by acting as electrodes. They have been shown to have a low limit of detection and exhibit a strong linearity with a fast readout time; however, the patch did not perform at the required level for more than four days due to biofouling [219]. Away from glucose monitoring, MNs have been developed for use as continuous monitors for alcohol in the body via enzyme-coupled arrays, as well as platinum- and gold-coated arrays for continuous monitoring of free cholesterol [220, 221]. Outside of the health care setting, continuous sweat monitoring has potential in elite athletes and sports teams. A wearable system has been developed to selectively and simultaneously measure metabolites of choice (e.g., lactate) and electrolytes (e.g., sodium), as well as pH and temperature. This device can transmit data wirelessly for real-time data analysis [222]. Other groups have explored wearable MN metabolite testing systems that would enable training programs to be tailored to, or by, each individual athlete [223, 224]. As wearable technology such as Fitbit and Apple Watch continue to grow commercially, there is potential for MNs to be incorporated into devices for everyday wear for continuous analysis, even in healthy users [225, 226]. However, the commercial potential of these wearable technologies relies on their ability to overcome potential problems, namely reliability, comfort, and cost [227].

MNs are not limited to the detection of molecules and electrolytes; they may also be used to assess electrical activity within the body. Electroencephalograms (EEGs) can assess electrical activity in the brain for diagnosis of diseases such as epilepsy or for brain imaging post–head injury. To do so, electrodes are attached to the patient, which requires extensive skin preparation, including the use of gels, and limiting the extent to which continuous monitoring can be put in place [228]. Silicon-based MN arrays can be used as "dry electrodes" with comparable results to the regular "wet electrode" [228]. MN electrodes for use in EEGs have also been successfully developed from SU-8 and have the potential to simultaneously measure other parameters, such as pH [229, 230]. MN-mediated EEGs have been shown to be painless, safe, blood-free, and with a relatively low associated cost [231]. Once a headset was designed to hold the electrode in place, the MN array was able to record brain activity for hours with very little physical or psychological stress [230]. Electric activity in other parts of the body can be analyzed too, particularly an electrocardiogram (ECG). Hollow MNs were used to lower the electrode–skin–electrode impedance, which enabled high signal-to-noise ratios [232]. However, the quality of the ECG reading greatly depends on the mechanical and temporal factors on the skin electrode surface [233].

39.7 FUTURE PERSPECTIVES FOR CLINICAL TRANSLATION AND INDUSTRIAL DEVELOPMENTS

It is clear that MNs are not limited to delivery of vaccines, as they are often portrayed, and may be soon recognized as a vital part of the global transdermal market, the value of which is expected to rise in excess of $80 billion by 2024 [234]. This continually expanding market is driven by technological advancements in transdermal drug delivery devices, particularly the third-generation technologies, such as iontophoresis, sonophoresis, and namely, MNs. MNs offer the potential to significantly increase the size of the transdermal market, with a report published in 2012 estimating the potential global market for MN-based delivery systems at just under $400 million [235].

In the past decade, there has been a substantial increase in the development of MN-based technologies, with growing interest by a number of industrial-based companies, with subsequent heavy investing in the development of such devices. Most interesting of note is Zosano Pharma, who develop transdermal delivery products based on Macroflux technology. Recently, in a move away from their initial focus on delivery of PTH for the management of postmenopausal osteoporosis, Zosano has recently announced successful results of a double-blind, placebo-controlled clinical trial focused on the delivery of zolmitriptan for the treatment of migraines using their Adhesive Dermally Applied Microarray intracutaneous system [236]. Previous technologies discussed in this chapter, such as Nanopass Technologies' MicronJet600 and Beckton-Dickonson's Soluvia, have been marketed successfully. However, these devices are based on silicon and metal MNs, respectively, and such materials employed in their design are subject to shortcomings, particularly silicon, which is not biodegradable and consequently prone to biofouling when implanted, with subsequent related skin problems [237]. Further concerns are poised as a result of inappropriate disposal of silicon or metal, which remain intact post–MN removal, which in turn has led most in the field to focus on MNs composed of FDA-approved biocompatible polymeric materials [238]. Initially, the hot polymer and carbohydrate melts used to make second-generation MNs resulted in the breakdown of biologics during fabrication [32]. Accordingly, the majority of recent research has focused on dissolving or hydrogel-forming MNs prepared from aqueous polymer blends [47, 56]. As such, the introduction of biocompatible polymeric MN devices has introduced a new era in the development of MN technology research, overcoming a number of limitations of previous MN designs. Thus, these technologies are envisaged to receive increased attention from pharma companies in the near future, principally due to the self-disabling nature of such systems. As illustrated in Figure 39.2D and E, these MNs will either dissolve or swell upon contact with the ISF, thus upon removal, insertion into another patient is practically impossible. Therefore, this will reduce transmission of infection by further preventing needle stick injuries associated with conventional needles. Disposal issues will also be avoided, as no "sharps" waste will be generated. These particular benefits could significantly affect health care in the developing world. Promisingly, the Prausnitz Group recently reported in 2017 the first successful partly blinded, placebo-controlled clinical trial of a dissolving MN vaccine patch for the prevention of seasonal influenza [109].

39.7.1 PRESCRIBER/PATIENT ACCEPTANCE OF MICRONEEDLES

As the body of literature supporting the use of MNs as a successful drug delivery platform to achieve clinically relevant applications continues to grow, the commercialization of a "true" MN product has come within reach. However, as with all novel medical devices, a number of barriers must be overcome prior to a MN-based product's successful implementation to market. It is now well recognized in modern health care settings that the input of the end user in the early development stage of new interventions cannot be underestimated. Such involvement, or lack thereof, can directly determine the success of a new device or innovation. Whether MN-based products are ultimately a commercial success will depend not only upon their ability to perform as designed but also their acceptability to patients and clinicians who administer them; therefore, these stakeholders should be included in the design process from the outset. The first study to gain an insight into end-user perspectives surrounding MN technology was conducted in 2011 by Birchall et al. [239], gathering views and opinions of the general public and health care professionals through mixed methods of focus groups and quantitative questionnaires. Participants of the preliminary study responded positively to the idea of MNs, highlighting key benefits such as reduced fear, pain, and needle stick injuries; increased acceptability by those affected by needle phobia; and the potential for self-administration. Potential concerns of the device such as effectiveness and how a patient would know the device had been applied properly were raised.

Mooney et al. used focus groups to explore children's views on MNs as an approach to drug delivery, but also for their potential role in monitoring purposes [240]. From the study, it was evident that children displayed disapproval of conventional blood sample means by needle and syringe, with pain, blood, and the imagery of traditional needle and syringes being particularly unfavorable aspects. In general, children displayed much greater acceptance of MNs upon visual examination and agreement that the device induced less fear compared to conventional hypodermic injection. Children highlighted some possible concerns, including potential allergy and potential inaccuracies in the measurements obtained by this novel technique; however, they further stated that such concerns would no longer be apparent upon receiving reassurance by their health care professional's approval and confidence in the novel method. Patient education and counseling were considered key for acceptance of this novel approach and highlighted the need for an alternative name, removing any reference to "needle" in the title due to the negative connotations associated with that term. The study concluded the need for proactive motivation to integrate end-user perspectives in the early stages of MN array design and development to meet the unique needs of this end-user group.

As possible prescribers for future MN-based systems, pediatricians are also key potential end users. The views of UK-based pediatricians by means of an online survey were investigated surrounding the potential use of MN technology within neonatal and paediatric care, particularly for MN-mediated monitoring [241]. Paediatricians widely agreed that an alternative monitoring technique to blood sampling in children was required. Furthermore, 83% of respondents believed there was a particular need in premature neonates. The consensus from this potential end-user group was overall positive in favor of MN technology and a MN-mediated monitoring approach. The findings of this study provide an initial indication of MN acceptability among a key potential end-user group. Furthermore, the concerns identified present a challenge to those working within the MN field to provide solutions to further improve this technology.

Elderly patients are suggested as another key demographic to avail of the benefits of MN technology, with this population receiving the majority of prescription medicines worldwide. Quinn et al. considered the use of MNs in those aged over 65 years, investigating the variability of insertion into aging skin, together with the practicality and acceptability of the novel technology [242]. As part of the study, seven subjects over the age of 65 years were asked to apply hydrogel-forming MNs (devoid of drug) to their ventral forearms, and breach of the stratum corneum layer was confirmed by optical coherence tomography. Insertion depths recorded in each case were similar to a comparative group, aged 20 to 30 years. However, skin recovery occurred at a slower rate in the older subjects, as measured using transepidermal water loss. The overall impression of MN technology in the elderly focus groups was positive, with participants from both groups identifying various benefits to MN-mediated drug delivery, such as the potential for controlled release resulting in reduced dosing frequency with subsequent improved adherence and, additionally, as an alternative route of delivery where oral or injectable medication was impractical. As in previous studies, concerns surrounding the technology were also raised, focused in this instance predominantly around practical issues associated with age-related functional decline, including reduced dexterity and changes in skin condition. Interestingly, despite an acknowledgement of the key benefits of the technology, a reluctance to change from their established conventional therapy was highlighted, which could present a potential barrier for successful implementation of MNs in place of existing therapy of other chronic conditions.

Qualitative studies such as those discussed here demonstrate the complex and multifaceted nature of end-user acceptance. Thus, when appropriately planned to capture the necessary demographics, these will undoubtedly aid the industry in taking the necessary action to address concerns and develop informative labeling and patient counseling strategies to ensure safe and effective use of MN-based devices. Marketing strategies will also be vital in achieving maximum market share relative to existing and widely accepted conventional delivery systems.

Previous studies have shown that patients can successfully apply MNs to their own skin following instruction provided by pharmacist counseling in conjunction with a patient information leaflet (PIL) [7]. However, in order to gain acceptance with regulatory bodies, and in parallel with this work, both the FDA and the UK's Medicines and Healthcare Products Regulatory Agency (MHRA) have specified the need for a method of confirmation that correct MN application has been achieved. One way in which this could be addressed is through visual feedback mechanisms incorporated within the MN design. The use of a pressure-sensitive film has been employed to inform volunteers whether or not they had applied an appropriate amount of pressure to successfully insert an MN into their own skin [8]. Despite this reassurance from both academic and clinical settings, substantial marketing and public education may be required with regard to the use and safety of such novel technology in order for it to be widely accepted as a self-administration device. Consideration must also be afforded to the packaging of MN-based products to ensure the items are suitably protected in transport, the product as a whole is patient friendly, easy to use, and can be easily disposed of. The packaging should provide mechanical protection and may also need to provide moisture and light protection if the MN system contains drug or excipients subject to degradation.

39.7.2 PATIENT SAFETY

Further long-standing regulatory guideline concerns pertaining to patient safety require addressing. The skin is resident to an abundance of antigen-presenting cells; therefore, it is crucial that the MN-mediated intradermal delivery of biomolecules does not unintentionally elicit immune responses to nonvaccine biological agents, such as insulin. Additionally, it is vital that the materials and formulation excipients utilized in the fabrication of MNs does not result in any local or systemic adverse reactions. However, while mild erythema is common with traditional transdermal patches, it still may be cause of concern to patients post–MN removal; therefore, patient education may be essential to ensure awareness that full recovery of skin barrier function will occur within a matter of hours and any reddening of the skin will similarly be transient, regardless of how long the MNs are in place [237]. Furthermore, it is highly unlikely that MNs would ever be applied to exactly the same position on the skin's surface due to the small size of the microprojections, and therefore it is likely that MN-based systems will have favorable safety profiles, especially in comparison to that of conventional hypodermic needles. Currently, polymeric MN-based systems are gathering attention within research and industry, and subsequently in relation to patient safety, deposition of polymer within human skin from dissolving MNs, and to a lesser extent that of hydrogel-forming MNs are of particular interest. While the majority of polymers typically employed in MN manufacture are biocompatible FDA-approved pharmaceutical excipients, such materials have never been utilized for intradermal administration. As a result, regulators may request information on if, and how much, polymer remains in the skin post–MN removal. This is unlikely to be an issue for one-off vaccine administration; however, many therapeutics currently under investigation proposed for MN-mediated delivery are for chronic conditions, thus requiring continual repeated applications. Recently, one study investigated the effect of repeat application of polymeric MNs to immuno-competent, hairless mice [243]. MNs were repeatedly applied to mice in the same application site over a number of weeks, and promisingly, over the entirety of the study duration, no detrimental effects to the integrity of skin barrier or protective function were observed. Consequently, this study provides preliminary firm evidence that warrants the assessment of repeated polymeric MN array applications in larger animal models and, ultimately, in human subjects, as recently investigated by Al-Kasasbeh et al. [244]. In this study hydrogel-forming MNs were repeatedly applied to the upper arm of 11 human volunteers aged between 24 and 39 years, over a five-day period. The safety of repeated MN application was assessed by measuring skin barrier integrity via transepidermal water loss and the presence of systemic inflammatory biomarkers (C-reactive protein, interleukin 1-β, tumor necrosis factor-α, immunoglobulin G, and immunoglobulin E) via blood sampling. The results demonstrated that repeat hydrogel-forming MN application does not lead to prolonged skin reactions or prolonged disruption of skin barrier function. Furthermore, concentrations of systemic inflammation biomarkers were all found to be within the normal range. These results provide some positive preliminary evidence of longer-term polymeric MN safety for regulators, though future studies will likely be required with a greater experiment duration to fully appease regulators.

The development of local skin and systemic infection as a result of possible microbial infiltration through transient micropores created following MN application presents another concern. The risk of infection as a result of microbial infiltration into the skin following MN application has been proven to be negligible [245]. The skin is an immunocompetent organ, in which large numbers of antigen-presenting cells are present; therefore, it is capable of capturing foreign microbes prior to the formation of infection should such microbes infiltrate the aqueous channels formed by MNs [246]. Reassuringly, to date, in line with these hypotheses there have been no reported cases of local or systemic infection as a result of MN application. While the current best practice for hypodermic injections involves preparation of the skin by cleansing prior to puncture, it is known that in many cases that such guidance is not strictly observed [247]. This recommended guidance may also be applied to MN application; however, ideally this would not need to be performed, as this inconvenient step adds unnecessary complexity to the process and may deter patients' acceptance of the device. As such, it will require consideration by regulatory bodies to deem the necessity of this of this cleansing step based on available evidence. Furthermore, the need for MN product sterility has been questioned. Various sterilization methods have been stipulated for solid MN products; however, their destructive nature results in detrimental effects upon MN mechanical integrity, thus affecting insertion. Such methods include e-beam, gamma irradiation, microwave radiation, and wet/dry heat sterilization. In contrast, low-dose gamma radiation has been shown to not result in significant changes to polymeric MNs' mechanical strength or swelling capacity [248]. Early negotiations between key stakeholders in academia, industry, and regulatory bodies have already begun, with it being suggested that low-bioburden manufacturing to GMP standards may be satisfactory to ensure patient safety, thus removing the need for continuous line sterile manufacturing [248].

39.7.3 Regulatory Acceptance of Microneedles

Industrialization of MN array technology has been driven principally as a result of the collaboration between key stakeholders from within the clinical, academic, and industrial settings. However, industrial scale-up of manufacturing and microfabrication processes present the largest barrier to implementation to market. Currently, MNs can be manufactured through many microfabrication methods, often requiring multiple stages. Scale-up to industrial manufacturing for mass production will require a focused strategic plan, particularly in regard to the vast number of small-scale production methods described in the literature [99]. Consequently, companies wanting to move forward with this type of MN product may need to invest substantial initial funding in order to facilitate the effective development and optimization of reliable and reproducible mass production line methods. As detailed within this chapter, MNs have been tested for diagnostic fluid sampling. Perhaps, with further optimization, an MN sampling device could be used in the diagnosis of viral infections and, as a result, prove instrumental in the fight against future pandemics. As this MN design could be CE marked as a medical device rather than a drug product, reduced regulatory requirements could mean that pharmaceutical companies may be willing to invest in such a device prior to investing in a drug containing an MN product. Importantly, the initial up-front costs of scaled-up manufacture could be offset by achieving faster market commercialization. As a result, the infrastructure would be in place for the future manufacture of drug-containing MNs.

In addition, robust guidance is needed in order to fully classify MN-based products; however, it has been suggested that they will likely fall under the medical device category for monitoring/diagnostic applications, and as a "combination product" (drug and device) or "drug product" for the delivery of drugs or vaccines [181, 249]. Once this distinction is clarified, this may allow for the adaptation of current quality control methods that will be needed for MNs, as traditional methods of quality control may not be entirely suited to MN products, as they are inherently different from both transdermal patches and hypodermic needles. Further classification of MNs with respect to if they are a transdermal or intradermal product may hold key answers to how MNs will be produced and the minimum GMP standards required. These questions may only be answered upon retrospective analysis of postmarketing surveillance findings. However, until then, both industrial and academia must strive to provide practical and appropriate solutions to address such issues in order to drive MN technology successfully from bench to bedside.

Though there are currently reasonable barriers to the translation of MNs to the clinic, studies which focus on collaboration between academia, industry, health care professionals, and patients have begun to address and provide answers to the concerns discussed earlier. The results from these studies cautiously suggest that with the appropriate education, MNs are an attractive drug delivery device for both prescribers and patients [7, 239, 241, 242], with favorable safety profiles [243–245], which have the potential to be manufactured on a large scale [250]. If all remaining concerns can be suitably addressed to meet the needs of both regulators and patients, the goal of bringing an MN-based product to the transdermal market will soon become a reality.

REFERENCES

[1] Dharadhar S, Majumdar A, Dhoble S, Patravale V. Microneedles for transdermal drug delivery: a systematic review. Drug Dev Ind Pharm 2019;45:188–201.
[2] Donnelly RF, Singh TRR, Morrow DIJ, Woolfson AD. Microneedle-Mediated Transdermal and Intradermal Drug Delivery. Chichester: John Wiley & Sons; 2012.
[3] McConville A, Hegarty C, Davis J. Mini-review: Assessing the potential impact of microneedle technologies on home healthcare applications. Medicines 2018;5:50.
[4] Gerstel MS, Place VA. Drug delivery device. US3964482A 1971.
[5] Henry S, McAllister DV, Allen MG, Prausnitz MR. Microfabricated microneedles: A novel approach to transdermal drug delivery. J Pharm Sci 1998;87:922–5.
[6] Donnelly RF, Singh TRR, Tunney MM, Morrow DIJ, McCarron PA, O'Mahony C, et al. Microneedle arrays allow lower microbial penetration than hypodermic needles in vitro. Pharm Res 2009;26:2513–22.

[7] Donnelly RF, Moffatt K, Alkilani AZ, Vicente-Pérez EM, Barry J, McCrudden MTC, et al. Hydrogel-forming microneedle arrays can be effectively inserted in skin by self-application: A pilot study centred on pharmacist intervention and a patient information leaflet. Pharm Res 2014;31:1989–99.

[8] Vicente-Pérez EM, Quinn HL, McAlister E, O'Neill S, Hanna L-A, Barry JG, et al. The use of a pressure-indicating sensor film to provide feedback upon hydrogel-forming microneedle array self-application in vivo. Pharm Res 2016;33:3072–80.

[9] Larrañeta E, Lutton REM, Woolfson AD, Donnelly RF. Microneedle arrays as transdermal and intra-dermal drug delivery systems: Materials science, manufacture and commercial development. Mater Sci Eng R Reports 2016;104:1–32.

[10] van der Maaden K, Jiskoot W, Bouwstra J. Microneedle technologies for (trans)dermal drug and vaccine delivery. J Control Release 2012;161:645–55.

[11] Ita K. Transdermal delivery of drugs with microneedles—Potential and challenges. Pharmaceutics 2015;7:90–105.

[12] Dang N, Liu TY, Prow TW. Nano- and microtechnology in skin delivery of vaccines. In: Skwarczynski M, Toth I, editors. Micro Nanotechnology in Vaccine Development. Oxford: Elsevier; 2017, p. 327–41.

[13] Roxhed N, Samel B, Nordquist L, Griss P, Stemme G. Painless drug delivery through microneedle-based transdermal patches featuring active infusion. IEEE Trans Biomed Eng 2008;55:1063–71.

[14] Tuan-Mahmood TM, McCrudden MTC, Torrisi BM, McAlister E, Garland MJ, Singh TRR, et al. Microneedles for intradermal and transdermal drug delivery. Eur J Pharm Sci 2013;50:623–37.

[15] Gardeniers JGE, Luttge R, Berenschot EJW, de Boer MJ, Yeshurun SY, Hefetz M, et al. Silicon micromachined hollow microneedles for transdermal liquid transport. J Microelectromechanical Syst 2003;12:855–62.

[16] Gupta J, Felner EI, Prausnitz MR. Minimally invasive insulin delivery in subjects with type 1 diabetes using hollow microneedles. Diabetes Technol Ther 2009;11:329–37.

[17] Harvey AJ, Kaestner SA, Sutter DE, Harvey NG, Mikszta JA, Pettis RJ. Microneedle-based intra-dermal delivery enables rapid lymphatic uptake and distribution of protein drugs. Pharm Res 2011;28:107–16.

[18] Quinn HL, Donnelly RF. Microneedle-mediated drug delivery. In: Donnelly RF, Singh TRR, Larrañeta E, McCrudden, ME, editors. Microneedles in Drug and Vaccine Delivery and Patient Monitoring. Chichester: John Wiley & Sons; 2018, p. 71–91.

[19] Donnelly RF, McCrudden MTC, Alkilani AZ, Larrañeta E, McAlister E, Courtenay AJ, et al. Hydrogel-forming microneedles prepared from "super swelling" polymers combined with lyophilised wafers for transdermal drug delivery. PLoS One 2014;9:111547.

[20] Badilescu S, Packirisamy M. BioMEMS: Science and engineering perspectives. Boca Raton: CRC Press, Taylor & Francis; 2011.

[21] Millard DR, Maisels DO. Silicon granuloma of the skin and subcutaneous tissues. Am J Surg 1966;112:119–23.

[22] Banks D. Microengineering, MEMS, and interfacing: A practical guide. Boca Raton: CRC Press, Taylor & Francis; 2006.

[23] Donnelly RF, Singh TRR, Woolfson AD. Microneedle-based drug delivery systems: Microfabrication, drug delivery, and safety. Drug Deliv 2010;17:187–207.

[24] Donnelly RF, Singh RT., Larrañeta E, McCrudden MTC. Microneedles for drug and vaccine delivery and patient monitoring. Chichester: John Wiley & Sons; 2018.

[25] Verbaan FJ, Bal SM, van den Berg DJ, Groenink WHH, Verpoorten H, Lüttge R, et al. Assembled microneedle arrays enhance the transport of compounds varying over a large range of molecular weight across human dermatomed skin. J Control Release 2007;117:238–45.

[26] Verhoeven M, Bystrova S, Winnubst L, Qureshi H, De Gruijl TD, Scheper RJ, et al. Applying ceramic nanoporous microneedle arrays as a transport interface in egg plants and an ex-vivo human skin model. Microelectron. Eng. 2012; 98:659–62.

[27] Pignatello R. Biomaterials applications for nanomedicine. Croatia: InTechOpen; 2011.

[28] Cai B, Xia W, Bredenberg S, Engqvist H. Self-setting bioceramic microscopic protrusions for transder-mal drug delivery. J Mater Chem B 2014;2:5992–8.

[29] Gittard SD, Narayan RJ, Jin C, Ovsianikov A, Chichkov BN, Monteiro-Riviere NA, et al. Pulsed laser deposition of antimicrobial silver coating on Ormocer®microneedles. Biofabrication 2009;1:41001.

[30] Navarro M, Michiardi A, Castaño O, Planell JA. Biomaterials in orthopaedics. J R Soc Interface 2008;5:1137–58.

[31] Finley J, Knabb J. Cutaneous Silica Granuloma. Plast Reconstr Surg 1982;69:340–3.

[32] Donnelly RF, Morrow DIJ, Singh TRR, Migalska K, Mccarron PA, O'mahony C, et al. Processing difficulties and instability of carbohydrate microneedle arrays. Drug Dev Ind Pharm 2009;35:1242–54.

[33] Hong X, Wei L, Wu F, Wu Z, Chen L, Liu Z, et al. Dissolving and biodegradable microneedle technologies for transdermal sustained delivery of drug and vaccine. Drug Des Devel Ther 2013;7:945–52.

[34] Markovsky E, Baabur-Cohen H, Eldar-Boock A, Omer L, Tiram G, Ferber S, et al. Administration, distribution, metabolism and elimination of polymer therapeutics. J Control Release 2012;161:446–60.

[35] Singh P, Carrier A, Chen Y, Lin S, Wang J, Cui S, et al. Polymeric microneedles for controlled transdermal drug delivery. J Control Release 2019;315:97–113.

[36] Cormier M, Johnson B, Ameri M, Nyam K, Libiran L, Zhang DD, et al. Transdermal delivery of desmopressin using a coated microneedle array patch system. J Control Release 2004;97:503–11.

[37] Verbaan FJ, Bal SM, van den Berg DJ, Dijksman JA, van Hecke M, Verpoorten H, et al. Improved piercing of microneedle arrays in dermatomed human skin by an impact insertion method. J Control Release 2008;128:80–8.

[38] Petlin DG, Tverdokhlebov SI, Anissimov YG. Plasma treatment as an efficient tool for controlled drug release from polymeric materials: A review. J Control Release 2017;266:57–74.

[39] Aghabegi Moghanjoughi A, Khoshnevis D, Zarrabi A. A concise review on smart polymers for controlled drug release. Drug Deliv Transl Res 2016;6:333–40.

[40] Natarajan JV., Nugraha C, Ng XW, Venkatraman S. Sustained-release from nanocarriers: A review. J Control Release 2014;193:122–38.

[41] Kim Y-C, Park J-H, Prausnitz MR. Microneedles for drug and vaccine delivery. Adv Drug Deliv Rev 2012;64:1547–68.

[42] Tsioris K, Raja WK, Pritchard EM, Panilaitis B, Kaplan DL, Omenetto FG. Fabrication of silk microneedles for controlled-release drug delivery. Adv Funct Mater 2012;22:330–5.

[43] Chen M-C, Ling M-H, Lai K-Y, Pramudityo E. Chitosan Microneedle Patches for Sustained Transdermal Delivery of Macromolecules. Biomacromolecules 2012;13:4022–31.

[44] Park JH, Allen MG, Prausnitz MR. Biodegradable polymer microneedles: Fabrication, mechanics and transdermal drug delivery. J Control Release 2005;104:51–66.

[45] Li W, Tang J, Terry RN, Li S, Brunie A, Callahan RL, et al. Long-acting reversible contraception by effervescent microneedle patch. Sci Adv 2019;5:8145.

[46] Mc Crudden MTC, Larrañeta E, Clark A, Jarrahian C, Rein-Weston A, Creelman B, et al. Design, formulation, and evaluation of novel dissolving microarray patches containing rilpivirine for intravaginal delivery. Adv Healthc Mater 2019;8:1801510.

[47] Donnelly RF, Singh TRR, Garland MJ, Migalska K, Majithiya R, McCrudden CM, et al. Hydrogel-forming microneedle arrays for enhanced transdermal drug delivery. Adv Funct Mater 2012;22:4879–90.

[48] Hardy JG, Larrañeta E, Donnelly RF, McGoldrick N, Migalska K, McCrudden MTC, et al. Hydrogel-Forming Microneedle Arrays Made from Light-Responsive Materials for On-Demand Transdermal Drug Delivery. Mol Pharm 2016;13:907–14.

[49] Migdadi EM, Courtenay AJ, Tekko IA, McCrudden MTC, Kearney M-C, McAlister E, et al. Hydrogel-forming microneedles enhance transdermal delivery of metformin hydrochloride. J Control Release 2018;285:142–51.

[50] Kearney MC, Caffarel-Salvador E, Fallows SJ, McCarthy HO, Donnelly RF. Microneedle-mediated delivery of donepezil: Potential for improved treatment options in Alzheimer's disease. Eur J Pharm Biopharm 2016;103:43–50.

[51] Courtenay AJ, McCrudden MTC, McAvoy KJ, McCarthy HO, Donnelly RF. Microneedle-mediated transdermal delivery of bevacizumab. Mol Pharm 2018;15:3545–56.

[52] Huang X, Brazel CS. On the importance and mechanisms of burst release in matrix-controlled drug delivery systems. J Control Release 2001;73:121–36.

[53] Lee K, Lee CY, Jung H. Dissolving microneedles for transdermal drug administration prepared by stepwise controlled drawing of maltose. Biomaterials 2011;32:3134–40.

[54] Liu S, Wu D, Quan YS, Kamiyama F, Kusamori K, Katsumi H, et al. Improvement of transdermal delivery of exendin-4 using novel tip-loaded microneedle arrays fabricated from hyaluronic acid. Mol Pharm 2016;13:272–9.

[55] Raphael AP, Crichton ML, Falconer RJ, Meliga S, Chen X, Fernando GJP, et al. Formulations for microprojection/microneedle vaccine delivery: Structure, strength and release profiles. J Control Release 2016;225:40–52.

[56] McCrudden MTC, Alkilani AZ, McCrudden CM, McAlister E, McCarthy HO, Woolfson AD, et al. Design and physicochemical characterisation of novel dissolving polymeric microneedle arrays for transdermal delivery of high dose, low molecular weight drugs. J Control Release 2014;180:71–80.

[57] Lee HS, Ryu HR, Roh JY, Park JH. Bleomycin-coated microneedles for treatment of warts. Pharm Res 2017;34:101–12.

[58] Pamornpathomkul B, Ngawhirunpat T, Tekko IA, Vora L, McCarthy HO, Donnelly RF. Dissolving polymeric microneedle arrays for enhanced site-specific acyclovir delivery. Eur J Pharm Sci 2018;121:200–9.

[59] National Institute for Health and Care Excellence. Insulin therapy in type 1 diabetes; 2016. Available from: https://cks.nice.org.uk/insulin-therapy-in-type-1-diabetes#!scenarioRecommendation:3

[60] Yang S, Feng Y, Zhang L, Chen N, Yuan W, Jin T. A scalable fabrication process of polymer microneedles. Int J Nanomedicine 2012;7:1415–22.

[61] Fukushima K, Ise A, Morita H, Hasegawa R, Ito Y, Sugioka N, et al. Two-layered dissolving microneedles for percutaneous delivery of peptide/protein drugs in rats. Pharm Res 2011;28:7–21.

[62] Hutton ARJ, Quinn HL, McCague PJ, Jarrahian C, Rein-Weston A, Coffey PS, et al. Transdermal delivery of vitamin K using dissolving microneedles for the prevention of vitamin K deficiency bleeding. Int J Pharm 2018;541:56–63.

[63] Zhang Y, Brown K, Siebenaler K, Determan A, Dohmeier D, Hansen K. Development of lidocaine-coated microneedle product for rapid, safe, and prolonged local analgesic action. Pharm Res 2012;29:170–7.

[64] Tan ML, Choong PFM, Dass CR. Recent developments in liposomes, microparticles and nanoparticles for protein and peptide drug delivery. Peptides 2010;31:184–93.

[65] Matiasevic D, Gershberg H. Studies on hydroxyproline excretion and corticosteroid-induced dwarfism: Treatment with human growth hormone. Metab Clin Expermimental 1966;2:720–9.

[66] Chen G, Jaffee EM, Emens LA. Immunotherapy and cancer therapeutics: A rich partnership. Cancer Immunother Immune Suppr Tumor Growth Second Ed 2013:415–32.

[67] Almeida AJ, Souto E. Solid lipid nanoparticles as a drug delivery system for peptides and proteins. Adv Drug Deliv Rev 2007;59:478–90.

[68] Singh R, Singh S, Lillard JW. Past, present, and future technologies for oral delivery of therapeutic proteins. J Pharm Sci 2008;97:2497–523.

[69] Bashyal S, Noh G, Keum T, Choi YW, Lee S. Cell penetrating peptides as an innovative approach for drug delivery; then, present and the future. J Pharm Investig 2016;46:205–20.

[70] Prüss-Üstün A, Rapiti E, Hutin Y. Estimation of the global burden of disease attributable to contaminated sharps injuries among health-care workers. Am J Ind Med 2005;48:482–90.

[71] Jamaledin R, Di Natale C, Onesto V, Taraghdari ZB, Zare EN, Makvandi P, et al. Progress in microneedle-mediated protein delivery. J Clin Med 2020;9:542.

[72] Bariya SH, Gohel MC, Mehta T a., Sharma OP. Microneedles: An emerging transdermal drug delivery system. J Pharm Pharmacol 2012;64:11–29.

[73] Tas C, Mansoor S, Kalluri H, Zarnitsyn VG, Choi S-O, Banga AK, et al. Delivery of salmon calcitonin using a microneedle patch. Int J Pharm 2012;423:257–63.

[74] Ng H-I, Fernando GJP, Kendall MAF. Induction of potent CD8+ T cell responses through the delivery of subunit protein vaccines to skin antigen-presenting cells using densely packed microprojection arrays. J Control Release 2012;162:477–84.

[75] Han M, Kim DK, Kang SH, Yoon H-R, Kim B-Y, Lee SS, et al. Improvement in antigen-delivery using fabrication of a grooves-embedded microneedle array. Sensors Actuators B Chem 2009;137:274–80.

[76] Kim Y-C, Quan F-S, Compans RW, Kang S-M, Prausnitz MR. Formulation and coating of microneedles with inactivated influenza virus to improve vaccine stability and immunogenicity. J Control Release 2010;142:187–95.

[77] Hooper JW, Golden JW, Ferro AM, King AD. Smallpox DNA vaccine delivered by novel skin electroporation device protects mice against intranasal poxvirus challenge. Vaccine 2007;25:1814–23.

[78] Daddona PE, Matriano JA, Mandema J, Maa YF. Parathyroid hormone (1–34)-coated microneedle patch system: Clinical pharmacokinetics and pharmacodynamics for treatment of osteoporosis. Pharm Res 2011;28:159–65.

[79] Roxhed N, Griss P, Stemme G. Membrane-sealed hollow microneedles and related administration schemes for transdermal drug delivery. Biomed Microdevices 2008;10:271–9.

[80] Davis SP, Martanto W, Allen MG, Prausnitz MR. Hollow metal microneedles for insulin delivery to diabetic rats. IEEE Trans Biomed Eng 2005;52:909–15.

[81] Ito Y, Hirono M, Fukushima K, Sugioka N, Takada K. Two-layered dissolving microneedles formulated with intermediate-acting insulin. Int J Pharm 2012;436:387–93.

[82] Liu S, Jin M, Quan Y, Kamiyama F, Katsumi H, Sakane T, et al. The development and characteristics of novel microneedle arrays fabricated from hyaluronic acid, and their application in the transdermal delivery of insulin. J Control Release 2012;161:933–41.

[83] Lee JW, Park J-H, Prausnitz MR. Dissolving microneedles for transdermal drug delivery. Biomaterials 2008;29:2113–24.

[84] Gomaa YA, Garland MJ, McInnes F, El-Khordagui LK, Wilson C, Donnelly RF. Laser-engineered dissolving microneedles for active transdermal delivery of nadroparin calcium. Eur J Pharm Biopharm 2012;82:299–307.

[85] McCrudden MTC, Torrisi BM, Al-Zahrani S, McCrudden CM, Zaric M, Scott CJ, et al. Laser-engineered dissolving microneedle arrays for protein delivery: Potential for enhanced intradermal vaccination. J Pharm Pharmacol 2015;67:409–25.

[86] Matsuo K, Yokota Y, Zhai Y, Quan Y-S, Kamiyama F, Mukai Y, et al. A low-invasive and effective transcutaneous immunization system using a novel dissolving microneedle array for soluble and particulate antigens. J Control Release 2012;161:10–7.

[87] Naito S, Ito Y, Kiyohara T, Kataoka M, Ochiai M, Takada K. Antigen-loaded dissolving microneedle array as a novel tool for percutaneous vaccination. Vaccine 2012;30:1191–7.

[88] Matsuo K, Hirobe S, Yokota Y, Ayabe Y, Seto M, Quan YS, et al. Transcutaneous immunization using a dissolving microneedle array protects against tetanus, diphtheria, malaria, and influenza. J Control Release 2012;160:495–501.

[89] Migalska K, Morrow DIJ, Garland MJ, Thakur R, Woolfson AD, Donnelly RF. Laser-engineered dissolving microneedle arrays for transdermal macromolecular drug delivery. Pharm Res 2011;28:1919–30.

[90] Ling M-H, Chen M-C. Dissolving polymer microneedle patches for rapid and efficient transdermal delivery of insulin to diabetic rats. Acta Biomater 2013;9:8952–61.

[91] Chen J, Qiu Y, Zhang S, Gao Y. Dissolving microneedle-based intradermal delivery of interferon-α-2b. Drug Dev Ind Pharm 2016;42:890–6.

[92] McCrudden MTC, Courtenay AJ, Donnelly RF. Microneedle-mediated Vaccine Delivery. In: Donnelly RF, Singh TRR, Larrañeta E, McCrudden MTC, editors. Microneedles for Drug and Vaccine Delivery and Patient Monitoring. Chichester: John Wiley and Sons; 2018, p. 93–127.

[93] Benecke O, DeYoung SE. Anti-Vaccine Decision-Making and Measles Resurgence in the United States. Glob Pediatr Heal 2019;6:1–5.

[94] Simonsen L, Kane A, Lloyd J, Zaffran M, Kane & M. In Focus Unsafe injections in the developing world and transmission of bloodborne pathogens: a review. Bull World Health Organ 1999;77:789–800.

[95] Giudice EL, Campbell JD. Needle-free vaccine delivery. Adv Drug Deliv Rev 2006;58:68–89.

[96] Huang CM. Topical vaccination: The skin as a unique portal to adaptive immune responses. Semin Immunopathol 2007;29:71–80.

[97] Lambert PH, Laurent PE. Intradermal vaccine delivery: Will new delivery systems transform vaccine administration? Vaccine 2008;26:3197–208.

[98] Al-Zahrani S, Zaric M, McCrudden C, Scott C, Kissenpfennig A, Donnelly RF. Microneedle-mediated vaccine delivery: Harnessing cutaneous immunobiology to improve efficacy. Expert Opin Drug Deliv 2012;9:541–50.

[99] Indermun S, Luttge R, Choonara YE, Kumar P, Du Toit LC, Modi G, et al. Current advances in the fabrication of microneedles for transdermal delivery. J Control Release 2014;185:130–8.

[100] Mistilis MJ, Joyce JC, Esser ES, Skountzou I, Compans RW, Bommarius AS, et al. Long-term stability of influenza vaccine in a dissolving microneedle patch. Drug Deliv Transl Res 2017;7:195–205.

[101] Mistilis MJ, Bommarius AS, Prausnitz MR. Development of a thermostable microneedle patch for influenza vaccination. J Pharm Sci 2015;104:740–9.

[102] Esser ES, Romanyuk AA, Vassilieva EV., Jacob J, Prausnitz MR, Compans RW, et al. Tetanus vaccination with a dissolving microneedle patch confers protective immune responses in pregnancy. J Control Release 2016;236:47–56.

[103] Sullivan SP, Koutsonanos DG, Del Pilar Martin M, Lee JW, Zarnitsyn V, Choi SO, et al. Dissolving polymer microneedle patches for influenza vaccination. Nat Med 2010;16:915–20.

[104] Edens C, Dybdahl-Sissoko NC, Weldon WC, Oberste MS, Prausnitz MR. Inactivated polio vaccination using a microneedle patch is immunogenic in the rhesus macaque. Vaccine 2015;33:4683–90.

[105] Edens C, Collins ML, Goodson JL, Rota PA, Prausnitz MR. A microneedle patch containing measles vaccine is immunogenic in non-human primates. Vaccine 2015;33:4712–8.

[106] Zhu Z, Ye X, Ku Z, Liu Q, Shen C, Luo H, et al. Transcutaneous immunization via rapidly dissolvable microneedles protects against hand-foot-and-mouth disease caused by enterovirus 71. J Control Release 2016;243:291–302.

[107] Pattani A, McKay PF, Garland MJ, Curran RM, Migalska K, Cassidy CM, et al. Microneedle mediated intradermal delivery of adjuvanted recombinant HIV-1 CN54gp140 effectively primes mucosal boost inoculations. J Control Release 2012;162:529–37.

[108] Mao QY, Wang Y, Bian L, Xu M, Liang Z. EV71 vaccine, a new tool to control outbreaks of hand, foot and mouth disease (HFMD). Expert Rev Vaccines 2016;15:599–606.

[109] Rouphael NG, Paine M, Mosley R, Henry S, McAllister DV., Kalluri H, et al. The safety, immunogenicity, and acceptability of inactivated influenza vaccine delivered by microneedle patch (TIV-MNP 2015): a randomised, partly blinded, placebo-controlled, phase 1 trial. Lancet 2017;390:649–58.

[110] Hirobe S, Azukizawa H, Hanafusa T, Matsuo K, Quan YS, Kamiyama F, et al. Clinical study and stability assessment of a novel transcutaneous influenza vaccination using a dissolving microneedle patch. Biomaterials 2015;57:50–8.

[111] Chu LY, Ye L, Dong K, Compans RW, Yang C, Prausnitz MR. Enhanced stability of inactivated influenza vaccine encapsulated in dissolving microneedle patches. Pharm Res 2016;33:868–78.

[112] McGrath MG, Vrdoljak A, O'Mahony C, Oliveira JC, Moore AC, Crean AM. Determination of parameters for successful spray coating of silicon microneedle arrays. Int J Pharm 2011;415:140–9.

[113] Vrdoljak A, McGrath MG, Carey JB, Draper SJ, Hill AVS, O'Mahony C, et al. Coated microneedle arrays for transcutaneous delivery of live virus vaccines. J Control Release 2012;159:34–42.

[114] Weldon WC, Zarnitsyn VG, Esser ES, Taherbhai MT, Koutsonanos DG, Vassilieva EV., et al. Effect of adjuvants on responses to skin immunization by microneedles coated with influenza subunit vaccine. PLoS One 2012;7:41501.

[115] Choi HJ, Bondy BJ, Yoo DG, Compans RW, Kang SM, Prausnitz MR. Stability of whole inactivated influenza virus vaccine during coating onto metal microneedles. J Control Release 2013;166:159–71.

[116] Koutsonanos DG, Esser ES, McMaster SR, Kalluri P, Lee JW, Prausnitz MR, et al. Enhanced immune responses by skin vaccination with influenza subunit vaccine in young hosts. Vaccine 2015;33:4675–82.

[117] Choi IJ, Kang A, Ahn MH, Jun H, Baek SK, Park JH, et al. Insertion-responsive microneedles for rapid intradermal delivery of canine influenza vaccine. J Control Release 2018;286:460–6.

[118] Quan FS, Kim YC, Song JM, Hwang HS, Compans RW, Prausnitz MR, et al. Long-term protective immunity from an influenza virus-like particle vaccine administered with a microneedle patch. Clin Vaccine Immunol 2013;20:1433–9.

[119] Kommareddy S, Baudner BC, Bonificio A, Gallorini S, Palladino G, Determan AS, et al. Influenza subunit vaccine coated microneedle patches elicit comparable immune responses to intramuscular injection in guinea pigs. Vaccine 2013;31:3435–41.

[120] Quan F-S, Kim Y-C, Vunnava A, Yoo D-G, Song J-M, Prausnitz MR, et al. Intradermal vaccination with influenza virus-like particles by using microneedles induces protection superior to that with intramuscular immunization. J Virol 2010;84:7760–9.

[121] Widera G, Johnson J, Kim L, Libiran L, Nyam K, Daddona PE, et al. Effect of delivery parameters on immunization to ovalbumin following intracutaneous administration by a coated microneedle array patch system. Vaccine 2006;24:1653–64.

[122] Prow TW, Chen X, Prow NA, Fernando GJP, Tan CSE, Raphael AP, et al. Nanopatch-targeted skin vaccination against West Nile Virus and Chikungunya Virus in Mice. Small 2010;6:1776–84.

[123] Corbett HJ, Fernando GJP, Chen X, Frazer IH, Kendall MAF. Skin vaccination against cervical cancer associated human papillomavirus with a novel micro-projection array in a mouse model. PLoS One 2010;5:13460.

[124] Hiraishi Y, Nandakumar S, Choi SO, Lee JW, Kim YC, Posey JE, et al. Bacillus Calmette-Guérin vaccination using a microneedle patch. Vaccine 2011;29:2626–36.

[125] Moon S, Wang Y, Edens C, Gentsch JR, Prausnitz MR, Jiang B. Dose sparing and enhanced immunogenicity of inactivated rotavirus vaccine administered by skin vaccination using a microneedle patch. Vaccine 2013;31:3396–402.

[126] Edens C, Collins ML, Ayers J, Rota PA, Prausnitz MR. Measles vaccination using a microneedle patch. Vaccine 2013;31:3403–9.

[127] Ma Y, Tao W, Krebs SJ, Sutton WF, Haigwood NL, Gill HS. Vaccine delivery to the oral cavity using coated microneedles induces systemic and mucosal immunity. Pharm Res 2014;31:2393–403.

[128] McNeilly CL, Crichton ML, Primiero CA, Frazer IH, Roberts MS, Kendall MAF. Microprojection arrays to immunise at mucosal surfaces. J Control Release 2014;196:252–60.

[129] Wang T, Wang N. Preparation of the multifunctional liposome-containing microneedle arrays as an oral cavity mucosal vaccine adjuvant-delivery system. Methods Mol. Biol. 2016;1404:651–67.

[130] Serpe L, Jain A, de Macedo CG, Volpato MC, Groppo FC, Gill HS, et al. Influence of salivary washout on drug delivery to the oral cavity using coated microneedles: An in vitro evaluation. Eur J Pharm Sci 2016;93:215–23.

[131] Laurent PE, Bonnet S, Alchas P, Regolini P, Mikszta JA, Pettis R, et al. Evaluation of the clinical performance of a new intradermal vaccine administration technique and associated delivery system. Vaccine 2007;25:8833–42.

[132] Flynn PM, Shenep JL, Mao L, Crawford R, Williams BF, Williams BG. Influence of needle gauge in mantoux skin testing. Chest 1994;106:1463–5.

[133] Schipper P, van der Maaden K, Romeijn S, Oomens C, Kersten G, Jiskoot W, et al. Repeated fractional intradermal dosing of an inactivated polio vaccine by a single hollow microneedle leads to superior immune responses. J Control Release 2016;242:141–7.

[134] Schipper P, van der Maaden K, Romeijn S, Oomens C, Kersten G, Jiskoot W, et al. Determination of depth-dependent intradermal immunogenicity of adjuvanted inactivated polio vaccine delivered by microinjections via hollow microneedles. Pharm Res 2016;33:2269–79.

[135] Van Der Maaden K, Trietsch SJ, Kraan H, Varypataki EM, Romeijn S, Zwier R, et al. Novel hollow microneedle technology for depth-controlled microinjection-mediated dermal vaccination: A study with polio vaccine in rats. Pharm Res 2014;31:1846–54.

[136] Morefield GL, Tammariello RF, Purcell BK, Worsham PL, Chapman J, Smith LA, et al. An alternative approach to combination vaccines: Intradermal administration of isolated components for control of anthrax, botulism, plague and staphylococcal toxic shock. J Immune Based Ther Vaccines 2008;6:1–11.

[137] Mikszta JA, Dekker JP, Harvey NG, Dean CH, Brittingham JM, Huang J, et al. Microneedle-based intradermal delivery of the anthrax recombinant protective antigen vaccine. Infect Immun 2006;74:6806–10.

[138] Mikszta JA, Sullivan VJ, Dean C, Waterston AM, Alarcon JB, Dekker III JP, et al. Protective immunization against inhalational anthrax: A comparison of minimally invasive delivery platforms. J Infect Dis 2005;191:278–88.

[139] Alarcon JB, Hartley AW, Harvey NG, Mikszta JA. Preclinical evaluation of microneedle technology for intradermal delivery of influenza vaccines. Clin Vaccine Immunol 2007;14:375–81.

[140] Laurent PE, Bourhy H, Fantino M, Alchas P, Mikszta JA. Safety and efficacy of novel dermal and epidermal microneedle delivery systems for rabies vaccination in healthy adults. Vaccine 2010;28:5850–6.

[141] Van Der Maaden K, Varypataki EM, Romeijn S, Ossendorp F, Jiskoot W, Bouwstra J. Ovalbumin-coated pH-sensitive microneedle arrays effectively induce ovalbumin-specific antibody and T-cell responses in mice. Eur J Pharm Biopharm 2014;88:310–5.

[142] Ding Z, Verbaan FJ, Bivas-Benita M, Bungener L, Huckriede A, van den Berg DJ, et al. Microneedle arrays for the transcutaneous immunization of diphtheria and influenza in BALB/c mice. J Control Release 2009;136:71–8.

[143] Ding Z, Van Riet E, Romeijn S, Kersten GFA, Jiskoot W, Bouwstra JA. Immune modulation by adjuvants combined with diphtheria toxoid administered topically in BALB/c mice after microneedle array pretreatment. Pharm Res 2009;26:1635–43.

[144] Bal SM, Ding Z, Kersten GFA, Jiskoot W, Bouwstra JA. Microneedle-based transcutaneous immunisation in mice with n-trimethyl chitosan adjuvanted diphtheria toxoid formulations. Pharm Res 2010;27:1837–47.

[145] Beran J, Ambrozaitis A, Laiskonis A, Mickuviene N, Bacart P, Calozet Y, et al. Intradermal influenza vaccination of healthy adults using a new microinjection system: A 3-year randomised controlled safety and immunogenicity trial. BMC Med 2009;7:1–15.

[146] Arnou R, Icardi G, De Decker M, Ambrozaitis A, Kazek MP, Weber F, et al. Intradermal influenza vaccine for older adults: A randomized controlled multicenter phase III study. Vaccine 2009;27:7304–12.

[147] Schagen SK, Zampeli VA, Makrantonaki E, Zouboulis CC. Discovering the link between nutrition and skin aging. Dermatoendocrinol 2012;4:298–307.

[148] CNN Business. The skincare industry is booming, fueled by informed consumers and social media 2019. Available at: https://edition.cnn.com/2019/05/10/business/skincare-industry-trends-beauty-social-media/index.html

[149] Orentreich DS, Orentreich N. Subcutaneous incisionless (subcision) surgery for the correction of depressed scars and wrinkles. Dermatologic Surg 1995;21:543–549.

[150] Fernandes D. Percutaneous collagen induction: An alternative to laser resurfacing. Aesthetic Surg J 2002;22:307–9.

[151] Fernandes D, Signorini M. Combating photoaging with percutaneous collagen induction. Clin Dermatol 2008;26:192–9.

[152] Aust MC, Reimers K, Kaplan HM, Stahl F, Repenning C, Scheper T, et al. Percutaneous collagen induction-regeneration in place of cicatrisation? J Plast Reconstr Aesthetic Surg 2011;64:97–107.

[153] Hassan KM, Benedetto AV. Facial skin rejuvenation: Ablative laser resurfacing, chemical peels, or photodynamic therapy? Facts and controversies. Clin Dermatol 2013;31:737–40.

[154] Gold MH, Biron JA. Treatment of acne scars by fractional bipolar radiofrequency energy. J Cosmet Laser Ther 2012;14:172–8.

[155] Rawlins JM, Lam WL, Karoo RO, Naylor IL, Sharpe DT. Quantifying collagen type in mature burn scars: A novel approach using histology and digital image analysis. J Burn Care Res 2006;27:60–5.

[156] Badran MM, Kuntsche J, Fahr A. Skin penetration enhancement by a microneedle device (Dermaroller ®) in vitro : Dependency on needle size and applied formulation. Eur J Pharm Sci 2009;36:511–23.

[157] Singh A, Yadav S. Microneedling: Advances and widening horizons. Indian Dermatol Online J 2016;7:244 – 254.

[158] Dermaroller®. Royal Derma Roller; 2015. Available from: https://www.consultingroom.com/Treatment/eDermastamp-eDS-Skin-Rejuvenation

[159] Soltani-Arabshahi R, Wong JW, Duffy KL, Powell DL. Facial allergic granulomatous reaction and systemic hypersensitivity associated with microneedle therapy for skin rejuvenation. JAMA Dermatology 2014;150:68–72.

[160] Hyochol A, Weaver M, Lyon D, Choi E, Fillingim R. A method to improve the efficacy of topical eflornithine hydrochloride cream. Physiol Behav 2017;176:139–48.

[161] Dhurat R, Sukesh M, Avhad G, Dandale A, Pal A, Pund P. A randomized evaluator blinded study of effect of microneedling in androgenetic alopecia: A pilot study. Int J Trichology 2013;5:6–11.

[162] Mohammed YH, Yamada M, Lin LL, Grice JE, Roberts MS, Raphael AP, et al. Microneedle enhanced delivery of cosmeceutically relevant peptides in human skin. PLoS One 2014;9:1–9.

[163] Lee HJ, Lee EG, Kang S, Sung JH, Chung HM, Kim DH. Efficacy of microneedling plus human stem cell conditioned medium for skin rejuvenation: A randomized, controlled, blinded split-face study. Ann Dermatol 2014;26:584–91.

[164] A. Machekposhti S, Soltani M, Najafizadeh P, Ebrahimi SA, Chen P. Biocompatible polymer microneedle for topical/dermal delivery of tranexamic acid. J Control Release 2017;261:87–92.

[165] Hirobe S, Otsuka R, Iioka H, Quan YS, Kamiyama F, Asada H, et al. Clinical study of a retinoic acid-loaded microneedle patch for seborrheic keratosis or senile lentigo. Life Sci 2017;168:24–7.

[166] Brown TJ, Alcorn D, Fraser JRE. Absorption of hyaluronan applied to the surface of intact skin. J Invest Dermatol 1999;113:740–6.

[167] Hiraishi Y, Nakagawa T, Quan YS, Kamiyama F, Hirobe S, Okada N, et al. Performance and characteristics evaluation of a sodium hyaluronate-based microneedle patch for a transcutaneous drug delivery system. Int J Pharm 2013;441:570–9.

[168] Lee SG, Jeong JH, Lee KM, Jeong KH, Yang H, Kim M, et al. Nanostructured lipid carrier-loaded hyaluronic acid microneedles for controlled dermal delivery of a lipophilic molecule. Int J Nanomedicine 2013;9:289–99.

[169] Liu S, Jin MN, Quan YS, Kamiyama F, Kusamori K, Katsumi H, et al. Transdermal delivery of relatively high molecular weight drugs using novel self-dissolving microneedle arrays fabricated from hyaluronic acid and their characteristics and safety after application to the skin. Eur J Pharm Biopharm 2014;86:267–76.

[170] Kim M, Yang H, Kim H, Jung H, Jung H. Novel cosmetic patches for wrinkle improvement: Retinyl retinoate- and ascorbic acid-loaded dissolving microneedles. Int J Cosmet Sci 2014;36:207–12.

[171] Lee C, Yang H, Kim S, Kim M, Kang H, Kim N, et al. Evaluation of the anti-wrinkle effect of an ascorbic acid-loaded dissolving microneedle patch via a double-blind, placebo-controlled clinical study. Int J Cosmet Sci 2016;38:375–81.

[172] Guyatt GH, Oxman AD, Ali M, Willan A, McIlroy W, Patterson C. Laboratory diagnosis of iron-deficiency anemia. J Gen Intern Med 1992;7:145–53.

[173] Cook JD. Diagnosis and management of iron-deficiency anaemia. Best Pract Res Clin Haematol 2005;18:319–32.

[174] Stange EF, Travis SPL, Vermeire S, Beglinger C, Kupcinkas L, Geboes K, et al. European evidence based consensus on the diagnosis and management of Crohn's disease: definitions and diagnosis. Gut 2006;55 Suppl 1:1–15.

[175] Schrauder MG, Strick R, Schulz-Wendtland R, Strissel PL, Kahmann L, Loehberg CR, et al. Circulating Micro-RNAs as potential blood-based markers for early stage breast cancer detection. PLoS One 2012;7:29770.

[176] New JP, Middleton RJ, Klebe B, Farmer CKT, de Lusignan S, Stevens PE, et al. Assessing the prevalence, monitoring and management of chronic kidney disease in patients with diabetes compared with those without diabetes in general practice. Diabet Med 2007;24:364–9.

[177] Wood E, Hogg RS, Yip B, Harrigan PR, O'Shaughnessy MV, Montaner JS. The impact of adherence on CD4 cell count responses among HIV-infected patients. JAIDS J Acquir Immune Defic Syndr 2004;35:261–8.

[178] Triggs E, Charles B. Pharmacokinetics and therapeutic drug monitoring of gentamicin in the elderly. Clin Pharmacokinet 1999;37:331–41.

[179] Gilman JT. Therapeutic drug monitoring in the neonate and paediatric age group. Clin Pharmacokinet 1990;19:1–10.

[180] Eilers R. Therapeutic drug monitoring for the treatment of psychiatric disorders. Clin Pharmacokinet 1995;29:442–50.

[181] Donnelly RF, Mooney K, Caffarel-Salvador E, Torrisi BM, Eltayib E, McElnay JC. Microneedle-mediated minimally invasive patient monitoring. Ther Drug Monit 2014;36:10–7.

[182] Hernández Arroyo MJ, Cabrera Figueroa SE, Sepúlveda Correa R, Valverde Merino M de la P, Iglesias Gómez A, Domínguez-Gil Hurlé A, et al. Impact of a pharmaceutical care program on clinical evolution and antiretroviral treatment adherence: a 5-year study. Patient Prefer Adherence 2013;7:729–39.

[183] Kang J-S, Lee M-H. Overview of therapeutic drug monitoring. Korean J Intern Med 2009;24:1–10.

[184] Lenzini P, Wadelius M, Kimmel S, Anderson JL, Jorgensen AL, Pirmohamed M, et al. Integration of genetic, clinical, and INR Data to refine warfarin dosing. Clin Pharmacol Ther 2010;87:572–8.

[185] Denus S de, Spinler SA, Miller K, Peterson AM. Statins and liver toxicity: A meta-analysis. Pharmacotherapy 2004;24:584–91.

[186] Hummel P. Psychometric Evaluation of the Neonatal Pain, Agitation, and Sedation Scale (n-Pass) Tool in Infants and Children Age One to Thirty-Six Months in the Post-Anesthesia Care Unit. Dissertation, Loyola University Chicago; 2014.

[187] Caffarel-Salvador E, Brady AJ, Eltayib E, Meng T, Alonso-Vicente A, Gonzalez-Vazquez P, et al. Hydrogel-forming microneedle arrays allow detection of drugs and glucose in vivo: Potential for use in diagnosis and therapeutic drug monitoring. PLoS One 2015;10:0145644.

[188] Carrigan SD, Scott G, Tabrizian M. Toward resolving the challenges of sepsis diagnosis. Clin Chem 2004;50:1301–14.

[189] Lomonte C, Forneris G, Gallieni M, Tazza L, Meola M, Lodi M, et al. The vascular access in the elderly: A position statement of the Vascular Access Working Group of the Italian Society of Nephrology. J Nephrol 2016;29:175–84.

[190] Brunner M, Derendorf H. Clinical microdialysis: Current applications and potential use in drug development. TrAC - Trends Anal Chem 2006;25:674–80.

[191] Leboulanger B, Guy RH, Delgado-Charro M B. Reverse iontophoresis for non-invasive transdermal monitoring. Physiol Meas 2004;25:35–50.

[192] Eltayib E, Brady AJ, Caffarel-Salvador E, Gonzalez-Vazquez P, Zaid Alkilani A, McCarthy HO, et al. Hydrogel-forming microneedle arrays: Potential for use in minimally-invasive lithium monitoring. Eur J Pharm Biopharm 2016;102:123–31.

[193] Kiang TKL, Schmitt V, Ensom MHH, Chua B, Häfeli UO. Therapeutic drug monitoring in interstitial fluid: a feasibility study using a comprehensive panel of drugs. J Pharm Sci 2012;101:4642–52.

[194] Singh TRR, Mcmillan H, Mooney K, Alkilani AZ, Donnelly RF. Microneedles for drug delivery and monitoring. In: Li X, Zhou Y, editors. Microfluidic Devices for Biomedical Applications. Cambridge, Elsevier; 2013, p. 185–230.

[195] Wang PM, Cornwell M, Prausnitz MR. Minimally invasive extraction of dermal interstitial fluid for glucose monitoring using microneedles. Diabetes Technol Ther 2005;7:131–41.

[196] Ólafsdóttir AF, Attvall S, Sandgren U, Dahlqvist S, Pivodic A, Skrtic S, et al. A clinical trial of the accuracy and treatment experience of the flash glucose monitor freestyle libre in adults with type 1 diabetes. Diabetes Technol Ther 2017;19:164–72.

[197] Courtenay AJ, Abbate MTA, McCrudden MTC, Donnelly RF. Minimally-invasive patient monitoring and diagnosis using microneedles. In: Donnelly RF, Singh TRR, Larrañeta E, McCrudden, MTC, editors. Microneedles for Drug and Vaccine Delivery and Patient Monitoring. Chichester: John Wiley & Sons; 2018, p. 207–34.

[198] Mukerjee EV, Collins SD, Isseroff RR, Smith RL. Microneedle array for transdermal biological fluid extraction and in situ analysis. Sensors Actuators A Phys 2004;114:267–75.

[199] Miller P, Moorman M, Manginell R, Ashlee C, Brener I, Wheeler D, et al. Towards an integrated microneedle total analysis chip for protein detection. Electroanalysis 2016;28:1305–10.

[200] Li CG, Lee CY, Lee K, Jung H. An optimized hollow microneedle for minimally invasive blood extraction. Biomed Microdevices 2013;15:17–25.

[201] Li CG, Joung H-A, Noh H, Song M-B, Kim M-G, Jung H, et al. One-touch-activated blood multidiagnostic system using a minimally invasive hollow microneedle integrated with a paper-based sensor. Lab Chip 2015;15:3286–92.

[202] Ranamukhaarachchi SA, Padeste C, Dübner M, Häfeli UO, Stoeber B, Cadarso VJ. Integrated hollow microneedle-optofluidic biosensor for therapeutic drug monitoring in sub-nanoliter volumes. Sci Rep 2016;6:29075.

[203] Romanyuk AV., Zvezdin VN, Samant P, Grenader MI, Zemlyanova M, Prausnitz MR. Collection of analytes from microneedle patches. Anal Chem 2014;86:10520–3.

[204] Chang H, Zheng M, Yu X, Than A, Seeni RZ, Kang R, et al. A swellable microneedle patch to rapidly extract skin interstitial fluid for timely metabolic analysis. Adv Mater 2017;29:1702243.

[205] Kiang T, Ranamukhaarachchi S, Ensom M. Revolutionizing therapeutic drug monitoring with the use of interstitial fluid and microneedles technology. Pharmaceutics 2017;9:43.

[206] Ng KW, Lau WM, Williams AC. Towards pain-free diagnosis of skin diseases through multiplexed microneedles: biomarker extraction and detection using a highly sensitive blotting method. Drug Deliv Transl Res 2015;5:387–96.

[207] Keum DH, Jung HS, Wang T, Shin MH, Kim Y-E, Kim KH, et al. Cancer detection: microneedle biosensor for real-time electrical detection of nitric oxide for in situ cancer diagnosis during endomicroscopy. Adv Healthc Mater 2015;4:1152.

[208] Song S, Na J, Jang MH, Lee H, Lee HS, Lim YB, et al. A CMOS VEGF sensor for cancer diagnosis using a peptide aptamer-based functionalized microneedle. IEEE Trans Biomed Circuits Syst 2019;13:1288–99.

[209] Miller PR, Xiao X, Brener I, Burckel DB, Narayan R, Polsky R. Microneedle-based transdermal sensor for on-chip potentiometric determination of K+. Adv Healthc Mater 2014;3:876–81.

[210] Do J, Lee S, Han J, Kai J, Hong C-C, Gao C, et al. Development of functional lab-on-a-chip on polymer for point-of-care testing of metabolic parameters. Lab Chip 2008;8:2113–20.

[211] Mandal A, Boopathy AV., Lam LKW, Moynihan KD, Welch ME, Bennett NR, et al. Cell and fluid sampling microneedle patches for monitoring skin-resident immunity. Sci Transl Med 2018;10:2227.

[212] Nayak S, Acharjya B. Mantoux test and its interpretation. Indian Dermatol Online J 2012;3:2–6.

[213] Jin J, Reese V, Coler R, Carter D, Rolandi M. Chitin microneedles for an easy-to-use tuberculosis skin test. Adv Healthc Mater 2014;3:349–53.

[214] Lee H-J, Choi H-J, Kim D-R, Lee H, Jin J-E, Kim Y-R, et al. Safety and efficacy of tuberculin skin testing with microneedle MicronJet600™ in healthy adults. Int J Tuberc Lung Dis 2016;20:500–4.

[215] Sun W, Araci Z, Inayathullah M, Manickam S, Zhang X, Bruce MA, et al. Polyvinylpyrrolidone microneedles enable delivery of intact proteins for diagnostic and therapeutic applications. Acta Biomater 2013;9:7767–74.

[216] Mir J, Zander DR. Minimally invasive allergy testing system. WO2007008824A2, 2011.

[217] Zimmermann S, Fienbork D, Stoeber B, Flounders AW, Liepmann D. A microneedle-based glucose monitor: fabricated on a wafer-level using in-device enzyme immobilization. Transducers; 12th Int. Conf. Solid-State Sensors, Actuators Microsystems. Dig. Tech. Pap. IEEE 2003; 99–102.

[218] Jina A, Tierney MJ, Tamada JA, McGill S, Desai S, Chua B, et al. Design, development, and evaluation of a novel microneedle array-based continuous glucose monitor. J Diabetes Sci Technol 2014;8:483–7.

[219] Lee SJ, Yoon HS, Xuan X, Park JY, Paik S-J, Allen MG. A patch type non-enzymatic biosensor based on 3D SUS micro-needle electrode array for minimally invasive continuous glucose monitoring. Sensors Actuators B Chem 2016;222:1144–51.

[220] Yoon H., Lee SJ, Park JY, Paik S-J, Allen MG. A non-enzymatic micro-needle patch sensor for freecholesterol continuous monitoring. IEEE 2014; 347–50.

[221] Mohan AMV, Windmiller JR, Mishra RK, Wang J. Continuous minimally-invasive alcohol monitoring using microneedle sensor arrays. Biosens Bioelectron 2017;91:574–9.

[222] Anastasova S, Crewther B, Bembnowicz P, Curto V, Ip HM, Rosa B, Yang GZ. A wearable multisensing patch for continuous sweat monitoring. Biosens Bioelectron 2016; 93:139–45.

[223] Vazquez P, O'Mahony C, Porta P, Zuliani C, Benito-Lopez F, Galvin P, Diamon D, O'Mathuna C. Microneedle platform for continuous monitoring of biomarkers in interstitial fluid, 2012. Microneedle platform for continuous monitoring of biomarkers in interstitial fluid. In: Microneedles 2012: 2nd International Conference on Microneedles. Cork, Ireland. 13–15 May 2012.

[224] Huang JT. Lactate measuring device and method for training adjustment in sports, 2015.

[225] Tay EH. Towards a wearable and wban-based health monitoring and automatic diagnosis system for low-cost personal healthcare in Qatar. Qatar Found Annu Res Forum Proc 2013;BIOP 06. US20150208970A1.

[226] Miller PR, Narayan RJ, Polsky R, Shin MH, Kim Y, Kim KH, et al. Microneedle-based sensors for medical diagnosis. J Mater Chem B 2016;4:1379–83.

[227] Sharma S, Saeed A, Johnson C, Gadegaard N, Cass AE. Rapid, low cost prototyping of transdermal devices for personal healthcare monitoring. Sens Bio-Sensing Res 2016; 13:104–8.

[228] Wang R, Jiang X, Wang W, Li Z. A microneedle electrode array on flexible substrate for long-term EEG monitoring. Sensors Actuators B Chem 2017;244:750–8.

[229] Stavrinidis G, Michelakis K, Kontomitrou V, Giannakakis G, Sevrisarianos M, Sevrisarianos G, et al. SU-8 microneedles based dry electrodes for Electroencephalogram. Microelectron Eng 2016;159:114–20.

[230] Arai M, Nishinaka Y, Miki N. Electroencephalogram measurement using polymer-based dry microneedle electrode. Jpn J Appl Phys 2015;54:06FP14.
[231] Wang L-F, Liu J-Q, Yan X-X, Yang B, Yang C-S. A MEMS-based pyramid micro-needle electrode for long-term EEG measurement. Microsyst Technol 2013;19:269–76.
[232] Yu LM, Tay FEH, Guo DG, Xu L, Yap KL. A microfabricated electrode with hollow microneedles for ECG measurement. Sensors Actuators A Phys 2009;151:17–22.
[233] O'Mahony C, Grygoryev K, Ciarlone A, Giannoni G, Kenthao A, Galvin P. Design, fabrication and skin-electrode contact analysis of polymer microneedle-based ECG electrodes. J Micromechanics Microengineering 2016;26:084005.
[234] Grand View Research. Transdermal drug delivery system market worth $81.4 billion by 2024; 2014. Available from: https://www.grandviewresearch.com/press-release/global-transdermal-drug-delivery-system-market
[235] Greystone Associates. Microneedles in Medicine: Technology, Devices, Markets and Prospects; 2010. Available from: https://www.businesswire.com/news/home/20101029005425/en/Research-Markets-Microneedles-Medicine—Technology-Markets
[236] Zosano Pharma. M207 Zolmitriptan; 2020.Available from: https://www.zosanopharma.com/
[237] Chow AY, Pardue MT, Chow VY, Peyman GA, Liang C, Perlman JI, et al. Implantation of silicon chip microphotodiode arrays into the cat subretinal space. IEEE Trans Neural Syst Rehabil Eng 2001;9:86–95.
[238] Hao Y, Li W, Zhou X, Yang F, Qian Z. Microneedles-Based Transdermal Drug Delivery Systems: A Review. J Biomed Nanotechnol 2017;13:1581–97.
[239] Birchall JC, Clemo R, Anstey A, John DN. Microneedles in clinical practice-an exploratory study into the opinions of healthcare professionals and the public. Pharm Res 2011;28:95–106.
[240] Mooney K, McElnay JC, Donnelly RF. Children's views on microneedle use as an alternative to blood sampling for patient monitoring. Int J Pharm Pract 2014;22:335–44.
[241] Mooney K, McElnay JC, Donnelly RF. Paediatricians' opinions of microneedle-mediated monitoring: a key stage in the translation of microneedle technology from laboratory into clinical practice. Drug Deliv Transl Res 2015;5:346–59.
[242] Quinn HL, Hughes CM, Donnelly RF. In vivo and qualitative studies investigating the translational potential of microneedles for use in the older population 2018:307–16.
[243] Vicente-Perez EM, Larraneta E, McCrudden MTC, Kissenpfennig A, Hegarty S, McCarthy HO, et al. Repeat application of microneedles does not alter skin appearance or barrier function and causes no measurable disturbance of serum biomarkers of infection, inflammation or immunity in mice in vivo. Eur J Pharm Biopharm 2017;117:400–7.
[244] Al-Kasasbeh R, Brady AJ, Courtenay AJ, Larrañeta E, McCrudden MTC, O'Kane D, et al. Evaluation of the clinical impact of repeat application of hydrogel-forming microneedle array patches. Drug Deliv Transl Res 2020;466:1–16.
[245] Donnelly RSTA AMM. Hydrogel-forming microneedle arrays exhibit antimicrobial properties: Potential for enhanced patient safety. Int J Pharm 2013;451:76–91.
[246] Zaric M, Lyubomska O, Touzelet O, Poux C, Al-Zahrani S, Fay F, et al. Skin dendritic cell targeting via microneedle arrays laden with antigen-encapsulated poly-D,L-lactide-co-glycolide nanoparticles induces efficient antitumor and antiviral immune responses. ACS Nano 2013;7:2042–55.
[247] World Health Organization. WHO best practices for injections and related procedures toolkit. Safe Injection Global Network (SIGN); 2010:1–51. Available from: https://www.who.int/infection-prevention/publications/best-practices_toolkit/en/
[248] McCrudden MTC, Alkilani AZ, Courtenay AJ, McCrudden CM, McCloskey B, Walker C, et al. Considerations in the sterile manufacture of polymeric microneedle arrays. Drug Deliv Transl Res 2015;5:3–14.
[249] Lutton REMM, Moore J, Larrañeta E, Ligett S, Woolfson AD, Donnelly RF. Microneedle characterisation: the need for universal acceptance criteria and GMP specifications when moving towards commercialisation. Drug Deliv Transl Res 2015;5:313–31.
[250] Lutton REM, Larrañeta E, Kearney MC, Boyd P, Woolfson AD, Donnelly RF. A novel scalable manufacturing process for the production of hydrogel-forming microneedle arrays. Int J Pharm 2015;494:417–29.

40 Clinical Testing of Microneedles for Transdermal Drug Delivery

Raja K. Sivamani, Gabriel C. Wu, Hongbo Zhai, and Howard I. Maibach
University of California, San Francisco, California

Boris Stoeber and Dorian Liepmann
University of California, Berkeley, California

CONTENTS

40.1 INTRODUCTION

Much research has been done in developing drug delivery methods different from traditional oral ingestion and hypodermic needle injections. Oral and subdermal delivery routes are successful methods of drug delivery, but have drawbacks that can affect efficacy and patient comfort. Orally ingested drugs pass through the acidic environment of the stomach and then are absorbed in the intestines. The acid in the stomach can degrade or denature many drugs and serves as one barrier in oral ingestion. When the drug passes through the stomach, it must be small enough to be absorbed through the intestinal wall. Larger drugs, like insulin, are not absorbed through the intestinal wall and are ineffective when taken orally. Once the drug passes through the intestinal wall, it then passes through the hepatic circulation, and the drug can be significantly cleared by the liver before passing onto the rest of the body. Only then can the drug take effect. As a result, the bioavailability of orally ingested drugs can be low. Also, because the drug must pass through the liver, drugs that have significant liver toxicity would not be suitable as an oral drug agent.

A major barrier to transdermal drug delivery is the stratum corneum, the 10- to 15-μm-thick outer layer of skin. Traditionally, hypodermic needles have been used to pierce through this barrier and deliver various types of drugs, vaccines, and treatments. Hypodermic needle injections allow for solubilized drugs to be delivered directly into or near the bloodstream. This method has an advantage over oral delivery in that it is effective for delivering drugs of larger sizes and the drugs do not have to pass through the liver and undergo metabolism before reaching systemic blood circulation. Although effective in drug delivery, a major drawback of hypodermic needles is that they cause pain, and many patients have needle phobia (1, 2). However, recent applications of semiconductor fabrication techniques led to the development of microneedles.

Microneedles are designed to pierce and successfully deliver injections past the stratum corneum, but are too short to stimulate the pain nerves (3, 4). Microneedles exist in two basic designs: in-plane and out-of-plane (Figure 40.1). In-plane microneedles have been integrated with circuitry, pumps, and sensors (5–7) and have been used in clinical tests to measure blood glucose levels (8). Reed and Lye (9) provide an extensive review of in-plane microneedle fabrication methods. In-plane microneedles are more easily integrated with electronic processes, but a disadvantage is that fabrication is restricted to one-dimensional arrays (9). Out-of-plane microneedles can be incorporated into two-dimensional arrays that allow for drug delivery over a greater area, similar in design to a "patch."

Out-of-plane microneedles have been fabricated in several designs. Solid microneedles have been shown to increase skin permeability (3). Hollow microneedles were subsequently developed so that fluid could be injected through them (10–13). Although most microneedles have been fabricated out of silicon, others have been fabricated from glass (11), metal (11), and polymers (11, 14). Stoeber and Liepmann (10) fabricated a microsyringe backing along with the microneedle array and measured *in vitro* dye injection depths of 75 to 100 μm. Some *in vivo* injection studies have been performed with out-of-plane microneedles, but few human studies have been done. Kaushik et al. (4) carried out the first human study to show that microneedles were painless upon insertion. Sivamani et al. (15) performed clinical injection studies and showed that microneedles helped compounds bypass the stratum corneum more quickly. Prausnitz (16) provides an overview of solid microneedle *in vivo* studies that investigate insulin permeability and vaccine delivery. McAllister et al. (11) used a single glass microneedle to inject insulin into diabetic rats and reduce their blood glucose by 70%. Gardeniers et al. (12) infused insulin into diabetic rats through a microneedle array and showed that it was comparable to subcutaneous insulin injection. Matsuda and Mizutani (14) implanted polymer microneedles for a month in rats to study the polymer degradation characteristics.

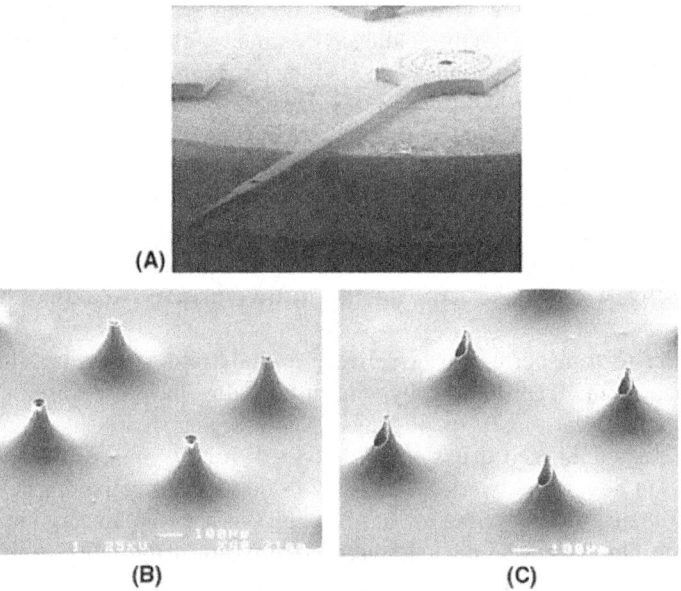

(A)

(B)   (C)

FIGURE 40.1   Silicon microneedles. (A) In-plane microneedle (5), (B) symmetric hollow microneedles, and (C) pointed hollow microneedles. The symmetric and pointed hollow microneedles are approximately 200 μm high with a lumen diameter of 40 μm.

Microneedles can serve as a painless drug delivery alternative because they are too short to stimulate pain nerve endings, but long enough to bypass the stratum corneum. One could imagine that an array of microneedles could be used to deliver painless vaccines to adults and children and that microneedle "patches" could be worn for continual painless delivery of drugs, such as insulin for diabetics. Clinical tests with microneedles were carried out by Kaushik et al. (4) and Sivamani et al. (15), showing their potential utility in humans.

40.2 CLINICAL STUDIES

Kaushik et al. (4) performed a pain study that asked volunteers to rate their pain when microneedles were inserted into their skin. When compared against a flat piece of silicon and a hypodermic needle, human subjects rated the microneedles to be similar to a flat piece of silicon. Both the microneedles and the smooth piece of silicon were rated as 0 on a 0 to 40 scale, suggesting that the microneedles were painless upon insertion.

Sivamani et al. (15) performed a clinical injection study to investigate if microneedles enhanced percutaneous penetration of methyl nicotinate. In their study they used two types of microneedles, as shown in Figures 40.1a and b and glued them onto a syringe, as shown in Figure 40.2. Methyl nicotinate is a vasodilator that has been used in many studies of percutaneous penetration (17–22). Methyl nicotinate–induced dilation of surface capillaries has been shown to follow circadian rhythms (23), with the maximum being at about noon and the minimum being at about midnight. Because of this, the experiments were carried out at the same times each day to make the results comparable to one another. Measurement of the blood flow through the skin capillaries was measured with a Laser Doppler Perfusion Monitor DRT-4 (Moor Instrument, Devon, England). Baseline blood flows of each volunteer were measured before application of the methyl nicotinate. In this way, each volunteers served as their own control.

Injections and topical applications of 0.1 M methyl nicotinate (Sigma, St. Louis, Missouri, USA) were administered to the volar forearms. Four treatments were carried out with each patient: topical application (TA), pointed microneedle injection (PMn), symmetric microneedle (SMn), and

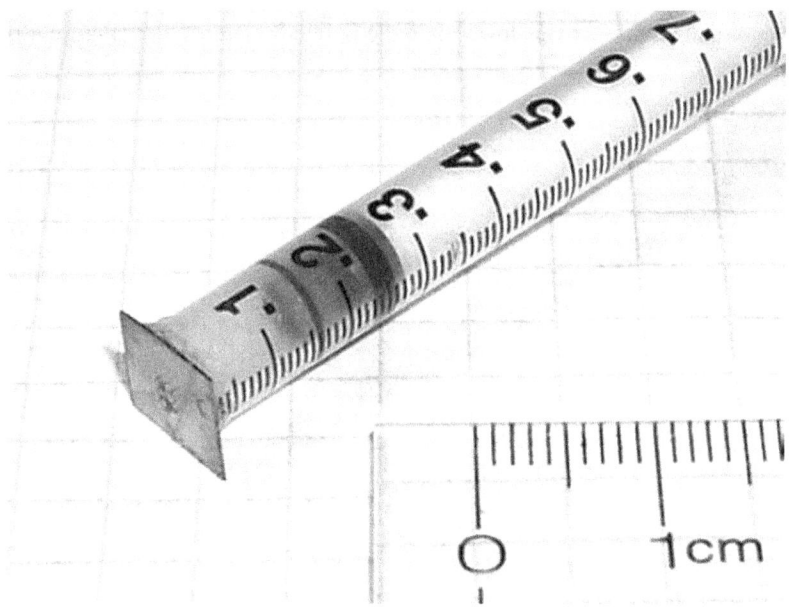

FIGURE 40.2 Microneedles on syringe. Eight-needle array of microneedles glued onto the tip of a syringe.

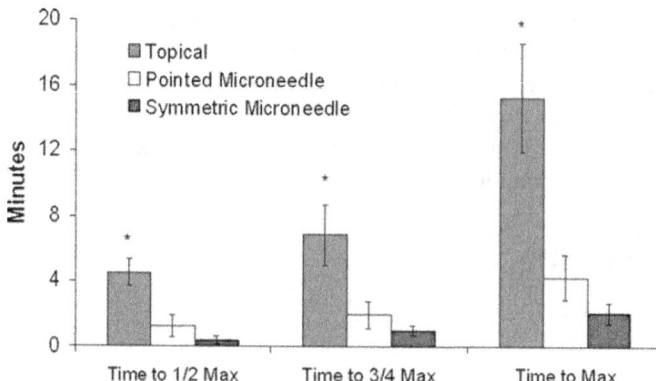

FIGURE 40.3 Time to reach maximum blood flux. Following 30-second treatments with methyl nicotinate, times to reach maximum flux were significantly longer for the topical treatment ($p < 0.05$). The pointed and the symmetric microneedle treatments were not statistically different in times to maximum blood flux.

microneedle control (MnC). The microneedle control refers to pressing an empty syringe/microneedle device on the arm. Each treatment was applied for 30 seconds over 1 cm^2.

Maximum blood fluxes and the time to reach maximum flux were measured. Both pointed and symmetric hollow microneedles (Figure 40.3) significantly decreased time to maximum blood flux compared to topical application of methyl nicotinate, but were statistically comparable to each other ($p = 0.09$). However, the pointed microneedle injections showed a higher maximum blood flux than symmetric microneedle injection or topical application (Figure 40.4). The symmetric microneedle and topical application of methyl nicotinate had similar maximum blood fluxes ($p = 0.07$).

Pointed and symmetric microneedles differ in the placement of the needle lumen (Figures 40.1a and b). The piercing and entry zone of the symmetric microneedle coincides with its lumen; in pointed microneedles, the lumen is offset from its piercing and entry zone. As a result, the symmetric microneedles may be more susceptible to clogging and have an increased resistance to fluid flow. Also, the pointed microneedle has a larger area for delivery and thereby lower resistance to fluid flow due to the elliptical structure of its lumen. This may explain why the symmetric microneedle–induced maximal blood flux was lower than the pointed microneedles (Figure 40.4). Both are

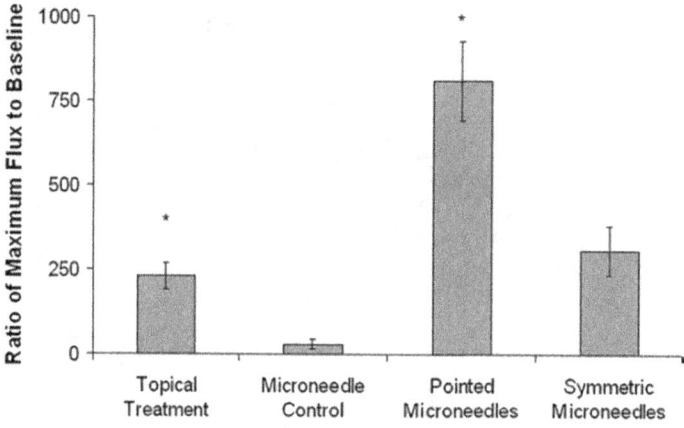

FIGURE 40.4 Percent increase over baseline at maximum blood flux. Following 30-second treatments with methyl nicotinate, maximum blood fluxes were compared to baseline blood fluxes, and pointed microneedles significantly increased the maximum blood flux over topical and symmetric microneedle treatments ($p < 0.05$). The microneedle control consisted of an empty microneedle syringe that was pressed onto the skin.

able to bypass the stratum corneum, as reflected in the decreased time to maximum blood flux (Figure 40.3), but the pointed needle may deliver more methyl nicotinate into the skin over the 30-second injection period. Hollow microneedles designed with a lumen different from the pierce and entry zone may increase drug injection efficacy.

All volunteers were asked to describe what they felt during the injection, and all responded by saying that they felt pressure but no pain, in agreement with Kaushik et al. (4).

These results show that hollow microneedles can painlessly bypass the stratum corneum during injections and deliver drugs to the skin capillaries in humans. Traditional hypodermic needle injections will continue to be advantageous in treatments requiring deeper penetration past the epidermis, like subdermal, muscular, or intravenous injections. However, hollow microneedles offer distinct advantages: they are painless and can reduce needle phobia in patients, are simpler to use than traditional injections, and can be integrated into devices for controlled, continuous drug delivery. Another advantage for hollow microneedles among transdermal drug delivery systems is the potential to inject large-sized protein formulations, such as sustained-release insulin formulations that range from 2 to 30 μm (24). The lumens of the hollow microneedle are 35 to 300 μm (10–13) and could successfully inject these formulations. Microneedles will be beneficial from a public health perspective too, because more people may be willing to receive vaccinations due to the increased convenience and comfort of the microneedle injection.

The design of the microneedle can affect how quickly drugs can be introduced through the needles. Microneedles can serve as a painless alternative to hypodermic vaccine injection and to administer drugs that may normally be administered in a topical manner. Revolutionary continuous and controlled drug therapies can be possible when pumps and sensors are mounted onto microneedle arrays.

Recent studies have evaluated the use of microneedles for multiple clinical application within immunology and dermatology.

Vaccinations have been explored as one possible application of microneedle technology. In fact, two pilot clinical studies have evaluated the use of microneedle-based delivery of vaccines in human participants (25, 26). In both studies microneedles that were shorter than 700 microns were used and compared against intramuscular vaccine delivery, and both studies showed that microneedle injections lead to as much immunogenicity as intramuscular injections. In both studies, pain was noted to be less with the microneedle-based delivery but local redness was increased in the microneedle injection group, suggesting that a sufficient immune response could be elicited from microneedle-based vaccinations. Further studies are needed, but both of these studies are promising.

Two studies evaluated if microneedles could assist with topical anesthesia. In one study, anesthesia was injected through hollow microneedles and achieved the same level of anesthesia as hypodermic needles (27). Moreover, 77% of participants preferred the self-administered microneedle injection rather than a hypodermic needle. In the other study, solid microneedles were used as a pretreatment on the forearm before applying topical 4% lidocaine and compared against the contralateral forearm with sham treatment (flat surface with no microneedles). The investigators found that pretreatment with microneedles enhanced topical anesthesia by 30 minutes in all participants and by 10 minutes in those that had greater pain sensitivity.

Finally, microneedles have been adapted for use in photodynamic therapy for actinic keratoses where topical 5-aminolevulinic acid is typically applied to the skin and allowed to incubate for one hour prior to exposing the skin to blue light. One study utilized a split-face design in 48 participants to show that the standard 60-minute incubation was comparable to microneedle pretreated skin that was incubated for only 20 or 40 minutes (29). Another study evaluated lowered incubation times of 10 and 20 minutes in a split-face design for the treatment of actinic keratoses (30). The 10-minute incubation did not show statistically significant improvement from the sham-treated side of the face (roller with no microneedles); However, the 20-minute incubation after microneedle treatment was significantly improved compared to the sham-treated side. The two studies suggest that microneedle pretreatment may enhance the transcutaneous penetration of 5-aminolevulinic acid and warrant more study in an expanded group of participants to better assess the role of microneedle pretreatment.

REFERENCES

1. Nir Y, Paz A, Sabo E, Potasman I. Fear of injections in young adults: prevalence and associations. Am J Trop Med Hyg 2003; 68(3):341–344.
2. Kleinknecht RA, Thorndike RM, Walls MM. Factorial dimensions and correlates of blood, injury, injection and related medical fears: cross validation of the medical fear survey. Behav Res Ther 1996; 34(4):323–331.
3. Henry S, McAllister DV, Allen MG, Prausnitz MR. Microfabricated microneedles: a novel approach to transdermal drug delivery. J Pharm Sci 1998; 8:922–925.
4. Kaushik S, Hord AH, Denson D, McAllister DV, Smitra S, Allen MG, Prausnitz MR. Lack of pain associated with microfabricated microneedles. Anesth Analg 2001; 92:502–504.
5. Zahn JD. Microfabricated Microneedles for Minimally Invasive Drug Delivery, Sampling and Analysis. Thesis, UC Berkeley and San Francisco.
6. Zahn JD, Deshmukh AA, Pisano AP, Liepmann D. Continuous on-chip micropumping through a microneedle. In: MEMS 2001: Proceedings of the 14th IEEE International Conference on Micro Electro Mechanical Systems, Interlaken, Switzerland, 2001: 503–506.
7. Chen J, Wise KD, Hetke JF, Bledsoe SC Jr. A multichannel neural probe for selective chemical delivery at the cellular level. IEEE Trans Biomed Eng 1997; 44(8):760–769.
8. Smart WH, Subramanian K. The use of silicon microfabrication technology in painless blood glucose monitoring. Diab Tech Ther 2000; 2(4):549–559.
9. Reed ML, Lye W-K. Microsystems for drug and gene delivery. Proc IEEE 2004; 92(1):56–75.
10. Stoeber B, Liepmann D. Fluid injection through out-of-plane microneedles. In: Proceedings of the International IEEE-EMBS Special Topic Conference on Microtechnologies in Medicine and Biology, 2000:34.
11. McAllister DV, Wang PM, Davis SP, Park J-H, Canatella PJ, Allen MG, Prausnitz MR. Microfabricated needles for transdermal delivery of macromolecules and nanoparticles: fabrication methods and transport studies. PNAS 2003; 100(24):13755–13760.
12. Gardeniers HJGE, Luttge R, Berenschot JW, de Boer MJ, Yeshurun SY, Hefetz M, van't Oever R, van den Berg A. Silicon micromachined hollow microneedles for transdermal liquid transport. J Microelectromech Syst 2003; 12(6):855–862.
13. Griss P, Stemme G. Side-opened out-of-plane microneedles for microfluidic transdermal liquid transfer. J Microelectromech Syst 2003; 12(3):296–301.
14. Matsuda T, Mizutani M. Liquid acrylate-endcapped biodegradable poly (ε-caprolactone-co-trimethylene carbonate). II. Computer-sided stereolithographic microarchitectural surface photoconstructs. J Biomed Mater Res 2002; 62(3):395–403.
15. Sivamani RK, Stoeber B, Wu GC, Zhai H, Liepmann D, Maibach H. Clinical microneedle injection of methyl nicorinate: stratum corneum penetration. Skin Res Technol 2005; 11(2):152–156.
16. Prausnitz MR. Microneedles for transdermal drug delivery. Adv Drug Del Rev 2004; 56:581–587.
17. Guy R, Wester RC, Tur E, Maibach HI. Noninvasive assessments of the percutaneous absorption of methyl nicotinate in humans. J Pharma Sci 1983; 72(9):1077–1079.
18. Guy RH, Tur E, Bjerke S, Maibach HI. Are there age and racial differences to methyl nicotinate-induced vasodilation in human skin? J Am Acad Derm 1985; 12(6):1001–1006.
19. Guy RH, Carlstrom EM, Bucks DAW, Hinz RS, Maibach HI. Percutaneous penetration of nicotinates: *in vivo* and *in vitro* measurements. J Pharm Sci 1986; 75(10):968–672.
20. Müller B, Kasper M, Surber C, Imanidis G. Permeation, metabolism and site of action concentration of nicotinic acid derivatives in human skin: correlation with topical pharmacological effect. Eur J Pharm Sci 2003; 20:181–195.
21. Boelsma E, Anderson C, Karlsson AMJ, Pnec M. Microdialysis technique as a method to study the percutaneous penetration of methyl nicotinate through excised human skin, reconstructed epidermis, and human skin *in vivo*. Pharm Res 2000; 17(2):141–147.
22. Caselli A, Hanane T, Jane B, Carter S, Khaodhiar L, Veves A. Topical methyl nicotinate- induced skin vasodilation in diabetic neuropathy. J Diab Comp 2003; 17:205–210.
23. Reinberg AE, Soudant E, Koulbanis C, Bazin R, Nicolai A, Mechkouri M, Touitou Y. Circadian dosing time dependency in the forearm skin penetration of methyl and hexyl nicotinate. Life Sci 1995; 57:1507–1513.
24. Takenaga M, Yamaguchi Y, Kitagawa A, Ogawa Y, Kawai S, Mizushima Y, Igarashi R. Optimum formulation for sustained-release insulin. Int J Pharm 2004; 271:85–94.

25. Levin Y, Kochba E, Shukarev G, Rusch S, Herrera-Taracena G, van Damme P. A phase 1, open-label, randomized study to compare the immunogenicity and safety of different administration routes and doses of virosomal influenza vaccine in elderly. Vaccine 2016; 34(44):5262–5272.

26. Rouphael NG, Paine M, Mosley R, et al. The safety, immunogenicity, and acceptability of inactivated influenza vaccine delivered by microneedle patch (TIV-MNP 2015): a randomised, partly blinded, placebo-controlled, phase 1 trial. Lancet. 2017; 390(10095):649–658.

27. Gupta J, Denson DD, Felner EI, Prausnitz MR. Rapid local anesthesia in humans using minimally invasive microneedles. Clin J Pain. 2012; 28(2):129–135.

28. Ornelas J, Foolad N, Shi V, Burney W, Sivamani RK. Effect of Microneedle Pretreatment on Topical Anesthesia: A Randomized Clinical Trial. JAMA Dermatol. 2016; 152(4):476–477.

29. Lev-Tov H, Larsen L, Zackria R, Chahal H, Eisen DB, Sivamani RK. Microneedle-assisted incubation during aminolaevulinic acid photodynamic therapy of actinic keratoses: a randomized controlled evaluator-blind trial. Br J Dermatol. 2017;176(2):543–545.

30. Petukhova TA, Hassoun LA, Foolad N, Barath M, Sivamani RK. Effect of Expedited Microneedle-Assisted Photodynamic Therapy for Field Treatment of Actinic Keratoses: A Randomized Clinical Trial. JAMA Dermatol. 2017; 153(7):637–643.

41 Delivery of Drugs, Vaccines, and Cosmeceuticals to Skin Using Microneedle Patches

Yasmine Gomaa
Alexandria University, Alexandria, Egypt

Mark R. Prausnitz[*]
Georgia Institute of Technology, Atlanta, Georgia

CONTENTS

41.1 Introduction 586
41.2 General Approaches of Drug Delivery to Skin Using Microneedle
Patches 586
41.3 Advantages of Microneedle Patches Over Conventional Drug
Delivery Routes 587
    41.3.1 Broad Applicability to Drugs Including Macromolecules 587
    41.3.2 Drug Delivery Targeted to Skin..588
    41.3.3 Simple Patch Application and Improved Patient Acceptance 588
    41.3.4 Improved Thermostability...588
    41.3.5 Avoidance of Sharps Waste 588
    41.3.6 Safety...589
    41.3.7 Single Use, Single Dose, No Reconstitution 589
    41.3.8 Mitigation of Pain and Needle Phobia 589
    41.3.9 Smaller Package Size 589
    41.3.10 Cost-Effective Manufacturing..589
41.4 Areas of Improvement in Microneedle Patches 589
    41.4.1 Incorporation of Delivery Feedback 590
    41.4.2 Reduction of Patch Wear Time on Skin..590
    41.4.3 Increased Dose of Encapsulated Drugs...590
    41.4.4 Improved Reproducibility of Microneedle Penetration
into Skin 590
41.5 Microneedle Patch Fabrication 591
    41.5.1 Microneedle Materials 591
    41.5.2 Microneedle Geometry 592
    41.5.3 Microneedle Patch Fabrication Methods 594
41.6 Assessment of Microneedle Penetration Into Skin...595
    41.6.1 Transcutaneous Electrical Resistance Measurements............................595

[*] Mark Prausnitz is an inventor of patents that have been or may be licensed to companies developing MNP-based products, a paid advisor to companies developing MNP-based products and is a founder/shareholder of companies developing MNP-based products, including Micron Biomedical. The resulting potential conflict of interest has been disclosed and is managed by the Georgia Institute of Technology and Emory University.

41.1 INTRODUCTION

Transdermal drug delivery (TDD) has existed since the first patch product was approved in 1979 to deliver drugs to the systemic circulation.[1] TDD is sometimes preferred over conventional oral drug delivery, as TDD avoids drug degradation in the gastrointestinal tract and liver. However, TDD is restricted to compounds that are able to permeate across the skin in amounts sufficient to reach therapeutic levels. In contrast, hypodermic needles broadly enable injection of drugs, but require expertise, cause pain, and generate biohazardous sharps waste.

MNPs combine the convenience of TDD and the effectiveness of hypodermic needles, while largely overcoming the individual limitations of both [1, 2]. MNPs can be administered by simply pressing onto the skin by hand to breach the upper layers of the skin barrier and thereby deliver drugs into the bloodstream through the underlying, highly vascularized dermis.

Although the idea of using MNPs was introduced and patented by ALZA Corporation in the 1970s [3], this technology was not demonstrated until microfabrication tools for making such small needles became available in the 1990s [1]. The first MN arrays reported in the literature were etched into a silicon wafer and developed for intracellular delivery *in vitro* [4]. These needles were inserted into cells and nematodes to increase molecular uptake and gene transfection. Use of MNPs for transdermal drug delivery was first reported by Henry et al. in the late 1990s, who demonstrated an increase by up to four orders of magnitude in skin permeability as a result of applying of 150-μm-long MNs to human skin *in vitro* [5]. Since then, research has been oriented toward the investigation of MN technology to deliver various compounds and development of new fabrication techniques utilizing different materials that have a wide range of MN architectures. As of the end of 2019, the MN field as a whole has generated more than 1000 peer-reviewed journal articles in different drug delivery fields and many more papers have been published since then.

In this chapter, we will discuss the advantages of MNPs over other dosage forms, specifically injections; limitations of MNPs and areas for improvement; MNP fabrication; and applications of MNPs. While MN technology has been studied in a variety of contexts, this chapter will focus on patches comprising solid MNs applied to the skin to administer drugs. Specifically, by "solid MNs," we refer to patch designs where the drug is either encapsulated within MNs or coated onto MNs. Information on the use of hollow MNs for injection, notably into the skin and the eye, and MNs for diagnostics can be found elsewhere [6–8].

41.2 GENERAL APPROACHES OF DRUG DELIVERY TO SKIN USING
MICRONEEDLE PATCHES

MNPs have been developed for delivery of drugs into the skin using a variety of mechanisms (Figure 41.1).

The first uses of MNPs to deliver drugs to the skin involved a two-step sequence [5, 10]. First, the MNP is applied to the skin and then removed, which creates an array of micropores

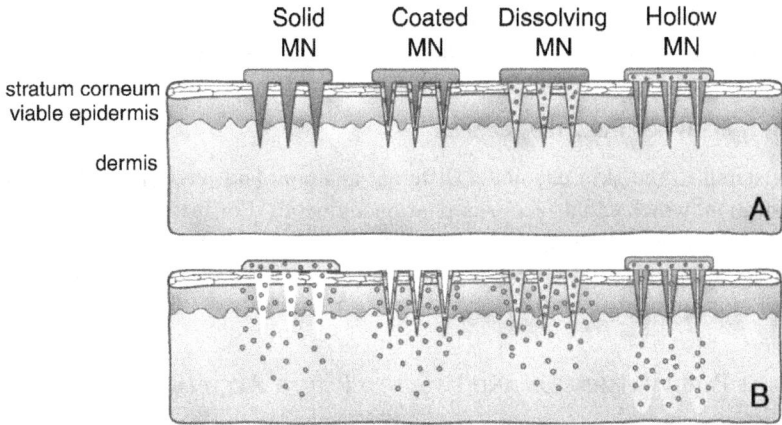

FIGURE 41.1 Methods of drug delivery to skin using microneedle patches. Microneedle patch application to skin (A). Drug delivery (B). Pretreatment with solid microneedles followed by diffusion of topically applied formulation through residual holes in skin (Solid MNs). Dissolution of drug coated onto microneedles after skin insertion (Coated MNs). Release of encapsulated drug in water-soluble or biodegradable materials in the skin upon microneedle dissolution (Dissolving MNs). Injection of liquid formulation through hollow microneedles. (Images reproduced with permission from Reference [9].)

in the skin. Second, a patch or topical formulation is applied to the porated skin surface and left in place so that drug could diffuse through the micropores into the skin. While this method is effective and is commonly used to facilitate delivery of cosmeceutical agents into the skin [11], this review will focus on next-generation MNPs that incorporate drug into the MNP.

MNPs can be fabricated to incorporate drug into the MNs matrix [12–14] so that the MN is a mixture of drug and excipients that provide the MN with mechanical strength, stabilize the drug during MNP fabrication and storage, facilitate MN dissolution, and provide other characteristics. A major advantage of this approach is that the MN dissolves in the skin, thereby releasing encapsulated drug, and leaves no sharps waste.

MNPs can also be fabricated to incorporate the drug as a coating on the surface of the MNs [15, 16]. In this case, the coating dissolves off the MNs in the skin, and the MNs generally remains intact. The coating formulation has similar functions as the formulation of dissolving MNs, except requirements for mechanical strength are generally reduced.

More recent literature has described MNs that serve as conduits for drug delivery from an external reservoir into the skin [17]. Such MNs have often been made of cross-linked hydrogel that swells in the skin, thereby providing a porous matrix through which the drug can diffuse from a reservoir in the patch backing.

41.3   ADVANTAGES OF MICRONEEDLE PATCHES OVER CONVENTIONAL DRUG DELIVERY ROUTES

MNPs have been developed to address limitations in drug delivery, notably enabling patients to self-administer drugs that would otherwise require injection, and, in some cases, to take advantage of unique capabilities of drug delivery targeted to the skin.

41.3.1   BROAD APPLICABILITY TO DRUGS INCLUDING MACROMOLECULES

Conventional transdermal delivery is limited to drugs with a molecular weight less than 500 Da, a dissociation constant (pKa) value between 6 and 9, a melting point less than 200°C, and an intermediate lipid–water partition coefficient [18–20]. MNs create holes of micron dimensions, which are orders of magnitude bigger than molecular dimensions of nanometers and therefore permit the transport of macromolecules as well as nanoparticles and microparticles [21].

41.3.2   DRUG DELIVERY TARGETED TO SKIN

Drugs administered to the skin encounter different anatomy and physiology than other routes of drug administration, which can affect drug pharmacokinetics. For instance, drugs administered to skin by suitably designed MNPs can reach the systemic circulation rapidly [22, 23], due to the rich capillary bed in the superficial dermis and effective lymphatic drainage from the skin. In addition, the rich milieu of immune cells in the skin render it a desirable target for vaccine delivery.

41.3.3   SIMPLE PATCH APPLICATION AND IMPROVED PATIENT ACCEPTANCE

MNPs can be administered by pressing onto the skin by hand or using a handheld applicator. This simple delivery method avoids the expertise needed for injections that limits patient access to medication and reduces adherence [24, 25]. In a recent clinical trial involving influenza vaccination by MNP, study participants were able to self-immunize after only brief training with audiovisual materials and without study investigator intervention [26]. In addition, the participants reported a strong preference for the MNPs compared to hypodermic injection. In other scenarios where self-administration may not be appropriate, administration by lesser-trained personnel can be used to increase access to otherwise-injectable medicines. This would be of great benefit, particularly in developing countries where not enough health care providers may be available [27]. Finally, drug administration by lesser-trained (and correspondingly lower-paid) personnel or by patient self-administration can provide cost savings [28].

41.3.4   IMPROVED THERMOSTABILITY

Many drugs need to be refrigerated during storage and transportation. This "cold chain" has costs and cannot always be maintained, especially in resource-constrained settings [29]. MNPs can provide increased drug stability at ambient and elevated temperatures, especially for biomolecules like proteins and vaccines. This thermostability can reduce overall costs and simplify the logistics of routine treatment and targeted interventions like vaccination campaigns [30–34].

Thermostabilization of influenza vaccine has received extensive attention in the MNP literature [30, 34–36]. Other vaccines have also been stabilized using MNP formulations, including measles, rubella, polio, and hepatitis B vaccines [37–40]. Drugs such as human growth hormone and parathyroid hormone have also been studied for their stability when formulated into MNPs [13, 33].

41.3.5   AVOIDANCE OF SHARPS WASTE

Unlike hypodermic needles, MNPs generate no or greatly reduced sharps waste, depending on the MNP design. For example, water-soluble MNs generate no sharps waste because the MNs dissolve away in the skin [41]. Moreover, MNPs are difficult to administer unintentionally and require specific expertise and equipment to reload with drug. This minimizes the risk of disease transmission due to accidental or intentional reuse of needles [27] and reduces or removes the cost and logistics of safe sharps disposal. Nondissolving (e.g., coated) MNs may be considered sharps waste, although they pose a different kind of hazard that is probably less than that posed by used hypodermic needles.

In all cases, used MNPs will need to be disposed of in a safe manner due to the residual bodily fluids (i.e., interstitial fluid of the skin) and/or residual drug in the MNPs. However, the amount of bodily fluid is likely to be small (i.e., less than the blood found on a used adhesive bandage) [6]. In some cases, drug residuals may not be of significant concern, but in other cases there may be dangers to others exposed to the residual drug, e.g., the drug is highly potent or a drug of abuse [42].

41.3.6 SAFETY

Because application of MNPs results in the creation of micropores in the stratum corneum to facilitate transdermal permeation of drugs, concomitant transport of other compounds or microorganisms is possible. This could be a safety concern, especially in immunocompromised patients. The safety of MNPs compared to traditional hypodermic needles has been the subject of many studies that have consistently indicated that the infection risk associated with skin application of MNPs is not likely to be greater than that associated with hypodermic needles [43, 44]. Cosmetic MN roller devices are used repeatedly (by the same person) and are not sterilized between uses, and this practice does not appear to cause infection; however, no studies have been performed to specifically address this question. Clinical trials and other human studies further support MNP safety, typically finding mild, transient erythema at the site of patch application as the most common reported side effect [26].

41.3.7 SINGLE USE, SINGLE DOSE, NO RECONSTITUTION

Vaccines are often available in multidose vials. This presentation can lead to vaccine wastage. For example, unused vaccines must be discarded when the vaccine expires before all of the doses are used, which is especially problematic in developing countries where funding for vaccines is limited [45]. Furthermore, unlike lyophilized drugs that need to be reconstituted before injection, drugs coated onto or encapsulated in MNPs do not need to be reconstituted before use, as they are "reconstituted" by the body fluids of the skin upon patch application. This simplifies administration and alleviates the need for expert personnel to perform reconstitution that, if done incorrectly, can lead to serious adverse medical consequences [46].

41.3.8 MITIGATION OF PAIN AND NEEDLE PHOBIA

MNPs are better accepted by patients because of reduced pain compared to injections [26]. People suffering from fear of hypodermic needles may not encounter this problem with MNPs given the small size of the needles and their arrangement in a patch. As a consequence, patient acceptability and adherence to MNP therapy is expected to be better than injection-based therapies, as indicated in numerous surveys of human subjects [26, 47, 48].

41.3.9 SMALLER PACKAGE SIZE

MNPs do not require large package space, especially if they have no applicator, reducing storage, transportation, and disposal costs. In contrast, injectable drugs require much more space, as they contain a large amount of water in addition to the active pharmaceutical ingredient and further require associated paraphernalia (i.e., needle, syringe, and vial).

41.3.10 COST-EFFECTIVE MANUFACTURING

Aseptic filling of vials and syringes is much more costly than manufacturing tablets. MNP manufacturing costs are likely to be competitive with injectable drugs, although probably not with tablets. A few companies have developed scaled-up MNP production facilities, but information on manufacturing cost is confidential. However, it is likely that large-scale manufacturing according to current Good Manufacturing Practice (cGMP) can be done in a cost-effective and reliable manner.

41.4 AREAS OF IMPROVEMENT IN MICRONEEDLE PATCHES

While MNPs have many advantages compared to other delivery methods, there are still areas for improvement to make drug delivery simpler, more reliable, and applicable to a larger set of drug classes.

41.4.1 Incorporation of Delivery Feedback

Patients can generally tell when they have successfully swallowed a pill or completed an injection. It would likewise be useful to have a means of assuring the patient of successful MNP application and delivery of drug payload. For example, feedback elements such as audible clickers or visible pressure-indicating sensor films have been incorporated into MNP designs [26, 49].

41.4.2 Reduction of Patch Wear Time on Skin

When a drug is coated on or encapsulated in MNs, MNPs are typically worn for minutes. In contrast, when MNs serve as conduits for drug diffusion into the skin from a reservoir (e.g., in the patch backing), the patch may need to be worn for hours or longer, which can be useful when slow drug release is desirable [17]. In some cases, reducing patch wear time on skin improves patient adherence by decreasing the risk of early patch removal [50]. Efforts to minimize wear time have focused on modification of MNP design and/or MN formulation. For instance, the rapid mechanical separation of a drug-loaded "arrowhead" from aMN shaft has enabled patch removal from skin as soon as 1 second after insertion (Figure 41.4g) [51]. MN formulation for faster dissolution has been aided by recognition that the drug and MN matrix do not need to be fully dissolved before patch removal; after they are sufficiently dissolved or hydrated so that the MNs coating or dissolving MNs matrix stays in the skin, the patch backing can be removed. For instance, rapid separation of MNs in skin was attained by including an effervescent formulation in the MNP backing, which upon contacting the skin interstitial fluid, sodium bicarbonate and citric acid in the MNP backing react to form carbon dioxide bubbles that weaken MN attachment to the patch backing and enable separation within 1 minute of skin insertion [52]. Another approach to reduce wear time is to minimize the amount of material to be dissolved and give the MN a large surface-to-volume ratio, achieved by thinner MNs or MN coatings [22]. However, this may need to be balanced with use of MNs of sufficient size to deliver a target dose and to have adequate mechanical strength.

41.4.3 Increased Dose of Encapsulated Drugs

The small size of MNPs generally limits the drug dose that can be delivered. Because coated and dissolving MNPs associate the drug with the MN, these patches can generally accommodate only up to 1 to 10 mg of drug. These MNs are attractive for vaccination given the typically small dose of vaccine (<0.1 mg). Larger doses may be achieved by using longer MNs or larger MNP areas, but these strategies are limited by pain and ergonomics of reliable MN penetration into skin [48].

Larger drug doses can be achieved by using MNPs to create conduits into the skin through which drug can be delivered over time. Skin pretreatment with MNPs followed by application of a topical formulation or patch, can deliver larger doses, but requires a two-step process, which some patients may consider cumbersome [1]. Cross-linked hydrogel MNs can be used as a drug pathway into the skin, but this method requires patients to wear a patch with in-dwelling MNs for extended periods of time. Optimal MNP design for a given application is thus influenced by the drug dose, importance of bolus vs. extended delivery, patient population, and other factors.

41.4.4 Improved Reproducibility of Microneedle Penetration into Skin

The inherent elasticity, irregular surface, and thickness variation of skin pose a challenge to the reproducibility of MNs penetration. It has been shown that the skin can deform around MNs, which results in either partial or incomplete piercing, depending upon MN length and other parameters [53]. The amount of drug delivered from the MNs into the skin corresponds directly to success and depth of insertion.

A variety of ways have been tested to overcome this limitation. One approach involves using longer MNs (i.e., approaching 1 mm in length) [54] or placing MNs atop micro-pedestals (making them, in effect, longer) to compensate for skin deformation [51]. However, longer needles are often associated with increased pain, making this approach less attractive, though it avoids the cost, size, and complexity of a high-velocity applicator, discussed later [55, 56]. Another approach is to localize the drug at the tip of the MNs, which obviates the need for full MN insertion into the skin [57].

Yet another approach involves the use of an applicator device, which provides reliable force and can increase insertion velocity. The increased strain rate associated with high-velocity insertion increases the skin's instantaneous stiffness, which avoids skin deformation during MN insertion [58]. Applicators can be an integral part of the MNP or supplied as a separate device for single or repeated use, respectively. These devices range from simple handheld applicators that either manually press MNs into the skin [55] or use a mechanically driven applicator [59–61] to more sophisticated electrically driven MNP applicators [53, 62]. The latter are more suitable for multiple use (e.g., repeated doses, multiple patients), whereas a mechanically driven applicator may be more cost-effective for single use [63]. In all cases, having an applicator adds cost and increases product size.

41.5   MICRONEEDLE PATCH FABRICATION

Optimal MN patch performance, cost, and utility depend on careful selection of MNP design specifications: materials, geometry, and fabrication process.

41.5.1   MICRONEEDLE MATERIALS

MNs have been made using a variety of different materials for delivering drug to the skin; a selection of MNs of various materials are shown in Figure 41.2.

The choice of materials for a MNP must satisfy multiple criteria that vary depending on patch design and patch components. The first MNs produced for drug delivery were made from silicon wafers using photolithography and deep reactive ion etching [5, 64]. Although silicon is attractive as a common microelectronics industry substrate with extensive processing experience, it is relatively

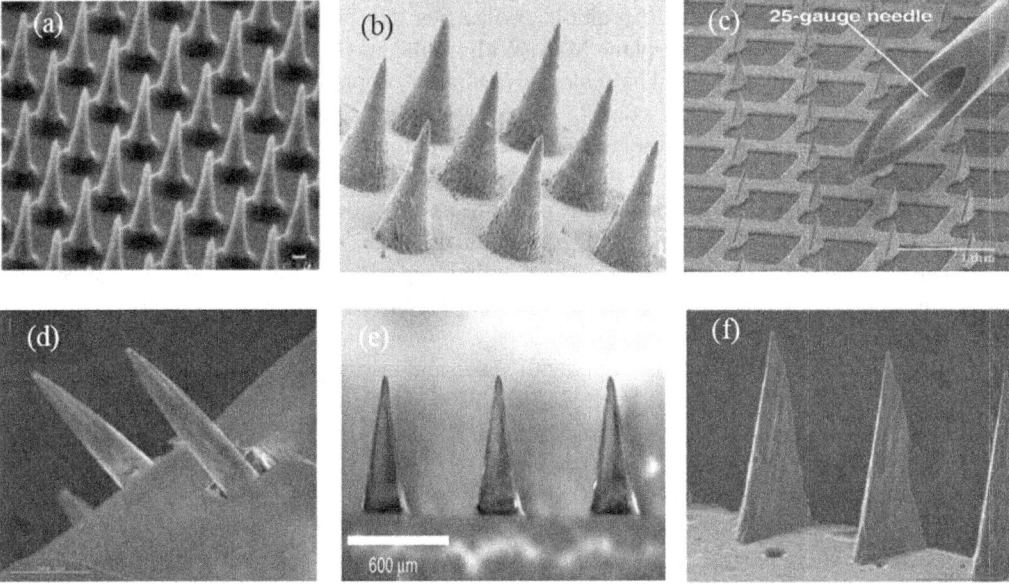

FIGURE 41.2   MNs made of different materials. (a) Silicon [64]. (b) Copolymer of methylvinylether and maleic anhydride [65]. (c) Titanium [59]. (d) Stainless steel [66]. (e) Carboxymethylcellulose [14]. (f) Maltose [67]. (Images reproduced with permission.)

expensive, fragile, unproven as a biocompatible material, and requires expensive microfabrication processes and cleanroom fabrication [63, 68, 69]. Metal MNs, either hollow or solid, are most commonly made of stainless steel [62, 70], titanium [59], palladium [71], or nickel [72]. Metal is often used to manufacture MNs, as it is mechanically strong, biocompatible, and can be produced cheaply through fabrication methods such as laser cutting [70, 73]. Metal is thus a good option for hollow MNs that require structural strength [74]; however, the small possibility of metal MNs breaking on insertion into the skin, leaving behind irretrievable pieces of metal, raises safety concerns [75].

Polymeric materials that have been efficiently fabricated into MNs include poly(methyl methacrylate) [76], poly-lactic acid [77], poly-glycolic acid [74], poly-lactic-co-glycolic acid [74], cyclic-olefin copolymer [78], polyvinylpyrrolidone [79], and sodium carboxymethylcellulose [14]. In addition, sugars such as galactose [80], maltose [67], and dextrin [81] have been used to fabricate MNs. These MNs proved superior over MNs made of other materials, as they are inexpensive, mostly biocompatible, and easily fabricated using micromolding processes that allow for mass MN production. Furthermore, the use of biodegradable and water-soluble polymers eliminates the risk of leaving biohazardous sharps waste in the skin: broken needles left embedded in the skin can safely degrade or dissolve. In addition, because of their viscoelastic properties, polymeric MNs may be less sensitive to shear-induced breakage, and drugs may be incorporated into biodegradable polymeric MNs for controlled drug delivery [68, 73, 74].

In some cases, MNs (and the backing) are made of swellable hydrogels that release encapsulated drug upon gel hydration. Materials such as poly(methyl vinyl ether-co-maleic acid) cross-linked with poly(ethylene glycol) have been used [17]. Work has also been done to develop MNs as slow-release devices made out of biodegradable polymers such as polylactic-co-glycolic acid and silk [73, 82].

41.5.2 MICRONEEDLE GEOMETRY

MN geometry is crucial for efficient MN-based drug delivery, because it influences the MNs' strength and ability to pierce the skin, and therefore the rate of drug delivery.

MNs have been developed with multiple geometries that can be divided initially into two major groups: in-plane and out-of-plane MNs. With in-plane MNs, the MN shafts or lumens are parallel to the substrate surface. The major advantage of in-plane MNs is that MN length can be easily and accurately controlled during the fabrication process [83]. Moreover, in-plane MN needle design and shape are adjustable and are beneficial for the integration of MNs with biosensors and micropumps [84]. However, it is very difficult to fabricate in-plane MN arrays with 2D geometry. In out-of-plane MNs, the lengths of the MNs protrude from the substrate surface; it is easier to fabricate out-of-plane MNs in 2D arrays. Furthermore, out-of-plane MNs have the major advantage of arranging MNs into an array so that the drug can be delivered over a larger surface area of the skin [63]. However, fabrication of out-of-plane MNs that are long and/or have a high aspect ratio is challenging [85].

MNs can be classified on the basis of overall shape and tip shape. Different MN shape designs have been proposed and fabricated, such as cylindrical, conical, pyramid, candle, spike, square, pentagonal, hexagonal, octagonal, and rocket shapes, or even more complex geometries [2, 85, 86]. Figure 41.3 shows some representative examples.

MNs typically range from 100 to 1000 μm in length and 50 to 300 μm in base diameter, with aspect ratios ranging between 2:1 and 10:1. Wider MNs and smaller aspect ratios provide increased strength that prevents MN fracture or, more typically, deformation [74, 90]. However, it is more difficult for wider MNs to penetrate deeply into the skin, which can reduce drug delivery efficiency and increase pain [55, 56, 91]. MN needle tip angles often range from 15 to 90 degrees, with various tip shapes like volcano, snake fang, cylindrical, conical, and tapered [83]. Some

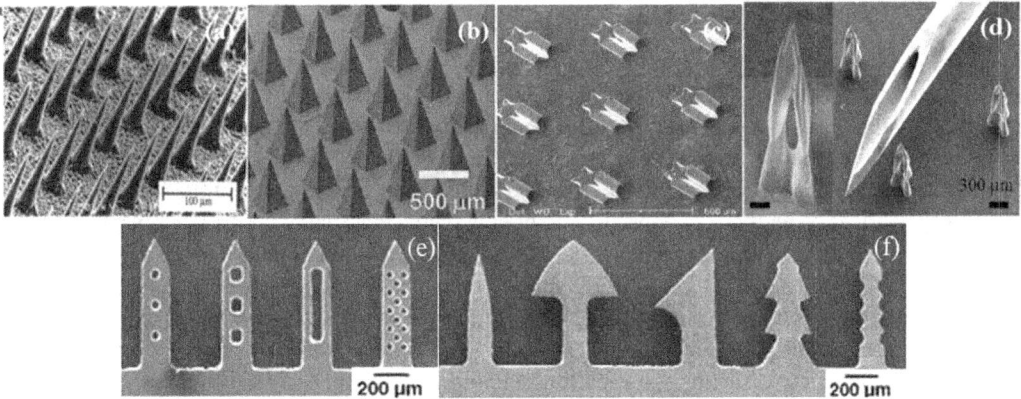

FIGURE 41.3 MNs made with different geometries. (a) Conical MNs [5]. (b) Pyramidal MNs [87]. (c) Star MNs [88]. (d) Merged tip MNs [89]. (e) Stainless steel MNs with "pockets" of different shapes and sizes etched through the MN shaft [2]. (f) Stainless steel MNs with complex shaft geometries [2]. (Images reproduced with permission.)

MNs taper continuously from a wide base to a sharp tip, which increases the mechanical strength needed to support polymer MNs [74, 90]. Other MNs have parallel walls along much of the shaft and only taper close to the tip; this design can often be strong enough for metal or silicon MNs [91]. Figure 41.4 shows representative images of MNs with different lengths, widths, needle tip angles, and shapes.

MNs are assembled into arrays that range in size typically from 10s to 10,000s of MNs. The array area is often in the range of 1 to 10 cm². This results in a wide range of MNs densities, where greater density (i.e., requiring thinner and therefore shorter MNs) can avoid the bed-of-nails effect by having sharper tips and stronger insertion forces [54, 90, 94]. Smaller densities of MNs make insertion into skin easier and accommodate wider and therefore longer MNs. Increasing MN array area accommodates more MNs (and therefore greater drug payload), but can increase pain [55, 56] and, more importantly, complicates MN insertion into nonplanar, deformable skin surfaces. The size of the MNP overall is typically larger than the MN array, in part to provide additional surface area for adhesive to adhere the patch to the skin and in part to make the patch sufficiently large for easy handling by patients.

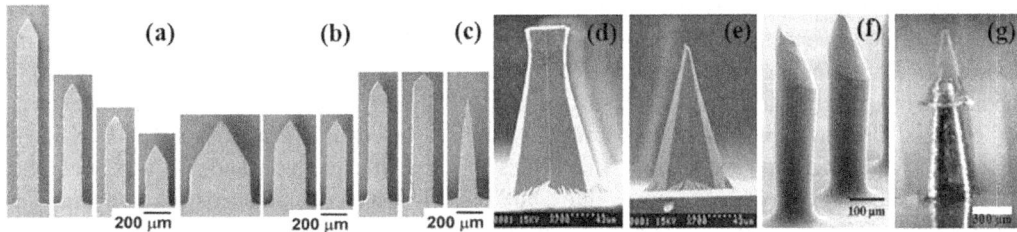

FIGURE 41.4 Scanning electron microscopy images of stainless steel MNs of different lengths (a), widths (b), and needle tip angles (c) [56]. MNs with different tip shapes (d–g): silicon MNs with flat (d) and sharp (e) tips [92], PGA MNs with bevelled (f) tips [74], and polyvinyl alcohol/sucrose separable arrowhead MNs on metallic shafts (g) [93]. (Images reproduced with permission.)

41.5.3   MICRONEEDLE PATCH FABRICATION METHODS

Since the 1990s, microfabrication technology has advanced immensely to the point that making MN-like structures is relatively straightforward. Techniques developed by the integrated circuit industry have made it possible to fabricate both solid and hollow MNs of different sizes and shapes with precise dimensions. Many additional methods have been developed to meet the needs of pharmaceutical manufacturing. A critical component of MNP manufacturing is fabrication of the MNs themselves [9, 95–97]. Fabrication methods of MNs depend greatly on the material of construction and MN type.

Reactive ion etching has been used to make MNs from silicon, notably sharp and short for vaccine delivery targeting the epidermis [5], where photolithography is employed to determine MNs spacing and base size parameters. The profile of the MNs as it tapers to a tip can be adjusted via plasma chemistry. This approach, while providing precision in MNs shape, can be costly and cumbersome to develop.

Photolithographic methods are also used in wet (e.g., in potassium hydroxide) etching of silicon to define MNs shapes along planes of silicon crystal [9, 95]; wet etching can also be used for metal MNs production (as when using acid) [98]. When etching metal MNs, the MNs are usually made in the plane of a metal sheet, creating one-dimensional linear arrays in the plane. The method can alternately etch two-dimensional arrays by etching in the plane and subsequently bending the MNs by 90 degrees. Conversely, in silicon etching, MNs generally protrude from the plane of the substrate. The metal wet etching method has been used to create MNs for use in clinical trials of drugs coating the MNs [22].

MNs can also be made with laser cutting [97]; metal MNs are produced in a manner similar to wet etching, except a laser (e.g., an Nd:YAG laser) "draws" and cuts the shapes with no need for a mask. MNs created with lasers may have rough edges that require removal with electropolishing. Inverse MN array molds have been made by "drilling" tapered holes in polymer sheets with laser ablation (e.g., with a CO_2 laser) [99].

Dissolving/polymeric MNs were initially fabricated using harsh conditions, such as UV photo curing, use of organic solvents, or elevated temperatures, where drug stability—especially in cases of biomacromolecular drugs such as proteins and DNA—was jeopardized [14, 73, 100, 101]. Furthermore, residual organic solvents and biodegradable materials themselves may lead to skin irritation [62]. An alternative way to make dissolving MNs, hydrogel MNs, and, in some cases, MNs for coating is micromolding by casting a liquid solution(s) onto an inverse mold (often made of polydimethyl siloxane) of the MNP [96]. After casting, the MNP needs to be dried before being removed from the mold, assembled into a patch, and placed in packaging. When a double casting is used, the first cast is often at least partially dried before applying the second cast. Rapid drying (e.g., using heat and/or vacuum) is desirable, but is often associated with loss of drug activity (especially for biological molecules and vaccines); drying conditions must therefore be optimized to maintain drug stability [30, 102, 103]. Air drying is typical, but lyophilization has also been used [103].

Different techniques have been demonstrated for coating MNs with molecules of varying molecular weights. The most commonly used coating method is dip coating [2, 104], where MNs are dipped into a coating solution of drugs and excipients. Those excipients have a major role in increasing the viscosity of the solution to ensure better adherence of the drug/excipients film on the MNs during drying and decreasing the MNs' surface tension to facilitate uniform coating. The latter can also be modulated by directly changing the MN surface properties. The coated film on the MNs should usually not go all the way to the base of the MN in order to limit the coating to the part of the MN that will be inserted in the skin upon application, which helps ensure optimal delivery and minimize drug loss.

Controlling the depth of MN dipping into a coating solution can localize coating, provided that surface tension–driven flow of solution up the MN shaft is considered [105]. One way to control the depth of the coating is to place a thin barrier film with an array of holes corresponding to the array of MNs over the coating solution that limits the depth to which the MN can be dipped (i.e., the MN dip is limited by MN length and film thickness). Undesirable capillary action of drugs up the MN can be mitigated by viscous formulations of coated drugs. Repeated dips can build thicker coatings and achieve higher loads of drugs, but may complicate (or in extreme cases, prevent) MN insertion [33]. Gas jets (e.g., nitrogen) can be used to force a drug coating solution that has been deposited onto the base substrate onto MNs and quickly dry the coating, particularly near the MN tips [106]. Spray coating and inkjet printing have also been used to deposit coating solution droplets onto MNs [107, 108].

Commercial facilities are currently translating lab-scale production of MNs to a larger manufacturing scale. In Singapore, the 3M corporation has utilized GMP manufacturing, producing arrays of tapered MNs ready for subsequent coating with drug formulations [109]. In Korea, hyaluronic acid MNPs for cosmeceutical applications have been produced, for example, by Raphas. Fabrication of these MNs takes place when two closely positioned surfaces are coated with liquid droplets; the surfaces then touch and are pulled away from each other, resulting in columns of fluid that produce arrays of tapered MNs when dry [110]. Other companies are also making hyaluronic and other cosmetic MNPs by other processes.

41.6 ASSESSMENT OF MICRONEEDLE PENETRATION INTO SKIN

Appropriate techniques to assure MN skin penetration and determine how MN geometry affects their penetration depth are crucial to evaluate MN design and drug delivery performance. Several techniques have been used to date.

41.6.1 Transcutaneous Electrical Resistance Measurements

The skin's electrical resistance lies predominantly in the stratum corneum, and any break in the integrity of the barrier leads to a decrease in skin impedance [111, 112]. Impedance spectroscopy is therefore a useful tool to determine skin barrier integrity after MN insertion [44, 113]. A strong correlation between skin impedance and skin permeability has been previously demonstrated: a decrease in skin impedance generally corresponds to an increase in skin permeability [114].

41.6.2 Transepidermal Water Loss Measurements

Healthy skin presents an effective barrier against water diffusion; damage to the skin barrier normally results in increased water loss by evaporation from the skin surface. Therefore, intact skin always has low basal transepidermal water loss (TEWL) values. Comparatively elevated values are an indication of tissue disruption [62, 66, 115]. Hence, TEWL measurements can be employed as an indirect method to investigate stratum corneum barrier integrity [116]. A closed-chamber, microclimate-controlled TEWL device has been demonstrated to track changes in human skin barrier function caused by the insertion of diverse MN arrays [117].

41.6.3 Labeling Micropores with Dye

This approach relies on visual or microscopic inspection of micropores created by MNs through application of a dye to the skin surface [53, 74, 118, 119]. In studies, dyes have been applied to skin pretreated with MNs, allowing infiltration of the dye into the channels created by the needles both *in vitro* and *in vivo*. The dye is then removed, and the skin is cleaned and observed. Dyes often used are trypan blue [74] and methylene blue [66, 120]. Dyes such as lissamine green [57], Evans blue [121], and sulphorhodamine B [121] can be also incorporated in dissolving MNs that, when inserted into the skin, dissolve, release the dye payload, and fill the created microconduits.

Uniformity of MN-created microchannels can be also characterized *in vivo* by calcein imaging studies [66]. The technique involves application of calcein solution to MN-pretreated skin for 30 seconds followed by removal of the dye and fluorescent imaging [122]. Image analysis is then performed using Fluoropore software, an image analysis tool that gives a value termed the "pore permeability index," representing the calcein flux into each pore.

41.6.4 HISTOLOGICAL EXAMINATION

Histological examination of MN-treated skin allows observations of MNs' ability to breach the stratum corneum barrier [66] and the depth of created channels [120]. However, these techniques are cumbersome; they involve taking a biopsy of the MN-treated skin followed by traditional histological sectioning of MN-treated skin and staining and then searching for skin sites where a MN has penetrated [115, 118, 123].

41.6.5 SCANNING ELECTRON MICROSCOPY

Creation of pores in MN-treated skin can be confirmed using scanning electron microscopy (SEM) [74]. This technique has limitations, as it involves lengthy dehydration processes that can result in altered skin structure and dimensional distortions. Most importantly, this technique cannot be utilized in an *in vivo* scenario. Generally, in cases where the technique requires MNs to be removed prior to application of the dye/marker, the inherent elasticity of the skin could cause a partial retraction of the tissue and provide an unreliable indication of the microchannel dimensions.

41.6.6 CONFOCAL LASER SCANNING MICROSCOPY

Confocal laser scanning microscopy (CLSM) is a well-established technique for obtaining high-resolution images from biological and other specimens [124]. It offers a noninvasive means for visualization of MN-created channels both *in vitro* and *in vivo* [125]. Furthermore, it allows development of depth penetration profiles of fluorescent permeants or microparticles by visualization of images parallel to the surface of the sample, at multiple depths, without the need for mechanical sectioning of the sample [126]. CLSM has been used to detect the dimensions of created microchannels by following the penetration depth profile of fluorescent microparticles through excised hairless rat skin samples treated with maltose or metallic MNs [66]. However, this method is severely limited by the fact that its maximum optical penetration depth is currently <0.25 mm into skin; it also relies on diffusion of a fluorescent dye [127]. As such, it is unable to provide information on MNs that may penetrate deeper than the epidermis or superficial dermis.

41.6.7 OPTICAL COHERENCE TOMOGRAPHY

Optical coherence tomography (OCT) is a noninvasive optical imaging technique currently capable of penetrating to tissue depths of approximately 2 mm. Therefore, OCT is a useful optical method for cross-sectional imaging of the epidermis and upper dermis *in vivo* [127]. No prior sample preparation is needed, thus removing the need for addition of a dye or radiolabeled marker to the system. OCT has been successfully used to visualize, in real time, polymeric MNPs while inserted into human skin *in vivo* [65], thus allowing for measurement of the exact depth of MN penetration. OCT has been investigated for studying the effect of varying MN geometric parameters—such as needle length and density, as well as application force—on resultant penetration characteristics (depth of MN penetration, width of pore created in the skin) of dissolving polymeric MNs *in vitro* [61]. Importantly, OCT could be successfully applied to follow *in situ* dissolution of dissolving MNs in real time [61].

41.7 COMBINING MICRONEEDLES WITH OTHER SKIN PERMEATION-ENHANCING STRATEGIES

A range of other enhancing techniques such as iontophoresis, electroporation, and use of drug carriers in combination with MNs to enhance drug delivery through MN-induced micropores have been investigated.

A significant increase in the transdermal permeation of small drugs and macromolecules was seen when combining MNs with iontophoresis [128–133]. An insulin delivery technology that combined skin pretreatment with short MNs and iontophoresis provided a continuous basal dose and on-demand bolus dosing [134]. A vaccine delivery device was capable of targeting electroporation to the dermis using an MN array coated with smallpox DNA vaccine, eliciting an antibody response similar to that against live virus [135].

Enhanced permeation of liposomes when combined with MN pretreatment of skin was demonstrated in several studies delivering either water-soluble or -insoluble drugs [136, 137]. Doxorubicin HCl and celecoxib co-loaded liposome delivery via MNs was found to be a promising strategy for skin tumor treatment, with targeting inhibition efficiency and negligible side effects [138]. Latex nanoparticles were able to cross the skin when applied to MN pretreated skin, suggesting the possibility of using nanoparticles to achieve controlled release of drug payload [64]. Solid lipid nanoparticle–loaded MNPs targeted lymph nodes where filarial nematodes reside in infected patients, leading to an effective therapy for lymphatic filariasis [139]. Several groups studied the properties of nanoparticles for optimal delivery in combination with MN pretreatment [126, 140]. Other research work has verified accumulation of the nanoparticles in the channels created by MNs [53, 141]. Nanosuspensions of cholecalciferol incorporated into dissolving MNs improved its transdermal delivery, suggesting that this combination therapy could be a promising strategy for transdermal delivery of other hydrophobic drugs [142]. A combination of more than two enhancement permeation approaches has also been studied: MN-induced microchannels in combination with iontophoresis resulted in efficient permeation of insulin-loaded nanovesicles [143].

41.8 APPLICATIONS OF MICRONEEDLE PATCHES

Delivery of dozens of different drugs via MNPs has been achieved in preclinical studies; a few of such efforts have progressed to evaluation in clinical trials. Studies have frequently compared drug pharmacokinetics, pharmacodynamics, and delivery with MNPs versus hypodermic injection to the muscle or subcutaneous space to determine if MNPs improve outcomes of drug administration (e.g., via faster uptake of drug into the bloodstream or increased vaccine immunogenicity).

41.8.1 VACCINES

Vaccine delivery is often targeted to the skin's abundant resident immunological cells, such that rapid diffusion away from the site of administration may not be desirable [82]. The extensive fluid transport from the skin to draining lymph nodes is another mechanism that can promote immune responses to skin vaccination. MN-based skin vaccination has enabled improved immune responses (compared to standard needle-and-syringe injection into muscle), as shown by vaccine dose sparing, greater longevity of immunity, greater breadth of immunity, and other features of the immune response [144–146]. Furthermore, compared to injection of liquid formulations, dry vaccines given by MNP may reside in the skin for a longer time due to slow clearance from the locally viscous environment created by MN excipients; slow release of vaccines has been shown to increase immunogenicity [82, 147].

Most vaccine clinical trials and much of the published literature on MNP use for vaccines have focused on the influenza vaccine [145]. Immune response in human subjects following influenza vaccination via MNs was observed in phase 1 clinical trials [26, 31, 148]. Several immunological advantages to MNP vaccination have been seen in animal (primarily murine) studies, including significant vaccine dose sparing. In one study, 1/100th of a dose of vaccine via MNP elicited an immune response similar to that following a full dose delivered intramuscularly [149]. Greater length and breadth of immunity, improved cellular immune responses, more rapid postinfection virus clearance from lungs, and isotype switching have been observed subsequent to MNP vaccination in comparison to intramuscular and subcutaneous injections of vaccine [144–146].

MNPs have also been tested for delivery of anthrax, Chikungunya virus, diphtheria, hepatitis B, hepatitis C, herpes simplex, human papillomavirus, inactivated poliovirus, measles, rubella, Ebola, rabies, rotavirus, plague, tetanus toxoid, tuberculosis, West Nile virus, and other vaccines [144–146, 150]. MNP vaccines have elicited both humoral and cellular immune responses in mice, rats, guinea pigs, rabbits, pigs, and macaques; these responses are frequently superior to responses following hypodermic injection of vaccine.

Delivering vaccine using extremely dense arrays of MNs (e.g., 10,000/cm^2) has demonstrated potent vaccine dose sparing, resulting from generation of a local milieu of immunogenic signals released due to epidermal cell death at the site of MNP insertion [151].

41.8.2 Drugs

Small-molecule and peptide drugs have progressed rapidly into clinical translation, though there is a relative paucity of information on use of MNs in these contexts in the literature. Advanced parathyroid hormone–related therapies for osteoporosis using MNPs have been through clinical trials with two different companies; one of these trials has entered phase 3 [152]. In these studies, patients have been able to self-administer MNPs. The drug absorbs quickly in comparison to subcutaneous injection, and improved clinical outcomes have been observed in terms of increased bone mass density [22]. Human studies using MNP delivery have also been conducted with zolmitriptan to treat migraines [153], insulin to treat diabetes [154], doxorubicin to treat basal cell carcinoma [155], glucagon to treat severe hypoglycemia [156], 5-aminolevulinic acid as part of photodynamic therapy of skin conditions [157], lidocaine for local anesthesia, and naltrexone to treat substance abuse disorders [10].

MN-assisted delivery of other drugs for systemic or local effect has also been studied in preclinical settings. Delivery of caffeine, galanthamine, ibuprofen, metronidazole, and theophylline for systemic effects has been evaluated [9, 158]. As noted earlier, drugs for photodynamic therapy and local anesthesia in the skin have been administered for a local effect, as has phenylephrine (near the anal sphincter) to treat fecal incontinence [159].

Insulin has received significant study for MNP delivery in bolus, basal, and glucose-responsive delivery forms [160, 161], as have other peptide and protein drugs. These include erythropoietin, low-molecular-weight heparin, oxytocin, leuprolide acetate, desmopressin, human growth hormone, levonorgestrel, salmon calcitonin, and, as mentioned earlier, parathyroid hormone [9, 158, 162, 163]. Plasmid DNA and siRNA have been administered using MNPs in several studies [164].

41.8.3 Cosmeceuticals

The scientific literature to date has primarily focused on medical applications of MNs. However, many cosmetic products based on MN technology are available for sale worldwide [165]. The first MN cosmetic products were introduced two decades ago. These take the form of a cylindrical drum roller that can be rolled across the skin, creating microscopic punctures with metal (and later polymer) MNs attached to the roller. Several such devices, such as Dermaroller designs, are currently available for cosmetic uses. Newer devices repeatedly apply a planar array of MNs to the skin, and sometimes incorporate electromechanical devices (e.g., Dermastamp). These devices are designed to trigger wound repair mechanisms in the skin (skin inflammation, proliferation, and remodeling) that promote collagen production and improve skin texture [166]. Other devices are often marketed for use with topical formulations: the MN device pretreats and porates the skin, and subsequent materials (e.g., glycolic acid peels and platelet-rich plasma) enter the skin more through the pores [137, 165, 167, 168].

Intradermal hyaluronic acid injections are widely used as cosmetic fillers, frequently to counteract the visual signs of skin aging. Dissolving MNs made of hyaluronic acid have been developed and marketed for similar cosmetic purposes. Unlike injections, MNPs can be used for self-administration of hyaluronic acid. These products have been gaining traction and popularity [169]. Recently, to camouflage visual contrast between hair strands and scalp skin, micropigment-encapsulated biodegradable MNs were developed that successfully delivered pigments, serving as a novel platform for scalp micropigmentation [170]. A combination technique involving MNs and fractional radiofrequency, known as microneedling fractional radiofrequency (MFR), has been the subject of several publications and is currently being tested in several clinical trials [171–173]. The dermal structure alteration caused by application of radiofrequency currents using insulated MNs is designed to stimulate neoelastogenesis and neocollagenesis [174].

With the increased interest in the cosmetic applications of MNs, several companies have commenced clinical trials. As of April 2021, 19 different clinical trials related to cosmetic applications of MNs have been reported at the U.S. National Institutes of Health's database of clinical trials at www.clinicaltrials.gov. Areas of investigation include the effects of MNs on skin scars, acne, vitiligo, signs of skin aging, wrinkles (including "crow's feet"), androgenic alopecia, texture, pigmentation, and cellulite.

41.9   FUTURE PERSPECTIVES

There is a great deal of excitement about and high expectations of the MN research field, evidenced by the increased number of research publications and groups working in this field over the past 20 years. However, the ultimate measure of impact of MNs is their translation into use in clinical medicine to benefit patients. Rigorous scientific and engineering development and evaluation are necessary; significant funding from the pharmaceutical industry willing to pay for product development and advanced clinical trials will also be required.

Two areas for MN research with far-reaching implications for human health can be highlighted. The first is the extent of benefits patients can expect from MNPs relative to more traditional technologies. The second is the development of low-cost, scalable, and reliable processes for MNP manufacturing. In animal models, vaccines delivered by MNPs are highly immunogenic, even at greatly reduced dosages; however, only limited studies to assess these findings in humans are available. The extent to which benefits observed in animal models and small-scale studies—for example, drug delivery to the skin that is appealing to patients; more rapid uptake into the bloodstream than traditional methods of drug administration—will persist in larger populations taking medication for longer periods of time, in contexts less rigorously controlled than a clinical trial needs further study. MNPs have proven popular in experimental settings and during formative evaluation activities like interviews and surveys, but it remains to be seen if people will prefer them in general and whether health care payers will be willing to invest in and pay for them.

Such questions are typical for the development of any innovative new medical technology. Their ubiquity, however, does not reduce the necessity to find answers through increased human experience in advanced clinical trials and evaluation of products developed for use in everyday clinical practice.

The first phase 3 human clinical trial is now underway, and more and more companies are investing in MN research and development, which is occurring in parallel with the growing success of MNs for cosmetic use. This suggests an increased confidence in the research community that patient acceptance and mass production of MNPs can be achieved. MNPs for medical applications are advancing closer to clinical practice, and the first approved medical products will likely be launched within several years.

41.10   CONCLUSION

Successful drug delivery with MNPs was first demonstrated approximately two decades ago. Since then, researchers have developed MN technologies that simplify administration of otherwise-injectable drugs to increase patient access to medicines and can improve drug pharmacokinetics and vaccine immunogenicity due to targeted drug delivery to the skin.

Numerous design objectives must be considered in order to create an optimal MNP. Critical design parameters like MN geometry and MN or MNP materials have significantly different effects and can be adjusted as needed. Drug formulations, patient populations, medical/public health goals, and other application-specific information will inform specific design objectives and their relative prioritization. Several issues must be considered during any MN conceptualization, design, or production process: drug stability in or on MNs, MNP application and insertion biomechanics, the fate of drug molecules in skin transported to capillaries for systemic distribution or to immune cells for vaccination, and MNP disposal after use.

MNPs can deliver drugs via coating or encapsulating drug onto or within MNs for release by dissolution in the skin; this approach has received significant attention in the literature and is being used in clinical trials for delivery of drugs, peptides, and vaccines. MNPs can also be designed to deliver drugs into skin by creating drug transport conduits in the skin; these can be residual holes created by pretreating skin with MNPs or by embedding porous (typically hydrogel) MNs in the skin.

Though the bulk of MNP technology commercialization and mass production to date has been for cosmetic applications, pharmaceutical applications are advancing through clinical trials, and cGMP manufacturing is being scaled up by many companies around the world. The union of robust commercialization programs with a strong research foundation will accelerate the development and use of MNPs for medical applications, including vaccination and drug delivery, in turn improving patient access and drug efficacy.

NOTE

1 Note that the term "drug" is used throughout this chapter to include therapeutic drugs as well as vaccines, cosmeceutical compounds, and other active materials being delivered.

REFERENCES

1. Prausnitz, M.R., Microneedles for transdermal drug delivery. Adv Drug Deliv Rev, 2004, **56**(5): p. 581–7.
2. Gill, H.S. and M.R. Prausnitz, Coated microneedles for transdermal delivery. J Control Release, 2007, **117**(2): p. 227–37.
3. Gerstel, M.S. and V.A. Place, Drug delivery device. US Patent number 3964482, 1976.
4. Hashmi, S., P. Ling, G. Hashmi, M. Reed, R. Gaugler, and W. Trimmer, Genetic transformation of nematodes using arrays of micromechanical piercing structures. Biotechniques, 1995, **19**(5): p. 766–70.
5. Henry, S., D.V. McAllister, M.G. Allen, and M.R. Prausnitz, Microfabricated microneedles: a novel approach to transdermal drug delivery. J Pharm Sci, 1998, **87**(8): p. 922–5.
6. Donnelly, R.F., K. Mooney, E. Caffarel-Salvador, B.M. Torrisi, E. Eltayib, and J.C. McElnay, Microneedle-mediated minimally invasive patient monitoring. Ther Drug Monit, 2014, **36**(1): p. 10–7.
7. Kim, Y.C., B. Chiang, X. Wu, and M.R. Prausnitz, Ocular delivery of macromolecules. J Control Release, 2014, **190**: p. 172–81.
8. Pettis, R.J. and A.J. Harvey, Microneedle delivery: clinical studies and emerging medical applications. Ther Deliv, 2012, **3**(3): p. 357–71.
9. Kim, Y.C., J.H. Park, and M.R. Prausnitz, Microneedles for drug and vaccine delivery. Adv Drug Deliv Rev, 2012, **64**(14): p. 1547–68.
10. Wermeling, D.P., S.L. Banks, D.A. Hudson, H.S. Gill, J. Gupta, M.R. Prausnitz, and A.L. Stinchcomb, Microneedles permit transdermal delivery of a skin-impermeant medication to humans. Proc Natl Acad Sci U S A, 2008, **105**(6): p. 2058–63.
11. Bhatnagar, S., K. Dave, and V.V.K. Venuganti, Microneedles in the clinic. J Control Release, 2017, **260**: p. 164–82.
12. Jeong, H.R., J.Y. Kim, S.N. Kim, and J.H. Park, Local dermal delivery of cyclosporin A, a hydrophobic and high molecular weight drug, using dissolving microneedles. Eur J Pharm Biopharm, 2018, **127**: p. 237–43.
13. Lee, J.W., S.O. Choi, E.I. Felner, and M.R. Prausnitz, Dissolving microneedle patch for transdermal delivery of human growth hormone. Small, 2011, **7**(4): p. 531–9.

14. Lee, J.W., J.H. Park, and M.R. Prausnitz, Dissolving microneedles for transdermal drug delivery. Biomaterials, 2008, **29**(13): p. 2113–24.

15. Widera, G., J. Johnson, L. Kim, L. Libiran, K. Nyam, P.E. Daddona, and M. Cormier, Effect of delivery parameters on immunization to ovalbumin following intracutaneous administration by a coated microneedle array patch system. Vaccine, 2006, **24**(10): p. 1653–64.

16. Ingrole, R.S.J. and H.S. Gill, Microneedle coating methods: A review with a perspective. J Pharmacol Exp Ther, 2019, **370**(3): p. 555–69.

17. Donnelly, R.F., T.R. Singh, M.J. Garland, K. Migalska, R. Majithiya, C.M. McCrudden, P.L. Kole, T.M. Mahmood, H.O. McCarthy, and A.D. Woolfson, Hydrogel-forming microneedle arrays for enhanced transdermal drug delivery. Adv Funct Mater, 2012, **22**(23): p. 4879–90.

18. Bos, J.D. and M.M. Meinardi, The 500 Dalton rule for the skin penetration of chemical compounds and drugs. Exp Dermatol, 2000. **9**(3): p. 165–69.

19. Shah, V.P., *Transdermal drug delivery system regulatory issues*, in *Transdermal Drug Delivery*, Guy R.H. and J. Hadgraft, Editors. 2003, Marcel Dekker Inc: New York. p. 361–67.

20. Meidan, V.M. and B.B. Michniak, Emerging technologies in transdermal therapeutics. Am J Ther, 2004, **11**(4): p. 312–16.

21. Shakeel, M., P. Dilnawaz, A.R. Ziyaurrrahman, B. Akber, and S. Bushra, Microneedle as a novel drug delivery system: a review. Int Res J Pharm, 2011, **2**(2): p. 72–7.

22. Daddona, P.E., J.A. Matriano, J. Mandema, and Y.F. Maa, Parathyroid hormone (1–34)-coated microneedle patch system: clinical pharmacokinetics and pharmacodynamics for treatment of osteoporosis. Pharm Res, 2011, **28**(1): p. 159–65.

23. Harvey, A.J., S.A. Kaestner, D.E. Sutter, N.G. Harvey, J.A. Mikszta, and R.J. Pettis, Microneedle-based intradermal delivery enables rapid lymphatic uptake and distribution of protein drugs. Pharm Res, 2011, **28**(1): p. 107–16.

24. Donnelly, R.F., K. Moffatt, A.Z. Alkilani, E.M. Vicente-Perez, J. Barry, M.T. McCrudden, and A.D. Woolfson, Hydrogel-forming microneedle arrays can be effectively inserted in skin by self-application: a pilot study centred on pharmacist intervention and a patient information leaflet. Pharm Res, 2014, **31**(8): p. 1989–99.

25. Norman, J.J., J.M. Arya, M.A. McClain, P.M. Frew, M.I. Meltzer, and M.R. Prausnitz, Microneedle patches: usability and acceptability for self-vaccination against influenza. Vaccine, 2014, **32**(16): p. 1856–62.

26. Rouphael, N.G., M. Paine, R. Mosley, S. Henry, D.V. McAllister, H. Kalluri, W. Pewin, P.M. Frew, T. Yu, N.J. Thornburg, S. Kabbani, L. Lai, E.V. Vassilieva, I. Skountzou, R.W. Compans, M.J. Mulligan, M.R. Prausnitz, and T.-M.S. Group, The safety, immunogenicity, and acceptability of inactivated influenza vaccine delivered by microneedle patch (TIV-MNP 2015): a randomised, partly blinded, placebo-controlled, phase 1 trial. Lancet, 2017, **390**(10095): p. 649–58.

27. Kermode, M., Unsafe injections in low-income country health settings: need for injection safety promotion to prevent the spread of blood-borne viruses. Health Promot Int, 2004, **19**(1): p. 95–103.

28. Lee, B.Y., S.M. Bartsch, M. Mvundura, C. Jarrahian, K.M. Zapf, K. Marinan, A.R. Wateska, B. Snyder, S. Swaminathan, E. Jacoby, J.J. Norman, M.R. Prausnitz, and D. Zehrung, An economic model assessing the value of microneedle patch delivery of the seasonal influenza vaccine. Vaccine, 2015, **33**(37): p. 4727–36.

29. Kartoglu, U. and J. Milstien, Tools and approaches to ensure quality of vaccines throughout the cold chain. Expert Rev Vaccines, 2014, **13**(7): p. 843–54.

30. Vrdoljak, A., E.A. Allen, F. Ferrara, N.J. Temperton, A.M. Crean, and A.C. Moore, Induction of broad immunity by thermostabilised vaccines incorporated in dissolvable microneedles using novel fabrication methods. J Control Release, 2016, **225**: p. 192–204.

31. Hirobe, S., H. Azukizawa, T. Hanafusa, K. Matsuo, Y.S. Quan, F. Kamiyama, I. Katayama, N. Okada, and S. Nakagawa, Clinical study and stability assessment of a novel transcutaneous influenza vaccination using a dissolving microneedle patch. Biomaterials, 2015, **57**: p. 50–8.

32. Pearson, F.E., C.L. McNeilly, M.L. Crichton, C.A. Primiero, S.R. Yukiko, G.J. Fernando, X. Chen, S.C. Gilbert, A.V. Hill, and M.A. Kendall, Dry-coated live viral vector vaccines delivered by nanopatch microprojections retain long-term thermostability and induce transgene-specific T cell responses in mice. PLoS One, 2013, **8**(7): p. e67888.

33. Ameri, M., P.E. Daddona, and Y.F. Maa, Demonstrated solid-state stability of parathyroid hormone PTH(1–34) coated on a novel transdermal microprojection delivery system. Pharm Res, 2009, **26**(11): p. 2454–63.

34. Mistilis, M.J., J.C. Joyce, E.S. Esser, I. Skountzou, R.W. Compans, A.S. Bommarius, and M.R. Prausnitz, Long-term stability of influenza vaccine in a dissolving microneedle patch. Drug Deliv Transl Res, 2017, **7**(2): p. 195–205.

35. Kim, Y.C., F.S. Quan, R.W. Compans, S.M. Kang, and M.R. Prausnitz, Stability kinetics of influenza vaccine coated onto microneedles during drying and storage. Pharm Res, 2011, **28**(1): p. 135–44.

36. Chen, X., G.J. Fernando, M.L. Crichton, C. Flaim, S.R. Yukiko, E.J. Fairmaid, H.J. Corbett, C.A. Primiero, A.B. Ansaldo, I.H. Frazer, L.E. Brown, and M.A. Kendall, Improving the reach of vaccines to low-resource regions, with a needle-free vaccine delivery device and long-term thermostabilization. J Control Release, 2011, **152**(3): p. 349–55.

37. Edens, C., M.L. Collins, J.L. Goodson, P.A. Rota, and M.R. Prausnitz, A microneedle patch containing measles vaccine is immunogenic in non-human primates. Vaccine, 2015. **33**(37): p. 4712–8.

38. Guo, L., Y. Qiu, J. Chen, S. Zhang, B. Xu, and Y. Gao, Effective transcutaneous immunization against hepatitis B virus by a combined approach of hydrogel patch formulation and microneedle arrays. Biomed Microdevices, 2013, **15**(6): p. 1077–85.

39. Kolluru, C., Y. Gomaa, and M.R. Prausnitz, Development of a thermostable microneedle patch for polio vaccination. Drug Deliv Transl Res, 2019, **9**(1): p. 192–203.

40. Joyce, J.C., T.D. Carroll, M.L. Collins, M.H. Chen, L. Fritts, J.C. Dutra, T.L. Rourke, J.L. Goodson, M.B. McChesney, M.R. Prausnitz, and P.A. Rota, A microneedle patch for measles and rubella vaccination is immunogenic and protective in infant rhesus macaques. J Infect Dis, 2018, **218**(1): p. 124–32.

41. Liu, L., Y. Wang, J. Yao, C. Yang, and G. Ding, A minimally invasive micro sampler for quantitative sampling with an ultrahigh-aspect-ratio microneedle and a PDMS actuator. Biomed Microdevices, 2016, **18**(4): p. 59.

42. Pastore, M.N., Y.N. Kalia, M. Horstmann, and M.S. Roberts, Transdermal patches: history, development and pharmacology. Br J Pharmacol, 2015, **172**(9): p. 2179–209.

43. Donnelly, R.F., T.R. Singh, M.M. Tunney, D.I. Morrow, P.A. McCarron, C. O'Mahony, and A.D. Woolfson, Microneedle arrays allow lower microbial penetration than hypodermic needles in vitro. Pharm Res 2009, **26**(11): p. 2513–22.

44. Gupta, J., H.S. Gill, S.N. Andrews, and M.R. Prausnitz, Kinetics of skin resealing after insertion of microneedles in human subjects. J Control Release, 2011, **154**(2): p. 148–55.

45. Sridhar, S., N. Maleq, E. Guillermet, A. Colombini, and B.D. Gessner, A systematic literature review of missed opportunities for immunization in low- and middle-income countries. Vaccine, 2014. **32**(51): p. 6870–9.

46. Clements, C.J., G. Larsen, and L. Jodar, Technologies that make administration of vaccines safer. Vaccine, 2004, **22**(15-16): p. 2054–8.

47. Arya, J., S. Henry, H. Kalluri, D.V. McAllister, W.P. Pewin, and M.R. Prausnitz, Tolerability, usability and acceptability of dissolving microneedle patch administration in human subjects. Biomaterials, 2017, **128**: p. 1–7.

48. Ripolin, A., J. Quinn, E. Larraneta, E.M. Vicente-Perez, J. Barry, and R.F. Donnelly, Successful application of large microneedle patches by human volunteers. Int J Pharm, 2017. **521**(1-2): p. 92–101.

49. Vicente-Perez, E.M., H.L. Quinn, E. McAlister, S. O'Neill, L.A. Hanna, J.G. Barry, and R.F. Donnelly, The use of a pressure-indicating sensor film to provide feedback upon hydrogel-forming microneedle array self-application in vivo. Pharm Res, 2016, 33(12): p. 3072–80.

50. Birchall, J.C., R. Clemo, A. Anstey, and D.N. John, Microneedles in clinical practice–an exploratory study into the opinions of healthcare professionals and the public. Pharm Res, 2011, **28**(1): p. 95–106.

51. Chu, L.Y. and M.R. Prausnitz, Separable arrowhead microneedles. J Control Release, 2011, **149**(3): p. 242–9.

52. Li, W., J. Tang, R.N. Terry, S. Li, A. Brunie, R.L. Callahan, R.K. Noel, C.A. Rodriguez, S.P. Schwendeman, and M.R. Prausnitz, Long-acting reversible contraception by effervescent microneedle patch. Sci Adv, 2019, **5**(11): p. eaaw8145.

53. Verbaan, F.J., S.M. Bal, D.J. van den Berg, J.A. Dijksman, M. van Hecke, H. Verpoorten, A. van den Berg, R. Luttge, and J.A. Bouwstra, Improved piercing of microneedle arrays in dermatomed human skin by an impact insertion method. J Control Release, 2008, **128**(1): p. 80–8.

54. Yan, G., K.S. Warner, J. Zhang, S. Sharma, and B.K. Gale, Evaluation needle length and density of microneedle arrays in the pretreatment of skin for transdermal drug delivery. Int J Pharm, 2010, **391**(1-2): p. 7–12.

55. Haq, M.I., E. Smith, D.N. John, M. Kalavala, C. Edwards, A. Anstey, A. Morrissey, and J.C. Birchall, Clinical administration of microneedles: skin puncture, pain and sensation. Biomed Microdevices, 2009, **11**(1): p. 35–47.

56. Gill, H.S., D.D. Denson, B.A. Burris, and M.R. Prausnitz, Effect of microneedle design on pain in human subjects. Clin J Pain, 2008, **24** (7): p. 585–94.

57. Fukushima, K., A. Ise, H. Morita, R. Hasegawa, Y. Ito, N. Sugioka, and K. Takada, Two-layered dissolving microneedles for percutaneous delivery of peptide/protein drugs in rats. Pharm Res, 2011, **28**(1): p. 7–21.

58. van der Maaden, K., E. Sekerdag, W. Jiskoot, and J. Bouwstra, Impact-insertion applicator improves reliability of skin penetration by solid microneedle arrays. AAPS J, 2014, **16**(4): p. 681–4.

59. Matriano, J.A., M. Cormier, J. Johnson, W.A. Young, M. Buttery, K. Nyam, and P.E. Daddona, Macroflux microprojection array patch technology: a new and efficient approach for intracutaneous immunization. Pharm Res, 2002, **19**(1): p. 63–70.

60. Verbaan, F.J., S.M. Bal, D.J. van den Berg, W.H. Groenink, H. Verpoorten, R. Luttge, and J.A. Bouwstra, Assembled microneedle arrays enhance the transport of compounds varying over a large range of molecular weight across human dermatomed skin. J Control Release, 2007, **117**(2): p. 238–45.

61. Donnelly, R.F., M.J. Garland, D.I.J. Morrow, K. Migalska, T.R.R. Singh, R. Majithiya, and A.D. Woolfson, Optical coherence tomography is a valuable tool in the study of the effects of microneedle geometry on skin penetration characteristics and in-skin dissolution. J Control Release, 2010, **147**(3): p. 333–41.

62. Bal, S.M., J. Caussin, S. Pavel, and J.A. Bouwstra, In vivo assessment of safety of microneedle arrays in human skin. Eur J Pharm Sci, 2008, **35**(3): p. 193–202.

63. van der Maaden, K., W. Jiskoot, and J. Bouwstra, Microneedle technologies for (trans) dermal drug and vaccine delivery. J Control Release, 2012, **161**(2): p. 645–55.

64. McAllister, D.V., P.M. Wang, S.P. Davis, J.H. Park, P.J. Canatella, M.G. Allen, and M.R. Prausnitz, Microfabricated needles for transdermal delivery of macromolecules and nanoparticles: fabrication methods and transport studies. Proc Natl Acad Sci USA, 2003, **100**(24): p. 13755–60.

65. Donnelly, R.F., R. Majithiya, T.R.R. Singh, D.I.J. Morrow, M.J. Garland, Y.K. Demir, k. Migalska, E. Ryan, D. Gillen, C.J. Scott, and A.D. Woolfson, Design, optimization and characterization of polymeric microneedle arrays prepared by a novel laser-based micromoulding technique. Pharm Res, 2011, **28**(1): p. 41–57.

66. Li, G., A. Badkar, H. Kalluri, and A.K. Banga, Microchannels created by sugar and metal microneedles: characterization by microscopy, macromolecular flux and other techniques. J Pharm Sci, 2010, **99**(4): p. 1931–41.

67. Li, G., A. Badkar, S. Nema, C.S. Kolli, and A.K. Banga, In vitro transdermal delivery of therapeutic antibodies using maltose microneedles. Int J Pharm, 2009, **368**(1-2): p. 109–15.

68. Banga, A.K., Microporation applications for enhancing drug delivery. Expert Opin Drug Deliv, 2009, **6**(4): p. 343–54.

69. Arora, A., M.R. Prausnitz, and S. Mitragotri, Micro-scale devices for transdermal drug delivery. Int J Pharm, 2008. **364**(2): p. 227–36.

70. Martanto, W., S.P. Davis, N.R. Holiday, J. Wang, H.S. Gill, and M.R. Prausnitz, Transdermal delivery of insulin using microneedles in vivo. Pharm Res, 2004, **21**(6): p. 947–52.

71. Chandrasekaran, S., J.D. Brazzle, and A.B. Frazier, Surface micromachined metallic microneedles. J MEMS, 2003, **12**(3): p. 281–88.

72. Davis, S.P., W. Martanto, M.G. Allen, and M.R. Prausnitz, Hollow metal microneedles for insulin delivery to diabetic rats. IEEE Trans Biomed Eng, 2005, **52**(5): p. 909–15.

73. Park, J.H., M.G. Allen, and M.R. Prausnitz, Polymer microneedles for controlled-release drug delivery. Pharm Res, 2006, **23**(5): p. 1008–19.

74. Park, J.H., M.G. Allen, and M.R. Prausnitz, Biodegradable polymer microneedles: fabrication, mechanics and transdermal drug delivery. J Control Release, 2005, **104**(1): p. 51–66.

75. Martanto, W., J.S. Moore, T. Couse, and M.R. Prausnitz, Mechanism of fluid infusion during microneedle insertion and retraction. J Control Release, 2006, **112**(3): p. 357–61.

76. Moon, S.J. and S.S. Lee, A novel fabrication method of a micro-needle array using inclined deep x-ray exposure. J Micromech Microeng, 2005, **15**(5): p. 903–11.

77. Han, M., D.K. Kim, H.K. Seong, H.R. Yoon, B.Y. Kim, S.S. Lee, K.D. Kim, and H.G. Lee, Improvement in antigen delivery using fabrication of a grooves-embedded microneedle array. Sensor Actuat B-Chem, 2009, **137**(1): p. 274–80.

78. Lippmann, J.M., E.J. Geiger, and A.P. Pisano, Polymer investment molding: Method for fabricating hollow, microscale parts. Sensor Actuat A- Phys, 2007, **134**(1): p. 2–10.

79. Sullivan, S.P., D.G. Koutsonanos, M. Del Pilar Martin, J.W. Lee, V. Zarnitsyn, S.O. Choi, N. Murthy, R.W. Compans, I. Skountzou, and M.R. Prausnitz, Dissolving polymer microneedle patches for influenza vaccination. Nat Med, 2010, **16**(8): p. 915–20.

80. Donnelly, R.F., D.I. Morrow, T.R. Singh, K. Migalska, P.A. McCarron, C. O'Mahony, and A.D. Woolfson, Processing difficulties and instability of carbohydrate microneedle arrays. Drug Dev Ind Pharm, 2009, **35**(10): p. 1242–54.

81. Ito, Y., J. Yoshimitsu, K. Shiroyama, N. Sugioka, and K. Takada, Self-dissolving microneedles for the percutaneous absorption of EPO in mice. J Drug Target, 2006, **14**(5): p. 255–61.

82. DeMuth, P.C., Y. Min, D.J. Irvine, and P.T. Hammond, Implantable silk composite microneedles for programmable vaccine release kinetics and enhanced immunogenicity in transcutaneous immunization. Adv Healthc Mater, 2014. **3**(1): p. 47–58.

83. Ashraf, M.W., S. Tayyaba, and N. Afzulpurkar, Micro electromechanical systems (MEMS) based microfluidic devices for biomedical applications. Int J Mol Sci, 2011, **12**(6): p. 3648–704.

84. Gardeniers, H.J.G.E., R. Luttge, E.J.W. Berenschot, M.J. de Boer, S.Y. Yeshurun, M. Hefetz, R. van 't Oever, and A. van den Berg, Silicon micromachined hollow microneedles for transdermal liquid transport. J Microelectromech Syst, 2003, **12**(6): p. 855–62.

85. Ashraf, M.W., S. Tayyaba, A. Nisar, N. Afzulpurkar, D.W. Bodhale, T. Lomas, A. Poyai, and A. Tuantranont, Design, fabrication and analysis of silicon hollow microneedles for transdermal drug delivery system for treatment of hemodynamic dysfunctions. Cardiovasc Eng, 2010, **10**(3): p. 91–108.

86. Ashraf, M.W., S. Tayyaba, N. Afzulpurkar, and A. Nisar, Fabrication and analysis of tapered tip silicon microneedles for mems based drug delivery system. Sensors and Transducers Journal, 2010, **122**(11): p. 158–73.

87. Park, J.H., S.O. Choi, S. Seo, Y.B. Choy, and M.R. Prausnitz, A microneedle roller for transdermal drug delivery. Eur J Pharm Biopharm, 2010, **76**(2): p. 282–89.

88. Zhang, W., J. Gao, Q. Zhu, M. Zhang, X. Ding, X. Wang, X. Hou, W. Fan, B. Ding, X. Wu, and S. Gao, Penetration and distribution of PLGA nanoparticles in the human skin treated with microneedles. Int J Pharm, 2010, **402**(1-2): p. 205–12.

89. Lim, J., D. Tahk, J. Yu, D.H. Min, and N.L. Jeon, Design rules for a tunable merged-tip microneedle. Microsyst Nanoeng, 2018, **4**: p. 29.

90. Ita, K., Reflections on the insertion and fracture forces of microneedles. Curr Drug Deliv, 2017. **14**(3): p. 357–63.

91. Davis, S.P., B.J. Landis, Z.H. Adams, M.G. Allen, and M.R. Prausnitz, Insertion of microneedles into skin: measurement and prediction of insertion force and needle fracture force. J Biomech, 2004, **37**(8): p. 1155–63.

92. Wei-Ze, L., H. Mei-Rong, Z. Jian-Ping, Z. Yong-Qiang, H. Bao-Hua, L. Ting, and Z. Yong, Super-short solid silicon microneedles for transdermal drug delivery applications. Int J Pharm, 2010, **389**(1-2): p. 122–29.

93. Chu, L.Y. and M.R. Prausnitz, Separable arrowhead microneedles. J Control Release, 2011, **149**(3): p. 242–49.

94. Crichton, M.L., A. Ansaldo, X. Chen, T.W. Prow, G.J. Fernando, and M.A. Kendall, The effect of strain rate on the precision of penetration of short densely-packed microprojection array patches coated with vaccine. Biomaterials, 2010, **31**(16): p. 4562–72.

95. Indermun, S., R. Luttge, Y.E. Choonara, P. Kumar, L.C. du Toit, G. Modi, and V. Pillay, Current advances in the fabrication of microneedles for transdermal delivery. J Control Release, 2014, **185**: p. 130–8.

96. Lee, J.W., M.R. Han, and J.H. Park, Polymer microneedles for transdermal drug delivery. J Drug Target, 2012, **21**: p. 211–23.

97. McAllister, D.V., P.M. Wang, S.P. Davis, J.H. Park, P.J. Canatella, M.G. Allen, and M.R. Prausnitz, Microfabricated needles for transdermal delivery of macromolecules and nanoparticles: fabrication methods and transport studies. Proc Natl Acad Sci U S A, 2003, **100**(24): p. 13755–60.

98. Madou, M.J., ed. *Fundamentals of Microfabrication and Nanotechnology.* 3rd ed. 2011, CRC Press: Boca Raton, Florida.

99. Tu, K.-T. and C.-K. Chung. *Fabrication of biodegradable polymer microneedle array via CO_2 laser ablation.* in *10th IEEE International Conference on Nano/Micro Engineered and Molecular Systems.* 2015. Xi'an, China.

100. Migalska, K., D.I. Morrow, M.J. Garland, R. Thakur, A.D. Woolfson, and R.F. Donnelly, Laser-engineered dissolving microneedle arrays for transdermal macromolecular drug delivery. Pharm Res, 2011, **28**(8): p. 1919–30.

101. Chu, L.Y., S.O. Choi, and M.R. Prausnitz, Fabrication of dissolving polymer microneedles for controlled drug encapsulation and delivery: Bubble and pedestal microneedle designs. J Pharm Sci, 2010, **99**(10): p. 4228–38.

102. Mistilis, M.J., J.C. Joyce, E.S. Esser, I. Skountzou, R.W. Compans, A.S. Bommarius, and M.R. Prausnitz, Long-term stability of influenza vaccine in a dissolving microneedle patch. Drug Deliv Transl Res, 2016, 7(2): p. 195–205.

103. Qiu, Y., G. Qin, S. Zhang, Y. Wu, B. Xu, and Y. Gao, Novel lyophilized hydrogel patches for convenient and effective administration of microneedle-mediated insulin delivery. Int J Pharm, 2012, **437**(1-2): p. 51–6.

104. Cormier, M., B. Johnson, M. Ameri, K. Nyam, L. Libiran, D.D. Zhang, and P. Daddona, Transdermal delivery of desmopressin using a coated microneedle array patch system. J Control Release 2004, **97**(3): p. 503–11.

105. Haj-Ahmad, R., H. Khan, M.S. Arshad, M. Rasekh, A. Hussain, S. Walsh, X. Li, M.W. Chang, and Z. Ahmad, Microneedle Coating Techniques for Transdermal Drug Delivery. Pharmaceutics, 2015, **7**(4): p. 486–502.

106. Raphael, A.P., M.L. Crichton, R.J. Falconer, S. Meliga, X. Chen, G.J. Fernando, H. Huang, and M.A. Kendall, Formulations for microprojection/microneedle vaccine delivery: Structure, strength and release profiles. J Control Release, 2016, **225**: p. 40–52.

107. McGrath, M.G., A. Vrdoljak, C. O'Mahony, J.C. Oliveira, A.C. Moore, and A.M. Crean, Determination of parameters for successful spray coating of silicon microneedle arrays. Int J Pharm, 2011, **415**(1-2): p. 140–9.

108. Uddin, M.J., N. Scoutaris, P. Klepetsanis, B. Chowdhry, M.R. Prausnitz, and D. Douroumis, Inkjet printing of transdermal microneedles for the delivery of anticancer agents. Int J Pharm, 2015, **494**(2): p. 593–602.

109. Duan, D., C. Moeckly, J. Gysbers, C. Novak, G. Prochnow, K. Siebenaler, L. Albers, and K. Hansen, Enhanced delivery of topically-applied formulations following skin pre-treatment with a hand-applied, plastic microneedle array. Curr Drug Deliv, 2011, **8**(5): p. 557–65.

110. Lee, K. and H. Jung, Drawing lithography for microneedles: a review of fundamentals and biomedical applications. Biomaterials, 2012, **33**(30): p. 7309–26.

111. Yamamoto, T. and Y. Yamamoto, Electrical properties of the epidermal stratum corneum. Med Biol Eng, 1976, **14**(2): p. 151–58.

112. Prausnitz, M.R., The effects of electric current applied to the skin: a review for transdermal drug delivery. Adv Drug Deliv Rev, 1996, **18**(3): p. 395–425.

113. Lanke, S.S., C.S. Kolli, J.G. Strom, and A.K. Banga, Enhanced transdermal delivery of low molecular weight heparin by barrier perturbation. Int J Pharm, 2009. **365**(1-2): p. 26–33.

114. Karande, P., A. Jain, and S. Mitragotri, Relationships between skin's electrical impedance and permeability in the presence of chemical enhancers. J Control Release, 2005, **110** (2): p. 307–13.

115. Badran, M.M., J. Kuntsche, and A. Fahr, Skin penetration enhancement by a microneedle device (Dermaroller®) in vitro: Dependency on needle size and applied formulation. Eur J Pharm Sci, 2009, **36**(4-5): p. 511–23.

116. Roskos, K.V. and R.H. Guy, Assessment of skin barrier function using transepidermal water loss: effect of age. Pharm Res, 1989, **6**(11): p. 949–53.

117. Gomaa, Y.A., D.I. Morrow, M.J. Garland, R.F. Donnelly, L.K. El-Khordagui, and V.M. Meidan, Effects of microneedle length, density, insertion time and multiple applications on human skin barrier function: assessments by transepidermal water loss. Toxicol In Vitro, 2010, **24**(7): p. 1971–8.

118. Wang, P.M., M. Cornwell, J. Hill, and M.R. Prausnitz, Precise microinjection into skin using hollow microneedles. J Invest Dermatol, 2006, **126**(5): p. 1080–87.

119. Oh, J.H., H.H. Park, K.Y. Do, M. Han, D.H. Hyun, C.G. Kim, C.H. Kim, S.S. Lee, S.J. Hwang, S.C. Shin, and C.W. Cho, Influence of the delivery systems using a microneedle array on the permeation of a hydrophilic molecule, calcein. Eur J Pharm Biopharm, 2008, **69**(3): p. 1040–45.

120. Kalluri, H. and A.K. Banga, Formation and closure of microchannels in skin following microporation. Pharm Res, 2011, **28**(1): p. 82–94.

121. Lee, K., C.Y. Lee, and H. Jung, Dissolving microneedles for transdermal drug administration prepared by stepwise controlled drawing of maltose. Biomaterials, 2011, **32**(11): p. 3134–40.

122. Kolli, C.S. and A.K. Banga, Characterization of solid maltose microneedles and their use for transdermal delivery. Pharm Res, 2008, **25**(1): p. 104–13.

123. Widera, G., J. Johnson, L. Kim, L. Libiran, K. Nyam, P.E. Daddona, and M. Cormier, Effect of delivery parameters on immunization to ovalbumin following intracutaneous administration by a coated microneedle array patch system. Vaccine, 2006, **24**(10): p. 1653–64.

124. Alvarez-Román, R., A. Naik, Y.N. Kalia, H. Fessi, and R.H. Guy, Visualization of skin penetration using confocal laser scanning microscopy. Eur J Pharm Biopharm, 2004, **58**(2): p. 301–16.

125. Bal, S., A.C. Kruithof, H. Liebl, M. Tomerius, J. Bouwstra, J. Lademann, and M. Meinke, In vivo visualisation of microneedle conduits in human skin using laser scanning microscopy. Laser Phys Lett, 2010, **7**(3): p. 242–46.

126. Gomaa, Y.A., M.J. Garland, F.J. McInnes, R.F. Donnelly, L.K. El-Khordagui, and C.G. Wilson, Microneedle/nanoencapsulation-mediated transdermal delivery: mechanistic insights. Eur J Pharm Biopharm, 2014, **86**(2): p. 145–55.
127. Fercher, A.F., Optical coherence tomography – development, principles, applications. Z Med Phys, 2010, **20**(4): p. 251–76.
128. Garland, M.J., E. Caffarel-Salvador, K. Migalska, A.D. Woolfson, and R.F. Donnelly, Dissolving polymeric microneedle arrays for electrically assisted transdermal drug delivery. J Control Release, 2012, **159**(1): p. 52–9.
129. Lin, W., M. Cormier, A. Samiee, A. Griffin, B. Johnson, C.L. Teng, G.E. Hardee, and P.E. Daddona, Transdermal delivery of antisense oligonucleotides with microprojection patch (Macroflux) technology. Pharm Res, 2001, **18**(12): p. 1789–93.
130. Wu, X.M., H. Todo, and K. Sugibayashi, Enhancement of skin permeation of high molecular compounds by a combination of microneedle pretreatment and iontophoresis. J Control Release, 2007, **118**(2): p. 189–95.
131. Vemulapalli, V., Y. Yang, P.M. Friden, and A.K. Banga, Synergistic effect of iontophoresis and soluble microneedles for transdermal delivery of methotrexate. J Pharm Pharmacol, 2008, **60**(1): p. 27–33.
132. Ronnander, J.P., L. Simon, and A. Koch, Transdermal Delivery of Sumatriptan Succinate Using Iontophoresis and Dissolving Microneedles. J Pharm Sci, 2019, **108**(11): p. 3649–56.
133. Noh, G., T. Keum, J.E. Seo, S. Bashyal, N.S. Eum, M.J. Kweon, S. Lee, D.H. Sohn, and S. Lee, Iontophoretic Transdermal Delivery of Human Growth Hormone (hGH) and the Combination Effect of a New Type Microneedle, Tappy Tok Tok((R)). Pharmaceutics, 2018, **10**(3).
134. Qin, G., Y. Gao, Y. Wu, S. Zhang, Y. Qiu, F. Li, and B. Xu, Simultaneous basal-bolus delivery of fast-acting insulin and its significance in diabetes management. Nanomedicine, 2012, **8**(2): p. 221–27.
135. Hooper, J.W., J.W. Golden, A.M. Ferro, and A.D. King, Smallpox DNA vaccine delivered by novel skin electroporation device protects mice against intranasal poxvirus challenge. Vaccine, 2007, **25**(10): p. 1814–23.
136. Qiu, Y., Y. Gao, K. Hu, and F. Li, Enhancement of skin permeation of docetaxel: a novel approach combining microneedle and elastic liposomes. J Control Release, 2008, **129**(2): p. 144–50.
137. Badran, M.M., J. Kuntsche, and A. Fahr, Skin penetration enhancement by a microneedle device (Dermaroller) in vitro: dependency on needle size and applied formulation. Eur J Pharm Sci, 2009, **36**(4-5): p. 511–23.
138. Ahmed, K.S., X. Shan, J. Mao, L. Qiu, and J. Chen, Derma roller(R) microneedles-mediated transdermal delivery of doxorubicin and celecoxib co-loaded liposomes for enhancing the anticancer effect. Mater Sci Eng C Mater Biol Appl, 2019, **99**: p. 1448–58.
139. Permana, A.D., I.A. Tekko, M.T.C. McCrudden, Q.K. Anjani, D. Ramadon, H.O. McCarthy, and R.F. Donnelly, Solid lipid nanoparticle-based dissolving microneedles: A promising intradermal lymph targeting drug delivery system with potential for enhanced treatment of lymphatic filariasis. J Control Release, 2019, **316**: p. 34–52.
140. Zhang, W., B. Ding, R. Tang, X. Ding, X. Hou, X. Wang, S. Gu, L. Lu, Y. Zhang, S. Gao, and J. Gao, Combination of microneedles with PLGA nanoparticles as a potential strategy for topical drug delivery. Curr Nanosci, 2011, **7**(4): p. 545–51.
141. Pearton, M., C. Allender, K. Brain, A. Anstey, C. Gateley, N. Wilke, A. Morrissey, and J. Birchall, Gene delivery to the epidermal cells of human skin explants using microfabricated microneedles and hydrogel formulations. Pharm Res, 2008, **25**(2): p. 407–16.
142. Vora, L.K., P.R. Vavia, E. Larraneta, S.E.J. Bell, and R.F. Donnelly, Novel nanosuspension-based dissolving microneedle arrays for transdermal delivery of a hydrophobic drug. J Interdisc Nanomed, 2018, **3**(2): p. 89–101.
143. Chen, H., H. Zhu, J. Zheng, D. Mou, J. Wan, J. Zhang, T. Shi, Y. Zhao, H. Xu, and X. Yang, Iontophoresis-driven penetration of nanovesicles through microneedle-induced skin microchannels for enhancing transdermal delivery of insulin. J Control Release, 2009, **139**(1): p. 63–72.
144. Marshall, S., L.J. Sahm, and A.C. Moore, The success of microneedle-mediated vaccine delivery into skin. Hum Vaccin Immunother, 2016, 12(11): 2975–83.
145. Skountzou, I. and R.W. Compans, Skin immunization with influenza vaccines. Curr Top Microbiol Immunol, 2015, **386**: p. 343–69.
146. Suh, H., J. Shin, and Y.C. Kim, Microneedle patches for vaccine delivery. Clin Exp Vaccine Res, 2014, **3**(1): p. 42–9.

147. Joyce, J.C., H.E. Sella, H. Jost, M.J. Mistilis, E.S. Esser, P. Pradhan, R. Toy, M.L. Collins, P.A. Rota, K. Roy, I. Skountzou, R.W. Compans, M.S. Oberste, W.C. Weldon, J.J. Norman, and M.R. Prausnitz, Extended delivery of vaccines to the skin improves immune responses. Journal of controlled release: official journal of the Controlled Release Society, 2019, **304**: p. 135–45.

148. Fernando, G.J.P., J. Hickling, C.M. Jayashi Flores, P. Griffin, C.D. Anderson, S.R. Skinner, C. Davies, K. Witham, M. Pryor, J. Bodle, S. Rockman, I.H. Frazer, and A.H. Forster, Safety, tolerability, acceptability and immunogenicity of an influenza vaccine delivered to human skin by a novel high-density microprojection array patch (Nanopatch). Vaccine, 2018, **36**(26): p. 3779–88.

149. Fernando, G.J., X. Chen, T.W. Prow, M.L. Crichton, E.J. Fairmaid, M.S. Roberts, I.H. Frazer, L.E. Brown, and M.A. Kendall, Potent immunity to low doses of influenza vaccine by probabilistic guided micro-targeted skin delivery in a mouse model. PLoS One, 2010, **5**(4): p. e10266.

150. Liu, Y., L. Ye, F. Lin, Y. Gomaa, D. Flyer, R. Carrion, Jr., J.L. Patterson, M.R. Prausnitz, G. Smith, G. Glenn, H. Wu, R.W. Compans, and C. Yang, Intradermal immunization by Ebola virus GP subunit vaccines using microneedle patches protects mice against lethal EBOV challenge. Sci Rep, 2018, **8**(1): p. 11193.

151. Depelsenaire, A.C., S.C. Meliga, C.L. McNeilly, F.E. Pearson, J.W. Coffey, O.L. Haigh, C.J. Flaim, I.H. Frazer, and M.A. Kendall, Colocalization of cell death with antigen deposition in skin enhances vaccine immunogenicity. J Invest Dermatol, 2014, **134**(9): p. 2361–70.

152. Radius Health, Inc. 2019. Efficacy & Safety of Abaloparatide-Solid Microstructured Transdermal System in Postmenopausal Women with Osteoporosis. https://clinicaltrials.gov/ct2/show/NCT04064411.

153. Zosano Pharma Corporation. 2017. A Study to Evaluate the Long-Term Safety of M207 in the Acute Treatment of Migraine (ADAM). https://clinicaltrials.gov/ct2/show/NCT03282227.

154. Kochba, E., Y. Levin, I. Raz, and A. Cahn, Improved insulin pharmacokinetics using a novel microneedle device for intradermal delivery in patients with type 2 diabetes. Diabetes Technol Ther, 2016, **18**(9): p. 525–31.

155. SkinJect, Inc. 2018. Open-Label Dose Escalation Trial to Evaluate Dose Limiting Toxicity and Maximum Tolerated Dose of Microneedle Arrays Containing Doxorubicin (D-MNA) in Basal Cell Carcinoma. https://clinicaltrials.gov/ct2/show/NCT03646188.

156. Zosano Pharma Inc. 2015. Safety and Efficacy of ZP-Glucagon to Injectable Glucagon for Hypoglycemia. https://clinicaltrials.gov/ct2/show/NCT02459938.

157. DUSA Pharmaceuticals, Inc. 2015. Microneedle Lesion Preparation Prior to Aminolevulinic Acid Photodynamic Therapy (ALA-PDT) for AK on Face. https://clinicaltrials.gov/ct2/show/NCT02632110.

158. Quinn, H.L., M.C. Kearney, A.J. Courtenay, M.T. McCrudden, and R.F. Donnelly, The role of microneedles for drug and vaccine delivery. Expert Opin Drug Deliv, 2014, **11**(11): p. 1769–80.

159. Baek, C., M. Han, J. Min, M.R. Prausnitz, J.H. Park, and J.H. Park, Local transdermal delivery of phenylephrine to the anal sphincter muscle using microneedles. J Control Release, 2011, **154**(2): p. 138–47.

160. Yu, J., Y. Zhang, Y. Ye, R. DiSanto, W. Sun, D. Ranson, F.S. Ligler, J.B. Buse, and Z. Gu, Microneedle-array patches loaded with hypoxia-sensitive vesicles provide fast glucose-responsive insulin delivery. Proc Natl Acad Sci U S A, 2015, **112**(27): p. 8260–5.

161. Narayan, R.J., Transdermal delivery of insulin via microneedles. J Biomed Nanotechnol, 2014, **10**(9): p. 2244–60.

162. Gomaa, Y.A., M.J. Garland, F. McInnes, L.K. El-Khordagui, C. Wilson, and R.F. Donnelly, Laser-engineered dissolving microneedles for active transdermal delivery of nadroparin calcium. Eur J Pharm Biopharm, 2012, **82**(2): p. 299–307.

163. Li, W., R.N. Terry, J. Tang, M.R. Feng, S.P. Schwendeman, and M.R. Prausnitz, Rapidly separable microneedle patch for the sustained release of a contraceptive. Nat Biomed Eng, 2019, **3**(3): p. 220–29.

164. McCaffrey, J., R.F. Donnelly, and H.O. McCarthy, Microneedles: an innovative platform for gene delivery. Drug Deliv Transl Res, 2015, **5**(4): p. 424–37.

165. McCrudden, M.T., E. McAlister, A.J. Courtenay, P. Gonzalez-Vazquez, T.R. Singh, and R.F. Donnelly, Microneedle applications in improving skin appearance. Exp Dermatol, 2015, **24**(8): p. 561–6.

166. Fernandes, D., Minimally invasive percutaneous collagen induction. Oral Maxillofac Surg Clin North Am, 2005, **17**(1): p. 51–63, vi.

167. Sharad, J., Combination of microneedling and glycolic acid peels for the treatment of acne scars in dark skin. J Cosmet Dermatol, 2011, **10**(4): p. 317–23.

168. Nofal, E., A. Helmy, A. Nofal, R. Alakad, and M. Nasr, Platelet-rich plasma versus CROSS technique with 100% trichloroacetic acid versus combined skin needling and platelet rich plasma in the treatment of atrophic acne scars: a comparative study. Dermatol Surg, 2014, **40**(8): p. 864–73.

169. Hiraishi, Y., T. Nakagawa, Y.S. Quan, F. Kamiyama, S. Hirobe, N. Okada, and S. Nakagawa, Performance and characteristics evaluation of a sodium hyaluronate-based microneedle patch for a transcutaneous drug delivery system. Int J Pharm, 2013, **441**(1-2): p. 570–9.
170. Lahiji, S.F., D.J. Um, Y. Kim, J. Jang, H. Yang, and H. Jung, Scalp Micro-Pigmentation via Transcutaneous Implantation of Flexible Tissue Interlocking Biodegradable Microneedles. Pharmaceutics, 2019, **11**(11).
171. Kim, S.T., K.H. Lee, H.J. Sim, K.S. Suh, and M.S. Jang, Treatment of acne vulgaris with fractional radiofrequency microneedling. J Dermatol, 2014, **41**(7): p. 586–91.
172. Gold, M., M. Taylor, K. Rothaus, and Y. Tanaka, Non-insulated smooth motion, micro-needles RF fractional treatment for wrinkle reduction and lifting of the lower face: International study. Lasers Surg Med, 2016, **48**(8): p. 727–33.
173. Jeon, I.K., S.E. Chang, G.H. Park, and M.R. Roh, Comparison of microneedle fractional radiofrequency therapy with intradermal botulinum toxin a injection for periorbital rejuvenation. Dermatology, 2013, **227**(4): p. 367–72.
174. Hantash, B.M., A.A. Ubeid, H. Chang, R. Kafi, and B. Renton, Bipolar fractional radiofrequency treatment induces neoelastogenesis and neocollagenesis. Lasers Surg Med, 2009, **41**(1): p. 1–9.

42 Microneedle Dermatotoxicology

Boen Wang
Lynbrook High School, San Jose, California

CONTENTS

42.1 INTRODUCTION

Microneedles (MNs), minimally invasive devices designed to painlessly penetrate the stratum corneum, were developed and patented in 1976 as a means for more efficient transdermal drug delivery (Ma and Wu 2017). Subsequent advancement in MN technology and manufacturing led to the development of several MN types, including hollow, solid, dissolving, coated, and hydrogel forming (Nguyen and Park 2018). Hollow MNs deliver drugs through a channel in a similar manner to hypodermic needles, while solid MNs are more frequently used in pretreatment to enhance skin permeability before application of a topical product. Dissolving MNs are constructed from a biodegradable polymer or polysaccharide with therapeutic molecules contained within; coated MNs contain the drug formulation on the outside surface of the needles. Lastly, hydrogel-forming MNs are composed of expanding material with an active agent attached to the baseplate (Nguyen and Park 2018). The following briefly states the promising potential applications of MNs, including dermal and intrascleral drug delivery, vaccine administration, blood and interstitial fluid extraction, and numerous uses in cosmetics (Ma and Wu 2017; Ramaut et al. 2018). All will eventually increase in use, should they be well tolerated by most users.

MNs allow delivery of higher-molecular-weight and hydrophilic drugs that would otherwise be unable to significantly diffuse across the stratum corneum. In contrast to enteral drug delivery, dermal drug delivery avoids stomach degradation and hepatic first-pass metabolism, while it may also produce higher drug concentrations in the dermis and other target tissues. MN transdermal drug delivery is a continually growing field with increasing patents filed every year for numerous drugs.

Here, we briefly discuss a few of the many studies involving MN drug delivery. Badran et al. (2009) demonstrated effective penetration of radiolabeled mannitol, a hydrophilic drug expected to have poor penetration into the stratum corneum, in full-thickness human skin grafts when combined with microneedling. Dhurat et al. found enhanced effectiveness of minoxidil in men with androgenetic alopecia when used in conjunction with micronneedling in comparison to conventional minoxidil treatment; they also demonstrated effectiveness of MN and minoxidil combination therapy in patients failing to respond to conventional minoxidil treatment (Dhurat and Mathapati 2015; Dhurat et al. 2013). Jiang et al. (2009) demonstrated effective intrascleral delivery of microparticles via MNs. With possible drug diffusion to surrounding tissues like the choroid, retina, and ciliary body, intrascleral drug delivery via MNs has the potential to treat posterior eye disease such as glaucoma and macular degeneration (Jiang et al. 2009).

In 2020, the first new drug application for a pharmaceutical microneedle patch, Qtrypta, was submitted to the Food and Drug Administration (FDA) by Zosano Pharma. The patch is a titanium microneedle with a coated zolmitriptan for acute migraine treatment.

While most MN vaccination studies focus on delivery of influenza antigen, many other applications exist for MN vaccines. MN delivery of vaccines releases antigenic material into the viable dermis, which has shown stronger immunological reactions when compared to muscle, the delivery target of traditional hypodermic needles (Engelke et al. 2015). A multicenter, randomized, open-label study in 978 healthy adults showed intradermal influenza vaccine delivered by microinjection systems to convey a noninferior humoral response against three influenza strains and two superior humoral responses to both A strains (H1N1, H3N2) (Leroux-Roels et al. 2008). Similar studies on influenza vaccination demonstrated comparable or superior responses when compared to responses from conventional intramuscular vaccination (Kenney et al. 2004; Van Damme et al. 2009). Other studies demonstrated effective levels of neutralizing antibodies in 100% of measles-vaccinated nonhuman primates compared to 75% of subcutaneously vaccinated nonhuman primates (Joyce et al. 2018). In a phase 1, partly blinded, controlled trial, the authors found no significant statistical difference in antibody titers among groups vaccinated with health care–administered intramuscular hypodermic needle influenza vaccine, health care–administered MN influenza vaccination patch, and self-administered MN influenza-vaccination patch, suggesting a possible future for self-administered vaccines (Rouphael et al. 2017). Chiefly, MNs have application in global health vaccination due to the ability for non-climate-controlled distribution and the potential for self-administration. In addition, MNs eliminate sharps, biohazardous waste, painful injections, and potential needle stick injuries present in vaccines administered via hypodermic needles.

Development of optimized hollow MNs has resulted in additional potential applications, including blood and interstitial fluid (ISF) extraction (Kiang et al. 2017; Li et al. 2013). When paired with biosensors and other microsystems, MNs have the potential for glucose and drug monitoring (Kiang et al. 2017). While experiments with MN-integrated biosensors have yielded encouraging results, extensive preclinical and clinical trials are needed before implementation as point-of-care devices for ISF collection, drug concentration assessment, or dosing in real time (Kiang et al. 2017).

Dermal microneedling has proven an effective therapy for atrophic acne scars and skin rejuvenation (Kim et al. 2011). Although the exact mechanism is unknown, MN puncture possibly disrupts older collagen strands and promotes damaged collagen removal (Fabbrocini et al. 2009). In addition, rolling with multiple MNs to promote new collagen and elastin deposition, known as collagen induction therapy, has become a popular practice in treating disfiguring scars and rhytides and rejuvenating skin (Fabbrocini et al. 2009; Aust et al. 2008).

Other methods used to improve the clinical appearance of acne scarring such as laser resurfacing pose potential risks associated with a disrupted skin epidermal barrier. Cho et al. (2012) showed microneedling to lead to improved grade of acne scars and global assessment of large pores in more than 70% of 30 tested patients. Kim et al. (2011) compared the effects of microneedling versus intense pulsed light (IPL) therapy for skin rejuvenation, finding significantly higher levels of collagen in microneedling when evaluated via caliper, microscopic examination, Western blot analysis for type I collagen, and enzyme-linked immunosorbent assay (ELISA) for total collagen content.

42.2   MATERIALS AND METHODS

To assess the safety profile of the growing applications of microneedles, we searched "micronee-dles" with key terms including "safety," "side effect," "toxicology," "adverse effect," "adverse event," "infection," "dermatitis," "granuloma," "scarring," and "hyperpigmentation" in scientific databases such as PubMed. The information presented in this review (updated as of July 2020) is compiled from other literature, original studies, and reports of adverse effects in patients and volunteers.

42.3   ADVERSE EVENTS AND PREVENTION

Perhaps the most extensive use of MNs in any one application occurs with collagen-induction therapy. Consequently, most discussion of adverse events and normal postprocedural expectations involve this application.

Common contraindications to MN collagen-induction therapy include active acne; herpes labia-lis or other active current infection such as impetigo or warts; patients on anticoagulant therapy such as warfarin and heparin or with other blood dyscrasias; patients with extreme keloid scarring tendency; and patients on chemotherapy, radiotherapy, or high doses of corticosteroids (Fernandes 2005; Singh and Yadav 2016).

Prior to MN collagen-induction therapy, patients should use a cleanser to remove any makeup or debris before applying any topical aesthetic cream or gel to the treatment area (Alster and Graham 2018). Alster and Graham (2018) typically apply a compounded 30% lidocaine cream for 20 to 30 minutes before removal with water-soaked gauze and alcohol prep immediately before therapy. In the healthy patient without treatment contraindications, typical postprocedural expectations in collagen induction therapy with MNs include pinpoint bleeding, bruising, erythema, and irritation (Fernandes 2005).

Fernandes (2005) outlines a predicted appearance timeline and general recommendations fol-lowing percutaneous collagen induction. Patients may note a bruised skin appearance with a swollen face following collagen induction therapy with a minimal, temporary ooze of serum. He recom-mends soaking skin with saline swabs for one to two hours followed by treatment with a tea tree oil cleanser, while also encouraging patients to use topical vitamin A and vitamin C cream or oil to enhance healing. Other authors recommend the use of hyaluronic acid gel in the first four hours posttreatment followed by 1% hydrocortisone cream or nonallergenic moisturizing cream after four hours (Alster and Graham 2018). However, it is important that patients use only topical products approved for intradermal use, as inappropriate topical formula in conjunction with MN therapy increases the potential for allergic and irritant reactions.

Vitamin A is known to aggravate flush and cause dry, flaky skin. Patients should thoroughly wash the face until serum, blood, and oil are removed to prevent any minor eschar formation, as minor eschars may result in the development of milia or pustules. Skin should look less dramatic following day 1, with moderate flush on day 4 to 5 and few visible signs postprocedure day 7. Patients should avoid unapproved topical formulations for at least 24 hours and refrain from direct sun exposure for at least 10 days. Fernandes advises at least one month in between retreat-ment with MNs, while Alster and Graham (2018) recommend biweekly intervals until the desired outcome is achieved.

Despite potential uses and existence for over four decades, MNs are yet to be fully integrated into the medical system. The following discussion investigates potential side effects of MNs, including infection, irritation and irritant contact dermatitis, allergic contact dermatitis, hyperpigmentation, abnormal scarring, and irritant and allergic granulomas. We also consider the potential for pho-toirritation/phototoxicity, photoallergic contact dermatitis, nonimmunologic contact urticaria, and immunologic contact urticaria. For a summary of literature documenting adverse events with MNs, see Table 42.1.

TABLE 42.1

Literature documenting MN adverse reactions in human patients

Adverse Reaction Type	Author(s) and Year	Number of Patients	Additional Details
Infection	Aust et al. (2008)	2	2/480 patients developed herpes simplex infection
	Torezan et al. (2013)	1	1/10 patients developed infection based on symptoms
	Cunha et al. (2017)	1	*Microsporum canis* infection of bilateral arms and legs
Irritant Contact Dermatitis (ICD)	Cercal Fucci-da-Costa + Reich Camasmie (2018)	1	Suspected irritation to arnica-based cream
Allergic Contact Dermatitis (ACD)	Yadav + Dogra (2016)	1	"Rail track appearance" of adverse reaction with positive patch test to nickel
Allergic/Irritant Granulomas 1	Soltani-Arabshahi et al. (2014)	3	2 patients with granulomatous reaction, systemic symptoms and + 1 reaction to Vita C serum; 1 patient with granulomatous reaction and no systemic symptoms
Irregular Scarring	Pahwa et al. (2012)2	1	"Tram tracking" appearance over temporal area, zygomatic arch, and forehead
	Dogra et al. (2014)2	2	2/36 patients presented with a "tram trek" adverse event; 1/2 "tram trek" patients withdrawn from study
Postinflammatory	Dogra et al. (2014)	5	5/36 patients; 3/5 patients withdrew from study; 2/5 patients improved with photoprotection
hyperpigmentation	Sharad (2011)	4	4/36 patients with more transient hyperpigmentation
	Majid (2009)	1	1/37 patients with transient hyperpigmentation

42.3.1 INFECTION

The stratum corneum serves many purposes, including as a physical and chemical defense against microorganisms. Microchannels formed during MN therapy have the potential to facilitate access of microorganisms and increase susceptibility to infection. Gupta et al. (2011) evaluated the kinetics of stratum corneum resealing in MN versus hypodermic needles, finding faster resealing in MN-treated skin. Others evaluated skin resealing kinetics with MNs, with studies describing closure times as rapid as 15 minutes (Bal et al. 2010), with other studies finding closure within 2 (Gupta et al. 2011), 8 to 24 (Haq et al. 2009), and 24 hours (Kelchen et al. 2016). Donnelly et al. (2009) evaluated microbial penetration in hypodermic needles versus MN-induced holes in Silescol membranes and neonate porcine skin and demonstrated significantly lower penetration of *Candida albicans, Pseudomonas aeruginosa,* and *Staphylococcus epidermidis* across viable epidermis in MN versus hypodermic needle puncture. Vicente-Perez et al. (2017) evaluated the effect of MN patches on mice, testing for biomarkers of inflammation and infection, weight, and several other variables and found no detectable levels of TNF-α among mice and no statistically significant increase in C-reactive protein, immunoglobulin G, or interleukin 1-beta in MN-tested mice in comparison to control mice, regardless of formulation type, needle density, number of applications, or mouse gender ($p > 0.05$ in all cases). In addition, mice in all study and control groups demonstrated increased weight over the course of the study. Collectively, the authors were unable to detect infection or any variable indicative of an infection across all tested mice.

Aust et al. (2008) performed a retrospective analysis of 480 patients with fine wrinkles, lax skin, scarring, and striae gravidarum treated with percutaneous collagen induction using the Medical Roll-CIT with topical vitamin A and C cosmetic creams for a minimum of 4 weeks postoperatively. Two patients developed herpes simplex infection following a full-face needling that was successfully treated with acyclovir.

In a pilot split-face study comparing conventional methyl aminolevulinate-photodynamic therapy (PDT) with microneedling-assisted PDT on actinically damaged skin, 1 of 10 patients developed an infection on the MN-treated side 7 days posttreatment, determined by signs and symptoms of high local temperature, redness, pain, and crusts; however, the patient responded well to cephalosporin treatment (Torezan et al. 2013).

Cunha et al. (2017) document a case of tinea corporis that emerged in corresponding locations of Dermaroller (540 stainless steel microneedles of 0.5 mm length) use approximately 3 weeks after start of her home MN therapy for bilateral scarring of her arms and legs. Potassium hydroxide examination of the lesions was positive for fungus, with lesion culture growing *Microsporum canis*. While the patient confirmed skin cleaning prior to and sanitation of the MN device before and after therapy, inadequate sterilization of the patient's skin and MN device cannot be excluded. The patient experienced complete resolution after treatment with oral terbinafine and topical sertaconazol at 5-week follow-up.

Leatham et al. (2018) document facial autoinoculation of varicella via a home microneedling roller device. A healthy woman with a distant history of primary varicella zoster virus (VZV) infection and no prior shingles vaccination reported grouped lesions over her chest, which she presumed to be an acneiform eruption. The patient self-treated the area with an at-home microneedling roller device and used the device over her face to reduce appearance of rhytides. On presentation, the patient had "grouped, eroded papules and vesicles on the right T4 dermatome" and "eroded papules on the forehead, lateral cheeks, many located at spaced distances." Polymerase chain reaction (PCR) yielded positive results for VZV. The patient was started on oral valacyclovir and was free of lesions and experienced no postherpetic neuralgia at 6 weeks.

42.3.2 IRRITANT DERMATITIS

Irritant dermatitis (ID) is an eczematous-like reaction occurring from contact with a chemical, biologic, or physical agent (Tan et al. 2014). Reaction severity depends upon the physicochemical property of the agent and the degree of activation of the innate immune system (Tan et al. 2014). Keratinocytes, comprising 95% of epidermal cells, are responsible for the production of the majority of cytokines likely responsible for the ensuing erythema and edema (Tan et al. 2014). In contact with any agent, there is the potential for ID; however, it is likely that disruption of the stratum corneum provides increased susceptibility to a particular irritant. MNs are most frequently manufactured from nonirritating metal, polymer, silicon, and glass, none of which are particularly common irritants (Nguyen and Park 2018). However, irritation following a procedure may result from the MNs themselves or any substance used in conjunction.

Cercal Fucci-da-Costa and Reich Camasmie (2018) document likely ID due to skin rejuvenation MN therapy over the patient's dorsal hands with 10 applications with a 0.5-mm Dermaroller. Following her MN therapy, the patient inadvertently applied arnica-based cream and developed yellowish papules compatible with MN perforation sites on an erythematous base 48 hours after arnica cream application. The authors attributed the lesions to ID from the arnica-based cream due to the sparing of MN-treated areas in which the cream was not applied and the patient's improvement 72 hours post–topical corticosteroid treatment.

Assessment of postprocedural erythema allows a rough estimate of the irritation incurred during the procedure; however, the degree of postprocedural erythema is likely dependent on factors such as MN application site, amount of MN applications, MN length and type, combination therapy with topical products, and variability between skin types.

Bal et al. (2008) applied MN arrays (200, 300, or 400 μm solid metal MN arrays and 300 or 550 μm hollow metal MN arrays) using a standardized electrical applicator to the forearms of 18 human volunteers and measured redness using skin color assessment and laser Doppler imaging. Longer needle lengths resulted in greater irritation, evidenced by the 400 μm solid MNs, resulting in significantly greater change in redness in comparison to the 200 μm solid MNs ($P < 0.001$). Lastly, they concluded 15 minutes post-application as the maximum change in redness, with minimal irritation lasting less than two hours for all MNs.

Gill et al. (2008) investigated the safety of single, longer MN lengths (480, 700, 960, and 1450 μm) on the volar forearm of healthy human volunteers, finding decreasing erythema over 2 hours in all subjects with no excessive erythema self-reported by research subjects when contacted at 24 hours.

Han Tae et al. (2012) used a chromameter to measure posttreatment erythema following MN therapy using 150 and 250 μm MN rollers over one side of the face of healthy human volunteers and found recovery time to baseline erythema to be 24 hours in the 5-application group and 48 hours in the 10-application group and a significant difference in the erythema index ratio between the two groups after 24 hours ($p = 0.002$). Conversely, they did not find a significant difference between the erythema index ratio of the 150 and 200 μm MN roller groups, although the mean erythema index ratios were higher in the 250 μm MN roller group.

42.3.3 Allergic Contact Dermatitis

Allergic contact dermatitis (ACD) is a type IV hypersensitivity reaction requiring prior sensitization and re-exposure to the allergen (Mowad et al. 2016). In the sensitization phase, the unprocessed chemical allergen, known as a hapten, penetrates the lower levels of the epidermis, where it is engulfed by a Langerhans cell and later presented to T cells (Marks and deLeo 2016). Upon subsequent exposure to the allergen, cell-mediated immune response results in an eczematous-like lesion. As previously mentioned, microneedling disrupts the stratum corneum, increasing the ability of molecules, possibly allergens, to enter the dermis.

Yadav and Dogra (2016) identified a potential case of ACD occurring as a result of a 1.5-mm titanium-coated, stainless steel microneedling device for the treatment of atrophic acne facial scars. Other than a local anesthetic applied one hour before and completely cleaned with normal saline and betadine, no serum or chemical was applied before, during, or after the procedure. The patient developed erythema and edema over the next 2 days, which gradually subsided. Simultaneously, the patient developed vesiculopustular lesions and erythematous papules arranged linearly along the lines of the microneedling device, giving a "rail track appearance." Lesions cleared in 4 weeks with 5 days of 30 mg oral prednisone and followed by mild topical corticosteroids, and after three months, she was patch-tested with both nickel sulfate (5% in petroleum) and titanium (10% in petroleum) with readings taken at 48 and 96 hours. The patient demonstrated a negative reaction to titanium and tiny vesiculopustular lesions and intense erythema, extending beyond the margins at 48 hours in response to nickel.

Of note Pahwa et al. (2012) and Dogra et al. (2014) document cases of "tram tracking" and "tram trek" scarring, respectively. It is unclear whether Yadav and Dogra's documentation of a "rail track"–appearing reaction represents a similar or distinct entity. However, the former authors were unable to attribute the scarring to a particular allergen or irritant, so these cases are discussed in the section, "Irregular Scarring."

42.3.4 Allergic/Irritant Chronic Inflammatory Reactions and Granulomas

Granulomatous inflammation is most commonly characterized by a collection of histiocytes (macrophages) surrounding an antigenic center, which may occasionally be necrotic; however, granulomatous inflammation encompasses presentations ranging from a well-organized granuloma to loose aggregates of epithelioid cells mixed with other inflammatory cells (Shah et al. 2017).

Granulomas may develop with or without immunologic modulation in the case of granulomatous hypersensitivity and foreign-body granulomas, respectively (Epstein 1989). Dermal granulomatous hypersensitivity has been associated with intradermal tattooing of red dyes with metallic elements and injection of dermal fillers such as hyaluronic acid and poly-L-lactic acid (PLA).

Pratsou and Gach (2013) report two females who underwent a facial microneedling procedure with a trained practitioner using a CE-marked, FDA-registered device (192 stainless steel MNs 1.5 mm long and 0.25 mm wide) coupled with skin cleansing and topical anesthetic cream. Within 24 hours, both developed significant lymphadenopathy, and the older sister developed pinpoint erythema, malaise, and headache. Systemic antibiotics were unhelpful, as the older sister's condition worsened with a "florid erythematous papular rash over her face" that spread to her trunk and limbs. The patient gradually improved over 2 weeks with systemic and topical corticosteroid treatment. Biopsy of lesions showed a nonspecific, chronic inflammatory infiltrate. Patch testing yielded a positive reaction to nickel sulphate (D4++), which was a known allergy to the patient. The authors were unable to attribute the reaction to her allergy, as the MN device contained up to 0.006% sulfur and 8% nickel bound to surgical-grade stainless steel (per the manufacturer)—an amount thought to pose little or no risk in short-term contact with nickel-sensitive individuals.

Soltani-Arabshahi et al. (2014) document three cases of granulomatous MN therapy reactions. The first two presented after Dermapen MN therapy followed by a high dose of lipophilic vitamin C (Vita C Serum; Sanítas Skincare) applied to the skin at the same medical spa. The Dermapen fraction microneedling device (Dermapen, LLC) is estimated to penetrate the skin anywhere from 0.25 to 2.00 mm. Both patients developed a progressive erythematous rash over the face in addition to systemic reactions, including arthralgias of varying intensity. In both cases, biopsy of indurated papules showed foreign body–type granulomatous reaction with focal, polarizable material present in giant cell cytoplasm. Patch testing both patients showed +1 reaction to Vita C Serum, while patch testing with Vita C Serum in five healthy volunteers yielded negative reactions. Both patients had persistent, mildly indurated, erythematous papules and plaques at nine months follow-up. The last of three patients presented following three microneedling procedures, two in which a gel product (Boske Hydra-Boost Gel; Boske Dermaceuticals) and one in which Vital Pigment Stabilizer (Dermapen, LLC) were applied before microneedling. While the patient did not have systemic symptoms, she did present with a progressively worsening erythematous rash that developed papular features, with a biopsy showing a similar granulomatous reaction. The last patient declined patch testing and demonstrated resolution at 3 weeks.

To limit chances of granuloma formation, patients should use only those products that are approved for intradermal use and prescribed by the physician in the immediate postprocedural time period. Alster and Graham (2018) typically allow patients to resume makeup application 2 days postprocedure and active skin care products 5 to 7 days after therapy.

42.3.5 IRREGULAR SCARRING

Pahwa et al. (2012) reported "tram tracking," or multiple discrete papular scars in a linear pattern in the horizontal and vertical directions, in a 25-year-old woman one month after treatment with a dermal rolling device (192 needles, 2 mm long) for management of acne scarring. Scarring was predominantly located over the temporal area, zygomatic arch, and forehead of the patient, who slightly improved with topical silicone gel at six months follow-up. They were unable to attribute the atypical scarring to an allergen or irritant.

Dogra et al. (2014) reported 2/36 patients undergoing MN therapy using a Dermaroller (192 fine microneedles, 1.5 mm in length and 0.1 mm in diameter) for atrophic acne scars to have a similar "tram trek" adverse effect. One patient developed severe tram-trek scarring over the malar prominence and was forced to withdraw; however, the patient improved with topical tretinoin. The second patient developed less severe tram trek scarring over the forehead and completed the study.

It is possible that the "tram trek" scarring may be a result of excessive force during the microneedling procedure over bony prominences of the patient's faces.

42.3.6 POST-INFLAMMATORY HYPERPIGMENTATION

Postinflammatory hyperpigmentation (PIH) is a hypermelanosis resulting from dermal inflammation or injury, most commonly in people of color (Davis and Callender 2010). The inflammation may be endogenous in the case of primary dermatoses or exogenous from external insults like trauma or physical injury (Epstein 1989). While the pathogenesis is not completely known, PIH is believed to result from increased production of melanin or increased release of melanin due to melanocyte-stimulating signals such as cytokines and various other inflammatory mediators (Davis and Callender 2010).

Dogra et al. (2014) found 5/36 patients to present with PIH following two to three treatments of MN therapy for post-acne scarring. Of the five patients, three had severe hyperpigmentation forcing them to withdraw from the study, while the other two gradually improved with photoprotection.

Sharad (2011) and Majid (2009) reported more transient PIH in 4/36 patients and 1/37 patients, respectively, in similar studies on MN therapy using a Dermaroller (192 fine microneedles, 1.5 mm in length and 0.25 mm in diameter) for atrophic scarring. Each previously mentioned case of hyperpigmentation featured Fitzpatrick type III or greater skin, except for one patient of unspecified type. To date, the amount of adverse hyperpigmentation reactions remain minimal and are possibly a result of improper ultraviolet (UV) protection following the procedure (Ramaut et al. 2018).

As in other skin resurfacing skin techniques, microneedling PIH is seen more commonly in skin of color. However, the risk of hyperpigmentation is thought to be lower when compared to other dermabrasive techniques such as chemical peels and lasers (Cohen and Elbuluk 2016). We strongly recommend the use of test spots, postprocedural use of at least SPF 30 sunscreen, and avoidance of UV exposure both prior and after MN therapy to minimize the chance of posttherapy dyspigmentation. Please see Cohen and Elbuluk (2016) for an in-depth review of the uses and efficacy of MNs in skin of color.

42.3.7 OTHER ADVERSE EFFECTS TO CONSIDER

Lastly, other potential reactions of which MN users should be aware include photoirritation, photoallergy, nonimmunologic contact urticaria (NICU), and immunologic contact urticaria (ICU).

Phototoxic or photoirritant reactions are evoked from the combination of an exogenous or endogenous compound and UV irradiation (Ibbotson 2014). Phototoxic reactions most often appear similar to an acute sunburn; however, they occasionally present with urticarial, eczematous, lichenoid, or, rarely, pigmentary changes (Maibach and Honari 2014). In contrast, photoallergy requires a prior sensitization to the chemical in the presence of UV radiation and an additional exposure in which there is a cell-mediated immune response and clinical presentation of the photoallergy (Ibbotson 2014). Photoallergic reactions most often present with eczematous-like changes (Maibach and Honari 2014).

Contact urticaria comprises a group of inflammatory reactions ranging from itching, burning, and tingling to systemic anaphylaxis (Gimenez-Arnau and Maibach 2014). Contact urticaria can be divided into NICU and ICU, with the two separate entities distinguished by immunologic memory in the case of ICU, but no required prior sensitization in NICU (Gimenez-Arnau and Maibach 2014). ICU and NICU are distinct in mechanism and etiology, but have very subtle, if any, difference in their clinical presentation (Gimenez-Arnau and Maibach 2014; Lahti 2000).

There is little to no current literature documenting photoirritation, photoallergy, NICU, or ICU resulting from MN therapy; however, we believe they are important conditions of which to be aware with the potential growth of MN use in the future.

42.4 CONCLUSION

Of all MN applications, the growth of MN use in the cosmetics industry for skin rejuvenation in the spa or the home setting raises the most concern. As previously mentioned, skin rejuvenation with MNs or collagen-induction therapy represents the most extensive use of MNs in any one therapy of all potential MN applications. In addition, skin rejuvenation is frequently performed outside of the medical setting, which also increases the chance of adverse events, especially those stemming from improper sterilization or the coupling with inappropriate topical products. We advise patients to understand contraindications for use and follow posttherapy guidelines, especially when seeking therapy outside of the medical setting.

Ramaut et al. (2018) systematically reviewed the MN literature and its potential application in atrophic acne scars, skin rejuvenation, hypertrophic scars, keloids, striae distensae, androgenetic alopecia, melasma, and acne vulgaris. They generally favored MN therapy due to minimal side effects with shorter recovery periods and similar results when compared to other treatments.

We believe MNs may be a relatively safe alternative and, in some circumstances, a superior option to many conventional therapies. However, further research and experience are needed to clarify the most appropriate and safe way to utilize this technology. When their use enters the medical domain, past marketing data will be invaluable in better understanding their toxicologic potential.

REFERENCES

Arya, J.; Henry, S.; Kalluri, H.; McAllister, D. V.; Pewin, W. P.; Prausnitz, M. R. Tolerability, usability and acceptability of dissolving microneedle patch administration in human subjects. Biomaterials 2017, *128, 1–7.*

Bao, L.; Zong, H.; Fang, S.; Zheng, L.; Li, Y. Randomized trial of electrodynamic microneedling combined with 5% minoxidil topical solution for treating androgenetic alopecia in Chinese males and molecular mechanistic study of the involvement of the Wnt/β-catenin signaling pathway. Journal of Dermatological Treatment 2020. *22, 1–7.*

Cervantes, J.; Hafeez, F.; Badiavas, E. V. Erythematous Papules after Microneedle Therapy for Facial Rejuvenation. Dermatologic Surgery 2019, *45(10), 1337–1339.*

Choi, S. Y.; Ko, E. J.; Yoo, K. H.; Han, H. S.; Kim, B. J. Effects of hyaluronic acid injected using the mesogun injector with stamp-type microneedle on skin hydration. Dermatologic Therapy 2020, *33(6), e13963*

Eisert, L.; Zidane, M.; Waigandt, I.; Vogt, P. M.; Nast, A. Granulomatous reaction following microneedling of striae distensae. JDDG: Journal Der Deutschen Dermatologischen Gesellschaft 2019, *14(4), 443–445.*

Hirobe, S.; Azukizawa, H.; Hanafusa, T.; Matsuo, K.; Quan, Y.-S.; Kamiyama, F.; et al. Clinical study and stability assessment of a novel transcutaneous influenza vaccination using a dissolving microneedle patch. Biomaterials 2015, *57, 50–58.*

Liu, S.; Zhang, S.; Duan, Y.; Niu, Y.; Gu, H.; Zhao, Z.; et al., Transcutaneous immunization of recombinant Staphylococcal enterotoxin B protein using a dissolving microneedle provides potent protection against lethal enterotoxin challenge. Vaccine 2019, *37(29), 3810–3819.*

Liu, T. M.; Sun, Y. M.; Tang, Z. Y.; Li, Y. H., Microneedle fractional radiofrequency treatment of facial photoageing as assessed in a split-face model. Clinical and Experimental Dermatology 2019, *44(4), 96–102.*

Rouphael, N. G.; Paine, M.; Mosley, R.; Henry, S.; McAllister, D. V.; Kalluri, H.; et. al. The safety, immunogenicity, and acceptability of inactivated influenza vaccine delivered by microneedle patch (TIV-MNP 2015): a randomised, partly blinded, placebo-controlled, phase 1 trial. The Lancet 2017, *390(10095), 649–658.*

Stojadinovic, O.; Morrison, B.; Tosti, A. Side effects of Platelet Rich Plasma and Microneedling. Journal of the American Academy of Dermatology 2019, *82(2), 501–502.*

Wang, C.; Sun, T.; Li, H.; Li, Z.; Wang, X. Hypersensitivity Caused by Cosmetic Injection: Systematic Review and Case Report. Aesthetic Plastic Surgery 2020, *45, 263–272.*

Zhu, D. D.; Zhang, X. P.; Zhang, B. L.; Hao, Y. Y.; Guo, X. D. Safety Assessment of Microneedle Technology for Transdermal Drug Delivery: A Review. Advanced Therapeutics 2020, *2000033.*

43 Transdermal Transport by Sonophoresis

Laurent Machet
Université de Tours, France

Alain Boucaud
Transderma Systems, Rue Giraudeau, Tours, France

CONTENTS

43.1 INTRODUCTION

Phonophoresis or sonophoresis is the term given to the use of ultrasound as a physical enhancer of percutaneous absorption of drugs. The skin provides an essential barrier function that effectively limits exchanges with the external environment in both directions: reduction of penetration of exogenous compounds and reduction of transepidermal losses. The main barrier property of the skin is due to the stratum corneum (SC), the outermost layer of the skin, that is a 10- to 20-μm-thick membrane composed of compact stacking of cornified keratinocytes that are separated by highly ordered intercellular lipid bilayers.

Topical or systemic administration of drugs through the skin needs to overcome this barrier. However, significant transdermal transport of high-molecular-weight molecules is quite impossible with conventional chemical enhancers. Physical enhancers have therefore been investigated to create wider pathways through the epidermis, using electric voltage, a process known as electroporation (1), or by using ultrasound, a process referred to as sonophoresis (or phonophoresis). On the other hand, the use of powerful techniques to overcome the skin barrier is limited by potential damage to the skin (1, 2).

The use of ultrasound as a transdermal transport enhancer, i.e., sonophoresis or phonophoresis, became very popular in sports medicine for local treatment of minor injuries and is believed both to accelerate functional recovery and to increase transdermal transport of topically applied drugs, especially nonsteroidal antiinflammatory drugs (3, 4). Using 1 to 3 MHz ultrasound, the extent of the drug transport enhancement still remains fairly low or is not even significant in some studies, as pointed out in a Cochrane systematic review published in 2014 (5). However, the feasibility of making the skin permeable to treatments such as insulin (6–8) or low-molecular-weight heparin (9) by using low-frequency ultrasound has increased the interest for the application of this noninvasive method in human medicine (1, 10–13).

43.2   PHYSICAL CHARACTERISTICS OF ULTRASOUND

Ultrasound is generated by a piezoelectric crystal transducer, which converts electric power into a mechanical oscillation generating an acoustic wave. After its emission, the wave is transmitted in an aqueous coupling medium (air or gas are bad transmitter media for ultrasound) placed between the transducer and the skin. This wave is partially reflected by the skin, while the other part penetrates and propagates through the skin with a direction parallel to the direction of oscillation. During its propagation, the wave is partially scattered and absorbed by the medium, resulting in attenuation of the emitted wave. An increase in temperature of the exposed medium is thus induced by the conversion of the ultrasound energy into heat.

The effects of ultrasound on the skin in terms of tolerance and efficacy of transdermal transport are directly related to the different ultrasound parameters i.e., frequency, intensity, and mode and time of application of the emitted wave.

43.2.1   FREQUENCY

The frequency f of the emitted wave depends on the size and the geometry of the ultrasound transducer. The frequency range of ultrasound is generally defined as higher than 20 kHz. In-depth penetration of the acoustic wave into the skin is inversely proportional to the frequency; hence, the biological effects of high-frequency ultrasound are mainly located at the skin surface (i.e., stratum corneum and epidermis), while low-frequency ultrasound may interact with deeper located structures (i.e., dermis, hypodermis, and muscles). Frequencies ranging from 0.8 to 2 MHz were first used (3, 14), then higher frequencies ranging from 3 to 20 MHz were investigated, with the idea of concentrating the acoustic energy on the SC (15, 16). Finally, low-frequency ultrasound (20 to 150 kHz) has been shown to enhance transdermal transport more effectively (6–9, 17).

43.2.2   MODE

The ultrasound waves can be emitted continuously (continuous mode) or in a sequential mode, for example, 0.1 second applied every second (discontinuous or pulsed mode). Pulsed mode is used in preference to continuous mode in order to avoid faster and more intense rises in temperature in or at the skin surface.

43.2.3   INTENSITY

Intensity I is equal to $I = c \times E$, where E is the emitted acoustic energy (E) and c is the speed of the ultrasound wave in the medium. In human soft tissues the value of c is ~1500 m/sec. The energy E depends on the density of the propagation medium (ρ), the total pressure (p) equal to the sum of the atmospheric pressure, and the pressure created by the ultrasonic wave: $E = p^2 / \rho c^2$. The intensity usually used in sonophoresis ranges from 0.5 to 2 W/cm^2, and the increase in pressure is approximately 0.2 bar, with an intensity of 1 W/cm^2 in water (18).

43.3 ULTRASOUND-ENHANCED PERCUTANEOUS ABSORPTION: PHARMACOKINETIC DATA

43.3.1 MEDIUM- AND HIGH-FREQUENCY PHONOPHORESIS

43.3.1.1 *In vitro* Studies

In vitro studies have been performed in the last three decades to quantify the increase in cutaneous permeability induced by ultrasound (Table 43.1). Differences between studies are related to ultrasound conditions (frequency, continuous or pulse mode, duration, intensity), monitoring (or not) of

TABLE 43.1

***In vitro* Studies of High- and Medium-Frequency Phonophoresis across Rat, Mice, or Human Skin (list is not limitative)**

Author and Year (Ref.)	F (kHz)	I (W/cm²)	Mode	Duration (minutes)	Molecule	Membrane	Effect
Vyas 1995 (81)	20000	3	P	15	Diclofenac	Mice skin	×2–30 enhancement
Machet 1996 (39)	3300	3	C	10	Digoxin	Hairless mice skin	Flux ×3, but heating resulted in the same effect
Meidan 1998 (20)	3300 1100	2.25	C	240	Hydrocortisone	Rat skin	×2.2 enhancement ×1.8
Meidan 1998 (74)	1100	2	C	5	Sucrose Mannitol Hydrocortisone	Rat skin	×4.5 enhancement ×4.1 ×7.7
Pelucio-Lopes 1993 (40)	1100	1.5	C	20	Azidothymidine	Human skin	Flux ×1 with a cooling coil
Hikima 1998 (21)	1100	4.3	C	10–30	Prednisolone	Hairless mouse skin	×2–5
Machet 1998 (41)	1100	1.5	C	20	Mannitol Estradiol Hydrocortisone	Hairless mice skin Human skin	Flux ×1 with a cooling coil Flux × 1 with a cooling coil
Brucks 1989 (38)	1000	1	C	240	Ibuprofen	Human epidermis	×3 enhancement
Mitragotri 1995 (22)	1000	2	C	300	7 molecules	Human epidermis	Flux ×13 estradiol, ×5 testosterone, ×4 cortisol, ×1.5 butanol, ×1.2 caffeine.
Johnson 1996 (23)	1000	1.4	C	1440	4 molecules with chemical enhancer	Human epidermis	Flux ×1 and ×75
Mitragotri 2001 (24)	1000	2	C	300	5 molecules	Human stratum corneum	×2–15 enhancement
Liao 2016 (82)	1000	2	P	5	Diclofenac	Rat skin	×1.1 enhancement ×1.3 enhancement with microbubbles

the increase in temperature induced by ultrasound within the donor compartment, control (or not) of the integrity of the skin by clinical and histological studies, and the origin of the membranes used (isolated epidermis, controlled skin thickness using a dermatome, or full-thickness skin). It can be concluded that the increase in percutaneous flux still remains moderate (enhanced ratio generally between 1 and 5) when ultrasound is applied over a short time (5 to 15 minutes) (19, 20). Increasing the exposure time from 10 to 60 minutes has been reported to result in a twofold to fivefold increase in transdermal diffusion of prednisolone *in vitro* with continuous application of 1 MHz ultrasound at 4.3 W/cm² (21). Interestingly, in the latter study no ultrasound-induced transdermal transport was found after removing the SC, demonstrating that ultrasound modified SC permeability. With longer exposure of skin to ultrasound (up to 20 hours), providing periodic replacement of donor and receptor compartment solutions to ensure sufficient dissolved gas concentrations and hence to maintain the cavitation activity, permeability may be increased across isolated epidermal sheets from 1 to 13 (22, 23). This was explained by the enhancement of diffusivity of the drug within the SC rather than an increase in the partition coefficient (24). However, it must be emphasized that these latter *in vitro* operating conditions are far from being applicable *in vivo*.

43.3.1.2   *In vivo* Studies

Studies conducted with various animal species have generally shown a significant effect of ultrasound on transdermal transport (Table 43.2). The technique became popular in humans in the United States (14). The efficacy of the technique overall is believed to be explained both by the physical effect of ultrasound itself on subcutaneous injured tissues and by enhancement of transdermal transport (4, 5). However, *in vivo* controlled studies have provided conflicting results (4, 5, 25) (Table 43.3).

In summary, it is clear that high- and medium-frequency ultrasound can increase both *in vitro* and *in vivo* transdermal transport of medium-sized molecules (<500 Da) that are currently used in clinical practice without ultrasound. Increasing locoregional diffusion of nonsteroidal antiinflammatory drugs twofold to tenfold in synovial tissue or muscles may be specifically helpful in sports medicine. However, when it does exist, such enhancement remains moderate or needs a long time exposure to ultrasound, making the use of this range of frequency for systemic transdermal delivery questionable.

TABLE 43.2
In vivo Studies of High- and Medium-Frequency Phonophoresis in Animals

Author and Year (Ref.)	F (kHz)	I (W/cm²)	Mode	Duration (minutes)	Molecule	Animal	Effect
Vyas 1995 (83)	20000	3	P	15	Diclofenac	rats	Reduction in provoked paw edema
Bommannan 1992 (15)	2000 10000 16000	0.2	C	20	Salicylic acid	guinea pigs	Urinary excretion increase at 10 MHz (×4)and 16 MHz (×2.5) but not at 2
Griffin 1963 (84)	1000	1–3	C	5	Cortisol	swine	Intramuscular concentration ×3
Levy 1989 (85)	1000 1000	1.5 3	C P	3 5	D-mannitol	rats	Increased diffusion ×5–20
Asano 1997 (48)	1000	1–2.5	P C	10–19 10	Indomethacin	rats	Mild increase in blood concentrations
Liao 2016 (82)	1000	2	P	5	Diclofenac	Rat	Reduction in provoked arthritis 70% with ultrasound 90% with ultrasound and microbubbles

TABLE 43.3

***In vivo* Studies of High- and Medium-Frequency Phonophoresis in Humans**

Author and Year (Ref.)	F (kHz)	I (W/cm²)	Mode	Duration (minutes)	Molecule	Number of Patients	Effect
Benson 1991 (86)	3000	1	C	5	Nicotinates	10	Nonsignificant
McElnay 1993 (87)	3000	1	C	5	Nicotinate	10	Vasodilatation ×1.7
Benson 1988 (88)	750–3000	1–1.5	C P	5	Prilocaine lignocaine	11	Significant increase in duration of anesthesia
Benson 1989 (89)	750–3000	1.5	C	5	Benzydamine	10	Nonsignificant
Williams 1990 (90)	1100	0.25	C	5	Anesthetic drugs	6	Nonsignificant
Griffin 1967 (91)	1000	0–3	C	5	Hydrocortisone	102	Reduced pain (68% vs. 28%)
Ciccone 1991 (92)	1000	1.5	P	5	Salicylate	40	Nonsignificant
Cagnie 2003 (4)	1000	1.5	C	5	Ketoprofen	10	×10 enhancement transport in synovial tissue; however, no enhancement in fat
McElnay 1985 (25)	870	2	P	5	lignocaine	10	Nonsignificant
McElnay 1986 (93)	870	2	P	5	Fluocinolone acetonide	12	Nonsignificant
Durmus 2014 (94)	1000	1.5	?	10	Capsaicin plus ultrasound versus capsaicin plus sham ultrasound	21 20	Significant decrease of pain in the ultrasound group as compared with placebo group
Coskun Benlidayi 2018 (95)	1000	1	C	5	Ibuprofen gel plus ultrasound versus ibuprofen cream plus ultrasound	30 31	Significant decrease of pain in both groups and more pronounced in the gel group

43.3.2 LOW-FREQUENCY SONOPHORESIS

This range of frequency has been investigated more intensively in recent years *in vitro* (Table 43.4), in some animal species *in vivo* (Table 43.5), and in humans (Table 43.6).

43.3.2.1 *In vitro*

Using a 20-kHz ultrasound probe, diffusion of low-molecular-weight molecules across epidermal sheets was increased from 2- to 5000-fold (26). Moreover, the synergistic action of a chemical enhancer such as sodium lauryl sulfate has been shown with low-molecular-weight molecules (27). Although statistically significant, the enhancement ratio remains relatively low in some *in vitro* studies performed on mouse skin (28), especially for hydrophilic drugs (29). A significant increase was also demonstrated using 350-μm-thickness human dermatomed skin, including the epidermis and upper dermis, with enhancement ratios of 4 and 34 for caffeine and fentanyl, respectively, during sonication, and the lag time was shortened (30). Moreover, by using 20-kHz ultrasound, it was shown that large molecules such as poly l-lysine (51 kDa) could be delivered through human heat-stripped skin with an exponential enhancement of the drug transport with ultrasound exposure time (31).

TABLE 43.4

In vitro **Studies of Low-Frequency Phonophoresis across Rat, Mice, or Human Skin**

Author and Year (Ref.)	F (kHz)	I (W/cm²)	Mode	Duration (minutes)	Molecule	Membrane	Effect
Ueda 1995 (17)	150	0.111	C	60	9 molecules	Hairless rat skin	Flux ×2–15
Ueda 1996 (62)	150	0.111	C	60	Benzoate sodium	Hairless rat skin	×7 enhancement
					Deuterium oxide		×4 enhancement
Monti 2001 (29)	40	0.44	C	240	Caffeine	Hairless mice skin	×4 enhancement
					Morphine		×10 enhancement
Mitragotri 19956 (22)	20	0.125	P	300	7 molecules	Human epidermis	Flux ×3 (estradiol), ×80 (cortisol), ×113 (water), ×400 salicylic acid), ×5000 (sucrose)
Zhang 1996 (96)	20	0.2	P	120	Vasopressin	Human epidermis	Kp = 1 10⁻⁵ cm/h with ultrasound Kp = 0 without ultrasound
Fang 1999 (28)	20	0.1–0.3	P	240	Clobetasol	Hairless mice	×1.9–4 enhancement
			C	240	17-propionate		×1.5–5.9 enhancement
Mitragotri 2000 (57)	20	1.6–14	P	90	Mannitol	Pig skin	×10 enhancement
Mitragotri 2001 (9)	20	7	P	10	Low-molecular-weight heparin	Pig skin	×21 enhancement
Boucaud 2001 (30)	20	2..5	P	60	Caffeine	Human skin	×4 enhancement
					Fentanyl		×34
	20	2.5	C	10	Caffeine		×1
					Fentanyl		×4
Manikkath 2017 (97)	20	7-8	P	30	Ketoprofen	Mice	×52 enhancement
					Ketoprofen plus dendrimer		×80 up to 1369

TABLE 43.5

In vivo **Studies of Low-Frequency Phonophoresis in Animals**

Author and Year (Ref.)	F (kHz)	I (W/cm²)	Mode	Duration (minutes)	Molecule	Animal	Effect
Tachibana 1993 (98)	48	0.17	C	5	Lidocaine	mice	Increased pain threshold
Mitragotri 1995 (7)	20	0.225	P	60	Insulin	rats	Marked decrease in blood glucose level
Mitragotri 1995 (22)	20	0.125	P	300	Salicylic acid	rats	Flux ×300
Mitragotri 2000 (99)	20	7	P	2	Mannitol	rats	×33 enhancement
					Inulin		×20 enhancement
					Glucose		×65 enhancement
Mitragotri 2001 (9)	20	7	P	2	Dalteparin	rats	Anti-Xa activity
Boucaud 2002 (7)	20	2.5	P	15	Insulin	rats	Marked decrease in blood glucose level
Boucaud 2001 (100)	20			15		pigs	Marked decrease in blood glucose level
Smith 2003 (32)	20	0.1	P	20	Insulin	rats	Marked decrease in blood glucose level
				60			

TABLE 43.6

In vivo **Studies of Low-Frequency Phonophoresis in Humans**

Author and Year (Ref.)	F (kHz)	I (W/cm²)	Mode	Duration (minutes)	Molecule	Number of Patients	Effect
Cagnie 2003 (4)	100	?	P	5	Ketoprofen	9	×14 enhancement transport in synovial tissue but no enhancement in fat
Kost 2000 (35)	20	10	P	2	Glucose	7	Increased reverse transport of glucose
Maruani 2010 (101)	36	2.72	P	5	Betamethasone 17-valerate alone or with ultrasound	15	Increased blanching test
Maruani 2010 (102)	36	2.72 3.50	P	5	Histamine	10	Increased dose-dependent size of the histamine-induced papules and of dermal edema measured with ultrasonography

43.3.2.2 *In vivo*

Enhancement of low-weight molecules has been demonstrated with a higher order of magnitude than that observed with medium- or high-frequency ultrasound (Table 43.5). Moreover, particular attention was drawn by Tachibana, who first demonstrated the transdermal diffusion of a macromolecule (insulin, 6 kDa) across hairless mice skin exposed to 48-kHz ultrasound applied for 5 minutes *in vivo*, resulting in a marked decrease (~80%) in glycemia (6). *In vivo* transdermal delivery of insulin was then confirmed by Mitragotri in 1995 using a 20-kHz ultrasound probe applied for 60 minutes (7) and by our group with a shorter application time of 15 minutes in hairless rats (Figure 43.1) (8). Using a homemade ultrasound device (cymbal arrays), Smith et al. (32) reported a 70% decrease in blood glucose concentration in Sprague-Dawley rats exposed to insulin and

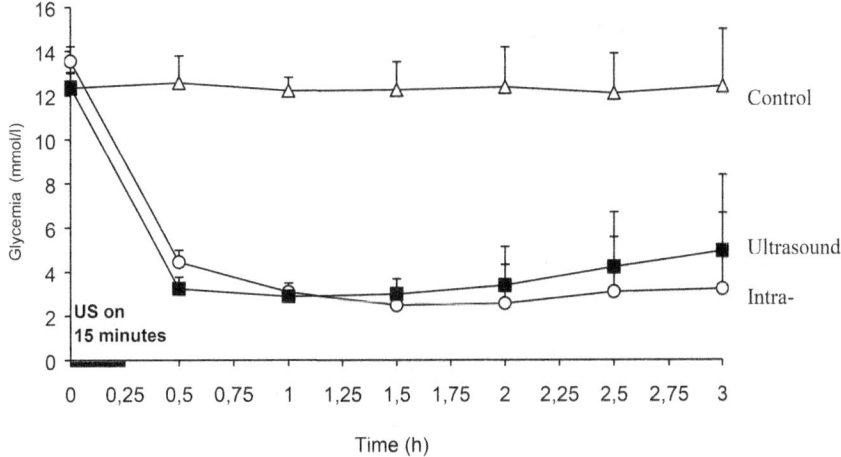

FIGURE 43.1   *In vivo* sonophoresis of insulin (20 kHz, pulsed mode, 2.5 W/cm², 15 minutes): decrease in glycemia of rats exposed to ultrasound is similar to the decrease in glycemia of rats treated with 0.5 IU intramuscular injection of insulin (mean values and standard deviation, 4 animals in each curve). (Redrawn from reference 8.)

20-kHz ultrasound at 100 W/cm² for 60 minutes. This was confirmed in pigs (100 to 140 lb) (33). Transdermal delivery of macromolecules with conserved biological activity was confirmed with ultrasound-induced transdermal delivery of low-molecular-weight heparin (9), demonstrating measurable systemic anti-Xa activity.

In summary, low-frequency ultrasound is able to overcome the skin barrier and could ultimately contribute to valuable therapeutic devices. The extent of enhancement is greater with passively low-penetrating drugs, suggesting that ultrasound interacts with the lipid bilayers of the SC (see Section 5.1) (22). Another field of application for ultrasound-induced skin permeability is the noninvasive quantitative assessment of blood concentration of glucose using reverse skin permeability of glucose (34). After the exposure of the skin of diabetic patients to 20-kHz ultrasound at 10 W/cm² for two minutes (50% duty cycle), fairly good correlation was found between glucose concentrations found in extracted fluids and in blood (35) using a vacuum pump to extract dermal interstitial fluid.

43.4 MECHANISM OF ACTION OF ULTRASOUND ON TRANSDERMAL TRANSPORT

The main modes of action of ultrasound-enhanced transport can be briefly summarized as follows: the propagation of ultrasonic waves in a medium induces two main physical consequences, i.e., heating and cavitation. These mechanisms are linked, as cavitation provokes local heating (36). Moreover, cavitation itself can create violent microjets that can dramatically affect adjacent material as metal, and in the present case the SC. Overall the consequence is an increase in skin permeability by increasing fluidity of intercellular lipids and by partial removal of intercellular fluid and possibly some corneocytes, resulting in enlarged intercellular spaces and in the creation of aqueous channels though the SC that can persist after the end of sonication.

43.4.1 HEATING

Several phenomena explain the increase in temperature within and at the skin surface exposed to ultrasound. Increase in temperature may be excessive, and it is possible to use an aqueous gel, which decreases reflection, or to use an ultrasound-pulsed mode or a low focused ultrasound wave, which decreases energy density, and to decrease the length and/or the intensity of the sonication.

43.4.1.1 Heating at the Skin Surface

Using 1-MHz ultrasound, Miyazaki et al. (37) showed a rise of 6°C for a fairly low intensity of 0.25 W/cm² and 12°C for an intensity of 0.75W/cm². Moreover, despite the use of a cooling coil, an 11°C increase occurred in the donor compartment using 1-MHz ultrasound in continuous mode for 4 hours (38). We obtained increases of 15°C to 30°C at intensities ranging from 1 to 3 W/cm² (39). Moreover, when heating with an electric resistance, we obtained an equivalent increase in percutaneous flow (Figure 43.2). Our findings obtained with a cooling system did not show any significant increase in percutaneous diffusion rates of various molecules with molecular weight of 138 to 781 Da (azidothymidine, digoxin, hydrocortisone, mannitol, estradiol, salicylic acid) (40, 41). Increase in temperature is thus one of the major factors that can explain the increase in percutaneous absorption in the frequency range from 1 to 3 MHz and in continuous mode. However, a threefold increase was observed with a larger molecule, vasopressin V-2 antagonist (molecular weight 1014 da) (42), demonstrating that heating is not the only mechanism of action of medium frequency.

Using lower-frequency ultrasound (20 kHz, 10 to 30 W/cm²) and monitoring the temperature, percutaneous flow of hydrocortisone was quadrupled through cellulose membranes and the temperature was increased threefold (25°C to 75°C), whereas the diffusion flux measured was close to that of controls at similar temperatures (43). By contrast, using lower intensities on hairless rat

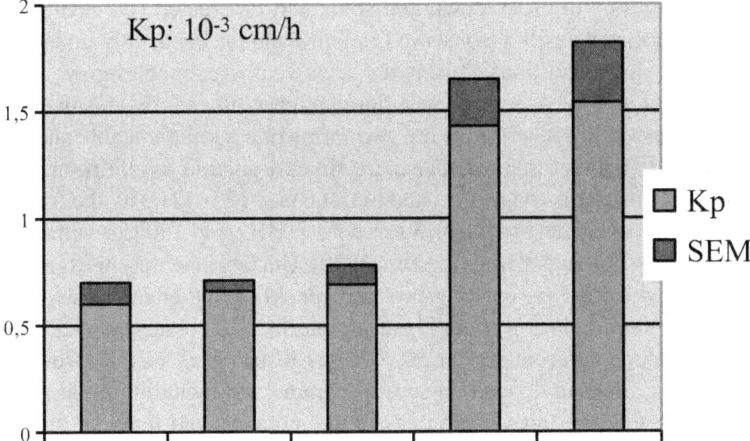

FIGURE 43.2   High-frequency phonophoresis of digoxin. Ultrasound (3.3 kHz, 3W/cm²) provoked an increase both in transdermal transport and temperature in donor compartment. Similar heating outside the skin with an electrical resistance resulted in similar increase in transdermal transport. (Redrawn from reference 39.)

skin (17) and in isolated epidermal sheets (7), the rise in temperature in the donor compartment was less and cannot explain the 10- to 100-fold increases in percutaneous absorption. Merino et al. (44) reported an increase in temperature of 20°C of mannitol solution exposed to 20 kHz at 15 W/cm² for 2 hours. However, only 25% of the transdermal transport enhancement was attributable to this rise in temperature. The same group also studied the migration of a hydrophilic tracer (calcein) by using confocal microscopy and compared with adequate heating control, again showing a greater efficacy of 20 kHz ultrasound than simple heating (45).

43.4.1.2   Heating within the Skin

When an ultrasound wave penetrates through the skin or other structure, it decreases gradually as it propagates. This phenomenon of attenuation is explained by three mechanisms i.e., absorption, reflection, and dispersion, and it depends on the frequency of the wave and the density and heterogeneity of the structure. Part of this ultrasound energy is finally converted into heat. Due to its heterogeneity, the attenuation coefficient of the skin is four times higher than that of other soft tissues (46, 47). It is known that in-depth penetration of ultrasound is inversely proportional to frequency: 50% of energy penetrates up to 10 cm beneath the SC using 90-kHz ultrasound, whereas the same amount of energy only penetrates to 2 cm using 1-MHz ultrasound. In-depth transmission might support vasodilatation of dermal capillaries allowing systemic diffusion. Asano et al. (48) showed an increase of 6°C at 1 W/cm² and an increase of 11°C at 2 W/cm² by introducing a thermal probe beneath the skin of rats exposed to ultrasound (1 MHz, 1 to 2 W/cm², continuous mode). Using a 20-kHz ultrasound probe, the intradermal temperature measured *in vivo* just beneath sonicated skin increases only by a few degrees Celsius during sonication (2, 49).

43.4.2   Cavitation

43.4.2.1   Description

Cavitation is the production of microbubbles in a liquid when a large negative pressure is applied to it. When a medium is exposed to ultrasound, the transmitted waves alternatively compress and stretch its molecular structure. If a sufficiently large negative pressure is applied to the liquid so that the distance between the molecules exceeds the critical molecular distance necessary to hold the liquid intact, the liquid will break down and voids will be created i.e., cavitation bubbles will form. Acoustic cavitation can easily be observed in liquid media, especially under high ultrasound intensity and low-frequency conditions. During the negative phase, bubbles grow around their equilibrium radius. However, the pressure in the medium increases during the positive phase, causing a reduction in the bubbles' radius size. There are two forms of cavitation: stable and unstable. Stable cavitation corresponds to bubbles that oscillate many times around its equilibrium radius (resonance radius Rr expressed in µm). Rr is roughly related to frequency (F in kHz) by the following equation: $F \times Rr = 3000$. Thus the resonance radius is 3 µm with 1 MHz and 150 µm with 20 kHz. The size of observed bubbles may be greater in living tissue (50). Unstable cavitation exists for a very short length of time, during which the gas cavity grows very quickly and then implodes, producing a local rise in temperature. When implosion occurs near an interface, it creates a shock wave and violent microjets that can damage adjacent structures, even as resistant as metal. Growth and decrease in bubble size and their lifespan depend on several parameters, including intensity and frequency of the ultrasound field, external pressure, viscosity, gas content, and temperature of the coupling medium. The occurrence of cavitation in water is facilitated by the presence of dissolved gas and needs to increase intensity when increasing frequency (18, 51).

The occurrence and consequences of cavitation have been studied in living cells and tissues (52–54) with possible applications for the destruction of cancers (55, 56) and permeation of cell membranes (57).

43.4.2.2 Implications in Transdermal Transport

The major role played by cavitation in ultrasound-mediated transdermal transport is supported by a series of experiments conducted *in vitro*:

1. The need to keep dissolved gas in the medium to form nuclei of cavitation (22, 58)
2. The possibility of permeating cell membranes *in vitro* (59) and the skin *in vivo* (60) is enhanced in the presence of artificial cavitation nuclei
3. The demonstration of pores created at the skin surface by ultrasound (42) and within the SC (49, 61, 62)
4. The demonstration of multiple pits induced by bubble implosion on gelatin gels (58) or aluminum foils exposed to ultrasound and the correlation with intensity and skin conductivity (63, 64)
5. Dose–response curves of skin conductivity enhancement with cavitation (65)

43.4.2.2.1 Cavitation Outside the Skin

Implosion of bubbles near the SC surface induced by cavitation can create localized damage, justifying systematic morphological studies. Small cavities of a few micrometers in size, which could correspond to the impact of cavitation bubbles on the SC surface resulting in microjets and shock waves, have indeed been shown using scanning electron microscopy (Figure 43.3) (41, 62, 66). Craterlike images of 5 to 15 µm in size were also reported in hairless mice exposed to 1-MHz ultrasound at 4.3 W/cm² *in vitro* (21). Scanning electron microscopic examination of rat skin after *in vivo* exposure to 150-kHz ultrasound demonstrated 100- to 150-µm lesions on the SC surface (67), corresponding to the size of the bubbles induced by stable cavitation at 20 kHz (18). Similarly, pits provoked by 20-kHz ultrasound application on aluminum foil (63, 68) probably corresponded to the same phenomenon, and interestingly, the numbers of pits increased with intensity and reduction in the distance between the skin and the probe. Cellular membrane disruption and intercytoplasmic and intracytoplasmic vacuoles have been demonstrated in fish without significant increase in temperature within the skin (69), and these lesions were not observed when cavitation in the donor compartment was suppressed using degassed water, indicating that these lesions originate from cavitation outside the skin.

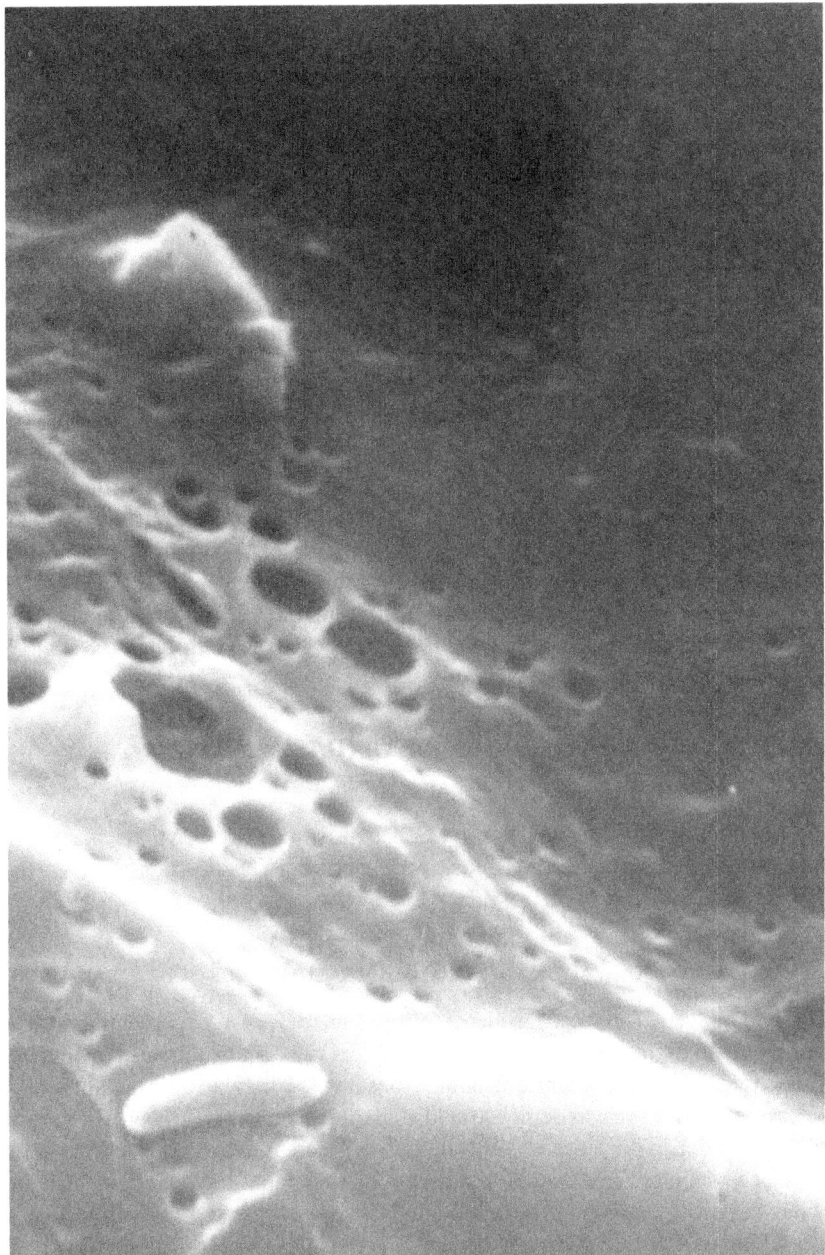

FIGURE 43.3 Numerous holes at the stratum corneum surface corresponding to cavitation occurring at skin interface.

43.4.2.2.2 Cavitation within the Skin

Indirect proof of cavitation has been demonstrated in isolated epidermis *in vitro* after incubating the epidermis with fluorescein, resulting in bleaching of fluorescence, probably secondary to the production of hydroxyl radicals induced by cavitation (22). Theoretically, cavitation is possible within the SC because of the presence of dissolved oxygen and nitrogen and the presence of lacunae between corneocytes (70). The aqueous contents of sweat channels, whose diameter are approximately

5 μm, makes it highly probable that cavitation could occur within it *in vivo* with medium-frequency ultrasound, but this is less probable with low-frequency ultrasound because of the greater size of the bubbles. The existence of dissolved gas at depth in living tissue can allow the development of cavitation bubbles (50). We demonstrated epidermal and dermal damage in mice using low-frequency ultrasound, including muscle and vessel necrosis highly suggestive of undesirable in-depth cavitation, using ultrasound parameters that are not far from those used in sonophoresis (2).

43.4.3 MISCELLANEOUS

Independent of cavitation and heating, ultrasound waves provoke a rise in pressure in liquid medium in the donor compartment. The relative contribution of this flow has been estimated to represent 0.02% at 1 W/cm^2 and 2% at 100 W/cm^2 and is thus negligible (18). Phonophoresis of mannitol across pig skin *in vitro* was found to be the same when ultrasound was applied before application of mannitol or simultaneously, suggesting no significant effect of convection in ultrasound-induced transdermal transport (68). On the other hand, we did not evidence any changes in glucose blood levels of rats when ultrasound was applied before the application of insulin, while marked hypoglycemia was observed when ultrasound and insulin were applied simultaneously (8).

In conditions of negligible temperature rise and absence of cavitation, mechanical stress has shown evidence of intercellular widening induced by transverse (shear) waves (71, see Section 5.1).

The boundary layer of water immediately adjacent to membranes in studies carried out *in vitro* is less well mixed and constitutes an additional resistance to diffusion through the skin. This can be reduced by acoustic streaming (18).

43.5 BIOLOGICAL CONSEQUENCES OF ULTRASOUND APPLICATION ON SKIN

SC lipids are essential to skin barrier integrity. Hence, it is possible to hypothesize that ultrasound can affect lipid fluidity either by heating, shock waves, or microjets and moreover provokes partial removal of lipids from SC.

43.5.1 REMOVAL OR MODIFICATION OF STRATUM CORNEUM LIPIDS

In a model of lipid bilayers using low-frequency ultrasound, defects were observed using an atomic-force microscope, with diameters of 10 to 100 nanometers (72). Intercellular lipid content was measured in hairless rat skin *in vitro* after ultrasound exposure (150 kHz) in a surfactant solution (Tween 20). Lipid release from the skin was demonstrated, and this increased with length of time of exposure to 150-kHz ultrasound. Lipid release was correlated with increased skin conductivity and enhanced transport of polar molecules (73). Similarly, sebaceous gland debulking was demonstrated on histological sections of hairless rat skin exposed to low-intensity ultrasound (74). Moreover, removal of 30% of the total amount of SC lipids was demonstrated using 20-kHz ultrasound (15 W/cm^2, duty cycle 0.1 to 0.9 for 2 hours) in pigs, a species with less prominent sebaceous glands (45).

43.5.2 IMAGING PATHWAY OF SONOPHORETIC TRANSPORT

As seen in Section 4.2.2.1, pits secondary to cavitation on the skin surface have been shown with both medium- and low-frequency ultrasound (21, 41, 49). Nevertheless, whether these craterlike lesions are a possible pathway for transdermal transport remains uncertain. The following section will report on evidence for possible in-depth pathways.

43.5.2.1 High- and Medium-Frequency Ultrasound

The migration of a tracer (lanthanum) has been demonstrated between intercorneocyte spaces after exposure to high-frequency ultrasound (10 to 16 MHz) and the tracer reached the dermis (16).

Widening of intercellular spaces was observed (75), with some desmosomal alteration, but these modifications were transient. The assumption that intercellular cavities were secondary to cavitation is doubtful, since the occurrence of cavitation is uncertain at the frequency and intensity used (18). It is thus more likely that widening of the intercellular space was secondary to mechanical stress causing disruption of the lipid bilayers. This is supported by a further study carried out on fish below the cavitational threshold at 3 MHz and 2 W/cm^2, which demonstrated intensity dose-dependent intercellular widening, while cavitation was undetectable (71). The maximum disorganization affecting the outer layers of the epidermis was found with a 45-degree angle of the incidence radiation, suggesting a role of a transverse wave in the occurrence of cell-to-cell disruption.

43.5.2.2 Low-Frequency Ultrasound

Human SC exposed to 168 kHz at 1.2 W/cm^2 for 15 minutes was examined with epifluorescence microscopy: 20 micrometer cavities were seen and considered to be the consequence of cavitation. As expected, the attenuation coefficient of SC was increased and assumed to be induced by multiplication of cell-to-cell interfaces, intercellular lipids, and entrapped air pockets (61). Confocal images were used to trace sonophoresis (20 kHz) of a hydrophobic and fluorescent compound and showed a marked but spatially discontinuous increase in transepidermal transport. The areas made permeable could not be identified to detect the anatomic structure, but there was focal in-depth penetration of the tracer, whereas despite being located within ultrasound field, adjacent areas did not display any penetration of the tracer. These modifications were restricted to a 1 cm^2 surface below the ultrasound probe (45). In a study combining low-frequency sonophoresis with tape stripping or oleic acid as a chemical enhancer, the penetration of lanthanum nitrate solution through an intercellular pathway was evidenced using transmission electron microscopy (66).

43.5.2.3 Dual-Frequency Ultrasound

Dual-frequency ultrasound, utilizing 20-kHz and 1-MHz wavelengths simultaneously, was found to significantly enhance the size of localized transport regions (LTRs) in both *in vitro* and *in vivo* models (76). The flux of 4 kDa dextran was 3.5- and 7.1-fold greater using 20 kHz + 1 MHz at 6 and 8 minutes, respectively, compared to the use of 20 kHz alone.

43.5.3 SKIN TOLERANCE TO ULTRASOUND

High-intensity focused ultrasound (HIFU) is used to treat and destroy tumors (77). High-intensity ultrasound (in general greater than 5 W/cm^2) can produce coagulation necrosis in biological tissue, and this is the phenomenon mainly exploited in the HIFU ablation technique. In contrast, low-intensity ultrasound (0.125 to 3 W/cm^2) leads to nondestructive heating and can be used for other clinical applications. However, some studies performed on excised skin have used intensities greater than 15 W/cm^2. Therefore, special attention has to be paid to tolerance of skin exposed to medium- and low-frequency ultrasound in the conditions used in transdermal transport studies. As seen earlier, parameters such as intensity, frequency, mode, and duration of ultrasound exposure are of importance, since it is expected that cavitation again can be a key issue in damaging living cells. With medium- and high-frequency ultrasound (1 to 3 MHz) and intensities ranging from 2 to 3 W/cm^2, we observed macroscopic changes in human skin *in vitro* (39). Histological studies have shown multiple areas of keratinocyte necrosis, with epidermal detachment, edema, and degeneration of collagen fibers in the upper part of the dermis, whereas heating alone produced no histological alterations (39, 48, 74). Transmission electron microscopy additionally revealed alterations of intracytoplasmic organites (39), and holes could be demonstrated on the skin surface using scanning electron microscopy (cf. Section 5.1) (41).

In vitro experiments using hairless mice skin exposed to low-frequency ultrasound (20 kHz continuous mode for 4 hours) showed epidermal and dermal lesions despite relatively low intensity (0.2 W/cm^2). Lesions were less marked using pulsed mode (28). Using human skin *in vitro*, we observed normal appearance of skin exposed to 2.5 W/cm^2 and dose-dependent severity of skin lesions, again greater with continuous mode, from 4 W/cm² to 20 W/cm². Similarly, a dose-dependent increase in temperature in the donor compartment was measured, varying from 33°C to 65°C (2). Comparable findings were reported in dogs (49). Experiments were also carried out *in vivo* with hairless rat skin exposed to 2.5 W/cm². Immediately after sonication, macroscopic and microscopic appearance was normal. However, overt macroscopic and microscopic lesions occurred 24 hours later, thus demonstrating delayed constitution of ultrasound-induced lesions (Figure 43.4) (2).These lesions were not expected to be induced by heating of the donor compartment, since the increase was moderate. Moreover, similar heating with an electrical resistance produced no lesions. Additionally, lesions were not provoked by diffusion of heated water through the skin, since the same ultrasound protocol, applied with a plastic film interposed between the ultrasound and the skin, resulted in the same epidermal and dermal lesions. Finally, the increase in temperature was moderate (+3°C), contrasting with the severity of vessel and muscle necrosis, suggesting probable in-depth cavitation (2). However, hairless mouse skin, and particularly the SC, is thinner than human skin, and this could explain why the human skin threshold tolerance to ultrasound is higher *in vitro*, and probably also *in vivo*, since preliminary findings in two human volunteers showed an absence of immediate or delayed cutaneous lesions after sonication (5 W/cm², pulse duration 1.6 seconds, 25% duty cycle, 15 minutes) (78). Ultrasound exposure (20 kHz, 10 W/cm², 50% duty cycle, 2 minutes) was well tolerated in seven diabetic patients *in vivo* (35). We conducted a double-blind, randomized, controlled

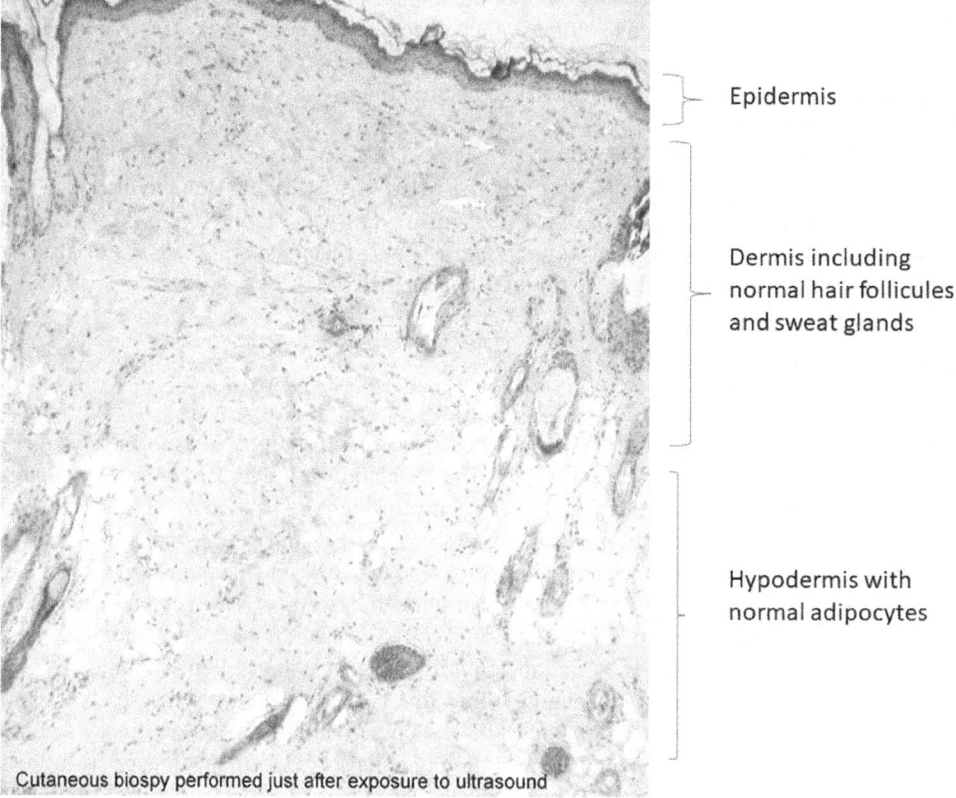

Epidermis

Dermis including normal hair follicules and sweat glands

Hypodermis with normal adipocytes

Cutaneous biospy performed just after exposure to ultrasound

FIGURE 43.4 (a) Normal aspect just after exposure to ultrasound. (b) Epidermal necrosis (black asterisks) with sub-epidermal detachement (black arrows), collagen damages (white dashed arrows) and neutrophilic polymorphonuclear infiltrate with some pycnotic cells (white arrows) in the dermis 48 hours after exposure to ultrasound, consistent with burn. (c) Vascular lesion (black arrows) deeply located at the dermo-hypodermal junction showing congestion and early thrombosis, eccrine sweat duct showing epithelial alterations (white arrows), and adipocytes necrosis (disappearance of the cell nucleus, black asterisks), consistent with deep burn.

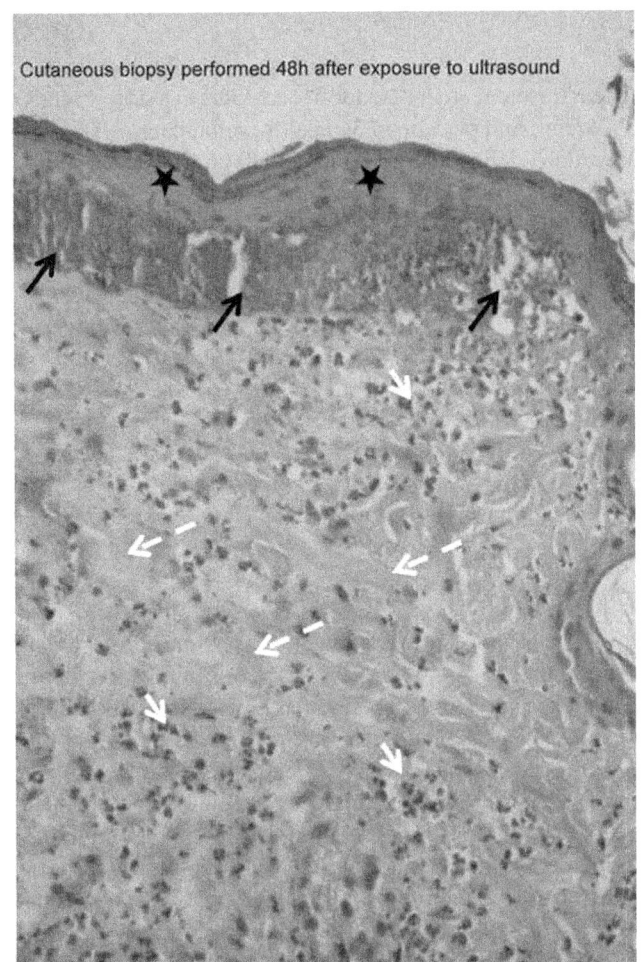

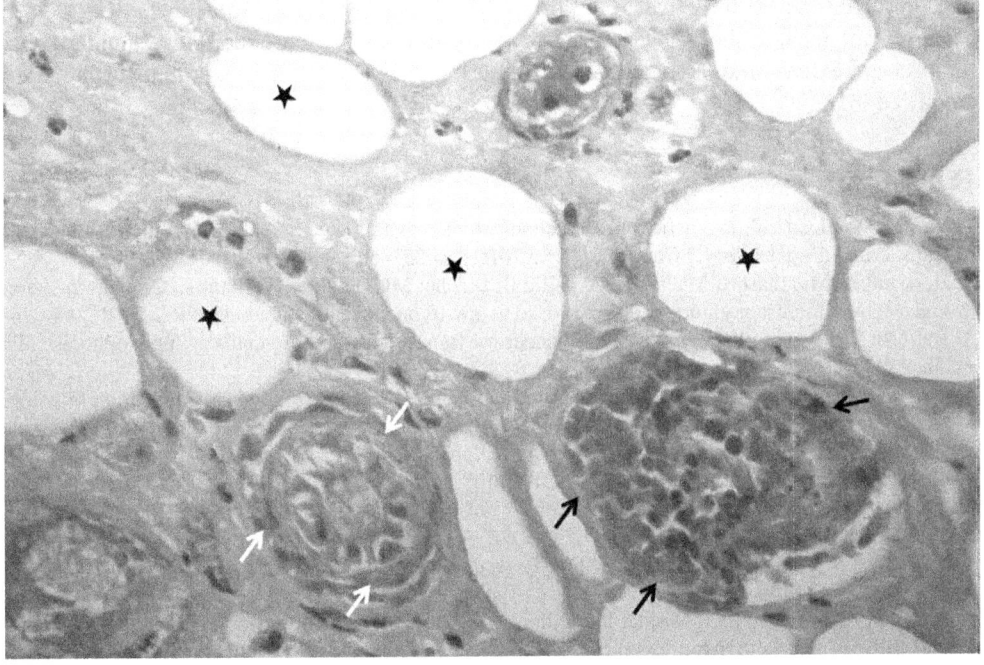

FIGURE 43.4 (*Continued*)

study using pulse-mode ultrasound at 36 kHz for five minutes in a step procedure of increasing dosage, from 1.57 to 3.50 W/cm², and placebo in 34 healthy volunteers (79). The primary outcome was toxic effects of the procedure, defined as a pain score >40 on a 0- to 100-mm visual analogue scale or necrosis. Erythema (scored from 0 to 3 in severity) was also evaluated. We found no pain score >38 and no skin necrosis with either ultrasound or placebo. Erythema was systematically observed immediately after ultrasound exposure, but after 1 day, we observed only three cases. The most frequent adverse effect was tinnitus.

43.6   STABILITY OF DRUGS EXPOSED TO ULTRASOUND

Possible degradation of drugs due to ultrasound has been checked *in vitro* using ultrasound at high intensity, and no degradation occurred with poly l-lysine (31), insulin (8), fentanyl, or caffeine (30). Persistent *in vivo* biological activity of insulin and low-molecular-weight heparin is also in accordance with the absence of significant degradation in the conditions used (7–9).

43.7   PROSPECTS: IS PAINLESS NEEDLE-FREE INJECTION A REALISTIC GOAL?

There is no doubt that ultrasound can markedly increase transdermal transport *in vitro* and *in vivo* in animals and humans (1, 6–13, 60, 62, 78, 80, 81). Findings published between 1990 and 2010 were encouraging, especially for diabetes therapy, as it was possible to decrease glucose blood levels in animals *in vivo* (6, 7) and monitor it using inverse sonophoresis (35). The daily dose of insulin required to treat an adult diabetic patient is usually between 30 and 60 IU, and the amount delivered to animals is about 0.5 to 1 IU for a short period. Thus repeated pulses over the day would theoretically make possible the administration of a daily dose. However, 19 years after Mitragotri's first paper, no ultrasound device is used to deliver insulin in humans perhaps because (1) human barrier skin is more difficult to overcome with ultrasound than animal skin, (2) sonicating 1 cm² of a rat weighing 500 g is expected to be much more effective than sonicating 1 cm² of a 60-kg human, and (3) there are technology problems to proposing a small ultrasound device powerful enough to deliver the ultrasound intensity necessary to achieve drug delivery. Other problems include short- and long-term safety in humans, reproducibility, standardization of the process, extension of sonicated area, and cost. Thus there is no doubt that further studies are required (81).

REFERENCES

1. Wong TW. Electrical, magnetic, photomechanical and cavitational waves to overcome skin barrier for transdermal drug delivery. J Control Release 2014; 193:257–69.
2. Boucaud A, Montharu J, Machet L, Arbeille B, Machet MC, Patat, F, Vaillant L. Clinical, histologic, and electron microscopy study of skin exposed to low-frequency ultrasound. Anat Rec 2001; 264, 114–9.
3. Byl NB. The use of ultrasound as an enhancer for transcutaneous drug delivery: phonophoresis. Phys Ther 1995; 75, 539–53.
4. Cagnie B, Vinck E, Rimbaut S, Vanderstraten G. Phonophoresis versus topical application of ketoprofen: comparison between tissue and plasma levels. Phys Ther 2003; 83, 707–12.
5. Ebadi S, Henschke N, Nakhostin Ansari N, Fallah E, van Tulder MW. Therapeutic ultrasound for chronic low-back pain. Cochrane Database Syst Rev. 2014 Mar 14; (3), CD009169.
6. Tachibana K, Tachibana S. Transdermal delivery of insulin by ultrasonic vibration. J Pharm Pharmacol 1991; 43, 270–71.
7. Mitragotri S, Blankschtein D, Langer R. Ultrasound-mediated transdermal protein delivery. Sciences 1995; 269, 850–3.
8. Boucaud A, Garrigue MA, Machet L, Vaillant L, Patat F. Effect of sonication parameters on transdermal delivery of insulin to hairless rats. J Control Release 2002; 81, 113–19.
9. Mitragotri S, Kost J. Transdermal delivery of heparin and low-molecular weight heparin using low frequency ultrasound. Pharm Res 2001; 18, 1151–56.

10. Azagury A, Khoury L, Enden G, Kost J. Ultrasound mediated transdermal drug delivery. Adv Drug Deliv Rev 2014; 72, 127–43.

11. Polat BE, Hart D, Langer R, Blankschtein D. Ultrasound-mediated transdermal drug delivery: mechanisms, scope, and emerging trends. J Control Release 2011; 152, 330–48.

12. Ita K. Recent progress in transdermal sonophoresis. Pharm Dev Technol 2017; 22, 458–66.

13. Seah BC, Teo BM. Recent advances in ultrasound-based transdermal drug delivery. Int J Nanomedicine 2018; 13, 7749–63.

14. Pottenger FJ, Karalfa BL. Utilization of hydrocortisone phonophoresis in United States army physical therapy clinics. Military Medicine 1989; 154, 355–58.

15. Bommannan D, Okuyama H, Stauffer P, Guy RH. Sonophoresis. I. The use of high-frequency ultrasound to enhance transdermal drug delivery. Pharm Res 1992; 9, 559–64.

16. Bommannan, D, Menon GK, Okuyama H, Elias PM, Guy RH. Sonophoresis. II. Examination of the mechanism(s) of ultrasound-enhanced transdermal delivery. Pharm Res 1992; 9, 1043–47.

17. Ueda H, Sugibayashi K, Morimoto Y. Skin penetration-enhancing effect of drugs by phonophoresis. J Control Release 1995; 37, 291–97.

18. Simonin, JP. On the mechanisms of *in vitro* and *in vivo* phonophoresis. J Control Release 1995; 33, 125–41.

19. Meidan VM, Walmsley AD, Irwin WJ. Phonophoresis- is it a reality ? Int J Pharm 1995; 118, 129–49.

20. Meidan VM, Docker MF, Walmsley AD, Irwin WJ. Phonophoresis of hydrocortisone with enhancers: an acoustically defined model. Int J Pharm 1998; 170, 157–68.

21. Hikima T, Hirai Y, Tojo K. Effect of ultrasound application on skin metabolism of prednisolone 21-acetate. Pharm Res 1998; 15, 1680–83.

22. Mitragotri S, Blankschtein D, Langer R. A Mechanistic study of ultrasonically-enhanced transdermal drug delivery. J Pharm Sci 1995; 84, 697–706.

23. Johnson M, Mitragotri S, Patel A, Blankschtein, D, Langer, R. Synergistic effects of chemical enhancers and therapeutic ultrasound on transdermal drug delivery. J Pharm Sci 1996; 85, 670–79.

24. Mitragotri S. Effect of therapeutic ultrasound on partition and diffusion coefficient in human stratum corneum. J Control Release 2001; 71, 23–29.

25. McElnay, JC, Matthews MP, Harland R, McCafferty DF. The effect of ultrasound on the percutaneous absorption of lignocaine. Br J Clin Pharmacol 1985; 20, 421–24.

26. Mitragotri S, Blankschtein D, Langer R. Transdermal drug delivery using low-frequency sonophoresis. Pharm Res 1996; 13, 411–20.

27. Mitragotri S, Ray D, Farell H, Tang H, Yu B, Kost J, Blankstein D, Langer R. Synergistic effect of ultrasound and sodium lauryl sulfate on transdermal drug delivery. J Pharm Sci 2000; 89, 892–900.

28. Fang JY, Fang CL, Sung KC, Chen HY. Effect of low frequency ultrasound on the *in vitro* percutaneous absorption of clobetasol 17-propionate. Int J Pharm 1999; 191, 33–42.

29. Monti D, Gianelli R, Chetoni P, Burgalassi S. Comparison of the effect of ultrasound and of chemical enhancers on transdermal permeation of caffeine and morphine through hairless mouse skin *in vitro*. Int J Pharm 2001; 229, 131–37.

30. Boucaud A, Machet L, Arbeille B, Machet MC, Sournac M, Mavon A, Patat F, Vaillant L. *In vitro* study of low-frequency ultrasound-enhanced transdermal transport of fentanyl and caffeine across human and hairless rat skin. Int J Pharm 2001; 228, 69–77.

31. Weimann LJ, Wu J. Transdermal delivery of poly l-lysine by sonomacroporation. Ultrasound Med Biol 2002; 28, 1173–80.

32. Smith NB, Lee S, Shung KK. Ultrasound-mediated transdermal *in vivo* transport of insulin with low-profile cymbal arrays, Ultrasound Med Biol 2003; 29, 1205–10.

33. Park EJ, Werner J, Smith NB. Ultrasound mediated transdermal insulin delivery in pigs using a lightweight transducer. Pharm Res. 2007; 24, 1396–401.

34. Mitragotri S, Coleman M, Kost J, Langer, R. Transdermal extraction of analytes using low-frequency ultrasound. Pharm Res 2000; 17, 466–70.

35. Kost J, Mitragotri S, Gabbay R, Pisko M, Langer R. Transdermal monitoring of glucose and other analytes using ultrasound. Nature Med 2000; 6, 347–50.

36. Holt RG, Roy RA. Measurements of bubble-enhanced heating from focused MHz-frequency ultrasound in a tissue-mimicking material. Ultrasound Med Biol 2001; 27, 1399–1412.

37. Miyasaki S, Mizuoka H, Oda M, Takada M. External control of drug release and penetration: enhancement of the transdermal absorption of indomethacin by ultrasound irradiation. J Pharm Pharmacol 1991; 43, 115–16.

38. Brucks R, Nanavaty M, Jung D, Siegel F. The effect of ultrasound on ibuprofen through human epidermis. Pharm Res 1989; 6, 697–701.

39. Machet L, Pinton, J, Patat F, Arbeille B, Pourcelot L, Vaillant L. *In vitro* phonophoresis of digoxin across hairless mice and human skin: thermal effect of ultrasound. Int J Pharm 1996; 133, 39–45.

40. Pelucio-Lopes C, Machet L, Vaillant L, Patat F, Letiecq M, Furet Y, Lorette G. Phonophoresis of azido-thymidine (AZT) ex vivo across human and hairless mice skin. Int J Pharm 1993; 96, 249–52.

41. Machet L, Cochelin N, Patat, F., Arbeille, B., Machet, M.C, Lorette, G., Vaillant L. *In vitro* phonopho-resis of mannitol, oestradiol and hydrocortisone across hairless mouse and human skin. Int J Pharm 1998;165, 169–74.

42. Machet L, Cochelin N, Patat F, Pelucio-Lopes C, Pourcelot L, Lorette G, Vaillant L. Phonophoresis of vasopressin ex vivo across hairless mouse and human skin. Eur J Dermatol 1995; 5, 441.

43. Julian TN, Zentner GM. Mechanism for ultrasonically enhanced transmembrane solute permeation. J Control Release 1990; 12, 77–85.

44. Merino G, Kalia YN, Delagado-Charro, MB, Potts RO, Guy RH. Frequency and thermal effects on the enhancement of transdermal transport by sonophoresis, J Control Release 2003; 88, 85–94.

45. Alvarez-Roman R, Merino G, Kalia YN, Naik A, Guy RH. Skin permeability enhancement by low frequency sonophoresis: lipid extraction and transport pathways. J Pharm Sci 2003; 92, 1138–46.

46. Goss SA, Fritzell L, Dunn, F. Comprehensive compilation of empirical ultrasonic properties of mam-malian tissues. J Acoust Soc Am 1978; 64, 423–57.

47. Goss SA, Johnson RL, Dunn F. Ultrasonic absorption and attenuation of high frequency sound in mam-malian tissue. Ultrasound Med Biol 1979; 5, 181–86.

48. Asano J, Suisha F, Takada M, Kawasaki N, Myasaki S. Effect of pulsed output ultrasound on the trans-dermal absorption of indomethacin from an ointment in rats. Biol Pharm Bull 1997; 20, 288–91.

49. Singer AJ, Homan CS, Church AL, McClain SA. Low-frequency sonophoresis: pathologic and thermal effects in dogs. Acad Emerg Med 1998; 5, 35–40.

50. Ter Haar GR, Daniels S. Evidence for ultrasonically induced cavitation *in vivo*. Phys Med Biol 1981; 26, 1145–49.

51. Esche R. Untersuchungen der Schwingungskavitation in Flüssigkeiten. Acustica 1952; 2, 208–18.

52. Carstensen, EL, Gracewski S, Dalecki D. The search for cavitation *in vivo*. Ultrasound Med Biol 2000; 26, 1377–85.

53. Poliachik SL, Chandler WL, Mourad PD, Ollos RJ, Crum LA. Activation, aggregation and adhesion of platelets exposed to high-intensity focused ultrasound. Ultrasound Med Biol 2001; 27, 1567–76.

54. Fan Z, Chen D, Deng CX. Characterization of the dynamic activities of a population of microbubbles driven by pulsed ultrasound exposure in sonoporation. Ultrasound Med Biol. 2014; 40, 1260–72.

55. Huber PE, Debus J. Tumor toxicity *in vivo* and radical formation *in vitro* depend on the shock wave-induced cavitation dose. Radiat Res 2001; 156, 301–09.

56. Cochran, SA, Prausnitz MR. Sonoluminescence as an indicator of cell membrane disruption by acoustic cavitation. Ultrasound Med Biol 2001; 27, 841–51.

57. Liu J, Lewis TN, Prausnitz MR. Non-invasive assessement and control of ultrasound-mediated mem-brane permeabilization. Pharm Res 1998; 15, 918–24.

58. Ueda H, Mutoh M, Seki T, Kobayashi D, Morimoto Y. Acoustic cavitation as an enhancing mechanism of low-frequency sonophoresis for transdermal drug delivery. Biol Pharm Bull. 2009; 32, 916–20.

59. Greenleaf WJ, Bolander ME, Sarkar G, Goldring MB, Greenleaf JF. Artificial cavitation nuclei signifi-cantly enhance acoustically induced cell transfection. Ultrasound Med Biol 1998; 24, 587–95.

60. Bhatnagar S, Kwan JJ, Shah AR, Coussios CC, Carlisle RC. Exploitation of sub-micron cavitation nuclei to enhance ultrasound-mediated transdermal transport and penetration of vaccines. J Control Release. 2016; 238, 22–30.

61. Wu J, Chappelow J, Yang J, Weimann L. Defects generated in human stratum corneum specimens by ultrasound. Ultrasound Med Biol 1998; 24, 705–10.

62. Lee KL, Zhou Y. Quantitative evaluation of sonophoresis efficiency and its dependence on sonication parameters and particle size. J Ultrasound Med. 2015; 34, 519–26.

63. Tehara T, Mitragotri S, Kost J, Langer R. Dependance of low-frequency sonophoresis on ultrasound parameters; distance of the horn and intensity. Int J Pharm 2002; 235, 35–42.

64. Tang H, Wang CC, Blankschtein D, Langer R. An investigation of the role of cavitation in low-frequency ultrasound-mediated transdermal drug delivery. Pharm Res 2002; 19, 1160–69.

65. Tezel A, Sens A, Mitragotri S. Investigations of the role of cavitation in low-frequency sonophoresis using acoustic spectroscopy. J Pharm Sci 2002; 91, 444–53.

66. Lee SE, Choi KJ, Menon GK, Kim HJ, Choi EH, Ahn SK, Lee SH. Penetration pathways induced by low-frequency sonophoresis with physical and chemical enhancers: iron oxide nanoparticles versus lan-thanum nitrates. J Invest Dermatol. 2010; 130, 1063–72.

67. Yamashita N, Tachibana K, Ogawa K, Tsujita N, Tmita A. Scanning electron microscopic evaluation of the skin surface after ultrasound exposure. Anat Rec 1997; 247, 455–61.

68. Mitragotri S, Farell J, Tang H, Terahara T, Kost J, Langer R. Determination of threshold energy dose for ultrasound-induced transdermal transport. J Control Release 2000; 63, 41–52.

69. Frenkel V, Kimmel E, Iger Y. Ultrasound-cavitation damage to external epithelia of fish skin. Ultrasound Med Biol 1999; 25, 1295–1303.

70. Menon GK, Elias PM. Morphologic basis for a pore-pathway in mammalian stratum corneum. Skin Pharmacol 1997; 10, 235–46.

71. Frenkel V, Kimmel E, Iger Y. Ultrasound-induced intercellular space widening in fish epidermis. Ultrasound Med Biol 2000; 26, 473–80.

72. Malghnani MS, Yang J, Wu J. Generation and growth of bilayer defects induced by ultrasound. J Acoust Soc Am. 1998; 103, 1682–85.

73. Ueda H, Ogihara M, Sugibayashi K, Morimoto Y. Change in the electrochemical properties of skin and the lipid packing in stratum corneum by ultrasonic irradiation. Int J Pharm 1996; 37, 217–24.

74. Meidan VM, Docker MF, Walmsley AD, Irwin WJ. Low intensity ultrasound as a probe to elucidate the relative follicular contribution to total transdermal absorption. Pharm Res 1998; 15, 85–92.

75. Menon GK, Bommannan DB, Elias PM. High-frequency sonophoresis: permeation pathways and structural basis for enhanced permeability. Skin Pharmacol 1994; 7, 130–39.

76. Schoellhammer CM, Srinivasan S, Barman R, Mo SH, Polat BE, Langer R, Blankschtein D. Applicability and safety of dual-frequency ultrasonic treatment for the transdermal delivery of drugs. J Control Release. 2015; 202, 93–100.

77. Mauri G, Nicosia L, Xu Z, Di Pietro S, Monfardini L, Bonomo G, Varano GM, Prada F, Della Vigna P, Orsi F. Focused ultrasound: tumour ablation and its potential to enhance immunological therapy to cancer. Br J Radiol 2018; 91, 20170641.

78. Machet L, Boucaud A. Phonophoresis: efficiency, mechanisms and skin tolerance. Int J Pharm 2002; 243, 1–15.

79. Maruani A, Vierron E, Machet L, Giraudeau B, Halimi JM, Boucaud A. Tolerance of low-frequency ultrasound sonophoresis: a double-blind randomized study on humans. Skin Res Technol. 2012; 18, 151–56

80. Merino G, Kalia YN, Guy RH. Ultrasound-enhanced transdermal transport. J Pharm Sci 2003; 92, 1125–37.

81. Zhang Y, Yu J, Kahkoska AR, Wang J, Buse JB, Gu Z. Advances in transdermal insulin delivery. Adv Drug Deliv Rev. 2019; 139, 51–70.

82. Liao AH, Chung HY, Chen WS, Yeh MK. Efficacy of combined ultrasound-and-microbubbles-mediated diclofenac gel delivery to enhance transdermal permeation in adjuvant-induced rheumatoid arthritis in the rat. Ultrasound Med Biol 2016; 42, 1976–85.

83. Vyas SP, Singh R, Asati RK. Liposomally encapsulated diclofenac for sonophoresis induced systemic delivery. J. Microencapsulation 1995; 12, 149–54.

84. Griffin, JE, Touchstone JC. Ultrasonic movement of cortisol into pig tissue. I -Movement into skeletal muscle. Am J Phys Med 1963; 42, 77–85.

85. Levy L, Kost J, Meshulam Y, Langer R. Effect of ultrasound on transdermal drug delivery to rats and guinea pigs. J Clin Invest 1989; 83, 2074–78.

86. Benson HAE, Mc Elnay JC, Harland R, Hargraft J. Influence of ultrasound on the percutaneous absorption of nicotinates esters. Pharm Res 1991; 8, 204–09.

87. McElnay JC, Benson HAE, Harland R, Hadgraft J. Phonophoresis of methyl nicotinate : a preliminary study to elucidate the mechanism of action. Pharm Res 1993; 10, 1726–31.

88. Benson HAE, Mc Elnay JC, Harland R. Phonophoresis of lignocaine and prilocaine from Emla cream. Int J Pharm 1988; 44, 65–69.

89. Benson HAE, Mc Elnay JC, Harland R. Use of ultrasound to enhance percutaneous absorption of benzydamine. Phys Ther 1989; 69, 113–18.

90. Williams AR. Phonophoresis : an *in vivo* evaluation using three topical anaesthetic preparations. Ultrasonics 1990; 28, 137–41.

91. Griffin JE, Echternach JL, Price RE, Touchstone JC. Patients treated with ultrasonic driven hydrocortisone and with ultrasound alone. Phys Ther 1967; 47, 595–601.

92. Ciccone CD, Leggin BG, Callamaro JJ. Effects of ultrasound and trolamine salicylate phonophoresis on delayed-onset muscle soreness. Phys Ther 1991; 71, 666–78.

93. McElnay JC, Kennedy TA, Harland R. Enhancement of the percutaneous absorption of fluocinolone using ultrasound. Br J Clin Pharmac 1986; 21, 609–10.

94. Durmus D, Alayli G, Goktepe AS, Taskaynatan MA, Bilgici A, Kuru O. Is phonophoresis effective in the treatment of chronic low back pain? A single-blind randomized controlled trial. Rheumatol Int. 2013; 33, 1737–44.

95. Coskun Benlidayi C I, Gokcen N, Basaran S. Comparative short-term effectiveness of ibuprofen gel and cream phonophoresis in patients with knee osteoarthritis. Rheumatol Int. 2018; 38, 1927–32.

96. Zhang I, Shung KK, Edwards DA. Hydrogels with enhanced mass transfer for transdermal drug delivery. J Pharm Sci 1996; 85, 1312–16.

97. Manikkath J, Hegde AR, Kalthur G, Parekh HS, Mutalik S. Influence of peptide dendrimers and sonophoresis on the transdermal delivery of ketoprofen. Int J Pharm. 2017; 521, 110–19.

98. Tachibana K, Tachibana S 1993. Use of ultrasound to enhance the local anesthetic effect of topically applied lidocaine. Anesthesiology 78, 1091–96.

99. Mitragotri S., Kost, J.. Low-frequency sonophoresis: an non invasive method of drug delivery and diagnostics. Biothechnol. Prog. 2000; 16, 488–92.

100. Boucaud A, Machet L, Garrigue MA, Vaillant L, Patat F. A practical use of low frequency ultrasound for rapid and reproducible transdermal delivery of insulin. Ultrasonics Symposium, IEEE 2001; pp. 1327–30.

101. Maruani A, Boucaud A, Perrodeau E, Gendre D, Giraudeau B, Machet L. Low-frequency ultrasound sonophoresis to increase the efficiency of topical steroids: a pilot randomized study of humans. Int J Pharm. 2010; 395, 84–90.

102. Maruani A, Vierron E, Machet L, Giraudeau B, Boucaud A. Efficiency of low-frequency ultrasound sonophoresis in skin penetration of histamine: a randomized study in humans. Int J Pharm. 2010; 385, 37–41.

44 Effect of Tape Stripping on Percutaneous Penetration and Topical Vaccination

Howard I. Maibach
University of California, San Francisco, California

Myeong Jun Choi
Charmzone Research and Development
Center, Wonju, Kongwon-do, Korea

Harald Löffler
Philipp University of Marburg, Marburg, Germany

CONTENTS

44.1 INTRODUCTION

The skin protects the body from unwanted environmental effects. The stratum corneum (SC), only 10 to 30 μm thick, provides a barrier to the percutaneous penetration of drugs and macromolecules (1). Despite major research and development efforts in topical/transdermal systems and the advantages of these routes, low SC permeability remains a major limit for the usefulness of the topical approach (2, 3). To increase permeability, chemical and physical approaches have been examined to decrease barrier properties. Physical approaches for skin penetration enhancement such as stripping (4–12), iontophoresis (13), and electroporation (13, 14) have been evaluated. In addition, penetration enhancers and vesicle systems have been used to enhance permeability (15–17). Tape stripping is commonly used to disrupt the epidermal barrier to enhance the delivery of applied drug and biological macromolecules.

Tape stripping is putatively simple, inexpensive, and minimally invasive. The number of tape strips needed to remove the SC varies with age, gender, anatomical site, skin condition, and possibly ethnicity (18). Tape stripping has been used in the dermatological and pharmaceutical fields to measure SC mass and thickness (4–6), to investigate percutaneous penetration of topically applied

639

drug *in vivo* (7–9), and to disrupt skin barrier function (19). Also, this technique has been used to collect SC lipids and protein samples (4, 20) and to detect proteolytic activity associated with the SC (21), quantitatively estimate enzyme levels and activities in the SC (22) and allows detection of metal in the SC (23, 24). Tape stripping has been used to disrupt the skin barrier before percutaneous peptide and DNA immunization (25–28). In addition, tape stripping is of sufficient utility to have been proposed by the Food and Drug Administration (FDA) as part of a standard method to evaluate bioequivalence of topical dermatological dosage forms (29).

This chapter reviews the stripping method and its application on the penetration enhancement into the SC and topical vaccination and defines restrictions and drawbacks.

44.2   SKIN BARRIER FUNCTION

The SC is a permeability barrier that depends upon the presence of a unique mixture of lipids in the SC's intercellular domains. The SC consists of keratin-filled cells, the corneocytes, entirely surrounded by crystalline lamellar lipid regions. The composition and thickness of the SC lipids strongly differ depending on animal species (30). The major lipid classes in the SC are ceramides (CERs), cholesterol (CHOL), and free fatty acids (FFAs). Both qualitative and quantitative compositions of the barrier lipids are important in maintaining an efficient skin barrier.

These lipids exist as a continuous lipid phase, occupying about 20% of the SC volume, arranged in multiple lamellar structures. All CERs and fatty acids found in the SC are rod and cylindrical in shape; this physical attribute makes them suitable for the formation of highly ordered gel-phase membrane domains. The CHOL is capable of either fluidizing membrane domains or of enhancing rigidity, depending on the physical properties of the other lipids and the proportion of CHOL relative to the other components (31). Intracellular lipids that form the only continuous domain in the SC are required for a competent barrier.

Efforts have been undertaken to characterize the lipid lamellar regions. Based on freeze-fracture electron microscopy, differential scanning calorimetry, and x-ray diffraction studies, the lipids appear arranged as lamellar structures, whose organization is strongly dependent on lipid composition (1). Human lipids are organized in two lamellar phases with a periodicity of approximately 13 and 6 nm, respectively. SC lipids, CERs, CHOL, and FFAs form the orthorhombic lateral packing, a densely packed structure. However, in equimolar mixtures prepared for CHOL and CERs, the major lipid fraction forms a lamellar phase (hexagonal lateral packing) with a periodicity of 12.8 nm. The addition of FFAs to CER/CHOL mixtures induced a transition from a hexagonal to orthorhombic lateral packing (32).

Diseases such as atopic dermatitis, psoriasis, and contact dermatitis are associated with barrier dysfunction. Most skin disorders that have a diminished barrier function present a decrease in total CER content, with some differences in their pattern (33–35). Pilgram et al. (36) reported that in cases of diseased skin, an impaired barrier function is related to an altered lipid composition and organization. In atopic dermatitis SC, they found that in comparison with healthy SC, the presence of the hexagonal lattice (gel phase) is increased with respect to the orthorhombic packing (crystalline phase). From lipid composition studies of atopic skin, intercellular lipids, especially CERs, play an important role in the barrier function and lipid organization. The lipid differences may be partially due to secondary increased cell turnover, rather than a primary cause-and-effect relationship.

44.3   STRIPPING FACTORS

When tape stripping is employed, several factors are important for standardization: (1) number of strips, (2) types and size of tapes, (3) the pressure applied to the strip prior to stripping and the peeling force applied for removal, and (4) anatomic sites. Some parameters are summarized in Table 44.1. We compared the experimental method, i.e., the type and size of tape, pressure and time applied on the skin, and number of strips on the stripping. Stripping data vary according to experimental conditions.

TABLE 44.1
Comparison of Tape Stripping Methods

Type of Tape (brand name)	Number of Strippings	Size	Applied Pressure	Applied Time (sec)	References
D-Square (CuDerm)	40	25 mm	10 kPa	2	(6)
Transpore (3M)	40		10 kPa	2	(6)
Micropore (3M)	40		10 kPa	2	(6)
D-Square (CuDerm)	16	25 mm	80 g/cm³	5	(9)
Leukoflex (Beiersdorf)	18–20	1.5 × 5 cm	Soft pressure		(20)
3M invisible (3M)	7		Controlled condition	10	(59)
Adhesive 6204 (3M)	10	2 × 10 cm		2	(22)
Scotch Book tape 845 (3M)	20		By rubbing six times		(60)
Scotch (3M)	7		1 kg rubber weight was rolled over it 10 times		(61)
Scotch 600 (3M)	2–5	4 cm	By rubbing with finger three movements		(62)
Blenderm (3M)	6	4 cm²			(63)
Transpore (3M)	20	2.5 × 5 cm	Firm pressure		(8)
Transpore (3M)	10	5 × 5 cm			(7)
Teasfilm (Beiersdorf)	20	4 cm²			(19)
D-Square (CuDerm)	16	25 mm	0.365 N/cm²		(64)
D-Square (CuDerm)	25	25 mm	Uniform pressure	5	(65)
Tesa (Beiersdorf)	20	1.5 × 2.0 cm	2 kg pressure	10	(15)
D-Square (CuDerm)	20	3.8 cm²	Uniform pressure	5	(4)

Tape stripping is employed with different adhesive tape, size, number of strips, and the pressure applied to the strip prior to stripping and the peeling force applied for removal.

Dreher et al. (4) improved the method by quantifying the mass of human SC removed by each strip utilizing a colorimetric protein assay. With this method, Bashir et al. (6) determined the physical and physiological effect of SC tape stripping, utilizing tapes with different physicochemical properties: D-Square (CuDerm, Dallas, Texas), Transpore (3M, St. Paul, Minnesota), and Micropore (3M, St. Paul, Minnesota). They demonstrated differences in the mean transepidermal water loss (TEWL) values between the tapes. Mean TEWL increased significantly as the deeper layers of the SC were reached by tape stripping for D-Square and Transpore but not for Micropore. Therefore, D-Square and Transpore tapes induce a significant increase in the TEWL, while Micropore tape did not. The TEWL value differed depending on the tapes and the amount of SC removed.

The number of tape strips to remove SC differs according to experimental conditions (Table 44.1). As the number of tape strips increased, TEWL value also increased. A proposed FDA bioequivalence guideline recommends 10 tape strips after drug application. Weerheim and Ponec (20) reported that the average numbers of tapes *in vivo* could be 18 to 20 strips to remove the SC completely. However, this number is not universal; in some individuals, 40 adhesive tape strips, regardless of the type of tape, do not disrupt the SC barrier to water (6).

44.4 TAPE STRIPPING VERSUS PERCUTANEOUS ABSORPTION AND PENETRATION

Percutaneous absorption and penetration is a complex physical and physiological process. This process initiates a series of absorption, distribution, and excretion that is influenced by numerous factors. Percutaneous absorption of drug depends mainly on the permeability coefficient of the drug, which is affected by drug polarity, molecular size, the vehicle in which the drug is applied, and the skin barrier. Other important factors are application conditions (nonocclusion or occlusion) and skin integrity, which is affected by disease and trauma, body site, and age (3, 12, 32, 37–40).

The intercellular lipid domain is a major pathway for the permeation of most drugs through the SC and acts as a major barrier for penetration. As a consequence of its hydrophobic nature, the SC barrier allows the penetration of lipid-soluble molecules more readily than water-soluble. Generally, small, nonpolar, lipophilic molecules are the most readily absorbed, while high water solubility confers less percutaneous absorptive capacity through normal skin (41).

Tape stripping is mainly used to measure drug concentration and its concentration profile across the SC. The SC is progressively removed by serial adhesive tape strippings and, consequently, percutaneous absorption and penetration is significantly increased in stripped skin (Table 44.2). Benfeldt et al. (7, 8) reported that in a microdialysis experiment, salicylic acid was increased in tape-stripped skin in humans and hairless rats at 157- and 170-fold, respectively. Morgan et al. (41) reported that in a microdialysis experiment, tape stripping increased penciclovir absorption by 1300-fold and acyclovir absorption by 440-fold. Although tape stripping increased the penetration of some drugs (42–46), this is not universal (47, 48). Physiological and pathological factors affect drug transport across the living human skin. Bos and Meinardi (49) suggested the 500-Da rule for the skin penetration of chemical compounds and drugs. This size limit may be changed by skin abnormalities such as atopic dermatitis and disrupted skin.

In addition to organic drugs, tape striping increased the penetration of biological macromolecules such as peptide and DNA into viable skin (25–28). Topically applied oligonucleotides (ONs)

TABLE 44.2
In Vivo Drug Penetration Studies in Barrier-Perturbed Skin

Barrier Perturbation	Species	Drug	Penetration Ratio[a]	Reference
None			1	
Tape stripping	Human	Hydrocortisone	2	(37)
	Human (occlusion)	Hydrocortisone	32.7	(37)
	Human	Low-molecular-weight heparin	1	(48)
	Human	Methylprednisolone aceponate	91.5	(45)
	Human	Salicylic acid	157	(8)
	Human	Penciclovir	1,300	(41)
	Human	Acyclovir	440	(41)
	Hairless guinea pig	Benzoic acid	2.1	(47)
	Hairless guinea pig	Hydrocortisone	3	(47)
	Rat	Nicotinic acid	10.8	(43)
	Rat	Cortisone	2.5	(43)
	Rat	Salicylic acid	0.8–46	(44)
	Hairless rat	Oligonucleotide	24–166	(14)
	Hairless rat	Salicylic acid	170	(7)
	Hairless mouse	Nitroglycerin	9.0	(46)
	Hairless mouse	Enoxacin	7.5	(42)

[a] Penetration ratio varies among drugs and species investigated. Most studies used traditional radiolabeling techniques, where the penetration is measured as total drug absorption over 4 to 10 days. In the case of salicylic acid, the study defined the cutaneous penetration and systemic absorption during 20-minute intervals over a period of four hours after drug administration.

and DNA do not penetrate normal human SC. But removal of SC by tape stripping leads to extensive penetration of ONs and DNA throughout the epidermis. Regnier et al. (14) compared ON penetration through intact and stripped hairless rat skin. Stripping increased ON concentration by one or two orders of magnitude (24- to 166-fold increase) (Table 44.2). In case of plasmid DNA, Yu et al. (50) reported that transfer gene activity depends on the number of strippings. They applied a CMV-CAT expression plasmid to the stripped area and found that the transfer gene expression was higher in the murine skin samples stripped five times prior to DNA application compared with those stripped three times prior to DNA application. This result indicated that abrasion of the skin prior to DNA application could improve cutaneous gene transfer and expression. Taken together, tape stripping is commonly used to enhance the delivery of chemical drugs and biological macromolecules.

44.5   TAPE STRIPPING AND TOPICAL VACCINATION

Why is the skin a major target for topical vaccination? The skin, an active immune surveillance site, is rich in potent antigen-presenting dendritic cells (DCs) such as Langerhans cells (LCs) in the epidermis. The LCs play a key role in the immune response to antigenic materials. Skin accessibility makes it an easy target for vaccination. Thus, skin is an attractive target site for topical vaccination and has become the focus of intense study for the induction of antigen-specific immune responses (51, 52). Wang et al. (53) observed that protein penetrates the SC barrier following occlusion by patch application, but immune responses generated in this way are Th2 predominant. This immune response does not elicit the cytotoxic T-lymphocytes (CTL) response that is important in preventing and therapy against viral infections and tumors.

In addition to disruption of the epidermal barrier, stripping enhances *in vitro* T-cell–mediated immune response (54). Tape stripping is immunostimulatory and results in the production and release of IL-1α, IL-1β, TNF-α, IL-8, IL-10, and INF-γ (26, 54, 55). Skin barrier disruption by tape stripping also increases costimulatory molecule expression (CD86, CD54, CD40, and MHC class II) and the antigen-presenting capacity of epidermal DCs (26, 56). In addition, tape stripping facilitates the generation of Th1 immune responses and stimulates LC migration to cutaneous lymph nodes (56).

Seo et al. (25) reported that topical application of tumor-associated peptide onto the SC barrier disrupted by tape stripping in mice induces a protective antitumor response *in vivo* and *in vitro*. They investigated the induction of CTL response on tape-stripped earlobes of C57/BL6 mice by application of CTL epitope peptide onto the SC. The optimal condition of CTL response was observed 12 and 24 hours after tape stripping at peptide doses of 48 and 96 μg per mouse. On the other hand, CTL induction was virtually absent when peptide was applied to intact skin (Table 44.3). Kahlon et al. (56) reported optimization of topical vaccination for the induction of CTL with peptide and protein antigens. They found that tape stripping significantly enhanced antigen-specific antibody (protein) and CTL responses (peptide and protein) measured at three and two weeks following immunization, respectively (Table 44.3). Stripping resulted in prolonged CTL responses at least two months after a single immunization. These results suggest that stripping can be widely used in inducing immune responses with topical vaccination *in vivo*.

In addition to peptide and protein antigen, tape stripping increased the humoral and cellular immune responses of topical DNA antigens (27, 28). Comparing the immune response with and without stripping, topical application without stripping induced a weak antibody response and did not elicit a sufficient CTL response. In contrast, topical application of this vaccine with stripping induced strong antibody responses and elicited substantial CTL responses. There was a significant difference between the results of topical application with and without stripping (27, 52).

To confirm the protective effect of topical vaccination, Watabe et al. (28) and Seo et al. (25) used an influenza and melanoma mouse model, respectively. Watabe et al. (28) investigated the

TABLE 44.3

Comparison to CTL Activity of Peptide, Protein, and DNA Immunization with and without Stripping

Antigen	Immunization	Specific lysis (%)
Peptide	Intact skin	11.0
	Stripped skin[a]	80.0
	Stripped skin + cholera toxin[b]	70.0
Protein[c]	Intact skin	8.0
	Stripped skin	46.0
DNA[d]	Intact skin	12.7
	Stripped skin	37.0

[a] Cervical lymph node cells (effectors) obtained from mice immunized 10 days earlier with tyrosinase-related protein 2 peptide (VYDFFVWL, 96 μg per mouse) either through intact earlobes or earlobes tape-stripped 12 hours earlier were subjected to CTL assay using L^{kb} target cells pulsed with tyrosinase peptide. The CTL assays were performed at an effector-to-target ratio of 10.

[b] C57BL/6 mice were immunized on the ear with 25 μg ovalbumin peptide (SIYRYYGL) and 25 μg cholera toxin following tape stripping. Mice were boosted in a similar fashion at one week and sacrificed at two weeks. Ovalbumin-expressing EG7 cells were used as the target and CTL assays were performed at an effector-to-target ratio of 50. The ear skin on the dorsal and ventral side was tape-stripped 10 times (using Scotch Brand 3710 adhesive tape).

[c] C57BL/6 mice were immunized on the ear with 250 μg ovalbumin protein and 25 μg cholera toxin following tape stripping. Mice were boosted in a similar fashion at one week and sacrificed at two weeks. Ovalbumin-expressing EG7 cells were used as the target and CTL assays were performed at an effector-to-target ratio of 50. The ear skin on the dorsal and ventral side was tape-stripped 10 times (using Scotch Brand 3710 adhesive tape).

[d] BALB/c mice were immunized with plasmid DNA–coded influenza M protein. Lymphoid cells from each immunized group were restimulated for five days using influenza M peptide–pulsed syngenic spleen cells. The peptide-pulsed p815 cells were used as targets. The CTL assays were performed at an effector-to-target ratio of 80. Fast-acting adhesive glue (Alon Alfa) was smeared on a glass slide to cover the mouse. After an interval of 20 to 30 seconds, the slide was ripped off.

efficacy of a topical DNA vaccine that expressed the matrix gene of the influenza virus using a mouse model. They topically applied plasmid DNA onto the stripped skin on days 0, 7, and 14. After the third immunization, the mice were challenged with 5LD$_{50}$ of influenza virus. Thirteen of 20 mice (65%) survived when they were topically immunized with plasmid DNA that expressed the matrix gene. When the mice were immunized with inactivated virus topically, only 18% of mice were protected and all mice were dead at seven days after virus inoculation in the case of the unimmunized control group. These results suggest that the topical administration of DNA vaccine induces a protective immunity against influenza challenge. Seo et al. (25) investigated the efficacy of topical peptide vaccination for tumor immunotherapy. Mice were immunized twice with tumor-associated peptide at barrier-disrupted skin and were challenged with B16 melanoma tumor cells. The B16 tumor cells were virtually completely rejected after epitope peptide immunization via a disrupted barrier. Also when tumor-bearing mice were treated with epitope peptide on tape-stripped skin, tumor cells regressed with peptide application, and 100% of the mice survived for one month and 95% for over 60 days. However, mice treated with peptide application to intact skin died after 34 days. Thus, topical immunization provides a simple, nonadjuvant system and a noninvasive means of inducing potent antitumor immunity that may be exploited for cancer immunotherapy in humans.

44.6 UNANSWERED QUESTIONS

Surber et al. (57) reviewed the standardized tape stripping technique; many factors remain to be investigated. As shown in Table 44.1, the types and sizes of tapes utilized equally affect the method and the pressure applied to the strip prior to stripping. A proposed FDA guideline describes serial tape stripping to determine the amount of drug within the skin. In this guideline, the first tape strip is discarded, the drug is extracted from the remaining pooled strips, and the quantified amount is expressed as a mass per unit area. From the guidelines, it is impossible to express the amount of drug substance per unit mass of SC and to determine the proportion of the SC that has been sampled by the tape stripping method. Although tape stripping is relatively simple to execute, there are many opportunities for experimental artifacts to develop. Tape stripping samples have high surface-to-volume ratio, and losses by evaporation can be significant even for chemicals with relatively low volatility. In addition, the tape stripping experiment is unsuitable for volatile chemicals (58). Considering the current application of the tape stripping method, topical vaccination and clinical trials for the determination of bioequivalence of topical dermatological products could be improved by stripping standardization.

44.7 CONCLUSION

Tape stripping is commonly used to disrupt the epidermal barrier, to enhance the delivery of drugs, and to obtain information about SC function. In addition, this technique is of sufficient utility to have been proposed by the FDA as part of a standard method to evaluate the bioequivalence of topical dermatological dosage forms. Application of this technique is greatly increasing in various dermatological and pharmaceutical fields. Considering the current application of the tape stripping method, clinical trials for the determination of bioequivalence of topical dermatological products could be improved with tape stripping standardization.

REFERENCES

1. Bouwstra JA, Honeywell-Nguyen PL, Gooris GS, Ponec M. Structure of the skin barrier and its modulation by vesicular formulations. Prog Lipid Res 2003; 42:1–36.
2. Rojanasakul Y. Antisense oligonucleotide therapeutics: drug delivery and targeting. Adv Drug Del Rev 1996; 18:115–131.
3. White PJ, Gray AC, Fogarty RD, Sinclair RD, Thuminger SP, Werther GA, Wraight CJ. C-5 propyne-modified oligonucleotides penetrate the epidermis in psoriatic and not normal human skin after topical application. J Invest Dermatol 2002; 118:1003–1007.
4. Dreher F, Arens A, Hostynek JJ, Mudumba S, Ademola J, Maibach, HI. Colorimetric method for quantifying human stratum corneum removed by adhesive tape stripping. Acta Derm Venereol 1998; 78:186–189.
5. Kalia YN, Albert I, Naik A, Guy RH. Assessment of topical bioavailability in vivo: the importance of stratum corneum thickness. Skin Pharmacol Appl Skin Physiol 2001; 14:82–86.
6. Bashir SJ, Chew AL, Anigbogu A, Dreher F, Maibach HI. Physical and physiological effects of stratum corneum tape stripping. Skin Res Technol 2001; 7:40–48.
7. Benfeldt E, Serup J. Effect of barrier perturbation on cutaneous penetration of salicylic acid in hairless rats: in vivo pharmacokinetics using microdialysis and non-invasive quantification of barrier function. Arch Dermatol Res 1999; 291:517–526.
8. Benfeldt E, Serup J, Menne T. Effect of barrier perturbation on cutaneous salicylic acid penetration in human skin: in vivo pharmacokinetics using microdialysis and non-invasive quantification of barrier function. Br J Dermatol 1999; 140:739–748.
9. Potard G, Laugel C, Schaefer H, Marty JP. The stripping technique: in vitro absorption and penetration of five UV filter on excised fresh human skin. Skin Pharmacol Appl Skin Physiol 2000; 13:336–344.
10. Rougier A, Dupuis D, Lotte C, Maibach HI. Stripping method for measuring percutaneous absorption in vivo. In: Broncugh RL, Maibach HI, eds. Percutaneous Absorption. Drug-Cosmetics-Mechanism-Methodology. New York: Marcel Dekker, 1999:375–394.

11. Schwindt DA, Wilhelm KP, Maibach HI. Water diffusion characteristics of human stratum corneum at different anatomical sites in vivo. J Invest Dermatol 1998; 111:385–389.
12. Rougier A, Dupuis D, Lotte C, Roguet R, Wester RC, Maibach HI. Regional variation in percutaneous absorption in man: measurement by the stripping method. Arch Dermatol Res 1986; 278:465–469.
13. Regnier V, Preat V. Localization of a FITC-labeled phosphorothioate oligonucleotide in the skin after topical delivery by iontophoresis and electroporation. Pharm Res 1998; 15:1596–1602.
14. Regnier V, Tahiri A, Andre N, Lemaitre M, Le Doan T, Preat V. Electroporation-mediated delivery of 3′-protected phosphodiester oligonucleotides to the skin. J Control Release 2000; 67:337–346.
15. Verma DD, Verna S, Blume G, Fahr A. Particle size of liposomes influences dermal delivery of substances into skin. Int J Pharm 2003; 258:141–151.
16. Magnusson BM, Walters KA, Roberts MS. Veterinary drug delivery: potential for skin penetration enhancement. Adv Drug Deliv Rev 2001; 50:205–227.
17. Chattaraj SC, Walker RB. Penetration enhancer classification. In: Smith EW, Maibach HI, eds. Percutaneous Penetration Enhancers. Boca Raton, Florida: CRC Press, 1995:5–20.
18. Palenske J, Morhenn VB. Changes in the skin's capacitance after damage to the stratum corneum in humans. J Cutan Med Surg 1999; 3:127–131.
19. Fluhr JW, Dickel H, Kuss O, Weyher I, Diepgen TL, Berardesca E. Impact of anatomical location on barrier recovery, surface pH and stratum corneum hydration after acute barrier disruption. Br J Dermatol 2002; 146:770–776.
20. Weerheim A, Ponec M. Determination of stratum corneum lipid profile by tape stripping in combination with high-performance thin-layer chromatography. Arch Dermatol Res 2001; 293:191–199.
21. Beisson F, Aoubala M, Marull S, Moustacas-Gardies AM, Voultoury R, Verger R, Arondel V. Use of the tape stripping technique for directly quantifying esterase activities in human stratum corneum. Anal Biochem 2001; 290:179–185.
22. Mazereeuw-Hautier J, Redoules D, Tarroux R, Charveron M, Salles JP, Simon MF, Cerutti I, Assalit MF, Gall Y, Bonafe JL, Chap H. Identification of pancreatic type I secreted phospholipase A2 in human epidermis and its determination by tape stripping. Br J Dermatol 2000; 142:424–431.
23. Cullander C, Jeske S, Imbert D, Grant PG, Bench G. A quantitative minimally invasive assay for the detection of metals in the stratum corneum. J Pharm Biomed Anal 2000; 22:265–279.
24. Hostynek JJ, Dreher F, Nakada T, Schwindt D, Anigbogu A, Maibach HI. Human stratum corneum absorption of nickel salts. Investigation of depth profiles by tape stripping in vivo. Acta Derm Venereol 2001; 212:11–18.
25. Seo N, Tokura Y, Nishijima T, Hashizume H, Furukawa F, Takigawa M. Percutaneous peptide immunization via corneum barrier-disrupted murine for experimental tumor immunoprophylaxis. Proc Natl Acad Sci USA 2000; 97:371–376.
26. Takigawa M, Tokura Y, Hashizume H, Yagi H, Seo N. Percutaneous peptide immunization via corneum barrier-disrupted murine for experimental tumor immunoprophylaxis. Ann NY Acad Sci 2001; 941:139–146.
27. Liu LJ, Watabe S, Yang J, Hamagima K, Ishii N, Hagiwara E, Onari K, Xin KQ, Okuda K. Topical application of HIV DNA vaccine with cytokine-expression plasmids induces strong antigen-specific immune responses. Vaccine 2001; 20:42–48.
28. Watabe S, Xin KQ, Ihata A, Liu LJ, Honsho A, Aoki I, Hamajima K, Wahren B, Okuda K. Protection against influenza virus challenge by topical application of influenza DNA vaccine. Vaccine 2001; 19:4434–4444.
29. Shah VP, Flynn GL, Yacobi A, Maibach HI, Bon C, Fleischer NM, Franz TJ, Kaplan LJ, Kawamoto J, Lesko LJ, Marty JP, Pershing LK, Schaefer H, Sequeira JA, Shrivastara SP, Wilkin J, Williams RL. Bioequivalence of topical dermatological dosage forms—methods of evaluation of bioequivalence. Pharm Res 1999; 15:167–171.
30. Hammond SA, Tsonis C, Sellins K, Rushlow K, Scharton-Kersten T, Colditz I, Glenn GM. Transcutaneous immunization of domestic animals: opportunities and challenges. Adv Drug Deliv Rev 2000; 43:45–55.
31. Wertz PW. Lipids and barrier function of the skin. Acta Derm Venereol 2000; 208:7–11.
32. Bouwsta JA, Honeywell-Nguyen PL. Skin structure and mode of action vesicles. Adv Drug Deliv Rev 2002; 54:s41–s55.
33. Matsumoto M, Umemoto N, Sugiura H, Uehara M. Difference in ceramide composition between "dry" and "normal" skin in patients with atopic dermatitis. Acta Derm Venereol 1999; 79:246–247.
34. Okamoto R, Arikawa J, Ishibashi M, Kawashima M, Takagi Y, Imokawa G. Sphingo-sylphosphorylcholine is upregulated in the stratum corneum of patients with atopic dermatitis. J Lipid Res 2003; 44:93–102.

35. Macheleidt O, Kaiser HW, Sandhoff K. Deficiency of epidermal protein-bound omega-hydroxyceramides in atopic dermatitis. J Invest Dermatol 2002; 119:166–173.
36. Pilgram GS, Vissers DC, van der Meulen H, Pavel S, Lavrijsen SP, Bouwstra JA, Koerten HK. Aberrant lipid organization in stratum corneum of patients with atopic dermatitis and lamellar ichthyosis. J Invest Dermatol 2001; 117:710–717.
37. Feldmann RJ, Maibach HI. Penetration of ^{14}C hydrocortisone through normal skin. Arch Dermatol 1965; 91:661–666.
38. Feldmann RJ, Maibach HI. Regional variations in percutaneous penetration of ^{14}C cortisol in man. J Invest Dermatol 1967; 48:181–183.
39. Wester RC, Maibach HI. Cutaneous pharmacokinetics: 10 steps to percutaneous absorption. Drug Metab Rev 1983; 14:169–205.
40. Rougier A, Lotte C, Maibach HI. In vivo percutaneous penetration of some organic compounds related to anatomic site in man: predictive assessment by the stripped method. J Pharm Sci 1987; 76:451–454.
41. Morgan CJ, Renwick AG, Friedmann PS. The role of stratum corneum and dermal vascular perfusion in penetration and tissue levels of water-soluble drugs investigated by microdialysis. Br J Dermatol 2003; 148:434–443.
42. Fang JY, Hong CT, Chiu WT, Wang YY. Effect of liposomes and niosomes on skin permeation of enoxacin. Int J Pharm 2001; 219:61–72.
43. Bronaugh RL, Stewart RF. Methods for in vitro percutaneous rat absorption studies V: penetration through damaged skin. J Pharm Sci 1985; 74:1062–1066.
44. Murakami T, Yoshioka M, Okamoto I, Yumoto R, Higashi Y, Okahara K, Yata N. Effect of ointment bases on topical and transdermal delivery of salicylic acid in rats: evaluation by skin microdialysis. J Pharm Pharmacol 1998; 50:55–61.
45. Günther C, Kecskes A, Staks T, Täuber U. Percutaneous absorption of methyprednisolone aceponate following topical application of Advantan lotion on intact, inflamed and stripped skin of male volunteers. Skin Pharmacol Appl Skin Physiol 1998; 11:35–42.
46. Higo N, Hinz RS, Lau DTW, Benet LZ, Guy RH. Cutaneous metabolism of nitroglycerin in vitro. II. Effect of skin condition and penetration enhancement. Pharm Res 1992; 9:303–306.
47. Moon KC, Wester RC, Maibach HI. Diseased skin models in the hairless guinea pig: in vivo percutaneous absorption. Dermatologica 1990; 180:8–12.
48. Xiong GL, Quan D, Maibach HI. Effect of penetration enhancers on in vitro percutaneous absorption of low molecular weight heparin through human skin. J Control Release 1996; 42:289–296.
49. Bos JD, Meinardi MMHM. The 500-Dalton rules for the skin penetration of chemical compounds and drugs. Exp Dermatol 2000; 9:165–169.
50. Yu WH, Kashari-Sabet M, Liggit D, Moore D, Heath TD, Debs RJ. Topical gene delivery to murine skin. J Invest Dermatol 1999; 112:390–375.
51. Babiuk S, Baca-Estrada M, Babiuk LA, Ewen C, Foldvari M. Cutaneous vaccination: the skin as an immunologically active tissue and the challenge of antigen delivery. J Control Release 2000; 66:199–214.
52. Choi MJ, Maibach HI. Topical vaccination of DNA antigens: topical delivery of DNA antigens. Skin Pharmacol Appl Skin Physiol 2003; 116:271–282.
53. Wang L, Lin JY, Hsieh KH, Lin PW. Epicutaneous exposure of protein antigen induces a predominant Th-2 like response with high IgE production in mice. J Immunol 1996; 156:670–678.
54. Nishijima T, Tokura Y, Imokawa G, Seo N, Furukawa F, Takigawa M. Altered permeability and disordered cutaneous immunoregulatory function in mice with acute barrier disruption. J Invest Dermatol 1997; 109:175–182.
55. Nickoloff BJ, Naidu Y. Perturbation of epidermal barrier function correlates with initiation of cytokine cascade in human skin. J Am Acad Dermatol 1994; 30:535–546.
56. Kahlon R, Hu Y, Orteu CH, Kifayet A, Trudeau JD, Tan R, Dutz JP. Optimization of epicutaneous immunization for the induction of CTL. Vaccine 2003; 21:2890–2899.
57. Surber C, Schwarb FP, Smith EW. Tape-stripping technique. In: Broncugh RL, Maibach HI, eds. Percutaneous Absorption. Drug-Cosmetics-Mechanism-Methodology. New York: Marcel Dekker, 1999:395–409.
58. Reddy MB, Stinchcomb AL, Guy RH, Bunge AL. Determining dermal absorption parameters in vivo from tape strip data. Pharm Res 2002; 19:292–298.
59. Fernandez C, Nielloud F, Fortune R, Vian L, Marti-Mestres G. Benzophenone-3: rapid prediction and evaluation using non-invasive methods of in vivo human penetration. J Pharm Biomed Anal 2002; 28:57–63.

60. Alberti I, Kalia YN, Naik A, Bonny JD, Guy RH. In vivo assessment of enhanced topical delivery of terbinafine to human stratum corneum. J Control Release 2001; 71: 319–327.

61. Wissing SA, Muller RH. Solid lipid nanoparticles as carrier for sunscreens: in vitro release and in vivo skin penetration. J Control Release 2002; 81:225–233.

62. Betz G, Nowbakht P, Imboden R, Imanidis G. Heparin penetration into and permeation through human skin from aqueous and liposomal formulations in vitro. Int J Pharm 2001; 228:147–159.

63. Couteau C, Perez-Cullel N, Connan AE, Coiffard LJM. Stripping method to quantify absorption of two sunscreens in human. Int J Pharm 2001; 222:153–157.

64. Chatelain E, Gabard B, Surber C. Skin penetration and sun protection factor of five UV filters: effect of the vehicle. Skin Pharmacol Appl Skin Physiol 2003; 16:28–35.

65. Simonsen L, Petersen MB, Benfeldt E, Serup J. Development of an animal model for skin penetration in hairless rats assessed by mass balance. Skin Pharmacol Appl Skin Physiol 2002; 15:414–424.

45 Transcutaneous Delivery of Drugs by Electroporation

Shivakumar H. Nanjappa
KLE College of Pharmacy, Bengaluru, India

S. Narasimha Murthy
The University of Mississippi School of Pharmacy, Mississippi

CONTENTS

45.1 INTRODUCTION

The skin is the protective barrier that prevents the entry of foreign material and pathogens into the human body. The human skin acts as a formidable barrier for the percutaneous absorption of drugs as well (Rai et al., 2010). Generally, the skin is known to be relatively more permeable to lipophilic drugs than hydrophilic drugs. From the drug delivery perspective, the skin is composed of two distinct layers, namely the outer epidermis and inner dermis (Escobar-Chavez et al., 2009). The outer epidermis, in turn, consists of two layers: the outer stratum corneum, which is a nonviable layer of the epidermis, and the inner viable epidermis. The human stratum corneum is typically made of 10 to 15 layers of cells termed corneocytes that act as a rate-controlling barrier for the absorption of therapeutic agents. The corneocytes are the dead, flattened, keratin-filled cells. The corneocytes are surrounded by an intercellular lipid bilayered matrix composed of ceramides, free fatty acids, cholesterol, and cholesterol sulfate. The dermal region of the skin houses different skin appendages such as hair follicles, sweat glands, and apocrine glands.

To overcome the barrier properties of the stratum corneum, attempts have been made to enhance skin permeation using chemical penetration enhancers (Shivakumar and Murthy, 2010). The chemical skin penetration enhancers are known to primarily act by increasing the solubility of the permeant in the stratum corneum or by disrupting the lipid domain of the skin. Considering the limitations of skin penetration enhancers in enhancing the permeation of therapeutic macromolecules, physical enhancement techniques such as sonophoresis, iontophoresis, and electroporation have been explored (Prausnitz, 1999). Sonophoresis enhances the transport of drug molecules through the skin under the influence of ultrasound. Transient cavitation is thought to be the principal mechanism of low-frequency ultrasound that would induce extensive disruption of stratum corneum lipids to enhance drug permeation through the skin. Generally, the enhancement in drug transport was known to increase with the decrease in ultrasound frequency (Meidan and Michniak, 2010). However, the application of ultrasound was known to only reduce the lag time without significantly increasing the drug delivery through the skin (Cullander and Guy, 1992).

Iontophoresis is an electrically mediated technique that promotes the transport of charged ions through the skin under the applied voltage or constant current by electrorepulsion and electro-osmosis (Pliquett and Weaver, 1996). The principal mechanism of iontophoresis is electrorepulsion that involves the enhancement of the permeation of ions through the skin by an electrode bearing the same polarity. Moreover, iontophoresis was found to induce electro-osmosis by promoting bulk transport of solvent along with the ions. Studies in the past indicate that iontophoresis involves electrically mediated transport that happens through aqueous pore pathways withoutalteration in the stratum corneum structure (Dinh et al., 1993). The technique has been explored to enhance the transdermal permeation of several charged permeants, including peptides and oligonucleotides, which otherwise need to be delivered only via the invasive parenteral route (Banga et al., 1999). However, iontophoresis was found to be more efficacious in enhancing the transport of low-molecular-weight ions compared to charged therapeutic macromolecules (Prausnitz, 1999). The technique has been successfully used in clinics for the last couple of decades in dermatology and dentistry for the delivery of several hydrophilic low-molecular-weight therapeutic agents.

45.2 ELECTROPORATION

Electroporation was initially used in molecular biology as a tool for gene transfection in which brief electrical pulses were used to create pores in the cell membranes that would promote the entry of DNA or other macromolecules (Treco and Selden, 1995). The technique was found to be a viable physical strategy to enhance the permeability of human skin that is composed of multilayer intercellular lipids analogous to the cell membrane (Figure 45.1). The technique has been

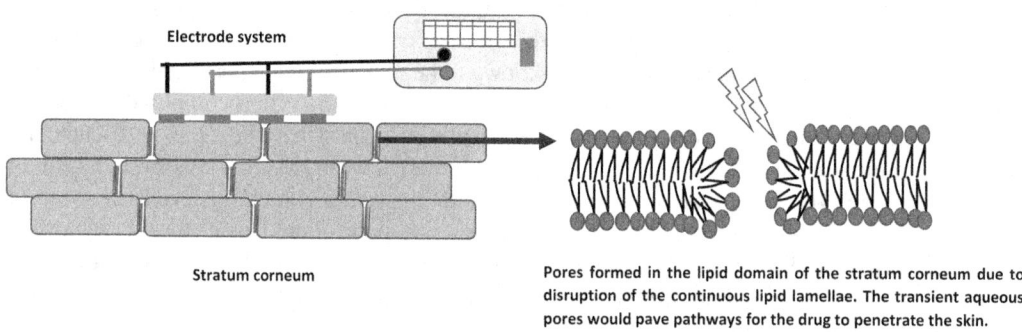

FIGURE 45.1 Illustration of skin electroporation. The skin electrodes are connected to the power source for application of the electrical pulses. The electrical pulses applied on the stratum corneum would lead to formation of pores in the intercellular lipid domains.

extensively explored to enhance the transdermal delivery of therapeutic macromolecules in particular that continues to be a challenging task. Dermal electroporation involves the application of high-voltage short electrical pulses to induce transient pores in the lipid domains of the stratum corneum (Prausnitz et al., 1999).

The process of transdermal electroporation involves the application of high-voltage pulses to induce transient pores in the stratum corneum of the skin leading to an increase in drug transport with a quicker onset and is normally associated with insignificant or minor skin damage (Hu et al., 2010). The technique is said to induce the creation of new aqueous pore pathways in the lipid bilayers of the stratum corneum of the skin (Denet et al., 2004). The pores created on the application of high-voltage electrical pulses are known to be small (measuring less than about 10nm), scanty (involving 0.1% of the application area), and transient (lasting from microseconds minutes). The electrical conductance of the lipid bilayers is said to be rapidly increased by several-fold on the application of electrical pulses. This short-duration, high-voltage electrical pulse is found to be more effective in enhancing transdermal transport of therapeutic agents when compared to long-duration, low-voltage pulses, as in the case of iontophoresis (Banga et al., 1999).

45.3 MECHANISM OF TRANSDERMAL DRUG DELIVERY BY ELECTROPORATION

The structural and biological makeup of the stratum corneum makes it an attractive substrate for electroporation. Electroporation is known to occur when the transdermal voltage applied exceeds a few hundred millivolts (mV), typically for the duration from $10\mu s$ to 100ms. The stratum corneum is composed of about 100 lipid bilayers in series that would require approximately 100 V pulses, for electroporation at about 1 V per bilayer, in order to get perturbed (Prausnitz et al., 1993). Electroporation is known to induce the rearrangement of the stratum corneum lipid bilayers of the skin and provide an electrophoretic driving force to enhance skin permeation on the application of high-voltage pulses (Prausnitz et al., 1999). The transient pores induced by the technique would rapidly and reversibly increase skin permeability. The electrical breakdown or recovery of the human epidermal membrane during electroporation is known to depend on the magnitude and duration of the applied voltage (Inada et al., 1994: Weaver 1993).

Different mechanisms are known to govern molecular transport through the skin by electroporation (Denet et al., 2004).

45.3.1 ENHANCED DIFFUSION

In vitro studies have revealed that higher skin permeabilization is evident during the application of electrical pulses. In addition, skin stays permeabilized over a prolonged duration; significantly increasing the passive transport of substrates. The increased transport due to post-pulse diffusion was quite evident even with neutral molecules or when the drug is added after pulsing or by reversing the electrode polarity. For small-molecular-weight compounds with molar mass less than 1000 Da, significant enhancement in the transport has been reported (Prausnitz, 1999).

45.3.1.1 Electrophoresis

Electrophoresis is the major driving force involved in the transport of charged ions during the application of high-voltage pulses (Pliquett 1999;Prausnitz et al., 1993;Weaver et al., 1999). The extent of electrokinetic transport of therapeutic agents depends on the total duty cycle of the electrical pulses, duration of the pulses, and ionic mobility of the drug ions.

45.3.1.2 Electro-osmosis

Electro-osmosis is responsible for the delivery of neutral molecules and even oppositely charged molecules across the skin during the application of electrical pulses. The direction of electro-osmosis depends on the surface charge of the skin. Generally, at pH higher than isoelectric point of the skin (pI), the skin is known to carry a net negative charge and the direction of electro-osmosis is from anode to cathode (Vanbever et al., 1998a). The relative contribution of electro-osmosis compared to electrokinesis is many-fold lesser. However, in the case of neutral molecules and molecules with a low charge to mass ratio, electro-osmosis would be the predominant mode of drug transport during pulse application.

45.4 FACTORS AFFECTING DRUG DELIVERY BY ELECTROPORATION

Several factors such as electrical parameters, physicochemical properties of the drug, and formulation factors are known to affect drug delivery during electroporation (Denet et al., 2004; Singhal and Kalia, 2017).

45.4.1 ELECTRICAL PROTOCOL

The electrical parameters include pulse waveform, voltage, pulse duration, pulse rate, and electrode polarity and design.

45.4.1.1 Pulse Waveform

Generally, explored waveforms include exponentially decaying pulses and square wave pulses. In exponential decay pulse, the set voltage decays over some time with a long voltage–time profile. The advantage of decaying pulses would be the ability to maintain long-lasting skin permeabilization, thereby promoting electrophoretic mobility. There are varied reports regarding the superiority of the type of waveform in terms of drug delivery efficiency (Denet et al., 2004; Vanbever et al., 1996a). *In vivo* studies have indicated that a square waveform is known to be more tolerant, as it did not induce any inflammation or necrosis (Dujardin et al., 2002).

45.4.1.2 Pulse Voltage, Pulse Duration, Pulse Number, and Pulse Rate

The drug transport across the skin can be controlled by monitoring the pulse voltage, pulse duration, pulse number, and pulse rate. A typical voltage applied during electroporation would usually range between 50 and150 V, although higher voltages have been employed during *in vitro* studies (Banga and Prausnitz, 1998). Generally, the drug transport across the skin is known to increase with increasing the pulse voltage, but less sharply at high pulse voltages.

For instance, the amount of terazosin hydrochloride delivered across rat skin was found to increase linearly with an increase in the voltage applied during electroporation (Sharma et al., 2000). Likewise, the flux usually increases linearly with an increase in pulse duration and pulse numbers. Similarly, an increase in the pulse length was found to increase the driving force required to transport the molecule across the skin (Weaver and Chizmadzhev,1996). Moreover, the pulse rate increases the transdermal delivery too. In addition, the onset time is reduced with an increase in pulse duration and rate. Studies in the past have indicated that a short duration (sub-µsec pulses) usually produced a high density of smaller pores, while longer pulses resulted in less dense, larger pores in the stratum corneum. The application of shorter pulses using large-area electrodes was found to be a safer option than larger pulses using small area electrodes. The amount of terazosin hydrochloride transported across the skin was found to increase linearly with pulse length and the number of pulses (Sharma et al., 2000).

The transdermal flux of calcein, a model fluorescent marker, was found to be a function of pulse length, pulse rate, electrode polarity, waveform, and total pulsing time (Prausnitz et al., 1993). It was observed that the transport number of the marker that ranged between 10^{-5} and 10^{-2} was found to depend on the voltage applied, while independent of pulse length, pulse rate, or waveform. Electroporation studies in the past have revealed that few low-voltages, long-duration pulses (50V, 200ms) were found to be more efficient to deliver the drug across the skin than many high-voltage, short-duration pulses (Vanbever et al., 1996a). However, long-duration pulses tend to cause significant local heating within the skin that could result in potential skin irritation.

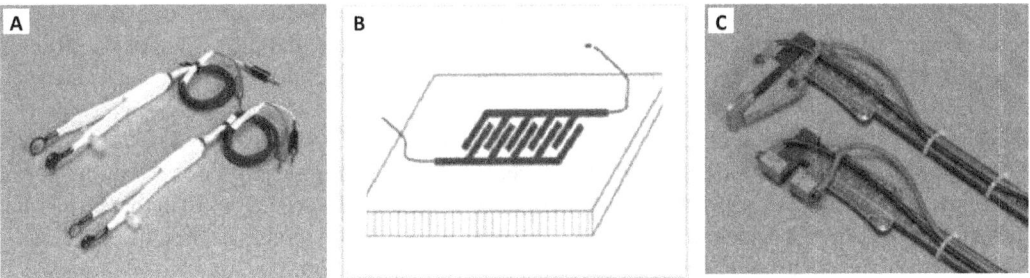

FIGURE 45.2 Different types of electrodes used in skin electroporation. (A) Tweezertrode. (B) Meander electrodes. (C) Caliper electrodes.

45.4.1.3 Electrode Polarity and Design

The polarity of the electrode usually affects the electrophoretic transport during electroporation. The efficiency of drug transport is determined by the design of electrodes as it affects the distribution and intensity of the electrical field around the application area (Denet et al., 2004). Few of the electrodes that are used in skin electroporation are shown in Figure 45.2. The meander electrodes that consist of an array of interweaving electrode fingers are commonly used for *in vivo* applications (Zhang and Rabussay 2002). These electrodes enable the electric field to get localized in the superficial skin layers, thereby preventing the undesirable effects in the underlying tissues. Inert electrodes such as those made of platinum are preferred to active electrodes such as silver/silver chloride, as thelatter normally induce pH shifts in the reservoir. The other electrodes used for skin electroporation are caliper, plate, tweezer, or clip electrodes (Heller et al., 2007). A novel plate electrode was employed to enable transgene expression by optimizing the electroporation parameters. The novel electrode contains four plates that grip a skin fold and are so aligned to allow pulses in two electric field orientations at a 90-degree angle to be applied without removing the electrode from the skin. The electrode demonstrated the potential for an easier and reproducible electrically mediated cutaneous plasmid delivery. Pulse application (eight pulses of 1000V/cm of 100 μs) with these electrodes were found to be well tolerated in patients for electrochemotherapy. The immediate effect observed was marks of the electrodes on the skin that disappeared within a few minutes, an unpleasant sensation due to muscle contraction, and transient erythema (Sersa et al., 2003).

A microelectrode comprising a microfabricated copper electrode array was designed to minimize the pain sensation during electroporation (Wong et al., 2006). Generally, the pain level during electroporation is said to depend on the dimension of the electrode, the contact area with the skin, and the distance between the electrodes. The smaller the electrode–skin contact area, the lesser was the pain sensation in the human study. For effective drug delivery, the electric threshold for a microelectrode array (skin contact area of 44 mm^2) was found to be comparable to that for a larger electrode. The microelectrode was able to deliver a significant number of chemotherapeutic agents through the skin by electroporation in clinical settings without causing any discomfort. An "in-skin electroporation" with microneedle electrode array was used for electroporation in hairless rats (Yan et al., 2010). The in-skin electroporation was found to display a much higher skin penetration and was minimally invasive. Preliminary preclinical studies have indicated that the microneedle array could be clinically feasible for the application of electrical pulses after applying a topical product following microneedle pretreatment.

45.4.2 PHYSICOCHEMICAL PROPERTIES OF THE DRUG AND FORMULATION ATTRIBUTES

Generally, the physicochemical properties of the drug such as surface charge, lipophilicity, and molecular weight affect drug transport during electroporation.

Electrophoresis appears to be the main underlying mechanism involved in the transport of ions across highly permeabilized skin by electroporation. In this context, the pKa value of the drug is said to determine the fraction of drug ionized at the prevalent pH and therefore the efficiency of drug transport during electroporation. Even though the transport of the neutral molecules across the skin by passive diffusion occurs during electroporation, the effect is relatively less compared to electrophoresis and passive diffusion. For instance, the transdermal transport of charged ions (protoporphyrin IX) using electrodes bearing similar charge was found to be higher than the uncharged moiety (protoporphyrin IX methyl ester) or ions bearing the opposite charge (Sen et al., 2002a). Skin, known to bear a net negative charge under physiological conditions, is found to be permselective to cations (Vanbever et al., 1998a).

The effect of the partition coefficient of the permeant in passive diffusion has been established (Barry, 2002). Theoretically, as the created new aqueous pathways or electropores are hydrophilic, the transport across the electropores is relatively more efficient for hydrophilic molecules than the lipophilic molecules.

The molecular weight of the permeant is known to influence the transdermal transport by electroporation. Generally, both electrokinetic and passive diffusion mediated transport during electroporation are inversely proportional to the molecular weight (Lombry et al., 2000). Particularly, the electrokinesis depends on the charge-to-mass ratio. The electrophoresis efficiency of a molecule decreases with a decrease in the charge-to-mass ratio. However, electroporation appears to be the only promising physical enhancement technique that has the potential to improve the permeation of therapeutic agents with a molecular mass as high as 40kDa.

The composition of the drug reservoir is generally known to affect drug delivery during electroporation. The drug transport was reported to increase nonlinearly with an increase in the drug concentration during electroporation (Denet et al., 2004). The pH shift induced by the electrodes may require the use of a buffer in the formulation of the drug reservoir. The other ions present in the drug reservoir such as the buffer ions, counterions, and the ions from the skin are known to compete with the permeant during electroporation. Hence, the key factors that need due consideration in the formulation of the drug reservoir would include selection of the appropriate pH and composition of the buffer.

45.5   ADVANTAGES AND LIMITATIONS OF ELECTROPORATION

Transdermal electroporation enables enhanced drug permeation across the skin compared to passive drug transport. The technique has a proven ability to deliver therapeutic macromolecules across the skin (Becker and Kuznetsov, 2008). Due to the dramatic increase in the skin permeability, electroporation-mediated transdermal transport is characterized by a reduced lag time. As the electrical parameters can be precisely controlled, the technique allows tailored preprogrammed drug delivery. Moreover, the technique permits rapid cessation of the drug delivery by the termination of the therapy. Besides, the technique is found to be effective on all cell types and species (Nickoloff, 1995). Above all, the technique is minimally invasive and not sensitizing and therefore considered more patient compliant (Preat and Vanbever, 2003). However, in case the electrical parameters are not optimized, the pores induced may be too large or may fail to close, causing cell damage or rupture (Weaver, 1995). The other drawback of the technique is that the material that moves in and out of the cell during electroporation is nonspecific.

45.6   APPLICATIONS OF ELECTROPORATION

The dramatic and reversible increase in the skin permeability on electroporation has been exploited to enhance the topical and transdermal drug delivery. The technique that is known to temporarily permeabilize the stratum corneum barrier to drug transport is therefore likely to broaden the drugs that otherwise may be unsuitable for topical or transdermal delivery (Escobar-Chavez et al., 2009). Electroporation has been reported to increase transdermal drug transport and shorten the lag time in the case of several permeants. A variety of therapeutic macromolecules, vaccines, genes, and proteins have been used as substrates for dermal and transdermal delivery.

Skin electroporation is known to increase the transdermal transport of a number of compounds that range from the low-molecular-weight (<1000 Da) therapeutic agents such as doxepin (Sameta et al., 2010), fentanyl (Vanbever et al., 1996a), piroxicam (Murthy et al., 2004), timolol (Denet and Preat, 2003), and terazosin (Sharma et al., 2000) to moderately sized drugs (<10 kDa) that include cyclosporine A (Wang and Krishnan, 1998) and human parathyroid hormone (Medi and Singh, 2003). Electroporation has been reported to enhance the transport of several drug molecules as indicated in Table 45.1.

Most importantly, electroporation is found to be a valuable technique to deliver therapeutic macromolecules like luteinizing hormone–releasing hormone (Riviere et al., 1995) and heparin (Prausnitz et al., 1995). The technique is also capable of enhancing the transdermal delivery of several compounds that range in solubilities from low (buprenorphine [Bose et al., 2001] to high (terazosin) [Sharma et al., 2000]). Electroporation has been employed to deliver drugs bearing a charge like fentanyl (anionic)[Vanbever et al., 1996a] or neutral molecules (mannitol [Vanbever et al., 1998a]). Flux enhancement for neutral and charged permeants that usually ranged in molar mass from 18 to 12,000 Da was found vary from 1 to 4 (Prausnitz, 1999).

TABLE 45.1
Application of Electroporation to Enhance the Transdermal Delivery of Drugs

Sl. No.	Therapeutic Molecule	Electrical Protocol	Skin Model	Log Enhancement Ratio	Reference
1	Alniditan	5 pulses of 200V for 500 ms.	Full-thickness abdominal skin of hairless rats	2	Jadoul et al., 1998
2	Atenolol	10 pulses of 400V for 10 ms.	Isolated human stratum corneum	2	Denet et al., 2003
3	Buprenorphine	20 pulses of 500 V for 10 ms	Full-thickness human skin	0	Bose et al., 2001
4	Domperidone	5 pulses of 250V for 700ms	Full-thickness abdominal skin of hairless rats	2	Jadoul et al., 1997
5	Fentanyl	Exponential decaying pulses 5 pulses of 150V for 300ms	Full-thickness abdominal skin of hairless rats	2	Vanbever et al., 1996a,b
6	Methotrexate	180 pulses of 150 V, 0.2 ms at 1 Hz	*In vivo* studies in mice	1	Wong et al., 2006
7	Metoprolol	5 pulses of 620 ms increased from 250 V	Abdominal hairless rat skin	3	Vanbever and Preat, 1995
8	Nalbuphine	20 pulses 300 V of 200 ms	Nude mouse skin	1	Huang et al., 2005
9	Sodium nonivamide	20 pulses 300 V of 200 ms	Nude mouse skin	1	Fang et al., 2002
10	Tetracaine HCl	400 pulses 130 V for 0.4 ms	Full-thickness rat abdominal skin	1	Hu et al., 2000
11	Terazosin hydrochloride	5 pulses of 88 V for 40 ms.	Full-thickness hairless rat skin	1	Sharma et al., 2000
12	Timolol	10 pulses of 400V for 10 ms.	Isolated human stratum corneum	1	Denet et al., 2003
13	5 Fluorouracil	20 pulses of 300V for 200ms	Nude mouse skin	2	Fang et al., 2004

45.6.1 DELIVERY OF SMALL MOLECULES

Electroporation was found to increase the *in vitro* transdermal permeation of fentanyl compared to passive transport (Vanbever et al., 1996a). A few exponential decaying pulses were found to be more effective in increasing the drug permeation compared to high-voltage, short-duration pulses. The study indicated that the transport of fentanyl through the skin could be controlled by appropriate voltage, pulse duration, and number of the exponentially decaying pulses. Rapid transport during pulsation was thought to be due to electrophoresis and diffusion through the highly permeabilized hairless rat skin (Vanbever et al., 1996b). The skin content of fentanyl indicated that electroporation was found to rapidly load the viable part of skin with the drug. Further, fentanyl was transdermally administered to hairless rats by application of high-voltage pulses following which the pharmacokinetics and pharmacodynamics were assessed (Vanbever et al., 1998b). Fentanyl plasma concentration reached one-third the maximum plasma concentration (~30ng/mL) in 30 minutes after electropulsation. Deep analgesia and supraspinal effects induced indicated that the antinociceptive activity was found to last for an hour. However, the magnitude of the effects was found to depend on the electrical parameters employed during electroporation.

Nalbuphine is a narcotic analgesic that needs to be administered multiple times in a day as an injection, as it exhibits a short half-life and low bioavailability. The electroporation-mediated transdermal permeation of hydrophilic drug and its four lipophilic pro-drugs were investigated (Sung et al., 2003). The effect of varying the electrical parameters like pulse voltage, duration of pulse, and pulse number were systematically investigated across barriers like hairless mouse skin, stratum corneum stripped skin, delipidized skin,and furry Wistar rat skin to elucidate the mechanisms underlying the electroporation-mediated transdermal delivery. The amount of drug permeated was found to increase at higher pulse voltage, duration, and pulse numbers irrespective of the polarity of the permeant, indicating the multiple mechanisms contributing to enhancement of transdermal transport. Electroporation of hairless mouse skin resulted in a flux of 164.13 ± 25.31 nmol.cm^{-2} that was much higher compared to the passive flux that amounted to 51.16 ± 5.50 nmol.cm^{-2}.

The effect of different electrical parameters influencing transdermal delivery of terazosin hydrochloride across hairless rat skin was reported (Sharma et al., 2000). It was observed that the pulse voltage, pulse length, and pulse number were the three important parameters that contributed to the enhancement in the drug transport in the same sequence. Five or more exponentially decaying pulses at 88 ± 2.5V with a decay time constant of 20ms was needed to obtain significant enhancement in drug delivery. Substantial enhancement in drug delivery was possible at lower applied voltages using electrodes with a larger surface area.

Timolol is a hydrophilic beta-blocker used in the management of hypertension, arrhythmias, and angina pectoris. The feasibility of electroporation to enhance the transdermal permeation of timolol was assessed *in vitro* across human stratum corneum (Denet and Preat, 2003). The technique was found to increase the transdermal permeation of timolol by three orders of magnitude with lag times of a few minutes. About 10electrical pulses of 400 V lasting 10 ms resulted in a flux of 24µg. cm^{-2}h^{-1} that was about fivefold compared to passive diffusion (5µg/cm^{2}h^{-1}). Timolol transport was found to be influenced by electrical parameters such as voltage, pulse duration, donor composition, and position of electrode. The enhanced transport of timolol was attributed to the long-lasting permeabilization of the skin that was evident in the decrease in the impedance due to the structural changes in the stratum corneum. Further, a steady-state flux of 40 ± 14 µg.cm^{-2}h^{-1} was obtained following electroporation across human stratum corneum that was much higher than the passive diffusion, which was found to be 3 ± 2µg.cm^{-2}h^{-1} (Denet et al., 2003). The cumulative amount of timolol transported [1]by electroporation at 21 hours was found to be 483 ± 46 µg.cm^{-2}h^{-1}.

Electroporation was found to increase the permeation of metoprolol across full-thickness rat skin compared to diffusion through untreated skin (Vanbever et al., 1994). The cumulative amount of drug transported in four hours was found to increase linearly with the applied pulse voltage. The cumulative amount of drug permeated was also found to increase linearly with the pulse time.

However, voltage was found to be more effective in controlling the amount of drug delivered by electroporation compared to the pulse time. Further, in another study it was observed that application of electrical pulses was found to enhance the permeation of metoprolol across hairless rat skin by nearly 1000-fold compared to untreated skin (Vanbever and Preat, 1995). The quantity of drug permeated increased linearly to the voltage when five pulses of 620ms were applied in the increasing order from 74 to 250V. Likewise, the amounts of metoprolol increased linearly as the pulse duration of five single pulses of 100 V was increased from 80 to 700 ms. It was concluded that application of low-voltage, long-duration pulses proved to be more efficient to increase the transdermal delivery of metoprolol than high-voltage, short-duration pulses.

Electroporation has been utilized to increase the percutaneous penetration of doxepin and its hydroxypropyl-β-cyclodextrin (HPCD) complex across porcine epidermis (Sammeta et al., 2010). The amount of drug retained in the epidermis did not differ significantly for doxepin or its complex following electroporation. However, when drug-loaded epidermis was subjected to release studies, the release reached a plateau within 2.5 days for doxepin, while in case of the complex, the release was prolonged for 5 days. Slow dissociation of the drug from the complex was responsible for the prolonged release of doxepin from the epidermis. Pharmacodynamic studies in hairless rats indicated the long-lasting analgesic activity of the drug when complexed with cyclodextrin.

The effect of electroporation on the transdermal permeation of tetracaine hydrochloride was investigated in side-by-side diffusion cells (Hu et al., 2000). Square wave pulses with a voltage of 130V, a pulse time of 0.4s, and pulse frequency of 40 pulses per minute were found to increase the transdermal transport of tetracaine hydrochloride. The transdermal flux of tetracaine at 0.25 hour, following the application of 400 pulses, was found to be 54.60 ± 6.0 $\mu g.cm^{-2}.h^{-1}$ that was much higher compared to passive diffusion, which was 8.2 ± 0.5 $\mu g.cm^{-2}.h^{-1}$. The study indicated that flux of tetracaine was found to increase upon increase in the pulse number.

A new *in vivo* real-time monitoring system based on fluorescent doxorubicin and fentanyl was proposed to assess the transdermal and topical delivery following electroporation (Blagus et al., 2013). Amplitudes of pulses ranging from 70 to 570 V were delivered across mouse skin using noninvasive multiarray electrodes. Patches soaked with the fluorescent compounds were applied to the skin before and after electroporation. Transdermal delivery of the compounds was found to increase with the amplitude up to amplitude of 360V, while it reduced at higher amplitudes. Topical delivery was found to increase with the amplitude that further increased on tape stripping. Analgesic activity of fentanyl that was determined by measuring the cornea reflex, pinna reflex, muscle reflex, tail, and withdrawal latency found to be less pronounced at the electric pulses with the amplitude of 570 V than at 360 V.

The effect of electrical parameters during electroporation on delivery of alniditan, a hydrophilic antimigraine drug, was explored (Jadoul et al., 1998). The transdermal flux of the drug was found to be increased by nearly two fold on application of electroporation. The drug permeation was found to depend on electrical voltage, pulse duration, and number of pulses. Application of high-voltage pulses was found to increase the transdermal delivery of the drug. The drug transport during and after pulsing were found to be crucial during electroporation. Creation of a drug reservoir during pulsing later increased skin permeability in high drug flux during the *in vitro* experiments. Electroporation was found to be more efficient than iontophoresis to increase the drug transport across the full-thickness abdominal skin.

45.6.2   DELIVERY OF MACROMOLECULES

Electroporation has been used to enhance the transport of macromolecules as well (Lombry et al., 2000). The higher the molecular weight of the permeant, the the transport. It was proved that for transdermal and topical delivery by skin electroporation, the higher molecular weight cutoff for the permeants has be less than 40 kDa. In addition, electroporation has been a promising technique to enhance the transdermal delivery of drugs encapsulated in vesicles or particles, which may or may not bear a charge (Banga and Prausnitz, 1998).

Cyclosporin A is a neutral lipophilic undecapeptide that is used in the treatment of psoriasis. The drug is found to be toxic if administered systemically to treat this condition. At the same time, yclosporin A is unsuitable for topical delivery considering its high molecular weight (1203 Da) and lipophilicity (logP = 2.92). Electroporation, when applied as a single pulse, was found to increase the transdermal delivery of cyclosporinA by three to four times compared to passive when rat skin was used as a barrier (Wang et al., 1998).When multiple pulses (25 pulses of 10ms each) of 200V were applied, a sixtyfold increase in the permeation was observed when compared to passive. *In vitro* experiments indicated that the drug delivered to the skin was found to be bound to the skin, while a fraction of the drug was found to leave the skin into the receptor compartment. The high skin retention of cyclosporin A was found to be beneficial in the treatment of psoriasis.

"Electroincorporation" is a technique where the drug encapsulated in vesicles or particles would be delivered into the skin by application of electrical pulses that usually cause breakdown of the stratum corneum barrier (Hofmann et al., 1995). The technique involves placing the particles directly on the skin followed by application of electrical pulses directly on top of the particles. The electric field is applied using the electrode that is known to hamper the barrier properties of the stratum corneum. Following the breakdown of the stratum corneum, the electrophoresis or the applied pressure is believed to drive the particles into the skin. Electroincorporation was accomplished using a "meander electrode" manufactured by Genetronics (San Diego, California, USA). The specialized electrode consists of interweaving electrode fingers that are coated on a plastic film backing that allows easy placement of the particles on the skin under the electrode. Electrodes shaped like calipers are available that can be easily integrated into a device or used to pulse the back of the animals. Particles of 0.2, 4.0, and 45 μm were said to be embedded in hairless mouse skin when electroporated with three exponential decay pulses with amplitude of 120V and pulse length of 1.2ms. Pressure-mediated electroporation has been used to deliver Lupron Depot (euprolide acetate) microspheres into hairless rats and human skin that was xenografted on immunodeficient nude mice (Banga et al., 1999).

The effect of electroporation on the penetration of estradiol from aqueous solution and ultra-deformable liposomes into human epidermis was investigated (Essa et al., 2004). The electroporation protocol involved application of five pulses of 100V each for 100ms with a spacing of 1 minute. Electroporation failed to alter the size of unilamellar ultra-deformable liposomes constituted of phosphatidyl choline and sodium cholate. Electroporation of the neutral lipophilic estradiol increased the transdermal permeation, as well as skin deposition, compared to the passive. The enhancement was ascribed to the structural changes induced in the skin by high-voltage pulses that led to the formation of microchannels. The *in vitro* permeation studies indicated that ultra-deformable liposomes failed to increase estradiol penetration compared with passive. The failure to increase the skin penetration was attributed to the relatively large liposomal size, and the ability of phosphatidyl choline that was added during or after pulsing expedited the skin barrier repair.

Attempts were made to enhance the transport of fluorescein-labeled insulin across porcine epidermis (Sen et al., 2002b). The study was based on the premise that anionic lipids could enhance the transport of macromolecules up to 10 kDa in size. It was the charge and not the type of phosphatidyl head group that was found to determine the electroporation-mediated transdermal transport. It was also proved that the phospholipids with saturated acyl chains enhance the transport of macromolecules better than those with unsaturated chains. The transport studies were performed in a vertical diffusion cell apparatus in which the porcine epidermis was sandwiched between the donor and receptor compartment. Negative pulses (100 V, 1 ms pulses at pulse width of 1 Hz) were applied across the epidermis using platinum electrodes. When electroporation was applied in presence of 1,2-dimyristol-3-phosphatidyl serine, a twentyfold enhancement in the transport of insulin was observed. It was also observed that in the absence of phospholipids, about half of the insulin transported was seen in the receiver, while half of the insulin remained in the epidermis. On the other hand, when phospholipid was present in the donor, all the transported insulin was detected in the receptor. Fluorescence microscopy revealed that the insulin transport was found to occur mainly through the lipid domains that surround the corneocytes. The studies indicted the possibility of delivering therapeutic amounts of insulin by transdermal electroporation.

Attempts were made to deliver fluorescein-labeled antisense oligodeoxynucleotides across human skin by electroporation (Zewert et al., 1995). High-voltage pulses were delivered (pulse time was varied from 1.0 to 2.2 ms) on heat-stripped stratum corneum sandwiched in a side-by-side permeation chamber. The concentration of oligodeoxynucleotides in the donor was 25 mM, while the fluorescence of the receptor solution was measured in a spectrofluorometer. The transport of oligodeoxynucleotides was found to increase when the applied voltage was increased from 69V to 80V but later plateaued. Florescence microscopy revealed that fluorescein-labeled oligodeoxy-nucleotide was deposited in certain localized areas in the skin. Attempts were made to elucidate the mechanism of transport of phosphonothioate oligonucleotide to enable topical delivery. It was observed that it took a few minutes to achieve therapeutic concentrations in viable tissues of the skin. The main mechanism of transport in the viable tissue of the skin during pulsing was identified to be electrophoresis, while the contribution of electroosmosis to the transport was found to be negligible (Regnier et al., 1999). Electrophoresis was thought to create a reservoir of oligonucleotide in the viable tissues of the skin within few minutes that in fact persisted within a therapeutic range for hours. Optimization of electroporation delivery indicated that phosphonothioate oligonucleotide could be delivered from a cathodal compartment with a low ionic strength in the donor. Attempts were also made to deliver 15-mer phosphodiester oligonucleotide into hairless rat skin by electroporation. It was noted during the studies that tertiary-protected phosphodiesters were more suited for topical delivery by skin electroporation due to improved stability against skin nucleases.

Heparin is a macromolecule (5 to 30 kDa) that has been frequently used in clinics as an anticoagulant and as a prophylactic in thromboembolism. The macromolecule finds application in unstable angina, prevention of arteriopathies after angioplasty, and bypass surgeries. High-voltage pulses were applied to increase the transdermal transport of heparin (Prausnitz et al., 1995). Electric pulses ranging from 150V, 250 V, to 350V at a rate of 12 pulses per minute resulted in a flux ranging from 100 to 500 μg/cm²h. The studies indicated that heparin was transported 10times more efficiently by electroporation than by iontophoresis. The *in vitro* studies involving human skin demonstrated that electroporation had the ability to enhance the transdermal transport of heparin to meet the therapeutic rates (1 to 10 U/h.cm²). It was also observed during the studies the post-pulse electrical resistance in the presence of heparin (300 Ω) was much lower than its absence (400 Ω), indicating that heparin, being a charged macromolecule, could also act as macromolecular enhancer. Heparin was found to retain its biological activity as it gets transported across the skin. However, since the small heparin molecules were preferentially transported, the anticoagulant activity per unit transported was found to be reduced. It is likely that heparin, to its charge, could get trapped in the aqueous pathway, thereby stabilizing the transient disruption of the stratum corneum induced by electrical pulses.

When compared to all other chemical and physical enhancement techniques, the mechanism underlying electroporation is different, as it involves a temporary alteration of the barrier properties of the skin that is most often reversible. Electroporation has been used in combination with other enhancement strategies such as chemical enhancers, iontophoresis, and microneedles. The aim of the combination strategies is to expand the scope of transdermal delivery to deliver several macromolecules such as therapeutic peptides and proteins across the skin.

Electroporation was found to enhance the *in vitro* transdermal flux of luteinizing hormone–releasing hormone (LHRH) across human skin significantly compared to iontophoresis alone (Bommannan et al., 1994). The iontophoretic flux (0.27 ± 0.08 μg/h.cm²) of LHRH across the epidermis separated from human cadaver skin was increased by nearly sixfold (1.62 ± 0.05 μg/h.cm²) following a single electroporation pulse. The electrical pulse used was an exponential decaying type with initial amplitude of 1000V for 5ms. In combination with iontophoresis, electroporation was able to enhance LHRH permeation, thus demonstrating a pulsatile delivery. The ability of electroporation to enable a pulsatile transdermal delivery of LHRH was further demonstrated in an isolated perfused porcine skin flap model (Riviere et al., 1995). An electroporative exponential pulse of 500 V for 5 ms was applied before iontophoresis at a current density of 0.4 mA/cm^2 for 30 minutes. Application of a single pulse to start the experiment resulted in an almost threefold increase in LHRH following 30 minutes of iontophoresis. A rapid onset of LHRH delivery was noted in the first 10 minutes after the initial pulse. Moreover, nearly a fourfold increase in maximal LHRH concentration in the perfusate was observed following pulsation. The studies proved the ability of electroporation to generate a pulsatile transdermal delivery. In most instances, iontophoresis enables a constant baseline level of transport, while electroporation pulses were employed to provide a rapid infusion.

The combined effect of electroporation and iontophoresis on *in vitro* transdermal permeation of human parathyroid hormone was investigated (Medi and Singh, 2003). Iontophoresis (0.5 mA/cm^2) was found to significantly enhance ($P<0.05$) the transdermal permeation of parathyroid hormone compared to passive diffusion. Electrical pulses (100V, 200V, and 300V) significantly improved the transdermal permeation of the hormone compared to iontophoresis alone. Microscopic evidence revealed that the stratum corneum of the skin was perturbed on application of electrical pulses. However, the application of electrical pulses followed by iontophoresis was found to increase the transdermal flux of the hormone by several-fold. Similarly, *in vitro* permeation studies across human cadaver skin indicated that the combination of electroporation followed by iontophoresis was found to enhance the transdermal transport of parathyroid hormone by nearly seventeen fold (Chang et al., 2000).

Structures termed "microconduits" were hypothesized to be created in the stratum corneum of the skin when electroporation was carried out with low-toxicity keratolytic agents such as urea and sodium thiosulphate (Ilic et al., 1999). Incandescent and fluorescent microscopic observations and flow tests indicated the formation of microconduits. It was hypothesized that new aqueous pathways existing in the lipid domain of the stratum corneum would get combined with subsequent disruption of the keratin matrix resulting in dislodgement of the entire stacks of corneocytes creating the microconduits. A single microconduit measuring about 50μm in diameter was thought to enable volumetric flow at the rate of 0.01ml/sec under a pressure difference of 0.01 atm, indicating the possibility of the stratum corneum barrier getting disrupted.

The effect of different electroporation on the *in vitro* transdermal permeation of salmon calcitonin was studied across human cadaver skin in combination with iontophoresis (Chang et al., 2000). Application of pulses (15 pulses of 500V, 200ms) followed by iontophoresis was found to result in higher transdermal flux of calcitonin. Electroporation was found to be instrumental in shortening the lag phase of iontophoretic transdermal transport of calcitonin.

The synergistic effect of calcium chloride and electroporation of model permeants like calcein and fluorescein isothiocyanate (FITC)–dextran was reported (Tokudome and Sugibayashi, 2004). The change in the lamellar structure of the skin on electroporation and recovery of its barrier property was assessed by FTIT-ATR. Transepidermal water loss (TEWL) recovered to normal within two hours after electroporation, while the high TEWL values were maintained for longer periods after electroporation with calcium chloride. Electroporation in the presence of calcium chloride solution was found to alter the barrier property of the skin, and the compromised barrier property was maintained for prolonged periods after the combined treatment. The studies proved that the combination of calcium chloride was found to markedly enhance the permeation of low- and high-molecular-weight permeants.

In-skin electroporation with a microneedle electrode array was used to puncture the stratum corneum skin barrier and at the same time ensure application of the electrical pulses to the viable skin tissues (Yan et al., 2010). The macromolecules used as a model permeant were FITC-dextran (Mol wt: 4.3 kDa) for the *in vitro* experiments that used hairless rat skin as a barrier. The in-skin electroporation was found to display a much higher skin penetration of the fluorescent permeant compared to microneedle or on skin electroporation alone. Particularly, higher permeation of the fluorescent permeant was observed when higher voltages were used with longer pulse width. The quantity of lactate dehydrogenase leached from the skin was used to assess the cell damage in hairless rats, which indicated that the in-skin electroporation was minimally invasive. It was concluded that the technique could clinically be feasible by application of electrical pulses after applying a topical product following microneedle pretreatment.

45.6.3 Delivery of Genes

Electroporation is known to enhance both the uptake and expression of the delivered DNA. Investigation of skin as a target for DNA vaccination in a clinical setting appears to be a promising option due to the immunocompetent nature of the dermis, accessibility of the target, and ease of monitoring (Broderick et al., 2014). Studies have indicated that electroporation parameters like electrical field intensity, pulse length, pulse width, and plasmid formulation affect the efficiency of DNA delivery to the skin. Skin diseases such as lupus vulgaris, fungal infections, and herpes simplex viral infections can derive benefits from gene therapy. Owing to the ease of accessibility, skin appears to be an attractive target organ for gene therapy. Even though most work in the field of gene therapy has focused on viral gene transfer, problems associated with viral delivery have initiated the development of nonviral strategies based on lipid- or liposomal-mediated gene transfer. The application of the technique in gene delivery has been demonstrated in an *in vivo* study in which lacZ DNA was delivered to hairless mice. Extensive expression of the lacZ gene was observed in the dermis and the hair follicles three days after the treatment, when the skin was removed and stained with X-gal (Zhang et al., 1997).

The effects of electroporation pulse amplitude, pulse length, and pulse numbers on cutaneous plasmid DNA delivery was investigated by assessing the immune response in rabbits (Medi et al., 2005). After immunization, the serum samples and peripheral mononuclear cells were analyzed for humoral and cellular immunity. Following electroporation at 200 V and 300 V, the expression of transgene in the skin was found to be 48-fold and 129-fold, respectively, in two days compared to passive, though it was transient. *In situ* histological staining with X-gal indicated the localized expression of galactosidase upon electroporation. The studies conclusively indicated that electroporation-mediated cutaneous vaccine delivery significantly enhanced ($p < 0.05$) the humoral and cellular immune responses to hepatitis B compared to passive treatment and therefore could prove to be a potential alternative to the conventional invasive intradermal delivery.

The $CD8^+$ T lymphocyte response to prostate cancer DNA vaccine encoding prostate-specific antigen (PSA) following intradermal electroporation was assessed in a mouse model (Roos et al., 2006). A combination of high short and low long pulses (1125 V/cm, two pulses of 50 µs + 275 V/cm, eight pulses of 10 ms) was found to exhibit the highest potency in inducing the PSA-specific $CD8^+$ T cells. The studies indicated that the electroporation parameters need to be carefully optimized not only to enhance the transfection efficiency but to enhance the cellular immune response. The studies demonstrated the application of dermal electroporation for the delivery of a genetic DNA vaccine depending on antigen specific T-cell induction.

A skin electroporation pulse protocol was developed in order to optimize the gene delivery in mice (Roos et al., 2009). Pulse protocols as short as 240ms was found to generate a robust cellular immune response in mice. In this context, the time of pulse delivery was reduced tenfold compared to the previously published protocols for intradermal electroporation. A single vaccination using the optimized gene delivery was found to generate high and consistent protein expression *in vivo*. A single vaccination gel electroporation-mediated gene delivery was found to generate high and consistent protein expression in mice. The optimized electroporation gene delivery ensured generation of cytotoxic antigen specific T cells that expressed both IFNγ and CD107a.

Transcutaneous electroporation was utilized to deliver a peptide vaccine into the skin (Zhao et al., 2006). The K^b-binding OVA-peptide SIINFEKL was used as a model peptide to induce a peptide-specific cytotoxic T-lymphocyte response in mice. Initially, an anionic lipid 1,2-dimyristoyl-3-phosphatidylserine (DMPS) was added during *in vitro* electroporation into the donor compartment of Franz diffusion cell to prolong the retention of the peptide in the microchannels created.

Electroporation was able to deliver enough vaccine and oligonucleotide adjuvant needed to generate an equivalent amount of T-lymphocyte response as that induced by intradermal injection. Further, *in vivo* experiments in mice demonstrated the efficacy of the electroporation-induced peptide delivery to elicit a specific T-lymphocyte response in mice that was comparable to that of an intradermal vaccine injection.

The immune response of myristylated peptide administered by electroporation was assessed in a mouse model (Misra et al., 2000). The electroporation was found to elicit a higher response of the peptide compared to intradermal immunization. The studies indicated that electroporation could be useful means to target antigens to Langerhans cells or antigen-presenting cells of the skin. The antigen delivered to the skin was further likely to elicit an immune response that mainly depends on the extent of antigen presentation on skin dendritic cells or Langerhans cells. Perturbation of the stratum corneum domain of the skin was considered the underlying mechanism involved in transcutaneous delivery of antigens. The study with myristylated peptide clearly inferred that electroporation could be a promising technique for nonadjuvanted skin immunization, especially with low-molecular-weight, weakly immunogenic antigens.

45.7   SAFETY ISSUES WITH ELECTROPORATION

Application of electrical current would typically reduce the resistance of the skin. The extent of reduction in the skin resistance would be a function of the duration of current application and the density of electrical current used. The drop in the skin resistance often reflects the increased permeability of the skin due to changes in the skin microstructure (Banga et al, 1999). As electropulsation involves application of short-duration pulses, much higher voltages the technique can be applied without causing a sensation. The skin resistance of the human stratum corneum was found to completely recover to almost 90% of the pre-pulse value on application of single pulses of 90V. However, when pulses >130 V were applied, the skin resistance was found to recover to 50% of the pre-pulse values (Pliquett et al., 1995). The permeabilization of the skin was found to depend on the electrical exposure dose that is the product of pulse voltage and cumulative pulsing exposure time. The resistance of the skin was found to drop to 20% of the pre-pulse value when electroporation was applied at a dosage of 0.4V.s but was found to recover quickly.

The stratum corneum is known to exhibit much higher electrical resistance compared to other viable parts of the skin. Electrical pulse applied to the skin would be concentrated on the nonviable stratum corneum to induce electroporation (Banga et al., 1999). On the contrary, the electrical field would be less concentrated on the viable tissue of the skin. The reversibility of the permeation following electroporation indicated that the technique does not damage the skin. The skin toxicology of electroporated skin has been investigated *in vivo* in a pig model (Riviere et al., 1995). Pulses of 0, 250, 500, and 1000V were applied to the animals followed by iontophoresis (0, 0.2, and 2 mA/cm^2 for 30 minutes or 10 mA/cm^2 for 10 minutes) and observed for erythema, edema, or petechiae. The studies indicated that erythema increased immediately after electroporation with the increase in the voltage applied, though it was found to dissipate in five minutes. Even though the pulse voltage had no effect on edema or petechiae, microscopic changes such as focal intraepidermal edema was found to increase with the increase in the pulse voltage.

A sensation of pain during electroporation was observed due to application of electrical pulses that could cause excitation of the nerves and the underlying muscles. Increase in the pulse rate, pulse duration, or pulse voltage was found to enhance itching, tingling sensation, pricking muscle contraction, and outright pain (Pruasnitz, 1996).

Exponential decaying pulses were found to disorganize the stratum corneum lipid barrier of the skin by increasing the extent of hydration. In addition, a transient increase in the TEWL and blood flow were observed (Jadoul et al., 1999). The effect of square wave pulses on skin integrity was also assessed in hairless rats (Dujardin et al., 2002). The square wave pulses were found to induce a drastic decrease in skin resistance, increase in skin TEWL, and transiently decrease (less than five minutes) the blood flow. However, these changes were found to be mild and reversible. The pulses did not induce any inflammation or necroses.

The safety of electroporation-mediated cutaneous vaccine delivery was further demonstrated by the same research group in rabbits (Medi and Singh, 2006). Five electrical pulses of 10 ms each (100 V, 200V, and 300 V) were applied to the back of New Zealand white rabbits, and the skin treated was assessed for viability, macroscopic barrier property, irritation, and microscopic changes. The skin viability was not affected by application of electroporation. However, an increase in TEWL was evident due to skin barrier perturbation that resulted in skin irritation and erythema or edema. Microscopic studies indicated inflammatory responses in the epidermis after application of electrical pulses of 200 V and 300 V. Nevertheless, the changes induced by electroporation were reversed in a week, proving the safety of the technique.

Enhancement of dermal and epidermal regeneration is a prime goal in the treatment of different wounds. Exogenous application of growth factors to the wounds have displayed the potential to improve would healing (Escobar-Chavez et al., 2009). However, frequent application of large amounts of growth factor would be required to meet the therapeutically relevant concentrations at the application site. Gene therapy has demonstrated the potential to deliver growth factor deep within the wound, where it could be more effective and would be able to constantly replenish the growth factors destroyed by peptidases. The potential of electroporation to enhance the transfection efficiency has been explored to enhance the wound healing process (Ferguson et al., 2005). It was identified that electroporation parameters improve the efficiency of DNA transfection in cutaneous wounds and thereby wound healing. However, investigations are on to explore whether electroporation-assisted DNA transfection with plasmid expression vectors would be an effective treatment modality to enhance the wound healing process.

45.8   CLINICAL APPLICATIONS OF ELECTROPORATION

Electroporation has found its clinical application as a physical therapy for transcutaneous electrical stimulation (TENS) in the management of lower back pain, arthritis, and pain caused by neurological disorders and postoperative pain (Prausnitz, 1996). Waveforms can be designed to pass no net current in order to reduce irritation during clinical application. The Food and Drug Administration (FDA) has accepted TENS to induce a very low potential risk to patients. However, the potential applications of electroporation for transdermal and topical use have not been fully exploited for clinical applications. Skin electroporation has found its clinical relevance in the management of skin disorders, including skin cancers, dermal vaccinations, and systemic metabolic diseases. Clinical application of high-voltage pulses tends to induce minor and transient side effects like muscular contraction or erythema that are usually found to be reversible. The design of the electrodes and the pulsing protocol would the key to reducing the undesirable side effects. Further, application of local anesthesia in combination with short-pulse electroporation appears to be a promising approach to minimize discomfort related to electroporation in patients (Roos et al., 2009). Studies have indicated that application of topical anesthetic cream to induce local anesthesia has the potential to decrease the sensation of electroporation during clinical use.

45.9   CONCLUSION

Electroporation is an efficient method for enhancing transdermal and topical drug delivery that has expanded the range of compounds that could be delivered through the skin. The technique has been identified as a promising method for delivery of proteins, peptides, genes, and vaccine to the skin. Electroporation is one of the promising physical enhancement techniques that was found capable of delivering macromolecules ranging up to 40 kDa in size across the skin. Despite the advantages, there are hurdles for the technology to make into clinics, as the voltages employed could be often intolerable in some subjects. However, when combined with enhancement methods, the current strength employed in electroporation can be modulated to enable transdermal delivery to meet the therapeutic requirements and to render it more tolerable. In this context, there is a need to optimize the electrode design and the pulsing protocol to suit the clinical application. Despite innumerable challenges, we can be hopeful that the technique would be commercialized and would be able make into the market in the near future.

REFERENCES

Banga AK, Prausnitz MR. Assessing the potential of skin electroporation for the delivery of protein- and gene-based drugs. TIBTECH,1998, 16, 408–12.

Banga, AK,Bose, S,Ghosh, TK. Iontophoresis and electroporation: comparisons and contrasts. Int J Pharm.,1999, 179, 1–19.

Bose S, Ravis WR, Lin Y-J, Zhang L., Hofmann GA, Banga AK, Electrically assisted transdermal delivery of buprenorphine. J Cont Rel.,2001, 73, 197–203.

Barry BW. Drug Delivery routes in the skin: A novel approach. Adv Drug Del Rev,2002, 54, Suppl 1, S31–40.

Becker, SM, Kuznetsov AV. Thermal *in vivo* skin electroporation pore development and charged macromolecule transdermal delivery: A numerical study of the influence of chemically enhanced lower lipid phase transition temperatures. Int J Heat Mass Trans., 2008, 51, 2060–74.

Blagus T, Markelc B, Cemazar M, Kosjek T, Preat V, Miklavcic D, Sersa G. *In vivo* real-time monitoring system of electroporation mediated control of transdermal and topical drug delivery. J Control Release,2013, 172, 862–71.

Bommannan DB, Tamada J, Leung L, Potts RO. Effect of electroporation on transdermal iontophoretic delivery of luteinizing hormone releasing hormone (LHRH) *in vitro*. Pharm. Res.,1994, 11, 1809–14.

Broderick KE, Khan AS, Sardesai NY (Eds.). DNA vaccination in skin enhanced by electroporation. Methods Mol Biol.,2014, 1143,123–30.

Chang SL, Hofmann GA, Zhang L, Deftos LJ, Banga AK. The effect of electroporation on iontophoretic transdermal delivery of calcium regulating hormones. J Control Release,2000; 66(2–3):127–33.

Cullander C and Guy RH. Transdermal delivery of proteins and peptides. Adv Drug Del Rev.,1992, 8, 291–329.

Denet AR, Preat V, Transdermal delivery of timolol by electroporation through human skin, J Control Release,2003, 88, 253–62.

Denet AR, Ucakar B, Preat V. Transdermal delivery of timolol and atenolol using electroporation and iontophoresis in combination: A mechanistic approach. Pharm Res.,2003, 20(12), 1946–51.

Denet AR, Vanbever R, Preat V. Skin electroporation for transdermal and topical delivery. Adv Drug Deliv Rev.,2004, 56, 659–74.

Dinh SM, Luo CW, Berner B. Upper and lower limits of human skin electrical resistance in iontophoresis. AJChE J.,1993, 39, 2011–18.

Dujardin N, Staes E, Kalia Y, Clarys P, Guy R, Preat V. *In vivo* assessment of skin electroporation using square wave pulses J ContRelease,2002, 79, 219–27.

Escobar-Chavez JJ, Bonilla-Martinez D, Villegas-Gonzalez MA, and Revilla-Vazquez AL. Electroporation as an efficient physical enhancer for skin drug delivery. J Clin. Pharmacol.,2009, 49, 1262–83.

Essa EA, Bonner MC, Barry BW. Electrically assisted skin delivery of liposomal estradiol: phospholipid as damage retardant. J Control Release,2004, 95, 535–46.

Fang J-Y, Hwang T-L, Huang Y-B, Tsai Y-H. Transdermal iontophoresis of sodium nonivamide acetate: V. Combined effect of physical enhancement methods. Int J Pharm.,2002, 235, 95–105.

Fang J-Y, Fang J-Y, Hung Ch-F, Fang Y-P, Chan T-F. Transdermal iontophoresis of 5-fluorouracil combined with electroporation and laser treatment. Int J Pharm.,2004, 270, 241–49.

Ferguson M, Byrnes C, Sun L, et al. Wound healing enhancement: electroporation to address a classic problem of military medicine. World J Surg.,2005, 29, S55–S59.

Heller LC, Jaroszeski MJ, Coppola D, McCray AN, Hickey J and Heller R. Optimization of cutaneous electrically mediated plasmid DNA delivery using novel electrode.Gene Ther.,2007, 14(3), 275–80.

Hofmann GA, Rustrum WV, SuderKS. Electroincorporation of microcarriers as a method for the transdermal delivery of large molecules. Bioelectrochem. Bioenerg.,1995, 38, 209–22.

Hu L, Batheja P, Meiden V and Michniak-Kohn B. In: KulkarniVS, editor. Handbook on Non-Invasive Drug Delivery Systems, 2010; 95–118. New York, USA: Elsevier Inc.

Hu, Q,Liang, W,Bao, J,Ping, Q. Enhanced transdermal delivery of tetracaine by electroporation. Int J Pharm.,2000, 202, 121–24.

Huang JF, Sung KC, Hu O Y-P, Wang JJ, Lin YH, Fang JY. The effects of electrically assisted methods on transdermal delivery of nalbuphine benzoate and sebacoyl dinalbuphine ester from solutions and hydrogels. Int J Pharm.,2005, 297:162–71.

Ilic L, Gowrishankar TR, Vaughan TE, Herndon TO, Weaver JC. Spatially constrained skin electroporation with sodium thiosulphate and urea creates transdermal microconduits. J Cont. Release,1999, 61, 185–202.

Inada H., Ghanem AH., Higuchi WI. Studies on applied voltage and duration of human epidermal membrane alteration/recovery and the resultant effect on iontophoresis. Pharm Res.,1994, 11, 687–97.

Jadoul A, Bouwstra J, Preat V. Effects of iontophoresis and electroporation on the stratum corneum—review of the biophysical studies, Adv. Drug Deliv. Rev.,1999, 35, 89–105.

Jadoul A, Lecouturier, N, Mesens J., CaersW and Preat V. Transdermal alniditan delivery by skin electroporation J ContRelease,1998, 54, 265–72.

Jadoul A and Preat V. Electrically enhanced transdermal delivery of domperidone Int. J Pharm.,1997, 154, 229–34.

Lombry C, Dujardin N and Preat V. Transdermal delivery of macromolecules using skin electroporation. Pharm Res.,2000,17(1), 32–37.

Medi BM and Singh J. Electronically facilitated transdermal delivery of human parathyroid hormone. Int J Pharm,2003, 26, 25–33.

Medi BM and Singh J. Skin targeted DNA vaccine delivery using electroporation in rabbits II Safety. Int J Pharm.,2006, 308, 61–68.

Medi BM, Hoselton S, Marepalli RB, Singh J. Skin targeted DNA vaccine delivery using electroporation in rabbits I Efficacy. Int J Pharm.,2005, 294, 53–63.

Meidan V and Michniak BB. Ultrasound-based Technology for skin barrier permeabilization. In: Kulkarni VS, editor. Handbook on Non-Invasive Drug Delivery Systems. New York, USA: Elsevier Inc.2010; p 119–33.

Misra A, Ganga S, Upadhyay P. Needle-free non-adjunacted skin immunization by electroporation-enahnced transdermal delivery of diphtheria toxoid and a candidate peptide vaccine against hepatisis B virus. Vaccine,2000, 18, 517–23.

Murthy SN, Zhao YL, Sen A, Hui SW. Cyclodextrin enhanced transdermal delivery of piroxicam and carboxyfluorescein by electroporation. J ContRelease,2004, 99, 393–402.

Nickoloff JA. Preface. In Nickoloff JA, ed. Electroporation Protocols for Microorganisms. Totowa, NJ: Humana Press Inc.1995, 5–6.

Pliquett U and Weaver JC. Electroporation of human skin; simultaneous measurement of changes in the transport of two fluorescent molecules and in the passive electrical properties. BioelectrochemBioenerg.,1996, 39, 1–12.

Pliquett U, Langer R, Weaver, JC. Changes in the passive electrical properties of human stratum corneum due to electroporation. Biochim Biophys Acta.,1995, 1239, 111–21.

Pliquett U. Mechanistic studies of molecular transdermal transport due to skin electroporation. Adv Drug Deliv Rev.,1999, 35, 41–60.

Prausnitz MR. A practical assessment of transdermal drug delivery by skin elctroporation. Adv Drug Del Rev.,1999, 35, 61–76.

Prausnitz MR. The effect of electric current applied to skin: A review for transdermal drug delivery1996, 18, 395–425.

Potts RO, Guy RH. Predicting skin permeability. Pharm. Res.,1992, 9, 663–69.

Prausnitz MR, Bose VG, Langer R, Weaver JC. Electroporation of mammalian skin-a mechanism to enhance transdermal drug delivery. Proc Natl Acad Sci.,1993, 90, 10504–508.

Prausnitz MR., Edelman ER, Gimm JA, Langer R, Weaver JC. Transdermal delivery of heparin by skin electroporation. Biol Technol.,1995, 13, 1205–09.

Prausnitz MR. The effect of electric current applied to skin: A review for transdermal drug delivery,1996, 18, 395–425.

Prausnitz M.R. A practical assessment of transdermal drug delivery by skin elctroporation. Adv. Drug Del. Rev,1999, 35, 61–76.

Preat V, Vanbever R. Skin eletroporation for transdermal and topical drug delivery. In: Transdermal Drug Delivery, 2003, 27–54. Mercer Dekker Inc: New York.

Rai V, Ghosh I, Bose S, Silva SMC, Chandra P, Michniak-Kohn B. A transdermal review on permeation of drug formulations, modifier compounds and delivery methods. J Drug Del Sci Tech.,2010, 20(2), 75–87.

Regnier V, De Morre N, Jadoul A, Preat V. Mechanisms of a phosphorothioate oligonucleotide delivery by skin electroporation. Int JPharm., 1999, 184, 147–56.

Riviere JE, Monterio-Riviere NA, Rogers RA., Bommannan D, Tamada J.A, Potts RO. Pulsatile transdermal delivery of LHRH using electroporation drug delivery and skin toxicology J Control Release,1995, 36, 229–33.

Roos AK., Eriksson F, Walters DC, Pisa P, King AD. Optimization of skin electroporation in mice to increase tolerability of DNA vaccine delivery to patients. Mol Therapy,2009, 17(9), 1637–42.

Roos AK, Moreno S, Leder C, Pavlenko M, King A, Pisa P. Enhancement of cellular immune response to a prostate cancer DNA vaccine by intradermal electroporation. Mol Therapy,2006, 13(2), 320–27.

Sammeta, SM,Vaka, SR,MurthySN. Transcutaneous electroporation mediated delivery of doxepin-HPCD complex: A sustained release approach for treatment of postherpetic neuralgia. J. Control Release,2010, 142, 361–67.

Sen A, Zhao Y, Zhang L, Hui SW. Enhanced transdermal transport by electroporation using anionic Lipids. J Control Release, 2002a, 82, 399–405.

Sen A, Daly ME, Hui SW. Transdermal insulin delivery using lipid enhanced electroporation. Biochemica et Biophysica Acta,2002b, 1564, 5–8.

Sersa G, Cemazar M, Rudolf Z. Electrochemotherapy: advantages and drawbacks in treatment of cancer patients. Cancer Ther.,2003, 1, 133–42.

Sharma A, Kara M, Smith R, Krishnan TR. Transdermal drug delivery using electroporation. I. Factors influencing in-vitro delivery of terazosin hydrochloride in hairless rats. J Pharm Sci., 2000,89, 528–35.

Shivakumar HN, Murthy SN. Topical and transdermal delivery. In: Kulkarni VS, editor. Handbook on Non-Invasive Drug Delivery Systems, New York, USA: Elsevier Inc.2010; p. 1–38.

Singhal M, Kalia YN. Skin Permeation and Disposition of Therapeutic and Cosmeceutical Compounds, Iontophoresis and Electroporation. Ed. Kenji Sugibayashi Tokyo: Springer Japan; 2017. p. 165–82.

Sung KC, Fang J-Y, Wang JJ, Hu OY-P. Transdermal delivery of nalbuphine and its prodrugs by electroporation. Eur J Pharm Sci.,2003,18, 63–70.

Tokudome T, Sugibayashi K. Mechanism of the synergic effects of calcium chloride and electroporation on the in vitro enhanced skin permeation of drugs J Cont Release, 2004, 95, 267–74.

Treco DA, Selden RF. Nonviral gene therapy. Mol Med Today,1995, 1, 314–21.

Vanbever R, Preat V. Factors affecting transdermal delivery of metoprolol by electroporation. BioelectrochemBioenerg.,1995, 38, 223–28.

Vanbever R, Leroy MA, Preat V, Transdermal permeation of neutral molecules by electroporation, J Control Release,54, 1998a, 243–50.

Vanbever R, Langers G, Montmayeur S, Preat V. Transdermal delivery of fentanyl: rapid onset of analgesia using skin electroporation. J Control Release, 1998b, 50, 225–35

Vanbever R, LeBoulenge E, Preat V. Transdermal delivery of fentanyl by electroporation: I. Influence of electrical factors.Pharm Res.,1996a, 13, 559–65.

Vanbever R, LeBoulenge E, Preat V. Transdermal delivery of fentanyl by electroporation: II. Influence of electrical factors.Pharm Res.,1996b, 13, 1360–66.

Vanbever R, Lecouturier N, Preat,V. Transdermal delivery of metoprolol by electroporation. Pharm Res.,1994, 11, 1657–62.

Wang Su, Kara M, Krishnan TR. Transdermal delivery of cyclosporin-A using electroporation. J Cont Rel.,1998, 50, 61–70.

Weaver JC Electroporation theory: concepts and mechanisms. In Nickoloff JA, ed. Electroporation Protocols for Microorganisms. Totowa, NJ: Humana Press Inc., 1995, 1–26.

Weaver JC, Chizmadzhev Y. Electroporation Biological Effects of Electromagnetic Fields. CRC Press, Boca Raton, NY, 1996; pp. 247–74.

Weaver JC. Electroporation: A general phenomenon for manipulating cells and tissues. J Cell Biochem.,1993, 51, 426–35.

Weaver JC, Vaughan TE, Chizmadzhev Y. Theory of electrical creation of aqueous pathways across skin transport barriers. Adv Drug Deliv Rev.,1999, 35, 21–39.

Wong TW, Chen CH, Huang CC, Lin CD, Hui SW. Painless electroporation with a new needle-free microelectrode array to enhance transdermal drug delivery. J Control Release, 2006, 110, 557–65.

Yan K, Todo H, Sugibayashi K. Transdermal drug delivery by in-skin electroporation using a microneedle array. Int J Pharm.,2010, 397, 77–83.

Zewert TE, Pliqett UF, Langer R, Weaver JC. Transdermal transport of DNA antisense oligonucleotides by electroporation. BiochemBiophys Res Comm.,1995, 212(2), 286–92.

Zhang L, Li L, An ZL, Hoffman RM, Hofmann GA, In vivo transdermal delivery of large molecules by pressure mediated electroincorporation and electroporation: a novel method for drug and gene therapy, Bioelectrochem Bioenerg.,1997, 42, 283–92.

Zhang L, Rabussay DP. Clinical evaluation of safety and human tolerance of electrical sensation induced by electric fields with non-invasive electrodes. Bioelectrochemistry,2002, 56, 233–36.

Zhao YL, Murthy SN, Manjili MH, Guan LJ, Sen A, Hui SW. Induction of cytotoxic T-lymphocytes by electroporation enhanced needle-free skin immunization. Vaccine, 2006, 24(9), 1282–90.

46 Iontophoresis in Penetration Enhancement

Taís Gratieri
Universidade de Brasília, Brasília, Brazil

Yogeshvar N. Kalia
University of Geneva, Geneva, Switzerland

CONTENTS

46.1 INTRODUCTION

Iontophoresis is a noninvasive technique that employs a mild electric current to enhance molecular penetration into or through biological tissues (Kalia et al. 2004). The proof of concept that the application of a mild electric field could drive molecules across the skin dates from 1900, but it was only in the past 25 years that the first prefilled transdermal iontophoretic patch systems employing this technology reached the market. Although these devices were not commercially successful, considerable progress was made in understanding the potential of the technology, patch design, the selection of drug candidates, and even broadening the range of potential application sites to tissues other than the skin (Gratieri et al. 2017).

Several complex mathematical models have been developed to interpret the effects of electric field application on the skin and iontophoretic transport either in terms of electrical/formulation parameters or as a function of permeant properties (Gratieri and Kalia 2013). The complexity of such models arises from the fact that the skin, especially the stratum corneum, has an extremely heterogeneous structure in terms of composition and organization. To date, there is no single predictor capable of theoretically elucidating the cutaneous permeation profile of a drug under the influence of the electric field. Proposed iontophoretic transport mechanisms help us to understand better the influence of experimental variables on delivery and show us how to achieve optimized conditions for effective therapy. Therefore, this chapter presents elementary concepts and iontophoretic transport mechanisms. The focus is to interpret the fundamental equations that have been used as a theoretical background for experimental research in the field of cutaneous iontophoretic drug delivery and to explain current strategies to further improve iontophoretic drug delivery, rather than to provide a complete theoretical framework. The evolution of the technology from the first commercial devices to current applications is briefly reviewed and discussed in the last section.

46.2 BASIC IONTOPHORETIC THEORIES

46.2.1 FIRST COMPONENT: PASSIVE PERMEATION

Iontophoresis is an active enhancement technique that can be used to improve topical or transdermal transport when passive delivery is not sufficient for a therapeutic effect, either because of poor bioavailability or inadequate input kinetics.

In steady-state conditions, transdermal drug flux following the passive application of a drug formulation can be described by Fick's law of diffusion (Scheuplein 1976):

$$J_{Passive} = \frac{Q}{A \, t} = \frac{D \, c_{s,m}}{h} \cdot \frac{c_v}{c_{s,v}} \tag{46.1}$$

where Q is the amount of drug that penetrates the biological barrier, A is the area of the membrane to which the formulation is applied, t is the time, D is the drug diffusion coefficient in the membrane of h thickness, $c_{s,m}$ and $c_{s,v}$ are the drug solubility in the membrane and vehicle, respectively, and c_v is the concentration of drug dissolved in the vehicle.

According to this equation, the flux can be increased either by increasing drug concentration in the formulation, thereby altering the degree of saturation, $c_v/c_{s,v}$, which is related to the thermodynamic activity, or by modifying the drug diffusion coefficient, D, in the membrane, a kinetic process. Nonetheless, for many molecules, increasing permeation by increasing drug concentration is only valid until a certain level after which a plateau is reached. A last resort with respect to influencing the thermodynamic aspects would be to modify the drug's physicochemical properties by synthesizing pro-drugs; alternatively, a switch to "kinetic" strategies would be required to facilitate molecular diffusion through the membrane and thereby alter the drug permeability coefficient (K_p) (Potts and Guy 1992; Scheuplein 1976):

$$K_p = \frac{DK_m}{h} \tag{46.2}$$

where K_m is the membrane/vehicle partition coefficient of the drug, given by $c_{s,m}/c_{s,v}$. These "kinetic" strategies effecting changes in the biological membrane to enhance drug delivery can be either physical, compromising the membrane integrity (Dragicevic and Maibach 2018), or chemical, modifying the formulation or incorporating permeation enhancers (Pham et al. 2016), either way influencing the permeability coefficient.

Iontophoresis, instead of deliberately altering membrane barrier properties, adds an external physical force (a mild electric potential gradient across a biological barrier) to increase drug diffusion, maintaining most of the membrane barrier characteristics unviolated. So, the passive drug diffusion described by Fick's law of diffusion is complemented by two other component transport mechanisms: electromigration (EM) and electroosmosis (EO).

46.2.2 IONTOPHORESIS

Iontophoresis involves the application of a low-intensity electrical current provided by a battery or a power source. The current is distributed through the conductive formulation and the skin by two electrodes maintained in separate anodal (+) and cathodal (−) compartments (Kalia et al. 2004). The drug formulation is placed in one compartment based on the drug's polarity (Figure 46.1). The other electrode, called the return or indifferent electrode, is placed anywhere on the skin to close the circuit, with the possibility of being placed on a distal part to the treated area.

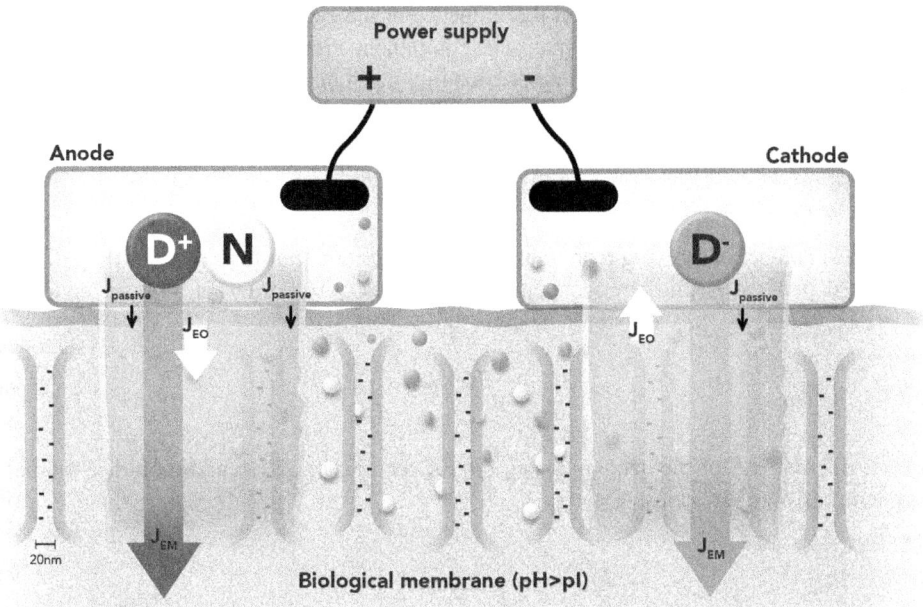

FIGURE 46.1 Schematic representation of iontophoresis, including the representation of transient pores created in the skin during current application. The anodal compartment is used to deliver cationic (D⁺) or neutral (N) drugs, while the cathodal compartment is used to host negatively charged drug molecules (D⁻). Application of an electric potential causes a current to flow through the circuit, generating the enhanced passive ($J_{passive}$), electromigration (J_{EM}), and electro-osmosis (J_{EO}) flux components accompanied by ion migration towards and out of the skin (represented by small circles).

In simple terms, the EM flux component refers to the drug electromigration towards the skin, while the EO component refers to a solvent flow to and from the skin. EO flow is in the direction of counter-ion movement, which tries to enable neutralization of the membrane charge. At physiological conditions, the skin is negatively charged (isoelectric point of ~4-4.5); hence, cation transport and the delivery of neutral molecules is facilitated in the anode-to-cathode direction (Pikal 1992).

Assuming that each phenomenon is independent, the total drug permeation flux is composed of three processes (Nernst–Planck theory) (Kasting 1992):

$$J_{Total} = J_{Passive} + J_{EM} \pm J_{EO} \tag{46.3}$$

where J_{Total} is the total flux, $J_{Passive}$ is the passive flux, and J_{EM} and J_{EO} are the fluxes resulting from EM and EO, respectively. If the drug is placed in the anode compartment, total flux is assisted by the EO component, but if the drug is negatively charged and placed in the cathodal compartment, then EO will hinder electrotransport.

46.2.2.1 Electromigration

Electromigration refers to the ordered ion movement under an applied electric field. The electromigratory flux of a drug is related to the component current flow i_d in a process that can be described by Faraday's law (Delgado-Charro and Guy 2001; Kalia et al. 2004; Phipps and Gyory 1992; Phipps et al. 1989; Sage and Riviere 1992):

$$J_d^{EM} = \frac{1}{A \, F \, z_d} \cdot i_d \tag{46.4}$$

where A is the cross-sectional area under the influence of the electric field, F is Faraday's constant (Coulombs/mole), and z_d is the drug valence. The component current flow of the drug can be related to the applied current I (Amperes) and a proportionality constant, the transport number of the drug, t_d, which represents the drug efficiency as a charge carrier:

$$J_{EM} = \frac{I\,t_d}{A\,F\,z_d} \tag{46.5}$$

As the transport number of the drug represents the current fraction transported by the drug ($0 < t_d < 1$), it is not only dependent on the physicochemical properties of the drug but also on the other ions present in the system:

$$t_d = \frac{c_d\,\mu_d}{\sum c_i \mu_i} \tag{46.6}$$

where μ_d is the mobility of the drug and c_i and μ_i are the concentration and mobility of other ions in the system, respectively. Consequently:

$$J_{EM} = \left(\frac{1}{z_d F}\right)\frac{u_d c_d}{\displaystyle\sum_{n=0}^{i} u_i c_i}\cdot I_D \tag{46.7}$$

where I_D is the applied current density ($= I/A$); therefore, by analyzing the EM mechanism, drug delivery can be basically influenced by current density, the drug valence, and the drug's ability to function as a charge carrier in relation to the other ions in the system.

46.2.2.2　Electroosmosis

Electroosmosis, the second component of iontophoretic delivery, can be described as a fluid flow that occurs when a voltage difference is imposed across a charged membrane (Pikal 1992). Principles of nonequilibrium thermodynamics were used to describe how the application of pressure and a potential difference across a membrane generates current and volume flows (Pikal 1992). The two flow phenomena can be expressed as:

$$Volume\ flow = L_{11}\ \Delta Pressure + L_{12}\ (-\Delta Potential)$$

$$Current\ flow = L_{21}\ \Delta Pressure + L_{22}\ (-\Delta Potential) \tag{46.8}$$

The flows are related to their causal or conjugate forces by the corresponding Onsager coefficients, L_{ij}; L_{11} represents the volume flow due to a pressure gradient, and L_{22} is the current flow due to the applied potential difference, which is equal to the conductance. The cross coefficients Lij describe interaction terms; L_{12} defines how the application of a potential difference across a membrane will create a volume flow. In an iontophoretic experiment, when an electric field is applied across the skin, $\Delta Pressure = 0$, therefore, the volume flow ($\mu l/cm^2/h$) can also be expressed by the product of the ratio of the Onsager coefficients (L_{12}/L_{22}) and the current density (Kalia et al. 2004).

$$Volume\ flow = \frac{L_{12}}{L_{22}}\cdot I_D = electroosmotic\ flow \tag{46.9}$$

In these conditions, a specific volume of solvent penetrates the skin from the anode, carrying dissolved cations or neutral molecules and, conversely, a specific volume of interstitial liquid is extracted from the skin towards the cathode, opposing the movement of anions but also extracting endogenous molecules, which is the theoretical basis for reverse iontophoresis. Reverse iontophoresis is basically a process of noninvasive sampling, which is not the focus of this chapter but has been described in other publications (Bouissou et al. 2009; Degim et al. 2003; Delgado-Charro and Guy 2001, 2003; Djabri et al. 2009; Giri et al. 2017, 2019; Sieg et al. 2003). In practical terms, this volume of solvent permeating the skin carries along with it dissolved molecules irrespective of their molecular weight but proportional to their concentration in the solvent.

The lack of direct correlation between J_{EO} and molecular weight and the existence of a correlation between drug electrophoretic mobility and t_d, and hence J_{EM}, is the reason why there was a consensus that higher-molecular-weight species, such as peptides and proteins, would rely almost exclusively on the EO component during iontophoresis application. Even though this theory has been challenged by a series of experiments demonstrating protein electromigration (Banerjee et al. 2019; Cazares-Delgadillo et al. 2007; Dubey and Kalia 2010; Dubey et al. 2011), a recent study showed that EO was the main mechanism involved in the delivery of the largest protein delivered through the intact stratum corneum so far, i.e., cetuximab a 152-kDa monoclonal antibody (Lapteva et al. 2020).

EO can also be defined as a solvent velocity, V_w, in which case, it is equivalent to a permeability coefficient with corresponding units, e.g., cm/h:

$$J_{EO} = V_w \cdot c_d \tag{46.10}$$

where V_w is the linear velocity of the solvent flow and c_d is the concentration of the drug in the vehicle (Pikal 1992).

46.2.3 Total Iontophoretic Flux

Following the mathematical representation of each component transport mechanism, the equations can be rearranged depending on the parameter to be analyzed. The passive contribution to the total iontophoretic flux can be represented as the product of the drug permeability coefficient, K_p, and the concentration in the formulation, and this gives:

$$J_{Total} = \left[K_p + v_w \right] . c_d + \frac{I \ t_d}{A \ F \ z_d} \tag{46.11}$$

Still other rearrangements are possible:

$$J_{Total} = k_p . c_d + (I_D)_{\Delta P = 0} \left[\left(\frac{L_{12}}{L_{22}} \right) . c_d + \frac{t_d}{F \ z_d} \right] \tag{46.12}$$

where volume flow is given by the product of the ratio of the Onsanger coefficients $\left(\frac{L_{12}}{L_{22}} \right)$ and the current density (I_D) when a potential is applied at constant pressure; this last representation shows that both EO and EM should be proportional to the applied current density (Kalaria et al. 2018).

46.2.4 Strategies to Further Enhance Iontophoretic Delivery

46.2.4.1 Establishing Relative Contributions of the Component Electrotransport Mechanisms

In the process of optimizing iontophoretic delivery of a specific drug candidate, information regarding the relative contribution of each delivery component can be useful. Several experiments have been performed isolating and analyzing the role of passive transport, EM, and EO to cutaneous delivery (Kalaria et al. 2012; Lapteva et al. 2020). For this, generally, a passive permeation experiment is performed and the obtained $J_{passive}$ subtracted from the J_{total} from an iontophoretic experiment. However, the magnitude of the passive component is most likely increased during iontophoresis because transient reorientation of the stratum corneum proteins and lipids in the presence of the electric field may alter membrane diffusivity, enhancing the passive permeability (Pikal 1992). Both *in vitro* and clinical studies demonstrate a drop in skin impedance with the current application, which may last a few up to 24 hours after therapy termination (Curdy et al. 2000, 2002; Kalia et al. 1996; Turner et al. 1997). Therefore, such transient membrane structural changes possibly have an effect on the passive component, but due to the nature of these "pathways," they would favor the transport of more hydrophilic molecules, which typically present poor or negligible passive permeation. Even so, the contribution of the passive component is generally minor compared to the other two components, and a possible underestimation of the passive role would not affect the enhancement strategy to be adopted.

The effect of electrical or formulation parameters will ultimately depend on the relative contributions of EM and EO. An experimental method to measure the electroosmotic contribution is by co-iontophoresing an electroosmotic marker with the molecule of interest. Such a marker must be neutral, hydrophilic, and preferably present a negligible passive transdermal transport so the contribution to transport is null and all the iontophoretic transport is due to electrically induced convective solvent flow. Acetaminophen and mannitol are commonly used as EO "markers," and the flux used to report on EO solvent flow from anode to cathode and hence estimate the EO contribution to the total drug transport (Lapteva et al. 2020). During iontophoresis, the linear velocity (V_w) of the current-induced water flow (cm/h) across the skin can be estimated using (Pikal, 1992):

$$V_w = \frac{J_M}{c_M} \tag{46.13}$$

where J_M and c_M are the flux and donor concentration of the marker, respectively. EO contribution to drug transport may be obtained by multiplying V_w by its concentration in the donor solution (c_D) [Equation (46.10)] (Marro et al. 2001). There should be no interaction between the marker and the molecule of interest. Even so, the importance of co-iontophoresing the two species is that certain molecules may interact with the skin diminishing, or even abolishing, EO. Control experiments using the same conditions but applying only the marker can be compared to co-iontophoresis experiments to provide the magnitude and significance of a possible electroosmotic flow inhibition. Results can be analyzed by calculating the inhibition factor (IF) (del Rio-Sancho et al. 2017):

$$IF = \frac{[Q_{M,\,control}]}{[Q_{M,\,drug}]} \tag{46.14}$$

where $Q_{M,\,control}$ is the amount of marker transported after an iontophoretic experiment of only the marker in the donor solution and $Q_{M,\,drug}$ is the corresponding quantity in the presence of the drug.

The inhibitory effect on EO by some positively charged peptides and proteins has been demonstrated (Bayon and Guy 1996; Delgado Charro et al. 1995; del Rio-Sancho et al. 2017; Schuetz et al. 2006). Iontophoretic experiments showed that while their hydrophobic surface regions participate in van der Waals–type interactions in the transport pathways, cationic amino acid side chains neutralize fixed negative charge sites in the skin. Still, the degree of EO inhibition may vary according to the molecule and skin ionization state. Co-iontophoresis of acetaminophen and μ-conotoxin CnIIIC (MW = 2375.73), a peptide antagonist of the $Na_v1.4$ sodium channel, with a net positive charge of 3.9 at pH 5.6 (experiment), showed an almost sevenfold reduction in the EO contribution (del Rio-Sancho et al. 2017), while co-iontophoresis of lysozyme (MW = 14.3 kDa) and the same marker produced a IF >12 (Dubey and Kalia 2014). Interestingly, EO inhibition seemed to be more influenced by the degree of ionization of the negatively charged binding sites in the skin than by the total positive net charge of the permeant, as IFs were higher closer to physiological pH values (IF of 12.0, 15.7, and 16.0 at pH 5, 6, and 7.15, respectively). Increasing skin pH increases skin ionization (pI 4 to 4.5), while at the same time lowering lysozyme net charge (pI 9.32). Therefore, at the highest

EO inhibition condition (pH 7.15), lysozyme had the lowest net charge (7.7), but the skin had more negatively charged binding sites, which was significant for EO inhibition (Dubey and Kalia 2014). If an increase in the total current does not produce sufficient delivery to elicit the desired effect, the molecule simply might not be a good candidate for iontophoresis, as skin binding might be too important an effect in limiting drug electrotransport (Dubey and Kalia 2014).

46.2.4.2 Increasing Total Current and Current Density

The total current (and hence the charge passed) can be increased by extending the application time or augmenting current density.

Even though it might seem logical to expect the same permeation under conditions of equivalent charge, in which lower current densities are compensated by longer application times, experiments have demonstrated current density may affect the drug distribution profile (Santer et al. 2018). A recent ocular iontophoresis study using the entire eye globe *ex vivo* demonstrated at constant charge (30 mA·min/cm²; 1.44 C), but with different application times and current densities (20 min at 1.5 mA/cm² and 5 min at 6 mA/cm²), the total delivery for both conditions was statistically equivalent, but not the drug distribution in the ocular compartments, i.e., the longer treatment time of 20 minutes enabled increased drug deposition in the deep ocular tissues (Santer et al. 2018). Extrapolating these results to cutaneous drug delivery, one might assume higher current densities could be useful for epidermal targeting, avoiding systemic distribution in short-time delivery of active cosmetic ingredients. Even though there might be a linear relationship between deposited amounts and increases in current density, the total drug transported may not be directly proportional to the total current. This was observed in the delivery of conotoxin CnIIIC, cited earlier (del Rio-Sancho et al. 2017). Even though this peptide binds in the skin, generating more complex interpretations of transport mechanisms, regression analysis confirmed deposition increased linearly with the current density ($r^2 = 0.99$). Still, the total amount of peptide deposited was not directly proportional to total current, as ~30 µg/cm² was deposited after 15 minutes of 0.5 mA/cm² (0.45C), while only ~22 µg/cm² were deposited after 30 minutes of 0.3mA/cm² (0.54C) (del Rio-Sancho et al. 2017). Indeed, the equations presented to describe iontophoretic transport mechanisms relate to drug flux in steady-state conditions; these may be achieved faster under higher current densities; hence, total delivered amounts or drug distribution may vary in conditions of the same total charge (Coulombs) but different current densities and application times.

In cases where there is a linear correlation between flux and current density, increasing current density may be sufficient to increase drug delivery, attaining a complete control over input kinetics and enabling therapy individualization (Abla et al. 2005; Kalaria et al. 2012, 2014, 2018; Patel et al. 2009). Nevertheless, the tissue resistance to current flow, given by Ohm's law, limits the maximal current density applied:

$$I = \frac{V}{R} \tag{46.15}$$

where V is the potential difference measured across the tissue in volts, and R is the resistance of the tissue in Ohms. Hence, the higher the aqueous content of a tissue, the lower the resistance and the higher the tolerability towards current application, explaining why I_D of 6 mA.cm⁻² is tolerable for the sclera (Santer et al. 2018), but not for the skin, in which the value of 0.5 mA.cm⁻² has been considered the higher safe current density to be applied. Above this value, unwanted cutaneous effects can occur, ranging from tickling sensations to erythema and discomfort (Ledger 1992). Still, when flux increase by only altering electronic parameters is not sufficient to achieve therapeutic levels, chemical modification of the molecule may be a promising alternative.

46.2.4.3 Pro-Drug Synthesis

The pro-drug strategy has been widely used to increase drug lipophilicity (improving K_m) rendering satisfactory cutaneous passive permeation. Monoester and diester derivatives of corticosteroid esters are routinely used to mask hydroxyl groups and so facilitate partition into the intercellular lipid matrix in the stratum corneum (e.g., triamcinolone acetonide and betamethasone dipropionate).

Conversely, the pro-drug strategy to further enhance iontophoretic delivery aims at improving a drug's ability to efficiently transport the electric current (improving t_d) and effectively migrate towards the skin (Figure 46.2). Hence, besides increasing hydrophilicity and aqueous solubility, imparting a charge to the molecule is extremely beneficial.

A cationic pro-drug of ketoprofen, the ester ketoprofen choline chloride, has been synthesized following this rationale showing five times higher flux after anodal iontophoresis than cathodal iontophoresis of ketoprofen across human epidermis skin (Lobo and Yan 2018). Also, a series of amino acid ester pro-drugs of acyclovir, an antiviral for the treatment of herpes simplex virus infections, were produced (ACV-X, where ACV = acyclovir and X = Arg, Gly, Ile, Phe, Trp, and Val) (Chen et al. 2016a). ACV has poor oil/water solubility, which limits its partitioning into the highly lipidic intercellular space in the keratinized stratum corneum. Exactly as described, the amino acid moieties are intended to improve the molecule hydrophilicity and consequently molecule t_d.

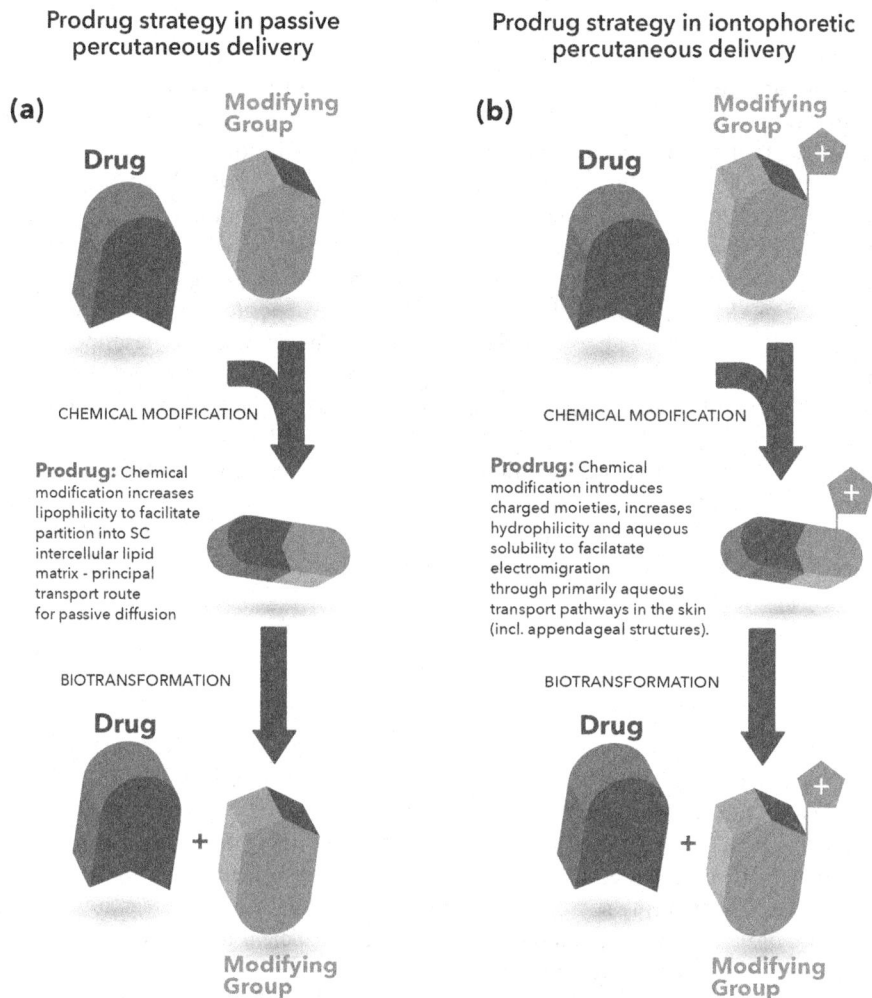

FIGURE 46.2 Schematic representations illustrating the different rationale for using pro-drugs to improve (a) passive and (b) iontophoretic transport into and across the skin. (Adapted and reproduced with permission from Chen et al. 2016a.)

Then, to exert the therapeutic effect, amino acid moieties of ACV pro-drugs must be cleaved by skin esterases, exposing the ACV terminal hydroxyl group for phosphorylation by viral thymidine kinase and human phosphorylase, as ACV triphosphate is the active form that inhibits viral DNA replication (Gnann et al. 1983). Indeed, synthesized pro-drugs ACV-Trp, ACV-Phe, ACV-Ile, ACV-Val, ACV-Gly, and ACV-Arg had solubility enhancements of 6, 33, 38, 48, 56, and >90-fold (by molar concentration), respectively, as compared to ACV, which could be attributed to the effect of hydrogen-bonded solvation of the ionizable group(s). Such solubility increments facilitated their formulation, as they were prepared in aqueous solution at a patient-friendly pH 5.5. As expected, the passive diffusion of ACV and ACV-X pro-drugs into and across porcine skin from 5 mM aqueous solutions was negligible after two hours; neither skin retention nor cumulative permeation was quantifiable. Iontophoresis resulted in therapeutically relevant drug amounts in the skin. The highest skin deposition of either the pro-drug or the ACV already biotransformed were achieved with the di-protonated pro-drug, ACV-Arg (785.9 ± 78.1 nmol/cm^2), which had the highest charge–mass ratio, highest solubility, and lowest log D (5.24×10^3, >820 mM, -6.08, respectively) among the six pro-drugs; therefore, its electromigration was presumably the highest under a given electric potential gradient. Iontophoresis of the two aromatic amino acid ester pro-drugs, ACV-Trp and ACV-Phe, led to the lowest skin deposition of ACV species (156.1 ± 76.3 and 249.8 ± 81.4 nmol/cm^2, respectively). Conversely to ACV-Arg, they had the lowest charge–mass ratios and solubilities and higher log D (2.43×10^3, 51.3 mM, -0.73, and 2.69×10^3, 304.4 mM, -1.22, for ACV-Trp and ACV-Phe, respectively) and thus presumably had lower electric mobility (Chen et al. 2016a).

Another notable aspect of the pro-drug strategy is that pro-drugs for iontophoresis may be designed for either topical or transdermal delivery based on the stability of the linkage to the charged moiety. Comparatively stable pro-drugs might have a higher probability of reaching the systemic circulation during iontophoresis. In contrast, enzymatically labile pro-drugs would be more likely to undergo hydrolysis earlier during cutaneous transit and release an uncharged parent drug that would be retained within the membrane. This was observed with the acyclovir pro-drugs, as total delivery of ACV-Arg, the most biolabile pro-drug, was dominated by ACV deposition, while a higher absolute amount and percentage of the applied ACV-Ile, the most enzymatically stable pro-drug, permeated across the skin as a function of time (Chen et al. 2016a). Further biodistribution studies demonstrated that while passive delivery of ACV or penciclovir from marketed cream and ointment formulations after application for 60 minutes resulted in modest cutaneous deposition, mainly in the stratum corneum or superficial viable epidermis, iontophoresis of ACV-Ile or ACV-Arg for only 10 minutes at 0.25 mA/cm^2 resulted in, respectively, twelvefold and twentyfold higher deposition of ACV species, but at deeper skin layers (100 to 200 µm) (Figure 46.3), corresponding to the basal epidermis and adjacent area, the target region for delivery where the virus would be found (Chen et al. 2016b).

The concept that pro-drug enzymatic stability leads to deeper drug penetration may even apply to biological barriers other than the skin. The ocular iontophoretic delivery of ACV-Gly, one of the ACV pro-drugs with the highest relative enzymatic stability in ocular tissues (half-life from 1.58 ± 0.13 to 5.54 ± 0.82 hours in the choroid/retina and vitreous humor extracts, respectively), showed considerable delivery of ACV species to the choroid/retina and vitreous humor (5.7 ± 2.3 and 11.7 ± 3.7 nmol/cm^2, respectively) after only five minutes transscleral iontophoresis to intact porcine eye globes (Chen and Kalia 2018). Nonetheless, other less intuitive aspects may also need to be considered such as the influence of polar surface area, dipole moment, charge, and possible tissue interactions, e.g. melanin binding in ocular delivery (Santer et al. 2018). This was observed after short-duration transscleral iontophoretic delivery of four triamcinolone acetonide (TA) amino acid ester prodrugs (TA-AA) (alanine, Ala; arginine, Arg; isoleucine, Ile and lysine, Lys) using whole porcine eye globes *in vitro*. Results showed TA-Ala had a similar ocular biodistribution profile to TA-Lys, even though TA-Lys was more enzymatically stable in the ocular tissues than TA-Ala and had net difference in charge, being dicationic, while TA-Ala was monocationic. Such results were attributed to the presence of localized charge centers on the molecular surface, which increased

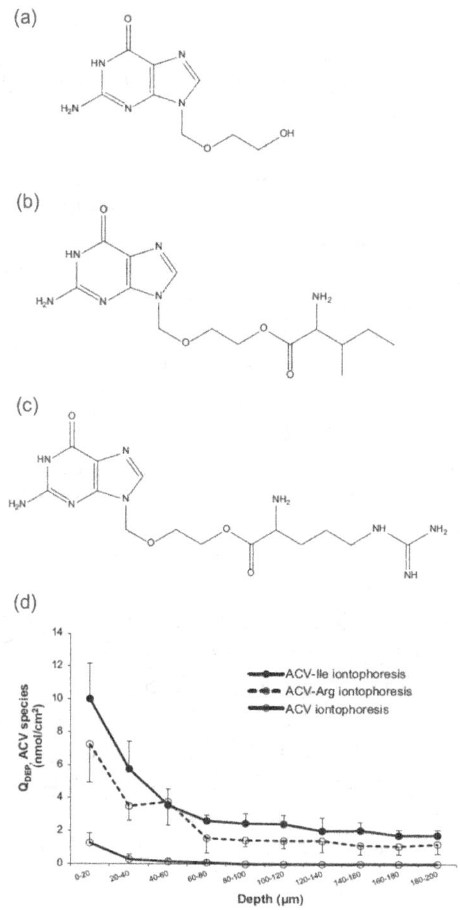

(a)

(b)

(c)

(d)

FIGURE 46.3 Chemical structure of (a) ACV, (b) ACV-Ile, and (c) ACVArg. (d) represents cutaneous biodistribution of ACV and ACV-X following iontophoresis of ACV, ACV-Arg, or ACVIle (5 mM) in 10 mM MES buffer (pH 5.5) at 0.25 mA/cm^2 for five minutes as a function of position to a depth of 200 μm. (Mean ± SD; $n = 5$). (Adapted and reproduced with permission from Chen et al. 2016b.)

the propensity of interaction with negative charges in the tissue and hindered electromigration (Figure 46.4). Indeed, the dipole moment, which indicates the localization of the positive charge in TA-Lys, was almost double that of TA-Ala (84 and 40, respectively), and the highest degree of melanin binding was confirmed for TA-Lys (Santer et al. 2018).

46.2.4.4 Nanoencapsulation

Attempts to further increase iontophoretic drug delivery by incorporating drugs in charged nanoparticles have obtained contradictory results (Malinovskaja-Gomez et al. 2016, 2017; Takeuchi et al. 2017). Nanoparticles with average diameters of approximately 100 nm have much larger hydrodynamic sizes than most of the proteins iontophoresed until now (e.g., cytochrome c has a molecular weight of 12.4 kDa and a Stokes radius of 1.7 nm [La Verde et al. 2017]). Such nanoparticles would also be larger than transient "nano-pores" created under the influence of the electric field, which has estimated ~20 nm of pore radii (Aguilella et al. 1994). As would be expected considering such dimensions, no improvement in drug delivery has been

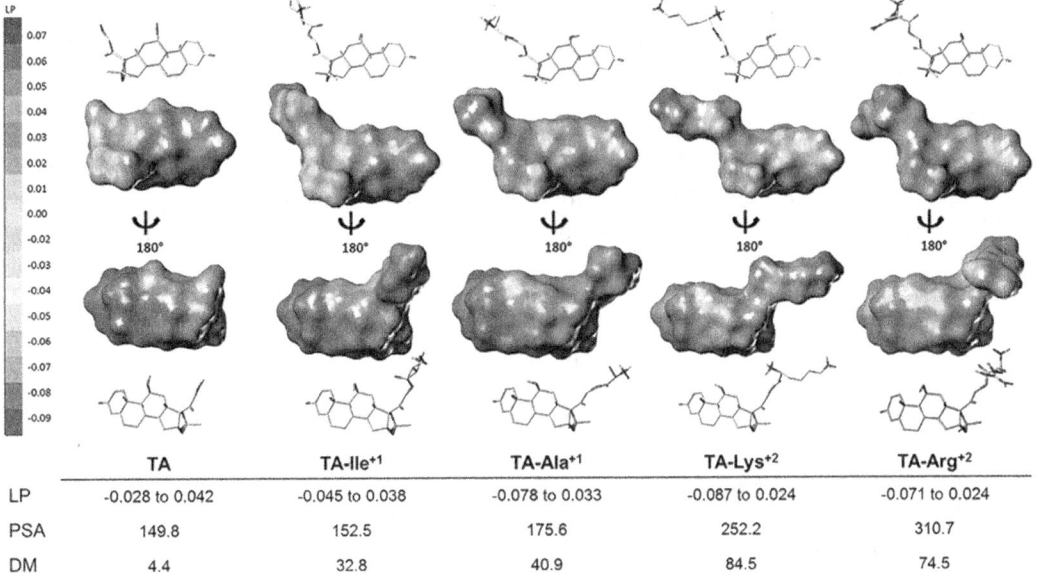

	TA	TA-Ile^{+1}	TA-Ala^{+1}	TA-Lys^{+2}	TA-Arg^{+2}
LP	-0.028 to 0.042	-0.045 to 0.038	-0.078 to 0.033	-0.087 to 0.024	-0.071 to 0.024
PSA	149.8	152.5	175.6	252.2	310.7
DM	4.4	32.8	40.9	84.5	74.5

FIGURE 46.4 Lipophilic surface potentials of TA, TA-Ile, TA-Ala, TA-Lys, and TA-Arg depicted on the minimized molecular conformations of the charged forms of the molecules. The lipophilicity scale ranges from most hydrophilic (−0.09, blue) to most lipophilic (0.07 brown) parts of the surface. LP: minimum/maximum lipophilicity values for each TA entity, PSA: polar surface area and DM: dipole moment, are listed in the table beneath the structures. (Reproduced with permission from Santer et al. 2018.)

observed from nano-encapsulating drugs into negatively charged lipid vesicles compared to free drug formulation (Bernardi et al. 2016; Malinovskaja-Gomez et al. 2017). Also, confocal laser scanning images of porcine skin after *in vitro* iontophoresis of negatively charged fluorescent PLGA nanoparticles loaded with a negatively charged drug were not able to confirm deeper nanoparticle distribution in the skin (Malinovskaja-Gomez et al. 2016). Intriguingly, cathodal iontophoresis of liposomes containing ovalbumin as a model antigen, even though not capable of increasing ovalbumin skin penetration when compared to the free drug, delivered higher protein amounts when silver nanoparticles were added to the formulation. Such nanoparticles were stabilized by Ag counter-ions, with borate and nitrate present in the dispersion; therefore, a negative zeta potential was presented. The authors have hypothesized that silver penetration, being a metal ion, may have facilitated the transport of electric current across the skin (Bernardi et al. 2016). Still, the relative contributions of EM and EO were not evaluated. Another possibility is that silver ions interact with negative skin residues, hindering EO, which would benefit cathodal delivery.

Anodal iontophoresis of positively charged nanoparticles, however, has been shown to lead to nanoparticle accumulation within the appendageal structures under the influence of the electric field. This has been observed with chitosan-coated nanoparticles, even though iontophoresis application resulted in a relatively modest drug delivery enhancement (1.9-fold) in comparison to passive nanoparticle delivery (Takeuchi et al. 2017). Noticeably, even though positively charged, electrophoretic mobility of chitosan-coated PLGA nanoparticles was approximately one-third of the uncoated negatively charged nanoparticle, comparing modulus values (Takeuchi et al. 2017). Again, it could be reasonable to assume that EO may play a significant role in driving nanoparticles to accumulate within appendageal structures. Still, previous studies have demonstrated that chitosan may also interact with negatively charged skin residues, hindering EO (Taveira et al. 2009). Thus, the determination of the relative contributions of EM and EO could be useful for rationally improving formulation efficiency. In such cases, other types of EO "markers" that could simulate only "electroosmotic follicle accumulation enhancement" would be necessary. Even though pilosebaceous units may represent a pathway of less fixed negative charges compared to the stratum corneum, which could mean a smaller volume of solvent flowing towards deeper skin (Lapteva et al. 2020), the hypothesis of nanoparticle electroosmotic follicle accumulation enhancement has been corroborated by other studies. Iontophoresis has been recently employed in an attempt to further enhance the delivery to squamous cell carcinoma of 5-fluorouracil from a type of immunoliposomes, functionalized with cetuximab, an anti-EGFR antibody (Petrilli et al. 2018). The formulation was developed to allow co-administration of the antibody and the chemotherapeutic agent. The authors assumed the lack of 5-fluorouracil recovery from the stratum corneum in all the experiments performed was strong evidence of drug penetration through the appendages, resulting in a higher accumulation in comparison to passive delivery. Still, liposomal encapsulation reduced drug skin penetration compared with the free drug in solution. One of the hypotheses for this was the interaction between the components of the developed nanoformulation and the skin, altering membrane lipophilicity and hence, K_m, decreasing the drug permeation.

Interestingly, functionalized liposomes doubled drug delivery to the viable epidermis, compared with control liposomes, which could be explained by the presence of cetuximab receptors in the viable epidermis. Also, *in vivo* iontophoretic topical treatment, performed in EGFR-overexpressing squamous cell carcinoma xenograft animal models, was more effective than subcutaneous treatment to control tumor growth and reduce cell proliferation, probably because of the better drug distribution throughout the tumor area achieved with iontophoresis in comparison to the subcutaneous injection. Besides, iontophoresis of nanoformulations could control systemic drug exposure, as drug amounts in the receptor chamber following iontophoresis of liposomes were reduced in comparison to drug solution (Petrilli et al. 2018).

46.3   IONTOPHORESIS EVOLUTION

The rationale for the use of iontophoresis in the first fully integrated system or with a disposable patch connected to a reusable controller was to provide a fast-burst release of small, potent molecules. Examples include lidocaine, for topical anesthesia (Iontocaine, IOMED, Inc., UT, USA; Lidosite, Vyteris, Inc., NJ, USA); fentanyl, for pain control (Ionsys, Alza Corporation, CA, USA); and sumatriptan succinate, for migraine treatment (Zecuity, NuPathe, Inc., PA, USA). By then, there was a general understanding that, besides the hydrophilic/charged character, the molecular weight for ideal iontophoresis candidates would be limited to 500 Da (Guy et al. 2000). Indeed, all three drugs had low molecular weight, were readily ionizable, and had good aqueous solubility (lidocaine 234.34 Da, fentanyl 336.47 Da, and sumatriptan succinate 413.49 Da). However, later on, the electrotransport of small to moderately sized proteins was demonstrated. In 2007 cytochrome c, a 12.4-kDa protein, was delivered noninvasively across intact skin. These results led to the belief that there would be a correlation between EM flux across the skin and electrophoretic mobility, which could be measured by capillary zone electrophoresis (CZE) (Chang and Bodmeier 1998). The idea was that the molecular charge could compensate for the higher molecular weight. Further studies on the electrotransport of ribonuclease A (Dubey and Kalia 2010) and ribonuclease T1 (Dubey et al. 2011) provided further support for this hypothesis; however, the surprising results obtained with lysozyme (Dubey and Kalia 2014) suggested that the charge-to-mass ratio and hence electric mobility alone might not be sufficient to predict protein electrotransport across the skin (Figure 46.5) and showed that three-dimensional structures and the spatial distribution of physicochemical properties across the protein surface must also be considered, primarily because the complex three-dimensional

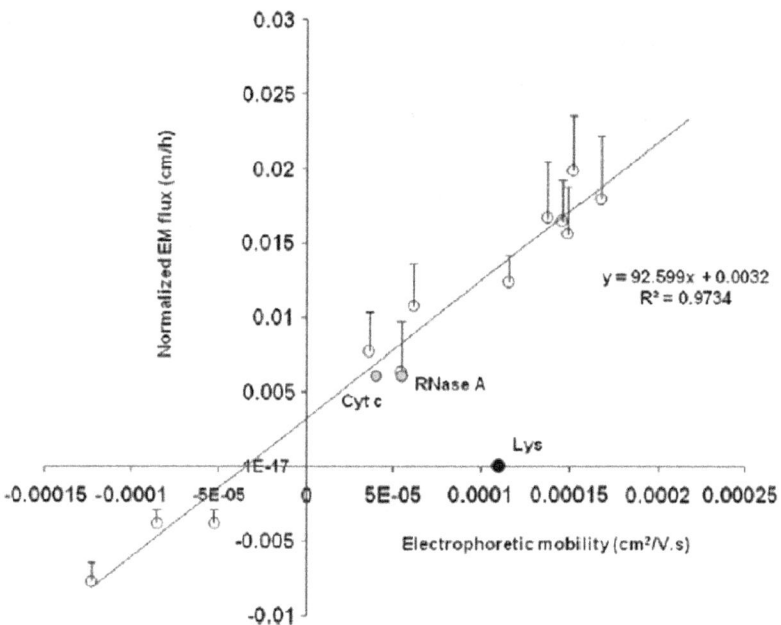

FIGURE 46.5 Correlation between normalized EM flux (J_{norm}-EM, cm/h) and electrophoretic mobility (ui, cm^2/V·s) for a series of small molecules, dipeptides, Cyt c and RNase A. The flux of lysozyme (0.7 mM) is much lower than that expected based on its electrophoretic mobility (J_{norm}-EM = 92.599 ui + 0.003, r^2 = 0.97). This indicates that electrophoretic mobility alone is not sufficient to predict iontophoretic permeation. (Reproduced with permission from Dubey and Kalia 2014.)

structure of proteins can facilitate interactions with cutaneous transport pathways. As previously discussed, localized charge centers may be inconvenient even for the transport of small molecules (Santer et al. 2018).

As mentioned before, iontophoresis was clinically first used to provide a fast-burst release enabling therapeutic drug concentrations to be reached more quickly and hence reducing the time required for the onset of pharmacological action. Still, other features of iontophoresis might be even more relevant in distinguishing it from other technologies for permeation enhancement. One such aspect is the complete external control of delivery kinetics, easily achieved for delivery of molecules that have an insignificant passive permeability. In a delimited area, modulating current parameters, i.e., duration, intensity, and profile; permeated amounts; and penetration depths can be controlled. For example, this has been achieved for polypharmacotherapy with the simultaneous delivery of more than one drug (Cazares-Delgadillo et al. 2016). Another equally relevant aspect of controlling delivery kinetics is delivery efficiency. Recent studies have demonstrated that in a situation where EM was the dominant mechanism for delivery (>80%), input parameters could be controlled, achieving remarkable delivery efficiencies, an equally relevant aspect for a transdermal system that may be the decisive factor for the pharmaceutical industry (Kalaria et al. 2018). Co-iontophoresis of pramipexole (PRAM; dopamine agonist) and rasagiline (RAS; MAO-B inhibitor) achieved delivery efficiencies of ~29% and ~25%, respectively, which corresponded to thirty-eightfold and twenty-sevenfold increases over passive diffusion (Kalaria et al. 2018). Linear correlation of skin deposition and permeation with increased current densities is demonstrated in Figure 46.6. Transport and drug delivery efficiencies of both drugs are shown in Table 46.1.

TABLE 46.1

Transport and Drug Delivery Efficiencies of PRAM and RAS as a Function of Applied Current Density[a]

Current (mA/cm^2)	% Transport Efficiency[b]		% Delivery Efficiency	
	PRAM	RAS	PRAM	RAS
0.15	3.05	3.01	10.1	10.3
0.3	2.99	2.69	19.8	18.1
0.5	2.58	2.3	29.0	25.8

[a] 20 mM PRAM and 20 mM RAS in 25 mM MES (pH 5.3) with 26 mM sodium metabisulfite.

[b] Transport efficiency = transport number (t_D) × 100%.

Source: Adapted and reproduced with permission from Kalaria et al. 2018.

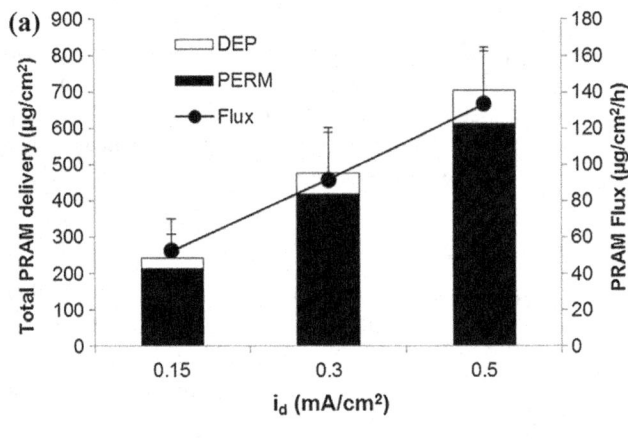

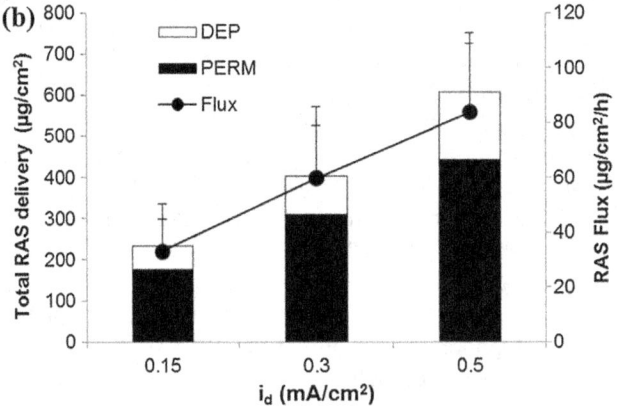

FIGURE 46.6 Total delivery (skin deposition + permeation) and steady-state fluxes of (a) PRAM and (b) RAS at different current densities after six hours of co-iontophoresis with a donor concentration of 20 mM of each drug in 25 mM MES pH 5.3 with 26 mM sodium metabisulfite. (Adapted and reproduced with permission from Kalaria et al. 2018.)

Moreover, the capability to target specific tissues minimizing systemic distribution (Petrilli et al. 2018), allied with the low levels of irritation at the application site with the use of low current densities, has made iontophoresis very appealing not only for the pharmaceutical but also for the cosmetic industry, which has already launched cosmetic devices for iontophoresis application. As desired for topical dermatological therapies, delivery should be controlled for the active to cross the stratum corneum and reach the viable epidermis in therapeutic amounts but to avoid entry into the circulatory system in the dermis, so that possible side effects are reduced (del Rio-Sancho et al. 2017). Even though some permeation is attained in the dermis, results have demonstrated a local enhanced topical delivery to subjacent muscle (Gratieri et al. 2014), by which, controlling the delivered dose, it might be possible to restrict relevant systemic distributed amounts. Besides, as iontophoresis increases skin penetration through the routes of least electric resistance, targeted appendageal delivery can be achieved employing appropriate formulations, which may be beneficial for the treatment of many dermatological disorders, e.g., alopecia (Gelfuso et al. 2013, 2015) and acne (Kurokawa et al. 2017). Advantages, disadvantages, and limitations of iontophoresis from the topical dermatological/cosmetic perspective are presented in Table 46.2.

Most cosmetic devices launched follow the same rationale and are similar to any other iontophoretic patch (Figure 46.7a), i.e., a flexible patch adhesive to the skin containing some active ingredient that would ideally have its skin retention increased. Still, different forms of iontophoretic applicators currently on the market have been designed to be moved manually over the skin (Figure 46.7b). Some of these miniaturized devices can even perform both sonophoresis and iontophoresis, separately or simultaneously (Park et al. 2019). The possible disadvantage of these types of devices might be the imprecision over the total cosmetic active ingredient delivered because of the lack of control of the area subjected to iontophoretic current. Generally, the iontophoresed area, for the calculation of current density, is assumed to be the one corresponding to the microcontroller area directly in contact with the skin. However, depending on the amount of formulation applied and the extent to which the formulation is spread, the current might be dispersed beyond the microcontroller's limits. Thus, current density control is not precise, is challenging to establish, and may vary depending on device movement. Rapid movements could simulate a condition of "turning on and off" the electric current application depending on the location of the device, i.e., the skin region under the current influence would be "on," while the skin not directly in contact with the device at that moment would be "off."

TABLE 46.2

Main Advantages and Disadvantages/Limitations of Iontophoresis for Topical Dermatological/Cosmetic Purposes

	Advantages	Disadvantages/ Limitations
Dermatological/ Cosmetic Formulation	Noninvasive	Only for hydrophilic drugs
	Skin remains intact	Current limited to 0.5 mA/cm^2
	Controlled delivery	High costs
	Higher drug penetration across the stratum corneum	May need long application periods for some molecules
	Rapid onset and offset	Difficult to cover large areas
	Targeted delivery: reduction of possible toxic effects	
	Possibility of follicle targeting	

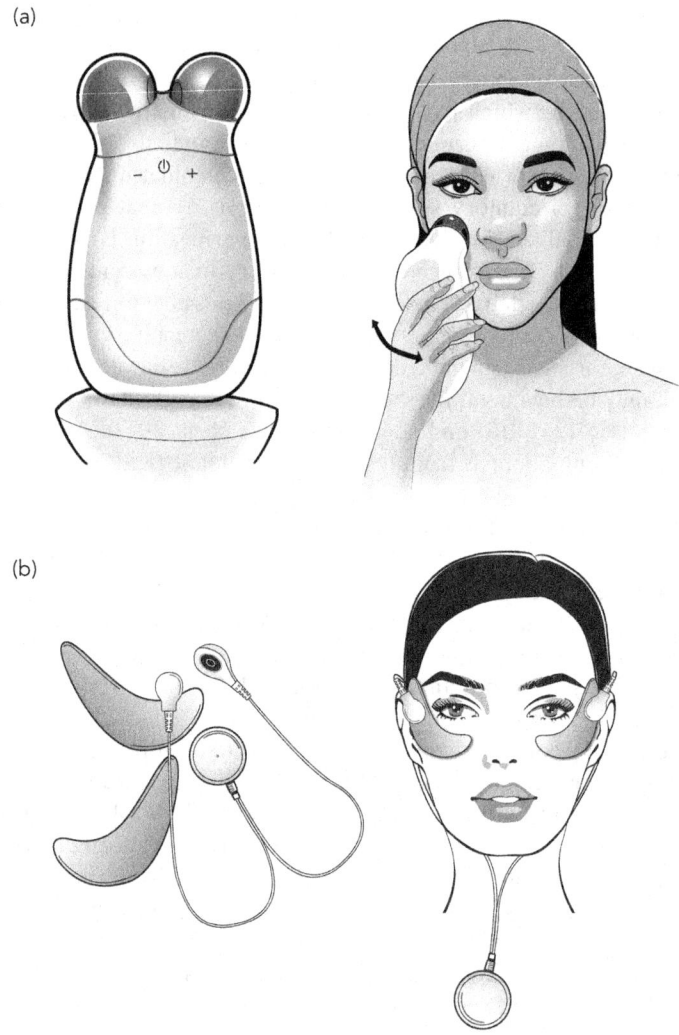

FIGURE 46.7 Representation of cosmetic iontophoretic devices applied on the skin: (a) mobile device applicator and (b) active iontophoretic patch device.

Such a form of application could be compared to pulsed current iontophoresis, which has so far failed to demonstrate conclusive evidence of advantages over constant current application (Malinovskaja-Gomez et al. 2017).

46.4 CONCLUSION

Iontophoresis has proven itself to be capable of quickly and effectively delivering significant amounts of drug and active ingredients in a controlled manner to the upper layers of the skin through an intact stratum corneum without compromising skin physiology. In the past few years, overall comprehension of the technique, the underlying transport mechanisms, and the variables affecting drug transport have all been increased. This is reflected by the evolution of the strategies to further increase drug delivery, which evolved from simply altering electrical and formulation parameters to effectively synthesizing better drug candidates. The evolution of patches and microcontrollers for current application allied with a new pool of drug candidates might broaden the significance of iontophoresis in the drug delivery market.

REFERENCES

Abla, N., A. Naik, R. H. Guy, and Y. N. Kalia. 2005. Contributions of electromigration and electroosmosis to peptide iontophoresis across intact and impaired skin. Journal of Controlled Release 108 (2-3):319–330.

Aguilella, V., K. Kontturi, L. Murtomaki, and P. Ramirez. 1994. Estimation of the pore-size and charge-density in human cadaver skin. Journal of Controlled Release 32 (3):249–257.

Banerjee, A., R. Chen, S. Arafin, and S. Mitragotri. 2019. Intestinal iontophoresis from mucoadhesive patches: A strategy for oral delivery. Journal of Controlled Release 297:71–78.

Bayon, A. M. R., and R. H. Guy. 1996. Iontophoresis of nafarelin across human skin in vitro. Pharmaceutical Research 13 (5):798–800.

Bernardi, D. S., C. Bitencourt, D. S. C. da Silveira, E. L. C. M. da Cruz, M. A. Pereira-da-Silva, L. H. Faccioli, and R. F. V. Lopez. 2016. Effective transcutaneous immunization using a combination of iontophoresis and nanoparticles. Journal of Nanomedicine and Nanotechnology 12 (8):2439–2448.

Bouissou, C. C., J. P. Sylvestre, R. H. Guy, and M. B. Delgado-Charro. 2009. Reverse iontophoresis of amino acids: Identification and separation of stratum corneum and subdermal sources in vitro. Pharmaceutical Research 26 (12):2630–2638.

Cazares-Delgadillo, J., A. Ganem-Rondero, V. Merino, and Y. N. Kalia. 2016. Controlled transdermal iontophoresis for poly-pharmacotherapy: Simultaneous delivery of granisetron, metoclopramide and dexamethasone sodium phosphate in vitro and in vivo. European Journal of Pharmaceutical Sciences 85:31–38.

Cazares-Delgadillo, J., A. Naik, A. Ganem-Rondero, D. Quintanar-Guerrero, and Y. N. Kalia. 2007. Transdermal delivery of cytochrome c-a 12.4 kda protein-across intact skin by constant-current iontophoresis. Pharmaceutical Research 24 (7):1360–1368.

Chang, C. M., and R. Bodmeier. 1998. Low viscosity monoglyceride-based drug delivery systems transforming into a highly viscous cubic phase. International Journal of Pharmaceutics 173 (1-2):51–60.

Chen, Y., I. Alberti, and Y. N. Kalia. 2016a. Topical iontophoretic delivery of ionizable, biolabile aciclovir prodrugs: A rational approach to improve cutaneous bioavailability (vol 99, pg 103, 2016). European Journal of Pharmaceutics and Biopharmaceutics 102:19–19.

Chen, Y., and Y. N. Kalia. 2018. Short-duration ocular iontophoresis of ionizable aciclovir prodrugs: A new approach to treat herpes simplex infections in the anterior and posterior segments of the eye. International Journal of Pharmaceutics 536 (1):292–300.

Chen, Y., T. Zahui, I. Alberti, and Y. N. Kalia. 2016b. Cutaneous biodistribution of ionizable, biolabile aciclovir prodrugs after short duration topical iontophoresis: Targeted intraepidermal drug delivery. European Journal of Pharmaceutics and Biopharmaceutics 99:94–102.

Curdy, C., Y. N. Kalia, F. Falson-Rieg, and R. H. Guy. 2000. Recovery of human skin impedance in vivo after iontophoresis: Effect of metal ions. AAPS PharmSciTech 2 (3).

Curdy, C., Y. N. Kalia, and R. H. Guy. 2002. Post-iontophoresis recovery of human skin impedance in vivo. European Journal of Pharmaceutics and Biopharmaceutics 53 (1):15–21.

Degim, I. T., S. Ilbasmis, R. Dundaroz, and Y. Oguz. 2003. Reverse iontophoresis: A non-invasive technique for measuring blood urea level. Pediatric Nephrology 18 (10):1032–1037.

del Rio-Sancho, S., C. Cros, B. Coutaz, M. Cuendet, and Y. N. Kalia. 2017. Cutaneous iontophoresis of mu-conotoxin cniiic-a potent na(v)1.4 antagonist with analgesic, anaesthetic and myorelaxant properties. International Journal of Pharmaceutics 518 (1-2):59–65.

Delgado-Charro, M. B., and R. H. Guy. 2001. Transdermal iontophoresis for controlled drug delivery and non-invasive monitoring. STP Pharma Sciences 11 (6):403–414.

Delgado-Charro, M. B., and R. H. Guy. 2003. Transdermal reverse iontophoresis of valproate: A noninvasive method for therapeutic drug monitoring. Pharmaceutical Research 20 (9):1508–1513.

Delgadocharro, M. B., A. M. Rodriguezbayon, and R. H. Guy. 1995. Iontophoresis of nafarelin - effects of current-density and concentration on electrotransport in-vitro. Journal of Controlled Release 35 (1):35–40.

Djabri, A., W. van't Hoff, P. Brock, I. C. K. Wong, R. H. Guy, and M. B. Delgado-Charro. 2009. Non-invasive assessment of renal function via transdermal reverse iontophoresis of iohexol: A pilot study. Therapeutic Drug Monitoring 31 (5):617–617.

Dragicevic, N., and H. Maibach. 2018. Combined use of nanocarriers and physical methods for percutaneous penetration enhancement. Advanced Drug Delivery Reviews 127:58–84.

Dubey, S., and Y. N. Kalia. 2010. Non-invasive iontophoretic delivery of enzymatically active ribonuclease a (13.6 kda) across intact porcine and human skins. Journal of Controlled Release 145 (3):203–209.

Dubey, S., and Y. N. Kalia. 2014. Understanding the poor iontophoretic transport of lysozyme across the skin: When high charge and high electrophoretic mobility are not enough. Journal of Controlled Release 183:35–42.

Dubey, S., R. Perozzo, L. Scapozza, and Y. N. Kalia. 2011. Noninvasive transdermal iontophoretic delivery of biologically active human basic fibroblast growth factor. Molecular Pharmacology 8 (4):1322–1331.

Gelfuso, G. M., M. A. D. Barros, M. B. Delgado-Charro, R. H. Guy, and R. F. V. Lopez. 2015. Iontophoresis of minoxidil sulphate loaded microparticles, a strategy for follicular drug targeting? Colloid Surface B 134:408–412.

Gelfuso, G. M., T. Gratieri, M. Delgado-Charro, R. H. Guy, and R. F. V. Lopez. 2013. Iontophoresis-targeted, follicular delivery of minoxidil sulfate for the treatment of alopecia. Journal of Pharmaceutical Sciences 102 (5):1488–1494.

Giri, T. K., S. Chakrabarty, and B. Ghosh. 2017. Transdermal reverse iontophoresis: A novel technique for therapeutic drug monitoring. Journal of Controlled Release 246:30–38.

Giri, T. K., B. Ghosh, P. Bose, S. Saha, and A. Sarkar. 2019. Extraction of levetiracetam for therapeutic drug monitoring by transdermal reverse iontophoresis. European Journal of Pharmaceutical Sciences 128:54–60.

Gnann, J. W., N. H. Barton, R. J. Whitley, T. W. Chang, and W. L. Rock. 1983. Acyclovir - mechanism of action, pharmacokinetics, safety and clinical-applications. Pharmacotherapy 3 (5):275–283.

Gratieri, T., and Y. N. Kalia. 2013. Mathematical models to describe iontophoretic transport in vitro and in vivo and the effect of current application on the skin barrier. Advanced Drug Delivery Reviews 65 (2):315–29.

Gratieri, T., E. Pujol-Bello, G. M. Gelfuso, J. G. de Souza, R. F. V. Lopez, and Y. N. Kalia. 2014. Iontophoretic transport kinetics of ketorolac in vitro and in vivo: Demonstrating local enhanced topical drug delivery to muscle. European Journal of Pharmaceutics and Biopharmaceutics 86 (2):219–226.

Gratieri, T., V. Santer, and Y. N. Kalia. 2017. Basic principles and current status of transcorneal and trans-scleral iontophoresis. Expert Opinion on Drug Delivery 14 (9):1091–1102.

Guy, R. H., Y. N. Kalia, M. B. Delgado-Charro, V. Merino, A. Lopez, and D. Marro. 2000. Iontophoresis: Electrorepulsion and electroosmosis. Journal of Controlled Release 64 (1-3):129–132.

Kalaria, D. R., P. Patel, V. Merino, V. B. Patravale, and Y. N. Kalia. 2014. Controlled iontophoretic delivery of pramipexole: Electrotransport kinetics in vitro and in vivo. European Journal of Pharmaceutics and Biopharmaceutics 88 (1):56–63.

Kalaria, D. R., P. Patel, V. Patravale, and Y. N. Kalia. 2012. Comparison of the cutaneous iontophoretic delivery of rasagiline and selegiline across porcine and human skin in vitro. International Journal of Pharmaceutics 438 (1-2):202–208.

Kalaria, D. R., M. Singhal, V. Patravale, V. Merino, and Y. N. Kalia. 2018. Simultaneous controlled iontophoretic delivery of pramipexole and rasagiline in vitro and in vivo: Transdermal polypharmacy to treat parkinson's disease. European Journal of Pharmaceutics and Biopharmaceutics 127:204–212.

Kalia, Y. N., A. Naik, J. Garrison, and R. H. Guy. 2004. Iontophoretic drug delivery. Advanced Drug Delivery Reviews 56 (5):619–658.

Kalia, Y. N., L. B. Nonato, and R. H. Guy. 1996. The effect of iontophoresis on skin barrier integrity: Non-invasive evaluation by impedance spectroscopy and transepidermal water loss. Pharmaceutical Research 13 (6):957–960.

Kasting, G. B. 1992. Theoretical-models for iontophoretic delivery. Advanced Drug Delivery Reviews 9 (2-3):177–199.

Kurokawa, I., N. Oiso, and A. Kawada. 2017. Adjuvant alternative treatment with chemical peeling and subsequent iontophoresis for postinflammatory hyperpigmentation, erosion with inflamed red papules and non-inflamed atrophic scars in acne vulgaris. Journal of Dermatology 44 (4):401–405.

La Verde, V., P. Dominici, and A. Astegno. 2017. Determination of hydrodynamic radius of proteins by size exclusion chromatography. Bio-Protocol 7 (8).

Lapteva, M., M. A. Sallam, A. Goyon, D. Guillarme, J. L. Veuthey, and Y. N. Kalia. 2020. Non-invasive targeted iontophoretic delivery of cetuximab to skin. Expert Opinion in Drug Delivery 17 (4):589–602.

Ledger, P.W. 1992. Skin biological issues in electrically enhanced transdermal delivery. Advanced Drug Delivery Reviews 9 (2–3):307.

Lobo, S., and G. Yan. 2018. Improving the direct penetration into tissues underneath the skin with iontophoresis delivery of a ketoprofen cationic prodrug. International Journal of Pharmaceutics 535 (1-2):228–236.

Malinovskaja-Gomez, K., S. Espuelas, M. J. Garrido, J. Hirvonen, and T. Laaksonen. 2017. Comparison of liposomal drug formulations for transdermal iontophoretic drug delivery. European Journal of Pharmaceutical Sciences 106:294–301.

Malinovskaja-Gomez, K., H. I. Labouta, M. Schneider, J. Hirvonen, and T. Laaksonen. 2016. Transdermal iontophoresis of flufenamic acid loaded PLGA nanoparticles. European Journal of Pharmaceutical Sciences 89:154–162.

Marro, D., Guy, R. H., Delgado-charro, M. B. 2001. Characterization of the iontophoretic permselectivity properties of human and pig skin. J Control Release. 70(1-2):213–217.

Park, J., H. Lee, G. S. Lim, N. Kim, D. Kim, and Y. C. Kim. 2019. Enhanced transdermal drug delivery by sonophoresis and simultaneous application of sonophoresis and iontophoresis. AAPS PharmSciTech 20 (3):96.

Patel, S. R., H. Zhong, A. Sharma, and Y. N. Kalia. 2009. Controlled non-invasive transdermal iontophoretic delivery of zolmitriptan hydrochloride in vitro and in vivo. European Journal of Pharmaceutics and Biopharmaceutics 72 (2):304–309.

Petrilli, R., J. O. Eloy, F. P. Saggioro, D. L. Chesca, M. C. de Souza, M. V. S. Dias, L. L. P. daSilva, R. J. Lee, and R. F. V. Lopez. 2018. Skin cancer treatment effectiveness is improved by iontophoresis of EGFR-targeted liposomes containing 5-fu compared with subcutaneous injection. Journal of Controlled Release 283:151–162.

Pham, Q. D., S. Bjorklund, J. Engblom, D. Topgaard, and E. Sparr. 2016. Chemical penetration enhancers in stratum corneum - relation between molecular effects and barrier function. Journal of Controlled Release 232:175–187.

Phipps, J. B., and J. R. Gyory. 1992. Transdermal ion migration. Advanced Drug Delivery Reviews 9 (2-3):137–176.

Phipps, J. B., R. V. Padmanabhan, and G. A. Lattin. 1989. Iontophoretic delivery of model inorganic and drug ions. Journal of Pharmaceutical Sciences 78 (5):365–369.

Pikal, M. J. 1992. The role of electroosmotic flow in transdermal iontophoresis. Advanced Drug Delivery Reviews 9 (2–3):201–237.

Potts, R. O., and R. H. Guy. 1992. Predicting skin permeability. Pharmaceutical Research 9 (5):663–669.

Sage, B. H., and J. E. Riviere. 1992. Model systems in iontophoresis transport efficacy. Advanced Drug Delivery Reviews 9 (2–3):265–287.

Santer, V., Y. Chen, and Y. N. Kalia. 2018. Controlled non-invasive iontophoretic delivery of triamcinolone acetonide amino acid ester prodrugs into the posterior segment of the eye. European Journal of Pharmaceutics and Biopharmaceutics 132:157–167.

Scheuplein, R. J. 1976. Permeability of skin - review of major concepts and some new developments. Journal of Investigative Dermatology 67 (5):672–676.

Schuetz, Y. B., P. A. Carrupt, A. Naik, R. H. Guy, and Y. N. Kalia. 2006. Structure-permeation relationships for the non-invasive transdermal delivery of cationic peptides by iontophoresis. European Journal of Pharmaceutical Sciences 29 (1):53–59.

Sieg, A., R. H. Guy, and M. B. A. Delgado-Charro. 2003. Reverse iontophoresis for noninvasive glucose monitoring: The internal standard concept. Journal of Pharmaceutical Sciences 92 (11):2295–2302.

Takeuchi, I., T. Takeshita, T. Suzuki, and K. Makino. 2017. Iontophoretic transdermal delivery using chitosan-coated plga nanoparticles for positively charged drugs. Colloid Surface B 160:520–526.

Taveira, S. F., A. Nomizo, and R. F. V. Lopez. 2009. Effect of the iontophoresis of a chitosan gel on doxorubicin skin penetration and cytotoxicity. Journal of Controlled Release 134 (1):35–40.

Turner, N. G., Y. N. Kalia, and R. H. Guy. 1997. The effect of current on skin barrier function in vivo: Recovery kinetics post-iontophoresis. Pharmaceutical Research 14 (9):1252–1257.

47 Vehicles and Topical Therapy

Christian Surber
University Hospital Zurich, Zürich, Switzerland

CONTENTS

47.1 PARTICULARITY OF TOPICAL THERAPY

Topical therapies offer a unique advantage in that products (Figure 47.1) for treatment are applied directly to the affected skin, resulting in a local, prolonged, and intimate contact of product and skin. Therefore, ingredients forming the vehicle play a crucial role in the absorption of actives. They are able to transiently decrease the skin barrier function by various mechanisms. Some active-free vehicles show substantial clinical effects, e.g., commonly used vehicle ingredients (petrolatum, glycerin, dimethicone) have demonstrated efficacy in skin barrier repair and symptom relief in steroid-responsive conditions. Hence, vehicle ingredients of topical products may evolve intrinsic effects that may be clinically substantial.

47.2 VEHICLE TERMINOLOGIES

A rich vocabulary used by regulatory bodies, industry, scientists, health care professionals, patients, and consumers has evolved to describe the vehicle of topical products. Vehicle formats are often associated with the conveyance of specific effects (Figure 47.2).

47.3 METAMORPHOSIS OF THE VEHICLE

The format of topical products containing volatile vehicle ingredients may change dramatically after application onto the skin (Figure 47.3a and b). It becomes obvious that vehicles on the skin after application may be very different from vehicles in their primary container. Conclusions referring to effects originating from the vehicle format in the primary container are not possible. The paradigm—often disseminated for topical corticosteroids—that ointments are more potent than creams and creams are more potent than lotions is not generally valid.

47.4 VEHICLE CHOICE

Adjusted vehicle polarity and viscosity lead to an optimal contact between the vehicle and affected skin and allow an uncomplicated application and distribution on the skin (Figure 47.4).

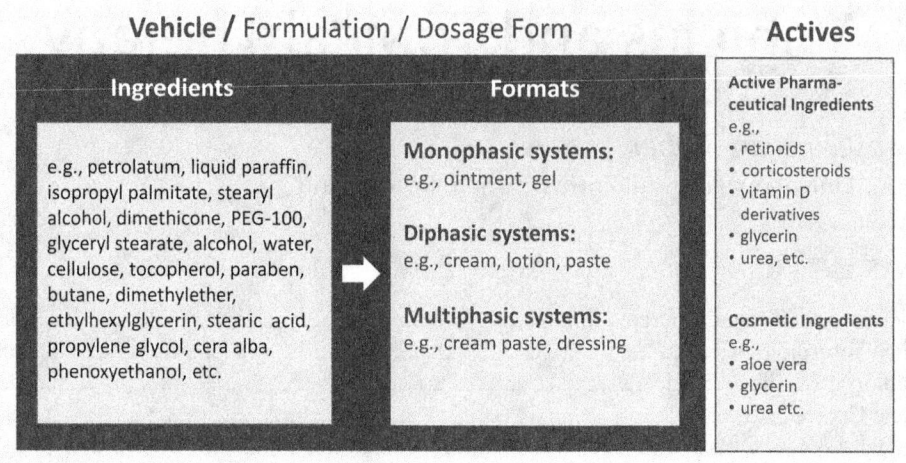

FIGURE 47.1 Topical dermatologic products are typically composed of an active and a vehicle, ranging widely in their physicochemical and textural nature. They are applied to diverse body surfaces of different properties (wet/dry, mucous/nonmucous, healthy/diseased) and sizes. The nature of the vehicle should be adapted to the nature of the skin to be treated to optimize application and contact of product with skin (see Figure 47.4). All vehicles are made of vehicle ingredients. Depending on their physicochemical nature and the manufacturing process, a three-dimensional structural matrix or typical vehicle format evolves, e.g., monophasic (ointment), biphasic (cream), or tri-/multiphasic systems (cream paste). For all formats, both lipophilic and hydrophilic forms exist. Some formats are defined in pharmacopoeias. Note that differences between pharmacopoeias exist (1, 2). The vehicle has the task of keeping an active stable and making it bioavailable, i.e., releasing and delivering it to the target site once applied to the skin. Also note that certain ingredients may act as vehicle ingredient, active pharmaceutical ingredient, or cosmetic ingredient (e.g., glycerin).

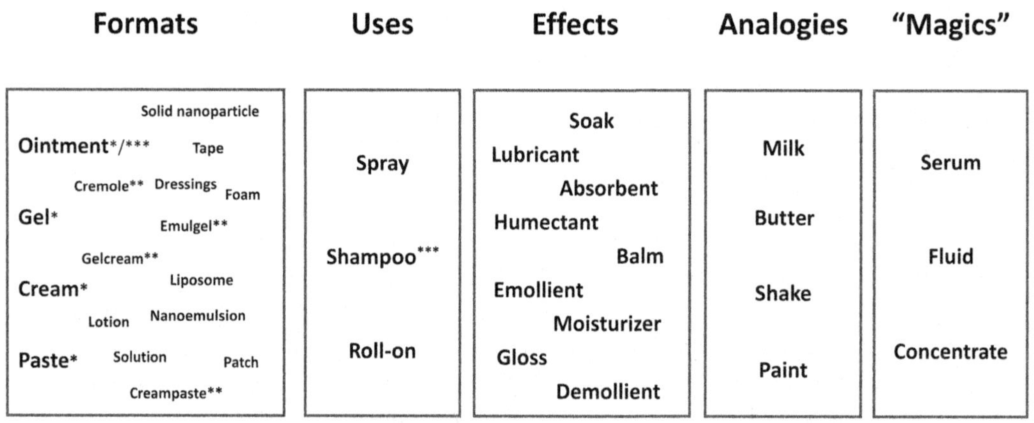

Formats	Uses	Effects	Analogies	"Magics"
Solid nanoparticle Ointment*/*** Tape Cremole** Dressings Foam Gel* Emulgel** Gelcream** Liposome Cream* Lotion Nanoemulsion Paste* Solution Patch Creampaste**	Spray Shampoo*** Roll-on	Soak Lubricant Absorbent Humectant Balm Emollient Moisturizer Gloss Demollient	Milk Butter Shake Paint	Serum Fluid Concentrate

FIGURE 47.2 Widely used terms to describe topical vehicles may be grouped according to their formats, uses, effects, analogies, or "magic" effects. The various designations describe large product groups (e.g., gel, hydrogel, lipogel, emulgel and gelcream, or moisturizer and emollient, etc.), which can be very different in their composition and properties. It is not possible to derive the properties from designations without knowing their exact composition. Colloquial expressions, personal experience, and recommendations have shaped our perceptions and expectations of product vehicles. Quality (translucent/sticky), effect (cooling/occlusive), and use/target (young skin/diseased skin) are often associated with distinct product formats (gel/ointment). *Designations of pharmacopeias (1, 2). **Format combinations are often created for marketing purposes. ***Origin and history of vehicle designations have shaped the meaning and perception of vehicles, e.g., the designation "ointment" derives from the word "anointment"—the application of oil (lipophilic) in a religious ceremony. The designation "shampoo" comes from the Indian language and means "to massage in."

(a)

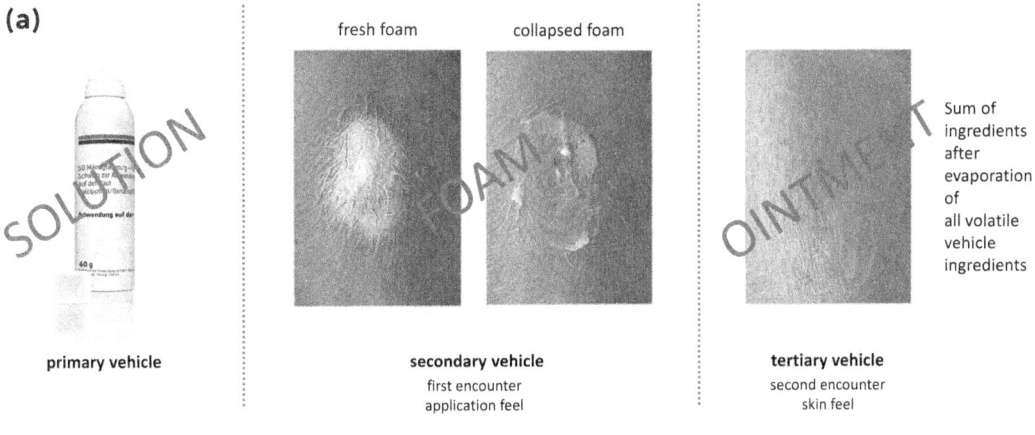

(b)

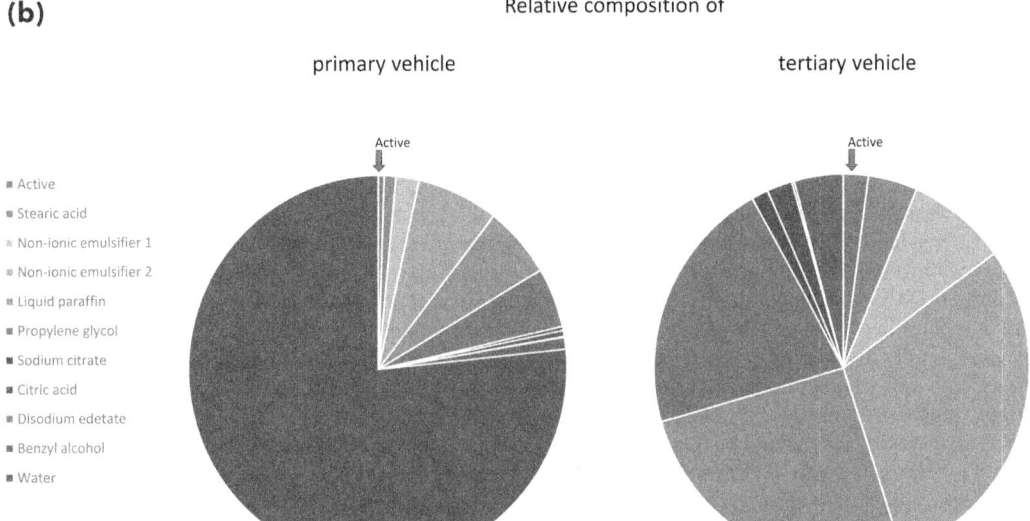

FIGURE 47.3 (**a**) Many topical products contain significant amounts of volatile vehicle ingredients (e.g., water, ethanol, propylene glycol, short-chained hydrocarbons) evaporating once applied onto the skin. After application, the sum of vehicle ingredients, and hence the vehicle format, may change dramatically. This phenomenon is coined the metamorphosis of the vehicle. It is often observed and generates a patient or consumer perception that is described as "the product is well absorbed." To illustrate this phenomenon concisely, the application of a pressurized product is presented. The primary vehicle is housed in the primary container. It ensures stability of actives during shelf-life. The secondary vehicle delivers the first product encounter with the skin and conveys the application feel. The tertiary vehicle delivers the second encounter with the skin and conveys the skin feel. The latter represents the sum of ingredients after evaporation of all volatile vehicle ingredients. In terms of designations, the product format changes from a solution (in the pressurized can) that is sprayed onto the skin to form a foam that collapses to become an ointment. (**b**) During the metamorphosis, the composition of the vehicle ingredients may change dramatically. It is obvious that the physicochemical sphere for an active in the vehicle alters. As a consequence, permeation of an active through skin may decrease (due to precipitation) or increase (due to supersaturation) (3). Effects originating from specific vehicle ingredients are documented (e.g., propylene glycol may be considered an absorption enhancer, petrolatum has an occlusive effect). However, it remains difficult to assign quantitative effect information to a single vehicle ingredient if it is part of a complex formulation with many other vehicle ingredients, some of which may evaporate after application.

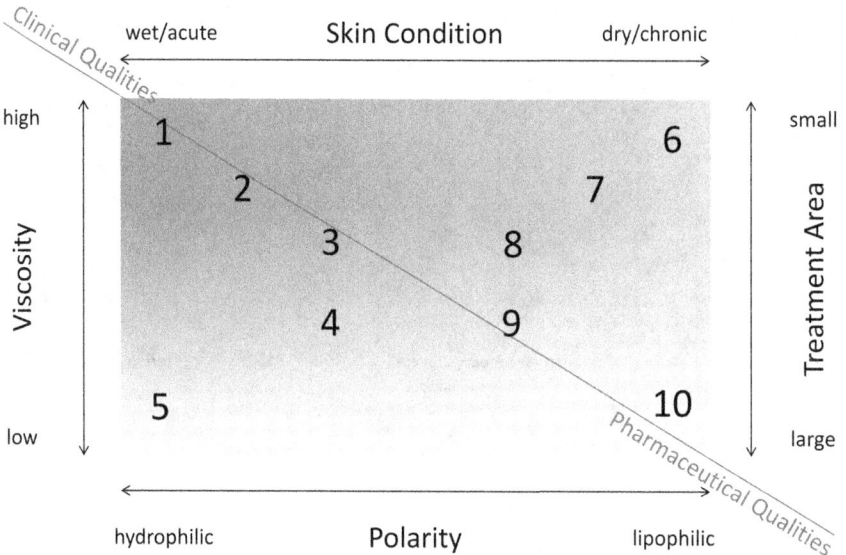

FIGURE 47.4 The vehicle choice is based on the nature of the vehicle (polarity and viscosity) and the nature of the dermatosis (treatment area and skin condition). Polarity (x-axis, bottom) and viscosity (y-axis, left) are relevant pharmaceutical vehicle qualities to consider. Hydrophilic vehicles are more suitable for wet/acute skin conditions, and lipophilic vehicles are more suitable for dry/chronic skin conditions (x-axis, top). Low-viscosity vehicles are more suitable for larger skin areas, whereas high-viscosity vehicles are more suitable for smaller skin areas (y-axis, right). Typical vehicle formats are (1) cross-linked hyaluronic acid gel (cubed water); (2) hydro-gel, hydrophilic ointment; (3) o/w-cream; (4) o/w- or hydro-lotion; (5) aqueous solution; (6) lipstick; (7) lipo-gel, lipophilic ointment; (8) w/o-cream; (9) w/o- or lipo-lotion; (10) lipophilic solution (oil). The diagram allows one to relate pharmaceutical and clinical qualities. A sensory evaluation of product polarity and viscosity by the health care professional, patient, and consumer is usually sufficient to make the right choice. To ensure therapy adherence, the patient's preference for particular vehicle textures, practicability of therapy modalities, and prescription of adequate amounts of product are crucial. To increase cosmetic acceptance, visible skin areas should be treated in such a way that it does not worsen the skin's aspect. Facial skin should not be treated with too lipophilic (greasy) vehicles to prevent shining, and the scalp is usually treated with solutions containing glycerin as a humectant. Vehicles on intertriginous skin should not increase friction. Vehicles with a high proportion of rapidly evaporating ingredients may be difficult to spread. The washability of a vehicle can be clinically relevant (skin and wound cleansing). Suitability of a vehicle predominantly depends on the physicochemical properties of the vehicle ingredients (hydro-/lipophilic, emulsifying) and not on the vehicle format.

47.5 PRACTICAL ASPECTS

To avoid treatment failures, explicit instructions on quantity to be applied per area and time should be given. This requires that areas of disease involvement and amount of product that can realistically be used and still be physically acceptable to the patient treating himself or herself at home has been estimated. A realistic application quantity is rarely more than 5 mg/cm^2. For semi-solid vehicles, the fingertip unit (400 to 500 mg) and for more liquid vehicles a mechanical dosage aid (e.g., pump with weight data per pump stroke), both with dosing tables and instructions, have proven value. The frequency of administration and duration of treatment are often determined on an individual basis.

Typical therapy modalities have been developed to avoid adverse effects (corticosteroids, retinoids). Patients apply medicated product on a daily basis only until symptoms improve (corticosteroids) or irritation occurs (retinoids) and then reduce application frequency. On days without medicated treatment, nonmedicated products are recommended. Localized and systemic adverse effects may occur. Almost any component of a topical product may sensitize or irritate; notable examples include vehicle ingredients (propylene glycol), preservatives, fragrances, or actives (corticosteroids). Patients with chronic wounds (incontinence-associated dermatosis, leg ulcer) appear to be particularly susceptible. Extensive, frequent, and/or long-term application of topical products with small molecular actives (salicylic acid, crotamiton, imiquimod) may lead to considerable systemic absorption. Due to a different body weight–to–body surface ratio, this hazard is increased in newborns, infants, and children. Dermatological products are grouped into three different regulatory categories. Medicinal products and medical devices are used for diseased skin, and cosmetics are used to protect and to keep the skin in good condition. For medicinal products and medical devices, disease-related claims are allowed, whereas for cosmetics, they are not allowed. The effect of medicinal products is based on pharmacological and immunological principles, and the effect of medical devices is based on nonpharmacological and nonimmunological principles. The demarcation between diseased and nondiseased skin is fluent (xerotic vs. dry skin), and, accordingly, all three product categories may be used for gradually similar skin conditions. Terms like cosmeceutical—a word created from *cosmetics* and *pharmaceuticals*—and cosmetic active—analogous to the regulatory term *active pharmaceutical ingredient*—or claims such as "for atopic-prone skin" are used in an attempt to valorize specific products of the category "cosmetics." This is sometimes a source of confusion, debate, and regulatory intervention.

REFERENCES

1. USP 41 (1.5.2019). <1151> Pharmaceutical Dosage Forms.
2. European Pharmacopoeia 9.0 (1.1.2017). Semi-Solid Preparations for Cutaneous Application.
3. Surber C, Knie U. Metamorphosis of Vehicles: Mechanisms and Opportunities. Curr Probl Dermatol. 2018;54:152–165.

48 The Role of *In Vitro* Skin Models in Optimization of Dermal Drug Delivery

Gøril Eide Flaten and Nataša Škalko-Basnet
University of Tromsø The Arctic University of Norway, Tromsø, Norway

Željka Vanić
University of Zagreb, Zagreb, Croatia

CONTENTS

48.1 INTRODUCTION

Although the skin offers a readily accessible surface for potential drug absorption and its structure is well defined, successful (trans)dermal therapy remains a challenge (Lam and Gambari, 2014).

Well-defined skin models, able to identify and evaluate the properties of the formulation crucial for the success of (trans)dermal therapy, are expected to shorten the developmental stage, assist in optimization, and reduce the need for animal and human studies.

The "golden standard" skin penetration model is the *in vivo* test in humans. However, due to ethical and cost concerns, *in vivo* human studies are strongly discouraged in the early stages of formulation development (Planz et al., 2016). Moreover, due to intravariability and inter-variability in subjects, the formulation features might be overseen and valuable information lost (Ilić et al., 2017). The use of *in vivo* animal models has been the main alternative to the *in vivo* studies until the prohibition of animal testing for toxicological concerns of cosmetic ingredients (EU, 76/768/EEC, February 2003) emphasized the need for other alternatives (Van Gele, et al., 2011). Excised animal skin has shown to be an attractive alternative approach, offering collection of a large number of data. However, availability of human skin is often restricted, and *ex vivo* animal skin was proposed as a suitable replacement. The most widely used technique to assess drug penetration through *ex vivo* human/animal skin is the Franz diffusion cell (Patel et al., 2016). Among the potential animal species to serve as skin donors, pig skin has been found to be the most reliable, considering the human/animal correlation due to similarities in histology, hair density, and skin thickness (Sintov, 2017). Newborn pig skin has also been proposed, since a good flux correlation of lipophilic substances has been confirmed for newborn pig and human skin (Cilurzo et al., 2007). However, pig *stratum corneum* (SC) comprises lipids organized in a hexagonal lattice in contrast to the orthorhombic organization of human SC (Silva Garcia Praça et al., 2018). In general, the penetration through animal skin is higher compared to human, and the findings need to be evaluated with precautions (Schaefer et al., 2008).

Human skin equivalents are increasingly used as an alternative to animal models. The early work relied on the use of normal human keratinocytes (NHKs) proliferating and differentiating on de-epidermized dermis (so-called living skin equivalent) as a model for skin irritancy (Ponec, 1992). The model was improved through inclusion of the supporting membranes to grow the NHKs into the reconstructed human epidermis. Finally, the models become commercially available as the models representing the human epidermis (EpiSkin®, EpiDerm®, SkinEthic®) or full-thickness skin (Phenion®) (Van Gele et al., 2011). Unfortunately, these skin models frequently exhibit much higher permeability than human and animal skin (Henning et al., 2009) and are better fitted as the models in the early phases of drug and drug formulation development (Mathes et al., 2014).

It is important to consider that different skin models do not possess the active dermal microcirculation, which is responsible for systemic drug absorption (Schaefer et al., 2008). To overcome this limitation, skin penetration studies using excised human/animal skin have been conducted in a flow-through Franz diffusion cell system. The acceptor medium, composed of a tissue culture medium, continuously flows under the skin, permitting the evaluation of the effect of microcirculation (Selzer et al., 2013). However, in this model the perfusion through the dermal layer cannot be assured, which is another parameter that can affect skin penetration of drugs, compounds, and xenobiotics (Lane, 2013). Some skin diseases, such as chronic wounds, are sensitive to perfusion, which can increase tissue oxygenation, thus favoring faster healing (Desmet et al., 2018). Therefore, exploring the effect of perfusion in skin penetration studies might be useful to develop effective localized therapy. Both *ex vivo* and *in vitro* skin penetration studies using the Franz diffusion cell do not include the subcutaneous fatty tissue, which needs to be removed from the skin membrane before the start of the experiment.

These limitations encouraged researchers to find an alternative *in vitro* and *ex vivo* models. Several *in vitro* skin models have been developed, which are discussed in more detail in this chapter. Those models offer advantages particularly for screening in the early stages of drug discovery or formulation development. To simplify the prediction of skin permeability, the silicone membranes (Oliveira et al., 2010), the ceramide-derived parallel artificial membrane permeability assay (PAMPA) (Sinko et al., 2012), and the phospholipid vesicle–based permeation assay (PVPA) (Engesland et al., 2013) have been proposed as suitable alternatives. However, it is important to consider their limitations, since the correlation between *in vitro* and *in vivo* data remains rather limited (Abd et al., 2016).

We aim to provide a nonbiased overview of the currently available *in vitro* models with the potential to be used in the topical formulation development. The models most widely used in the skin irritancy and toxicity studies are not prioritized, and the focus is formulation optimization.

48.2 THE SKIN AS A BARRIER

The anatomy and physiology of the skin, particularly the barrier properties of the skin, have been summarized in various extensive reviews (Bouwstra et al., 2003; Bouwstra and Ponec, 2006; Groen et al., 2011; Hadgraft, 2001; Jepps et al., 2013; Mathes et al., 2014; Van Gele at al., 2011). In brief, the SC is considered the main contributor to the skin barrier properties (Baroni et al., 2012; Menon et al., 2012), while the role of the full epidermis should not be neglected (Andrews et al., 2013). Drug/active substance transport through the skin usually occurs through the epidermal penetration pathway or through skin appendages (Bolzinger et al., 2012; Schaefer et al., 2008). The mode of transport is predominantly by passive diffusion; therefore, the nonviable skin models mimic this process only to a limited extent.

Metabolism that occurs particularly in the living parts of the epidermis is rather difficult to mimic by any *in vitro* modeling. In addition, the residence time of a molecule in the dermis is rather short (Souto, 2005). Moreover, the dermis includes permeable capillaries driving the molecule to the microcirculation upon exiting the epidermis. Considering the drugs/active substances of interest for (trans)dermal therapy, the lipophilicity of the molecule plays a crucial role. A very lipophilic molecule able to overcome the SC barrier will be "stopped" by the aqueous interface beneath the horny layer.

In dermatopharmacokinetics, the permeation of drugs through the skin is often presented as an infinite sink (Lam and Gambari, 2014). The final potential of the drug (penetrant) can be increased (transdermal therapy) or limited (dermal therapy) by the right choice of a carrier/vehicle. Therefore, the penetrant's partitioning into skin, diffusivity through the skin, and exposure at the skin surface determine the permeability of a penetrant. However, by tailoring the vehicle features, it is possible to overcome the penetrant's limitations and optimize the therapy (Chittenden, et al., 2014).

48.3 UTILIZING THE CARRIER/VEHICLE TO TAILOR SKIN PENETRATION

Carriers/vehicles for active substances/drugs can be utilized to control the effectiveness and acceptability of skin formulations. By choosing the right carrier, we can control the (trans)dermal delivery. To be specific, we used the term percutaneous/dermal absorption to describe the passage of various compounds across the skin. The penetration was defined as the entry of a substance into a particular skin layer, whereas the permeation represents the penetration from one layer into another (Bolzinger et al., 2012). Although most of the studies have been focused on the permeation of drugs, it is important to follow the potential unwanted penetration of the cosmetics, as well as occupational exposure. By understanding the interplay between the vehicle, skin, and drug, it is possible to control the drug release, its penetration through the SC, permeation through the skin layers, potential drug deposition inside the skin, or the absorption into systemic circulation (Daniels and Knie, 2007). Many vehicles can affect the physical state and permeability of the skin through the hydration effect or an alteration of the skin temperature. Occlusive and lipophilic vehicles such as paraffin, fats, and oils reduce water loss and increase the skin moisture content, thus promoting the drug penetration. The water-in-oil (W/O) emulsions are less occlusive than the lipid materials, but more occlusive than the oil-in-water (O/W) emulsions. On the contrary, hydrogels comprising a high water content may improve the hydration level of the skin. Stahl et al. (2011) studied the permeability of ibuprofen from various vehicles and reported a rapid increase of ibuprofen permeability from the gel formulation within the first four hours, followed by a deposition of the drug inside the skin, while W/O emulsion exhibited a longer lag time than hydrogel but enabled the transdermal delivery of ibuprofen. Rather extensive work has been done on the role of penetration enhancers such as ethanol, propylene glycol, and oleic acid. They are commonly used as humectants or parts of an oily or aqueous phase of the formulation, enhancing the penetration of many substances into and through the skin. In addition, the substances such as phospholipids, terpenes, and nonionic surfactants are used as building blocks for various nanosized drug delivery systems. Among the most studied are liposomes, ethosomes, propylene glycol liposomes, invasomes, niosomes, and microemulsions (Dragicevic-Curic et al., 2008; Tavano et al., 2011). Nanoparticles able to pass via hair follicles may enhance drug percutaneous absorption (Raber et al., 2014). The penetration of drug/active substances into and across the skin will be also affected by the size and surface properties (lipophilicity, surface charge) of the drug carriers. Regarding the vesicle-based nanosystems, it has been demonstrated that decreasing the system's size improves the delivery of a drug into and across the skin (Elsayed et al., 2007). However, microparticles and larger vesicles act as the drug reservoirs on the skin surface, assuring the prolonged drug release. Considering the surface charge of vesicles, negatively charged liposomes have been shown to enhance the skin penetration of a drug to a greater extent than positively charged and neutral liposomes (Gillet et al., 2011a). The rigidity/elasticity of a vesicle's membranes has been proven to affect the deposition of the drug onto and inside the skin. Conventional liposomes and especially polyethylene glycol (PEG)–coated liposomes with rigid membranes have been demonstrated to accumulate drug inside the SC (Knudsen et al., 2012). Deformable (elastic) liposomes containing edge activators (single-chain surfactants) in the bilayers were proposed as a nanosized delivery system able to squeeze between narrow pores and transport encapsulated drugs deeper into and through the skin (Cevc, 2004; Cevc and Blume, 1992, 2001). Although no consensus was reached on whether the vesicles indeed penetrated in an intact form through the skin, the deformable vesicles have evolved from the first and second (Transferosomes) into the third generation of hyperadaptable vesicles for improved peripheral skin conditions, inflammation, and pain (Cevc, 2012, Ternullo et al., 2018).

For example, the skin permeability of meloxicam formulated in deformable liposomes (Duangjit et al., 2014) was affected by the vesicle surface properties. The effect of the edge activators and hydroxypropyl-beta-cyclodextrins on the skin disposition of itraconazole was confirmed by Alomrani et al. (2014).

Most of the vehicles used in pharmaceutical and cosmeceutical formulations are complex mixtures comprising more than one component; therefore, the choice can be made to tailor cumulative or synergistic effects on skin penetration (Chittenden et al., 2014).

Predicting penetration of a drug/active ingredient into and through the skin can be modeled by various means. The mathematical models of skin permeability, although rather simple, offer a possibility to determine the key parameters affecting skin permeability (Mitragotri et al., 2011). The rather extensive overview of numerical methods for diffusion-based modeling of skin permeation is provided by Frasch and Barbero (2013) and Naegel and co-workers (2013) and is not covered in this chapter.

The most commonly applied mathematical models rely on the quantitative structure–permeability relationship and mechanistic models (Chen et al., 2013; Lee et al., 2010). Although certain useful information can be gained through mathematical modeling (Sugibayashi et al., 2010), it is important to consider that to determine the effect of the carrier/vehicle, interplay between the vehicle and drug, as well as formulation type, more complex models, closer to *in vivo* situations, are required.

48.4 ARTIFICIAL *IN VITRO* SKIN MODELS

In vitro skin penetration of pharmaceutical or cosmetic ingredients, as well as formulations destined for topical treatment, is usually evaluated in human or animal tissue. However, there are both ethical and practical difficulties related to the use of biological tissues in addition to disadvantages such as high intraindividual and interindividual variations. This is particularly a challenge related to diseased skin that most of the topical drug formulations are developed for. The variability both between donors and within the same donor may thus be an issue when interpreting experimental data. Therefore, it is of high importance to identify artificial, robust, and reproducible models to study skin permeation (Flaten et al., 2015).

Further, understanding the physicochemical determinants of vehicle–membrane interaction is critical in selecting the optimal penetration enhancers and effective formulation design (Flaten et al., 2015; Oliveira et al., 2012a). Even the optimal *in vitro* modeling of human skin penetration requires a relevant *in vitro/in vivo* correlation and assurance that the influence of membranes and equipment is taken into consideration (Zsikó et al., 2019). Recently, skin equivalents has been proposed as an alternative to animal experiments in the development of dermal drugs and cosmetics (Mori et al., 2017).

However, most of the research still relies on the simplified artificial model membranes that could offer a fast and reproducible alternative to study the basic physicochemical mechanisms of drug permeation and would thus enable an initial screening approach to narrow down the selection of the formulations to be evaluated using a more biologically intact model. In this way they would serve in improving the efficiency in the optimization of new topical formulations.

Most of the artificial models used to mimic healthy, and to a less extent compromised skin, are relying either on phospholipid mixture models or various types of diffusion cells (de Jagar et al., 2006). Several attempts have been made to develop closer-to-*in vivo* models, such as those based on chromatographic methods, non-lipid-based models (e.g., PAMPA and silicone membranes), and lipid-based models, as simple alternative models for predicting dermal absorption (Flaten et al., 2015).

In the lipid-based category, the following models are identified as the most commonly used, among others:

1. Skin-PAMPA (Sinko et al., 2009)
2. Skin–phospholipid vesicle–based permeation assay (PVPA) mimicking the SC (Engesland et al., 2013)
3. SC substitute (SCS) with synthetic SC lipids (de Jager et al., 2006)
4. Membranes designed to study the impact of ceramide species (Ochalek, et al., 2012a)

48.4.1 CHROMATOGRAPHIC METHODS

Chromatographic systems are used to estimate the permeability coefficients of different substances. The systems offer a determination of the main interactions between the substances and biological membranes (hydrophobic, steric, electronic contributions) and have the advantages of chromatographic techniques, including the reproducibility, speed, and automation (Hidalgo-Rodriguez et al., 2013). Examples of such types of systems are liposome electrokinetic chromatography (Wang et al., 2009) and biopartitioning micellar chromatography (Escuder-Gilabert et al., 2003; Waters et al., 2013). However, considering the optimization of the formulations intended for administration onto the skin and the drug penetration effects of various additives and carriers/vehicles, these systems offer a quite limited potential compared to other *in vitro* models and are therefore not further covered in this chapter.

48.4.2 NON-LIPID-BASED MODEL MEMBRANES

48.4.2.1 PAMPA

The Parallel Artificial Membrane Permeability Assay (PAMPA) model, first introduced as a rapid *in vitro* model for assessing transcellular intestinal permeability (Kansy et al., 1998), was further developed by Ottaviani et al. (2006) towards a model mimicking the skin barrier. The model consisted of an artificial membrane composed of 70% silicone oil and 30% isopropyl myristate coated on a hydrophobic polyvinylidene fluoride filter and was shown to be able to determine human skin permeation for a selection of model drugs in accordance with the available literature. A positive correlation was also established between the membrane retention of the compounds and SC/water partition coefficients. This model has been further exploited in combination with *in silico* methods in a combined approach to predict the skin penetration and distribution of model substances (Ottaviani et al., 2007). The model has been proposed as a suitable model for differentiating highly permeable compounds, since the model seemed to be able to distinguish between the compounds trapped in the barrier and compounds not retained in the barrier. The capacity of the detection of a substance retained in the barrier mimicking the SC could be useful to assess the effects of the formulations (Ottaviani et al., 2006). Further, the model has been used in the initial lead compound selection of synthesized steroids and standard corticosteroids (Dobričić et al., 2014; Markovic et al., 2012), as well as in studying the effect of the vehicles on the permeation of drugs (Karadzovska and Riviere, 2013). Karadzovska et al. (2013) tested a selection of drugs in different vehicles. The permeability data obtained from the PAMPA model were compared with the data from the porcine skin diffusion experiments. The non-lipid-containing PAMPA model performed better than a lipid-containing skin–PAMPA model and other synthetic membranes, namely the Strat-M membrane (further described in the section on lipid-based models). However, both the PAMPA and Strat-MTM showed potential in predicting absorption, as well as discriminating between the different vehicles (Karadzovska et al., 2013).

48.4.2.2 Silicone Model Membranes

The poly(dimethylsiloxane) (PDMS) or silicone membranes have been used for decades for screening of the effects of different vehicles and assessing their impact on the overall mechanisms of drug transport across the human skin (Oliveira et al., 2011). In 1970 Nakano and Patel used silicone membranes to study the release of salicylic acid from five ointment bases. The *in vitro* release pattern from various bases was found to be in an agreement with the *in vivo* data reported in the literature, enabling identification of the most promising ointment bases (Nakano and Patel, 1970). Several studies determining the effect of various additives on the skin penetration of a drug have been performed utilizing this model. Dias et al. (2007) conducted a study on a wide selection of vehicles (mineral oil, isopropyl myristate, oleic acid, decanol, octanol, butanol, ethanol, propylene glycol, glycerin, and water, as well as their mixtures) on the permeation of caffeine, salicylic acid, and benzoic acid. For example, the effect of both hydrophilic and lipophilic vehicles (water, ethanol, propylene glycol, mineral oil, Miglyol 812) on the penetration of ibuprofen has been studied (Watkinson et al., 2009a,b, 2011). The studies focused on the molecular mechanism of interactions between different vehicles (ethanol, isopropyl myristate, dimethyl isosorbide, PEG 200 and PEG 400 and Transcutol P) with the model membranes through the thermodynamics, and kinetic analyses of the uptake, membrane partitioning, and transport studies of a model compound have also been conducted (Oliveira et al., 2010, 2011, 2012a,b).

Although these membranes could be used to predict the skin permeability of the lipophilic compounds, it has been suggested that they could not be used for the hydrophilic compounds (Miki et al., 2015). This was revealed in a study by Uchida et al. (2016) examining the efficacy of a silicone membrane as a substitute for human skin to determine the skin permeation parameters of the drugs differing in lipophilicity and molecular weight. Thus for the hydrophilic compounds, such as antipyrine and caffeine, calculated partition parameter (KL) values were almost 100-fold lower for the silicone membrane than for the human and hairless rat skin, while permeability coefficient (P) values for the silicone membrane were similar to those in human and hairless rat skin. Conversely, for the lipophilic drug (n-butyl paraben and flurbiprofen), KL values for the silicone membrane were similar to or tenfold higher than those achieved in human and hairless rat skins, while P values for the silicone membrane were almost 100-fold higher than those in human and hairless rat skins. Interestingly, the permeation parameters of the drugs with Mw between 151 (methyl p-aminobenzoate) and 234 (lidocaine) and log Ko/w values from 1.10 (aminopyrine) to 2.81 (propyl paraben) for the silicone membrane and human or hairless rat skin showed a significant correlation, meaning that the silicone membranes can be applied to assess the permeability of these model compounds. Nevertheless, for the other drugs, based on their lipophilicity, underestimation or overestimation of permeability relative to those in human skin or hairless rat skin can be expected. To improve the model and permit testing of a wider spectra of drugs, the PDMS and PEG 6000 copolymer-impregnated membrane has been developed. The improved model has so far only been tested using the drugs in the aqueous solutions (Miki et al., 2015); whether the model can be used to assist in formulation development remains to be confirmed.

48.4.3 LIPID-BASED MODEL MEMBRANES

48.4.3.1 PAMPA

The skin–PAMPA model comprising synthetic certramides, cholesterol, stearic acid, and silicon oil, was introduced as an improvement of the original pure solvent-based PAMPA membrane, described earlier (Sinko et al., 2009, 2012). Although the certramides are structurally different from ceramides, their comparable molecular mass and hydrogen acceptor/donor capacity enable them to act as the lipid constituents in the PAMPA sandwich membrane, together with cholesterol, stearic acid, and silicone oil (Sinko et al., 2009, 2012).

The permeability data obtained for a selection of the model drugs tested on the skin–PAMPA model were correlated with the human skin penetration data obtained from the different skin databases. The skin–PAMPA model was shown to exhibit rather poor correlation with the epidermis, but good correlation with the full-thickness skin (Sinko et al., 2012). The skin–PAMPA model has been further evaluated and compared to mammalian skin and in silico models (Alonso et al., 2019; Luo et al., 2016; Zhang et al., 2019). The skin–PAMPA model has shown to be much more permeable compared to human skin, however, the permeability values determined on skin–PAMPA overall show a good linear correlation with data obtained using both pig ear and mammalian skin (Luo et al., 2016; Zhang et al., 2019).

Compatibility between the PAMPA barrier and lipophilic solvents/penetration enhancers, as well as topical formulations containing nonionic emulsifiers, has been confirmed (Balázs et al., 2016; Köllmer et al., 2019). Furthermore, the effect of drug permeation in the presence of penetration enhancers evaluated in the skin–PAMPA model correlated well with the permeability data obtained in human skin (Balázs et al., 2016). The model has also shown to be able to discriminate between different formulations, as well as rank them according to permeation of the selected drug comparably to what was observed in human skin (Karadzovska et al., 2013; Luo et al., 2016; Tsinman and Sinko, 2013;). In the study by Tsinman and Sinko (2013), a modified version of the skin–PAMPA model was applied to evaluate different ibuprofen-containing skin formulations: silicone-based gel, silicone and acrylic copolymer, and one commercially available formulation. In the simple penetration experiments, the modified skin–PAMPA models were able to distinguish between the different formulations, and the ranking of the tested formulations according to the flux was in an agreement with the penetration through human epidermis.

Moreover, the skin–PAMPA model has been further proposed as a useful tool to evaluate and classify transdermal patches by modifying the setup so that the traditional donor compartment was replaced by the patch to be tested (Vizserálek et al., 2015)

48.4.3.2 Phospholipid Vesicle–Based Permeation Assay

The PVPA was originally introduced as a liposome-based barrier model for estimation of intestinal permeability, with the potential to perform in a medium- to high-throughput screening format (Flaten, et al. 2006b, 2009). The PVPA consists of a tight layer of liposomes on a filter support, thus mimicking the cells of biological barriers (Figure 48.1) (Flaten, et al. 2006a,b). By changing the lipid composition of the liposomes, the PVPA barriers could be modified to mimic the other biological barriers, including the skin (Berben et al., 2018; Engesland et al., 2013; Naderkhani et al., 2014). The first PVPA models mimicking the SC barrier of the skin were introduced by Engesland et al. (2013); thereafter several modified versions have been described (Engesland et al., 2013, 2016; Ma et al. 2017; Palac et al., 2014; Shakel et al., 2019; Zhang et al., 2016). All proposed PVPA models

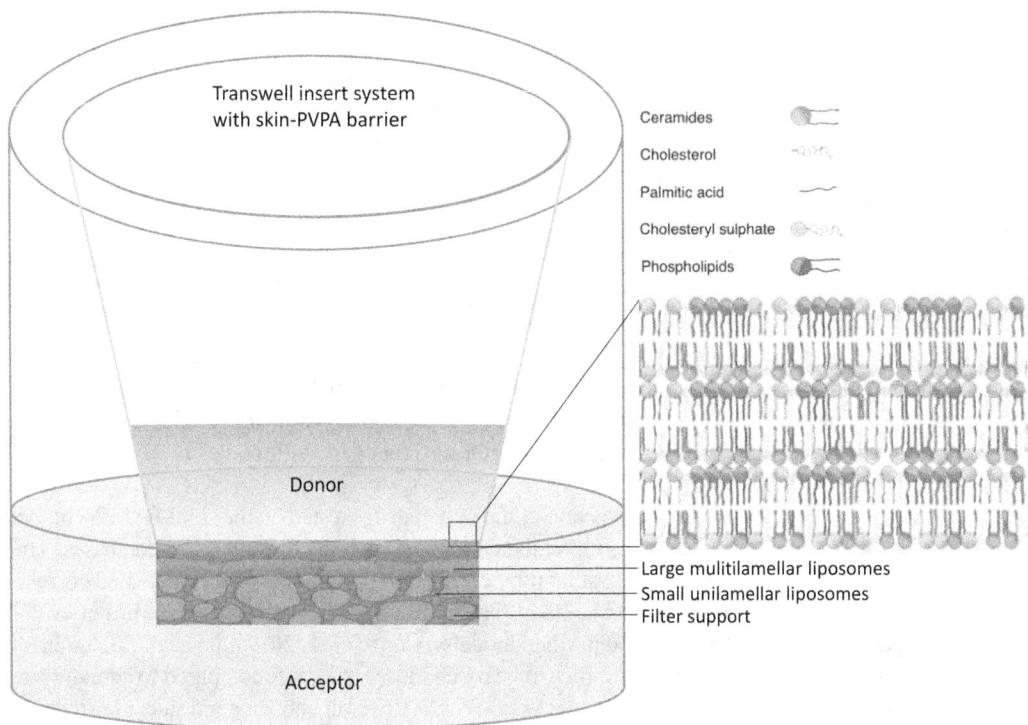

FIGURE 48.1 Schematically explained structure and lipid composition of the skin–PVPA barrier consisting of liposomal vesicles deposited into the pores (small unilamellar vesicles) and on top (larger multilamellar vesicles) of the filter support. The sketch of the structure is based on the structural characterization studies showing that both smaller unilamellar and bigger multilamellar structures could be found in the barrier after freeze–thaw cycling.

(Source: Flaten et al. 2006a.)

for estimating skin penetration could be divided into two main categories: the simple skin–PVPA model comprising cholesterol and egg phospholipids (Engesland et al., 2013, 2016; Palac et al., 2014; Zhang et al., 2016) and the more complex and biological mimicking skin–PVPAs containing all the main lipid classes found in the skin (ceramides, cholesterol, free fatty acids, and cholesteryl sulphate) (Engesland et al., 2013., 2016; Shakel et al., 2019; Palac et al., 2014;; Ma et al., 2017).

When comparing the permeability of a selection of drugs, a similar ranking was observed between the skin–PVPA models and animal skin penetration models and calculated *in silico* values (Engesland et al., 2013; Zhang et al., 2016). In addition, the skin–PVPAs were compared to the reconstructed human skin model EpiSkin®. The skin–PVPAs demonstrated the ability to distinguish between drug solutions and liposomal formulations and were found to be superior to EpiSkin®, considering their abilities to identify the effects of formulations on permeability in early drug development, ease of use, efficiencies, and cost-effectiveness (Engesland et al., 2015). In a subsequent study, the skin–PVPA models were used to evaluate the effect of vesicle carrier on skin penetration. Different liposome formulations, including conventional, deformable, and propylene glycol liposomes, were explored, and the permeation of the drug was shown to be clearly affected by the lipid composition and increased in the presence of penetration enhancers and edge activators, as expected (Palac et al., 2014). PVPA models have also been successfully used to explore the penetration-enhancing effect of menthol and the mechanism behind it (Ma et al., 2017), as well as demonstrated to be compatible with relevant cosolvents in topical formulations such as ethanol, DMSO, oleic acid, and cremophor (Shakel et al., 2019; Zhang et al., 2016).

Engesland and co-workers (2013) revealed that the barrier function of the PVPA model could be modified in a controlled manner. Therefore, the PVPA models for compromised skin were developed providing reproducible and consistent results. Importantly, the distinction could be made between the barriers mimicking compromised and healthy skin. The skin–PVPA models thus also have the potential to provide permeation predictions when investigating drugs or cosmeceuticals intended for various compromised skin conditions (Engesland et al., 2016).

48.4.4 *Stratum corneum* (SC) Substitute

Bouwstra and colleagues developed the SC substitute (SCS) consisting of a porous material covered with the synthetic SC lipids that closely mimics the SC lipid organization and SC barrier function (de Jager et al., 2006). The steady-state flux of the moderately hydrophobic to moderately lipophilic model compounds through the SCS and human SC has been shown to be similar (de Jager et al., 2006; Groen et al., 2008). The SCS thus may function as a standardized and reliable percutaneous penetration model. Another major advantage of the SCS is that the composition of the synthetic SC lipid mixtures can be easily modified. This allows studying the relationship between the lipid composition, lipid organization, and barrier function in one single model.

All this information was used to unravel the effect of lipid composition and additives such as penetration enhancers and moisturizers on changes in lipid organization and permeation. The SCS has thus been extensively used to study the effect of changes in the lipid composition both in respect to the lipid organization and on its barrier function (Groen et al., 2011; Mojumdar et al., 2014; Uche et al., 2019; Uchiyama et al., 2016).

The function of the different changes in lipid composition in diseased skin has also been studied, and modification to the original SCS been made to mimic lipid organization and composition in dry and diseased skin, with an emphasis on atopic dermatitis (Basse et al., 2013).

48.4.5 Others

Ochalek et al. (2012a) proposed SC lipid model membranes designed to study the impact of ceramide species and lipid composition on the drug diffusion and penetration. The effect of chain length of ceramides on the permeability of drugs and water through the barriers was studied to elucidate the reason for altered barrier properties in patients with atopic eczema or psoriasis (Pullmannová et al., 2017) and the influence of cholesterol depletion and separation of the model membrane accessed (Sochorová et al., 2019). These membranes have also been used to investigate the impact of transdermal penetration enhancers on the permeation of the model drugs. The enhancer exhibited a pronounced effect on the barrier properties of SC lipid model membranes, and the effect depended on the type of ceramides present in the barrier (Čuříková et al., 2017; Ochalek, et al., 2012b).

The Strat-M is synthetic barrier model that is composed of multiple layers of polyether sulfone, creating a morphology similar to human skin, including a very tight surface layer. Its porous structure could be impregnated with a proprietary blend of the lipids, thus adding skinlike properties to the barrier (Karadzovska et al., 2013; Zsikó et al., 2019). The flux of a model drug in the presence of different penetration enhancers through StratM barriers containing lipids in ratios similar to what is found in the SC correlated well with the results obtained in human cadaver skin (Haq et al., 2018). Further, the StratM was combined with lanoline to provide lipidic components similar to the lipidic matrix in the skin. By comparing the permeability obtained from the lanoline-covered barrier with the pig skin model, it was demonstrated that similar absorption was estimated for the model substances in those two models (Carrer et al., 2018).

Recently, an artificial SC model based on self-assembled organogelators, prepared from stearic acid, tristearin, or sorbitan tristearate, and gelled in squalene, have been proposed as a potential artificial *in vitro* skin model for assessment of permeation (Maretti et al., 2019).

48.5   TISSUE CULTURE–DERIVED SKIN EQUIVALENTS

Tissue culture–derived skin equivalents have become increasingly important as an alternative to animal and human skin for the testing of percutaneous absorption, phototoxicity, corrosivity, and irritancy of dermal and cosmetic formulations. The equivalences are composed of several layers of human cells in a culture spread over a polymeric matrix. Such a design allows incorporation of the various cell types to form a structure of targeted composition and complexity (Abd et al., 2016; Capallere et al., 2018; Godin and Touitou, 2007). These reconstructed skin equivalents are intended to mimic the epidermis (reconstructed human skin epidermis models) or full human skin (living skin equivalents). Reconstructed human skin epidermis models are commercially available as SkinEthic and EpiDerm®, while EpiSkin®, GraftSkin®, EpiDermFT®, and Pheninon® represent living skin equivalents (Abd et al., 2016; Netzlaff et al., 2005; Van Gele et al., 2011).

Numerous studies have compared the efficacy of the tissue culture–derived skin models with *ex vivo* human and animal skin models. Overall, the reconstructed epidermis equivalents have been proven to be more permeable than *ex vivo* human skin. However, they are more consistent in permeability and responsiveness than human skin, which is highly variable. The relatively weak barrier function of the tissue-cultured models is considered to be their major limitation and is a consequence of the impaired desquamation and the presence of unkeratinized microscopic foci (Netzlaff et al., 2005). Therefore, these models are not recommended for studying the permeation of lipophilic drugs. For instance, the permeation of terbinafine and clotrimazole (hydrophobic drugs) through the GraftSkin® and SkinEthic® was more than 800-fold higher than through the human skin, while the flux of salicylic acid (hydrophilic drug) was similar to that obtained with the human skin (Schmook et al., 2001). The increased permeability of the tissue-cultured models was also demonstrated by Schäfer-Korting et al. (2008). In a study by Zghoul et al. (2001), a five times higher flux for flufenamic acid (hydrophobic drug) was found with the EpiDerm® in comparison to *ex vivo* human skin. However, the model was shown able to distinguish the drug permeation profiles from the different topical formulations, i.e., ointment and solution. Similarly, EpiDerm® was found to be suitable for evaluation of liposomes differing in size and bilayer elasticity (Babu et al., 2009). Comparison of EpiSkin® with the PVPA artificial skin model in the evaluation of topical nanoformulations demonstrated that the reconstructed human epidermis was able to detect only minor differences between the examined liposomal formulations encapsulating drugs of different molecular weights and lipophilicity in comparison to the PVPA model (Engesland et al., 2015).

Currently, the use of reconstructed skin models is approved by guidelines of Organisation for Economic Co-operation and Development (OECD) for skin corrosion, acute skin irritation, and phototoxicity testing (Küchler et al., 2013; Lin et al., 2019). However, none of these models is yet approved for skin absorption testing. Moreover, additional work is required to validate the various models, especially the living skin equivalents, although they may be useful for *in vitro* screening (Abd et al., 2016). The relatively high cost and data reproducibility also limit their use in assessment of dermal formulations (Flaten et al., 2015).

Attempts have been made to utilize skin-on-chip devices as a state-of-the-art platform to study skin penetration. The organotypic cultures are cultivated in the chips to mimic human skin, and by measuring the transepithelial electrical resistance, information on the diffusion properties of tested substances is gained (Lukács et al., 2019; Mohammadi et al., 2016).

48.6   *EX VIVO* ANIMAL SKIN MODELS

Most of the permeability studies are performed using a static Franz diffusion cell method. It consists of donor and receptor chambers between which the animal model membrane is positioned so that the SC is facing the donor compartment where the examined formulation is applied, while the dermis (full-thickness skin) is touching the receptor compartment. For determining the skin (membrane) integrity, OECD Guidance Document 28 (2004) recommends measuring transepidermal water loss (TEWL), electrical resistance, or the use of tritiated water as a permeation marker. Although TEWL measurements have the advantage in that no solutions have to be added to perform the barrier integrity test, Netzlaff et al. (2006a) have proven that TEWL measurement cannot detect small changes in the SC that could still influence drug diffusion. Therefore, calculation of the permeability coefficient is still a more precise method. The experiments could be done so that the donor chamber is left opened (nonocclusive conditions) or covered (occlusive conditions) to permit or escape drying or hydration of the skin surface (Schaefer et al., 2008). The composition of the receptor medium, which is continuously stirred during the experiment, should be chosen to mimic *in vivo* conditions; however, it should also ensure sufficient solubility of the drug. The experiments are usually performed at $32 \pm 1°C$. The addition of the solubility-increasing compounds to the receptor fluid (ethanol or PEG) may alter the barrier function of the skin due to a possible back-diffusion to the skin, particularly if ethanol is used at a higher concentration (40%). To reduce this risk, PEG-20-oleyl ether (6%) and bovine or porcine serum albumin are recommended, since they do not destabilize the integrity of the skin (Moser et al., 2001). It is important to consider that possible enzymatic degradation and microbiological contamination of the biological material might occur. Therefore, addition of preservatives such as sodium azide or ethanol could be beneficial, as long they do not have an effect on the barrier properties of skin by changing the lag time and duration of the experiment (Henning et al., 2009).

To quantify the skin penetration and deposition, the skin extraction measurements (Rastogi and Singh, 2001), horizontal stripping and sectioning (de Jalón et al., 2001), quantitative autoradiography, and spectroscopic methods (Pirot et al., 1997) can be employed. The tape stripping method has been widely used in both *in vivo* (Dick et al., 1997) and *in vitro (ex vivo)* evaluations of topical formulations on human (Cambon et al., 2001; Wagner et al., 2001) and animal (Raber et al., 2014) skin. A velocity should be kept constant throughout the procedure. A slowing down or stopping of the procedure could lead to an increase in the SC amount adhered on the tape strip, whereas an increase in speed could result in a reduced amount of corneocytes. The detached tape strips contain both the amount of corneocytes and the corresponding amount of the penetrated formulation, which can be determined by conventional analytical procedures. It has been proven that different types of formulations can strongly affect the amount of SC removed with every tape strip. For example, after application of an ethanolic solution, the adhesion of the horny layer to the tape strips is increased, while after application of an oily formulation, the adhesion to the tape is decreased. Therefore, for the comparison of the drug penetration from various drug formulations, it is crucial that the amount of formulation detected on the single tape strip is directly related to the standardized real position in the horny layer (Lademann et al., 2009).

48.6.1 PORCINE SKIN

Domestic pig skin is recognized as the most appropriate animal model due to the numerous anatomical, histological, and physiological similarities with human skin such as the epidermal thickness, dermal-epidermal thickness ratio, resemblance in hair follicle, and blood vessel density in the skin, as well as the content of SC glycosphingolipids, ceramides, dermal collagen, and elastin (Dick and Scott, 1992; Godin and Touitou, 2007). Although pig ear skin exhibits hair follicles larger than those of humans, the porcine ear skin represents a more suitable *in vitro* model for analysis of the penetration and storage of topically applied substances in the hair follicles than excised human skin, mainly due to the fact that the human skin contracts after removal. Namely, restretching of the skin to its original size mainly stretches the interfollicular fibers, while the fibers around the hair follicles remain contracted. In contrast to excised human skin, pig ear tissue does not contract when the cartilage is not removed (Lademann et al., 2010). Pig skin is readily obtained as a waste product from animals slaughtered for food. The comparison of drug permeability using human and pig skin has demonstrated a good correlation, particularly for lipophilic substances, while skin from rodents generally exhibited higher permeation rates (Dick and Scott, 1992). In addition, pig skin exhibits less donor variability than human skin (Barbero and Frasch, 2009). Most of the literature reports on the use of pig ears in *ex vivo* permeation studies do not specify the age of the animal. It is important that ears have not been scalded or flamed after animal sacrificing because such a pretreatment completely destroys the integrity of the epidermis. The central region of the outer side of the porcine ear has been recommended because of the similarity with human skin layers (Meyer et al., 2006).

Various drug formulations, including creams, ointments, lotions, (micro)emulsions, microparticles, and colloidal drug delivery systems (nanosystems), have been assessed using *ex vivo* pig skin models (Flaten et al., 2015). It would extend beyond the scope of this chapter to enlist all literature reporting on the use of *ex vivo* pig skin to optimize different formulations; therefore, only some are mentioned here. For example, Scognamiglio et al. (2013) evaluated the penetration potential of deformable liposomes and ethosomes containing resveratrol using freshly excised pig ear. The deformable liposomes decreased the amount of resveratrol accumulated in the dermis as compared to ethosomes. Full-thickness porcine ear skin has been used for optimization of the nanostructured lipid carriers containing minoxidil or finasteride (Gomes et al., 2014) or polyamide nanocapsules containing sunscreen filters (Hanno et al., 2012). Senyigit et al. (2010) performed permeation studies using full-thickness porcine ear skin to determine the epidermal accumulation of clobetasol from lecithin/chitosan nanoparticles. The skin deposition of quercetin from W/O microemulsion and its percutaneous delivery was determined using the full-thickness porcine ear skin (Vicentini et al., 2008).

The W/O vehicle was found to be the superior to other vehicles (O/W and amphiphilic bases) when assessed on dermatomed porcine abdominal skin (0.7 mm thick) (Nagelreiter et al., 2013). Dermatomed dorsal porcine skin was also used in the optimization of microemulsion composition for transdermal delivery of testosterone (Hathout et al., 2010).

Newborn pig skin has attracted considerable attention as a model for dermal formulations (Cilurzo et al., 2007). However, the diversity in the thickness of newborn pig skin regarding the age of the animal from only 1 day old (~1.2 kg) (Manconi et al., 2011b; Mura et al., 2009) to 40 days old (~20 kg) needs to be considered (Wang et al., 2014).

48.6.2   Other *Ex Vivo* Animal Skin Models: Rodents, Snake, and Bovine Udder

Primate, mouse, rat, guinea pig, rabbit, bovine (udder), and snake models have also been proposed as *ex vivo* animal models. However, the primate research is almost inaccessible, and often too expensive, so rodent skin is often used as a replacement for pig skin. The use of rodent skin requires ethical permission, since it is obtained from a living animal and is not a by-product like pig skin. In addition, the hairless species are also available: nude mice, hairless rats, and hairless guinea pigs in which the absence of hair coat mimics the human skin better than hairy skin. The rodent exhibits an extremely high density of hair follicles, leading to an obligatory hair removal prior to formulation administration (Godin and Touitou, 2007). The guinea pig skin is therefore considered a more appropriate rodent surrogate for human skin studies (Barbero and Frasch, 2009).

The effect of the size of self-assembled nanoparticles on the effectiveness of transdermal delivery of minoxidil was assessed using several *ex vivo* rodent models (Shim et al., 2004). When using hairy guinea pig skin, the permeation of the drug in 40-nm-sized nanoparticles was 1.5-fold higher in the epidermis than that of 130-nm-sized nanoparticles. This influence of the nanoparticle size was not observed in hairless guinea pigs, thus showing that the follicular route is the main penetration pathway for the minoxidil-loaded nanoparticles, whereas the permeation was promoted with decreasing the size of the nanoparticles. The full-thickness abdominal rat skin was applied to optimize a microemulsion formulation proposed for the treatment of skin fungal infections (Butani et al., 2014). A microemulsion comprising 5% isopropyl myristate and 35% mixture (3:1, Tween 80:propylene glycol) exhibited twofold higher drug permeation of amphotericin B into the skin as compared to a plain drug solution. Rabbit skin can also be used as an animal skin model. The full-thickness skin from the inner side of albino rabbit ear was used to compare ketotifen skin permeability from the two types of vesicles: deformable liposomes and ethosomes (Elsayed et al., 2006).

Although not commonly used, shed snake skin can also serve as an alternative skin model; the snakes molt periodically, and a single animal can provide repeated sheds, thus eliminating interindividual variability seen in other animal models. Moreover, removal is injury-free and no chemical or heat pretreatment is required (Itoh et al., 1990). Moreover, since it is not a living tissue, storage at room temperature for relatively long periods of time is feasible (Haigh and Smith, 1994). However, the lack of hair follicles could influence drug permeability (Godin and Touitou, 2007). Therefore, this model is not appropriate for investigating dermal absorption of drugs that penetrate the skin via the follicular route. When the shed snake membrane was compared with hairless mouse and human as models to evaluate the permeability of 5-fluorouracil in formulations comprising different penetrating enhancers, it become evident that human skin cannot be replaced by snake skin (Rigg and Barry, 1990). Ngawhirunpat et al. (2008) confirmed that the skin metabolisms in snake and shed snake skin were significantly different from human skin.

48.7 *EX VIVO* HUMAN SKIN MODELS

Human skin is the most relevant model for evaluating the effect of formulation components on (trans)dermal drug delivery. Human skin can originate from various sources, mostly from plastic surgery (Godin and Touitou, 2007). However, the use of human skin is very restricted by the ethical permissions and laboratory facilities, and only a limited number of laboratories have access to human skin. In addition, human skin permeability varies greatly between the specimens taken from the same or different anatomical sites of the same donor (27% variance *in vivo* and 43% *in vitro*, respectively). Even greater variations (45% *in vivo* and 66% *in vitro*, respectively) are reported between the specimens from different subjects or different age groups (Haigh and Smith, 1994). These variations are contributed to differences in the lipid composition, skin thickness, or hydration, which are affected by body site, sex, race, age, and disease (Barbero and Frasch, 2009). The metabolism and biotransformation of chemicals applied to the skin after excision of the tissue from the donor can also affect model suitability (Haigh and Smith, 1994).

Various topical formulations have been evaluated on *ex vivo* human skin, and selected relevant studies are discussed here in more detail. For example, Zhao et al. (2009) evaluated nanoparticles incorporated in hydrofluoroalkane foam for enhanced dermal delivery of tocopherol acetate using full-thickness human skin. Optimization of a gel vehicle for dermal delivery of epicatechin has been performed on full-thickness human cadaver skin obtained from the back region of Caucasian subjects. Ultrez 10 gel was confirmed to promote the penetration and retention of epicatechin in the upper layers of human cadaver viable skin (Suppasrivasuseth et al., 2006). Typically, skin was used to compare two or more nanocarriers or vehicles. For example, Dubey et al. (2007) compared the penetration potential of methotrexate-containing ethosomes with the conventional liposomes using dermatomed (500 µm thickness) human cadaver skin and concluded that ethosomes enhanced the transdermal flux of the drug and decreased the lag time across the skin. In another study, full-thickness breast skin obtained after cosmetic surgery was used for the estimation of celecoxib skin delivery by ethosomes conventional liposomes and deformable liposomes. An increased skin accumulation of the drug has been determined for ethosomes and deformable liposomes (Bragagni et al., 2012). The full-thickness human abdominal skin was utilized to optimize temoporfin-loaded vesicles destined for photodynamic therapy of cutaneous diseases: invasomes (Dragicevic-Curic et al., 2009a), flexosomes (Dragicevic-Curic et al., 2010), and liposomes-in-gel formulations (Dragicevic-Curic et al., 2009b).

48.8   SKIN PERFUSION MODELS

Although they can be considered *ex vivo* human skin models due to their specific features, we have categorized this separately. To more closely mimic the conditions within the living skin, skin perfusion models have been proposed as the closest to *in vivo* animal or human studies. Skin perfusion models are composed of a surgically prepared portion of skin panni, also called a flap, involving the active circulation of the dermis layer, skin metabolism, and the presence of subcutaneous fatty tissue (Patel et al., 2016). These models offer the advantage of perfusion with a tissue–culture medium by cannulization of one of the vessels in the skin panni. To confirm and monitor flap perfusion during skin penetration experiments, dermofluorimetry is the most used technique (Black et al., 2001). Miland and colleagues (2008) proposed a less invasive technique, dynamic infrared thermography (DIRT), which was also used to differentiate between well-perfused and less perfused areas (Miland et al., 2008). Additionally, methods used in *in vivo/ex vivo* investigations, e.g., mass balance, surface washings, tape stripping, are applicable to be utilized in the skin perfused model (Schaefer et al., 2008). Several animal specimens have been used to obtain skin perfusion models, such as pig, mouse, and rat. The first studies were performed with a perfused ear model, which showed high permeability and was later used only as a tool to predict penetration through premature neonate skin (Schaefer et al., 2008). The perfused cow udder (Kietzmann et al., 1993), pig forelimb (Wagner et al., 2003), and isolated perfused pig skin flap (obtained from pig abdomen) (Riviere et al., 1986) were also used as perfused models. The perfused bovine udder skin (BUS) model comprises the isolated udders continuously perfused via the left and right external pudendal arteries with an oxygenated nutrient solution (Pittermann et al., 2013). Comparison with *ex vivo* human and porcine skin has demonstrated that bovine udder skin is well-correlated, but also a less variable barrier against caffeine, benzoic acid, testosterone, and flufenamic acid penetration (Netzlaff et al., 2006b). This model enables the comparison of the dermal penetration, metabolism, and absorption of the substances after topical administration. A good correlation with *in vivo* studies has been obtained when testing dermal absorption of organophosphates, steroids, benzoic acid, and caffeine on the isolated perfused pig skin flap (Carver et al., 1989). Wester and collaborators (1998) also found similar dermal absorption of other compounds between the pig skin perfusion model and *in vivo* studies on humans. However, the limitations of using animal skin also applies for skin perfusion models.

The isolated perfused human skin flap (IPHSF) has been used to study (trans)dermal penetration (Ternullo et al., 2017a,b). The model was used to directly compare the skin penetration enhancement potential of three lipid-based nanocarriers (CLs, DLs, and SLNs) incorporating either calcein or rhodamine, markers of different lipophilicities. The confocal laser scanner microscopy (CLSM) technique was used to follow the penetration profiles. The penetration profiles were directly compared to established skin penetration models such as cellophane membrane and full-thickness pig/human skin in the Franz diffusion cell (Ternullo et al., 2017b). The model was proven to be a valuable tool in skin penetration studies, as well as in optimization of dosage forms/delivery systems for skin therapy.

With the development of microfluidics and organ-on-a-chip concept, skin equivalents emerged as a novel type of perfused skin model. They are not yet widely studied due to the limited access to technology; however, Mori et al. (2017) confirmed the feasibility of a skin equivalent containing vascular channels (perfusion conditions) as a model for studying vascular absorption. The results suggested that this skin equivalent can be used for skin-on-a-chip applications, including drug development, cosmetics testing, and studying skin biology.

In summary, the advantages and limitations of the most commonly used *in vitro/ex vivo* models are provided in Table 48.1.

TABLE 48.1

Advantages and Limitations of Most Common Skin Models Used for Optimization of Topical Formulation

Skin Model	Advantages	Limitations
Silicone model membranes	Reproducible Low cost Storage	Non-lipid based Low resemblance to SC Non-biological origin
PAMPA	Reproducible Prolonged storage capabilities Low cost	Synthetic lipids/non-lipid based Lipid organization not characterized/Low resemblance to SC Non-biological origin
PVPA	Reproducible Lipid composition easily modified Relatively low cost Storage	Lipid organization not characterized Nonbiological origin
SCS	Mimicking SC lipid organization Steady-state flux similar to human SC Reproducible Lipid composition easily modified Relatively low cost	Not used in formulation optimization yet Nonbiological origin
Reconstructed human skin equivalents	Consistence in permeability in comparison to human skin	More permeable than human skin Questionable barrier function High cost
Pig ear	Easily obtained (waste from slaughter) Similarity with human skin	Age of animal influences skin thickness Removal of hairs (skin damage) Storage
Newborn pig	Thickness of the SC is similar to human horny layer	Higher number of hairs than in humans Different anatomical sites: abdomen, back Difference in the skin thickness; newborn and older animals Storage
Mouse	Small size, uncomplicated handling Hairless species available	Ethical permission Very thin skin, highly permeable High density of hair follicles Removal of hairs (skin damage)
Rat	Small size, uncomplicated handling Hairless species available	Ethical permission Thin skin, more permeable than human High density of hair follicles Removal of hairs (skin damage)
Guinea pig	Similar permeability to human and pig ear skin Hairless species available	Ethical permission High density of hair follicles Removal of (skin damage)
Rabbit	Ears as waste from slaughter Similar permeability to guinea pig	Ethical permission High density of hair follicles Removal of hairs (skin damage)
Shed snake	Single animal provides repeated sheds Multiple samples from one shed Storage at room temperature	Absence of hair follicles Differences in skin metabolism, compared to human skin Absence of living epidermis and dermis
Bovine udders	Easily obtained (waste from slaughter) BUS comparable to living skin Multiple samples from one animal	One donor enables testing of only one sample (BUS) Weaker barrier to some drugs than pig skin Storage

(Continued)

TABLE 48.1 (*Continued*)

Advantages and Limitations of Most Common Skin Models Used for Optimization of Topical Formulation

Skin Model	Advantages	Limitations
Human	The most relevant model	Ethical permission
		Higher intervariability and intravariability than with porcine ear skin
		Different sources: age, sex, race, plastic surgery, amputation, cadaver
		Different anatomical parts: abdomen, tight, breast, back, etc.
		Storage

BUS, perfused bovine udder skin; *PAMPA*, parallel artificial membrane permeability assay; *PVPA*, phospholipid vesicle–based permeation assay; *SC*, stratum corneum; *SCS*, stratum corneum substitute.
Source: Modified from Flaten et al. (2015), with permission from Elsevier.

48.9   CONCLUSION

Localized skin therapy of dermal diseases, as well as potential transdermal drug delivery, are in the pipelines of many pharmaceutical industries, However, restrictions in the use of animals in optimization of pharmaceutical as well as cosmeceutical formulations destined for the administration onto the skin lead to a search for alternative skin penetration models. Recent years have seen an increase in the number and variety of models offering a possibility for rapid screening and faster optimization of skin formulations; however, their limitations need to be taken into account. The choice of the most applicable *in vitro* model should be based on the interplay between availability, ease of the use, cost, and respective limitations.

REFERENCES

Abd, E., Yousef, S.A., Pastore, M.N. et al. 2016. Skin models for the testing of transdermal drugs. Clin. Pharmacol. 8, 163–76.
Alomrani, A.H., Shazly, G.A., Amara, A.A. et al. 2014. Itraconazole-ghydroxypropyl-β-cyclodextrin loaded deformable liposomes: *in vitro* skin penetration studies and antifungal efficacy using *Candida albicans* as model. Colloids Surf. B: Biointerfaces 121: 74–81.
Alonso, C., Carrer, V., Espinosa, S. et al. 2019. Prediction of the skin permeability of topical drugs using in silico and *in vitro* models. Eur. J. Pharm. Sci. 136: 104945.
Andrews, S.N., Jeong, E., Prausnitz, M.R. 2013. Transdermal delivery of molecules is limited by full epidermis, not just stratum corneum. Pharm. Res. 30:1099–109.
Babu, S., Fan, C., Stepanskiy, L., et al. 2009. Effect of size at the nanoscale and bilayer rigidity on skin diffusion of liposomes. J. Biomed. Mater. Res. A 91: 140–48.
Balázs, B., Vizserálek, G., Berkó, S. et al. 2016. Investigation of the efficacy of transdermal penetration enhancers through the use of human skin and a skin mimic artificial membrane. J. Pharm. Sci. 105: 1134–40.
Barbero, A.M., Frasch, H.F. 2009. Pig and guinea pig skin as surrogates for human *in vitro* penetration studies: a quantitative review. Toxicol. *In Vitro* 23: 1–13.
Baroni, A., Buommino, E., De Gregorio, V., et al. 2012. Structure and function of the epidermis related to varrier properties. Clin. Dermatol. 30: 257–62.
Basse, L. H., Groen, D., Bouwstra. J.A. 2013. Permeability and lipid organization of a novel psoriasis stratum corneum substitute. Int. J. Pharm. 457: 275–82.
Berben, P., Bauer-Brandl, A., Brandl, M. et al. 2018. Drug permeability profiling using cell-free permeation tools: Overview and applications. Eur. J. Pharm. Sci. 119: 219–33.
Black, C.E., Huang, N., Neligan, P.C. et al. 2001. Effect of nicotine on vasoconstrictor and vasodilator responses in human skin vasculature. Am. J. Physiol. Regul. Integr. Comp. Physiol. 281: 1097–104.

Bolzinger, M.-A., Briançon, S., Pelletier, J., et al. 2012. Penetration of drugs through skin, a complex-rate controlling membrane. Curr. Opin. Colloid Interface Sci. 17: 156–65.

Bouwstra, J.A., Honey-Nguyen, P.L., Gooris, G.S., et al. 2003. Structure of the skin barrier and its modulation by vesicular formulations. Progress Lipid Res. 42: 1–36.

Bouwstra, J.A., Ponec, M. 2006. The skin barrier in healthy and diseased state. Bioch. Biophys. Acta 1758: 2080–95.

Bragagni, M., Mennini, N., Maestrelli, F., et al. 2012. Comparative study of liposomes, transfersomes and ethosomes as carriers for improving topical delivery of celecoxib. Drug Deliv. 19: 354–61.

Butani, D., Yewale, C., Misra, A. 2014. Amphotericin B topical microemulsion: formulation, characterization and evaluation. Colloids Surf. B: Biointerfaces 116: 351–58.

Capallere, C., Plaza, C., Meyrignac, C. et al. 2018. Property characterization of reconstructed human epidermis equivalents, and performance as a skin irritation model. Toxicol. *In Vitro* 53: 45–56.

Cambon, M., Issachar, N., Castelli, D., et al. 2001. An *in vivo* method to assess the photostability of UV filters in a sunscreen. J. Cosmet. Sci. 52: 1–11.

Carrer, V., Guzmán, B., Martí, M., et al. 2018. Lanolin-based synthetic membranes as percutaneous absorption models for transdermal drug delivery, Pharmaceutics 10(3): 73.

Carver, M.P., Williams, P.L., Riviere, J.E. 1989. The isolated perfused porcine skin flap III. Percutaneous absorption pharmacokinetics of organophosphates, steroids, benzoic acid, and caffeine. Toxicol. Appl. Pharmacol. 97: 324–37.

Cevc, G. 2004. Lipid vesicles and other colloids as drug carriers on the skin. Adv. Drug Deliv. Rev. 56: 675–711.

Cevc, G. 2012. Rational design of new product candidates: The next generation of highly deformable bilayer vesicles for noninvasive, targeted therapy. J. Control. Release 160: 135–46.

Cevc, G., Blume, G. 1992. Lipid vesicles penetrate into intact skin owing to the transdermal osmotic gradients and hydration force. Biochim. Biophys. Acta 1104: 226–32.

Cevc, G., Blume, G. 2001. New, highly efficient formulation of diclofenac for the topical, transdermal administration in ultradeformable drug carriers, Transfersomes. Biochim. Biophys. Acta 1514: 191–205.

Chen, L., Han, L., Lian, G. 2013. Recent advances in predicting skin permeability of hydrophilic solutes. Adv. Drug Deliv. Rev. 65: 295–305.

Chittenden, J.T., Brooksm J.D., Riviere, J.E. 2014. Development of a mixed-effect pharmacokinetic model for vehicle modulated *in vitro* transdermal flux of topically applied penetrants. J. Pharm. Sci. 103: 1002–12.

Cilurzo, F., Minghetti, P., Sinico, C. 2007. Newborn pig skin as model membrane in *in vitro* drug permeation studies: a technical note. AAPS PharmSciTech 8: A94.

Čuříková, B., Procházková, A.K., Filková, B. et al. 2017. Simplified stratum corneum model membranes for studying the effects of permeation enhancers, Int. J. Pharm. 534: 287–96.

Daniels, R., Knie, U. 2007. Galenics of dermal product - vehicles, properties and drug release. JDDG 5: 369–83.

de Jager, M., Groenink, W., Bielsa, I. et al. 2006. A novel *in vitro* percutaneous penetration model: evaluation of barrier properties with p-aminobenzoic acid and two of its derivatives. Pharm. Res. 23: 951–60.

de Jalón, E.G., Blanco-Príeto, M.J., Ygartua, P., et al. 2001. Topical application of acyclovir-loaded microparticles: quantification of the drug in porcine skin layers. J. Control. Release 75: 191–97.

Desmet, C.M., Préat, V., Gallez, B. 2018. Nanomedicines and gene therapy for the delivery of growth factors to improve perfusion and oxygenation in wound healing. Adv. Drug Deliv. Rev. 129: 262–84.

Dias, M., Hadgraft, J., Lane, M.E. 2007. Influence of membrane-solvent-solute interactions on solute permeation in model membranes. Int. J. Pharm. 336,: 108–14.

Dick, I.P., Blain, P.G., Williams, F.M. 1997. The percutaneous absorption and skin distribution of lindane in man. I. *In vivo* studies. Hum. Exp. Toxicol. 16: 645–51.

Dick, I.P., Scott, R.C. 1992. Pig ear skin as an in-vitro model for human skin permeability. J. Pharm. Pharmacol. 44: 640–45.

Dobričić, V., Marković, B., Nikolić, K., et al. 2014. 17beta-carboxamide steroids–*in vitro* prediction of human skin permeability and retention using PAMPA technique. Eur. J. Pharm. Sci. 52: 95–108.

Dragicevic-Curic, N., Gräfe, S., Gitter, B., et al. 2010. Surface charged temoporfin-loaded flexible vesicles: *in vitro* skin penetration studies and stability. Int. J. Pharm. 384: 100–08.

Dragicevic-Curic, N., Scheglmann, D., Albrecht, V., et al. 2008. Temoporfin-loaded invasomes: development, characterization and *in vitro* skin penetration studies. J. Control. Release 127: 59–69.

Dragicevic-Curic, N., Scheglmann, D., Albrecht, V., et al. 2009a. Development of different temoporfin-loaded invasomes-novel nanocarriers of temoporfin: characterization, stability and *in vitro* skin penetration studies. Colloids Surf. B Biointerfaces 70: 198–206.

Dragicevic-Curic, N., Winter, S., Stupar, M., et al. 2009b. Temoporfin-loaded liposomal gels: viscoelastic properties and *in vitro* skin penetration. Int. J. Pharm. 373: 77–84.

Dubey, V., Mishra, D., Dutta, T., et al. 2007. Dermal and transdermal delivery of an anti-psoriatic agent via ethanolic liposomes. J. Control. Release 123: 148–54.

Duangjit, S., Pamornpathomkul, B., Opanasopit, P., et al. 2014. Role of the charge, carbon chain length, and content of surfactant on the skin penetration of meloxicam-loaded liposomes. Int. J. Nanomedicine 9(1): 2005–17.

Elsayed, M.M.A., Abdallah, O.Y., Naggar, V.F., et al. 2006. Deformable liposomes and ethosomes: mechanism of enhanced skin delivery. Int. J. Pharm. 322: 60–66.

Elsayed, M.M.A., Abdallah, O.Y., Naggar, V.F., et al. 2007. Lipid vesicles for skin delivery of drugs: Reviewing three decades of research. Int. J. Pharm. 332: 1–16.

Engesland, A., Škalko-Basnet, N., Flaten, G.E., 2015. PVPA and EpiSkin® in assessment of drug therapies destined for skin administration. J. Pharm. Sci. 104: 1119–27.

Engesland, A., Skar, M., Hansen, T., et al. 2013. New applications of phospholipid vesicle-based permeation assay: permeation model mimicking skin barrier. J. Pharm. Sci. 102: 1588–600.

Engesland, A., Škalko-Basnet, N., Flaten, G.E. 2016. In vitro models to estimate drug penetration through the compromised stratum corneum barrier. Drug Devel. Ind. Pharm. 42: 1742–51.

Escuder-Gilabert, L., Martínez-Pla, J. J., Sagrado, S., et al. 2003. Biopartitioning micellar separation methods: modelling drug absorption. J. Chrom. B. 797: 21–35.

Flaten, G.E., Awoyemi, O., Luthman, K., et al. 2009. The phospholipid vesicle-based permeability assay: 5. Development towards an automated procedure for high throughput permeability screening. JALA 14: 12–21.

Flaten, G.E., Bunjes, H., Luthman, K., et al. 2006a. Drug permeability across a phospholipid vesicle based barrier 2. Characterization of barrier structure, storage stability and stability towards pH changes. Eur. J. Pharm. Sci. 28: 336–43.

Flaten, G.E., Dhanikula, A.B., Luthman, K., et al. 2006b. Drug permeability across a phospholipid vesicle based barrier: A novel approach for studying passive diffusion. Eur. J. Pharm. Sci. 27: 80–90.

Flaten, G. E., Palac, Z., Engesland, A., et al. 2015. In vitro skin models as a tool in optimization of drug formulation. Eur. J. Pharm. Sci. 75: 10–24.

Frasch, H.F., Barbero, A.M. 2013. Application of numerical methods for diffusion-based modelling of skin permeation. Adv. Drug Deliv. Rev. 65: 208–20.

Gillet A., Compere P., Lecomte F. et al. 2011a. Liposome surface charge influence on skin penetration behaviour. Int. J. Pharm. 411: 223–31.

Godin, B., Touitou, E. 2007. Transdermal skin delivery: predictions for humans from in vivo, ex vivo and animal models. Adv. Drug Deliv. Rev. 59: 1152–61.

Gomes, M.J., Martins, S., Ferreira, D., et al. 2014. Lipid nanoparticles for topical and transdermal application for alopecia treatment: development, physicochemical characterization, and in vitro release and penetration studies. Int. J. Nanomedicine 9(1): 1231–42.

Groen, D., Gooris, G.S., Ponec, M., et al. 2008. Two new methods for preparing a unique stratum corneum substitute. Bioch. Biophys. Acta 1778: 2421–29.

Groen, D., Poole, D.S., Gooris, G.S., et al. 2011. Investogating the barrier function of skin lipid models with varying compositions. Eur. J. Pharm. Biopharm. 79: 334–42.

Hadgraft, J. 2001. Skin, the final frontier. Int. J. Pharm. 224: 1–18.

Haigh, J.M., Smith, E.W. 1994. The selection and use of natural and synthetic membranes for in vitro diffusion experiments. Eur. J. Pharm. Sci. 2: 311–30.

Hanno, I., Anselmi, C., Bouchemal, K. 2012. Polyamide nanocapsules and nano-emulsions containing Parsol(R) MCX and Parsol(R) 1789: in vitro release, ex vivo skin penetration and photo-stability studies. Pharm. Res. 29: 559–73.

Haq, A., Goodyear, B.; Ameen, D., et al. 2018. Strat-M® synthetic membrane: Permeability comparison to human cadaver skin. Int. J. Pharm. 547: 432–37.

Hathout, R.M., Woodman, T.J., Mansour, S., et al. 2010. Microemulsion formulations for the transdermal delivery of testosterone. Eur. J. Pharm. Sci. 40: 188–96.

Henning, A., Schaefer, U.F., Neumann, D. 2009. Potential pitfalls in skin permeation experiments: influence of experimental factors and subsequent data evaluation. Eur. J. Pharm. Biopharm. 72: 324–31.

Ilić, T., Pantelić, I., Lunter, D. et al. 2017. Critical quality attributes, in vitro release and correlated in vitro skin permeation-in vivo tape stripping collective data for demonstrating therapeutic (non)equivalence of topical semisolids: A case study of "ready-to-use" vehicles. Int. J. Pharm. 528: 253–67.

Itoh, T., Xia, J., Magavi, R., et al. 1990. Use of shed snake skin as a model membrane for in vitro percutaneous penetration studies: comparison with human skin. Pharm. Res. 7: 1042–47.

Jepps, O.G., Dancik, Y., Anissimov, Y.G., et al. 2013. Modeling the human skin barrier – Towards a better understanding of dermal absorption. Adv. Drug Deliv. Rev. 65: 152–68.

Kansy, M., Senner, F., Gubernator, K. 1998. Physicochemical high throughput screening: Parallel artificial membrane permeation assay in the description of passive absorption processes. J. Med. Chem. 41: 1007–10.

Karadzovska, D., Brooks, J.D., Monteiro-Riviere, N.A., et al. 2013. Predicting skin permability from complex vehicles. Adv. Drug Deliv. Rev. 65: 265–77.

Karadzovska, D., Riviere, J.E. 2013. Assessing vehicle effects on skin absorption using artificial membrane assays. Eur. J. Pharm. Sci. 50: 569–76.

Kietzmann, M., Löscher, W., Arens, D., et al. 1993. The isolated perfused bovine udder as an *in vitro* model of percutaneous drug absorption skin viability and percutaneous absorption of dexamethasone, benzoyl peroxide, and etofenamate. J. Pharmacol. Toxicol. Methods 30: 75–84.

Knudsen, N.Ø., Rønholt, S., Salte, R.D., et al. 2012. Calcipotriol delivery into the skin with PEGylated liposomes. Eur. J. Pharm. Biopharm. 81: 532–39.

Köllmer, M., Mossahebi, P., Sacharow, E. et al. 2019. Investigation of the compatibility of the skin PAMPA model with topical formulation and acceptor media additives using different assay setups. AAPS PharmSciTech, 20: 89.

Küchler S, Strüver K, Friess W. 2013. Reconstructed skin models as emerging tools for drug absorption studies. Expert Opin. Drug Metab. Toxicol. 9: 1255–63.

Lademann, J., Jacobi, U., Surber, C., et al. 2009. The tape stripping procedure–evaluation of some critical parameters. Eur. J. Pharm. Biopharm. 72: 317–23.

Lademann, J., Richter, H., Meinke, M., et al., 2010. Which skin model is the most appropriate for the investigation of topically applied substances into the hair follicles? Skin Pharmacol. Physiol. 23: 47–52.

Lam, P.L., Gambari, R. 2014. Advanced progress of microencapsulation technologies: *In vivo* and *in vitro* models for studying oral and transdermal drug deliveries. J. Control. Release 178: 25–45.

Lane, M.E. 2013. Skin penetration enhancers. Int. J. Pharm. 447: 12–21.

Lee, P.H., Conradi, R., Shanmugasundram, V. 2010. Development of an in silico model for human skin permeation based on a Franz cell skin permeability assay. Bioorg. Med. Chem. Lett. 20: 69–73.

Lin, Y.C., Hsu, H.C., Lin, C.H., et al. 2019. Testing method development and validation for *in vitro* Skin Irritation Testing (SIT) by Using Reconstructed Human Epidermis (RhE) Skin Equivalent - EPiTRI®. In: Kojima H, Seidle T. and Spielmann H. eds., Alternatives to Animal Testing, 8–18. Springer, Singapore.

Lukács B., Bajza A., Kocsis, D. 2019. Skin-on-a-chip device for ex vivo monitoring of transdermal delivery of drugs—design, fabrication, and testing. Pharmaceutics 11: 445.

Luo, L., Patel, A., Sinko, B. et al. 2016. A comparative study of the *in vitro* permeation of ibuprofen in mammalian skin, the PAMPA model and silicone membrane. Int. J. Pharm. 505: 14–19.

Ma, M., Di, H-J., Zhang, H. et al. 2017. Development of phospholipid vesicle-based permeation assay models capable of evaluating percutaneous penetration enhancing effect. *Drug Develop*. Ind. Pharm. 43: 2055–63.

Manca, M.L., Manconi, M., Nacher, A. et al. 2014. Development of novel diolein-niosomes for cutaneous delivery of tretinoin: Influence of formulation and *in vitro* assessment. Int. J. Pharm. 477: 176–86.

Manconi, M., Sinico, C., Caddeo, C., et al. 2011b. Penetration

Maretti, E., Rustichelli, C., Miselli, P., et al. 2019. Self-assembled organogelators as artificial stratum corneum models: key-role parameters for skin permeation prediction. Int. J. Pharm. 557: 314–28.

Markovic, B.D., Vladimirov, S.M., Cudina, O.A., et al. 2012. A PAMPA assay as fast predictive model of passive human skin permeability of new synthesized corticosteroid C-21 esters. Molecules 17: 480–91.

Mathes, S.H., Ruffner, H., Graf-Hausner, U. 2014. The use of skin models in drug development. Adv. Drug Del. Rev. 69-70: 81–102.

Menon, G.K., Cleary, G.W., Lane, M.E. 2012. The structure and function of the stratum corneum. Int. J. Pharm. 435: 3–9.

Meyer, W., Schönnagel, B., Fleischer, L.G. 2006. A note on integumental (1–>3)(1–>6)beta-D-glucan permeation, using the porcine ear skin model. J. Cosmet. Dermatol. 5: 130–34.

Miki, R., Ichitsuka, Y., Yamada, T. et al. 2015. Development of a membrane impregnated with a poly(dimethylsiloxane)/poly(ethylene glycol) copolymer for a high-throughput screening of the permeability of drugs, cosmetics, and other chemicals across the human skin. Eur. J. Pharm. Sci. 66: 41–49.

Miland, Å.O., de Weerd, L., Weum, S., et al. 2008. Visualising skin perfusion in isolated human abdominal skin flaps using dynamic infrared thermography and indocyanine green fluorescence video angiography. Eur. J. Plast. Surg. 31: 235–42.

Mitragotri, S., Anissimov, Y.G., Bunge, A.L. et al. 2011. Mathematical models of skin permeability: An overview. Int. J. Pharm. 418: 115–29.

Mohammadi, M.H., Heidary Araghi, B., Beydaghi, V. et al. 2016. Skin diseases modeling using combined tissue engineering and microfluidic technologies. *Adv. Healthc. Mater.* 5: 2459–80.

Mori, N., Morimoto, Y., Takeuchi, S. 2017.Skin integrated with perfusable vascular channels on a chip. Biomaterials 116: 48–56.

Moser, K., Kriwet, K., Naik, A., et al. 2001. Passive skin penetration enhancement and its quantification *in vitro*. Eur. J. Pharm. Biopharm. 52, 103–12.

Mojumdar, E.H., Kariman, Z., van Kerckhove, L., et al. 2014. The role of ceramide chain length distribution on the barrier properties of the skin lipid membranes. Biochim. Biophysic. Acta 1838: 2473–83.

Mura, S., Manconi, M., Sinico, C., et al. 2009. Penetration enhancer-containing vesicles (PEVs) as carriers for cutaneous delivery of minoxidil. Int. J. Pharm. 380: 72–79.

Naderkhani, E., Isaksson, J., Ryzhakov, A., et al. 2014. Development of a biomimetic phospholipid vesicle-based permeation assay for the estimation of intestinal drug permeability. J. Pharm. Sci. 103: 1882–90.

Naegel, A., Heisig, M., Wittum, G. 2013. Detailed modeling of skin penetration-An overview. Adv. Drug. Deliver. Rev. 65: 191–207.

Nagelreiter, C., Raffeiner, S., Geyerhofer, C., et al. 2013. Influence of drug content, type of semi-solid vehicle and rheological properties on the skin penetration of the model drug fludrocortisone acetate. Int. J. Pharm. 448: 305–12.

Nakano, M., Patel, N.K. 1970. Release, uptake, and permeation behavior of salicylic acid in ointment bases. J. Pharm. Sci. 59: 985–88.

Netzlaff, F., Lehr, C.-M., Wertz, P.W., et al. 2005. The human epidermis models EpiSkin, SkinEthic and EpiDerm: an evaluation of morphology and their suitability for testing phototoxicity, irritancy, corrosivity, and substance transport. Eur. J. Pharm. Biopharm. 60: 167–78.

Netzlaff, F., Kostka, K.H., Lehr, C.M., et al. 2006a. TEWL measurements as a routine for evaluating the integrity of epidermis sheets in static Franz type diffusion cells *in vitro*. Limitations shown by transport data testing. Eur. J. Pharm. Biopharm. 63: 44–50.

Netzlaff, F., Schaefer, U.F., Lehr, C.-M., et al. 2006b. Comparison of bovine udder skin with human and porcine skin in percutaneous permeation experiments. Altern. Lab. Anim. 34: 499–513.

Ngawhirunpat, T., Opanasopit, P., Rojanarata, T., et al. 2008. Evaluation of simultaneous permeation and metabolism of methyl nicotinate in human, snake, and shed snake skin. Pharm. Dev. Technol. 13: 75–83.

Ochalek, M., Heissler, S., Wohlrab, J., et al. 2012a. Characterization of lipid model membranes designed for studying impact of ceramide species on drug diffusion and penetration. Eur. J. Pharm. Biopharm. 81: 113–20.

Ochalek, M., Podhaisky, H., Ruettinger, H.-H., et al. 2012b. SC lipid model membranes designed for studying impact of ceramide species on drug diffusion and permeation, part III: influence of penetration enhancer on diffusion and permeation of model drugs. Int. J. Pharm. 436: 206–13.

OECD. 2004. Guidance document for the conduct of skin absorption studies number 28. In OECD Series on Testing and Assessment.

Oliveira, G., Beezer, A.E., Hadgraft, J., et al. 2010. Alcohol enhanced permeation in model membranes. Part I. Thermodynamic and kinetic analyses of membrane permeation. Int. J. Pharm. 393: 61–67.

Oliveira, G., Beezer, A.E., Hadgraft, J., et al. 2011. Alcohol enhanced permeation in model membranes. Part II. Thermodynamic analysis of membrane partitioning. Int. J. Pharm. 420: 216–22.

Oliveira, G., Hadgraft, J., Lane, M.E. 2012a. The role of vehicle interactions on permeation of an active through model membranes and human skin. Int. J. Cosmet. Sci. 34: 536–45.

Oliveira, G., Hadgraft, J., Lane, M.E. 2012b. The influence of volatile solvents on transport across model membranes and human skin. Int. J. Pharm. 435: 38–49.

Ottaviani, G., Martel, S., Carrupt, P.A. 2006. Parallel artificial membrane permeability assay: a new membrane for the fast prediction of passive human skin permeability. J. Med. Chem. 49: 3948–54.

Ottaviani, G., Martel, S., Carrupt, P.-A. 2007. In silico and *in vitro* filters for the fast estimation of skin permeation and distribution of new chemical entities. J. Med. Chem. 50: 742–48.

Palac, Z., Engesland, A., Flaten, G.E., et al. 2014. Liposomes for (trans)dermal drug delivery: the skin-PVPA as a novel *in vitro* stratum corneum model in formulation development. J. Liposome Res. 24: 313–22.

Patel, P., Schmieder, S., Krishnamurthy, K. 2016. Research techniques made simple: drug delivery techniques, part 2: commonly used techniques to assess topical drug bioavailability. J. Invest. Dermatol. 136: 434–9.

Pirot, F., Kalia, Y.N., Stinchcomb, A.L., et al. 1997. Characterization of the permeability barrier of human skin *in vivo*. Proc. Natl. Acad. Sci. U S A 94: 1562–67.

Pittermann, W., Hildebrandt, C., Prinz, A., et al. 2013. Comparative study of the skin tolerability of hand disinfectants using the BUS model. Hyg. Med. 38: 134–41.

Planz, V., Lehr, C-M., Windbergs, M. 2016. *In vitro* models for evaluating safety and efficacy of novel technologies for skin drug delivery. J. Control. Release 242: 89–104.

Ponec, M. 1992. *In vitro* cultured human skin cells as alternatives to animals for skin irritancy screening. Int. J. Cosmet. Sci. 14: 245–64.

Pullmannová, P., Pavlíková, l., Kováčik, A. et al. 2017. Permeability and microstructure of model stratum corneum lipid membranes containing ceramides with long (C16) and very long (C24) acyl chains. Biophysic. Chem. 224: 20–31.

Raber, A.S., Mittal, A., Schafer, J. et al. 2014. Quantification of nanoparticle uptake into hair follicles in pig ear and human forearm. J. Control. Release 179: 25–32.

Rastogi, S.K., Singh, J. 2001. Lipid extraction and transport of hydrophilic solutes through porcine epidermis. Int. J. Pharm. 225: 75–82.

Rigg, P.C., Barry, B.W. 1990. Shed snake skin and hairless mouse skin as model membranes for human skin during permeation studies. J. Invest. Dermatol. 94: 235–40.

Riviere, J.E., Bowman, K.F., Monteiro-Riviere, N.A., et al. 1986. The isolated perfused porcine skin flap (IPPSF). I. A novel *in vitro* model for percutaneous absorption and cutaneous toxicology studies. Fund. Appl. Toxicol. 7: 444–53.

Schaefer, U.F., Hansen, S., Schneider, M., et al. 2008. Models for skin absorption and skin toxicity testing In: Ehrhardt, K., Kim, K-J. (Eds), Drug Absorption Studies. Springer, New York, pp. 3–33.

Schäfer-Korting, M., Mahmoud, A., Lombardi Borgia, S. et al. 2008. Reconstructed epidermis and full-thickness skin for absorption testing: Influence of the vehicles used on steroid permeation. ATLA 36: 441–52.

Schmook, F.P., Meingassner, J.G., Billich, A. 2001. Comparison of human skin or epidermis models

Scognamiglio, I., De Stefano, D., Campani, V. et al., 2013. Nanocarriers for topical administration of resveratrol: a comparative study. Int. J. Pharm. 440: 179–87.

Selzer, D., Abdel-Mottaleb, M.M.A., Hahn, T., et al. 2013. Finite and infinite dosing: Difficulties in measurements, evaluations and predictions. Adv. Drug Deliv. Rev. 65: 278–94.

Senyigit, T., Sonvico, F., Barbieri, S., et al. 2010. Lecithin/chitosan nanoparticles of clobetasol-17-propionate capable of accumulation in pig skin. J. Control. Release 142: 368–73.

Shakel, Z., Nunes, C., Costa Lima, S.A., et al. 2019. Development of a novel human stratum corneum model, as a tool in the optimization of drug formulations. Int. J. Pharm. 569:118571

Shim, J., Seok Kang, H., Park, W-S., et al. 2004. Transdermal delivery of mixnoxidil with block copolymer nanoparticles. J. Control. Release 97: 477–84.

Silva Garcia Praça, F., Silva Garcia Medina, W., Eloy, J.O. et al. 2018. Evaluation of critical parameters for *in vitro* skin permeation and penetration studies using animal skin models. Eur. J. Pharm. Sci. 111: 121–32.

Sinko, B., Garrigues, T.M., Balogh, G.T. et al. 2012. Skin-PAMPA: a new method for fast prediction of skin penetration. Eur. J. Pharm. Sci. 45: 698–707.

Sinko, B., Kokosi, J., Avdeef, A., et al. 2009. A PAMPA study of the permeability-enhancing effect of new ceramide analogues. Chem. Biodiversity 6: 1867–74.

Sintov, A.C. 2017. Cumulative evidence of the low reliability of frozen/thawed pig skin as a model for *in vitro* percutaneous permeation testing. Eur. J. Pharm. Sci. 102: 261–63.

Sochorová, M., Audrlická, P., Červená, M. et al. 2019. Permeability and microstructure of cholesterol-depleted skin lipid membranes and human stratum corneum. J. Colloid Interface Sci. 535: 227–38.

Souto, E.B. 2005. SLN and NLC for Topical Delivery of Antifungals. Institute of Pharmacy, Freie Universität, Berlin.

Stahl, J., Wohlert, M., Kietzmann, M. 2011. The effect of formulation vehicles on the *in vitro* percutaneous permeation of ibuprofen. BMC Pharmacol. 11: 12.

Sugibayashi, K., Todo, H., Oshizaka, T., Owada, Y. 2010. Mathematical model to predict skin concentration of drugs: toward utilization of silicone membrane to predict skin concentration of drugs as an animal testing alternative. Pharm. Res. 27: 134–42.

Suppasrivasuseth, J., Bellantone, R.A., Plakogiannis, F.M., et al. 2006. Permeability and retention studies of (-)epicatechin gel formulations in human cadaver skin. Drug Dev. Ind. Pharm. 32: 1007–17.

Tavano, L., Alfano, P., Muzzalupo, R., et al. 2011. Niosomes vs microemulsions: new carriers for topical delivery of Capsaicin. Colloids Surf. B Biointerfaces 87: 333–39.

Ternullo, S., Basnet, P., Holsæter, A.M., et al. 2018. Deformable liposomes for skin therapy with human epidermal growth factor: The effect of liposomal surface charge. Eur. J. Pharm. Sci. 125: 163–71.

Ternullo, S., de Weerd, L., Eide Flaten, G., et al. 2017a. The isolated perfused human skin flap model: A missing link in skin penetration studies? Eur. J. Pharm. Sci. 96: 334–41.

Ternullo, S., de Weerd, L., Holsæter, A.M., et al. 2017b. Going skin deep: A direct comparison of penetration potential of lipid-based nanovesicles on the isolated perfused human skin flap model. Eur. J. Pharm. Biopharm. 121: 14–23.

Tsinman, K., Sinko, B. 2013. A high throughput method to predict skin penetration and screen topical formulations. Cosmetics Toiletries 128: 192–99.

Uche, L.E., Gooris, G.S., Bouwstra, J.A., et al. 2019. Barrier capability of skin lipid models: effect of ceramides and free fatty acid composition. Langmuir 35: 15376–88.

Uchida, T., Yakumaru, M., Nishioka, K., et al. 2016. Evaluation of a silicone membrane as an alternative to human skin for determining skin permeation parameters of chemical compounds. Chem. Pharm. Bull. 64: 1338–46.

Uchiyama, M., Oguri, M., Mojumdar, E.H., et al. 2016. Free fatty acids chain length distribution affects the permeability of skin lipid model membranes. Biochem. Biophys. Acta 1858: 2050–59.

Van Gele, M., Geusens, B., Brochez, L., et al. 2011. Three-dimensional skin models as tools for transdermal drug delivery: challenges and limitations. Expert Opin. Drug Deliv. 8: 705–20.

Vicentini, F.T.M.C., Casagrande, R., Verri Jr, W.A., et al. 2008. Quercetin in lyotropic liquid crystalline formulations: physical, chemical and functional stability. AAPS PharmSciTech 9: 591–96.

Vizserálek, G., Berkó, S., Tóth, G. et al. 2015. Permeability test for transdermal and local therapeutic patches using Skin PAMPA method. Eur. J. Pharm. Sci. 76: 165–72.

Wagner, H., Kostka, K-H., Lehr, C-M., et al. 2001. Interrelation of permeation and penetration parameters obtained from in vitro experiments with human skin and skin equivalents. J. Control. Release 75: 283–95.

Wagner, S.M., Nogueira, A.C., Paul, M., et al. 2003. The isolated normothermic hemoperfused porcine forelimb as a test system for transdermal absorption studies. J. Artif. Organs 6: 183–91.

Wang, J., Guo, F., Ma, M., et al. 2014. Nanovesicular system containing tretinoin for dermal targeting delivery and rosacea treatment: a comparison of hexosomes, glycerosomes and ethosomes. RSC Adv. 4: 45458–66.

Wang, Y., Sun, J., Liu, H. et al. 2009. Predicting skin permeability using liposome electrokinetic chromatography. Analyst 134: 267–72.

Waters, L.J., Shahzad, Y., Stephenson, J. 2013. Modelling skin permeability with micellar liquid chromatography. Eur. J. Pharm. Sci. 50: 335–40.

Watkinson, R.M., Guy, R.H., Hadgraft, J., et al. 2009a. Optimisation of cosolvent concentration for topical drug delivery II: influence of propylene glycol on ibuprofen permeation. Skin Pharmacol. Physiol. 22: 225–30.

Watkinson, R.M., Guy, R.H., Oliveira, G., et al. 2011. Optimisation of cosolvent concentration for topical drug delivery III–influence of lipophilic vehicles on ibuprofen permeation. Skin Pharmacol. Physiol. 24: 22–26.

Watkinson, R.M., Herkenne, C., Guy, R.H., et al. 2009b. Influence of ethanol on the solubility, ionization and permeation characteristics of ibuprofen in silicone and human skin. Skin Pharmacol. Physiol. 22: 15–21.

Wester, R.C., Melendres, J., Sedik, L., et al. 1998. Percutaneous absorption of salicylic acid, theophylline, 2, 4-dimethylamine, diethyl hexyl phthalic acid, and p-aminobenzoic acid in the isolated perfused porcine skin flap compared to man in vivo. Toxicol. Appl. Pharmacol. 151: 159–65.

Zghoul, N., Fuchs, R., Lehr, C-M., et al. 2001. Reconstructed skin equivalents for assessing percutaneous drug absorption from pharmaceutical formulations. ALTEX 18: 103–06.

Zhang, H., Zhu, X., Shen, J., et al. 2016. Characterization of a liposome-based artificial skin membrane for in vitro permeation studies using Franz diffusion cell device, J. Liposome Res. 27: 302–11.

Zhang, Y., Lane, M.E., Hadgraft, J., et al. 2019. A comparison of the in vitro permeation of niacinamide in mammalian skin and in the Parallel Artificial Membrane Permeation Assay (PAMPA) model. Int. J. Pharm. 556: 142–49.

Zhao, Y., Moddaresi, M., Jones, S.A., et al. 2009. A dynamic topical hydrofluoroalkane foam to induce nanoparticle modification and drug release in situ. Eur. J. Pharm. Biopharm. 72: 521–28.

Zsikó, S., Cutcher, K., Kovács, A. 2019. Nanostructured lipid carrier gel for the dermal application of lidocaine: comparison of skin penetration testing methods. Pharmaceutics 11: 310.

49 Effects of Phospholipids on Skin

Use of Primary Human Keratinocytes and Fibroblasts as 2D Cell Culture Models

Claudia Vater and Victoria Klang
University of Vienna, Vienna, Austria

CONTENT

49.1 CORE MESSAGE

Human primary keratinocytes and fibroblasts are classic 2D cell culture models that are highly useful for the assessment of the skin compatibility of cosmetic and pharmaceutical formulation compounds. The skin compatibility of phospholipid-based nanoemulsions was investigated using different cytotoxicity assays. Agreement between results of the different tests was good; the overall cell viability of both keratinocytes and fibroblasts was far higher for the tested lecithin-based formulations than for the control stabilized by sodium dodecyl sulfate. The effect of the formulations on wound healing can be investigated by scratch assays using human primary fibroblasts. First results indicate suitable properties of phospholipid-based formulations.

49.2 INTRODUCTION

Phospholipids are known to be versatile surface-active agents that can be used for the production of a range of cosmetic or pharmaceutical formulations. Among others, vesicular systems, submicron-sized emulsions, lipid nanoparticles, or lyotropic liquid crystalline mesophases (*microemulsions*) can be produced using different derivatives of phosphatidylcholine [1–5].

In general, phospholipids are assumed to be among the most eudermic options in formulation development even for sensitive target areas such as mucosae or skin. *In vivo* application studies have nonetheless indicated certain negative effects on the state of the skin barrier during regular use, at least for lysophosphatidylcholine mixtures [6]. Although these effects were reversible, our aim was to evaluate the biocompatibility of different commercially available phospholipid mixtures in aqueous and multiphase systems. To this end, *in vitro* 2D cell culture methods were established in our lab. Despite modern alternatives to these classic techniques, they have their rightful spot to evaluate effects of individual formulation compounds or entire formulations on human tissues. An obvious advantage is a more time- and cost-efficient workflow when compared to the more complex 3D culture models [7, 8].

Evaluation of biocompatibility using cell culture systems is a vital step when developing new formulations. A wide variety of established cell lines are available for research purposes. A common example are different murine cell lines, which are easily available and very robust; they can be passaged without limitation [9, 10]. These advantages render them useful for standard biocompatibility tests in preliminary studies. However, results obtained with immortalized cell lines may not reflect the actual *in vivo* situation. It is the general opinion that cytotoxicity tests *in vitro* are more convincing when performed with cells homologous to human tissue. Thus, appropriate cell lines for cytotoxicity and tolerance tests concerning human skin are human dermal fibroblasts and human epidermal keratinocytes [11, 12]. The present chapter summarizes our work and recent findings in context with the use of human primary skin cells—epidermal keratinocytes and dermal fibroblasts—for evaluation of the cytotoxic potential of formulation compounds. In particular, the effect of surfactants on skin was evaluated and set into context with recent skin penetration and permeation studies using these surfactants.

49.3   METHODOLOGICAL ASPECTS AND OUTCOMES

For our experiments, the following approach was taken, which is discussed in the next sections.

49.3.1   Isolation of Primary Skin Cells

For the isolation of primary keratinocytes and fibroblasts, skin of healthy female and male donors aged between 20 and 65 years is used as obtained during plastic surgery. Approval of the internal ethics committee of the involved medical facility is required; in our case, this is accounted for by the Medical University of Vienna.

Skin used for the isolation of cells stems from abdomen, back, or breast of surplus skin. There is also the possibility to isolate keratinocytes from neonatal foreskin; however, these cells are more prone to expression of psoriasis-associated markers, which might cause problems, especially in organotypic cultures [13]. Furthermore, neonatal skin cells exhibit significantly faster healing rates in experimentally induced wounds *in vitro* when compared with skin cells derived from adult skin [14]. Thus, the use of skin cells derived from adult skin is recommended for all regular experiments.

Superficial skin strips from adult skin are incubated in dispase II in phosphate buffered saline (PBS) overnight at 4°C. The epidermis is separated mechanically and then digested with trypsin and DNase I for 30 minutes at 37°C. Keratinocytes are cultured in a serum-free keratinocyte growth medium (KGM-2); for details see [15, 16].

As for the isolation of fibroblasts, dermal specimens are incubated in a fibroblast isolation enzyme working solution diluted in distilled water for approximately 4 hours while shaking at 37°C. Afterwards, the suspension is filtered and washed with PBS, then filtered again. The cell suspension is spun down, and cells are washed with Dulbecco's Modified Eagle's Medium (DMEM), then spun down again. The supernatant is removed, and the cells are resuspended in medium (DMEM supplemented with 10% fetal bovine serum [FBS] and 1%

TABLE 49.1

Final Supplement Concentrations after Addition to the Medium

Bovine pituitary extract	0.004 mL/mL
Epidermal growth factor (recombinant human)	0.125 ng/mL
Insulin (recombinant human)	5.000 μg/mL
Hydrocortisone	0.330 μg/mL
Epinephrine	0.390 μg/mL
Transferrin (recombinant human)	10.00 μg/mL
$CaCl_2$	0.060 mM

penicillin-streptomycin), then plated in a culture flask. A more detailed description of these isolation procedures can be found in the literature [15–17].

49.3.2 CULTIVATION

In general, the cultivation of primary keratinocytes is more challenging than the cultivation of fibroblasts. Compared to fibroblasts, keratinocytes are more prone to apoptosis when cell density is too low or to differentiation and senescence when cell density is too high [18].

Keratinocytes can be cultured following two main approaches. The classic method developed by Rheinwald and Green [19] is based on the use of serum-containing media and a feeder layer of lethally irradiated mouse fibroblasts. A more recent approach refrains from using feeder cells, but instead relies on serum-free media that are low in calcium. When using these serum-free media, the chances of contamination with other cells such as fibroblasts or melanocytes is reduced. Thus, this is recommended when the objective is to study the properties of keratinocytes alone. To achieve a satisfying growth rate, the serum-free media have to be mixed with supplements. In case of the medium used in our laboratory, KGM-2, these supplements are provided in an additional supplement pack. The final supplement concentrations after addition to the medium are given in Table 49.1.

Using this medium, keratinocytes are cultured at 37°C in a 5% CO_2 humidified environment. The medium should be changed every 48 hours until about 70% confluency is achieved. Then cells are split in a ratio of 1:7 to 1:10.

For cultivation of fibroblasts, it is possible to use conventional media like DMEM or RPMI-1640, mixed with 10% FBS and 1% penicillin-streptomycin. After isolation, it is possible to add 15% FBS for the first passages to boost cell growth.

The typical phenotype of epidermal keratinocytes and dermal fibroblasts is shown in Figure 49.1.

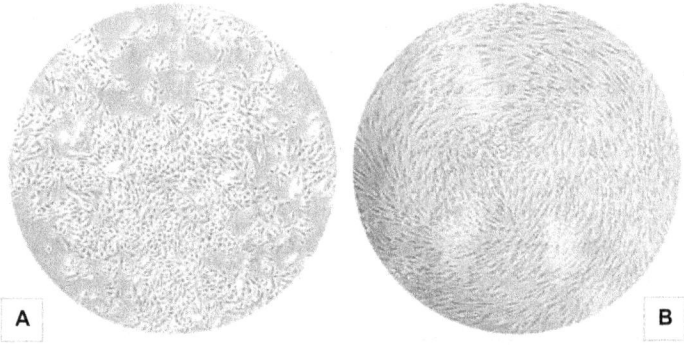

FIGURE 49.1 Microscopic images of primary human keratinocytes (A) and fibroblasts (B); magnification 100×, Nikon Diaphot 300.

49.3.3   Cytotoxicity Assays: Effect of Nanoemulsions on Skin Cell Viability

The goal of our current studies is to investigate the skin compatibility of individual additives or to evaluate new dermal formulations. For aqueous formulations with low viscosity, such as phospholipid-based submicron emulsions, or *nanoemulsions*, evaluation in cell viability assays is possible. To this end, we deployed two established cell viability assays: the EZ4U assay and BrdU assay.

The combination of these two cytotoxicity assays delivers important information about cell viability, but also about the cells' ability to proliferate. This is of particular interest when targeting wound healing properties.

The Biomedica EZ4U cell proliferation kit assay is a modification of the MTT test based on 3-(4,5-dimethylthiazol-2-yl)-2,5-diphenyltetrazolium bromide. The assay scans for mitochondrial damage in cells and therefore correlates directly with cell viability [20].

The BrdU assay is a tool for the quantitative measurement of DNA replication. It measures the amount of the pyrimidine analogon BrdU being incorporated into DNA instead of thymidine [21]. Cellular incorporation of BrdU can be detected by anti-BrdU–specific antibodies following membrane permeabilization via enzyme-linked immunosorbent assay (ELISA).

For both assays, primary cells are suspended in a colorless culture medium at 10^4 cells per well for fibroblasts and 1.5×10^4 cells per well for keratinocytes. Then the cells are seeded on 96-well flat-bottom plates. After incubation for 24 hours at 37°C in a 5% CO_2 humidified environment, the formulation of interest is added to the culture at the desired concentration, e.g., 1 + 1 with sterile saline solution. After a specified incubation time, the formulation is removed from the culture plates. Plates are washed at least three times with colorless culture medium before adding the EZ4U substrate or BrdU labeling solution, respectively. Colorimetric staining of the cells and the supernatant are evaluated, e.g., with a multiwell plate reader at 450 nm in case of the EZ4U assay and at 370 nm in case of the BrdU assay, to quantify the respective reaction products. For more detailed information, see [16, 17].

Low viscosity of the formulation of interest is vital for the success of cell viability assays. The investigated submicron-sized emulsions were of the oil-in-water type, containing 10% w/w oil and 5% w/w of surfactant. Formulations containing phospholipid-type surfactants were evaluated in parallel to formulations stabilized by sodium dodecyl sulfate (SDS). For the oil phase, common cosmetic oils such as jojoba oil, medium-chain triglycerides, and sunflower oil were used.

Different incubation times were tested for comparative purposes. Since prolonged experiment times were found to be less informative due to reinstigated cell proliferation, shorter incubation times of a few hours only are recommended. The results of the cytotoxicity assays using an incubation time of two hours are given in Figure 49.2. Cell viability of both keratinocytes and fibroblasts was generally quite high after treatment with phospholipid-based nanoemulsions, especially when compared with the corresponding SDS-based formulations. The latter generally exhibited high cytotoxicity, basically leading to survival rates around 0%. It can be summarized that cell viability as observed with both the EZ4U and BrdU assay was significantly higher for the three tested lecithin-based nanoemulsions than for their counterparts containing SDS as surfactant ($p < 0.05$ in all cases).

In case of primary keratinocytes (Figure 49.2a), cell viability rates were comparable for all three lecithin-based nanoemulsions. Cell viability was observed to be generally high, with values over 80% in the case of the EZ4U assay and over 60% in the BrdU assay. With the EZ4U assay, the observed cell viability was generally higher than with the BrdU assay, but not to a statistically significant extent. In conclusion, results of the two different cytotoxicity assays were in good agreement for the keratinocyte cultures.

In the case of primary fibroblasts (Figure 49.2b), more differences between individual lecithin-based formulations were observed. The highest cell viability was observed for S75-mct (98% with EZ4U, 96% with BrdU), followed by S75-jojo (90% with EZ4U, 66% with BrdU) and S75-sun

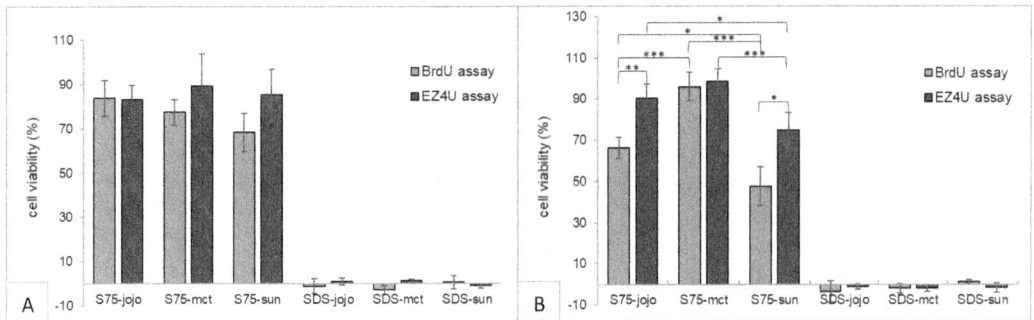

FIGURE 49.2 Cell viability of human epidermal keratinocytes (A) and dermal fibroblasts (B) after 2 hours of incubation with nanoemulsions. Data are expressed as % viability ± SD, $n = 4$ with 12 parallel experiments per formulation. Gray bars represent the results obtained by BrdU assays, black bars those obtained by EZ4U assays. S75: Lipoid S75 (soybean phospholipids with phosphatidylcholine content of 70% w/w); SDS: sodium dodecyl sulfate; jojo: jojoba oil; mct: medium-chain triglycerides; sun: sunflower oil. Nanoemulsions consisted of 5% w/w of surfactant (S75 or SDS), 10% w/w of oil component, and water. (Image reprinted from [17] with permission of Elsevier.)

(75% with EZ4U, 48% with BrdU). The results of the EZ4U assay indicate significantly lower fibroblast viability rates after treatment with S75-sun when compared to the corresponding formulations S75-jojo and especially S75-mct ($p \leq 0.05$ and $p \leq 0.001$). The results of the BrdU assay confirm this observation; significantly lower fibroblast viability was observed for S75-sun, with even larger differences to S75-jojo and especially S75-mct ($p \leq 0.001$). Thus, good agreement of the results obtained with the two different assays was confirmed for the fibroblast cultures despite differences in absolute values (tendency to higher absolute values in cell viability for EZ4U, which reach statistical significance in the case of S75-jojo and S75-sun).

49.3.4 INVESTIGATION OF WOUND HEALING USING SCRATCH ASSAYS

Taking these results one step further, Norway spruce resin and betulin were incorporated into phospholipid-based nanoemulsions to investigate their potential for wound healing applications. Since the described phospholipid-based formulations exhibited good compatibility with both epidermal and dermal human cells, they are promising candidates for stabilization of formulations to be used on sensitive or damaged skin. Formulations containing the previously mentioned wound healing agents are currently under investigation. Resin from Norway spruce (*Picea abies*) is known to have wound healing properties; ointments prepared from Norway spruce resin have been used in Scandinavia for centuries to treat acutely and chronically infected wounds [22]. Extract from birch bark (*Betula pendula*) has a long-lasting history as a traditional remedy to accelerate wound healing. Betulin is the main compound of these extracts and has been shown to accelerate wound healing *ex vivo* and *in vivo* [23]. At the moment, these formulations are being tested in cell viability assays and additional scratch assays *in vitro*. The latter is a simple, cost-efficient, and well-developed method to measure cell migration. After creating a standardized scratch in a cell monolayer, images are recorded at defined time intervals to observe and quantify cell migration during this simulated wound healing process [24]. Formulations can be applied after the scratch to analyze their effects on wound healing. Preliminary studies with nanoemulsions containing Norway spruce resin delivered promising results (Figure 49.3). After induction of an artificial injury to a confluent fibroblast monolayer and treatment with the test formulations, cell migration into the wound region was observed in regular intervals over 20 hours. First results indicated enhanced cell migration in the case of formulations with the test compound.

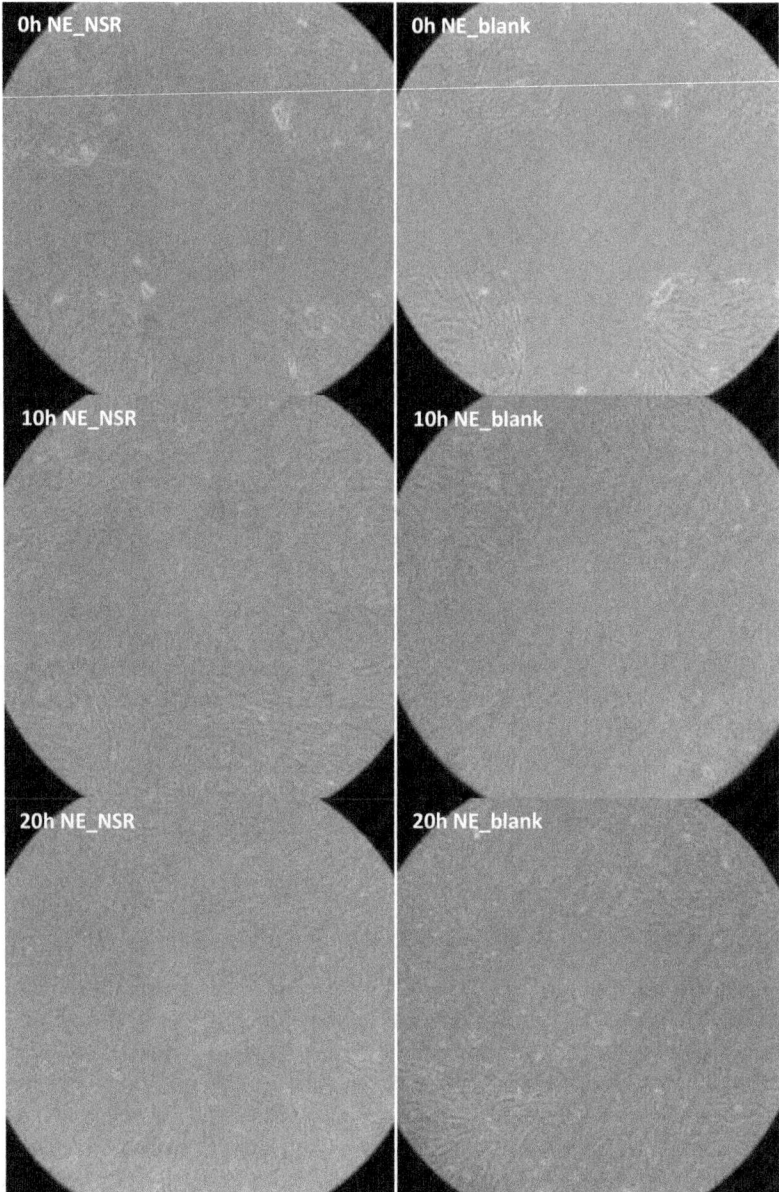

FIGURE 49.3 Microscopic images of the wound healing process observed on a confluent monolayer of primary fibroblasts after injury and subsequent treatment with either a test nanoemulsion with Norway spruce resin (NE_NSR) or a control nanoemulsion (NE_blank). Images represent time intervals directly after the treatment after 10 hours and after 20 hours. Magnification is 100× (Nikon Diaphot 300).

49.4   IMPORTANT EXPERIMENTAL PARAMETERS

During investigation of cosmetic or pharmaceutical formulations with cell viability assays of human primary cells, some important aspects should be considered. On the one hand, aspects related to the formulation's physicochemical properties play an important role for the success of the experiments. On the other hand, the experimental parameters related to the cells themselves, their treatment, and the duration of the experiment are of importance.

Regarding formulation properties, it is evident that only formulations with low viscosity that can be rinsed off easily are suitable for the envisioned experiments. Formulations with high viscosity such as thick oil-rich emulsion systems would exhibit increased stickiness to the cell layer; trying to wash them off with medium would be futile, and the growth area could be damaged in the attempt.

In regard to experimental parameters of the described cell culture experiments, human primary skin cells are generally more sensitive to external influences than cells derived from immortalized cell lines. Immortalized cell lines such as HaCaT keratinocyte cell lines or mouse fibroblast cell lines 3T3 or L929 are more robust in nature; they are a useful model to answer basic research questions [9]. However, more meaningful results are obtained by using primary cells homologous to human tissue for final studies. Cell density should be closely monitored, and experiment durations should be confined to a few hours.

49.5 COMPARISON TO OTHER METHODS

During the course of our studies, other techniques were deployed to assess the effect of different phospholipid-based nanoemulsions on skin barrier function. Thus, results of the *in vitro* cell culture experiments were confirmed in regard to their general implications.

Diffusion cell studies with porcine skin as a model membrane and a hydrophilic model drug were performed to compare nanoemulsions with different kinds of surfactants [16]. Results showed that formulations based on anionic surfactants were able to deliver the drug more efficiently through the model than skin formulations containing the amphiphilic lecithins or nonionic surfactants [16]. These findings are in line with the cytotoxicity results, as anionic surfactants exerted a stronger effect on skin cells *in vitro* and can thus be expected to also have a stronger impact on skin penetration of co-applied substances.

Furthermore, we compared the skin penetration of a lecithin mixture and the anionic SDS as basic aqueous formulations (liposomal/aqueous dispersions) [17]. *Ex vivo* skin penetration studies were conducted using attenuated total reflection–Fourier transform infrared (ATR-FTIR) spectroscopy in combination with tape stripping [25–27]. It was of interest to compare the penetration behavior of the two surfactants to obtain an idea of their skin irritation potential, since the latter is most likely linked to the spatial distribution of the surfactant in the stratum corneum [28]. The experiments showed a rapid decrease of the relative lecithin concentration with increasing skin depth, with traceable amounts only until about 15% of stratum corneum depth. In contrast, the more aggressive SDS penetrated into the stratum corneum in larger relative amounts and reached deeper stratum corneum layers [17]. This is in line with previous findings [29, 30]. Regarding the penetration of other formulation compounds such as cosmetic oils, these were only detectable in the outermost cell layers of the stratum corneum. The observed penetration behavior of the surfactants lecithin and SDS corresponds well with the diffusion cell and cell culture data. In summary, it can be concluded that SDS affects skin barrier function and the individual epidermal and dermal cells to a much stronger extent than lecithin-based surfactants. To investigate effects on a molecular level, analysis of human skin cells is currently being performed via atomic force microscopy. Thus, changes in cell morphology caused by the surfactants can be observed directly [31, 32].

49.6 CONCLUSION

The effect of phospholipid-based nanoemulsions on cell viability *in vitro* was investigated using human primary keratinocytes and fibroblasts. Cell viability was confirmed to be high for all investigated nanoemulsions stabilized by lecithin mixtures with both EZ4U and BrdU assays. In contrast, survival rates around 0% were observed for control formulations based on sodium dodecyl sulfate. Ongoing scratch assays using human primary fibroblasts aim to explore the potential of phospholipid-based nanoemulsions with and without additives for wound healing purposes.

ACKNOWLEDGEMENT

We would like to acknowledge the financial support of the Research Platform Characterisation of Drug Delivery Systems on Skin and Investigations of Involved Mechanisms, University of Vienna, and of the Phospholipid Research Center, Heidelberg, Germany. We would also like to thank Claudia Valenta for support and valuable discussions.

REFERENCES

1. V. Klang, C. Valenta, Lecithin-based nanoemulsions, J. Drug Deliv. Sci. Technol. 21 (2011) 55–76.
2. J. Li, X. Wang, T. Zhang, C. Wang, Z. Huang, X. Luo, Y. Deng, A review on phospholipids and their main applications in drug delivery systems, Asian J. Pharm. Sci. 10 (2015) 81–98.
3. P. van Hoogevest, A. Wendel, The use of natural and synthetic phospholipids as pharmaceutical excipients, Eur. J. Lipid Sci. Technol. 116 (2014) 1088–1107.
4. P. van Hoogevest, A. Fahr, Phospholipids in Cosmetic Carriers, in: Nanocosmetics, Springer International Publishing, 2019: pp. 95–140.
5. J.C. Schwarz, V. Klang, M. Hoppel, D. Mahrhauser, C. Valenta, Natural microemulsions: Formulation design and skin interaction, Eur. J. Pharm. Biopharm. 81 (2012) 557–562.
6. M. Wolf, V. Klang, T. Stojcic, C. Fuchs, M. Wolzt, C. Valenta, NLC versus nanoemulsions: Effect on physiological skin parameters during regular in vivo application and impact on drug penetration, Int. J. Pharm. 549 (2018) 343–351.
7. F. Netzlaff, C.M. Lehr, P.W. Wertz, U.F. Schaefer, The human epidermis models EpiSkin®, SkinEthic® and EpiDerm®: An evaluation of morphology and their suitability for testing phototoxicity, irritancy, corrosivity, and substance transport, Eur. J. Pharm. Biopharm. 60 (2005) 167–178.
8. S.H. Mathes, H. Ruffner, U. Graf-Hausner, The use of skin models in drug development, Adv. Drug Deliv. Rev. 69–70 (2014) 81–102.
9. B.G. Auner, M. Wirth, C. Valenta, Antioxidative activity and cytotoxicity of four different flavonoids for dermal applications, J. Drug Deliv. Sci. Technol. 15 (2005) 227–232.
10. A. Hafner, J. Lovri, I. Pepi, J. Filipovi-Grči, Lecithin/chitosan nanoparticles for transdermal delivery of melatonin, J. Microencapsul. 28 (2011) 807–815.
11. G. Kaur, J.M. Dufour, Cell lines: Valuable tools or useless artifacts., Spermatogenesis. 2 (2012) 1–5.
12. C. Wiegand, U.C. Hipler, Evaluation of biocompatibility and cytotoxicity using keratinocyte and fibroblast cultures, Skin Pharmacol. Physiol. 22 (2009) 74–82.
13. G. Tjabringa, M. Bergers, D. Van Rens, R. De Boer, E. Lamme, J. Schalkwijk, Development and validation of human psoriatic skin equivalents, Am. J. Pathol. 173 (2008) 815–823.
14. R. Mateu, V. Živicová, E.D. Krejí, M. Grim, H. Strnad, A. Vlek, M. Kolá, L. Lacina, P. Gál, J. Borský, K. Smetana, B. Dvoánková, Functional differences between neonatal and adult fibroblasts and keratinocytes: Donor age affects epithelial-mesenchymal crosstalk in vitro, Int. J. Mol. Med. 38 (2016) 1063–1074.
15. M. Mildner, C. Ballaun, M. Stichenwirth, R. Bauer, R. Gmeiner, M. Buchberger, V. Mlitz, E. Tschachler, Gene silencing in a human organotypic skin model, Biochem. Biophys. Res. Commun. 348 (2006) 76–82.
16. C. Vater, A. Adamovic, L. Ruttensteiner, K. Steiner, P. Tajpara, V. Klang, A. Elbe-Bürger, M. Wirth, C. Valenta, Cytotoxicity of lecithin-based nanoemulsions on human skin cells and ex vivo skin permeation: Comparison to conventional surfactant types, Int. J. Pharm. 566 (2019) 383–390.
17. C. Vater, V. Hlawaty, P. Werdenits, M. Anna Cichoń, V. Klang, A. Elbe-Bürger Funding, M. Wirth, C. Valenta Funding, Effects of lecithin-based nanoemulsions on skin: short-time cytotoxicity MTT and BrdU studies, skin penetration of surfactants and additives and the delivery of curcumin, Int. J. Pharm. 580 (2020).
18. T. Aasen, J.C.I. Belmonte, Isolation and cultivation of human keratinocytes from skin or plucked hair for the generation of induced pluripotent stem cells, Nat. Protoc. 5 (2010) 371–382.
19. J.G. Rheinwald, H. Green, Seria cultivation of strains of human epidemal keratinocytes: the formation keratinizin colonies from single cell is, Cell. 6 (1975) 331–343.
20. T. Mosmann, Rapid colorimetric assay for cellular growth and survival: Application to proliferation and cytotoxicity assays, J. Immunol. Methods. 65 (1983) 55–63.
21. H.G. Gratzner, Monoclonal antibody to 5-bromo- and 5-iododeoxyuridine: A new reagent for detection of DNA replication, Science. 218 (1982) 474–475.

22. J.J. Jokinen, A. Sipponen, Refined spruce resin to treat chronic wounds: rebirth of an old folkloristic therapy, Adv. Wound Care. 5 (2016) 198–207.
23. I. Steinbrenner, P. Houdek, S. Pollok, J.M. Brandner, R. Daniels, Influence of the oil phase and topical formulation on the wound healing ability of a birch bark dry extract, PLoS One. 11 (2016) 1–17.
24. C.-C. Liang, A.Y. Park, J.-L. Guan, In vitro scratch assay: a convenient and inexpensive method for analysis of cell migration in vitro, Nat. Protoc. 2 (2007) 329–333.
25. C.F. Goh, D.Q.M. Craig, J. Hadgraft, M.E. Lane, The application of ATR-FTIR spectroscopy and multi-variate data analysis to study drug crystallisation in the stratum corneum, Eur. J. Pharm. Biopharm. 111 (2017) 16–25.
26. B. Gotter, W. Faubel, R.H.H. Neubert, Optical methods for measurements of skin penetration, Skin Pharmacol. Physiol. 21 (2008) 156–165.
27. M. Hoppel, D. Baurecht, E. Holper, D. Mahrhauser, C. Valenta, Validation of the combined ATR-FTIR/tape stripping technique for monitoring the distribution of surfactants in the stratum corneum, Int. J. Pharm. 472 (2014) 88–93.
28. G. Mao, C.R. Flach, R. Mendelsohn, R.M. Walters, Imaging the distribution of sodium dodecyl sulfate in skin by confocal raman and infrared microspectroscopy, Pharm. Res. 29 (2012) 2189–2201.
29. M. Hoppel, E. Holper, D. Baurecht, C. Valenta, Monitoring the distribution of surfactants in the stratum corneum by combined ATR-FTIR and tape-stripping experiments, Skin Pharmacol. Physiol. 28 (2015) 167–175.
30. M. Wolf, M. Halper, R. Pribyl, D. Baurecht, C. Valenta, Distribution of phospholipid based formula-tions in the skin investigated by combined ATR-FTIR and tape stripping experiments, Int. J. Pharm. 519 (2017) 198–205.
31. C. Riethmüller, Assessing the skin barrier via corneocyte morphometry, Exp. Dermatol. 27 (2018) 923–930.
32. M. Soltanipoor, T. Stilla, C. Riethmüller, J.P. Thyssen, J.K. Sluiter, T. Rustemeyer, T.W. Fischer, S. Kezic, I. Angelova-Fischer, Specific barrier response profiles after experimentally induced skin irrita-tion in vivo, Contact Dermatitis. 79 (2018) 59–66.

50 Human Cadaver Skin Viability for *In Vitro* Percutaneous Absorption

Storage and Detrimental Effects of Heat Separation and Freezing

Ronald C. Wester, Julie Christoffel, Tracy Hartway, Nicholas Poblete, and Howard I. Maibach
University of California, San Francisco, California

James Forsell
Northern California Transplant Bank, San Rafael, California

CONTENTS

50.1 INTRODUCTION

Human cadaver skin is utilized in hospitals and research laboratories for various reasons. For nearly four decades, hospitals have banked skin for use as an effective temporary covering for burn wounds (1). Research laboratories also use cadaver skin to study the percutaneous absorption of drugs (2) and hazardous chemicals of environmental concern (3). Procedures such as heat treatment to separate epidermis from dermis are performed as part of the skin preparation for these studies. Human cadaver skin is not an easily obtained commodity, and storage for use becomes a necessity. Refrigerating and freezing skin are commonly done. With treatment and storage, skin viability has become a concern. This study determined human cadaver skin viability from the point of death through the time of storage and the effect of heat and freezing treatment.

50.2 MATERIALS AND METHODS

Human cadaver skin was obtained from the Northern California Transplant Bank (San Rafael, California, USA). All donors were Caucasian, aged 21 to 53 years, and both genders were represented. The time of a subject's death was recorded; skin was taken from the subject's thighs by use of a dermatome targeted to 500 micrometers. The skin was immediately placed in MEM-BSS and refrigerated at 4°C. The skin was then transported on ice to the laboratory and stored refrigerated at 4°C in Eagle's MEM-BSS with 50 µg/mL gentamicin until used.

Dermatomed skin samples were mounted in an *in vitro* assembly consisting of flow-through design glass diffusion cells (Laboratory Glass Apparatus, Inc., Berkeley, California). Eagle's MEM-BSS with gentamicin served as a receptor fluid, and the flow rate was 1.5 mL/hr. The receptor fluid was at 37°C, skin surface temperature at 32°C. Eagle's MEM contains glucose, and glucose metabolism to lactate in anaerobic energy metabolism was used as the measure of skin viability. Lactate production was determined using the Sigma Diagnostic Kit No. 826-UV (St. Louis, Missouri) and a Hitachi spectrophotometer (San Jose, California).

Dermatomed skin was used as stored in the refrigerator, frozen at −22°C for storage, or heat separated (60°C water for one minute) into epidermis and dermis.

50.3   RESULTS

Figure 50.1 shows lactate production from four human skin sources mounted in the diffusion system. Each data point represents 4-hour receptor fluid collection intervals over the 24-hour diffusion period. No chemical was dosed on the skin—just receptor fluid perfusing the skin. Lactate was produced by the skin sources over the full 24-hour period. The lactate curves rise in the early part of the period, where glucose is diffusing into the skin and lactate is diffusing out of the skin. Two skin sources reached steady state at about 12 hours; lactate from the other two skin sources continued to rise until the process was stopped at 24 hours.

Table 50.1 and Figure 50.2 give the cumulative lactate produced (mmol/L) for the 24-hour perfusion period. Human skin was either dermatomed skin or heat-separated epidermis used within the time period of 0.75 to 13 days after donor death. The number of skin samples from the number of skin donors for each time period are also listed. With dermatomed skin, refrigerated for only 0.75 day, the 24-hour cumulative lactate was a high of 19.8 ± 8.0 mmol/L. Lactate production

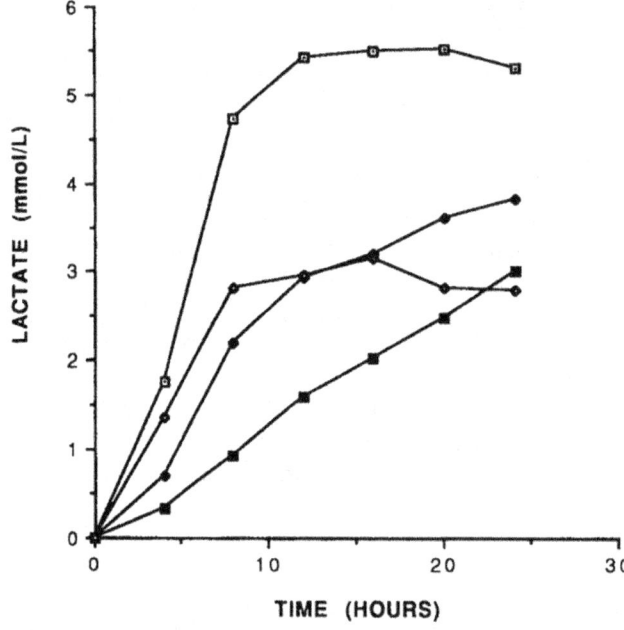

FIGURE 50.1   Lactate production from glucose (anaerobic energy metabolism) of four human skin sources perfused for 24 hours with Eagle's minimum essential media (MEM)–Earle's balanced salt solution (BSS) with 50 µg/mL gentamicin. An initial time delay is noted where glucose absorbs into skin and lactose perfuses out of skin.

TABLE 50.1

***In Vitro* Human Skin Viability: Glucose Energy Metabolism to Lactate**

Time after Death (Days)[a]	Dermatomed Skin		Heat-Separated Epidermis	
	Lactate[b] (mmol/L/24 hr)	Number[c]	Lactate[b] (mmol/L/24 hr)	Number[c]
0.75	$19.8 \pm 8.9^{d,e}$	6/2	$2.0 \pm 1.1^{e,f}$	3/1
2	5.9 ± 4.1^{d}	13/4	1.8 ± 0.8^{f}	8/3
3	8.0 ± 4.8	8/3	0.6 ± 0.5	6/2
4	6.5 ± 1.7	9/3	0.7 ± 0.4	6/2
6	6.8 ± 3.0	11/3	0.2 ± 0.1	5/2
8	4.6 ± 2.3	6/2	0.2 ± 0.1	3/1
13	2.0 ± 0.6	3/1	0.9 ± 0.4	3/1

[a] Stored refrigerated in Eagle's minimum essential media (MEM)–Earle's balanced salt solution (BSS) with 50 µm/mL gentamicin.

[b] Mean ± SD.

[c] Number of skin samples/number of human skin donors.

[d] $p < 0.000$.

[e] $p < 0.01$.

[f] $p < 0.007$.

decreased by day 2 ($p < 0.000$) and remained steady through day 8. Lactate production decreased further by approximately one-half between day 8 and day 13. Heat-separated epidermis lactate production was less than dermatomed skin ($p < 0.01$) at 2.0 ± 1.1 mmol/L. This level was maintained to the 2-day period, then decreased ($p < 0.007$) at day 3 and remained less than 1 mmol/L through the 13-day test period.

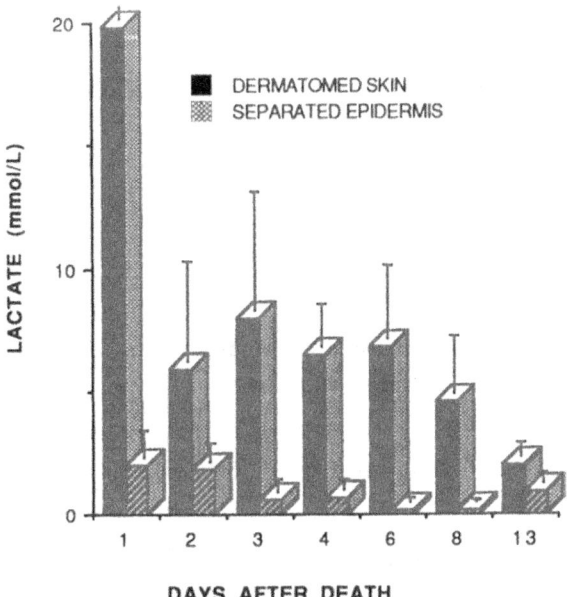

DAYS AFTER DEATH

FIGURE 50.2 Viability of human skin stored refrigerated at 4°C in Eagle's minimum essential media (MEM)–Earle's balanced salt solution (BSS) with 50 µg/mL gentamicin. Time indicated is that after donor's death.

TABLE 50.2

Heat Effect on Human Skin Simulating Epidermis Heat-Separation Procedure

	Lactate (mmol/L) Produced in 24 hr		
Source	Control Dermatomed Skin	Heat-Treated Skin[c]	Statistics
Number 1[a]	13.6 ± 1.5	1.5 ± 0.6	$p < 0.000$
Number 2[b]	7.4 ± 4.0	0.7 ± 0.14	$p < 0.04$

[a] Male, 21, thigh skin, used 69 hours after death ($n = 3$).
[b] Female, 30, thigh skin, used 39 hours after death ($n = 3$).
[c] Heated for one minute in 60°C water.

Dermatomed skin was heat-treated at 60°C for one minute to simulate the heat-separation procedure to produce epidermis separated from dermis (but no separation was performed) (Table 50.2). Lactate production decreased significantly ($p < 0.000$ and $p < 0.04$) for both heat-treated skin samples. Therefore, heating to separate epidermis from dermis damages viability. In another study (Table 50.3), lactate production was determined in heat-separated epidermis and dermis. The cumulative lactate production was much less than intact dermatomed skin, again showing the detrimental effect of heat separation on skin viability.

Table 50.4 shows replicates from six dermatomed skin and heat-separated epidermis samples that were frozen at –22°C. The process of freezing was detrimental to skin viability of dermatomed skin ($p < 0.04$). Separated epidermis was not significantly different between refrigerated and frozen ($p > 0.05$) because the heat-separation process to get the epidermal layer had already been detrimental to skin viability.

50.4   CONCLUSION

It is logical that prolonged life and improved quality for stored skin is desirable for any transplant situation (4). During *in vivo* percutaneous absorption and transdermal delivery, the skin is viable and does metabolize glucose for energy, and metabolism does extend to other enzymes and other chemicals (5, 6). Understanding and maintaining human cadaver skin viability place the skin use closer to the *in vivo* situation. This study shows that, in a sustaining media, skin can be energy viable for up to 8 days. Harvesting the skin and use within a day of donor death gives the highest

TABLE 50.3

Viability of Dermatomed Human Skin and Heat-Separated Epidermis and Dermis

	Lactate (mmol/L/24 hr) Production		
Time (hr)	Dermatomed skin[a]	Epidermis[a]	Dermis[a]
29	9.7 ± 2.3[b]	1.5 ± 0.4[b]	0.9 ± 0.4[b]

Note: Note that epidermis plus dermis does not equal intact skin.

[a] Mean ± SD; male age 25, thigh skin. Epidermis and dermis separated after heat treatment for one minute in 60°C water.
[b] $p < 0.004$.

TABLE 50.4

Freezing Effect of Human Skin on Energy Metabolism

	Lactate Production (mmol/L/24 hr)			
	Dermatomed Skin		**Heat-Separated Epidermis**	
Skin Sample	**Refrigerated[a]**	**Frozen[a,b]**	**Refrigerated**	**Frozen[b]**
1	12.2 ± 2.1	0.1 ± 0.1	1.0 ± 0.08	0.19 ± 0.13
2	2.4 ± 0.7	0.4 ± 0.3	1.5 ± 0.6	0.18 ± 0.13
3	7.4 ± 4.0	2.6 ± 0.4	–	–
4	9.7 ± 2.3	2.4 ± 0.5	1.5 ± 0.4	2.1 ± 0.2
5	9.5 ± 0.4	1.2 ± 0.04	0.2 ± 0.1	0.1 ± 0.05
6	27.5 ± 4.1	0.0	0.2 ± 0.1	0.0

[a] $p < 0.04$.
[b] Frozen 24 hours or longer.

viability. Our system gets the skin quickly into sustaining media and refrigeration; it is not known if a delay from harvest to storage will affect viability. Common practices of freezing skin for storage or heat treatment to separate epidermis from dermis can destroy skin viability. The effect of enzymatically separating skin is not known. Bhatt et al. (7) also showed that heat treatment of hairless mouse skin for separation purposes eliminates viability.

Cadaver skin viability can be maintained and monitored. Glucose utilization can be measured by conversion of [14C]glucose to $^{14}CO_2$ (8) or by lactate production (9), as shown here. The lactate production methodology does not require radioactivity use equipment.

ACKNOWLEDGMENT

We thank the Northern California Transplant Bank who supplied the skin and made this study possible. Special acknowledgment to George Kositzin for the extra effort to obtain the skin samples.

REFERENCES

1. May SR, DeClement FA. Skin banking. Part III. Cadaveric allograft skin viability. J Burn Care Rehab 1981; 2:128–141.
2. Wester RC, Maibach HI. Percutaneous absorption of drugs. Clin Pharmacokinet 1992; 3:253–266.
3. Wester RC, Maibach HI, Sedik L, Melendres J, Wade M. Percutaneous absorption of PCBs from soil: in vivo rhesus monkey, in vitro human skin, and binding to powdered human stratum corneum. J Toxicol Environ Hlth 1993; 39:375–382.
4. Hurst LN, Brown DH, Murray KA. Prolonged life and improved quality of stored skin grafts. Plast Reconstr Surg 1984; 73:105–109.
5. Wester RC, Noonan PK, Smeach S, Kosobud L. Pharmacokinetics and bioavailability of intravenous and topical nitroglycerin in the rhesus monkey: estimate of percutaneous first pass metabolism. J Pharm Sci 1983; 72:745–748.
6. Bronaugh RL, Stewart RF, Storm JE. Extent of cutaneous metabolism during percutaneous absorption of xenobiotics. Toxicol Appl Pharmacol 1989; 99:534–543.
7. Bhatt RH, Micali G, Galinkin J, Palicharla P, Koch R, West DP, Solomon LM. Determi- nation and correlation of in vitro viability for hairless mouse and human neonatal whole skin and stratum corneum/epidermis. Arch Dermatol Res 1997; 289:170–173.
8. Collier SW, Sheikh NM, Sakr A, Lichtin JL, Stewart RF, Bronaugh RL. Maintenance of skin viability during in vitro percutaneous absorption/metabolism studies. Toxicol Appl Pharmacol 1989; 99:522–533.
9. Kraeling MEK, Lipicky RJ, Bronaugh RL. Metabolism of benzocaine during percutaneous absorption in the hairless guinea pig: acetylbenzocaine formation and activity. Skin Pharmacol 1996; 9:221–230.

51 Determination of Percutaneous Absorption by *In Vitro* Techniques

Margaret E.K. Kraeling and Jeffrey J. Yourick
Food and Drug Administration, Laurel, Maryland

Disclaimer: This book chapter reflects the views of the authors and should not be construed to represent FDA's views or policies.

CONTENTS

51.1   INTRODUCTION

In vitro studies are widely used for determining the percutaneous absorption of chemicals that are dermally applied to or come in contact with skin. Safety evaluations of chemicals of concern often rely on *in vitro* studies using animal or human skin to obtain penetration information. The use of animal skin data must be carefully used when considering estimating human exposure due to skin absorption because of differences in structural and barrier properties of animal and human skin (1, 2).

In vitro absorption studies can also be used to determine skin metabolism of compounds after topical exposure to chemicals. The issue of metabolism may be important if a chemical is either metabolically activated or detoxified as it is absorbed through the skin, especially if the chemical has systemic toxicity potential. Doing metabolic studies requires viable skin, which makes the skin collection more complex and less flexible for study design. In addition, for the metabolism studies, skin viability must be maintained in the diffusion cell throughout the measurement period (3).

In 2004, the Organisation for Economic Co-operation and Development (OECD) adopted a guideline (OECD TG 428) for the testing of chemicals via *in vitro* skin absorption methods (4). This guideline was adopted to provide guidance for the measurement of skin absorption of a test substance topically applied to excised skin. It may be used in close association with OECD TG427 (5), which describes *in vivo* absorption testing of substances applied to skin. These two guideline documents from the OECD provide a basis to conduct both *in vitro* and *in vivo* dermal absorption studies via a harmonized study design. This allows skin absorption and penetration data to be more easily compared across laboratories and countries. The OECD TG428 for *in vitro* testing touches on many important elements of conducting these types of studies such as the skin source, design of diffusion cells, the receptor fluid, skin preparation and integrity, test substance application, test duration and data analysis. The OECD TG427 for *in vivo* skin absorption testing highlights elements such as selection of animal species, preparation of animal skin for dosing, test substance preparation and application to skin, skin washing, skin layer sampling and data analysis. Both skin absorption guidelines for *in vivo* and *in vitro* testing are further addressed in the subsequent OECD document on "Guidance Notes on Dermal Absorption, Series on Testing and Assessment, No. 154" (6). These guidance notes were mainly focused on addressing harmonized dermal absorption values for risk assessment of pesticides and biocides. Contained in this document is a valuable description of the "Triple Pack" testing approach that helps to provide better estimates of human dermal absorption than can be found by solely testing with animal skin. The European Food Safety Authority (EFSA) has recently released their "Guidance on Dermal Absorption" (7). This EFSA guidance is based on obtaining dermal absorption values for risk assessment of plant protection products and their residues. A framework is presented of a tiered approach to obtain dermal absorption values using human *in vitro* studies, rat *in vivo* and *in vitro* studies, and the "Triple Pack" approach. Each element of the study design is discussed, including data analysis and reporting, which should ideally help to decrease variability across laboratories and increase the quality of data used for human risk assessment.

51.2   PHYSIOCHEMICAL PROPERTIES RELATED TO ABSORPTION STUDY PLANNING AND DESIGN

It is important to know the partition coefficient, solubility, and properties of test chemicals to aid in the design of *in vitro* dermal absorption studies. The log of the octanol/water partition coefficient (log P) is used as an estimate of the percutaneous absorption properties of chemicals. Chemicals need some degree of lipophilicity to permeate through the stratum corneum layer. Some degree of water solubility is also needed for penetration through the more hydrophilic epidermal and dermal layers of skin. It has been determined that the ideal range for skin absorption occurs when a chemical has a log P value of between 1 and 3 (8). For example, when a series of homologous alcohols (C2 to C10) were topically applied to human skin, it was found that the smaller nonpolar alcohols had slower absorption rates than the larger, more lipophilic alcohols through the epidermal and dermal layers (9). The molecular weight, or sheer size, and chemical dimensions of a chemical may influence skin absorption. In general, the skin absorption of chemicals tends to decrease once the molecular weight reaches 500 daltons and above. (10)

51.3   DIFFUSION CELL DESIGN

In vitro guidelines generally allow for the use of either flow-through or Franz static diffusion cells. However, it should be noted that only the flow-through diffusion cells are able to maintain skin disc viability for a reasonable duration for testing. The flow-through cell design enables a stream of fluid (buffer, solvent, media, etc.) to be pumped at a low flow rate such as 1.5 mL/hour underneath the skin disc. To maintain skin disc viability, a cell culture type media is pumped through the receptor chamber throughout the study to maintain viable skin functions. It has been shown that skin disc viability can be maintained in flow-through cells for 24 hours (3). Most diffusion cells are manufactured out of Teflon or glass to minimize test chemical binding to the diffusion cell walls.

51.4   SOURCE OF SKIN

Human skin is the ideal skin to use instead of animal skin for the most human-relevant data for safety assessment. However, there are difficulties related to obtaining human skin, especially viable human skin, for *in vitro* absorption studies. It is easier to obtain human cadaver skin from tissue banks, but this skin cannot be considered as viable, since it is usually frozen after obtaining the sample. Therefore, animal skin is often used and is acceptable via guidelines such as OECD T428 when used for absorption and metabolism studies. Animal skin is generally thought to be more permeable to a wide range of chemicals than is human skin. After testing a limited number of chemicals, it was shown that rat and rabbit skin overpredict human skin absorption. However, pig, nonhuman primate, and hairless guinea pig skin are more predictive of human *in vivo* skin absorption than other animal species (2). Other studies have reviewed this subject and have concluded that pig and guinea pig skin are good skin models for use in predicting human *in vivo* absorption (11). A review by Todo in 2017 (12) addresses the advantages and disadvantages of using different species of animals for skin absorption studies. In many cases, the use of animal skin may provide a conservative estimate of human skin penetration for safety assessment purposes. The use of hairless animals is preferred, since it is easier to use a dermatome to produce a split-thickness skin disc to mount in the diffusion cell. Metabolism of topically applied compounds by animal skin may be different than human skin (see chapter 19).

51.5   VIABILITY OF SKIN

Skin metabolism can be measured when viable skin is used in absorption studies. Therefore, viable skin more realistically simulates actual dermal absorption scenarios than when using nonviable skin. The skin has a limited degree of metabolic capacity when compared to liver tissue, but skin can metabolically activate or detoxify a chemical as it passes through the skin (12). Phase II biotransformation pathways were tested in fresh, viable full-thickness human skin explants and found that skin explants have significant capacity for glucuronidation, sulfation, N-acetylation, catechol methylation, and glutathione conjugation (13). The hydrolysis product of the ultimate carcinogen formed from benzo(a)pyrene was identified in the diffusion cell receptor fluid following topical application of benzo(a)pyrene to viable hairless guinea pig skin (14). The skin has also been shown to have significant capability for conjugating percutaneously absorbed compounds. The glycine conjugates of benzoic (15) and salicylic acid (16) were observed in hairless guinea pig skin after absorption of the parent compounds. Substantial amounts of absorbed benzocaine were found to be acetylated in human and hairless guinea pig skin (15, 17). Viability of skin can be assessed by using the MTT assay (18, 19) (see chapter 19). Cadaver skin is also acceptable for use in a skin absorption study; however, the integrity of the barrier should be determined and fall within historical limits of a marker (tritiated water) (20) or by physical methods like transepidermal water loss (TEWL) or transepidermal electrical resistance (TEER) testing (4, 6). Since enzymatic activity is reduced or absent in cadaver skin, metabolism of the test compound can be determined in skin homogenates or tissue model constructs produced from primary human skin cells.

51.6   PREPARATION OF SKIN

A split-thickness preparation of skin should be used in diffusion cells unless full-thickness skin can be justified. A dermatome section containing the epidermis and upper papillary dermal layer (200 to 400 μm) most closely simulates the barrier layer of skin (20). Full-thickness skin can artificially retain absorbed compounds that bind or diffuse poorly through it (most lipophilic chemicals) (21). Preparation of an epidermal layer by separation of the epidermis and dermis using heat is effective for nonhairy skin (22, 23), but the viability of the skin may be destroyed.

51.7   RECEPTOR FLUID

A physiological buffer such as a balanced salt solution or tissue culture medium is needed to maintain viability of the skin for at least 24 hours (3). Bovine serum albumin (BSA) is sometimes added to increase the solubility of lipophilic compounds. Some protocols utilize solubilizing agents added to the receptor fluid to help partition lipophilic compounds; however, caution must be used, as the skin barrier can be damaged (24). It is preferable to use a physiological buffer even when metabolism is not measured to simulate *in vivo* conditions.

51.8   RECOVERY

Determination of total recovery of a test compound lends credibility to experimental results. Normal mass balance recovery of radiolabeled compounds in percutaneous absorption experiments should exceed 90%. However, high recovery values cannot be obtained for volatile compounds unless the evaporating material is trapped. Study recovery values less than 90% should be explained when other variables are encountered. The OECD guidance addresses variabilities of recovery (6).

51.9   DETERMINATION OF ABSORPTION

The determination of systemic absorption is sometimes a controversial issue in an *in vitro* diffusion cell study. Since the skin can sometimes serve as a reservoir for absorbed material, measurement of the absorbed compound appearing in the receptor fluid alone may not be an accurate determination of systemic skin absorption. Both skin and receptor fluid levels should be measured at the end of a study. If determination of systemic absorption is desired, it is not sufficient to simply measure only the receptor fluid levels. If significant amounts remain in skin, additional studies may be necessary to determine if the material in skin will eventually be systemically absorbed. Also, skin levels must be known in order to determine mass balance at the end of the experiment. Recoveries of at least 90% should be obtained unless the test compound is volatile.

Skin can be fractionated to observe localization in different layers. The stratum corneum layer can be removed from the surface of the skin by successive stripping with 13 or more pieces of cellophane tape (22). Individual variation has been reported in the number of strips necessary, presumably due to differences in the pressure applied to the tape and differences in the tape itself. The epidermal and dermal layers can be separated with heat, as previously described in the preparation of skin. The guidelines for skin absorption studies recommended by the European Union's Scientific Committee for Consumer Products (SCCP) require that material remaining in the viable skin levels (exclusive of stratum corneum) be considered systemically absorbed (24). The OECD guideline for *in vitro* skin absorption studies states that all material remaining in skin (including the stratum corneum) may need to be considered as systemically absorbed unless additional studies show that there is no eventual absorption (4, 6).

For example, in 2002, the safety of lawsone as a coloring agent in hair dye products was evaluated by the European Union's Scientific Committee on Cosmetic Products and Non-Food Products (SCCNFP) and concluded that lawsone was mutagenic and not suitable for use as a hair coloring agent. *In vitro* diffusion cell skin absorption studies were conducted to measure the extent of lawsone absorption through human skin (25). Lawsone skin absorption was determined from two hair coloring products and two shampoo products, all containing henna. Products remained on the skin for 5 minutes (shampoos) and 1 hour (hair color paste). For one of the henna hair paste products, 0.3% of the applied dose was absorbed into the receptor fluid in 24 hours, while 2.2% remained in the skin. For one of the henna shampoo products, 0.3% of the applied dose was absorbed into the receptor fluid at 24 hours, while 3.6% remained in the skin. Extended absorption studies conducted for 72 hours showed that a small but significant increase in lawsone levels occurred in the receptor fluid values, while all skin levels (stratum corneum, epidermis, and dermis) decreased significantly (Table 51.1 and 51.2).

TABLE 51.1

Penetration of Lawsone from a Commercial Henna Hair Paste (Product A) in 24 and 72 Hours

% of Applied Dose Penetrated

	24 Hours[1]	72 Hours[2]
Receptor Fluid	0.3 ± 0.1^a	0.5 ± 0.1^a
Stratum Corneum	1.6 ± 0.2^a	0.5 ± 0.1^a
Epidermis and Dermis	0.6 ± 0.1^a	0.3 ± 0.03^a
Total in Skin	2.2 ± 0.3^a	0.8 ± 0.1^a
Total Penetration	2.5 ± 0.3^a	1.3 ± 0.1^a
Wash	102.0 ± 3.3	93.1 ± 2.2
Recovery	105.1 ± 3.1	94.5 ± 2.2

[1] Values are the mean $\pm$ SEM of 11 replicates (two donors). Other 24-hour values are the mean $\pm$ SEM of six replicates (two donors). Lawsone applied dose was 1.51 ± 0.22 µg/cm^2.

[2] Values are the mean $\pm$ SEM of five replicates (one donor). Lawsone applied dose was 1.36 ± 0.03 µg/cm^2.

[a] Significantly different between the 24-hour and 72-hour values (t-test $p < 0.05$).

Source: Reference 5.

TABLE 51.2

Penetration of Lawsone from a Commercial Henna Shampoo (Product C) in 24 and 72 Hours

% of Applied Dose Penetrated

	24 Hours[1]	72 Hours[2]
Receptor Fluid	0.3 ± 0.02^a	0.4 ± 0.04^a
Stratum Corneum	2.4 ± 0.3^a	1.4 ± 0.2^a
Epidermis and Dermis	1.2 ± 0.2^a	0.5 ± 0.1^a
Total in Skin	3.6 ± 0.5^a	1.9 ± 0.2^a
Total Penetration	3.9 ± 0.5^a	2.3 ± 0.3^a
Wash	90.3 ± 3.0	82.0 ± 3.2
Recovery	94.7 ± 3.1	84.7 ± 3.4

[1] Receptor fluid values are the mean $\pm$ SEM of 24 replicates (three donors). Other 24-hour values are the mean $\pm$ SEM of 12 replicates (three donors). Lawsone applied dose was 1.08 ± 0.07 µg/cm^2.

[2] Values are the mean $\pm$ SEM of 12 replicates (three donors). Lawsone applied dose was 0.79 ± 0.14 µg/cm^2.

[a] Significantly different between the 24-hour and 72-hour values (t-test $p < 0.05$).

Source: Reference 25.

51.10   REPORTING OF ABSORPTION RESULTS

Absorption studies are usually conducted by applying the test compound under conditions that simulate topical exposure. In general, the results reported should include an absorption profile over time as measured from receptor fluid levels. The composite absorption profile should also include measurements of skin levels and recovery values to better calculate exposure. When test chemical remains in the skin (i.e., skin reservoir) at the end of the study, it may need to be determined on a case-by-case basis whether to include skin levels as absorbed material. To calculate a permeability constant (steady-state rate divided by applied concentration), an infinite dose is applied to the skin. Consumer-relevant exposure conditions require finite dosing, and therefore a steady-state absorption rate is not achieved. Finite dosing study absorption is usually expressed as a percent of the applied dose or as an absorption rate. These derived absorption values are specific for the dose applied and vehicle used and often cannot be easily extrapolated to other product types and consumer conditions of use.

51.11   CONCLUSION

For relevant *in vitro* skin absorption data, results from an *in vitro* method should come from a study design that simulates relevant consumer use conditions. It is preferable to use viable skin whenever possible, especially if metabolism is important. However, cadaver or certain types of animal skin is acceptable since adequate supplies of viable human skin are sometimes difficult to obtain. Absorption values for compounds obtained from animal skin generally exceed the permeability of these same compounds in human skin.

In *in vitro* skin absorption studies, absorption must be clearly defined. Not including skin levels at the end of a study can lead to differences in percutaneous absorption measurements and the resulting exposure calculations. For compounds that remain in the skin, it is recommended that extended skin absorption studies be conducted to determine the fate of those penetrated compounds.

REFERENCES

1. Bronaugh RL, Stewart RF, Congdon ER. Methods for *in vitro* percutaneous absorption studies IL Comparison of human and animal skin. Tox Appl Pharmacol 1982; 62:481–488.
2. Jung EC, Maibach HI. Animal models for percutaneous absorption, In: Shah VP, Maibach HI, Jenner J, eds. Topical Drug Bioavailability, Bioequivalenec, and Penetration, New York: Springer, 2014:21–40.
3. Collier SW, Sheikh NM, Sakr A, Lichtin JL, Stewart RF, Bronaugh RL. Maintenance of skin viability during *in vitro* percutaneous absorption/metabolism studies. Tox Appl Pharmacol 1989; 99:522–533.
4. OECD (Organisation for Economic Co-operation and Development). Test No. 428: Skin Absorption: *In Vitro* Method, OECD Guideline for the Testing of Chemicals, Section 4, OECD Publishing, Paris, 2004.
5. OECD (Organisation for Economic Co-operation and Development). Test No. 427: Skin Absorption: *In Vivo* Method, OECD Guideline for the Testing of Chemicals, Section 4, OECD Publishing, Paris, 2004.
6. OECD (Organisation for Economic Co-operation and Development). No. 156. Environmental Health and Safety Publications: Guidance Notes of Dermal Absorption. Environment Directorate. Joint Meeting of the Chemicals Committee and the Working Party on Chemicals, Pesticides and Biotechnology. Organisation for Economic Co-Operation and Development, Paris, August 2011.
7. EFSA (European Food Safety Authority). Guidance on Dermal Absorption. EFSA Journal 2017; 15(6):4873–4933.
8. Brain KR, Chilcot RP. Physicochemical factors affecting skin absorption, In: Chilcot RP, Price S, eds. Principles and Practice of Skin Toxicology, New York: John Wiley & Sons, Ltd, 2008:83–92.
9. Cross SE, Magnusson BM, Winckle G, Anissimov Y, Roberts MS. Determination of the effect of lipophilicity on the *in vitro* permeability and tissue reservoir characteristics of topically applied solutes in human skin layers. J Invest Dermatol 2003; 120(5):759–764.
10. Bos JD, Meinardi MMHM. The 500 dalton rule for the skin penetration of chemical compounds. Exp Dermatol 2000; 9:165–169.
11. Frasch HF, Barbero AM. A paired comparison between human skin and hairless guinea pig skin *in vitro* permeability and lag time measurements for 6 industrial chemicals. Cutan Ocul Toxicol 2009; 28:107–113.

12. Todo H. Transdermal permeation of drugs in various animal species. Pharmaceutics 2017; 9:33–44. doi: 10.3390/pharmaceutics9030033.
13. Manevski N, Swart P, Balavenkatraman KK, Bertschi B, Camenisch G, Kretz O, Schiller H, Walles M, Ling B, Wettstein R, Schaefer DJ, Itin P, Ashton-Chess J, Pognan F, Wolf A, Litherland K. Phase II metabolism in human skin: skin explants show full coverage for glucuronidation, sulfation, N-acetylation, catechol methylation, and glutathione conjugation. Drug Metab Dispos 2015; 43:126–139.
14. Ng KME, Chu I, Bronaugh RL, Franklin CA, Somers DA. Percutaneous absorption and drugs. Exp Dermatol 2000; 9:165–169.
15. Nathan D, Sakr A, Lichtin JL, Bronaugh RL. *In vitro* skin absorption and metabolism of benzoic acid, p-aminobenzoic acid, and benzocaine in the hairless guinea pig. Pharm Res 1990; 7:1147–1151.
16. Boehnlein J, Sakr A, Lichtin JL, Bronaugh RL. Metabolism of retinyl palmitate to retinol (vitamin A) in skin during percutaneous absorption. Pharm Res 1994; 11:1155–1159.
17. Kraeling MEK, Lipicky RJ, Bronaugh RL. Metabolism of benzocaine during percutaneous absorption in the hairless guinea pig. Acetylbenzocaine formation and activity. Skin Pharmacol 1996; 9:221–230.
18. Hood HL, Wickett RR, Bronaugh RL. The *in vitro* percutaneous absorption of the fragrance ingredient musk xylol. Fd Chem Toxicol 1996; 34:483–488.
19. Eppler AR, Kraeling, MEK, Wickett RR, Bronaugh RL. Assessment of absorption and irritation potential of arachidonic acid and glyceryl arachidonate using *in vitro* diffusion cell techniques. Fd Chem Toxicol 2007; 45(11):2109–2117.
20. Bronaugh RL, Stewart RF. Methods for *in vitro* percutaneous absorption studies VI. Preparation of the barrier layer. J Pharm Sci 1986; 75:487–491.
21. Bronaugh RL, Stewart RF. Methods for *in vitro* percutaneous absorption studies III. Hydrophobic compounds. J Pharm Sci 1984; 73:1255–1258.
22. Kraeling MEK, Zhou W, Wang P, Ogunsola O. *In vitro* skin penetration of acetyl hexapeptide-8 from a cosmetic formulation. Cutan Ocul Toxicol 2015; 34:46–52.
23. Kraeling MEK, Topping VD, Keltner ZM, Belgrave KR, Bailey KD, Gao X, Yourick JJ. *In vitro* percutaneous penetration of silver nanoparticles in pig and human skin. Reg Tox Pharm 2018; 95: 314–322.
24. SCCP. Opinion concerning basic criteria for the *in vitro* assessment of percutaneous absorption of cosmetic ingredients. Adopted by the Scientific Committee on Cosmetic Products and Non-Food Products Intended for Consumers During the 25th Plenary Meeting of 20 October 2003.
25. Kraeling MEK, Jung CT, Bronaugh RL. Absorption of lawsone through human skin. Cutan Ocul Toxicol 2007; 26: 45–56.

52 Stripping Method for Measuring Percutaneous Absorption *In Vivo*

André Rougier
Laboratoire Pharmaceutique, La Roche-Posay, Courbevoie, France

Claire Lotte
Laboratoires de Recherche Fondamentale, L'Oréal,
Aulnay sous Bois, France

Howard I. Maibach
University of California, San Francisco, California

CONTENTS

From a practical viewpoint, it remains difficult to draw valid conclusions from the literature concerning the absorption level of a given compound. This is essentially due to the diversity of techniques used, animal species (1, 2), anatomical location (3, 4), duration of application (1), dose applied (5, 6), and vehicle used (1, 7). Furthermore, because this kind of research has interested scientists from widely differing disciplines, each worker has chosen or adapted the methodology to elucidate a particular problem.

From a theoretical viewpoint, over the two past decades, considerable attention has been paid to the understanding of the mechanisms and routes by which chemical compounds may penetrate the skin. Without considering the different interpretation about mechanisms acting on percutaneous absorption, it is well established that the main barrier is the stratum corneum (3, 8, 9), which also acts as a reservoir for topically applied molecules (10, 11). Moreover, it is likely that at the early step of the absorption process, the interaction between the physicochemical properties of the drug, the vehicle, and the horny layer plays an important role in total absorption.

In the first part of this chapter, we hypothesize that the amount of chemical present in the stratum corneum at the end of application may represent the stratum corneum vehicle partitioning and could also reflect the rate of penetration of the chemical.

In the second part, we ascertain that this hypothesis is independent of the main factors likely to modify the absorption level of a compound, that is, contact time, dose applied, vehicle used, anatomical site involved, and animal species chosen.

52.1   *IN VIVO* RELATIONSHIP BETWEEN STRATUM CORNEUM CONCENTRATION AND PERCUTANEOUS ABSORPTION

We chose to test on the hairless rat 10 radiolabeled molecules with very different physicochemical properties and belonging to different chemical classes.

For each compound, a group of 12 female hairless Sprague-Dawley rats, aged 12 weeks, weighing 200 ± 20 g, was used. The molecules, dissolved in ethanol/water mixtures (chosen according to the solubility of the chemical), were applied on 1 cm^2 of dorsal skin for 30 minutes. The standard dose applied was 200 nmol cm^2. At the end of the application, the excess product on the treated area was rapidly removed by two washings with ethanol/water (95:5), followed by two rinsings with distilled water, and light drying with cotton wool.

The 12 animals were then divided into two groups (Figure 52.1). The animals of group 1, wearing collars to prevent licking, were placed individually in metabolism cages for four days. Urinary excretion was established by daily sampling of the urine and liquid scintillation counting (Packard

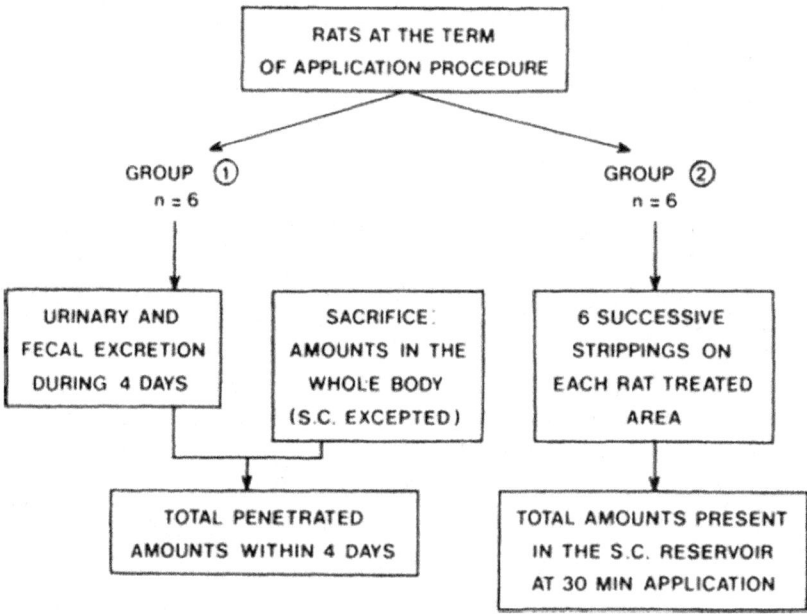

FIGURE 52.1 Procedures for determining total percutaneous absorption, within four days, and the stratum corneum reservoir at the end of application. (From Reference 12.)

Instruments 460 C). The feces were collected daily, pooled, and counted by liquid scintillation after lyophilization, homogenization, and combustion of the samples with an Oxidizer 306 (Packard Instruments).

After four days, the animals were sacrificed and a series of six strippings were carried out on the treated area to determine the amount of product not penetrated within 96 hours. The remaining skin of the treated area (epidermis and dermis) was sampled and counted by liquid scintillation after digestion in Soluene 350 (United Technology Packard). The carcasses were lyophilized and homogenized, and the samples were counted by liquid scintillation after combustion. The total amount of chemical penetrating within four days was then determined by adding the amounts found in the excreta (urine plus feces), in the epidermis and dermis of the application area, and in the entire animal body.

At the end of application and washing, the stratum corneum of the treated area of the animals from the second group was removed by six strippings, using 3M adhesive tape. The radioactivity on each strip was measured after complete digestion of the keratinic material in Soluene 350 (United Technology Packard), addition of Dimilume 30 (United Technology Packard), and liquid scintillation counting.

In our experimental conditions, the capacity of the stratum corneum reservoir for each compound has been defined as the sum of the amounts found in the first six strippings.

The percutaneous absorption results show (Figure 52.2) that after 96 hours there are large differences in the amounts of substances that have penetrated through the skin. Thus, one can observe that the most penetrating molecule, benzoic acid, penetrates 50 times more than dexamethasone.

When the compounds benzoic acid, acetylsalicylic acid, dehydroepian-drosterone, sodium salicylate, testosterone, hydrocortisone, and dexamethasone are classified according to a decreasing

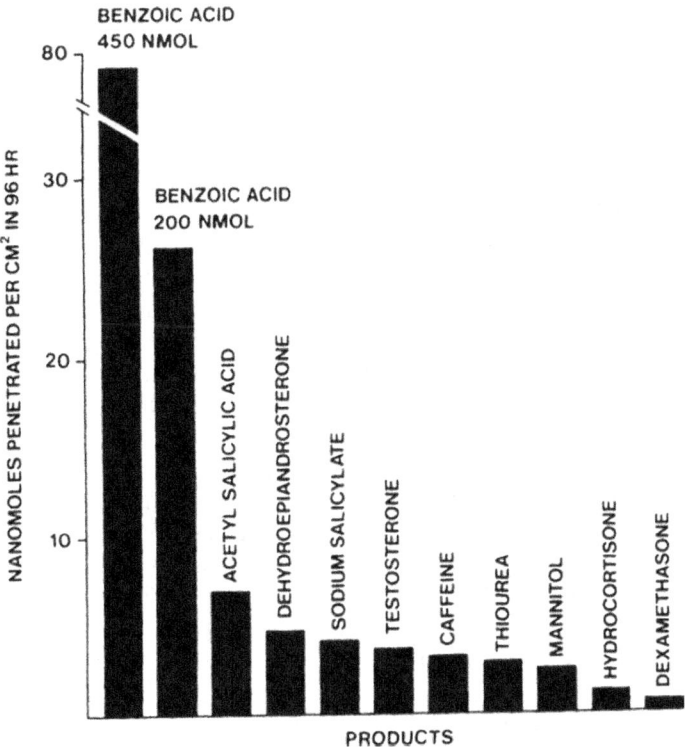

FIGURE 52.2   Percutaneous absorption levels of the tested compounds four days after their topical administration in the hairless rat. (From Reference 12.)

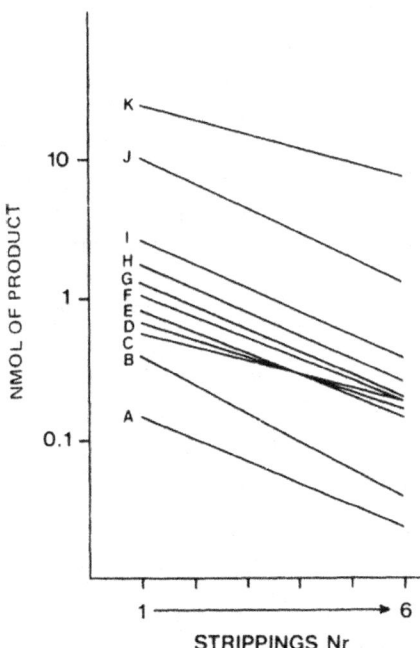

FIGURE 52.3 Distribution of the tested molecules within the horny layer of the dosed area, 30 minutes after their administration in the hairless rat: (A) dexamethasone, (B) hydrocortisone, (C) dehydroepiandrosterone, (D) testosterone, (E) mannitol, (F) thiourea, (G) caffeine, (H) sodium salicylate, (I) acetylsalicylic acid, (J) benzoic acid (200 nmol), and (K) benzoic acid (450 nmol). (From Rougier et al., unpublished data, 1983.)

order of penetration rate, we observe that this order is similar to that found in the literature concerning studies in humans (13, 14). Likewise, it is established that acetylsalicylic acid and salicylic acid have similar penetrating properties (14), whereas their sodium salts exhibit diminished penetration (8), and, indeed, we observed that sodium salicylate penetrates less than acetylsalicylic acid.

Figure 52.3 shows the concentrations of compounds present on each stripping of the dosed area of the animals of group 2 at the end of the application procedures. It is worth noting that, as in the *in vitro* results (15), *in vivo*, the substance concentration decreases inside the stratum corneum following an exponential relation. Considering the diversity of the compounds tested, it seems that this observation can be outlined as one of the factors governing percutaneous absorption.

As shown in Figure 52.4, independent of the physicochemical nature of the tested agent, there exists a highly significant linear correlation between the total amount of chemical penetration within four days (y) and the amount present in the stratum corneum at the end of the application time (x, 30 minutes; $r = 0.98$, $p < 0.001$).

From a theoretical viewpoint, this correlation sheds some light on a possible explanation of the stratum corneum barrier effect. A weak reservoir capacity would correspond to a weak penetration and therefore a strong barrier. Inversely, a high reservoir capacity corresponds to a high penetration and therefore a weak barrier effect. As a consequence, it is possible that barrier and reservoir functions of the horny layer may reflect the same physiological reality. From a practical viewpoint, the simple measurement of the amount of a chemical within the stratum corneum at the end of a 30-minute application gives a good predictive assessment of the total amount penetrating within four days.

As previously mentioned, the absorption level of molecules has been proved to be dependent on their application conditions. It was therefore important to ascertain that the "stripping method" was independent of the main factors able to modify the penetration level of a chemical, that is, application time, dose applied, vehicle used, and anatomical site involved.

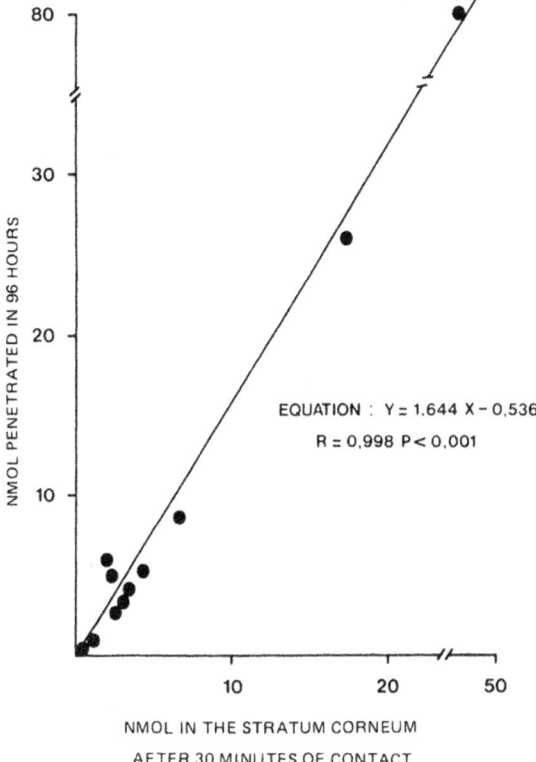

FIGURE 52.4 Relationship between the penetration level of the tested compounds after four days and their concentrations in the stratum corneum at the end of the application (30 minutes). (From Reference 12.)

52.2 INFLUENCE OF APPLICATION CONDITIONS ON THE RELATIONSHIP BETWEEN STRATUM CORNEUM CONCENTRATION AND PERCUTANEOUS ABSORPTION

52.2.1 INFLUENCE OF APPLICATION TIME

The duration of application of a compound may considerably influence the total amount absorbed. Moreover, the time of application of a substance may be closely related to its field of use.

Percutaneous absorption of four radiolabeled compounds—theophylline, nicotinic acid, acetyl-salicylic acid, and benzoic acid—was studied in the hairless rat. One thousand nanomoles of each compound was applied onto 1 cm² of dorsal skin during 0.5, 2, 4, and 6 hours, thus covering most of the usage conditions of the compounds topically applied. Total percutaneous absorption within four days for each compound and each application time was carried out as described in the foregoing section. The stratum corneum reservoir was assessed for each compound after an application time fixed at 30 minutes by stripping the treated area.

As shown in Figure 52.5, the penetration rate of the tested compounds is strictly proportional to the duration of application ($r = 0.98$, $p < 0.001$). From a theoretical viewpoint, this relationship provides evidence that, as in the *in vitro* studies (16, 17), a constant flux of penetration really does exist *in vivo*. This type of correlation having been found for four compounds with widely different physicochemical properties, it is reasonable to assume that it may constitute one of the laws of the *in vivo* percutaneous absorption phenomena. From a practical viewpoint, this linear relationship implies that the knowledge of the 4-day penetration of a compound applied for only 30 minutes has a predictive value for penetration resulting from longer application times.

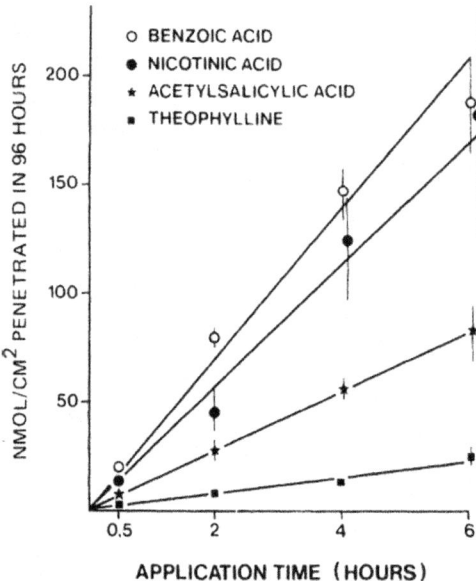

FIGURE 52.5 Relationship between the penetration levels of the tested compounds and the application time in the hairless rat. (From Reference 18.)

As discussed in the preceding section, with a 30-minute application, the total amount of compound recovered within the horny layer is strictly correlated with the amount that penetrated in a 4-day period. Figure 52.6 shows that this correlation is confirmed ($r = 0.99$, $p < 0.001$) for the four agents tested in this experiment. The total percutaneous absorption of a compound being directly linked to the duration of application (Figure 52.5), the simple knowledge of the reservoir effect of the stratum corneum for a chemical applied for 30 minutes allows the predictive assessment of its penetration resulting from longer application times. Thus, this only mildly invasive method offers

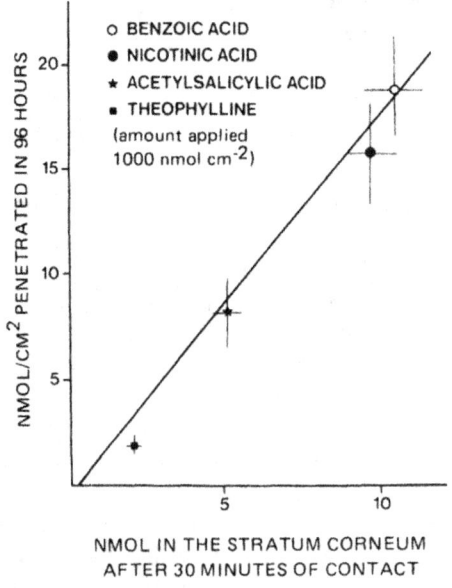

FIGURE 52.6 Correlation between the amount of chemical in the stratum corneum at the end of application (30 minutes) and its overall penetration within 4 days in the hairless rat. (From Reference 18.)

the advantages, when applied to humans, of reducing skin exposure and of immobilizing subjects only for a short period.

52.2.2   INFLUENCE OF DOSE APPLIED

In most medical and toxicological specialties, the administered dose is defined precisely. This has not always been the case in dermatotoxicology and dermatopharmacology. It is, however, well known that an increased concentration of an applied chemical on the skin increases percutaneous penetration (5, 6, 19), as does increasing the surface area treated or the application time. This question of concentration may have special significance in infants because the surface/body weight ratio is greater than in adults.

Percutaneous absorption of four radiolabeled compounds—theophylline, nicotinic acid, acetylsalicylic acid, and benzoic acid dissolved in ethylene glycol/Triton X-100 (90:10)—was studied in the hairless rat. For each compound, increasing doses from 125 to 1000 nmol were applied onto 1 cm² of dorsal skin for 30 minutes. For each compound and each dose, total percutaneous absorption within 4 days and the stratum corneum reservoir at the end of application time were assessed, as described in the preceding section.

As shown in Figure 52.7, within the limits of the concentrations used, there exists a linear dose–penetration relationship ($r = 0.98$, $p < 0.001$). However, it has been shown by Skog and Wahlberg (20) that when the applied concentration was increased, penetration was increased up to a certain point, at which a plateau was reached. Within the range of concentration used in the present study, this phenomenon does not appear. This tends to indicate that the horny layer is unaffected by the concentrated solutions, with the permeability constant being unaltered over the entire concentration range. When one considers the differences in physicochemical properties of the tested compounds, it seems that, at least for a range of concentrations, the linear relationship existing between dose applied and percutaneous absorption level might be taken as a general law.

Independently of the physicochemical nature of the chemical and whatever dose was administered, there is a highly significant correlation between the total amounts that penetrated over a 4-day period and the amounts recovered in the stratum corneum at the end of application time

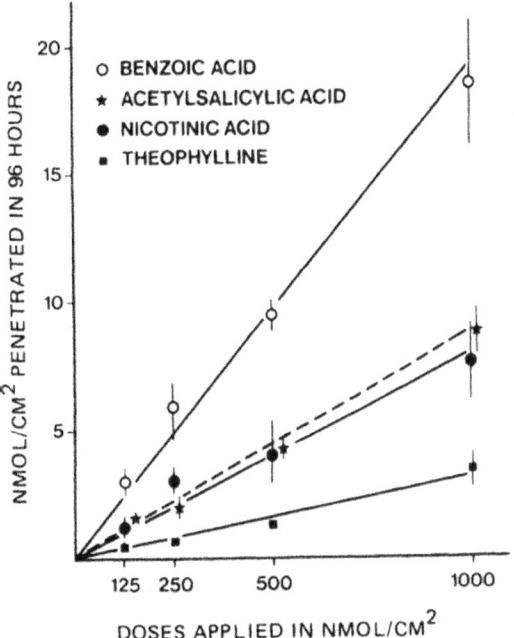

FIGURE 52.7   Relationship between dose applied and penetration rate of the tested compounds in the hairless rat. (From Rougier et al., unpublished data.)

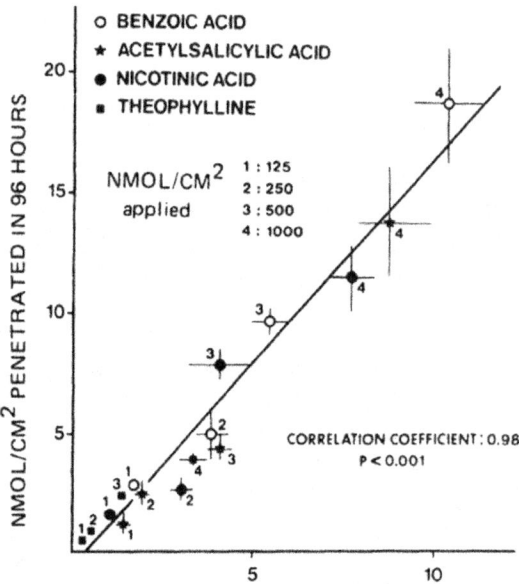

FIGURE 52.8 Influence of dose applied on the relationship between the level of penetration of the tested compounds after 4 days and their concentration in the stratum corneum at the end of application (30 minutes). (From Rougier et al., unpublished data.)

($r = 0.98$, $p < 0.001$) (Figure 52.8). From a toxicological viewpoint, the influence of applied concentration on the overall penetration of a drug can therefore be easily predicted using the stripping method. From a pharmacological viewpoint, Sheth et al. (21) have shown that the therapeutic efficacy of increasing doses of an antiviral (iododeoxyuridine) on herpes simplex infection can be predicted by the use of the stripping method.

52.2.3 INFLUENCE OF VEHICLE

In recent years, increasing attention has been devoted to the influence that the components of a vehicle may have on enhancing or hindering skin absorption of drugs. The effects of vehicles have been reviewed in detail by several authors (22–25). It is now well established that substances added to formulations as excipients and other factors, such as the physical form of the drug, affect not only its release and absorption but also its action. Unfortunately, few techniques can be used routinely to elucidate rapidly the role that a vehicle or a component in a vehicle may have on the overall absorption of a drug *in vivo*.

The influence of nine vehicles on the *in vivo* percutaneous absorption of [^{14}C]benzoic acid was studied in the hairless rat using the stripping method. Twenty microliters of each vehicle, containing 200 nmol of benzoic acid, were applied to 1 cm^2 of dorsal skin for 30 minutes. After this time, total percutaneous absorption and stratum corneum reservoir were assessed, as previously described.

As shown in Figure 52.9, although the vehicles used were simple in composition, the total amount of benzoic acid that penetrated over 4 days varied by a factor of 50, once more demonstrating the importance of vehicle in skin absorption. Figure 52.9 also shows the maximum solubility values (mg/mL) of benzoic acid in each vehicle. It is generally admitted that the release of a compound can be favored by the selection of vehicles having low affinity for that compound or by one in which it is least soluble (26, 27). As may be seen, the solubility of benzoic acid differed by a factor 30 between the least and the most efficient solvent medium (vehicles 4 and 6). However, we can see that there is a weak relationship between penetration level and maximum solubility of benzoic acid. For instance, the greatest penetration is not obtained with the vehicle in which benzoic acid is least soluble, and vice versa.

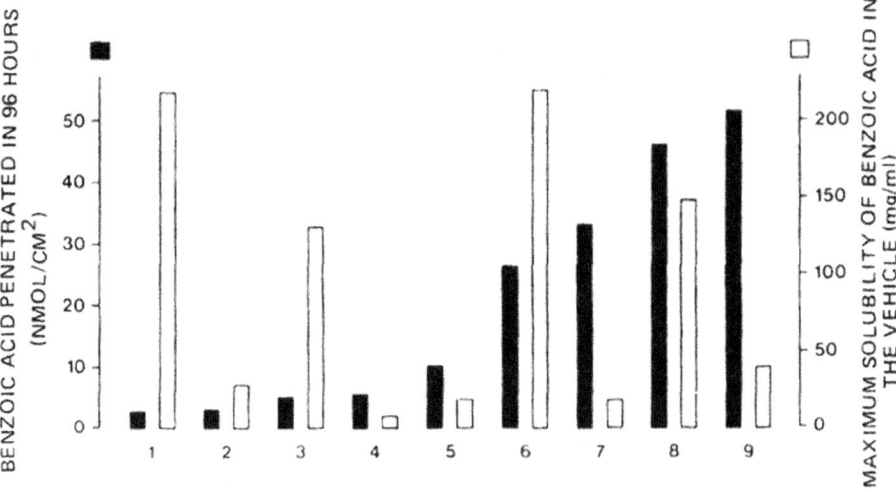

FIGURE 52.9 Comparative values of solubility of benzoic acid in the vehicles and corresponding percutaneous absorption levels: (1) propylene glycol/Triton X-100 (90:10), (2) glycerol/Triton X-100 (90:10), (3) ethylene glycol/Triton X-100 (90:10), (4) ethylene glycol/Triton X-100; 90:10)/water (40:60), (5) (propylene glycol/Triton X-100; 90:10)/water (40:60), (6) ethanol/water (95:5), (7) methanol/water (40:60), (8) ethanol/water (60:40), and (9) ethanol/water (40:60). (From Reference 28.)

Applied vehicles have the potential to either increase or decrease the quantity of water in the horny layer and, thereby, to increase or decrease penetration (29). It is interesting that the penetration of benzoic acid is enhanced by increasing the water content of the vehicles, whatever the organic phase (vehicles 1 and 5 and vehicles 6, 8, and 9).

As shown in Figure 52.10, independent of the vehicles' composition, the amount of benzoic acid found within the horny layer at the end of the application and the amount penetrating in 4 days are

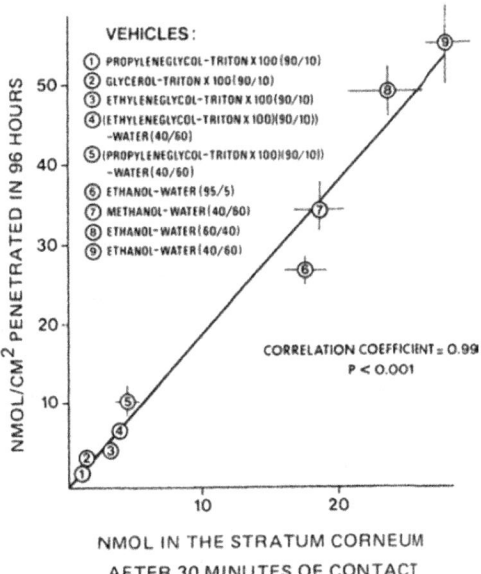

FIGURE 52.10 Influence of the tested vehicles on the relationship between the penetration level of benzoic acid within 4 days and its concentration in the stratum corneum at the end of application (30 minutes). (From Reference 28.)

linearly correlated ($r = 0.99$, $p < 0.001$). The influence of the vehicle composition on the *in vivo* penetration level of a chemical can therefore be easily predicted by simply stripping the treated area and measuring the amount engaged in the stratum corneum at the end of the application.

52.2.4 INFLUENCE OF ANATOMICAL SITE

Although all authors agree on the importance of anatomical location in percutaneous absorption, the literature contains relatively little information on the subject. Furthermore, general reviews dealing with this topic, among others (24, 30, 31), often give contradictory explanations of the differences in permeability observed from one site to another. Moreover, if it is clear that both *in vitro* (31) and *in vivo* (32–34), the anatomical location is of great importance, the connection between the differences observed, the structure of the skin, and the physicochemical nature of the penetrant remain obscure.

Percutaneous absorption of four radiolabeled compounds—acetylsalicylic acid, benzoic acid, caffeine, and benzoic acid sodium salt—was measured in humans on four body sites using the stripping method. For each substance and each location, a group of six to eight male Caucasian informed volunteers, aged 28 ± 2 years, was used. One thousand nanomoles of each compound were applied to an area of 1 cm² in 20 μL of ethylene glycol/water/Triton X-100 mixtures, the composition of which was chosen according to the solubility of each compound. After 30 minutes of contact, the excess substance in the treated area was rapidly removed as described earlier for the rat. On each patient, two strictly identical applications were performed in an interval of 48 hours. The first application, designed to measure the total penetration of the chemical involved, was made on the right-hand side of the body. For technical convenience, the compounds chosen for the test were ones that are quickly eliminated in the urine. By using data from the literature on the kinetics of urinary excretion of these substances (14, 35, 36), administered by different routes in various species, the total amounts penetrating within the following 4 days were deduced, after liquid scintillation counting, from the amounts excreted in the first 24-hour urine. These were, respectively, 75%, 50%, 75%, and 31% of the total quantities of benzoic acid sodium salt, caffeine, benzoic acid, and acetylsalicylic acid absorbed, respectively.

At the end of the second application, performed on the left-hand side of the body (contralateral site), the stratum corneum of the treated area was removed by 15 successive strippings (3M adhesive tape), and the radioactivity present in the horny layer was measured as previously described for the rat.

To make comparisons easier, Figure 52.11 expresses the permeability of each site to the various compounds in relation to that of the arm to benzoic acid sodium salt. This representation offers the advantage of simultaneously showing differences in permeability due to both the physicochemical properties of the penetrants and to the structural peculiarities of the areas where they were applied.

Skin permeability appears to be as follows: arm ≤ abdomen < postauricular < forehead. It is worth noting that whatever the compound applied, the forehead is about twice as permeable as the arm or the abdomen. It may be pointed out that this average ratio agrees well with those reported for the same areas with other compounds (32, 33).

A possible explanation of the higher penetration in areas where there are more sebaceous glands, such as the forehead, could be that absorption occurs through the follicles, rather than through the epidermis. In our opinion, it is difficult to reconcile the great disproportion, a factor of 50 to 100, existing between the number of sebaceous glands of the arm and the forehead (37, 38) and the relatively weak difference, a factor of two to three, observed in skin permeability between these two sites. As a consequence, if it is reasonable to assume that the follicular pathway plays a role in percutaneous absorption, it has to be reevaluated.

In the past, the sebum was believed to reduce absorption of hydrophilic compounds (39). This theory has since been disproved (40). As our results show (Figure 52.11), the same ratio, a factor of two, exists between permeability levels of areas such as the forehead, which is rich in sebum, and

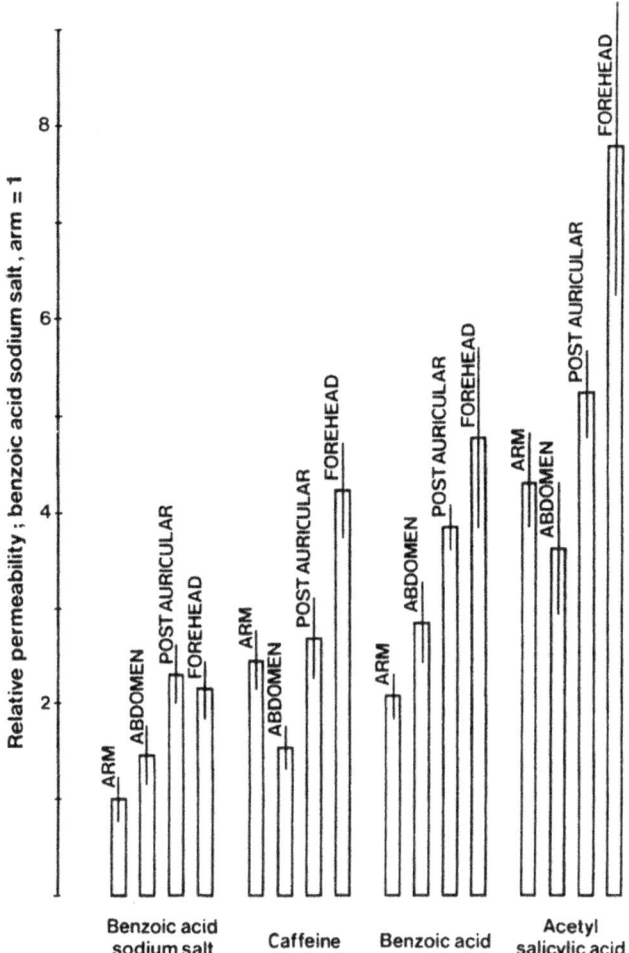

FIGURE 52.11 Influence of anatomical site on the total percutaneous absorption of the tested compounds (values expressed relatively to that of benzoic acid sodium salt applied on the arm). (From Reference 41.)

the arm, which has very little, to compounds with totally different lipid/water solubility, such as benzoic acid and its sodium salt.

Among the numerous applications of studies on the relationship existing between skin permeability and anatomical site, considerable attention has been given in recent years to finding favorable "windows" for transdermal treatment of systemic diseases. For various reasons, the postauricular area has been studied most often for scopolamine transdermal drug delivery (42, 43). According to Taskovitch and Shaw (44), in this area the closeness of the capillaries to the surface of the skin may promote resorption of substances and give the postauricular skin its good permeability. As our results show (Figure 52.11), whatever the compound applied, this area has a high level of permeability. Apart from caffeine, it is statistically higher than that of the arm or abdomen and often similar to that of the forehead.

As Figure 52.12 shows, the correlation between the amount of substance present in the stratum corneum at the end of a 30-minute application and the total amount absorbed within 4 days is confirmed in humans, whatever the factors involved in differences of permeability between sites ($r = 0.97$, $p < 0.001$). As a consequence, by simply measuring the quantity (x) of a chemical present in the stratum corneum at the end of the application, it is now possible to predict the total quantity

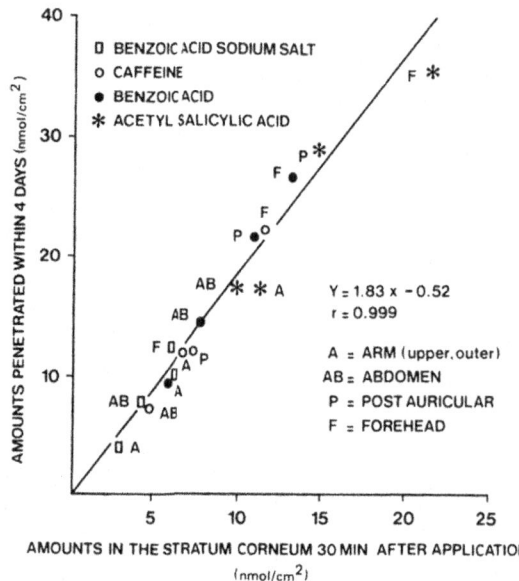

FIGURE 52.12   Correlation between total percutaneous absorption within 4 days and the amounts present in the stratum corneum at the end of the application time (30 minutes) for each compound and each anatomical site. (From Reference 24.)

(y) absorbed over a 4-day period. It should also be mentioned that this correlation curve is similar to that established in the rat (see Section 52.1), thus demonstrating that the relationship between the reservoir function of the horny layer and percutaneous absorption is independent of the animal species.

The consequences of such findings are obvious and far-reaching. They would make it easier to screen new drugs in animals and thus predict their toxicological or pharmacological implications. They would also circumvent some ethical difficulties of human experiments, particularly those using potentially toxic agents. It is self-evident that *in vivo* investigations with animals, and particularly humans, are preferable to *in vitro* methods. It is also obvious that the experimenter has a higher degree of responsibility when performing *in vivo* percutaneous absorption studies in humans. Moreover, the blood and urine analyses generally used in the *in vivo* methods involve severe technical problems because of the low concentrations that must be assayed. Radiolabeled compounds are detected with high sensitivity but imply ethical problems when applied to humans. For technical convenience, labeled compounds were used in our experiments. However, because of the relatively large amount of substance present in the stratum corneum at the end of the application, it should be possible, with the stripping method, to measure percutaneous absorption in both animals and humans by appropriate nonradioactive analytical techniques. When it is nevertheless essential to use labeled substances, this method makes it possible both to substantially reduce the level of radioactivity administered and to limit contact time.

REFERENCES

1. Tregear RT. The permeability of skin to molecules of widely differing properties. In: Rook A, Champion RH, eds. Progress in Biological Sciences in Relation to Dermatology. 2nd ed. London: Cambridge University Press, 1964:275–281.
2. Winkelmann RK. The relationship of structure of the epidermis to percutaneous absorption. Br J Dermatol 1969; 81(Suppl 4):11–22.
3. Marzulli FN. Barrier to skin penetration. J Invest Dermatol 1962; 39:387–393.

4. Lindsey D. Percutaneous penetration. In: Pillsbury DM, Livingood CS, eds. Proceedings of the 12th International Congress of Dermatology. Amsterdam: Exerpta Medica, 1963; 407–415.

5. Maibach HI, Feldmann RJ. Effect of applied concentration on percutaneous absorption in man. J Invest Dermatol 1969; 52:382.

6. Wester RC, Maibach HI. Relationship of topical dose and percutaneous absorption in rhesus monkey and man. J Invest Dermatol 1976; 67:518–520.

7. Poulsen BJ. Design of topical drug products: biopharmaceutics. In: Ariens EJ, ed. Drug Design. Vol. IV. New York: Academic Press, 1973:149–190.

8. Malkinson FD, Rothman S. Percutaneous absorption. In: Marchionini A, Spier HW, eds. Handbuch der Haut und Geschlecht Skrauberten, Normale und Pathologische de Haut, Vol. 1. Part 1. Berlin-Heidelberg: Springer-Verlag, 1963:90–156.

9. Stoughton RB. Percutaneous absorption. Toxicol Appl Pharmacol 1965; 7(Suppl 2):1–6.

10. Stoughton RB, Fritsh WF. Influence of dimethyl sulfoxide (DMSO) on human percutaneous absorption. Arch Dermatol 1964; 90:512–517.

11. Vickers CFH. Existence of a reservoir in the stratum corneum. Arch Dermatol 1963; 88:20–23.

12. Rougier A, Dupuis D, Lotte C, Roguet R, Schaefer H. *In vivo* correlation between stratum corneum reservoir function and percutaneous absorption. J Invest Dermatol 1983; 81:275–278.

13. Feldmann RJ, Maibach HI. Percutaneous penetration of steroids in man. J Invest Dermatol 1969; 52:89–94.

14. Feldmann RJ, Maibach HI. Absorption of some organic compounds through the skin in man. J Invest Dermatol 1970; 54:399–404.

15. Schaefer H, Stuttgen G, Zesch A, Schalla W, Gazith J. Quantitative determination of percutaneous absorption of radiolabeled drugs *in vitro* and *in vivo* in human skin. In: Mali JWH, ed. Current Problems in Dermatology. Basel: S. Karger, 1978:80–94.

16. Scheuplein RJ. Mechanism of percutaneous absorption: II. Transient diffusion and relative importance of various routes of skin absorption. J Invest Dermatol 1967; 48:79–88.

17. Treherne JE. Permeability of skin to some electrolytes. J Physiol 1956; 13:171–180.

18. Rougier A, Dupuis D, Lotte C, Roguet R. The measurement of the stratum corneum reservoir: a predictive method for *in vivo* percutaneous absorption studies: influence of application time. J Invest Dermatol 1985; 84:66–68.

19. Scheuplein RJ, Ross LW. Mechanism of percutaneous absorption of solvents deposited solids. J Invest Dermatol 1974; 62:353–360.

20. Skog E, Wahlberg JE. A comparative investigation of the percutaneous absorption of lethal compounds in the guinea pig by means of the radioactive isotopes ^{51}Cr, ^{58}Co, ^{65}Zn, ^{110m}Ag, ^{115m}Cd, ^{203}Hg. J Invest Dermatol 1964; 43:187–192.

21. Sheth NV, Keough MB, Spruance SL. Measurement of the stratum corneum drug reservoir to predict the therapeutic efficacy of topical iododeoxyuridine for herpes simplex virus infection. Annual Meeting of the American Federation of Clinical Research, Washington, DC, May 1986.

22. Barr M. Percutaneous absorption. J Pharm Sci 1962; 57:395–408.

23. Idson B. Biophysical factors in skin penetration. J Soc Cosmet Chem 1971; 22:615–620.

24. Idson B. Percutaneous absorption. J Pharm Sci 1975; 64:901–924.

25. Rothman S. Physiology and Biochemistry of the Skin. Chicago: University of Chicago Press, 1990.

26. Blank HI, Scheuplein RJ. The epidermal barrier. In: Rook A, Champion RH, eds. Progress in Biological Sciences in Relation to Dermatology. 2nd ed. London: Cambridge University Press, 1964:245–261.

27. Schutz E. Der Einflub von polyathylenglycol 400 auf die percutan resorption von Wirkstoffen. Archiv Exp Pathol Pharmakol 1957; 232:237–240.

28. Dupuis D, Rougier A, Roguet R, Lotte C. The measurement of the stratum corneum reservoir: a simple method to predict the influence of vehicles on *in vivo* percutaneous absorption. Br J Dermatol 1986; 115:233–238.

29. Shelley WB, Melton FM. Factors accelerating the penetration of histamine through normal intact skin. J Invest Dermatol 1949; 13:61–64.

30. Barry BW. Dermatological formulations: percutaneous absorption. In: Swarbrick J, ed. Drugs and Pharmaceutical Sciences. Vol. 18. New York: Marcel Dekker, 1983.

31. Scheuplein RJ. Site variation in diffusion and permeability. In: Jarrett A, ed. Physiology and Pathophysiology of the Skin. New York: Academic Press, 1979:1731–1752.

32. Feldmann RJ, Maibach HI. Regional variations in percutaneous penetration of ^{14}C cortisol in man. J Invest Dermatol 1967; 48:181–183.

33. Maibach HI, Feldmann RJ, Milby TH, Serat WF. Regional variations in percutaneous penetration in man. Arch Environ Health 1971; 23:208–211.

34. Wester RC, Maibach HI, Bucks DA, Aufrere MB. *In vivo* percutaneous absorption of paraquat from hand, leg and forearm of humans. J Toxicol Environ Health 1984; 14:759–162.

35. Bridges JW, French WR, Smith RL, Williams RT. The fate of benzoic acid in various species. Biochem J 1970; 118:47–51.

36. Bronaugh RL, Stewart RR, Congdon ER, Giles AL. Methods for *in vitro* percutaneous absorption studies. I. Comparison with *in vivo* results. Toxicol Appl Pharmacol 1982; 62:474–480.

37. Benfenati A, Brillanti F. Sulla distribuzione delle ghiandole sebaceenella cute del corpo umano. Arch Ital Dermatol 1939; 15:33–42.

38. Szabo, G. The regional frequency and distribution of hair follicles in human skin. In: Montagna W, Ellis RA, eds. The Biology of Hair Growth. New York: Academic Press, 1958:33–38.

39. Calvery HO, Draize JH, Lang EP. Metabolism and permeability of normal skin. Physiol Rev 1946; 26:495–540.

40. Blank HI, Gould E. Penetration of anionic surfactants into the skin. II Study of mechanisms which impede the penetration of synthetic anionic surfactants into skin. J Invest Dermatol 1961; 37:311–315.

41. Rougier A, Lotte C, Maibach HI. *In vivo* percutaneous penetration of some organic compounds related to anatomic site in man: predictive assessment by the stripping method. J Pharm Sci 1987.

42. Shaw JE, Chandrasekaran SK, Michaels AS, Taskovitch L. Controlled transdermal delivery, *in vitro* and *in vivo*. In: Maibach HI, ed. Animal Modes in Human Dermatology. Edinburgh, London: Churchill-Livingstone, 1975:136–146.

43. Shaw JE, Chandrasekaran SK, Campbell PS, Schmitt LG. New procedures for evaluating cutaneous absorption. In: Drill VA, Lazar P, eds. Cutaneous Toxicity. New York: Academic Press, 1977:83–94.

44. Taskovitch L, Shaw JE. Regional differences in morphology of human skin. Correlation with variations in drug permeability. J Invest Dennatol 1978; 70:217.

53 Tape Stripping
Technique and Applications

Rebekka Christmann, Anne S. Raber, and Ulrich F. Schaefer
Saarland University, Saarbrücken, Germany

Ana Melero
University of Valencia, Valencia, Spain

Brigitta Loretz
Helmholtz-Institute for Pharmaceutical Research
Saarland, Saarbrücken, Germany

CONTENTS

53.1　INTRODUCTION

The tape stripping (TS) technique enables the noninvasive, painless, and successive removal of the stratum corneum (SC) layer by layer, including fast skin recovery.

The SC (3 to 20 μm in thickness) consists of around 15 to 25 layers of dead corneocytes, which are connected via corneodesmosomes, embedded in an intercellular lipid matrix (Alikhan and

Maibach 2010; Honari and Maibach 2014; Haftek 2015). By applying successive adhesive tape strips (ASs) on the skin surface area, only dead cells embedded in lipid matrix are removed by adhering to the AS (Herkenne et al. 2008). TS in skin research has been used for several distinct readouts, which can be grouped into three application areas (Lindemann et al. 2003; Lademann et al. 2006; Breternitz et al. 2007; Weigmann et al. 2012):

1. Assessment of the barrier properties of the SC for drugs, cosmetics, and occupational chemicals
2. Investigation of skin biology in health and disease conditions
3. A way for standardized injury, enabling healing studies, vaccination, or increased delivery

When the method was first developed, the aim was to get insights on the SC barrier nature. Jan Wolf first mentioned the TS method to get superficial horny layer samples suitable for microscopy (Wolf 1940). Herman Pinkus a few years later found the technique appropriate to determine the thickness of the SC by a successive layer-by-layer removal via TS and observed the healing in subsequent biopsies (Pinkus 1951). The method itself consists of repetitive application of ASs on the skin surface and a quick peel-off. Upon identifying the possibility of SC to act as drug reservoir and barrier, over the decades many studies followed in refining and "standardizing" the method, adding more analytical possibilities to reveal more and more details on the complex skin structure. Dermatological formulation development in pharmacy and cosmetics and occupational toxicology uses TS as a standard method with various downstream analysis of different complexities. Current analytical detection limits allow the quantification of nonlabelled chemicals or endogenous molecules from the ASs. The removal of SC by TS also inspired studies on topical vaccination and delivery of macromolecules via the skin. For skin biology, diagnostics, and drug/chemical skin absorption, the TS method continues to be in use and functions often as a standard method, when newer, noninvasive methods are compared (e.g., spectroscopy). In contrast, the use of TS for controlled SC damage has lost importance since the advent of microneedles and ablative laser techniques appeared. This chapter focuses most on pharmaceutical investigations in the discussion of technical issues and examples of current studies. Nevertheless, a few selected examples of skin biology and pathophysiology are included in the last section, since skin condition is closely related to dermal delivery and similar analytics is or might be used.

53.2   THE TAPE STRIPPING METHOD

In general, the TS technique consists of the following steps (Wagner, et al. 2002; Melero et al. 2011; EMA 2018; Lademann et al. 2009; Surber, Schwarb, and Smith 2005)

1. Preparation of the skin surface area (hair removal, cleaning, marking of the application area)
2. Application of the formulation
3. Cleaning of the skin surface of excess formulation
4. Application of a AS, with a defined size
5. Pressing the AS on the skin surface with a roller, stamp, thumb, etc.
6. Fast removal of the AS with forceps
7. Determination of the SC amount adhered on the AS
8. Repetition of steps 3 to 7 until the desired amount of SC is removed
9. Analysis of the drug or substances of interest on the AS

To obtain only a reduced skin barrier, steps 2,3, and 9 are skipped.

The TS technique can be applied in vivo and in vitro, in human skin, as well as in nonhuman skin (e.g. animal: pig, mice). In this chapter, the method will only be discussed relating to human skin. More information and detailed TS technique protocols for in vitro and in vivo can be found at (Melero et al. 2011; Wagner, et al. 2000, 2002; EMA 2018; N'Dri-Stempfer et al. 2009). Since the results of the TS depend on many influencing parameters during the performance and the variety of conditions impede the comparison between published works, a standardization of the method is needed. Crucial parameters that can be a source of variation in the TS results (natural, e.g., anatomical region, age, gender, sex, time of day, presence of skin wrinkles, season or hydration state, as well as methodological factors), will be discussed systematically next.

53.3 TECHNICAL ISSUES: STANDARDIZATION OF THE TECHNIQUE AND CRITICAL PARAMETERS TO OBTAIN REPRODUCIBLE RESULTS

53.3.1 DECISIONS AND REQUIREMENTS BEFORE THE EXPERIMENT: IN VIVO AND IN VITRO STUDIES

The following questions are essential in the beginning: in vivo or in vitro, human or nonhuman (animal) subjects. In the case of in vivo experiments, human experiments are the gold standard, but animals are reasonably easier to obtain and the results can be scaled up to humans (Abd et al. 2016). Independent of the experimental setup, prior evaluation from an authorized ethical committee must be obtained, including informed consent signed by participants. Since in vivo testing in animals should be reduced to a minimum and replaced by other appropriate models, in vitro techniques are of great interest (Eskes and Zuang 2005). Ex vivo human skin is still considered the best surrogate for human volunteers.

Even for in vitro experiments, different experimental setups can be chosen. Diffusion cell, a setting that was developed to study drug permeation through the skin, consists of a donor (application of the formulation) and acceptor compartment (filled with buffer/acceptor solution) separated by excised skin as a membrane. Apart from the widely known static Franz diffusion cell (FDC), there are also flow-through diffusion cells available, facilitating better sink conditions. Sink conditions are mandatory for permeation studies to ensure that the permeation through the skin is not influenced by the solubility of the applied drug in the receptor solution. That means the highest concentration of the permeated drug during the experiment in the receptor solution must be below 10% of its saturation solubility in the receptor solution (WHO 2006).

Besides the diffusion cells, there is also a skin penetration model, the Saarbruecken Penetration Model (SB-M). Here, the formulation is applied on the excised skin, which is the only acceptor compartment, and the skin humidity is preserved by a soaked filter paper beneath it (Selzer et al. 2013a). After a predetermined time, the amount of drug in the skin can be determined in the SC by TS and in the underlying deeper skin layers by cutting with a cryomicrotome and subsequent analysis (Wagner et al. 2000).

The realization of sink conditions in a FDC can often only be achieved by supplementing with solubility enhancers. As a result, the SC properties can be altered by damage, saturation, and hydration. This issue also points out the importance of the in vitro setup chosen; in comparison to the FDC, nonphysiological skin hydration is prevented in the SB-M (Wagner et al. 2000, 2002; Selzer et al. 2013a).

Institutions such as the organization for economic co-operation and development (OECD), U.S. food and drug administration (FDA), and scientific committee on consumer safety (SCCS) provide guidelines containing general instructions on accepted techniques (OECD 2004a,b; SCCS 2018; WHO 2006; FDA 1997). TS is the most widely used experimental setup to determine the permeation of substances within the SC, equally feasible in vitro as well as in vivo (Brain, Walters, and Watkinson 2002).

While most human in vivo studies are performed on the volar forearm, in vitro studies most commonly utilize abdominal or breast skin obtained from surgery. It has to be considered here that the absorption rate through skin can be up to fortyfold different (Feldmann and Maibach 1967). Nevertheless, in vitro experiments have shown to be sufficient in predicting in vivo skin absorption

(Franz 1975; Wagner et al. 2000; Lehman, Raney, and Franz 2011; Hotchkiss et al. 1992; Wagner et al. 2002; Hotchkiss et al. 1990). Studies that evaluate the correlation between in vivo and in vitro experiments are rare. Ilic et al. compared the pig as the most used animal skin to human in vivo TS results (Ilić et al. 2017). Wagner et al. performed a study with direct comparison of in vivo and in vitro permeation and penetration on human abdominal skin. TS for drug analysis in SC was performed prior (in vivo) and after (in vitro) plastic surgery (Wagner et al. 2002). Invasiveness of skin samples for penetration studies is an obstacle for studies on volunteers. The TS procedure only or in combination with cyanoacrylate biopsy is less invasive. Few studies investigating the follicular route or delivery with hair follicles as the target have been performed as in vitro/in vivo correlations (Raber et al. 2014; Patzelt et al. 2008; Christmann et al. 2020).

53.3.2 Preparation of the Skin Surface Area

The application site of the in vivo TS procedure in humans must be carefully selected (Lademann et al. 2009; Breternitz et al. 2007). It should be free of hair and uneven areas (e.g., wrinkles, scars, tattoos). Instead of shaving, hair should be removed with scissors to avoid potential SC damage and removal (Lademann et al. 2009). Breternitz and co-workers compared the TS procedure in facial skin (cheek), back, forearm, and upper arm, finding statistically significant differences, with the facial skin the easiest application site to completely remove the SC, followed by the back, forearm, and upper arm (Breternitz et al. 2007). In agreement with those results, Löffler and co-workers found that the facial skin (forehead) SC could be removed faster in comparison to the back and, lastly, the forearm (Löffler, Dreher, and Maibach 2004). In addition, Raj et al. confirmed this by finding a higher SC amount on the forearm than on facial skin (cheek); they also studied the difference between ethnicities (Caucasian and Black African) without finding statistical significant differences (Raj et al. 2016). Bashir et al. studied the differences between the volar and the dorsal forearm; regardless of the AS type used, no significant difference was found in the amount of SC removed from both sides (Bashir et al. 2001). When performing in vitro experiments, the skin type selected and its treatment can be a source of variability in SC properties (e.g., human skin from cosmetic surgery, biopsies, cadaver skin) (Abd et al. 2016). If animal skin is used, the species will also influence the quality of the results. Porcine skin is most widely used and considered the best surrogate for human skin (Praça et al. 2018). The treatment of the excised skin is also a determining parameter in the case of in vitro experiments. There is a general agreement that excised human skin can be stored up to six months at −20°C, as −80°C storage produces cell damage (Barbero and Frasch 2016). Some authors recommend the use of 10% glycerol as a preservative (Küchler, Strüver, and Friess 2013), but the freezing procedure, even in presence of cryoprotectants, is not effective in the case of animal skin (Praça et al. 2018). Finally, the skin should be kept in appropriate storage material. Aluminum foil and Parafilm have been widely used. However, the use of Parafilm should be avoided, since incorporated hydrocarbons, like paraffin, can alter the skin barrier property.

53.3.2.1 Delimitation of the Stripping Area

To facilitate complete removal of the SC by means of TS in both the lateral and vertical directions, the stripping area must be perfectly delimited to assure that each AS contains only the layer below the previous AS. Different approaches have been applied both in vivo and in vitro, such as the use of a mask to cover the stripping area, in which an aluminum tape is stuck to the skin leaving a hole with a known diameter. The AS is applied onto the mask and the surrounding skin is not removed by the AS sides (Melero et al. 2011). Other authors prefer to mark the stripping area with a marker. In this case, the removal of skin layers can also include the one with the marked tissue. Therefore, the area has to be marked again after several ASs; also the marker ink must not interfere with the analytical method (Lademann et al. 2009). In addition, a possible lateral diffusion of the formulation should be taken into account and controlled by TS the area adjacent to the application area.

Weigmann et al. found a major impact on the lateral spreading of clobetasol propionate formulations due to different vehicles (Weigmann et al. 1999b). For a better investigation of the lateral spreading, concentric TS was developed by Gee et al. (2012). ASs of 3M were designed with concentric perforations to separate into a mid-circle of 8 mm (the same area as the application site) and three rings of 8 mm width. The penetration and TS study was performed to investigate the difference in lateral diffusion of three model actives (caffeine, hydrocortisone, and ibuprofen) on eight human volunteers. The three model drugs showed variation in the amount, depth, and lateral spreading in SC from the initial application site. The logP of the drugs affect the lateral spreading as well as the depth of penetration. In addition, the molecular weight and the solubility of the drug inside the moisture layer on the skin were suggested to have an effect on lateral spreading. Selzer et al. determined experimentally the lateral diffusion effect of flufenamic acid and caffeine in in vitro skin absorption experiments using FDCs and finite dose conditions, to incorporate it into mathematical models (Selzer et al. 2013b).

53.3.3 APPLICATION OF THE FORMULATION: INFINITE AND FINITE DOSING

Regarding the TS technique itself, the nature of the formulation under study will dramatically condition drug delivery but also the amount of SC adhered to the AS. The nature of the vehicle can influence the characteristics of the SC by modifying corneocyte hydration (Melero et al. 2011), cohesion between cells (Surber, Schwarb, and Smith 2005), lipid components of SC, and fluidity of the intercellular lipid matrix (Abd et al. 2016). In this sense, different vehicles have been designed to enhance or delay drug permeability (Melero et al. 2011; Ourique et al. 2011). These physiological changes in SC, as well as the influence of the vehicle on the adhesiveness of the AS, will affect the amount of SC removed by each AS compared to untreated skin (Lademann et al. 2009).

Another crucial parameter is the incubation time of the formulation—the longer it is, the more pronounced the effect. Apart from the influence of the vehicle itself on SC, the drug also will distribute within the SC layers as a function of time.

Finally, there are two possibilities in skin permeation experiments to apply the dose, infinite or finite, and that influences the drug penetration and permeation into and through the skin.

The commonly used method is the infinite-dose experiment, in which the applied drug amount is infinitely large and constant, so a change in the donor (applied drug) concentration over the incubation time due to diffusion or evaporation can be neglected (Brain, Walters, and Watkinson 2002). For permeation studies (detection of the applied drug in the acceptor solution), the main kinetic parameters derived from infinite-dose experiments are steady-state flux (equilibrium due to saturation of drug in SC) and the permeability coefficient.

Wagner et al. demonstrated that the drug amount in vitro detected in the SC (due to the saturation process) can be fitted to Michaelis-Menten kinetics (Wagner et al. 2000), allowing the determination of the drug amount in the SC during steady state and the time until half of the maximum drug amount in the steady state has been reached.

The much less studied case is the finite-dose experiment, which mimics the clinical relevance more realistically with very small applied volumes of formulation. Finite-dose experiments are defined in the OECD guideline 428 by the application of $\leq 10\mu l/cm^2$ of a liquid formulation to the skin (OECD 2004b). For semisolid formulations, values range from 1 to 10 mg/cm^2 (Rougier et al. 1983; Vickers 1963; Pershing, Corlett, and Jorgensen 1994).

In finite-dose experiments, the barrier damage or alteration of the SC due to formulation exposure is reduced and can be neglected. Since the low volume of formulation has a negligible effect on SC hydration, finite-dose experiments have the benefit for polar drugs to avoid the overestimation of the polar pathway. Limitations of poorly soluble drugs may become visible in finite-dose experiments when the depletion results in insufficient solubilization at the skin surface (Intarakumhaeng, Wanasathop, and Li 2018). Experimental finite-dose experiments are more challenging. Crucial for the correct calculation of the results and for mass balance is the application of a precisely defined amount of formulation to the skin. Suitable incubation time is less predictable because it should enable assessment of the depletion effect. Furthermore, a homogeneous distribution has to be ensured to minimize effects on the outcome (van de Sandt et al. 2004). It has to be taken into account that the small donor volume alone does not necessarily stand for a finite dose. The finite dose must demonstrate dose depletion kinetics resulting from absorption, volatilization, or precipitation of the solute of interest.

Different methods of calculation must be used for finite and infinite dosing. Infinite dosing experiments establish a steady state flux and are frequently presented as cumulative absorption to derive permeation coefficient K_p and lag time T_{lag} values. Analyzing the data as flux vs. time is essential to understand the true nature of the actual kinetics profile. Calculations for finite dosing are very complex and normally not done. Instead, peak flux and peak t are calculated for comparison (Selzer et al. 2017).

53.3.4 Cleaning of the Skin Surface of Excess Formulation

In this step, the removal of the formulation and cleaning procedure should be done carefully, because some formulations can degrade the SC in such a manner that it can be easily removed by gentle rubbing (e.g., Keratolytics; Alikhan and Maibach 2010). The cleaning procedure has to be fast and sufficient to avoid further formulation inside permeating or outside driving the SC. To reduce the influence of free formulation residues on the SC, discarding the first tape strips was a common procedure (Surber, Schwarb, and Smith 2005). However, today, a sufficient surface cleaning procedure with subsequent ASs, including mass balance calculations for finite dosing experiments, is recommended (EMA 2018; Lademann et al. 2009; N'Dri-Stempfer et al. 2009; Selzer et al. 2013b).

53.3.5 Adhesive Tape Strip: Application and Removal

The next step of the TS procedure is probably the most critical one regarding the experimental setup itself. Here, the ASs should be applied and removed in an even manner to reduce intra and inter differences of the investigator as well as of subjects. It must be highlighted at this point that the complete removal of the SC is desired and that it can be affected by different influences and parameters, which will be discussed in detail next.

53.3.5.1 Selection of the Adhesive Tape Strip

The AS selection is of the utmost importance. Some requirements regarding the AS are essential: It should be able:

1. To remove corneocytes
2. To not interfere with the drug or SC amount analysis
3. To be flexible to adapt to the skin surface
4. To be translucent to allow microscopic visualization
5. To cover the complete stripping skin surface area
6. To avoid undesired skin reactions for in vivo performance (apart from those expected by the technique itself)

Several types of AS have been used, including commercial and self-made (Lademann et al. 2009). Bashir and co-workers compared different types of ASs: D-Squame, Transpore (iso-octyl acrylate, methyl acrylic acid copolymer, colophony resin and ethylene vinyl acetate polyethylene copolymer), and Micropore (nonwoven rayon with an iso-octyl acrylate and acrylic copolymer) (Bashir et al. 2001). No significant differences in terms of amount of SC removed between the ASs were found; only a trend was shown, where the D-Squame tape removed the highest SC amount and Micropore the least. Interestingly, the Micropore tape showed no significant increase in transepidermal water loss (TEWL) up to 40 ASs, where the other ASs showed an increase after 20 and 30 ASs (Transpore and D-Squame, respectively). The authors concluded that the composition of the AS is able to remove the corneocytes in a similar manner, but not the intercellular matrix, thus explaining the similarities in the removed SC amount but the differences in the TEWL. Breternitz and co-workers also studied different tape types using D-Squame, Corneofix, and Blenderm tapes (Breternitz et al. 2007). The SC amount removed could not be quantified for Blenderm tapes due to interference with the analytical method, and D-Squame tapes removed a higher SC amount compared to Corneofix tapes. Significant differences for the TEWL were found in the following order: D-Squame > Blenderm > Corneofix. These findings support the thesis that different results cannot be compared regarding the used AS number; instead, the determination of SC amount in ASs is crucial not only for result comparisons but also as a SC removal endpoint indicator. Therefore, the selection of the AS as well as the endpoint indicator of SC removal should be carefully considered (Hahn et al. 2010).

53.3.5.2 Applying Force for Uniform Adhesiveness

The pressure that is applied on the AS after application on the skin surface and prior to removal has a major impact on the amount of SC removed. It is not only applied to adhere the AS on the skin surface but also to reduce the influence of wrinkles and furrows by stretching the skin. Unfortunately, many studies do not describe the method and pressure applied on AS, thus making comparisons between studies complicated.

Different methods for pressure application have been studied, e.g., stamp, thumb, and roller, and also models like the SB-M are available to standardize the applied pressure on ASs for in vitro investigations (Wagner et al. 2000). Higher pressure application as well as a longer duration remove a higher amount of SC (Breternitz et al. 2007; Löffler, Dreher, and Maibach 2004). This leads to the conclusion that the kind of pressure application and the duration have a major impact on the SC amount removed. A standardization of the pressure application during TS is necessary.

53.3.5.3 The Way the Adhesive Tape Strips Are Removed from the Skin Surface

This parameter has also been considered by several authors as a factor that can affect the results in an important manner. However, this factor is difficult to standardize and depends very much on the researcher performing the technique. Nevertheless, the recommendations are to apply always a constant removal velocity and strength to the applied strips (Lademann et al. 2009).

53.3.6 DETERMINATION OF THE STRATUM CORNEUM AMOUNT ADHERED ON THE ADHESIVE TAPE STRIP FOR CONCENTRATION–DEPTH PROFILES

TS results are mostly presented as concentration–depth profiles of the applied drug—here the concentration of the applied drug is plotted against the SC depth, which is calculated based on the amount of SC removed. The concentration–depth profiles depend on time and on the drug physicochemical properties (Selzer et al. 2013a).

In the beginning the amount of drug removed per AS was correlated to the AS number, not taking into account that the amount of SC adhered to each individual AS differs. The SC amount per AS not only differs between types of AS, operators, and volunteers, but also the amount of adhered SC decreases with increasing AS number. An explanation for this is the increasing cohesion between the cells in the deeper SC, leading to a decreasing and overall inconsistent amount of SC adhered to individual AS. Those findings lead to the necessity to determine the SC amount adhered to each individual AS to gain reliable concentration–depth profiles (Bashir et al. 2001; Lindemann et al. 2003). Various approaches were made to determine the amount of SC attached to the AS. The attempts can roughly be divided into AS destructive and nondestructive methods, where nondestructive methods are always superior to destructive ones, leaving the AS for further investigations, e.g., drug amount analysis.

Despite its drawbacks, an often used nondestructive approach is the gravimetric determination of the SC amount on the AS (Kalia, Pirot, and Guy 1996). The method is time consuming (measuring the AS before and after the procedure, discharging the static from the AS, etc.; Mohammed et al. 2012), and the SC amount determined is often overestimated due to exogenous (applied formulation) and endogenous (sebum, intestinal fluid) substances adhered on the AS (Lademann et al. 2009). Still the method is often used to determine the efficiency of other approaches.

Kalia, Pirot, and Guy combined the gravimetric approach with TEWL measurements by means of a linearized Fick's first law—the thickness of the remaining SC on the skin after each AS can be estimated (Kalia, Pirot, and Guy 1996). Especially after normalization to the SC thickness, interindividual differences can be eliminated. Kalia et al. demonstrated that independent of the overall SC thickness, by equal relative SC amount removal, the increase of TEWL is the same (Kalia et al. 2000). They also observed that in comparison to skin impedance (correlated to skin hydration), which decreases mostly after the removal of the first AS, a noticeable TEWL increase first occurs after a removal of 75% of the SC layer (6 to 8 µm). TEWL measurements can also be used to determine the total removal of SC (endpoint determination of the tape stripping procedure) (EMA 2018). However, Netzlaff et al. showed a missing discriminative power for the skin integrity of human heat-separated epidermis in in vitro studies (Netzlaff et al. 2006).

Dreher et al. determined the SC amount via the identification of sodium hydroxide–soluble proteins of the SC adhered on the AS after neutralization by a commercially available protein assay (similar to the Lowry assay), as a standard heat-separated epidermis was used (Dreher et al. 1998) (see also Bashir et al. 2001; Breternitz et al. 2007). Since the distribution of SC on removed AS is not always homogenous, the total analysis of the AS is preferable (Dreher et al. 2005).

Weigmann et al. determined the SC protein amount by pseudo-absorption at 430 nm, where the absorbance of the AS is only influenced by the scattering, reflection, and diffraction of the light by corneocyte aggregates. The drawbacks of this nondestructive method are that errors might occur when the "stack effect" of the SC on the AS is present (overlay of SC layers on one AS) and when the corneocyte aggregates are nonhomogenously distributed over the AS, since only a representative area of the AS is analyzed (Weigmann et al. 1999a). See also (Lindemann et al. 2003; Jacobi et al. 2005). To capture the inhomogeneities of SC distribution on a AS, a special spectrometer with a measuring area over 1 cm² is needed. For better performance and an automation of this approach, a corneocyte density analyzer based on a slide projector was developed (Lademann et al. 2006).

Marttin et al. determined the SC protein amount of the AS via the protein absorbance in the UV range at 278 nm, but the absorption is only characterized by a weak band, leading to an insensitive and unreliable method (Marttin et al. 1996; Lademann et al. 2009). Lindemann et al. stained the SC proteins adhered on a AS selectively with trypan blue, which can be detected at 652 nm (Lindemann et al. 2003).

Voegeli et al. introduced the infrared densitometry (IR-D) for the determination of SC protein amount per AS. The amount of SC is measured by the reduction of absorbance on AS at 850 nm. For an in-process implementation of the method, a novel infrared densitometer especially suitable for D-Squame disks with a diameter of 22 mm was developed (SquameScan 850A). By means of corresponding calibration curves, the SC protein amount per AS can be evaluated quickly and indirectly. Up to 45% of the AS area is analyzed, diminishing the influence of inhomogeneity of SC protein amount on the AS, a thermal denaturation of biomolecules is prevented, and the technique is nondestructive; additionally, the absorption value can be read directly from the display. Given that, this method is superior to a colorimetric assay determination of the SC protein amount even with a slightly less sensitivity (Voegeli et al. 2007; Raj et al. 2016). The method was further investigated by Hahn et al., and they proved the practicability of IR-D not only for in vitro skin stripping but also, more importantly, for determining the SC removal endpoint in vivo. In addition, they demonstrated the possible use of different ASs (Tesafilm kristall klar) (Hahn et al. 2010). Mohammed et al.

correlated the SC protein recovery via IR-D to the gravimetric approach, showing a good correlation and leading to the assumption that the IR-D method is superior due to being a faster and less accident-sensitive technique (Mohammed et al. 2012).

53.3.7 ANALYSIS OF THE DRUG OR SUBSTANCES OF INTEREST

Different methods can be used to analyze the amount of drug present in the samples, with high- performance liquid chromatography (HPLC) and mass spectrometry (MS) being the most widely used methods. The only requirements for the method selected are the ability to discriminate the drug from the other extracted components of the skin and a high sensitivity, because the stripped amounts are usually very low (Surber, Schwarb, and Smith 2005). To enhance the reliability of the analysis, pooling several ASs in the same extracting vial is recommended, especially in the deepest SC layers. The sequence for sample pooling should be determined for each drug and incubation time, as it depends on the penetration ability of each compound. Equally important to obtain reliable results is to develop an appropriate extracting method. Preferably, this method should not extract the glue of the ASs to avoid analytic interferences. A mass balance, extracting all the materials that were in touch with the drug, as well as all the collected ASs, should be done to assure that the 100 ± 15% of the applied drug is recovered through the extraction medium (SCCS 2018). Analysis can be performed from the extracted AS for quantification or directly on the AS, e.g., in combination with visualization to also gain spatial information. Figure 53.1 and Table 53.1 provide a summary of analytical methods and selected examples for their applications.

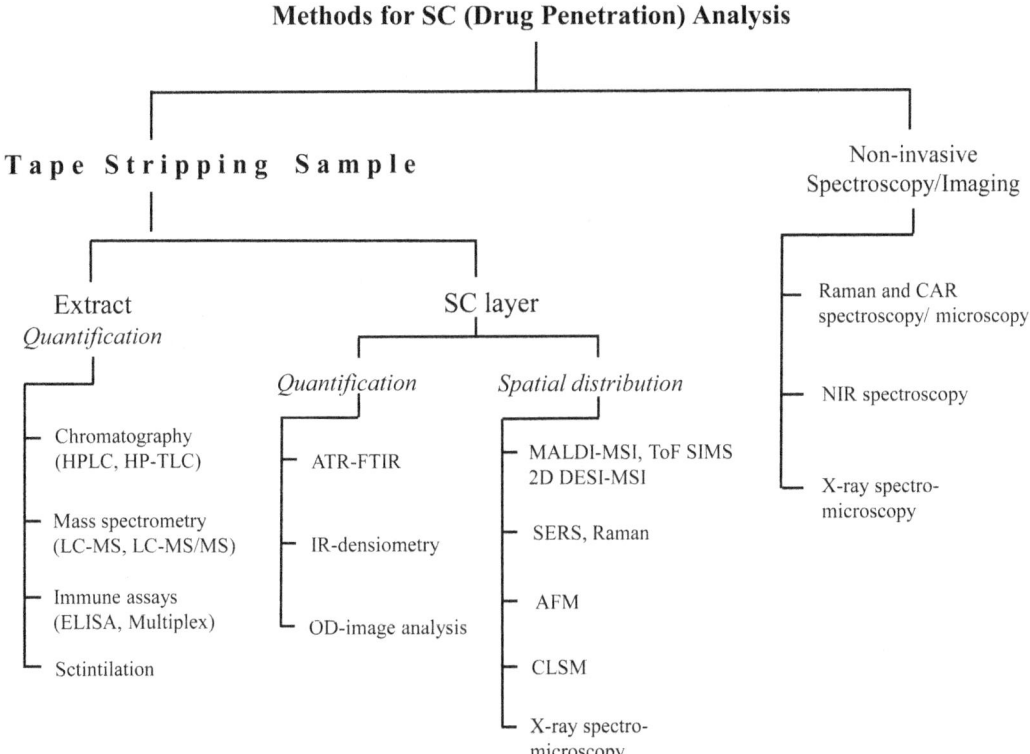

FIGURE 53.1 Overview of analytical methods applied in SC/skin investigations with a special focus on TS on noninvasive methods.

TABLE 53.1

Examples for Various Analytical Techniques from Tape Stripping Samples or Skin Cross-Sections for Depth Profiling

Analytical Technique	Application	Reference
LC-MS/MS (Liquid chromatography–tandem mass spectrometry)	Protein analysis for disease diagnostics	(Azimi et al. 2018)
ToF-SIMS (Time of flight–secondary ion mass spectrometry)	Analysis of skin lipid quantity and distribution from human skin in relation to aging	(Starr et al. 2016)
Thermal and spectroscopic analysis	Probing drug crystallization on pig skin	(Goh et al. 2019)
MALDI-MSI (Matrix-assisted laser desorption ionization–mass spectrometry imaging)	Skin distribution profiles in skin biopsy cross-sections of Jak inhibitors; lipid analysis in skin cross-sections	(Bonnel et al. 2018; Hart et al. 2011)
DESI-MSI (Desorption electrospray ionization–mass spectrometry imaging)	Concentration–depth profiles of cosmetic actives over larger skin areas	(Motoyama and Kihara 2017)
Raman spectroscopy	Analysis of lipid and protein signals of human in vivo AS extracts (for diagnostics)	(Janssens et al. 2014)
Raman microscopy	Analysis on skin biopsy cross-sections; development of a surrogate for correction of signal attenuation in skin depth	(Ashtikar et al. 2013; Ashtikar et al. 2017; Franzen et al. 2013; Franzen, Anderski, and Windbergs 2015)
SERS/TERS (Surface enhanced Raman scattering / tip-enhanced Raman scattering) and AFM (Atomic force microscopy)	Detection of invasome carriers in human skin; spin-coated coverslips replaced the tape for stripping to reduce signal interference from the adhesive	(Ashtikar et al. 2017)
CARS (Coherent anti-Stokes Raman scattering spectroscopy)	Used CARS in combination with 2-photon microscopy for nondestructive analysis of skin penetration of deuterated actives	(Chen, X. et al. 2015)
STXM (Scanning transmission x-ray microscopy)	Analysis of quantum dots or drug substances skin penetration depth in skin/reconstructed skin samples	(Nastiti, C. M. R. R. et al. 2019; Yamamoto et al. 2015; Yamamoto et al. 2017; Wanjiku et al. 2019)
AFM	Probing of corneocyte stiffness in various SC depth	(Milani et al. 2018)
SEM (Scanning electron microscopy)	Corneocytes morphology; biodegradable nanocarrier degradation in hair follicle plucks of rat skin	(Starr et al. 2016; Svenskaya et al. 2019)
CLSM (Confocal laser scanning microscopy) and MPT-FLIM (Multiphoton tomography–fluorescence lifetime imaging)	Probing size dependency of skin penetration pathway with fluorescent polystyrene particles; monitoring fluorescence-marked nanocarriers in rat skin punch biopsies; imaging of zinc oxide nanoparticle penetration in human skin samples and in vivo	(Zou et al., 2017; Svenskaya et al., 2019; Zvyagin et al., 2008; Roberts et al., 2011; Leite-Silva et al., 2013)
ELISA (Enzyme-linked immunosorbent assay)	Interleukin protein biomarker quantification in AS extracts as a diagnostic; analysis of endogenous antimicrobial peptides in relation to SC depth	(Berekméri et al. 2018; Clausen et al. 2018)
Multiplex immunoassay	From AS extracts for diagnostic biomarker identification	(Koppes et al. 2016)

53.4 TAPE STRIPPING TO ASSESS BIOEQUIVALENCE IN GENERIC TOPICALLY APPLIED DRUG PRODUCTS

The TS technique has been under discussion for several years for the assessment of bioequivalence (BE) of topically applied drug products to provide a faster, cheaper, and easier method compared to the gold-standard clinical endpoint studies, like the pharmacodynamic bioassay (vasoconstrictor assay), which can only be used for the BE assessment of topically applied glucocorticoids (FDA 1995). To show the possible utilization of TS for BE studies, TS was often compared to the pharmacodynamic bioassay of glucocorticoids (Pershing et al. 2002; Au, Skinner, and Kanfer 2010).

The technique enables the determination of drug concentration–time curves in the SC. This leads to the suggestion that two formulations with comparable SC drug concentration–time curves can be seen as bioequivalent, similar to the BE assessment of orally applied drug formulations (comparable plasma concentration–time curves). It is often referred to as the dermatopharmacokinetics (DPK) approach (Miranda et al. 2018; Shah et al. 1998; Pershing et al. 1992). In 1998 the FDA published a draft guidance called *Topical Dermatological Drug Products NDAs and ANDAs: In Vivo Bioavailability, Bioequivalence, In Vitro Release, and Associated Studies*, which recommended the DPK approach to prove the BE of topically applied drug products (FDA 1998; Shah et al. 1998). Unfortunately, the draft guidance in this form was not precise and adequate enough to determine the BE of topical drug products. Eventually, the withdrawal of the draft guidance followed in 2002 (FDA 2002). Major criticisms were:

1. Lack of reproducibility between laboratories
2. Lack of bioavailability assessment for drugs, where the SC is not the site of action
3. Lack of the method to distinguish between active and inactive (e.g., crystalized) drug amount (Yacobi et al. 2014)
4. The need for many volunteers to gain statistical power, which declines the economic benefit over clinical endpoint studies (N'Dri-Stempfer et al. 2008; Miranda et al. 2018)

Since then, a lot of effort has been put into the improvement and standardization of the DPK technique, even though the trend is heading more towards a "whole toolkit" instead of one "universal method" for the BE assessment of topical drug products (Yacobi et al. 2014). For example, Bunge and Guy, together with coworkers, developed a so-called "two-times method." The time points were restricted to only one uptake and one clearance time point, given that replicate measurements could be done in each subject, increasing the statistical power (reduction of volunteers up to 40%), in comparison to the multiple time points suggested by the FDA draft guidance. In comparison to the FDA draft guidance, where a standardized number of ASs was removed, a TS endpoint indicator was advised (Navidi et al. 2008; N'Dri-Stempfer et al. 2008, 2009). In 2018, the Committee for Medicinal Products for Human Use (CHMP) of the European Medicines Agency (EMA) published a draft guideline on the quality and equivalence of topical products, suggesting the DPK approach as a replacement for a therapeutic equivalence study for semisolid formulations. The guideline recommends a pilot study prior to the pivotal study to validate and define the procedure in detail and to demonstrate the statistical power to detect BE and non-BE products. It also demands one uptake and one clearance time point, replication in one volunteer, the gravimetric method for SC amount determination combined with TEWL measurements as endpoint indicator, and including mass balance (EMA 2018).

53.5 DEPTH PROFILES AS A RESULT OF TAPE STRIPPING: CHANCE FOR IN SILICO MODELING

Skin absorption experiments are complicated procedures, requiring an immense effort in terms of time and costs. In silico models to predict the absorption kinetics of a drug in skin are highly interesting.

Mathematical modeling requires physicochemical input parameters of the used drug, such as the molecular weight and the partition coefficient (Reddy, McCarley, and Bunge 1998). The partition coefficient is of great importance, as the lipophilic character of the SC leads to a poor partitioning of hydrophilic drugs in this layer. Smaller substances below 500 daltons are known to penetrate the SC more efficiently than larger substances (George 2005). Input parameters are commonly derived from infinite-dose experiments, as in a finite-dose experiment the steady state is not reached and the parameters change constantly over the incubation time (Anissimov and Roberts 2001). TS can determine drug concentration–SC depth profiles, which requires the normalization of the drug amount per AS to the amount of removed SC per AS.

Drug permeation and penetration results build the data basis for modeling and simulation in skin drug absorption. Thus, permeation (e.g., FDCs) and TS studies of high quality are an important source for skin absorption/penetration modeling. Important input parameters (D_{lip}:D_{cor} diffusivities in lipids and corneocytes, $K_{lip/w}$ lipid–water partition coefficient), as well as resulting lag time and drug permeability are experimental results that are needed for modeling (Hansen et al. 2008)

TS and FDC experiments can be performed without requirements for chemical modification due to the many useable quantification methods by which the permeated or extracted sample can be analyzed. Other noninvasive investigation techniques often remain limited in absolute quantification or may need drug modifications (e.g., fluorophore conjugation) or are limited for drugs with certain properties (e.g., spectrophotometric detectability against tissue background) like confocal fluorescence microscopy, confocal Raman microscopy. Methods like x-ray scanning microscopy are of interest and find first use in simulation, but are, at least so far, limited to smaller studies due to the high technical effort (expensive equipment, expert knowledge) (Schulz et al. 2017).

Thus, a major limitation in drug penetration simulation is the availability of high-quality experimental data for a large enough drug group representing structural diversity and obtained under a constant, reproducible protocol. Such a database would allow researchers first to set up and train (e.g., machine learning or artificial intelligence) a computer model with a broad drug/compound library before validation with a set of compounds not included in the setup/training as a quality control for the prediction. Important for achieving such a database are clear protocols/guidelines for performance of drug penetration/permeation experiments and data accessibility to allow the use of results across various laboratories and institutions.

Several models have been proposed, differing in the approach. Models use drug descriptors like molecular weight, logP, etc., to predict drug penetration based on structure–activity relationships (SARs). SAR models are build only on the drug; therefore, they do not represent vehicle or solvent effects. Pharmacokinetic or compartmental models define certain skin structures as uniform compartments and calculate transport rates at compartment borders. An excellent review on mathematical models is provided by Mitragoti in cooperation with most active groups in modeling (Mitragotri et al. 2011). For example, the brick-and-mortar structure of the SC, with mean dimensions found by microscopic observations, can be integrated in such a model; thus, to compute the pathway, a molecule has to penetrate into the SC. Naegel et al. developed a mathematical diffusion model, considering microscopic SC dimensions at a sub-compartmental scale to predict concentration–depth profiles for finite-dose application (Naegel et al. 2011). Binding to keratinocytes, reservoir formation and lateral diffusion are factors to consider at least for certain drugs with certain properties. Including all these parameters in computational simulation models is a still ongoing effort.

A recent article questioned the sensitivity of microscopic diffusion models for their sensitivity to input parameters (Wen, Koo, and Lape 2018). Models can be improved with larger databases. Independent of the direct research question that transdermal transport studies aim to answer, wherever possible, it should also be an aim to enlarge our database for transdermal transport with high-quality data suitable for modeling.

53.6   EXAMPLES FOR FURTHER APPLICATIONS OF TAPE STRIPPING AND RELATED METHODS

The following section highlights selected studies to illustrate the considerable variability the rather simple TS method allows in sample analysis and discusses briefly a few reference methods that appeared useful to produce comparable results of concentration–depth profiles in the skin.

Figure 53.1 provides an overview of analytical techniques used to investigate TS samples in a qualitative/quantitative form on the corneocyte layer or from the extract.

Increasing sensitivity of analysis methods allows the quantification of molecules from single AS, thus enhancing the quality of the concentration–depth profile. Early protocols worked with radiolabeled substances for sufficient sensitivity or sometimes pooled ASs for the analysis by chromatography. Compared to HPLC, analysis by liquid chromatography–MS (e.g., LC-MS, LC-MS/MS) profits from excellent sensitivity and specificity, allowing the measurement of substances in trace amounts in complex samples.

More advanced methods like 2D desorption electrospray immunization MS imaging (DESI-MSI), time of flight-secondary ion MS (ToF-SIMS), matrix-assisted laser desorption ionization, and MS imaging (MALDI-MSI) can be applied in skin research for specific tasks, e.g., for concentration–depth profiles of cosmetics (Motoyama and Kihara 2017), endogenous skin lipids (Starr et al. 2016), or investigating molecular distributions for larger skin areas in a reasonable time. Higher spatial resolution than DESI-MSI can be achieved by ToF-SIMS or MALDI-MSI. ToF-SIMS is a sensitive method but limited to the mM range. MALDI-MSI is an even more sensitive method and able to detect drug amounts in the μM range. Bonnel et al. showed the usability of the method for skin distribution profiles for drug molecules in skin biopsy cross-sections (Bonnel et al. 2018). They selected four drugs (ruxolitinib, tofacitinib, roflumilast, and LEO 29102) of varying physicochemical properties and also tested two formulations and compared the results of MALDI-MSI with classical TS, extraction, and UHPLC–tandem MS analysis. MALDI-MSI has a lower limit of quantification, which is also suitable to detect drugs in trace amounts in tissue. The drug roflumilast had problems in detection because it showed strong tissue binding and resulted in difficulties of drug extraction by the matrix, so the sensitivity of the method also depends on the tissue-binding ability of the drug.

Using thermal and spectroscopic probe-based microscopic methods, Goh et al. investigated the crystallization of ibuprofen when applied as a concentrated solution on pig skin (Goh et al. 2019). Drug crystal formation in SC layers mainly at 4 to 7 μm depth was investigated by transition temperature microscopic imaging and photothermal microspectroscopy of AS.

Quantification of endogenous molecules in the skin is also important, as it can be a denominator for the skin condition. Endogenous or exogenous proteins/peptides from AS can be measured by antibody-mediated methods and allow insights in their SC distribution in healthy or diseased states. Performing ELISA from a TS sample (extracts) enables the investigation of protein biomarkers. A few recent examples are summarized in Table 53.1.

Over the last several years the advances in spectroscopic and microscopic methods led to investigations of such methods as completely noninvasive techniques of skin investigation and penetration studies. Vibrational spectroscopy, comprising infrared and Raman spectroscopy, measures the vibrational energy from chemical bonds of compounds to create a "fingerprint" and thus measure (identify and quantify) in a label-free, nondestructive manner. However, the substrate needs to fulfill the criteria of unique spectral features and sufficient quantity to be detectable in complex tissue matrices. This requirement limits the number of substances that can be monitored without a label in some depth. Deuteration as a label is sometimes used to increase the sensitivity of Raman spectroscopy.

Ashtikar et al. summarized several critical issues for using Raman microscopy (Ashtikar et al. 2013). The penetration depth is limited to the top layers; for excised skin also, the water loss must be prevented. For cross-sections or biopsies, however, the penetration depth is sufficient. To correct the signal attenuation with depth, Franzen et al. introduced a surrogate mimicking the main skin components (Franzen et al. 2013). The measured signal decreased in the surrogate in correlation with depth, allowing researchers to develop an algorithm for compensation. In the following study, the same group quantified caffeine in human skin samples as a proof-of-concept study for possible depth profiling (Franzen, Anderski, and Windbergs 2015).

Spectroscopic real-time in vivo and ex vivo studies are explored as alternatives for drug profiling in SC and skin, but due to the discussed limitations and difficulties are still in the explorative phase and not (yet) replacing the traditional methods like TS. Instead, they are also used for the quantification and mapping of AS. AFM and tip-enhanced Raman scattering were used to detect invasomes in human skin samples (Ashtikar et al. 2017).

Rühl and co-workers developed a method to identify label-free drug compounds (demonstrated with dexamethasone) by soft x-ray spectromicroscopy inside excised human and animal skin and reconstructed human skin. By the local drug amount quantification, concentration–depth profiles with spatial resolution (70 nm) can be determined. The results gained from this method were in good agreement with a LC-MS/MS method, but with a higher spatial resolution (differences between SC and viable epidermis cannot be detected via LC-MS/MS analysis), even though the quantification limit in the LC-MS/MS method was lower (Yamamoto et al. 2015, 2017; Wanjiku et al. 2019).

Microscopy techniques like confocal laser scanning microscopy and two-photon microscopy also are used; however, they have a limited depth which is accessible, and fluorophores need to be selected to cope with the autofluorescence of human skin samples and appendix organs.

Some specialized forms of the conventional TS procedure or related sampling techniques for specific questions were also developed.

Some less conventional uses of the TS method are the isolation of microbes or specific skin cell types. TS was several times used for skin microbiome analysis, also looking for the depth of microbes (Röckl and Müller 1959; Zeeuwen et al. 2012). The surface microbiome can be sampled as efficiently with respective AS as it can be collected by the more traditionally used swapping (Ogai et al. 2018). Langerhans cells from human skin were isolated from AS of excised skin and cultivated as a human in vitro model for investigation of vaccination adjuvants (Tajpara et al. 2018).

Differential stripping is a combination of TS and cyanoacrylate skin surface biopsy to quantify substances in the skin appendices. Although hair follicles occupy a rather small fraction of the skin area, for some drugs or formulations, this route seems to be preferred. Imaging techniques to resolve spatial distribution or quantification of content in such skin appendage organs should provide some information on this sort of targeting. In differential stripping, first TS is applied to clean the surface of SC from the applied substance/formulation. Subsequently, cyanoacrylate biopsy with a glass slide or AS is performed to rip off the follicular casts and remaining corneocytes. The extraction of the ASs and the cyanoacrylate biopsy then allows the quantification of the follicular content vs. the SC content of the analyte (Teichmann et al. 2005). Raber A et al. showed an in vitro–in vivo correlation $r^2 = 0.987$ for the pig ear model (the most used animal in vitro model for hair follicle penetration studies) and the vellus hair follicle of in vivo human health volunteers' forearms in follicular delivery of model nanoparticles (Raber et al. 2014).

Sebutape is an AS with pores designed for the collection of sebum. Such sampling can investigate the effect of topical drugs on sebum production or the difference in the sebum of healthy vs. acne-prone persons (Camera et al. 2016). With Sebutape method of CuDerm Corporation, the AS changes color from white to transparent upon contact with sebum and allows grading of skin into dry/intermediate/oily upon comparison with a reference. Comparable ASs or pieces of filter paper can collect samples from the skin surface for profiling of samples by zero-volt paper spray ionization MS (zvPSI-MS) within short exposure times (Motoyama and Kihara 2017). Such a method cannot only measure sebum but also sweat and excreted degradation products.

53.7 CONCLUSION

The relatively uncomplicated and minimally invasive nature of in vivo TS (compared to other suggested methods for in vivo skin penetration/permeation studies) render it the contemporary standard method for penetration studies into the SC and maintain its place within dermal/transdermal delivery studies. Other suggested noninvasive approaches for achieving skin drug penetration profiles are mostly validated against TS. The method of skin TS is still in debate for BE testing for dermal delivery. However, the need for such a method of DPK research and lack of widely applicable methods is a driving force for continued studies.

Provided acceptance of available guidelines and proper experimental working and reporting occur, TS will generate valuable results in understanding the SC barrier function (maybe in the future even by in silico prediction). The number of analytical techniques applicable to analyze TS samples is large and highly sensitive in terms of chemical identification and/or spatial resolution. The selected examples presented in this chapter aimed to highlight the possibilities for TS applications. Thus, TS, in particular of the human skin and in vivo, has and will continue to contribute understanding in the dermal delivery of pharmaceutics, skin biology in health and disease states, and toxicology investigations.

REFERENCES

Abd, E., S. A. Yousef, M. N. Pastore, K. Telaprolu, Y. H. Mohammed, S. Namjoshi, J. E. Grice, and M. S. Roberts. 2016. "Skin Models for the Testing of Transdermal Drugs." Clinical Pharmacology: Advances and Applications 8: 163–176.

Alikhan, A., and H. I. Maibach. 2010. "Biology of Stratum Corneum: Tape Stripping and Protein Quantification." In Textbook of Aging Skin, edited by M. A. Farage, K. W. Miller, and H. I. Maibach, 401–407. Berlin, Heidelberg: Springer.

Anissimov, Y. G., and M. S. Roberts. 2001. "Diffusion Modeling of Percutaneous Absorption Kinetics: 2. Finite Vehicle Volume and Solvent Deposited Solids." Journal of Pharmaceutical Sciences 90 (4): 504–520.

Ashtikar, M., L. Langelüddecke, A. Fahr, and V. Deckert. 2017. "Tip-Enhanced Raman Scattering for Tracking of Invasomes in the Stratum Corneum." Biochimica et Biophysica Acta (BBA) - General Subjects 1861 (11, Part A): 2630–2639.

Ashtikar, M., C. Matthäus, M. Schmitt, C. Krafft, A. Fahr, and J. Popp. 2013. "Non-Invasive Depth Profile Imaging of the Stratum Corneum Using Confocal Raman Microscopy: First Insights into the Method." European Journal of Pharmaceutical Sciences 50 (5): 601–608.

Au, W. L., M. Skinner, and I. Kanfer. 2010. "Comparison of Tape Stripping with the Human Skin Blanching Assay for the Bioequivalence Assessment of Topical Clobetasol Propionate Formulations." Journal of Pharmacy & Pharmaceutical Sciences 13 (1): 11–20.

Azimi, A., M. Ali, K. L. Kaufman, G. J. Mann, and P. Fernandez-Penas. 2018. "Tape Stripped Stratum Corneum Samples Prove to Be Suitable for Comprehensive Proteomic Investigation of Actinic Keratosis." Proteomics. Clinical Applications, 13 (3): 1800084 (1–8).

Barbero, A. M., and H. F. Frasch. 2016. "Effect of Frozen Human Epidermis Storage Duration and Cryoprotectant on Barrier Function Using Two Model Compounds." Skin Pharmacology and Physiology 29 (1): 31–40.

Bashir, S. J., A.-L. Chew, A. Anigbogu, F. Dreher, and H. I. Maibach. 2001. "Physical and Physiological Effects of Stratum Corneum Tape Stripping." Skin Research and Technology 7 (1): 40–48.

Berekméri, A., A. Latzko, A. Alase, T. Macleod, J. S. Ainscough, P. Laws, M. Goodfield et al. 2018. "Detection of IL-36γ Through Noninvasive Tape Stripping Reliably Discriminates Psoriasis from Atopic Eczema." The Journal of Allergy and Clinical Immunology 142 (3): 988–991.

Bonnel, D., R. Legouffe, A. H. Eriksson, R. W. Mortensen, F. Pamelard, J. Stauber, and K. T. Nielsen. 2018. "MALDI Imaging Facilitates New Topical Drug Development Process by Determining Quantitative Skin Distribution Profiles." Analytical and Bioanalytical Chemistry 410 (11): 2815–2828.

Brain, K., K. A. Walters, and A. C. Watkinson. 2002. "Methods for Studying Percutaneous Absorption." In Dermatological and Transdermal Formulations. Vol. 24, edited by K. A. Walters, 195–267. New York, London: CRC Press:Informa Healthcare.

Breternitz, M., M. Flach, J. Präßler, P. Elsner, and J. W. Fluhr. 2007. "Acute Barrier Disruption by Adhesive Tapes Is Influenced by Pressure, Time and Anatomical Location: Integrity and Cohesion Assessed by Sequential Tape Stripping; a Randomized, Controlled Study." British Journal of Dermatology 156 (2): 231–240.

Camera, E., M. Ludovici, S. Tortorella, J.-L. Sinagra, B. Capitanio, L. Goracci, and M. Picardo. 2016. "Use of Lipidomics to Investigate Sebum Dysfunction in Juvenile Acne." Journal of lipid Research 57 (6): 1051–1058.

Chen, X., S. Grégoire, F. Formanek, J.-B. Galey, and H. Rigneault. 2015. "Quantitative 3D Molecular Cutaneous Absorption in Human Skin Using Label Free Nonlinear Microscopy." Journal of Controlled Release 200: 78–86.

Christmann, R. Thomas, C. Jager, N. Raber, A., S. Loretz, B. Schaefer, U., F. Tschernig, T. Vogt, T. Lehr, C.-M. 2020. "Nanoparticle Targeting to Scalp Hair Follicles: New Perspectives for a Topical Therapy for Alopecia Areata." Journal of Investigative Dermatology 140 (1): 243–246.e5

Clausen, M.-L., H.-C. Slotved, K. A. Krogfelt, and T. Agner. 2018. "Measurements of AMPs in Stratum Corneum of Atopic Dermatitis and Healthy Skin-Tape Stripping Technique." Scientific Reports 8 (1): 1666 (1–8)

Dreher, F., A. Arens, J. J. Hostýnek, S. Mudumba, J. Ademola, and H. I. Maibach. 1998. "Colorimetric Method for Quantifying Human Stratum Corneum Removed by Adhesive-Tape-Stripping." Acta Dermato-Venereologica 78 (3): 186–189.

Dreher, F., B. S. Modjtahedi, S. P. Modjtahedi, and H. I. Maibach. 2005. "Quantification of Stratum Corneum Removal by Adhesive Tape Stripping by Total Protein Assay in 96-Well Microplates." Skin Research and Technology 11 (2): 97–101.

EMA. 2018. "European Medicines Agency. CHMP/QWP/708282/2018 Draft Guideline on Quality and Equivalence of Topical Products." 1–36. Accessed March 1, 2019. https://www.ema.europa.eu/en/quality-equivalence-topical-products

Eskes, C., and V. Zuang. 2005. "Alternative (Non-Animal) Methods for Cosmetics Testing: Current Status and Future Prospects. A Report Prepared in the Context of the 7th Amendment to the Cosmetics Directive for Establishing the Timetable for Phasing Out Animal Testing." Alternatives to Laboratory Animals: ALTA 33(1): 1. Accessed June 12, 2019. https://doi.org/10.1177/026119290503301s19

FDA. 1995. "U.S. Food and Drug Administration. Guidance for Industry. Guidance Topical Dermatologic Corticosteroids: In Vivo Bioequivalence: Department of Health and Human Services." Accessed June 12, 2019. https://www.fda.gov/regulatory-information/search-fda-guidance-documents/topical-dermatologic-corticosteroids-vivo-bioequivalence

FDA. 1997. "U.S. Food and Drug Administration. Guidance for Industry. Nonsterile Semisolid Dosage Forms. Scale-up and Postapproval Changes: Chemistry, Manufacturing, and Controls; in Vitro Release Testing and in Vivo Bioequivalence Documentation. SUPAC-SS: Department of Health and Human Services. Center for Drug Evaluation and Research (CDER)." Accessed June 8, 2019. https://www.fda.gov/regulatory-information/search-fda-guidance-documents/supac-ss-nonsterile-semisolid-dosage-forms-scale-and-post-approval-changes-chemistry-manufacturing

FDA. 1998. "U.S. Food and Drug Administration. Guidance for Industry. Topical Dermatological Drug Product NDAs and ANDAs - in Vivo Bioavailability, Bioequivalence, in Vitro Release, and Associated Studies. Draft Guidance. Department of Health and Human Services. Center for Drug Evaluation and Research (CDER)." Accessed June 5, 2019. https://www.federalregister.gov/documents/1998/06/18/98-16141/draft-guidance-for-industry-on-topical-dermatological-drug-product-ndas-and-andasin-vivo

FDA. 2002. "U.S. Food and Drug Administration. Draft Guidance for Industry on Topical Dermatological Drug Product NDAs and ANDAs - in Vivo Bioavailability, Bioequivalence, in Vitro Release and Associated Studies; Withdrawal. Notice: Department of Health and Human Services." Federal Register 67 (96): 35122–35123.

Feldmann, R. J., and H. I. Maibach. 1967. "Regional Variation in Percutaneous Penetration of 14C Cortisol in Man." 48 (2): 181–83.

Franz, T. J. 1975. "Percutaneous Absorption. On the Relevance of in Vitro Data." Journal of Investigative Dermatology 64 (3): 190–195.

Franzen, L., J. Anderski, and M. Windbergs. 2015. "Quantitative Detection of Caffeine in Human Skin by Confocal Raman Spectroscopy - a Systematic in Vitro Validation Study." European Journal of Pharmaceutics and Biopharmaceutics 95:110–116.

Franzen, L., D. Selzer, J. W. Fluhr, U. F. Schaefer, and M. Windbergs. 2013. "Towards Drug Quantification in Human Skin with Confocal Raman Microscopy." European Journal of Pharmaceutics and Biopharmaceutics 84 (2): 437–444..

Gee, C. M., J. A. Nicolazzo, A. C. Watkinson, and B. C. Finnin. 2012. "Assessment of the Lateral Diffusion and Penetration of Topically Applied Drugs in Humans Using a Novel Concentric Tape Stripping Design." Pharmaceutical Research 29 (8): 2035–2046.

George, K. 2005. "A Two-Dimensional Mathematical Model of Non-Linear Dual-Sorption of Percutaneous Drug Absorption." Biomedical Engineering Online 4:40.

Goh, C. F., J. G. Moffat, Craig, D. Q. M., J. Hadgraft, and M. E. Lane. 2019. "Monitoring Drug Crystallization in Percutaneous Penetration Using Localized Nanothermal Analysis and Photothermal Microspectroscopy." Molecular Pharmaceutics 16 (1): 359–370. doi:10.1021/acs.molpharmaceut.8b01027.

Haftek, M. 2015. "Epidermal Barrier Disorders and Corneodesmosome Defects." Cell and Tissue Research 360 (3): 483–490.

Hahn, T., S. Hansen, D. Neumann, K.-H. Kostka, C.-M. Lehr, L. Muys, and U. F. Schaefer. 2010. "Infrared Densitometry: A Fast and Non-Destructive Method for Exact Stratum Corneum Depth Calculation for in Vitro Tape-Stripping." Skin Pharmacology and Physiology 23 (4): 183–192.

Hansen, S. Henning, A. Naegel, A. Heisig, M. Wittum, G. Neumann, D. Kostka, K.-H. Zbytovska, J. Lehr, C.-M. Schaefer, U. F. 2008. "In-silico model of skin penetration based on experimentally determined input parameters. Part I: Experimental determination of partition and diffusion coefficients." European Journal of Pharmaceutics and Biopharmaceutics 68 (2): 352–367.

Hart, P. J., S. Francese, E. Claude, M. N. Woodroofe, and M. R. Clench. 2011. "MALDI-MS Imaging of Lipids in Ex Vivo Human Skin." Analytical and Bioanalytical Chemistry 401 (1): 115–125.

Herkenne, C., I. Alberti, A. Naik, Y. N. Kalia, F.-X. Mathy, V. Préat, and R. H. Guy. 2008. "In Vivo Methods for the Assessment of Topical Drug Bioavailability." Pharmaceutical Research 25 (1): 87–103.

Honari, G., and H. I. Maibach. 2014. "Chapter 1 - Skin Structure and Function." In Applied Dermatotoxicology: Clinical Aspects, edited by H. I. Maibach and G. Honari, 1–10. Amsterdam: Academic Press.

Hotchkiss, S.A.M., M. A. Chidgey, S. Rose, and J. Caldwell. 1990. "Percutaneous Absorption of Benzyl Acetate Through Rat Skin in Vitro. 1. Validation of an in Vitro Model Against in Vivo Data." Food and Chemical Toxicology 28 (6): 443–447.

Hotchkiss, S.A.M., P. Hewitt, J. Caldwell, W. L. Chen, and R. R. Rowe. 1992. "Percutaneous Absoprtion of Nicotinic Acid, Phenol, Benzoic Acid and Triclopyr Butoxyethyl Ester Through Rat and Human Skin in Vitro: Further Validation of an in Vitro Model by Comparison with in Vivo Data." Food and Chemical Toxicology 30 (10): 891–899.

Ilić, T., I. Pantelić, D. Lunter, S. Đorđević, B. Marković, D. Ranković, R. Daniels, and S. Savić. 2017. "Critical Quality Attributes, in Vitro Release and Correlated in Vitro Skin Permeation-in Vivo Tape Stripping Collective Data for Demonstrating Therapeutic (Non)Equivalence of Topical Semisolids: A Case Study of "Ready-to-Use" Vehicles." International Journal of Pharmaceutics 528 (1-2): 253–267.

Intarakumhaeng, R., A. Wanasathop, and S. K. Li. 2018. "Effects of Solvents on Skin Absorption of Nonvolatile Lipophilic and Polar Solutes Under Finite Dose Conditions." International Journal of Pharmaceutics 536 (1): 405–413.

Jacobi, U., H.-J. Weigmann, J. Ulrich, W. Sterry, and J. Lademann. 2005. "Estimation of the Relative Stratum Corneum Amount Removed by Tape Stripping." Skin Research and Technology 11 (2): 91–96.

Janssens, M., J. van Smeden, G. J. Puppels, Lavrijsen, A. P. M., P. J. Caspers, and J. A. Bouwstra. 2014. "Lipid to Protein Ratio Plays an Important Role in the Skin Barrier Function in Patients with Atopic Eczema." British Journal of Dermatology 170 (6): 1248–1255.

Kalia, Y. N., I. Alberti, N. Sekkat, C. Curdy, A. Naik, and R. H. Guy. 2000. "Normalization of Stratum Corneum Barrier Function and Transepidermal Water Loss in Vivo." Pharmaceutical Research 17 (9): 1148–1150.

Kalia, Y. N., F. Pirot, and R. H. Guy. 1996. "Homogeneous Transport in a Heterogeneous Membrane: Water Diffusion Across Human Stratum Corneum in Vivo." Biophysical Journal 71: 2692–2700.

Koppes, S. A., R. Brans, S. Ljubojevic Hadzavdic, Frings-Dresen, M. H. W., T. Rustemeyer, and S. Kezic. 2016. "Stratum Corneum Tape Stripping: Monitoring of Inflammatory Mediators in Atopic Dermatitis Patients Using Topical Therapy." International Archives of Allergy and Immunology 170 (3): 1871–93.

Küchler, S., K. Strüver, and W. Friess. 2013. "Reconstructed Skin Models as Emerging Tools for Drug Absorption Studies." Expert Opinion on Drug Metabolism & Toxicology 9 (10): 1255–1263.

Lademann, J., A. Ilgevicius, O. Zurbau, H. D. Liess, S. Schanzer, H.-J. Weigmann, C. Antoniou, R. V. Pelchrzim, and W. Sterry. 2006. "Penetration Studies of Topically Applied Substances: Optical Determination of the Amount of Stratum Corneum Removed by Tape Stripping." Journal of Biomedical Optics 11 (5): 54026.

Lademann, J., U. Jacobi, C. Surber, H.-J. Weigmann, and J. W. Fluhr. 2009. "The Tape Stripping Procedure - Evaluation of Some Critical Parameters." European Journal of Pharmaceutics and Biopharmaceutics 72 (2): 317–323.

Lehman, P. A., S. G. Raney, and T. J. Franz. 2011. "Percutaneous Absorption in Man: In Vitro-In Vivo Correlation." Skin Pharmacology and Physiology 24 (4): 224–230.

Leite-Silva, V. R. Le Lamer, M. Sanchez, W. Y. Liu, D. C. Sanchez, W. H. Morrow, I. Martin, D. Silva, H. D. Prow, T. W. Grice, J. E. Roberts, M. S. 2013. "The effect of formulation on the penetration of coated and uncoated zinc oxide nanoparticles into the viable epidermis of human skin in vivo." European Journal of Pharmaceutics and Biopharmaceutics 84 (2): 297–308.

Lindemann, U., H.-J. Weigmann, H. Schaefer, W. Sterry, and J. Lademann. 2003. "Evaluation of the Pseudo-Absorption Method to Quantify Human Stratum Corneum Removed by Tape Stripping Using Protein Absorption." Skin Pharmacology and Applied Skin Physiology 16 (4): 228–236.

Löffler, H., F. Dreher, and H. I. Maibach. 2004. "Stratum Corneum Adhesive Tape Stripping: Influence of Anatomical Site, Application Pressure, Duration and Removal." British Journal of Dermatology 151 (4): 746–752.

Marttin, E. Neelissen-Subnel, M., T. De Haan, F., H. Boddé, H., E. 1996. "A critical comparison of methods to quantify stratum corneum removed by tape stripping." Skin Pharmacol. Appl. Skin Physiol. 9 (1) 69–77.

Melero, A., T. Hahn, U. F. Schaefer, and M. Schneider. 2011. "In Vitro Human Skin Segmentation and Drug Concentration-Skin Depth Profiles." In Permeability Barrier: Methods and Protocols. Vol. 763, edited by K. Turksen. Methods in Molecular Biology. Totowa, NJ: Humana Press.

Milani, P., J. Chlasta, R. Abdayem, S. Kezic, and M. Haftek. 2018. "Changes in Nano-Mechanical Properties of Human Epidermal Cornified Cells Depending on Their Proximity to the Skin Surface." Journal of Molecular Recognition 31 (9): e2722.

Miranda, M., J. J. Sousa, F. Veiga, C. Cardoso, and C. Vitorino. 2018. "Bioequivalence of Topical Generic Products. Part 1: Where Are We Now?" European Journal of Pharmaceutical Sciences 123:260–267.

Mitragotri, S., Y. G. Anissimov, A. L. Bunge, H. F. Frasch, R. H. Guy, J. Hadgraft, G. B. Kasting, M. E. Lane, and M. S. Roberts. 2011. "Mathematical Models of Skin Permeability: An Overview." International Journal of Pharmaceutics 418 (1): 115–129.

Mohammed, D., Q. Yang, R. H. Guy, P. J. Matts, J. Hadgraft, and M. E. Lane. 2012. "Comparison of Gravimetric and Spectroscopic Approaches to Quantify Stratum Corneum Removed by Tape-Stripping." European Journal of Pharmaceutics and Biopharmaceutics 82 (1): 171–174.

Motoyama, A., and K. Kihara. 2017. "Mass Spectrometry in Cosmetic Science: Advanced Ionization Techniques for Detecting Trace Molecules in or on Human Skin." Mass Spectrometry (Tokyo, Japan) 6 (Spec Iss 2): S0071.

Naegel, A., T. Hahn, U. F. Schaefer, C.-M. Lehr, M. Heisig, and G. Wittum. 2011. "Finite Dose Skin Penetration: A Comparison of Concentration-Depth Profiles from Experiment and Simulation." Computing and Visualization in Science 14 (7): 327–339.

Nastiti, C. M. R. R., Y. Mohammed, K. C. Telaprolu, X. Liang, J. E. Grice, M. S. Roberts, and H. A. E. Benson. 2019. "Evaluation of Quantum Dot Skin Penetration in Porcine Skin: Effect of Age and Anatomical Site of Topical Application." Skin Pharmacology and Physiology 14:1–10.

Navidi, W., A. Hutchinson, B. N'Dri-Stempfer, and A. L. Bunge. 2008. "Determining Bioequivalence of Topical Dermatological Drug Products by Tape-Stripping." Journal of Pharmacokinetics and Pharmacodynamics 35 (3): 337–348.

N'Dri-Stempfer, B., W. Navidi, R. H. Guy, and A. L. Bunge. 2008. "Optimizing Metrics for the Assessment of Bioequivalence Between Topical Drug Products." Pharmaceutical Research 25 (7): 1621–1630.

N'Dri-Stempfer, B., W. Navidi, R. H. Guy, and A. L. Bunge. 2009. "Improved Bioequivalence Assessment of Topical Dermatological Drug Products Using Dermatopharmacokinetics." Pharmaceutical Research 26 (2): 316–328.

Netzlaff, F., K.-H. Kostka, C.-M. Lehr, and U. F. Schaefer. 2006. "TEWL Measurements as a Routine Method for Evaluating the Integrity of Epidermis Sheets in Static Franz Type Diffusion Cells In Vitro. Limitations Shown by Transport Data Testing." European Journal of Pharmaceutics and Biopharmaceutics 63 (1): 44–50.

OECD. 2004a. "Guidance Document for the Conduct of Skin Absorption Studies. OECD Environmental Health and Safety Publications. Series of Testing and Assessment. No. 28." OECD, Paris.

OECD. 2004b. "Guideline for the Testing of Chemicals. Skin Absorption: In Vitro Method. 428." OECD, Paris, 1–8.

Ogai, K., S. Nagase, K. Mukai, T. Iuchi, Y. Mori, M. Matsue, K. Sugitani, J. Sugama, and S. Okamoto. 2018. "A Comparison of Techniques for Collecting Skin Microbiome Samples: Swabbing Versus Tape-Stripping." Frontiers in Microbiology 9:1–10.

Ourique, A. F., A. Melero, da Silva, C. d. B., U. F. Schaefer, A. R. Pohlmann, S. S. Guterres, C.-M. Lehr, K.-H. Kostka, and R.C.R. Beck. 2011. "Improved Photostability and Reduced Skin Permeation of Tretinoin: Development of a Semisolid Nanomedicine." European Journal of Pharmaceutics and Biopharmaceutics 79 (1): 95–101.

Patzelt, A., H. Richter, R. Buettemeyer, Huber, H. J. R., U. Blume-Peytavi, W. Sterry, and J. Lademann. 2008. "Differential Stripping Demonstrates a Significant Reduction of the Hair Follicle Reservoir In Vitro Compared to In Vivo." European Journal of Pharmaceutics and Biopharmaceutics 70 (1): 234–238.

Pershing, L. K., S. Bakhtian, C. E. Poncelet, J. L. Corlett, and V. P. Shah. 2002. "Comparison of Skin Stripping, In Vitro Release, and Skin Blanching Response Methods to Measure Dose Response and Similarity of Triamcinolone Acetonide Cream Strengths from Two Manufactured Sources." Journal of Pharmaceutical Sciences 91 (5): 1312–1323.

Pershing, L. K., J. L. Corlett, and C. Jorgensen. 1994. "In Vivo Pharmacokinetics and Pharmacodynamics of Topical Ketoconazole and Miconazole in Human Stratum Corneum." Antimicrobial Agents and Chemotherapy 38 (1): 90–95.

Pershing, L. K., B. S. Silver, G. G. Krueger, V. P. Shah, and J. P. Skelley. 1992. "Feasibility of Measuring the Bioavailability of Topical Betamethasone Dipropionate in Commercial Formulations Using Drug Content in Skin and a Skin Blanching Bioassay." Pharmaceutical Research 9 (1): 45–51.

Pinkus, H. 1951. "Examination of the Epidermis by the Strip Method of Removing Horny Layers. I. Observations on Thickness of the Horny Layer, and on Mitotic Activity After Stripping." The Journal of Investigative Dermatology 16 (6): 383–386.

Praça, F. S. G., Medina, W. S. G., J. O. Eloy, R. Petrilli, P. M. Campos, A. Ascenso, and Bentley, M. V. L. B. 2018. "Evaluation of Critical Parameters for In Vitro Skin Permeation and Penetration Studies Using Animal Skin Models." European Journal of Pharmaceutical Sciences 111: 121–132.

Raber, A. S., A. Mittal, J. Schäfer, U. Bakowsky, J. Reichrath, T. Vogt, U. F. Schaefer, S. Hansen, and C.-M. Lehr. 2014. "Quantification of Nanoparticle Uptake into Hair Follicles in Pig Ear and Human Forearm." Journal of Controlled Release 179 (1): 25–32.

Raj, N., R. Voegeli, A. V. Rawlings, S. Gibbons, M. R. Munday, B. Summers, and M. E. Lane. 2016. "Variation in Stratum Corneum Protein Content as a Function of Anatomical Site and Ethnic Group." International Journal of Cosmetic Science 38 (3): 224–231.

Reddy, M. B., K. D. McCarley, and A. L. Bunge. 1998. "Physiologically Relevant One-Compartment Pharmacokinetic Models for Skin. 2. Comparison of Models When Combined with a Systemic Pharmacokinetic Model." Journal of Pharmaceutical Sciences 87 (4): 482–490.

Roberts, M., S. Dancik, Y. Prow, T., W. Thorling, C., A. Lin, L., L. Grice, J., E. Robertson, T., A. König, K. Becker, W. 2011. "Non-invasive imaging of skin physiology and percutaneous penetration using fluorescence spectral and lifetime imaging with multiphoton and confocal microscopy." European Journal of Pharmaceutics and Biopharmaceutics 77 (3): 469–488.

Röckl, H., and E. Müller. 1959. "Beitrag Zur Lokalisation Der Mikroben Der Haut." Archiv für klinische u. experimentelle Dermatologie (209): 13–29.

Rougier, A., D. Dupuis, C. Lotte, R. Roguet, and H. Schaefer. 1983. "In Vivo Correlation Between Stratum Corneum Reservoir Function and Percutaneous Absorption." Journal of Investigative Dermatology 81 (3): 275–278.

SCCS. 2018. "(Scientific Committee on Consumer Safety) the SCCS Notes of Guidance for the Testing of Cosmetic Ingredients and Their Safety Evaluation. 10th Revision. SCCS/1602/18." SCCS.European Commission Health and Food Safety Directorate, Luxembourg.

Schulz, R., K. Yamamoto, A. Klossek, R. Flesch, S. Hönzke, F. Rancan, A. Vogt et al. 2017. "Data-Based Modeling of Drug Penetration Relates Human Skin Barrier Function to the Interplay of Diffusivity and Free-Energy Profiles." Proceedings of the National Academy of Sciences of the United States of America 114 (14): 3631–336.

Selzer, D., M. M. A. Abdel-Mottaleb, T. Hahn, U. F. Schaefer, and D. Neumann. 2013. "Finite and Infinite Dosing: Difficulties in Measurements, Evaluations and Predictions." Advanced Drug Delivery Reviews 65 (2): 278–294.

Selzer, D. Hahn, T. Naegel, A. Heisig, M. Kostka, K.-H. Lehr, C.-M. Neumann, D. Schaefer, U., F. Wittum, G. 2013. "Finite dose skin mass balance including the lateral part: Comparison between experiment, pharmacokinetic modeling and diffusion models." Journal of Controlled Release 165(2): 119–128.

Selzer, D. Schaefer, U., F. Lehr, C.-M. Hansen, S. 2017. "Basic Mathematics in Skin Absorption". In Percutaneous Penetration Enhancers. Drug Penetration Into/Through the Skin. Methodology and General Considerations. Vol, edited by N. Dragicevic and H. Maibach, 3-25. Springer Verlag Berlin, Heidelberg.

Shah, V. P., G. L. Flynn, A. Yacobi, H. I. Maibach, C. Bon, N. M. Fleischer, T. J. Franz et al. 1998. "Bioequivalence of Topical Dermatological Dosage Forms-Methods of Evaluation of Bioequivalence. AAPS/FDA Worshop Report." Pharmaceutical Research 15 (2): 167–171.

Starr, N. J., D. J. Johnson, J. Wibawa, I. Marlow, M. Bell, D. A. Barrett, and D. J. Scurr. 2016. "Age-Related Changes to Human Stratum Corneum Lipids Detected Using Time-of-Flight Secondary Ion Mass Spectrometry Following in Vivo Sampling." Analytical Chemistry 88 (8): 4400–4408.

Surber, C., F. P. Schwarb, and E. W. Smith. 2005. "Tape-Stripping Technique." In Percutaneous Absorption: Drugs, Cosmetics, Mechanisms, Methodology. Vol 155, edited by R. L. Bronaugh, N. Dragicevic, and H. I. Maibach. 4th, 399–410. Boca Raton: CRC Press.

Svenskaya, Y. I., E. A. Genina, B. V. Parakhonskiy, E. V. Lengert, E. E. Talnikova, G. S. Terentyuk, S. R. Utz, D. A. Gorin, V. V. Tuchin, and G. B. Sukhorukov. 2019. "A Simple Non-Invasive Approach Toward Efficient Transdermal Drug Delivery Based on Biodegradable Particulate System." ACS Applied Materials & Interfaces 11 (19): 17270–17282.

Tajpara, P., C. Schuster, E. Schön, P. Kienzl, M. Vierhapper, M. Mildner, and A. Elbe-Bürger. 2018. "Epicutaneous Administration of the Pattern Recognition Receptor Agonist Polyinosinic-Polycytidylic Acid Activates the MDA5/MAVS Pathway in Langerhans Cells." FASEB Journal 32 (8): 4132–4144.

Teichmann, A., U. Jacobi, M. Ossadnik, H. Richter, S. Koch, W. Sterry, and J. Lademann. 2005. "Differential Stripping: Determination of the Amount of Topically Applied Substances Penetrated into the Hair Follicles." Journal of Investigative Dermatology 125 (2): 264–269.

van de Sandt, J. J. M., J. A. van Burgsteden, S. Cage, P. L. Carmichael, I. Dick, S. Kenyon, G. Korinth et al. 2004. "In Vitro Predictions of Skin Absorption of Caffeine, Testosterone, and Benzoic Acid: A Multi-Centre Comparison Study." Regulatory Toxicology and Pharmacology 39 (3): 271–281.

Vickers, C.F.H. 1963. "Existence of Reservoir in the Stratum Corneum." Archives of Dermatology 88 (1): 20.

Voegeli, R., J. Heiland, S. Doppler, A. V. Rawlings, and T. Schreier. 2007. "Efficient and Simple Quantification of Stratum Corneum Proteins on Tape Strippings by Infrared Densitometry." Skin Research and Technology 13 (3): 242–251.

Wagner, H., K.-H. Kostka, C.-M. Lehr, and U. F. Schaefer. 2000. "Drug Distribution in Human Skin Using Two Different In Vitro Test Systems: Comparison with in Vivo Data." Pharmaceutical Research 17 (12): 1475–1481.

Wagner, H., K.-H. Kostka, C.-M. Lehr, and U. F. Schaefer. 2002. "Human Skin Penetration of Flufenamic Acid: In Vivo/In Vitro Correlation (Deeper Skin Layers) for Skin Samples from the Same Subject." Journal of Investigative Dermatology 118 (3): 540–544.

Wanjiku, B., K. Yamamoto, A. Klossek, F. Schumacher, H. Pischon, L. Mundhenk, F. Rancan et al. 2019. "Qualifying X-Ray and Stimulated Raman Spectromicroscopy for Mapping Cutaneous Drug Penetration." Analytical Chemistry 91 (11): 7208–7214.

Weigmann, H.-J., J. Lademann, H. Meffert, H. Schaefer, and W. Sterry. 1999a. "Determination of the Horny Layer Profile by Tape Stripping in Combination with Optical Spectroscopy in the Visible Range as a Prerequisite to Quantify Percutaneous Absorption." Skin Pharmacology and Applied Skin Physiology 12 (1-2): 34–45.

Weigmann, H.-J., J. Lademann, R. V. Pelchrzim, W. Sterry, T. Hagemeister, R. Molzahn, M. Schaefer, M. Linscheid, H. Schaefer, and V. P. Shah. 1999b. "Bioavailability of Clobetasol Propionate - Quantification of Drug Concentrations in the Stratum Corneum by Dermatopharmacokinetics Using Tape Stripping." Skin Pharmacology and Applied Skin Physiology 12: 46–53.

Weigmann, H.-J., S. Schanzer, C. Vergou, C. Antoniou, W. Sterry, and J. Lademann. 2012. "Quantification of the Inhomogeneous Distribution of Topically Applied Substances by Optical Spectroscopy: Definition of a Factor of Inhomogeneity." Skin Pharmacology and Physiology 25:118–123.

Wen, J., S. M. Koo, and N. Lape. 2018. "How Sensitive Are Transdermal Transport Predictions by Microscopic Stratum Corneum Models to Geometric and Transport Parameter Input?" Journal of Pharmaceutical Sciences 107 (2): 612–623.

WHO. 2006. "Environmental Health Criteria 235. Dermal Absorption." World Health Organization: Geneva.

Wolf, J. 1940. "Das Oberflächenrelief Der Menschlichen Haut." Z. mikr.-anat. Forsch. 47: 351–400.

Yacobi, A., V. P. Shah, E. D. Bashaw, E. Benfeldt, B. Davit, D. Ganes, T. Ghosh et al. 2014. "Current Challenges in Bioequivalence, Quality, and Novel Assessment Technologies for Topical Products." Pharmaceutical Research 31 (4): 837–846.

Yamamoto, K., R. Flesch, T. Ohigashi, S. Hedtrich, A. Klossek, P. Patoka, G. Ulrich et al. 2015. "Selective Probing of the Penetration of Dexamethasone into Human Skin by Soft X-Ray Spectromicroscopy." Analytical Chemistry 87 (12): 6173–6179.

Yamamoto, K., A. Klossek, R. Flesch, F. Rancan, M. Weigand, I. Bykova, M. Bechtel et al. 2017. "Influence of the Skin Barrier on the Penetration of Topically-Applied Dexamethasone Probed by Soft X-Ray Spectromicroscopy." European Journal of Pharmaceutics and Biopharmaceutics 118: 30–37.

Zeeuwen, P. L. J. M., J. Boekhorst, E. H. van den Bogaard, H. D. de Koning, P. M. C. van de Kerkhof, D. M. Saulnier, I. I. van Swam et al. 2012. "Microbiome Dynamics of Human Epidermis Following Skin Barrier Disruption." Genome Biology 13 (11):101(1–8).

Zou, Y. Celli, A. Zhu, H. Elmahdy, A. Cao, Y. Hui, X. Maibach, H. I. 2017. "Confocal laser scanning micros-copy to estimate nanoparticles' human skin penetration in vitro." International journal of nanomedicine 12: 8035–8041.

Zvyagin, A., V. Zhao, X. Gierden, A. Sanchez, W. Ross, J., A. Roberts, M., S. 2008. "Imaging of zinc oxide nanoparticle penetration in human skin in vitro and in vivo." Journal of biomedical optics 13 (6): 064031.

54 Blood Flow as a Technology in Percutaneous Absorption

The Assessment of the Cutaneous Microcirculation by Laser Doppler and Photoplethysmographic Techniques

Ethel Tur
Tel Aviv University, Tel Aviv, Israel

CONTENTS

54.1 INTRODUCTION

The search for blood flow measurement by optical techniques resulted 85 years ago with the innovation of photoplethysmography (1), substantiated and expanded by Hertzman (2). Laser Doppler techniques came forth 40 years later (3), followed by the manufacture of commercial devices (4, 5). These optical methodologies enable tracing the movement of red blood cells in the skin, which is useful in following percutaneous penetration, when the penetrant has an effect on blood vessels or on blood flow. In addition, physiology, anatomy, and even pathology of the skin can be studied. Moreover, laser Doppler flowmetry (LDF) measurements are applicable in the evaluation of internal diseases and conditions that affect the skin microvasculature.

The diverse application areas of the technique include tissues other than the skin, like the buccal, nasal, or rectal mucosa, as well as the intestine through an endoscope and kidney, liver, or lung intraoperatively. This chapter exclusively deals with cutaneous LDF and reviews only investigations where this method was used to measure skin blood flow. In each field of LDF investigation, knowledge has broadened in the last few years. In view of the large number of studies conducted in this area, it is impossible to review each and every one; therefore, we only attempt to demonstrate the possibilities of the technique.

After a review of some of the relevant basic considerations in experimental designs involving LDF, we discuss several conditions where LDF can be utilized. These include investigations of normal and diseased skin and the influence of the nervous system, environmental temperature, smoking, and pregnancy on skin blood flow. Studies of disease processes, severity, and treatment evaluation are then discussed, including hypertension, peripheral vascular disease, diabetes mellitus, and Raynaud phenomenon. We conclude with future possibilities and expectations.

54.2 THE METHOD OF LASER DOPPLER

54.2.1 BASIC PRINCIPLES

LDF is a noninvasive method that continuously follows the flow of red blood cells (6). It operates on the Doppler principle, employing a low-power helium–neon laser emitting red light at 632.8 nm. The radiation is transmitted via an optical fiber to the skin. The radiation is diffusely scattered, and its optical frequency is shifted by the moving red blood cells. The reflected light, being coherently mixed with another portion of the light scattered from static tissues, generates a Doppler beat signal in the photodetector output current. A quantitative estimation of the cutaneous blood flow derives from spectral analysis of the beat signal.

54.2.2 ADVANTAGES

As an objective, noninvasive, and real-time measurement technique, LDF is an attractive practical tool for estimating cutaneous blood flow. Besides, LDF is relatively simple, fast, and inexpensive and can provide information that supplements the results of various other techniques.

54.2.3 DISADVANTAGES

LDF is inferior in quantitating blood flow as compared to other techniques, such as the 133Xe washout technique. However, it is important to note that different methods measure different sections of the microvasculature. It is likely that the flux signal shown by LDF represents the large volume of red blood cells moving within the larger blood vessels, particularly the subpapillary plexus, rather than the much smaller volume of red blood cells residing within the nutritive capillaries. The depth of laser penetration in the wavelengths used is approximately 1 mm.

Therefore, in normal skin it is likely to include the subpapillary plexus, as well as the capillaries in the subpapillary dermis. In diseased skin, it may measure a different body of vessels; for instance, in psoriasis the epidermal ridges are elongated, and this may alter the relative contribution of superficial and deep blood flow to the laser Doppler signal. Another disadvantage of LDF is that results obtained by various instruments or by the same instrument in different people cannot be compared.

54.2.4 RECENT DEVELOPMENTS

Improvements of the laser Doppler technique offer new possibilities and present new findings. Progressions are illustrated by refinements such as computerization and the design of a probe holder, which allows repeated measurements over the same site before and after manipulations to the skin through a multichannel LDF instrument, which allows simultaneous measurements of several sites

(7). Another development is an integration-type LDF, equipped with a temperature-load instrument, allowing responses of the skin blood flow to cooling from 30°C to 10°C to be evaluated (8). But the most substantial development is laser Doppler imaging (scanning LDF) (9–12), which records the tissue perfusion in several thousand measurement points. A map of the spatial distribution of the blood flow is obtained in a short period of time.

Unlike LDF, which continuously records blood flow over a single point, laser Doppler imaging maps blood flow distribution over a specific area. Thus, the two methods do not compete with each other, but are rather complementary. Laser Doppler imaging has the advantage of operating without any contact with the skin surface, avoiding the influence of the pressure of the probe on tissue perfusion.

It can rapidly measure large areas of skin and allows simultaneous measurement of the extent of blood flow changes in abnormal areas of skin and estimates the area of these changes. Furthermore, objective evaluation of various interventions and therapeutic response may be obtained by serial scans.

54.3 CONCEPTS AND DESIGN OF EXPERIMENTAL STUDIES USING LDF

54.3.1 PLANNING AND PERFORMING LDF BLOOD FLOW MEASUREMENTS

Both static and dynamic LDF measurements can be used (13–15). Static studies, like baseline blood flow measurements, record only the steady-state blood flow, neglecting all transients. On the contrary, dynamic investigations can examine the competence of the blood vessels by following their response to triggers (12–14). Reactive hyperemia is an example for a dynamic test (12–14) recording the postocclusion time course of the blood flow. Other provocative methods examining the response to external triggers include cognitive tests (16), isotonic (17) and isometric tests (12), vasomotor reflexes (18, 19), intracutaneous needle stimulation (20), topical vasodilators (21), and thermal tests (12).

Some of these tests are vasoconstrictive (the isometric and cognitive tests and vasomotor reflexes), and some are vasodilative (the arterial postocclusive reactive hyperemia, intracutaneous needle stimulation, the thermal test, and the isotonic test).

To optimize skin blood flow response to the different tests, vasoconstrictive stimuli should be performed on a high-blood-flow site, whereas vasodilative stimuli should be performed on a low-blood-flow site. Consequently, the magnitude of the changes induced is maximized, providing a significant improvement in the quality of the data obtained. Moreover, vasoconstriction mediated by sympathetic stimulation, as in the cognitive test, should be provoked in the hands and feet, where the local blood supply is under a sympathetic vasoconstrictor control, and not in the face, which has a poor sympathetic vasoconstrictor supply (15).

Thus, to enhance the sensitivity of the measurements, the site tested should be carefully selected. For example, the fingers, being rich with microvascular arteriovenous anastomoses, are useful for vasoconstrictive tests, while the forearms are suitable for the vasodilative tests. The forearms have several advantages as a preferred site for vasodilative tests: (1) abundance of arterioles and capable of reactive hyperemia; (2) a local effect, rather than thermoregulatory reflexes (22), is responsible for thermally induced vasodilatation; and (3) little inconvenience is experienced by the subjects tested.

The appropriate test should also be carefully selected in order to adequately probe the relevant topic. Before reaching a conclusion, one should bear in mind that differences in experimental settings might lead to different results. For instance, in order to study differences between young and old patients, different tests were used when addressing different questions. When aiming to study the thermoregulatory responses to cold stress, vasoconstrictor responses to inspiratory gasp, contralateral arm cold challenge, and body cooling were measured (20), and differences were indeed found: elderly subjects had a diminished sympathetic vasoconstrictor response.

In contrast, in order to evaluate the penetration of drugs through aged skin, the erythema that results from topical application of methyl nicotinate was measured (23), and no differences were found between young and old subjects, indicating that microvascular reactivity to the applied stimulus was comparable.

54.3.1.1 Vasoconstrictive Test

For the isometric test, the site of blood flow measurement is the left middle fingertip. After establishing the baseline blood flow, it is continuously recorded when the subject squeezes a hard rubber ball in the right hand for 30 seconds. The subject then releases the grip, and the maximum decrease in blood flow is recorded. The hemodynamic response to the isometric hand grip exercise involves activation of the sympathetic nervous system, eliciting an increase in blood pressure, which is mainly dependent upon cardiac output (12).

For the cognitive test, the site of blood flow measurement is again the fingertip. The subject is requested to subtract 7 sequentially from 1000 for a two-minute period. Blood flow is monitored continuously. There is a rapid fall in the blood flow to the finger at the beginning of the mental arithmetic activity and a rapid recovery at the end. The maximum decrease in blood flow is registered. This decrease is a manifestation of a sudden increase in sympathetic activity (15).

The venoarteriolar reflex measures the ability to decrease flow during venous stasis (normally seen in the feet on dependency) and is assumed to be dependent on an intact sympathetic nerve function (24). The reflex occurs following increased venous pressure, which induces constriction of the arterioles followed by a decrease in skin blood flow. An increase of venous pressure can be achieved by occlusion with a cuff (for instance, at the base of the investigated finger) (25) or by lowering the leg below heart level (26–28). Usually, resting blood flow to the dorsum of the foot is measured with the patient resting in the supine position. Then standing flow is measured (or the flow after occlusion by a cuff), and the lowest reading over five minutes of standing is registered. The venoarteriolar reflex can be expressed as the percent decrease in skin blood flow on standing. The reaction is mediated by a sympathetic axon reflex, composed of receptors in small veins and resulting in an increase in precapillary resistance.

With the inspiratory gasp test, the subject is instructed to breathe in as deeply and quickly as possible and to hold the breath for 10 seconds. The percentage in reduction from the resting flow is calculated. This procedure records the sympathetic vasoconstrictor reflex (29).

54.3.1.2 Vasodilative Tests

For the cutaneous postischemic reactive hyperemia test, blood flow in the middle part of the flexor aspect of the forearms (or sometimes the proximal part of the finger) is recorded. The arm is then clamped in a pneumatic cuff and inflated to greater than 40 mmHg above systolic pressure for a period of one to five minute during which blood flow measurements are continuously recorded. The cuff is then deflated resulting in an increase in blood flow, which is recorded continuously, usually until the blood flow returns to baseline values. Any of the following parameters can be measured: (1) baseline flow; (2) peak flow above baseline flow; (3) the time required to reach the peak; (4) the ratio between the peak flow and the time required to reach it, expressing the ability of the tissue to respond to fast external triggers; (5) the time required to return to the blood flow at rest; and (6) the area under the response–time curve (12–14).

For the intracutaneous needle stimulation (injection trauma) test, testing blood flow is recorded, and then a needle is inserted, usually in the center of the probe holder, to a depth previously set by a needle guard. The blood flow reaches a peak within 15 minutes of injection and then gradually returns to normal over several hours, depending on the degree of trauma (18).

For the thermal test, resting blood flow is measured in the middle part of the flexor aspect of the left forearm, while the probe is mounted through a thermostat probe holder. The temperature setting of the thermistor is adjusted to 26°C. The temperature is maintained at 26°C for two minutes, before turning the setting to 28°C for the next two-minute period. This 2°C step sequence is repeated every two minutes until the temperature reaches 44°C. Blood flow is recorded at the end of each two-minute interval (12).

For the axon reflex vasodilator response, vasoactive substances such as substance P, capsaicin, or histamine are administered topically or intradermally (30–32). Alternatively, acetylcholine is administered with the aid of electrophoresis (27). The extent of the response is measured at several distances from the site of administration. The same procedure is followed for measuring the response to direct stimulation with a firm mechanical stroke with a dermograph (Lewis triple response) (27).

With the isotonic test, the subject squeezes a partially inflated blood pressure cuff with maximum effort, at which the pressure is recorded, and one-third of it is calculated. The subject is then instructed to grip the cuff at this value of one-third of the maximum pressure. This isotonic exercise causes vasodilatation, and an increase in skin blood flow results (16).

54.3.2 CHOOSING SUBJECTS

When comparing subjects or various groups of subjects, variations in population regarding sex (33, 34), age (20), and race (35) should be taken into account. Assuring that subjects match for these variables will decrease the variance within the results.

54.4 APPLICATIONS

LDF may be used to study the time course of circulatory changes caused by physiological or pathological processes, including changes caused by pharmacological substances. Internal and external factors, skin conditions, and general conditions that affect the skin are all candidates for LDF investigations.

54.4.1 SKIN PHYSIOLOGY, PHARMACOLOGY, AND PATHOLOGY

54.4.1.1 Percutaneous Penetration

LDF was applied for tracing the percutaneous penetration of vasoactive agents such as methyl nicotinate (6), prostacyclin (36), or methadone (37) and for studying variations in normal skin (6, 19). For instance, LDF assisted in evaluating the enhancement effect of ultrasound on skin penetration (38). Thus, spatial variations (19), percutaneous penetration enhancers (39), vehicle effect on percutaneous absorption (40), the appendage contribution to penetration (41), and age and racial differences (42) were all studied with LDF. A decreased percutaneous penetration was recorded in black subjects at various skin sites (43). Circadian differences in penetration kinetics of methyl and hexyl nicotinate were also demonstrated by LDF (44). On the other hand, LDF is not suitable for studying the percutaneous penetration of vasoconstrictive agents such as glucocorticoids (45).

Transdermal delivery utilizing iontophoresis was studied at different sites of the forearms and hands, and vasodilatation was site dependent (46). It was shown that cutaneous vascular responses to iontophoresis of vasoactive agents comprise nonspecific, current-induced hyperemia and specific effects of the administered drug (47).

54.4.1.2 UVB-Induced Erythema

The effect of ultraviolet (UV) light may be evaluated by LDF, but the technique was not adequate for individuals with dark skin (48).

The UVB-induced skin blood flow was monitored using the laser Doppler perfusion imaging technique. It was as sensitive as conventional LDF, but had the many advantages of measuring blood flow over large areas without contact with the skin surface (49). Laser Doppler perfusion imaging was also successfully used for phototesting (50).

54.4.1.3   Inflammation and Contact Dermatitis

Inflammation is well suited for LDF studies because of its marked vasoactive component. An increase in blood flow indicated the induction of erythema by topical application of *Staphylococcus aureus* superantigen on intact skin (51). This occurred with both healthy subjects and patients with atopic dermatitis, suggesting that the superantigen may exacerbate and sustain inflammation. The UV-induced inflammation was increased following topical application of estrogen (52), while hypnotic suggestion attenuated UV inflammation (53).

The effect of various topical steroid formulations on UV-induced inflammation was measured by LDF, and it enabled grading the potency of these topical corticosteroids (54).

LDF was also used to assess the effect of systemic antiinflammatory drugs, and it enabled grading of the effect of these drugs (55, 56). Prick tests with allergens and histamine may also be evaluated by LDF (57). Regional variations in response to histamine should be taken into consideration (58).

LDF is widely used for measuring the response to known irritants. Increased duration of exposure resulted in an increased response, and comparison between the back and forearm indicated a greater sensitivity on the back (59). The cumulative effect of subthreshold concentrations of irritants was indicated in studies with LDF (60). The vehicle effect on irritation was also studied by LDF, and the irritant effect depended on the vehicle (61).

The damage to the skin by repetitive washing (62) and the protective effect of barrier creams were also assessed by LDF (63), as well as the effect of treatment such as topical application of nonsteroidal antiinflammatory drugs in various vehicles (thus studying the vehicle effect as well) (64). LDF measurements also suggested an improvement of acute irritant contact dermatitis (ICD) with twice-daily application of cool compresses. No significant difference was found between the efficacy of physiologic saline or water compresses (65).

Nonimmunologic contact urticaria induced by benzoic acid was followed, and regional variations mapped by LDF (66), as was the suppressive effect of psoralen plus ultraviolet A (PUVA) treatment (67) and topical nonsteroidal antiinflammatory drugs (68). Regional variations, as well as age-related regional variations, in the response to histamine were found (69).

Patch tests for allergic contact dermatitis may be objectively evaluated with LDF, as were patch tests with calcipotriol ointment in various patients, including psoriasis patients (70).

Laser Doppler imaging was more suitable for the quantification of allergic contact dermatitis than the regular LDF, as readings with the latter are time consuming, and laser Doppler imaging is valuable for measuring the area of response (71). Both allergic contact dermatitis and ICD were studied with laser Doppler imaging (72). The technique allowed quantification of a subclinical pattern of the allergic inflammation (73).

54.4.1.4   Psoriasis

Psoriasis, with its increased blood flow near the skin surface, is a natural candidate for LDF studies. Several investigators aimed at studying the disease process, whereas others were interested in the effect of several therapeutic modalities. A recent publication concentrated on the question whether cutaneous blood vessels in psoriasis possess a generalized inherently abnormal response to neuropeptides (74). Calcitonin gene-related peptide (CGRP) was intradermally injected in three concentrations to uninvolved skin of psoriatic patients and to healthy controls. This resulted in an increase in blood flow, which did not differ between the two groups, thus indicating that in uninvolved psoriatic skin, the vasculature is not different from normal in its response to CGRP. Effects of treatment were assessed by LDF and compared to clinical evaluation methods (75).

Laser Doppler imaging allows rapid measurement of the area and the level of increase of blood flow in psoriatic plaques (9). Plaque severity can be assessed in terms of mean blood flow and area of increased blood flow simultaneously. The obtained scan image reveals the distribution and intensity of the rim of increased blood flow around the psoriatic plaque. This could be used in the study of early biochemical or immunological changes in the skin, before lesions become clinically observable. As an aid in evaluating phototherapy, a reduced sensitivity to both UVA and UVB was demonstrated in psoriasis plaques as compared to uninvolved skin, using the same instrument (10). The method also showed an improved response to PUVA treatment when calcipotriol was topically applied (76). Laser Doppler imaging was further used to demonstrate an abnormal thermal sensory response in psoriasis (77).

The application of LDF for the study of psoriasis, including evaluation of therapy has been extensively reviewed (78).

54.4.1.5 Atopic Dermatitis

In a study of dermographism, a significant reduction in the intensity of hyperemia was found in atopic dermatitis patients following pressure on the skin (79). The role of acetylcholine in the etiology of pruritus in atopic dermatitis was studied by injecting acetylcholine and monitoring the vascular reaction. The reaction in the patients started earlier and was longer than the control group, suggesting an etiological role (80).

54.4.1.6 Age, Chronic Venous Insufficiency, and Cutaneous Ulcers

In comparison to the skin of adults (average age 34.6 years), the skin of small children (average age 3.5 years) demonstrated an increased cutaneous blood perfusion as measured by LDF (81).

Differences between elderly and younger individuals and between the forehead and cheek were found utilizing LDF during cooling from 30°C to 10°C. In the forehead, the decrease in skin blood flow during cooling showed no marked quantitative change with age, but with aging, the rate of this decrease was reduced. In the cheek, on the other hand, the skin blood flow decreased markedly with aging, but no clear change was observed in the rate of this decrease (82).

Skin blood flow to the dorsum of the foot reduces with age, which might contribute to the attenuated cutaneous vasoreactivity to heat and ischemia in elderly people (83). Moreover, the response to heat is attenuated in the aged (84).

Laser Doppler flux is a product of the concentration of moving blood cells and the blood cell velocity. In an attempt to obtain more information about the cutaneous microcirculation in legs with venous ulcers and in healthy legs, the dynamics of the curves of the LDF, the concentration of moving blood cells, and the blood cell velocity were analyzed in patients with venous leg ulcers and in healthy subjects. The curves of the concentration of moving blood cells and the blood cell velocity were in opposite phase, reflecting the capillary blood flow. The greater amplitude of the LDF and the concentration of moving blood cells in legs with venous ulcers reflect the blood flow in anatomically altered capillaries in those legs (85).

The ability of the skin blood vessels to dilate in response to pilocarpine electrophoresis was assessed in patients with chronic venous insufficiency, but the microvasculature showed a normal capacity to vasodilate (86). The effect of external compression was also studied: compression increased the microcirculatory flow, which might be its mode of action in treating venous insufficiency (87).

In patients with venous ulcers, erythematous ulcer edges exhibited higher blood flow values than nonerythematous edges (88). Postural vasoregulation caused relative ischemia and reperfusion in venous leg ulcers, but the known mediators of reperfusion injury were not released, and therefore were not associated with the process (89). LDF was also used to monitor the effect of prostanoids on ischemic ulcers (90) and the effect of Crystacide on chronic venous insufficiency and venous hypertension associated with ulcerations (91). It was also utilized to monitor the effect of Venoruton on the prevention and control of flight microangiopathy and edema in subjects with varicose veins flying for more than 7 hours (92).

To evaluate different types of alternating pressure air mattresses for the prevention and treatment of pressure ulcers, LDF was used on the sacrum, heels, trochanters, and buttock over at least two alternating cycles. Results indicated significant differences between the products (93).

For further examples of the use of LFD in peripheral vascular disease, please refer to Section 54.4.2.2.

54.4.1.7 Pigmentary Lesions and Melanoma

LDF has a potential for use in oncology, being able to monitor the vascularization in tumors and adjacent skin. For instance, it may serve as an additional tool in the diagnosis of pigmentary skin lesions. Melanomas showed higher laser Doppler blood flow readings than basal cell carcinomas, and both showed higher readings than benign lesions (94). LDF was higher in the center of melanomas than in either the middle of melanocytic nevus or in neighboring healthy skin areas (95).

Laser Doppler imaging was used to delineate the boundaries of pigmented lesions (96) and was able to monitor blood flow following photodynamic therapy of nonmelanoma skin tumors (97).

54.4.1.8 Burns and Flaps

Surgical procedures such as liposuction (98) and flaps can be monitored (99) and their success predicted (100). Similarly, burn severity and treatment may be evaluated (101).

Laser Doppler perfusion imaging was used to measure the depth of burns (102). The instrument was useful if the effect of scanning distance, curvature of the tissue; thickness of topical wound dressings; and pathophysiological effects of skin color, blisters, and wound fluids were known and adjusted. Further studies proved it accurate to differentiate deep dermal from superficial partial-thickness burns in the extremities (103) and to determine the need for excision and grafting in advance of clinical judgment (104).

54.4.2 General Conditions and Diseases

External factors, as well as certain general conditions and diseases, may affect the skin or have an effect on its blood flow even when the skin itself is healthy, as demonstrated by the effect of cellular phones on skin blood flow (105).

54.4.2.1 Nervous System

Skin blood flow is centrally controlled by the autonomic system and takes part in the general regulatory mechanism. Autonomous activity was reflected in skin blood flow, which fluctuated in response to sympathetic modulation (106). Various vasodilating factors that control blood flow can be assessed by LDF (107).

Higher mental activity alters skin blood flow: During cognitive activity, skin blood flow to the finger decreases, but not to the molar region (15). The reason is that vasoconstriction in the finger is mediated by sympathetic stimulation, which controls the blood supply to the hands and feet, whereas the face has a poor sympathetic vasoconstrictor supply.

Sound stimuli also affect the skin microcirculation in sites rich with sympathetic innervations, as was demonstrated by LDF (108).

The effect of neural blockade at various spinal levels and general anesthesia was followed with LDF, and functions like respiratory movements were correlated (109).

LDF measurements in acral regions ranked the role of alpha-1 and alpha-2 adrenoceptors in mediating sympathetic responses (110). Alpha-2 adrenoceptors were more potent in increasing the cutaneous microvascular resistance and reducing the perfusion.

To study the mechanism of pain relief by vasodilator agents, LDF measurements were conducted following intradermal injection of various vasodilators and compared to the pain threshold (111). The pain threshold did not correlate with blood flow, indicating that the effect of vasodilators on primary afferent nociceptors is not related to the vasodilatory effect.

Laser Doppler measurement of patients with chronic fatigue syndrome showed peripheral cholinergic abnormalities in their vascular endothelium (112).

For further examples of the utilization of LDF for the study of the nervous system, please refer to Sections 54.3, 54.4.2.2, and 54.4.2.9.

54.4.2.2   Environmental Temperature

Emotional stress induced vasoconstriction after prolonged heating to 34°C, whereas after prolonged cooling to 22°C, vasodilatation was induced (113). The stress-induced decreased flow in warm subjects is probably neurally mediated, since it is preceded by increased skin sympathetic activity. But the increase of flow in cold subjects is more obscure. Different neural commands at different temperatures might be a possibility. Another possibility is that arteriovenous shunts receive a vaso-constrictor sympathetic input, whereas resistant vessels receive a vasodilator input. In cold subjects with high baseline vasoconstriction, the arteriovenous shunts are closed and unable to constrict any further, so only the vasodilatation in the resistance vessels is detected. In warm subjects, thermo-regulatory activity is low, the basal flow is high, and the arteriovenous shunts are open. When emo-tional stress occurs, the constrictor effect on the open arteriovenous shunts will be more pronounced and mask the vasodilatation in the resistance vessels. A study that examined effects of hyperoxia on thermoregulatory responses found that hyperoxia elicited an inhibitory effect on thermoregulatory skin blood flow (114).

Both LDF and laser Doppler imaging were utilized to correlate skin blood flow to temperature changes. The two did not correlate at sites with arteriovenous shunts (115).

Central thermoregulatory mechanisms affect the postural vasoconstrictor response. Following heating of the trunk with an electrical blanket, the postural fall in blood flow diminished in skin areas with relatively numerous arteriovenous shunts (plantar surface of the big toe) (116). In con-trast, areas with only few or no arteriovenous shunts (dorsum of the foot) displayed similar postural flows before and after heating. Therefore, partial release of sympathetic vasoconstrictor tone associ-ated with indirect heating appears to override the local postural control of cutaneous vascular tone in areas where arteriovenous anastomoses are relatively numerous. When measured at heart level, the indirect heating was accompanied by a significant increase in foot blood flow. Many experi-ments utilizing both LDF and other techniques support the view that this reflex thermoregulatory vasodilatation is mainly due to the release of sympathetic vasoconstrictor tone, induced by the elevated core temperature. The normal postural fall in foot skin blood flow was preserved within the skin temperature range of 26°C to 36°C, but at higher temperatures, it was markedly attenuated or even abolished (117). This might contribute to some of the problems of cardiovascular adaptations seen in hot environments.

The skin microcirculatory reaction to internally and externally applied cold stimuli was mea-sured by LDF. Results showed a decrease in the microcirculation after external stimulation, while no reaction was detected in response to internal stimulations. Repetitive stimulations evoked slow habituation (118).

The influence of room temperature on peripheral flow in healthy subjects and patients with peripheral vascular disease was followed by LDF (119). The flow was not affected much when the room temperature was increased from 24°C to 30°C; therefore, this range is suitable for skin blood flow studies. For temperatures higher than 30°C, the peripheral circulation increased. The relation-ship between skin flow and room temperature was linear in room temperatures between 23°C and 30°C, whereas between 3°C 0 and 35°C, it was curvilinear.

54.4.2.3   Flushing and Facial Pallor

Flushing, a transient reddening of the face and other body sites, is caused by vasodilatation, which may be provoked by many pharmacologic and physiologic reactions. Emotionally provoked blush-ing was recorded in the forehead by LDF. There was a sudden increase of blood flow, which returned to baseline value after approximately three minutes (120).

Other provoking factors are alcohol and conditions such as menopause, carcinoid, mastocytosis, or drugs like nicotinic acid (121). Flushing occurs after orchidectomy for carcinoma of the prostate, and LDF measurements correspond closely to the intensity of the attacks as experienced by the patients and also to the measurement of sweating by evaporimetry (122).

The LDF technique is appropriate for quantitative assessment of alcohol-provoked flushing. Comparing LDF to the change in molar thermal circulation index, a linear correlation was found between the two methods. Moreover, the LDF method was more specific and more sensitive (123).

The effects of various therapeutic modalities for facial flushing and rosacea were also studied. Systemic administration of nicotinic acids produces a generalized cutaneous erythema, partially mediated by prostaglandin biosynthesis. To further examine the mechanism, local cutaneous vasodilatation was studied following topical application of methyl nicotinate (124). Pretreatment with prostaglandin inhibitors (indomethacin, ibuprofen, and aspirin) significantly suppressed the erythemal response, while doxepin had no effect on this response. Arginine vasopressin was infused in high levels, comparable to those attained during physical stress, and a marked facial pallor in healthy men resulted (125). The pallor was objectively verified by LDF measurements, consistent with a fall in nutritional blood flow to the skin. In contrast, blood flow to the finger rose, indicating an increased blood flow through arteriovenous shunts. Thus, LDF assisted in determining that arginine vasopressin has a selective vasoactive effect in the skin.

54.4.2.4 Physical Activity

Cutaneous microvascular blood flow on the dorsum of the hand (nonglabrous skin) and on the finger pulp (glabrous skin) was measured by LDF. Endothelium-dependent vasodilation was assessed by an iontophoretic application of acetylcholine on the dorsum of the hand and by an induction of postocclusive reactive hyperemia on the finger pulp. Endothelium-independent vasodilation was assessed on the dorsum of the hand by iontophoretically applied sodium-nitroprusside. The acetylcholine evoked increase in LDF was significantly greater in the group of cyclists as compared with controls. In contrast, sodium-nitroprusside produced a significantly smaller response in the group of cyclists. Thus, a greater vasodilator capacity of endothelium in glabrous as well as in nonglabrous skin was demonstrated in the group of physically trained subjects. In addition, regular physical activity modified the reactivity of vascular smooth muscle cells (126). Another study using similar methods (acetylcholine, sodium nitroprusside, and postocclusive reactive hyperemia) found that athletes have higher endothelial activity than less trained individuals (127).

Another study found that postischemic LDF was significantly lower in nonathletic subjects than in athletes. In both groups the hyperemic stimulus significantly increased LDF. The flow reserve, estimated as peak/basal LDF, was significantly lower in control subjects than in athletes (128).

54.4.2.5 Smoking

Studies suggest an abnormality in capillary blood flow and its regulation in the skin as an immediate result of cigarette smoking, and a chronic effect as well (13). Cigarette smoking triggers the release of vasopressin: A significant correlation was found between the skin blood flow response to cigarette smoking and the plasma vasopressin levels after smoking (129). The vasopressin released may mediate some of the vasoconstriction, since pretreatment with a vasopressin antagonist reduced the nicotine-induced vasoconstriction in the skin, while vasopressin antagonist alone had no effect.

Calcium ions may play a role in the pathogenesis of the vasoconstriction caused by acute smoking. Elderly habitual smokers were given the calcium-channel blocker nifedipine and calcitonin, a hypocalcemizing hormone that has a vasoactive action. Both drugs prevented the LDF-measured vasoconstriction induced by cigarette smoking, indicating that the process is calcium mediated (130).

The vasodilatory response of the skin microvasculature was impaired in subjects who have smoked cigarettes for many years, involving both endothelium-dependent and endothelium-independent responses. Both acetylcholine- and sodium-nitroprusside induced skin blood flow increases were significantly attenuated in comparison with nonsmokers. Heart rate was also significantly blunted (131). Vascular responsiveness is altered even in light smokers compared to control subjects. The total hyperemic response was approximately 45% smaller in smokers compared to nonsmoker controls (132).

These and other studies illuminate some of the mechanisms involved in the changes of the microvascular bed in the skin of habitual smokers and reveal both acute and chronic changes. Chronic changes occur relatively early in a person's smoking history, but later they become more severe. It would be interesting to assess the correlation between these skin blood flow changes and the future development of peripheral vascular disease in a long-term study.

54.4.2.6 Pregnancy and Gestational Hypertension

Both normal and hypertensive pregnancy manifest microvascular changes. In gestational hypertension, baseline blood flow on the fingertip was lower than in normal pregnancy, but this measurement could not discriminate between these subjects and nonpregnant healthy controls (12). Provocative tests were then used (isometric test, cognitive test, reactive hyperemia test, and thermal test), and the isometric test gave the most discriminative results. The control group showed a larger decrease than both the normal pregnancy group and the gestational hypertension group. Gestational hypertension showed a larger decrease than the normal pregnancy group. The cognitive test and the postischemic reactive hyperemia allowed some degree of discrimination, whereas the thermal test did not show any abnormality in the pregnant groups. Thus LDF recording of the response to vasoactive stimuli may differentiate between groups of subjects with normal or hypertensive pregnancy and nonpregnant subjects. Normal pregnancy modifies the response of the skin microvasculature to some vasoactive stimuli, whereas gestational hypertension pushes that response back toward the nonpregnant state. However, the method cannot yet be applied as a diagnostic tool for the individual patient.

54.4.2.7 Hypertension

Hypertension is associated with, or even originates from, an increased total peripheral resistance. The skin microvasculature plays a role in this peripheral resistance, hence the importance of its investigation in hypertension.

The decrease of skin blood flow that follows smoking of two cigarettes was measured in hypertensive habitual smokers (133). The same measurements were done before any treatment and following intravenous administration of alpha-1 inhibition with doxazosin and beta-1 blockade with atenolol. Skin blood flow decreased under all these conditions, but the decrease was attenuated by doxazosin compared to atenolol. These findings indicate that selective alpha-1 adrenoceptors have a major effect on smoking-induced cutaneous vasoconstriction. In this respect, doxazosin is preferable to atenolol for the antihypertensive treatment of patients who smoke.

In hypertensive patients both the resting flow and the standing flow to the feet were significantly lower, but increased after nifedipine treatment (24). The venoarteriolar reflex was lower in hypertensive patients, improving after nifedipine treatment, but still below normal.

Side effects of treatments and their mechanisms may be studies by LDF. Following nifedipine treatment, a weaker venoarteriolar reflex was observed in patients who developed ankle edema, whereas before treatment their response did not differ from those who did not develop edema (134). In another study, calcium channel blockers of different chemical origins antagonized postural vasoconstriction in the skin of the dorsum of the foot, indicating altered postural capillary blood flow regulation (135). Fluid filtration to the extravascular compartment may then eventuate, which may explain ankle edema during treatment with calcium channel blockers.

The cutaneous postischemic reactive hyperemia response does not seem to differentiate between hypertensive patients and normotensive controls (14, 136). Thus, a few provocative tests were able to detect differences between hypertensive patients and controls, while other tests could not.

54.4.2.8 Peripheral Vascular Disease

The adequacy of skin blood flow in the ischemic extremity is an important determinant in the assessment of the severity of peripheral vascular disease. Old and young healthy volunteers were compared to patients with lower limb atherosclerosis and intermittent claudication and patients with lower limb atherosclerosis and critical ischemia (137). Elderly controls had higher flux values in the toe compared with claudicators, while claudicators had higher perfusion values than patients with critical ischemia.

Using the ratio between toe and finger flows narrows the range of the results, eliminating differences in cardiac output that occur from patient to patient; this method was able to distinguish between a group of healthy controls and a group of patients with peripheral vascular disease (138). The same technique was useful for evaluating patients with peripheral arterial disease and for distinguishing different etiologies of the disease (25). Patients with intermittent claudication, patients with rest pain, and those with critical foot ischemia had a significantly lower resting flow than normal. Healthy controls showed a reduction of skin blood flow on standing, which was smaller in patients with severe claudication. Patients with rest pain had higher skin blood flow values when standing, indicating a loss of the vasomotor tone and an increase of flow determined by gravity. The inverse effect of an increase in blood flow with standing was associated with the clinical improvement when the patients lowered their limbs (25).

Microcirculatory alterations in limbs with claudication were found, with early occurrence of microcirculatory compensation to atherosclerotic disease of increasing severity (139). The skin perfusion increased with dependency, which explains why patients obtain relief from pain with dependency.

Skin blood flow is an important determinant of healing of ulcers or an inevitable amputation. The baseline skin blood flow in patients with peripheral vascular disease was significantly lower than normal, and the pulse waves attenuated or absent (140). In indeterminate cases, the accuracy of the LDF method could be enhanced by the use of reactive hyperemia.

Using provocative tests, there was a correlation between the impairment of the LDF results and the gravity of the clinical picture, with significant differences being recorded between limbs with no sign of necrosis and limbs affected by slight necrosis (141). In patients with pain at rest, postischemic hyperemia was absent. Following therapy with intraarterial administration of naftidrofuryl, a statistically significant improvement in several LDF-assessed parameters was achieved, and treatment of four limbs with percutaneous transluminal angioplasty resulted in a completely normal test, matching the disappearance of all the symptoms caused by the peripheral occlusive arterial disease.

A reduction in the postischemic reactive hyperemia was found in patients with leg ulcers, with a sensitivity comparable to the measurements of distal systolic blood pressure (142). The healing effect of peripheral sympathectomy and pain relief were also monitored by LDF (143).

These studies again demonstrate that appropriate physiologic tests like hydrostatic pressure loading and postischemic reactive hyperemia test are more indicative of abnormalities than are static parameters like resting flow. LDF can also provide explanations to therapeutic effects, like that of CO_2 baths in occlusive arterial disease, where an increased skin blood flow and increased oxygen utilization were observed (144).

The microcirculation under compression bandages has been assessed by LDF, demonstrating flow changes related to the cuff pressure, making it possible to assess the microcirculation through intact bandages, without the need to place any sensors at the skin–bandage interface (145).

54.4.2.9 Diabetes Mellitus

Diabetes mellitus is the most illustrative disease for the application of skin blood flow measurements, with its microangiopathic changes serving as a natural target for LDF application to probe the disease's various aspects. Skin blood flow is affected in diabetes, either directly or via the nervous system, as exemplified by deficient responses in the fingertip that resemble premature aging

(146). LDF was widely used in studying the process of diabetes mellitus and the etiology of its various complications, in grading disease severity, predicting its outcome, and following treatment. Damage to the microcirculation in diabetes mellitus is responsible for a great number of its grave complications. The neuropathy that further affects the microcirculation adds to the diversity and complexity of the disease, making the exposure of its yet unsolved aspects even more intriguing and rewarding. An understanding of the mechanisms responsible for microvascular complications may help in developing new treatment modalities. Furthermore, detection of early functional changes in the microcirculation might identify patients at risk at a reversible stage.

The possibility of using the skin as a model for diabetic microangiopathy and its correlation to retinopathy and nephropathy is still under investigation.

A normal physiological fall in cutaneous blood flow following food ingestion was demonstrated by LDF measurements. This fall was attenuated in insulin-dependent diabetes mellitus (IDDM). These abnormalities of vasoconstriction in the peripheral microcirculation were present after eight years of diabetes and preceded the development of clinically apparent neuropathy or vascular disease (147). Using a thermal probe for provocation, blood flow values were lower than normal at 35 C, and this difference was even more pronounced at 4°C (148). Retinopathy and nephropathy were also associated with such a decrease.

Sympathetic neural dysfunction was indicated by a reduction of vasoconstrictor responses to contralateral arm cold challenge and body cooling and also to inspiratory gasp (20). Vascular disturbances measured on the dorsum of the hand seemed to be exaggerated by parasympathetic neuropathy (149).

Skin microvascular vasodilator response to both injection trauma and local thermal injury was impaired in IDDM, unrelated to diabetic control (18). This impairment in response to injury may be an important factor in the development of foot ulceration that often follows minor trauma. In order to investigate the mechanisms underlying the impaired hyperemia to local injury, substance P was intradermally injected and a reduced peak response was achieved in IDDM patients as compared to controls, whereas the response to capsaicin was the same (150). Following histamine blockade with chlorpheniramine, the response to capsaicin remained unaltered, while the response to substance P was reduced in both groups. Therefore, impaired skin hyperemia may represent decreased vascular reactivity to locally released substance P from peripheral nerve fibers.

Structural pathology in early diabetic neuropathy is best correlated to peroneal motor conduction velocity (151). Transcutaneous oxygen and LDF measurements were correlated with peroneal motor conduction velocity in IDDM patients, suggesting that hypoxia generates diabetic peripheral neuropathy and that in early neuropathy, therapeutic measures to improve blood flow might arrest its progress. Indeed, pentoxifylline treatment (400 mg three times daily) increased the skin blood flow in the lower extremity, as measured after three and six months of therapy (152).

Nociceptive C fibers were evaluated by measuring the axon reflex vasodilatation of the foot in response to electrophoresis of acetylcholine, to direct mechanical stroke with a dermograph, and to a deep inspiratory gasp (27). The flare was reduced only in patients with foot complications, and it correlated with the clinical diminution of pain sensation—both are components of nociceptive C fiber function. Reduction of the flare indicated an impairment of neurogenic inflammatory response, which, along with an impairment of the protective pain sensation, may be a contributory factor in the poor and slow healing of foot lesions of diabetic patients. Since sympathetic vasoconstrictor reflexes were present in most diabetic patients with foot ulceration, the role of autonomic neuropathy in ulcer development is questioned.

Similar results were obtained by measuring the flare induced by acetylcholine iontophoresis at various current strengths (153). Maximum flare response was reduced in neuropathic patients, especially those with a previous history of foot ulceration, suggesting that small fiber neuropathy affects ulcer development. The flare was also reduced in some patients with retinopathy without neuropathy, suggesting an early loss of small nociceptor C fibers, preceding large fiber neuropathy.

The curve of the hyperemic response plotted against current strength did not show a rightward shift, indicating that the abnormal response was due to axonal loss rather than to dysfunction. The flare did not correlate with the cardiac autonomic function.

Subjects at risk of developing non-insulin-dependent diabetes mellitus (NIDDM) who have fasting hyperglycemia exhibited decreased microvascular hyperemia, positively correlated with insulin sensitivity and negatively correlated with fasting plasma insulin concentrations (154). Thus, hyperinsulinemia as a result of insulin resistance may affect the microvascular function in the prediabetic state. Noncritically ischemic feet have a higher hyperemic response in comparison with critically ischemic feet (155).

The venoarteriolar response was lower in diabetic patients than in healthy controls, and lowest in patients with neuropathy (26). Both the increased skin blood flow and the impaired venoarteriolar reflex are causes of edema and may contribute to the thickening of capillary basement membranes detected in diabetes.

A hyperthermal LDF was developed to quantify autonomic dysfunction in the skin (156). The technique measures the time to induction of an increase of microcirculation following hyperthermia. Autonomic dysfunction was found in diabetic patients even with a short disease duration, suggesting that it was an early complication of NIDDM, even when the disease was well controlled.

Investigations of the sympathetic nervous function in NIDDM showed that deep breathing induced a decrease in skin blood flow (157). Many other neurovascular functional tests in experimental and human diabetes were studied (158).

Diabetes induces functional microvascular disturbances in the forearms. The cutaneous postischemic reactive hyperemia response was significantly lower than in nondiabetic controls (14). Retinopathy was a further factor in achieving more abnormal results. Evaluation of beraprost sodium treatment revealed a decreased effect when the severity of retinopathy and nephropathy increased (159).

A variety of treatment modalities were assessed by LDF, starting with simple physical measures like elastic stockings, through old and new medications, to evaluation of a combined kidney and pancreas transplantation. Elastic stockings repressed the deterioration of the microcirculation, as was shown by LDF studies (160). The effect of an angiotensin-converting enzyme inhibitor, captopril, was studied on IDDM (161). It improved skin blood flow, as measured with LDF using postocclusive reactive hyperemia response, and this was independent of its hypotensive effect.

In NIDDM, during insulin infusion foot blood flow was redistributed with an increase in capillary flow relative to arteriovenous shunt flow (162). Since blood that passes through arteriovenous shunts does not enter the capillary bed and plays no role in skin nutrition, this represents an improvement in the skin nutrition.

Hypoglycemia, but not hyperinsulinemia, caused a regional skin vasodilatation in healthy control subjects. Following a hyperinsulinemic euglycemic clamp, hypoglycemia was induced by a stepwise reduction in the intravenous glucose infusion. The increase in blood flow that was observed in healthy controls was absent in patients with non-insulin-dependent diabetes mellitus (163).

Defibrotide, an oral profibrinolytic drug, was given to non-insulin-dependent diabetic patients with microangiopathy. The microcirculation was evaluated by the venoarteriolar response and by the rise in skin blood flow following local heating—both decreased in diabetic patients. Following six months of treatment, patients in the new drug treatment group improved their microcirculatory parameters (venoarteriolar reflex) in association with an improvement in signs and symptoms (164). Calcium channel blockers were also evaluated with LDF (165).

A combined kidney and pancreas transplantation improved the skin microvascular reactivity; therefore, the possibility that transplantation could reverse or halt diabetic complications was studied (23). Skin blood flow at rest, postischemic reactive hyperemia, and venoarteriolar reflex at 2 and 38 months following transplantation were measured. The resting blood flow was higher

38 months following transplantation as compared to two months, but the delayed time to peak during hyperemia was even more impaired at 38 months. This is probably due to a disturbed function of the smooth muscle cells of the vessel wall and might indicate a progress of structural changes in spite of an improved metabolism. The venoarteriolar reflex was also impaired at both time points, probably due to neuropathy, since this reflex depends on an intact sympathetic nerve function. A trend for improvement in four out of five patients with the most impaired reflex was observed, but it did not reach statistical significance, but still may indicate that diabetic neuropathy can improve after transplantation (23). Laser Doppler perfusion imaging of patients with diabetic neuropathy showed skin vasodilation following topical application of methyl nicotinate at the forearm and foot levels, suggesting a potential of methyl nicotinate to increase blood flow and to prevent diabetic foot problems (166).

These and other studies indicate that LDF can be useful in the investigation of some diabetes pathophysiological mechanisms, disease severity, and the efficacy of its control.

54.4.2.10 Raynaud Phenomenon

The intermittent blanching that occurs in Raynaud phenomenon is believed to result from an active microvascular vasoconstriction and emptying. Therefore, LDF is useful for the investigation of the pathophysiological mechanisms underlying Raynaud phenomenon and for evaluating treatments.

To clarify the etiology of Raynaud phenomenon, three vasodilators were intravenously administered, and the response of CGRP was compared with that of endothelium-dependent adenosine triphosphate and the endothelium-independent prostacyclin (167). The first vasodilator induced an increase in blood flow in the hands of patients but not in healthy controls, which may reflect a deficiency of endogenous CGRP release in Raynaud phenomenon.

The role of the histaminergic and peptidergic axes in primary Raynaud phenomenon was also studied (29, 30). Digital blood flow response to intradermal injections of saline, histamine, histamine-releasing agent (compound 48/80), substance P, and CGRP was measured. No evidence of local deficiency in histamine release or in the response to histamine was found (30), even at low temperatures (29), and the patients reacted normally to the neuropeptides substance P (29, 30) and CGRP (30), providing a rationale for treating Raynaud phenomenon with vasoactive peptides.

Digital skin blood flow of both hands was measured during local heating of only one hand. Patients with Raynaud phenomenon showed a decreased digital blood flow during stepwise cooling in both hands, but the reaction in the cooled hand was more pronounced and more consistent (168). Patients with Raynaud phenomenon had an abnormal vascular response to temperature change (32). Studying the hyperemic response to local skin warming, the patients showed vasodilatation at lower skin temperatures than normal, independent of central sympathetic control. Knowledge of skin temperature is therefore important for the interpretation of blood flow studies in Raynaud phenomenon. Provocative testing (occlusion) under different degrees of finger and body cooling detected an increase in the number of fingers of patients exhibiting vasospasm as the severity of cooling increased (169).

Occupational exposure to vibrations causes Raynaud phenomenon. For prevention and treatment of vibration syndrome, an objective test was developed, combining LDF with finger cooling (170). It enabled the demonstration of significant differences among four groups: subjects without vibration exposure, subjects with exposure but with no signs of white fingers, subjects with few attacks, and subjects with frequent attacks.

In patients with Raynaud phenomenon suffering from scleroderma, blood flow decrease during cooling was similar to healthy controls, but the patients had a longer rewarming period (171). In such patients, when resting blood flow was very low, the postischemic reactive hyperemia response was absent (172). After warming the hand in warm water, the hyperemic response was restored and its magnitude corrected, but its time course was longer, with a delay to achieving maximum flow as compared to controls. This may be related to changes in the vessels themselves or to connective tissue sclerosis limiting the rate of response.

Provocative tests, which evoke sympathetic tone, like the isometric test, were studied in addition to temperature measurements in groups of patients with primary Raynaud phenomenon, systemic sclerosis, and undifferentiated connective tissue disease as compared to a control group (173). Considerable differences were found in both the level of vessels involved and the relative importance of local finger temperature and discrimination between various etiologies of Raynaud phenomenon was possible.

Cutaneous postocclusive reactive hyperemia enabled grading obstructive vascular disease in groups of patients with Raynaud phenomenon, but could not discriminate among individuals in the subgroups (174). Another provocative test, the cognitive test, detected two subgroups within the patients with Raynaud phenomenon (175). The first subgroup showed a reduction in blood flow similar to healthy controls, whereas the second showed a paradoxical increase, suggesting an organic etiology.

LDF was used to evaluate various treatment modalities in Raynaud phenomenon. Thus, a single topical application of minoxidil 5% solution to the fingers was ineffective (176). Ketanserin, an antagonist of the serotonin-2-(5-HT-2)-receptor, was given to nine patients with generalized scleroderma (177). Finger systolic pressure and LDF after cooling and rewarming of the finger did not improve. Thus, ketanserin in the doses used (20 mg three times a day in the first week and 40 mg three times a day for 4 weeks) was not effective in the treatment of Raynaud phenomenon in generalized scleroderma. When given to patients with primary Raynaud phenomenon, ketanserin normalized digital blood flow (178).

Pretreatment with alpha-adrenoceptor antagonists did not abolish this effect, suggesting that in contrast to the effects on the systemic circulation, the mechanism underlying digital vasodilatation after ketanserin does not involve alpha-adrenoceptor antagonism.

Application of the vasodilator hexyl nicotinate at various sites on the upper limb resulted in an increase in blood flow both in patients with Raynaud phenomenon (13 with primary Raynaud disease and 12 with systemic sclerosis and Raynaud phenomenon) and in normal subjects (179). Moreover, increasing the drug concentration increased flow rate.

The effect of nifedipine on perniosis was also studied. An increase in blood flow to a finger or a toe adjacent to a diseased one could be demonstrated after the drug intake (180).

54.4.2.11   Other Diseases

Several diseases, like leprosy, have distinct skin lesions, which may be followed up by LDF. Blood flow in lesions of leprosy paralleled the clinical appearance and histopathology of the lesions during treatment (181, 182). The amount of hyperemia was useful in monitoring the early changes of reversal reaction during chemotherapy.

LDF was also valuable in evaluating peripheral autonomic function in leprosy (183). The skin overlying Kaposi sarcoma was studied by LDF as well (184). In addition, LDF was used to investigate microvascular physiology in patients with sickle cell disease (185). Large local oscillations in skin blood flow to the arm were demonstrated, occurring simultaneously at sites separated by 1 cm, suggesting a synchronization of rhythmic flow in large domains of microvessels. The periodic flow may be a compensatory mechanism to offset the deleterious altered rheology of erythrocytes in sickle cell disease.

Changes in skin microvascular reactivity were demonstrated in hypertriglyceridemia (186), and even in Alzheimer disease (187, 188).

In a study involving a very low-cardiovascular-risk female population of 862 healthy females screened for cardiovascular risk factors, a significant correlation was observed between the weight of cardiovascular risks and the impairment of postischemic forearm skin reactive hyperemia. Thus, skin LDF may represent a valuable, simple, and noninvasive tool to assess and monitor microvascular function in future prospective observational and interventional studies (189).

54.5   CONCLUSION

The LDF method allows real-time analysis of a wide range of physiological and pathological processes, as well as pharmacological processes and percutaneous penetration.

It provides objective numerical data at various time points or at various skin sites. However, results obtained by LDF should not be interpreted as absolute values, but should rather serve as relative estimates. It should be noted that results obtained by different instruments or by the same instrument in different subjects cannot be compared. Furthermore, biological variations within the disease state can also produce discord between different studies. There is a need therefore for technical improvements, calibration standards, better probe designs, and more reproducible measuring procedures before LDF turns into a useful clinical tool. Improvements may lead to a wider use in the area of skin pharmacology, which naturally requires accuracy and repeatability.

An important development was laser Doppler imaging (scanning LDF) (28), which quickly and sequentially remotely scans the tissue perfusion in several thousand measurement points. A map of the spatial distribution of the blood flow is thus obtained. Unlike regular LDF, which continuously records the blood flow over a single point, laser Doppler imaging maps the blood flow distribution over a specific area. Thus, the two methods do not compete with each other, but are rather complementary. The laser Doppler imaging has the advantage of operating without any contact with the skin surface, and, therefore, it does not disturb the local blood flow. A software module was implemented in the laser Doppler imaging, resulting in a duplex mode for recording both spatial and temporal blood perfusion components (190). Another new device combines laser Doppler perfusion imaging and digital photography, with many clinical applications like evaluating grafts or treatment of leg ulcers (191). It has also been used for mapping the vulvar skin blood flow in psoriasis or lichen sclerosus with invasive neoplasia, demonstrating increased perfusion in vulvar cancer (192).

Other improvements in laser Doppler are the introduction of advanced computerization and the development of new probes, such as multisite probes allowing simultaneous measurements at several sites and multisubject probes allowing simultaneous measurements of several subjects. These developments are accompanied by multichannel LDF instruments capable of simultaneous collection of data from many independent probes. Finally, a new probe holder design (7) permits repeated measurements over the same site before and after manipulations to the skin.

Technical innovations have improved the accuracy and repeatability of LDF, allowing its use as a clinical tool. The studies published in the last years (193–197) clearly indicate that LDF is useful in diverse clinical and investigational areas.

REFERENCES

1. Molitor H, Kniazuk M. A new bloodless method for continuous recording of peripheral circulatory changes. J Pharmacol Exp Ther 1936; 57:6–18.
2. Hertzman AB. Photoelectric plethysmography of the fingers and toes in man. Proc Soc Exp Biol Med 1937; 37:529–534.
3. Stern MD. In vivo evaluation of microcirculation by coherent light scattering. Nature 1975; 254:56–58.
4. Holloway GA, Watkins DW. Laser Doppler measurement of cutaneous blood flow. J Invest Dermatol 1977; 69:306–309.
5. Nilsson GE, Tenland T, Oberg PA. A new instrument for continuous measurement of tissue blood flow by light beating spectroscopy. IEEE Trans Biomed Eng 1980; 27: 12–19.
6. Tur E. Cutaneous blood flow: laser Doppler velocimetry. Int J Dermatol 1991; 30: 471–476.
7. Braverman IM, Schechner JS. Contour mapping of the cutaneous microvasculature by computerized laser Doppler velocimetry. J Invest Dermatol 1991; 97:1013–1018.
8. Nagashima Y, Yada Y, Suzuki T, Sakai A. Development and clinical application of an integration type laser Doppler flowmeter equipped with temperature-load instrument for skin blood flow. Jpn J Appl Physiol 2001; 31:295–304.
9. Wardell K, Naver HK, Nilsson, GE, Wallin BG. The cutaneous vascular axon reflex characterized by laser Doppler perfusion imaging. J Physiol 1993; 460:185–199.

10. Speight EL, Essex TJH, Farr PM. The study of plaques of psoriasis using a scanning laser–Doppler velocimeter. Br J Dermatol 1993; 128:519–524.

11. Speight EL, Farr PM. Erythemal and therapeutic response of psoriasis to PUVA using high-dose UVA. Br J Dermatol 1994; 131:667–672.

12. Liu D, Svsanber K, Wang I, Andersson-Engels S, Svanberg S. Laser Doppler perfusion imaging: new technique for determination of perfusion of splanchnic organs and tumor tissue. Lasers Surg Med 1997; 20:473–479.

13. Tur E, Tamir A, Guy RH. Cutaneous blood flow in gestational hypertension and normal pregnancy. J Invest Dermatol 1992; 99:310–314.

14. Tur E, Yosipovitch G, Oren-Vulfs S. Chronic and acute effects of cigarette smoking on skin blood flow. Angiology 1992; 43:328–335.

15. Tur E, Yosipovitch G, Bar-On Y. Skin reactive hyperemia in diabetic patients. Diabetes Care 1991; 14:958–962.

16. Wilkin JK, Trotter K. Cognitive activity and cutaneous blood flow. Arch Dermatol 1987; 123:1503–1506.

17. Weinstein L, Janjan N, Droegemueller W, Katz MA. Forearm plethysmography in normotensive and hypertensive pregnant women. South Med J 1981; 74:1230–1232.

18. Low PA, Neumann C, Dyck PJ, Fealey RD, Tuck RR. Evaluation of skin vasomotor reflexes by using laser–Doppler velocimetry. Mayo Clin Proc 1983; 58:583–592.

19. Allen J, Frame JR, Murray A. Microvascular blood flow and skin temperature changes in the fingers following a deep aspiratory gasp. Physiol Meas 2002; 23:365–373.

20. Rayman G, Williams SA, Spencer PD, Smaje LH, Wise PH, Tooke JE. Impaired microvascular hyperaemic response to minor skin trauma in type I diabetes. Br Med J 1986; 292:1295–1298.

21. Mayrovitz NH, Smith J, Delgado M. Variability in skin microvascular vasodilatory responses assessed by laser Doppler imaging. Ostomy Wound Manage 1997; 43:66–70.

22. Khan F, Spence VA, Belch JJF. Cutaneous vascular responses and thermoregulation in relation to age. Clin Sci 1992; 82:521–528.

23. Roskos KV, Bircher AJ, Maibach HI, Guy RH. Pharmacodynamic measurements of methyl nicotinate percutaneous absorption: the effect of aging on microcirculation. Br J Dermatol 1990; 122:165–171.

24. Shami SK, Chittenden SJ. Microangiopathy in diabetes mellitus: II Features, complications and investigation. Diabetes Res 1991; 17:157–168.

25. Jorneskog G, Tyden G, Bolinder J, Fagrell B. Skin microvascular reactivity in fingers of diabetic patients after combined kidney and pancreas transplantation. Diabetologia 1991; 34:S135–S137.

26. Cesarone MR, Laurora G, Belcaro GV. Microcirculation in systemic hypertension. Angiology 1992; 43:899–903.

27. Belacro G, Nicolaides AN. Microvascular evaluation of the effects of nifedipine in vascular patients by laser–Doppler flowmetry. Angiology 1989; 40:689–694.

28. Belacro G, Nicolaides AN. The venoarteriolar response in diabetics. Angiology 1991;42:827–835.

29. Parkhouse N, Le Quesne PM. Impaired neurogenic vascular response in patients with diabetes and neuropathic foot lesions. N Engl J Med 1988; 318:1306–1309.

30. Wardell K, Naver HK, Nilsson GE, Wallin BG. The cutaneous vascular axon reflex characterized by laser Doppler perfusion imaging. J Physiol 1993; 460:185–199.

31. Bunker CB, Foreman JC, Dowd PM. Vascular responses to histamine at low-temperatures in normal digital skin and Raynaud's phenomenon. Agents Actions 1991; 33:197–199.

32. Bunker CB, Foreman JC, Dowd PM. Digital cutaneous vascular responses to histamine and neuropeptides in Raynaud's phenomenon. J Invest Dermatol 1991; 96:314–317.

33. Maurel A, Hamon P, Macquin-Mavier I, Largue G. Cutaneous microvascular flow studied by laser–Doppler. Presse Med 1991; 20:1205–1209.

34. Walmsley D, Goodfield MJD. Evidence for an abnormal peripherally mediated vascular response to temperature in Raynaud's phenomenon. Br J Rheumatol 1990; 29:181–184.

35. Gean CJ, Tur E, Maibach HI, Guy RH. Cutaneous responses to topical methyl nicotinate in black, oriental and caucasian subjects. Arch Dermatol Res 1989; 281:95–98.

36. Belch JJ, Mclaren M, Lau CS, Mackay IR, Bancroft A, McEwen J, Thompson JM. Cicaprost, an orally active prostacycline analogue: its effects on platelet aggregation and skin blood flow in normal volunteers. Br J Clin Pharmacol 1993; 35:643–647.

37. Drummond PD, de Silva-Rossdeutscher E. Transcutaneous iontophoresis of methadone provokes local flushing and thermal hyperalgesia. Inflamm Res 2003; 52:366–371.

38. McElnay JC, Benson HA, Harland R, Hadgraft J. Phonopheresis of methyl nicotinate: a preliminary study to elucidate the mechanism of action. Pharm Res 1993; 10:1726–1731.

39. Ryatt KS, Stevenson JM, Maibach HI, Guy RH. Pharmacodynamic measurement of percutaneous penetration enhancement in vivo. J Pharmacol Sci 1986; 75:374–377.

40. Guy RH, Tur E, Schall LM, Elamir S, Maibach HI. Determination of vehicle effects on percutaneous absorption by laser Doppler velocimetry. Arch Dermatol Res 1986; 278:500–502.

41. Tur E, Maibach HI, Guy RH. Percutaneous penetration of methyl nicotinate at three anatomical sites: evidence for an appendageal contribution to transport? Skin Pharmacol 1991; 4:230–234.

42. Guy RH, Tur E, Bjerke S, Maibach HI. Are there age and racial differences to methyl nicotinate-induced vasodilatation in human skin? J Am Acad Dermatol 1985; 12:1001–1006.

43. Berardesca E, Maibach HI. Racial differences in pharmacodynamic response to nicotinates in vivo in human skin: black and white. Acta Derm Venereol 1990; 70:63–66.

44. Reinberg AE, Soudant E, Koulbanis C, Bazin R, Nicolai A, Mechkouri M, Touitou Y. Circadian dosing time dependency in the forearm skin penetration of methyl and hexyl nicotinate. Life Sci 1995; 57:1507–1513.

45. Noon JP, Evans CE, Haynes WG, Webb DJ, Walker BR. A comparison of techniques to assess skin blanching following the topical application of glucocorticoids. Br J Dermatol 1996; 134:837–842.

46. Gardner-Medwin JM, Taylor JY, Macdonald IA, Powell RJ. An investigation into variability in microvascular skin blood flow and the responses to transdermal delivery of acetylcholine at different sites in the forearm and hand. Br J Clin Pharmacol 1997; 43:391–397.

47. Grossmann M, Jamieson MJ, Kellogg DL Jr, Kosiba WA, Pergola PE, Crandall CG, Shepherd AM. The effect of iontophoresis on the cutaneous vasculature: evidence for current-induced hyperemia. Microvasc Res 1995; 50:444–452.

48. Kollias N, Bager A, Sadiq I. Minimum erythema dose determination in individuals of skin types V and VI with diffuse reflectance spectroscopy. Photodermatol Photoimmunol Photomed 1994; 10:249–254.

49. Youn JI, Park SB, Park BS, Han WS. Comparative quantitative analysis of ultraviolet B-induced skin blood flow change using laser Doppler perfusion imaging technique. Photodermatol Photoimmunol Photomed 2000; 16:167–171.

50. Falk M, Ilias MA, Wardell K, Anderson C. Phototesting with a divergent UVB beam in the investigation of anti-inflammatory effects of topically applied substances. Photodermatol Photoimmunol Photomed 2003; 19:195–202.

51. Strange P, Skov L, Lisby S, Nielsen PL, Baadsgaard O. Staphylococcal enterotoxin B applied on intact normal and intact atopic skin induces dermatitis. Arch Dermatol 1996; 132:27–33.

52. Jemec GB, Heideheim M. The influence of sex hormones on UVB induced erythema in man. J Dermatol Sci 1995; 9:221–224.

53. Zacharie R, Oster H, Bjerring P. Effects of hypnotic suggestions on ultraviolet B radiation-induced erythema and skin blood flow. Photdermatol Photoimmunol Photomed 1994; 10:154–160.

54. Bjerring P. Comparison of the bioactivity of monetasone furoate 0.1% fatty cream, betamethasone dipropionate 0.05% cream and betamethasone valerate 0.1% cream in humans. Inhibition of UV-B-induced inflammation monitored by laser Doppler blood flowmetry. Skin Pharmacol 1993; 6:187–192.

55. Duteil L, Queille C, Poncet M, Czernielewski J. Processing and statistical analysis of laser Doppler data applied to the assessment of systemic anti-inflammatory drugs. J Dermatol Sci 1991; 2:376–382.

56. Denham KJ, Boutsiouki P, Clough GF, Church MK. Comparison of the effects of desloratadine and levocetirizine on histamine-induced wheal, flare and itch in human skin. Inflamm Res 2003; 52:424–427.

57. Nyren M, Ollmar S, Nicander I, Emtestam L. An electric impedance technique for assessment of wheals. Allergy 1996; 51:923–926.

58. Tur E, Aviram G, Zeltser D, Brenner S, Maibach HI. Regional variations of human skin blood flow responses to hitamine. Curr Probl Dermatol 1995; 22:50–66.

59. Dykes PJ, Black DR, York M, Dickens AD, Marks R. A step-wise procedure for evaluating irritant materials in normal volunteer subjects. Hum Exp Toxicol 1995; 14:204–211.

60. Tur E, Eshkol Z, Brenner S, Maibach HI. Cumulative effect of subthreshold concentrations of irritants in humans. Am J Contact Dermatitis 1995; 6:216–220.

61. Agner T. An experimental study of irritant effects of urea in different vehicles. Acta Derm Venereol (Stockh) 1992; 177:S44–S46.

62. Grunewald AM, Gloor M, Gehring W, Kleesz P. Damage to the skin by repetitive washing. Contact Dermatitis 1995; 32:225–232.

63. Marks R, Dykes PJ, Hamami I. Two novel techniques for the evaluation of barrier creams. Br J Dermatol 1989; 120:655–660.

64. Poelman MC, Piot B, Guyon F, Deroni M, Leveque JL. Assessment of topical nonsteroidal anti-inflammatory drugs. J Pharm Pharmacol 1989; 41:720–722.

65. Levin CY, Maibach HI. Do coll water or physiplogic saline compresses enhance resolution of experimentally induced irritant contact dermatitis? Contact Dermatitis; 45: 146–150.

66. Shriner DL, Maibach HI. Regional variations of non-immunologic contact urticaria. Functional map of the human face. Skin Pharmacol 1996; 9:312–321.

67. Larmi E. PUVA treatment inhibits non-immunologic immediate contact reactions to benzoic acid and methyl nicotinate. Int J Deramatol 1989; 28:609–611.

68. Johansson J, Lahti A. Topical non-steroidal anti-inflammatory drugs inhibit nonimmunologic immediate contact rections. Contact Dermatitis 1988; 19:161–165.

69. Tur E. Age-related regional variations of human skin blood flow response to histamine. Acta Derm Venereol 1995; 75:451–454.

70. Fullerton A, Avnstorp C, Agner T, Dahl JC, Olsen LO, Serup J. Patch test study with calcipotriol ointment indifferent patient groups, including psoriatic patients with and without adverse dermatitis. Acta Derm Venereol 1996; 76:194–202.

71. Quinn AG, McLelland J, Esex T, Farr PM. Quantification of contact allergic inflammation: a comparison of existing methods with a scanning laser Doppler velocimeter. Acta Derm Venereol 1993; 73:21–25.

72. Quinn AG, McLelland J, Esex T, Farr PM. Measurement of cutaneous inflammatory reactions using a scanning laser Doppler velocimeter. Br J Dermatol 1991; 125:30–37.

73. Stucker M,Auer T, Hoffman K, Altmeyer P. Two-dimensional blood flow determinations in allergic reactions using laser Doppler scanning. Contact Dermatitis 1995; 33:299–303.

74. Artemi P, Seale P, Satchell P, Ware S. Cutaneous vascular response to calcitonin gene related peptide in psoriasis and normal subjects. Australas J Dermatol 1997; 38:73–76.

75. Zachariae R, Oster H, Bjering P, Kragballe K. Effects of psychological intervention on psoriasis: a preliminary report. J Am Acad Dermatol 1996; 34:1008–1015.

76. Speight EL, Farr PM. Calcipotriol improves the response of psoriasis to PUVA. Br J Dermatol 1994; 130:79–82.

77. Yosipovitch G, Chan YH, Tay YK, Goh CL. Thermosensory abnormalities and blood flow dysfunction in psoriatic skin. Br J Dermatol 2003; 149:492–497.

78. Tur E, Tamir A, Tamir G, Brenner S. Psoriasis. In: Berardesca E, Elsner P, Maibach HI, eds. Bioengineering of the Skin: Cutaneous Blood Flow and Erythema. Part 2: Laser Doppler Velocimetry and Photoplethysmography. Boca Raton, Florida: CRC Press, 1995:123–131.

79. Hornstein OP, Boissevain F, Wittmann H. Non-invasive measurement of the vascular dynamics of dermographism—comparative study in atopic and non-atopic subjects. J Dermatol 1991; 18:79–85.

80. Vogelsang M, Heyer G, Hornstein OP. Acetylcholine induces different cutaneous sensations in atopic and non-atopic subjects. Acta Derm Venereol 1995; 75:434–436.

81. Fluhr JW, Pfisterer S, Gloor M. Direct comparison of skin physiology in children and adults with bioengineering methods. Pediatr Dermatol 2000; 17:436–439.

82. Nagashima Y, Yada Y, Suzuki T, Sakai A. Evaluation of the use of an integration-type laser–Doppler flowmeter with a temperature-loading instrument for measuring skin blood flow in elderly subjects during cooling load: comparison with younger subjects. Int J Biometeorol 2003; 47:139–147.

83. Van den Brande P, von Kemp K, De Coninck A, Debing E. Laser Doppler flux characteristics at the skin of the dorsum of the foot in young and in elderly healthy human subjects. Microvasc Res 1997; 53:156–162.

84. Kenney WL, Morgan AL, Farquhar WB, Brooks EM, Pierzga JM, Derr JA. Decreased active vasodilator sensitivity in aged skin. Am J Physiol 1997; 272:H1609–H1614.

85. Malanin K, Havu VK, Kolari PJ. Dynamics of cutaneous laser Doppler flux with concentration of moving blood cells and blood cell velocity in legs with venous ulcers and in healthy legs. Angiology 2004; 55:37–42.

86. Shami SK, Cheatle TR, Chittenden SJ, Scurr JH, Coleridge-Smith PD. Hyperaemic response in the skin microcirculation of patients with chronic venous insufficiency. Br J Surg 1993; 80:433–435.

87. Abu-Own A, Shami SK, Chittenden SJ, Farrah J, Scurr JH, Smith PD. Microangiopathy of the skin and the effect of leg compression in patients with chronic venous insufficiency. J Vasc Surg 1994; 19:1074–1083.

88. Schemeller W, Roszinski S, Huesmann M. Tissue oxygenation and microcirculation in dermatoliposclerosis with different degrees of erythema at the margins of venous ulcers. A contribution to hypodermitis symptoms. Vasa 1997; 26:18–24.

89. He CF, Cherry GW, Arnold F. Postural vasoregulation and mediators of reperfusion injury in venous ulceration. J Vasc Surg 1997; 25:647–653.

90. Gschwandtner ME, Koppensteiner R, Maca T, Minar E, Schneider B, Schnurer G, Ehringer H. Spontaneous laser Doppler flux distribution in ischemic ulcers and the effect of prostanoids: a crossover study comparing the acute action of prostaglandin E1 and iloprost vs saline. Microvasc Res 1996; 51:29–38.

91. Belcaro G, Cesarone MR, Nicolaides AN, Geroulakos G, Di Renzo A, Milani M, Ricci A, Brandolini R, Dugall M, Ruffini I, Cornelli U, Griffin M. Improvement of microcirculation and healing of venous hypertension and ulcers with Crystacide. Evaluation of free radicals, laser Doppler flux and PO2. A prospective-randomized controlled study. Angiology 2003; 54:325–330.

92. Cesarone MR, Belcaro G, Geroulakos G, Griffin M, Ricci A, Brandolini R, Pellegrini L, Dugall M, Ippolito E, Candiani C, Simeone E, Errichi BM, Di Renzo A. Flight microangiopathy on long-haul flights: prevention of edema and microcirculation alterations with Venoruton. Clin Appl Thromb Hemost 2003; 9:109–114.

93. Rithalia SV. Evaluation of alternating pressure air mattresses: one laboratory-based strategy. J Tissue Viability 2004; 14:51–58.

94. Tur E, Brenner S. Cutaneous blood flow measurements for the detection of malignancy in pigmented skin lesions. Dermatology 1992; 184:8–11.

95. Junger M, Steins A, Schlagenhauff B, Rassner G. Microcirculation of cutaneous melanoma. Hautarzt 1999; 50:848–852.

96. Ilias MA, Wardell K, Stucker M, Anderson C, Salerud EG. Assessment of pigmented skin lesions in terms of blood perfusion estimates. Skin Res Technol 2004; 10:43–49.

97. Wang I, Andersson Engels S, Nilsson GE, Wardell K, Svanberg K. Superficial blood flow following photodynamic therapy of malignant non-melanoma skin tumors measured by laser Doppler perfusion imaging. Br J Dermatol 1997; 136:184–189.

98. Gupta SC, Khiabani KT, Stephenson LL, Zamboni WA. Effect of liposuction on skin perfusion. Plast Reconstr Surg 2003; 112:1965.

99. Ribuffo D, Muratori L, Antoniadou K, Fanini F, Martelli E, Marini M, Messineo D, Trinci M, Scuderi N. A hemodynamic approach to clinical results in the TRAM flap after selective delay. Plast Reconstr Surg 1997; 99:1706–1714.

100. Place MJ, Witt P, Hendricks D. Cutaneous blood flow patterns in free flaps determined by laser Doppler flowmetry. J Reconstr Microsurg 1996; 12:355–358.

101. Niezgoda JA, Cianci P, Folden BW, Ortega RL, Slade JB, Storrow AB. The effect of hyperbaric oxygen therapy on a burn wound model in human volunteers. Plast Reconstr Surg 1997; 99:1620–1625.

102. Droog EJ, Steenbergen W, Sjoberg F. Measurement of depth of burns by laser Doppler perfusion imaging. Burns 2001; 27:561–568.

103. Riordan CL, McDonough M, Davidson JM, Corley R, Perlov C, Barton R, Guy J, Nanney LB. Non-contact laser Doppler imaging in burn depth analysis of the extremities. J Burn Care Rehabil 2003; 24:177–186.

104. Jeng JC, Bridgeman A, Shivnan L, Thornton PM, Alam H, Clarke TJ, Jablonski KA, Jordan MH. Laser Doppler imaging determines need for excision and grafting in advance of clinical judgment: a prospective blinded trial. Burns 2003; 29:665–670.

105. Monfrecola G, Moffa G, Procaccini EM. Non-ionizing electromagnetic radiations, emitted by a cellular phone, modify cutaneous blood flow. Dermatology 2003; 207:3–5.

106. Bernardi L, Hayoz D, Wenzel R, Passino C, Calciati A, Weber R, Noll G. Synchronous and baroceptor-sensitive oscillations in skin microcirculation: evidence for central autonomic control. Am J Physiol 1997; 273:H1867–H1878.

107. Ozbebit FY, Esen F, Gulec S, Esen H. Evaluation of forearm microvascular blood flow regulation by laser Doppler flowmetry, iontophoresis, and curve analysis: contribution of axon reflex. Microvasc Res 2004; 67:207–214.

108. Kolev OI, Nilsson G, Tibbling L. Influence of intense sound stimuli on skin microcirculation. Clin Auton Res 1995; 5:187–190.

109. Kano T, Shimoda O, Higashi K, Sadanaga M. Effects of neural blockade and general anesthesia on the laser Doppler skin blood flow waves recorded from the finger or toe. J Auton Nerv Syst 1994; 48:257–266.

110. Willette RN, Hieble JP, Sauermelch CF. The role of alpha adrenoceptor subtypes in sympathetic control of the acral-cutaneous microcirculation. J Pharmacol Exp Therap 1991; 256:599–605.

111. Mashimo T, Pak M, Choe H, Inagaki Y, Yamamoto M, Yoshiya I. Effects of vasodilators guanethidine, nicardipine, nitroglycerine, and prostaglandin E1 on primary afferent nociceptors in humans. J Clin Pharmacol 1997; 37:330–335.

112. Khan F, Kennedy G, Spence VA, Newton DJ, Belch JJ. Peripheral cholinergic function in humans with chronic fatigue syndrome, Gulf War syndrome and with illness following organophosphate exposure. Clin Sci (Lond) 2004; 106:183–189.
113. Elam M, Wallin BG. Skin blood flow responses to mental stress in man depend on body temperature. Acta Physiol Scan 1987; 129:429–431.
114. Yamashita K, Tochihara Y. Effects of hyperoxia on thermoregulatory responses during feet immersion to hot water in humans. J Physiol Anthropol Appl Human Sci 2003; 22:181–185.
115. Bornmyr S, Svensson H, Lilja B, Sundkvist G. Skin temperature changes and changes in skin blood flow monitored with laser Doppler flowmetry and imaging; a methodological study in normal humans. Clin Physiol 1997; 17:71–81.
116. Hassan AA, Rayman G, Tooke JE. Effect of indirect heating on the postural control of skin blood flow in the human foot. Clin Sci 1986; 70:577–582.
117. Hassan AA, Tooke JE. Effect of changes in local skin temperature on postural vasoconstriction in man. Clin Sci 1988; 74:201–206.
118. Kolev OI. Cutaneous microcirculatory reaction to externally and internally applied cold caloric stimuli and its habituation. Clin Auton Res 2003; 13:295–297.
119. Winsor T, Haumschild DJ, Winsor D, Mikail A. Influence of local and environmental temperatures on cutaneous circulation with use of laser Doppler flowmetry. Angiology 1989; 40:421–428.
120. Steurer J, Hoffman U, Bollinger A. Skin hyperemia in a habitual blusher. Vasa 1997; 26:135–136.
121. Tur E, Ryatt KS, Maibach HI. Idiopathic recalcitrant facial flushing syndrome. Dermatologica 1990; 181:5–7.
122. Frodin T, Alund G, Varenhorst E. Measurement of skin blood flow and water evaporation as a means of objectively assessing hot flushes after orchidectomy in patients with prostate cancer. The Prostate 1985; 7:203–208.
123. Wilkin JK. Quantitative assessment of alcohol-provoked flushing. Arch Dermatol 1986; 122:63–65.
124. Wilkin JK, Fortner G, Reinhardt LA, Flowers OV, Kilpatrick SJ, Streeter WC. Prostaglandins and nicotinate-provoked increase in cutaneous blood flow. Clin Pharmacol Ther 1985; 38:273–277.
125. Wiles PG, Grant PJ, Davies JA. The differential effect of arginine vasopressin on skin blood flow in man. Clin Sci 1986; 71:633–638.
126. Lenasi H, Strucl M. Effect of regular physical training on cutaneous microvascular reactivity. Med Sci Sports Exerc 2004; 36:606–612.
127. Kvernmo HD, Stefanovska A, Kirkeboen KA. Enhanced endothelial activity reflected in cutaneous blood flow oscillations of athletes. Eur J Appl Physiol 2003; 90:16–22.
128. Vassalle C, Lubrano V, Domenici C, L'Abbate A. Influence of chronic aerobic exercise on microcirculatory flow and nitric oxide in humans. Int J Sports Med 2003; 24:30–35.
129. Waeber B, Schaller MD, Nussberger J, Bussien JP, Hofbauer KG, Brunner HR. Skin blood flow reduction induced by cigarette smoking. Role of vasopressin. Am J Physiol 1984; 247:H895–H901.
130. Nicita-Mauro V. Smoking, calcium, calcium antagonists, and aging. Exp Gerontol 1990; 25:393–399.
131. Pellaton C, Kubli S, Feihl F, Waeber B. Blunted vasodilatory responses in the cutaneous microcirculation of cigarette smokers. Am Heart J 2002; 144:269–274.
132. Noble M, Voegeli D, Clough GF. A comparison of cutaneous vascular responses to transient pressure loading in smokers and non-smokers. J Rehabil Res Dev 2003; 40:283–288.
133. Lecerof H, Bornmyr S, Lilja B, De Pedis G, Hulthen UL. Acute effects of doxazosin and atenolol on smoking-induced peripheral vasoconstriction in hypertensive habitual smokers. J Hypertens Suppl 1990; 8:S29–S33.
134. Salmasi AM, BelcaroG, Nicolaides AN. Impaired venoarteriolar reflex as a possible cause for nifedipine-induced ankle oedema. Int J Cardiol 1991; 30:303–307.
135. Iabichella ML, Dell'Omo G, Melillo E, Pedrinelli R. Calcium channel blockers blunt postural cutaneous vasoconstriction in hypertensive patients. Hypertension 1997; 29:751–756.
136. Orlandi C, Rossi M, Finardi G. Evaluation of the dilator capacity of skin blood vessels of hypertensive patients by laser Doppler flowmetry. Microvasc Res 1988; 35:21–26.
137. Kvernebo K, Slagsvold CE, Stranden E, Kroese A, Larsen S. Laser Doppler flowmetry in evaluation of lower limb resting skin circulation. A study in healthy controls and atherosclerotic patients. Scand J Clin Lab Invest 1988; 48:621–626.
138. Winsor T, Haumschild DJ, Winsor D, Mikail A. Influence of local and environmental temperatures on cutaneous circulation with use of laser Doppler flowmetry. Angiology 1989; 40:421–428.
139. Cisek PL, Eze AR, Comerota AJ, Kerr R, Brake B, Kelly P. Microcirculatory compensation to progressive atherosclerotic disease. Ann Vasc Surg 1997; 11:49–53.

140. Karanfilian RG, Lynch TG, Lee BC, Long JB, Hobson RW. The assessment of skin blood flow in peripheral vascular disease by laser Doppler velocimetry. Am Surg 1984; 50:641–644.

141. Leonardo G, Arpaia MR, Del Guercio R. A new method for the quantitative assessment of arterial insufficiency of the limbs: cutaneous postischemic hyperemia test by laser Doppler. Angiology 1987; 38:378–385.

142. Kristensen JK, Karlsmark T, Bisgaard H, Sondergaard J. New parameters for evaluation of blood flow in patients with leg ulcers. Acta Derm Venereol 1986; 66:62–65.

143. Koman LA, Smith BP, Pollock FE Jr, Smith TL, Pollock D, Russel GB. The microcirculatory effects of peripheral sympathectomy. J Hand Surg Am 1995; 20:709–717.

144. Hartmann BR, Bassenge E, Pittler M. Effect of carbon dioxide-enriched water and fresh water on the cutaneous microcirculation and oxygen tension in the skin of the foot. Angiology 1997; 48:337–343.

145. Melhuish JM, Krishnamoorthy L, Bethaves T, Clark M, Williams RJ, Harding KG. Measurement of the skin microcirculation through intact bandages using laser Doppler flowmetry. Med Biol Eng Comput 2004; 42:259–263.

146. Stansberry KB, Hill MA, Shapiro SA, McNitt PM, Bhatt BA, Vinik AI. Impairment of peripheral blood flow responses in diabetes resembles an enhanced aging effect. Diabetes Care 1997; 20:1711–1716.

147. Rossi M, Lall K, Standfield N, Dornhorst A. Impaired vasoconstriction of peripheral cutaneous blood flow in Type 1 diabetic patients following food ingestion. Diabet Med 1998; 15:463–466.

148. Rendell M, Bergman T, O'Donnell G, Drobny E, Borgos J, Bonner F. Microvascular blood flow, volume and velocity measured by laser Doppler techniques in IDDM. Diabetes 1989; 38:819–824.

149. Bornmyr S, Svensson H, Lilja B, Sundkvist G. Cutaneous vasomotor responses in young type I diabetic patients. J Diabetes Complicat 1997; 11:21–26.

150. Boolell M, Tooke JE. The skin hyperaemic response to local injection of substance P and capsaicin in diabetes mellitus. Diabetic Med 1990; 7:898–901.

151. Young MJ, Veves A, Walker MG, Boulton AJM. Correlations between nerve function and tissue oxygenation in diabetic patients: further clues to the aetiology of diabetic neuropathy. Diabetologia 1992; 35:1146–1150.

152. Rendell M, Bamisedun O. Skin blood flow and current perception in pentoxifylline treated diabetic neuropathy. Angiology 1992; 43:843–851.

153. Walmsley D, Wiles PG. Early loss of neurogenic inflammation in the human diabetic foot. Clin Sci Colch 1991; 80:605–610.

154. Jaap AJ, Shore AC, Tooke JE. Relationship of insulin resistance to microvascular dysfunction in subjects with fasting hyperglycemia. Diabetologia 1997; 40:238–243.

155. Wall B. Assessment of ischemic feet in diabetes. J Wound Care 1997; 6:32–38.

156. Koltringer P, Langsteger W, Lind P, Klima G, Wakonig P, Eber O, Reisecker F. Autonomic neuropathies in skin and its incidence in non-insulin-dependent diabetes mellitus. Horm Metabol Res 1992; 26:S87–S89.

157. Valensi P, Smagghue O, Paries J, Velayoudon P, Nguyen TN, Attali JR. Peripheral vasoconstrictor responses to sympathetic activation in diabetic patients: relationship with rheological disorders. Metabolism 1997; 46:235–241.

158. Westerman RA, Low AM, Widdop RE, Neild TO, Delaney CA. Non-invasive tests of neurovascular function in human and experimental diabetes mellitus. In: Molinatti GM, Bar RS, Belfiore F, Porta M, eds. Endothelial Cell Function in Diabetic Microangiopathy. Problems in Methodology and Clinical Aspects, Vol 9, Karger, Basel, 1990:127.

159. Aso Y, Inukai T, Takemura Y. Evaluation of microangiopathy of the skin in patients with non-insulin-dependent diabetes mellitus by laser Doppler Flowmetry; microvasculatory responses to beraprost sodium. Diabetes Res Clin Pract 1997; 36:19–26.

160. Belcaro G, Laurora G, Cesarone MR, Pomante P. Elastic stockings in diabetic microangiopathy. Long-term clinical and microcirculatory evaluation. Vasa 1992; 21: 193–197.

161. Yosipovitch G, Schneiderman J, Erman A, Chetrit A, Milo G, Boner G, van Dijk DJ. The effect of an angiotensin converting enzyme inhibitor on skin microvascular hyperemia in microalbuminuric insulin-dependent diabetes mellitus. Diabet Med 1997; 14:235–241.

162. Flynn MD, Boolell M, Tooke JE, Watkins PJ. The effect of insulin infusion on capillary blood flow in the diabetic neuropathic foot. Diabet Med 1992; 9:630–634.

163. Aman J, Berne C, Ewald U, Tuvemo T. Cutaneous blood flow during a hypoglycaemic clamp in insulin-dependent diabetic patients and healthy subjects. Clin Sci Colch 1992; 82:615–618.

164. Belcaro G, Marelli C, Pomante P, Laurora G, Cesarone MR, Ricci A, Girardello R, Barsotti A. Fibrinolytic enhancement in diabetic microangiopathy with defibrotide. Angiology 1992; 43:793–800.

165. Rendell MS, Shehan MA, Kahler K, Bailey KL, Eckermann AJ. Effect of calcium channel blockade on skin blood flow in diabetic hypertension: a comparison of isradipine and atenolol. Angiology 1997; 48:203–213.

166. Caselli A, Hanane T, Jane B, Carter S, Khaodhiar L, Veves A. Topical methyl nicotinate induced skin vasodilation in diabetic neuropathy. J Diabetes Complications 2003; 17:205–210.

167. Shawket S, Dickerson C, Hazleman B, Brown MJ. Selective suprasensitivity to calcitonin-gene-related peptide in the hands in Raynaud's phenomenon. Lancet 1989; 2: 1354–1357.

168. Suichies HE, Aarnoudse JG, Wouda AA, Jentink HW, de Mul FF, Greve J. Digital blood flow in cooled and contralateral finger in patients with Raynaud's phenomenon. Comparative measurements between photoelectrical plethysmography and laser Doppler flowmetry. Angiology 1992; 43:134–141.

169. Allen JA, Devlin MA, McGrann S, Doherty CC. An objective test for the diagnosis and grading of vasospasm in patients with Raynaud's syndrome. Clin Sci 1992; 82:529–534.

170. Kurozawa Y, NasuY, Oshiro H. Finger systolic blood pressure measurements after finger cooling. Using the laser–Doppler method for assessing vibration-induced white finger. J Occup Med 1992; 34:683–686.

171. Kristensen JK, Englhart M, Nielsen T. Laser Doppler measurement of digital blood flow regulation in normals and in patients with Raynaud's phenomenon. Acta Derm Venereol 1983; 63:43–47.

172. Goodfiled M, Hume A, Rowell N. Reactive hyperemic responses in systemic sclerosis patients and healthy controls. J Invest Dermatol 1989; 93:368–371.

173. Engelhart M, Seibold JR. The effect of local temperature versus sympathetic tone on digital perfusion in Raynaud's phenomenon. Angiology 1990; 41:715–723.

174. Wollersheim H, Reyenga J, Thien T. Postocclusive reactive hyperemia of fingertips, monitored by laser Doppler velocimetry in the diagnosis of Raynaud's phenomenon. Microvasc Res 1989; 38:286–295.

175. Martinez RM, Saponaro A, Dragagna G, Santoro L, Leopardi N, Russo R, Tassone G. Cutaneous circulation in Raynaud's phenomenon during emotional stress. A morphological and functional study using capillaroscopy and laser Doppler. Int Angiol 1992; 11:316–320.

176. Whitmore SE, Wigley FM, Wise RA. Acute effect of topical minoxidil on digital blood flow in patients with Raynaud's phenomenon. J Rheumatol 1995; 22:50–54.

177. Engelhart M. Ketanserin in the treatment of Raynaud's phenomenon associated with generalized scleroderma. Br J Dermatol 1988; 119:751–754.

178. Brouwer RM, Wenting GJ, Schalekamp MA. Acute effects and mechanism of action of ketanserin in patients with primary Raynaud's phenomenon. J Cardiovasc Pharmacol 1990; 15:868–876.

179. Bunker CB, Lanigan S, Rustin MHA, Dowd PM. The effects of topically applied hexyl nicotinate lotion on the cutaneous blood flow in patients with Raynaud's phenomenon. Br J Dermatol 1988; 119:771–776.

180. Rustin MHA, Newton JA, Smith NP, Dowd PM. The treatment of chilblains with nifedipine: the results of a pilot study, a double-blind placebo-controlled randomized study and a long-term open trial. Br J Dermatol 1989; 120:267–275.

181. Agusni I, Beck JS, Potts RC, Cree IA, Ilias MI. Blood flow velocity in cutaneous lesions of leprosy. Int J Lepr Other Mycobact Dis 1988; 56:394–400.

182. Abbot NC, Beck JS, Feval F, Weiss F, Mobayen MH, Ghazi-Saidi K, Dowlati Y, Velayati AA, Stanford JL. Immunotherapy with Mycobacterium vaccae and peripheral blood flow in long-treated leprosy patients, a randomised, placebo-controlled trial. Eur J Vasc Endovasc Surg 2002; 24:202–208.

183. Wilder Smith A, Wilder Smith E. Electrophysiological evaluation of peripheral autonomic function in leprosy patients, leprosy contacts and controls. Int J Lepr Other Mycobact Dis 1996; 64:433–440.

184. Leu AJ, Yanar A, Jost J, Hoffman U, Franzeck UK, Bollinger A. Microvascular dynamics in normal skin versus skin overlying Kaposi's sarcoma. Microvasc Res 1994; 47:140–144.

185. Rodgers GP, Schechter AN, Noguchi CT, Klein HG, Nienhuis AW, Bonner RF. Periodic microcirculatory flow in patients with sickle-cell disease. N Engl J Med 1984; 311:1534–1538.

186. Tur E, Politi Y, Rubinstein A. Cutaneous blood flow abnormalities in hypertriglyceridemia. J Invest Dermatol 1994; 103:597–600.

187. Algotsson A, Nordberg A, Almkvist O, Winblad B. Skin vessel reactivity is impaired in Alzheimer's disease. Neurobiol Aging 1995; 16:577–582.

188. Maltz JS, Eberling JL, Jagust WJ, Budinger TF. Enhanced cutaneous vascular response in AD subjects under donepezil therapy. Neurobiol Aging 2004; 25:475–481.

189. Vuilleumier P, Decosterd D, Maillard M, Burnier M, Hayoz D. Postischemic forearm skin reactive hyperemia is related to cardiovascular risk factors in a healthy female population. J Hypertens 2002; 20:1753–1757.

190. Wardell K, Nilsson GE. Duplex laser Doppler perfusion imaging. Microvasc Res 1996; 52:171–182.

191. Bornmyr S, Martensson A, Svensson H, Nilsson KG, Wollmer P. A new device combining laser Doppler perfusion imaging and digital photography. Clin Physiol 1996; 16:535–541.
192. Saravanamuthu J, Seifalian AM, Reid WM, Maclean AB. A new technique to map vulva microcirculation using laser Doppler perfusion imager. Int J Gynecol Cancer 2003; 13:812–818.
193. Chen CT, Hsiu H, Fan JS, Lin FC, Liu YT. Complexity analysis of beat-to-beat skin-surface laser-Doppler flowmetry signals in stroke patients. Microcirculation 2015; 22 (5): 370–377
194. Hsiu H, Hsu WC, Wu YF, Hsu CL, Chen CY. Differences in the skin-surface laser Doppler signals between polycystic ovary syndrome and normal subjects. Microcirculation 2014; 21(2):124–130
195. Hsiu H, Hsu CL, Hu HF, Hsiao FC, Yang SH. Complexity analysis of beat-to-beat skin-surface laser-Doppler signals in diabetic subjects. Microvasc Res 2014; 93: 9–13
196. Hsiu H, Chen CT, Hung SH, Chen GZ, Huang YL. Differences in time-domain and spectral indexes of skin-surface laser-Doppler signals between controls and breast-cancer subjects. Clin Hemorheol Microcirc 2018; 69(3):371–381
197. Lin FC, Hsiu H, Chiu HS, Chen CT, Hsu CH. Characteristics of pulse-waveform and laser-Doppler indices in frozen-shoulder patients. Biomed Signal Processing and Control 2020; 56: In Press (Feb 2020).

55 Confocal Raman Microspectroscopy in the Assessment of Skin Barrier Function and Drug Penetration

Jacqueline Resende de Azevedo, Marie-Alexandrine Bolzinger, Stéphanie Briançon, and Yves Chevalier
University of Lyon, Université Claude Bernard Lyon 1, Villeurbanne, France

Yuri Dancik
Le Studium Loire Valley Institute of Advanced Studies, France
University of Tours, Tours, France

CONTENTS

55.1 INTRODUCTION

The outermost skin layer, the stratum corneum (SC), consists of corneocytes embedded in a lipid matrix. The intercellular lipids are mainly cholesterol, ceramides, and free fatty acids organized into multilamellar stacks of bilayers. The state of intercellular lipids strongly influences the permeability of drugs that diffuse through the intercellular pathway. Hence, the lipid organization in the SC is of primary importance for the control of drug delivery to the skin.

The molecular organization of SC lipids is still not firmly established. Three main structures have been described: (1) the orthorhombic phase, the densest organization with crystalline hydrocarbon chains and unequal distribution in the lattice, resulting in two different distances between lattice planes (0.37 nm and 0.41 nm); (2) the hexagonal phase with equally spaced crystallized hydrocarbon chains; (3) and the fluid lamellar phase, where the lipids are in a fluid (molten) state. The current view of lipid organization in SC at 32°C is a two-phase coexistence of the orthorhombic and hexagonal structures (Pilgram et al. 1999; Norlén 2001; Babita et al. 2006; Bouwstra and Ponec 2006; Bouwstra et al. 2007). An open question with respect to the lateral packing of lipids (Norlén 2001) is whether the lipid matrix is made of a single gel "phase" or several coexisting fluid and solid (crystalline and/or gel) phases. Another question that has been addressed is whether the barrier efficiency of the SC is related to the extents of the orthorhombic, hexagonal, and lamellar phases (Boncheva et al. 2008; Damien and Boncheva 2010; Groen et al. 2011).

Confocal Raman microspectroscopy (CRM) has become a major technique for the study of skin because of its non-destructive character and the possibility of monitoring the penetration of the drug and/or penetration enhancer, provided that characteristic Raman bands can be associated with the compounds (Förster et al. 2011a). Simultaneously, the spectroscopic method yields time structural information on the conformation changes of endogenous molecules in the skin induced by the absorption of a drug, a moisturizer, a penetration enhancer, or a change in environmental parameters such as temperature or relative humidity. When the Raman spectrometer is associated with a confocal microscope, it is called CRM. CRM provides three-dimensional spectroscopic information with the spatial resolution of an optical microscope.

In this chapter, we first briefly describe the principles of CRM and variants of it that have been used towards the investigation of the skin barrier. Then, we report on the use of CRM to study (1) the major intrinsic SC components and physical features that contribute to the skin barrier function and (2) the effects of age, hydration, and dermatological diseases on these intrinsic components and physical features. We then review the use of CRM to study skin absorption and penetration of drugs, as well as the effects of penetration enhancers, in human skin in vivo, ex vivo, and reconstructed human skin models.

55.2   PRINCIPLES OF CONFOCAL RAMAN MICROSPECTROSCOPY

CRM is based on the combined use of spectroscopic analysis and structural observation by optical microscopy. The characteristic features of this technique are the chemical analysis by spectroscopy and the three-dimensional mapping of the sample by microscopy. CRM brings about new possibilities and definite benefits over the classical methods for assessing skin absorption.

The several classical methods for assessing skin penetration of drugs (or any other kind of molecule) from a formulation containing them rely on in vitro measurements of passive diffusion of drugs through excised skin (Bronaugh and Maibach 1999). The diffusion of drugs through excised skin from a donor compartment containing the formulation to a receptor compartment containing a receiver fluid is measured. The permeation profile is a plot of the cumulated amount of drug that reaches the receptor fluid as a function of the duration of exposure to the formulation. The distribution of drug molecules inside the skin layers is more difficult to measure. In a classical Franz cell experiment, the cell is dismantled at the end of the experiment, the skin layers are separated, and an analysis of the drug accumulated within each layer is performed. This methodology generally yields the total amount of drug in the tissue and can also give the distribution of drug in the vertical direction (z-direction). Information pertaining to the spatial distribution in the horizontal direction (x,y plane) and the possible modification of the skin structure induced by absorption of compounds are missing. The usual method to obtain depth-dependent profiles of the drug content is the so-called tape stripping method; it is restricted to analysis in the SC. Chemical or spectroscopic analysis of histological sections of skin provide the distribution along the depth and one lateral direction.

These various methods (tape stripping, histological sectioning) accurately quantify permeant distribution, but they are destructive, involving hard manipulation of the skin samples (Touitou et al. 1998; Dancik et al. 2018), and are time-intensive. Moreover, time-resolved experiments (i.e., study of dynamic processes) are difficult to implement, and information on the possible perturbations of the structure of endogenous skin components is missing.

Spectroscopic methods associated with a microscope overcome the limitations reported earlier because they are non-destructive. They include infrared spectroscopy in attenuated total reflectance mode (ATR-IR) (Francoeur et al. 1990; Naik et al. 1995; Zhang et al. 2007a) and CRM. CRM has several advantages over IR microscopy, such as higher sensitivity, especially in media containing large amounts of water, and confocal microscopy that allows recording time-revolved 3D pictures of the distribution of spectral data inside skin. CRM measures vibrational frequencies of chemical bonds and parts of molecules. It allows distinguishing chemical species through their characteristic vibrations and provides fingerprints for the identification of substances without requiring any labeling or dyeing.

Raman spectroscopy is closely related to IR spectroscopy, since in both techniques the frequencies of molecular vibrations are measured. IR and Raman spectroscopy both measure the vibrational energy of molecules, but the interaction between the incident radiation and the compound differs. Raman spectroscopy is sensitive to polarizable chemical bonds, whatever their polarity, while IR absorption takes place for polar bonds for which the molecular vibration changes the dipole moment. IR requires a change in the dipole moment of the molecule upon absorption of light, whereas Raman relies on a change in the polarizability of the molecule. Therefore, the spectroscopic selection rules are different for both techniques. Symmetric molecules show Raman spectra, but not many IR bands. Most molecules present in the skin have both absorption bands in Raman and IR spectroscopy.

IR spectroscopy is a classical absorption technique where the absorbance or the attenuated reflectance of the sample is measured. Conversely, Raman spectroscopy relies on measurements of scattered light, specifically, light scattering by the sample. This makes an important difference between Raman and IR spectroscopy (Caspers et al. 2001). When using Raman spectroscopy, the sample is irradiated with an intense beam of monochromatic light from a laser. A very small part of the light (~1 photon out of 10^8) undergoes inelastic scattering from molecular vibrations, resulting in Stokes and anti-Stokes scattered light at frequencies different from the incident radiation. The frequency shifts correspond to the frequencies of the molecular vibrations; they are expressed as wavenumbers (cm^{-1}), as in IR spectroscopy.

The strong absorbance of water limits the application of IR spectroscopy to tissues containing water. Only thin samples can be analyzed in transmission mode, and small penetration depths are available in attenuated reflection mode. On the other hand, Raman absorbance of water is weak, and the frequency of the light can be chosen independently of the frequency range of the spectroscopic analysis. This is a definite advantage for a method relying on a scattering phenomenon. Therefore, the wavelength of the incident laser light for Raman analysis is selected such that the sample is transparent and there is no fluorescence that would disturb the analysis. In modern equipment, several laser wavelengths are available (from green light to infrared) as excitation light to match the various sample properties. The depth of penetration in the sample can reach several 10s of µm. Since visible light is used, a confocal optical microscope is associated for collecting 3D maps of Raman spectra with the spatial resolution of optical microscopy (0.2 to 0.5 µm in x,y plane; 0.5 to 1 µm in z-axis).

Assignment of peaks in the resulting spectra can be complex. There are many lists of Raman frequencies and assignments in the literature (Barry et al. 1992; Anigbogu et al. 1995; Förster et al. 2011a; Tfaili et al. 2012a). The Raman frequency assignments of the major vibrational modes for the SC of mammalian skin are given in Table 55.1.

The intensities of Raman bands are proportional to the concentration of species, so that semiquantitative or quantitative analyses can be done (Tfaili et al. 2012a). A close selection of appropriate conditions is achieved to study the skin, especially the excitation wavelength of the laser source (Tfaili et al. 2012b). Various excitation wavelengths in the visible or near-IR (from 532 nm to 1064 nm) are available as commercial sources; they are safe for in vivo measurements. Wavelengths of

TABLE 55.1

Raman Assignments of the Major Vibrational Modes for Stratum Corneum

Raman Wave Number (cm⁻¹)	Assignment
526	ν(S–S)
600	ρ(H)
623	ν(C=S)
644	ν(C=S); amide IV
746	ρ(CH$_2$) in phase
827	δ(CCH) aliphatic
850	δ(CCH) aromatic
883	ρ(CH$_2$); ν(C–C); ν(C–N)
931	ρ(CH$_3$) terminal; ν(C–C) of proteins α-helix
956	ρ(CH$_3$); δ(CCH) alkenic
1002	ν(C–C) aromatic ring
1031	ν(C–C) skeletal *cis* conformation
1062	ν(C–C) skeletal *trans* conformation
1082	ν(C–C) skeletal random conformation
1126	ν(C–C) skeletal *trans* conformation
1155	ν(C–C); δ(COH)
1172	ν(C–C)
1244	δ(CH$_2$) wagging; ν(C–N) amide III disordered
1274	ν(C–N); δ(NH) amide III of proteins α-helix
1296	δ(CH$_2$)
1336	not assigned
1385	δ(CH$_3$) symmetric
1421	δ(CH$_3$)
1438	δ(CH$_2$) scissoring
1552	δ(NH); ν(C–N) amide II
1585	ν(C=C) alkenic
1602	not assigned
1652	ν(C=O) amide I of proteins α-helix
1743	ν(C=O) amide I of lipids
1768	ν(COO)
2723	ν(C–H) aliphatic
2852	ν(C–H in CH$_2$) symmetric
2883	ν(C–H in CH$_2$) asymmetric
2931	ν(C–H in CH$_3$) symmetric
2958	ν(C–H in CH$_3$) asymmetric
3060	ν(C–H) alkenic
3280	ν(O–H) of H$_2$O

Abbreviations: δ = *Deformation;* ν = *Stretch;* ρ = *Rock.*
Source: *From Förster et al. 2011a, with permission.*

532 nm, 633 nm, and 785 nm were widely used to record Raman spectra inside skin. This parameter affects the scattered Raman intensity, possible fluorescence background, and signal attenuation with skin depth (Tfaili et al. 2012b). The actual *z*-depth in the sample is different from the optical path length because of the different refractive indices of the skin layers.

55.3 VARIANTS OF RAMAN SPECTROSCOPY

There are several variants of classical Raman spectroscopy besides the spontaneous Raman scattering technique where the spectrum acquisition is a direct measurement of the scattered light. Surface-enhanced Raman scattering (SERS) shows enhanced intensity for molecules located in the vicinity of metal particles. The sensitivity improvement requires the deposition of metal nanoparticles at the surface of the sample. SERS allows a specific analysis of the species present at the sample surface. Resonance Raman spectroscopy provides a selective spectrum of a molecule with high sensitivity when the frequency of the laser light of the Raman spectrometer is tuned to a UV-vis absorption band of the molecule. Coherent Raman spectroscopy (Min et al. 2011) relies on non-linear effects of two-photon absorption. A resonance occurs when the frequency difference between the two lights matches the frequency of the molecular vibration. A signal-to-noise ratio enhancement by several orders of magnitude is achieved when the resonance condition is met. However, such resonance methods are not spectroscopic methods because a single Raman frequency is measured at once. Coherent anti-Stokes Raman scattering (CARS) (Evans and Xie 2008) and stimulated Raman scattering (SRS) (Downes and Elfick 2010; Slipchenko et al. 2010) are the two major techniques. Several improvements of these techniques were recently introduced in order to increase the sensitivity an decrease the non-resonant background by epi-detection (Li et al. 2005); high-speed confocal microscopy data can be collected (Saar et al. 2010). Equipment for two-color microscopy has been designed (Lu et al. 2012). SRS appears more sensitive and accurate than CARS (Nandakumar et al. 2009; Freudiger et al. 2008). Such techniques allow time-resolved confocal microscopy measurements with high sensitivity at the selected vibration frequencies of the penetrant molecules. Determination of band shifts that are characteristic of interactions of penetrant molecules and skin components requires several measurements at different specific frequencies and merging them into a full spectrum. A recent SRS technique making use of modulation of excitation Raman frequencies and signal demodulation by Fourier transform allows the acquisition of several Raman bands at the same time, and possibly parts of the Raman spectra (Fu et al. 2012). SRS has been used to investigate the lipid distribution in skin (Klossek et al., 2017; Wanjiku et al., 2019), as well as the skin absorption of *trans*-retinol and propylene glycol (Saar et al. 2010), ketoprofen and ibuprofen (Saar et al. 2011), and retinoic acid (Freudiger et al. 2008). Near-infrared Fourier transform (NIRFT) Raman spectroscopy designates the use of a higher wavelength laser, typically 1064 nm, to probe skin (Barry et al. 1992; Williams et al. 1993; Anigbogu et al. 1995; Gniadecka et al. 1998; Schallreuter et al. 1999; Wohlrab et al., 2001; Knudsen et al. 2002; William et al. 2004; Naito et al. 2008). Advantages over lower, more conventional wavelengths such as 785 nm are deeper penetration of the incident light into the tissue and reduced signal attenuation due to scattering. However, in most NIR systems the laser powers are in the range of a few hundred mW, which may be unsafe for volunteers. Several NIR studies with volunteers have nonetheless been conducted (Knudsen et al. 2002; Schallreuter et al. 1999; Naito et al. 2008).

55.4 CHARACTERIZATION OF INTRINSIC HUMAN SKIN PARAMETERS RELATED TO DRUG PENETRATION

55.4.1 INSTRUMENTATION AND SETTINGS FOR STUDIES WITH VOLUNTEERS

Thanks to the non-invasiveness and non-destructiveness of the method, Raman spectroscopy lends itself to in vivo characterization of the basic composition and morphology of human skin, as well as tracking chemicals applied onto the skin and studying the ensuing effects on skin physiology and morphology. Measurements on volunteers require a Raman spectroscope certified for use with volunteers. Most published studies make use of the gen2-Skin Composition Analyzer (SCA), or its predecessor, the Model 3510 SCA, from RiverD International (Rotterdam, The Netherlands).

In vivo measurements on volunteers are most often performed on the volar forearm. RiverD's instruments incorporate a measurement stage containing a fused silica window onto which the volunteer can place his or her forearm. In addition to the forearm, the water composition of the cheek has been investigated by Egawa and Tagami (2008). Pudney et al. (2012) have described a Raman probe allowing investigation of areas of the body that are more difficult to access; e.g., the axilla, the scalp, and the mouth. However, this probe is not currently commercially available.

The 785-nm laser wavelength is generally used to obtain the "fingerprint region" spectra (400 to 1800 cm^{-1}) of the skin; this is also the region within which topically applied compounds are detected. With the RiverD instruments the "high wavenumber region" spectra (2500 to 4000 cm^{-1}) are acquired using a 671-nm laser. As described later, the high wavenumber region spectra are most often used to obtain the keratin and water intensities from which the skin water content–depth profile can be derived. For in vivo use, the RiverD instruments' laser powers are limited to 20 and 30 mW for the 785-nm and 671-nm laser, respectively. Integration times vary from one study to the next but are generally between 1 and 10 seconds. The skin depths investigated in vivo reach from the surface to either 20 or 40 μm into the skin in most studies. The selected depth increment is generally either 2 or 4 μm.

While the RiverD system utilizes two excitation wavelengths to obtain the fingerprint and high wavenumber region spectra, Chrit et al. (2005) demonstrated in vivo confocal spectra using a probe with one laser source (633 nm) that captures the entire frequency region, from 500 to 3600 cm^{-1}.

55.4.2 Tracking Intrinsic Skin Components and Physical Features

Along with the exceedingly complex biology of skin comes its highly complex barrier functions. There are four skin barriers: the physical, chemical, immunological, and microbial skin barrier (Niehues et al. 2018).

CRM has proven highly useful for investigation into the basic makeup and efficacy of the SC barrier. The major intrinsic constituents of skin contributing to and regulating the physical barrier function include water, natural moisturizing factor (NMF), protein (mainly keratin), and lipid compounds (for a comprehensive review, see Dancik et al. (2015)). Interindividual and intraindividual variability of human skin, age, exposure to water or moisturizers, environmental humidity, and dermatological pathologies are factors that may, individually or in concert, alter the amounts and physical organization of these constituents that strongly influence the absorption and penetration kinetics of topical compounds.

55.4.2.1 Total Water Content and Stratum Corneum Thickness

Caspers et al. (1998, 2000, 2001, 2003) showed that water content in the skin of volunteers could be tracked as a function of depth. The methodology they proposed relies on tracking the Raman bands of water and protein and integrating their respective intensities, 3350 to 3550 cm^{-1} (water) and 2910 to 2960 cm^{-1} (protein). The water content is obtained from the ratio of the water mass to the total tissue mass (consisting of water and dry material):

$$Water\ content = 100\% \times \frac{W}{P} \Big/ \left(\frac{W}{P} + R \right)$$

with W and P designating the water and protein integrated intensities and R a fixed water-to-protein signal proportionality constant. A typical water content–depth profile is shown in Figure 55.1. The Raman spectra were collected at different depths from the skin surface (0 μm) to 20 μm. The intensity of the stretching band of the O–H bond of water increases with depth into the skin. A sharp increase of the Raman band occurs when passing from the SC to the viable epidermis because the viable epidermis contains much more water (~70%) than SC. The water content at the skin surface is typically around 30%. Going deeper into the SC, the water content increases until a plateau value

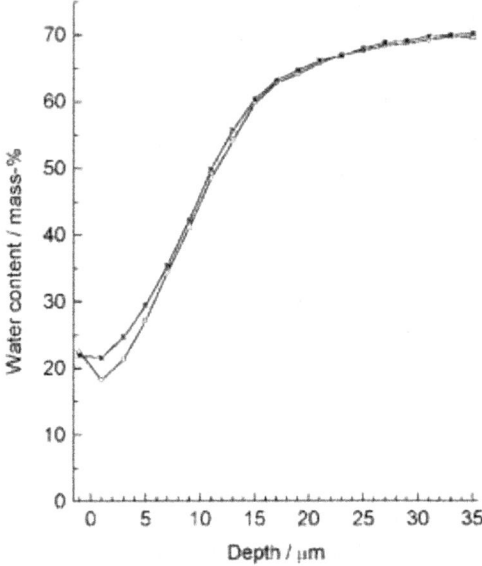

FIGURE 55.1 Consecutive in vivo water concentration profiles of the stratum corneum measured at one spot on the volar aspect of the arm: (o) from the skin surface towards the viable epidermis; (∗) from the viable epidermis to the skin surface. Experimental conditions: signal collection time; 3 seconds per data point; step size; 2 mm; laser power, 100 mW; excitation wavelength, 720 nm. (Reproduced from Caspers et al. 2000 with permission.)

of around 70% is reached. The discontinuity in the water content profile at the end of the SC water gradient yields an estimate of the location of the stratum corneum–stratum granulosum boundary and therefore the thickness of the SC (Caspers et al. 2001).

Caspers et al. (1998, 2001) provided a methodology for tracking intrinsic skin components crucial to its barrier function other than water. They showed semi-quantitative concentration (intensity)–depth profiles of the major constituents of NMF and some of its components, e.g., urea.

With the development of instrumentation designed for use with volunteers, a large number of publications illustrate the power of CRM for non-invasive investigation of human skin parameters. Several groups have proposed different algorithms for determination of the SC thickness from the water content–depth profiles obtained from volunteer studies. Egawa et al. (2007) used the first derivative of the water content profile to find the depth at which the rate of change of water content becomes almost zero, i.e., where the water content reaches an approximately constant value. Crowther et al. (2008) fitted average water content–depth profiles to a four-parameter Weibull model to determine the inflection point in the profile. Hancewicz et al. (2012) argued that no single method could be used for the variety of in vivo water content–depth profiles that can be obtained. They proposed a method that analyzes each given profile using five different logistic function models, yields a distribution of SC thickness values from inflection points, and determines the most likely value for each profile. To date, no consensus as to the most appropriate method has emerged. More recent studies have either fitted a model to the data (Dąbrowska et al. 2016) or approximated the SC thickness as the intercept of the two slopes in the water content–depth profile (Böhling et al. 2014; Mahrhauser et al. 2015; Binder et al. 2017; Richters et al. 2017; Sriram et al. 2018; Dancik et al. 2018; Bielfeldt et al. 2019). Through comparison with other techniques, a consensus has, however, emerged regarding the appropriateness of CRM for the estimation of the SC thickness. SC estimates by CRM are comparable to values obtained by optical coherence tomography (Crowther et al. 2008) and confocal reflectance microscopy (Hancewicz et al. 2012; Böhling et al. 2014). It should be noted, however, that the quality of comparisons depends on body site (Crowther et al. 2008; Böhling et al. 2014).

55.4.2.2 Types of Water Molecules

The general water band in the high wavenumber region is made up of a number of sub-bands assigned to differently bound water molecules. Vyumvuhore et al. (2013, 2015) showed that deconvolution of the total water Raman band (3100 to 3700 cm^{-1}) using its second derivative yielded sub-bands assigned to totally (primary) bound water (3210 cm^{-1}), partially bound water (3280 and 3345 cm^{-1}), and unbound or free water molecules (3470 cm^{-1}). Boireau-Adamezyk et al. (2014) also split the total water signal into three subtypes using a perpendicular drop-down cutoff integrating method, i.e., subdividing the total water band into three regions assigned to "bound," "intermediately mobile," and "mostly mobile" water types (Figure 55.2). The separation into several types refers to the state of binding of water molecules to neighboring protein and lipid constituents of the SC. Totally bound water molecules are tightly bound to the polar sites of SC protein; partially bound water molecules interact through only two or three out of the four hydrogen bonds, whereas unbound water molecules are not directly linked to other SC components.

In a series of papers, Darvin and Lademann's group illustrated the use of a methodology for studying the distribution of water types as a function of depth in the SC (Choe et al. 2016, 2018a, 2018b; Sdobnov et al. 2019). Arguing for greater precision than provided by the perpendicular drop-down cutoff integrating method, they deconvoluted the entire high wavenumber spectral region using 10 Gaussian functions. Among the obtained sub-bands, four are assigned to the different water types: the tightly hydrogen-bound water molecules (single donor–double acceptor around 3005 cm^{-1}), the strongly hydrogen-bound water (double donor–double acceptor around 3277 cm^{-1}), the weakly hydrogen-bound water (single donor–single acceptor around 3458 cm^{-1}), and the free water.

Identifying and tracking the water types is important for the characterization of water mobility in SC and delivery of topical compounds to skin (Boireau-Adamezyk et al. 2014) as well as differentiating between healthy and diseased skin (Vyumvuhore et al. 2013). Binding of water determines the flexibility and stiffness of the SC. Healthy skin contains about 33% of bound water (g water per 100 g tissue) (Vyumvuhore et al. 2013).

Direct measurement of water penetration in the skin by CRM requires replacing water of natural isotopic abundance by deuterated water, D$_2$O, which shows a Raman peak corresponding to the O–D stretching vibration at 2500 cm^{-1}, different from endogenous water and clearly distinguishable

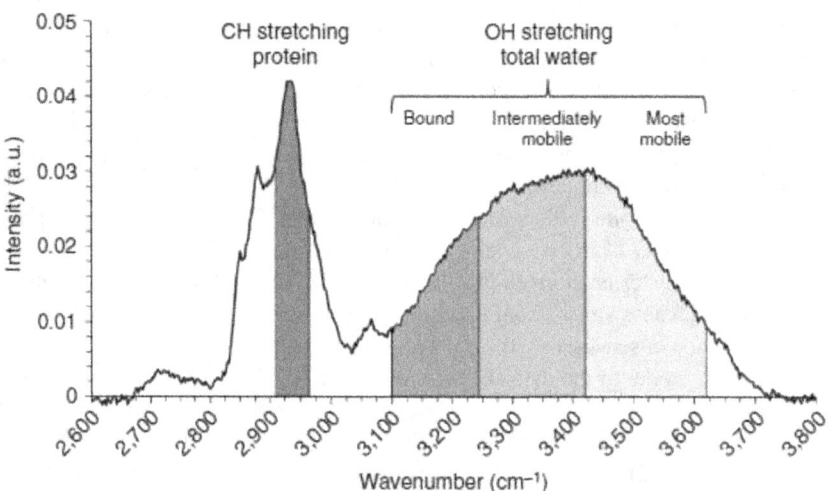

FIGURE 55.2 Raman confocal spectra in the high wavenumber region highlighting the bands of CH stretching and OH stretching that can be used for the calculation of water content and that of the water molecules in the three states based on their mobility. (Reproduced from Boireau-Adamezyk et al. 2014 with permission.)

in the spectra (Förster et al. 2011b). By applying emulsions and surfactant solutions made in deuterated water, the authors observed that water penetrated from the formulations into the SC, keeping a profile similar to that of endogenous water. Penetration of deuterated water in the SC after application of pure D_2O on skin under occlusive conditions was confirmed by Ashtikara et al. (2013).

55.4.2.3   Lipid Conformation and Lateral Packing

CRM has been proven useful in making fundamental observations related to lipid conformation and lateral packing order (Choe et al. 2016; Vyumvuhore et al. 2013, 2015).

Different Raman spectral manifestations of the conformational order of lipids can be drawn from experiments performed on thin films of lipids, such as in recent in vitro studies on ceramide films prepared from seven classes and subclasses of ceramides (Tfayli et al. 2010, 2012a). For example, intrachain conformational order information is obtained from the bands of C–C skeletal optical mode and the band of the twisting CH_2 group, whereas the CH_2 scissoring and stretching modes reflect the lateral packing of the lipid molecules, and the amide I band is used to evaluate the strength of H-bonds (Tfayli et al. 2012a). In vivo determination of lipids ordering by Raman spectroscopy is much more difficult (Tfayli et al. 2012b).

A nice example of in vivo skin imaging used SRS microscopy (**Section 3**) was provided by Saar et al. (2010). In vivo skin optical imaging of mouse skin was achieved by focusing on three vibration bands to image skin structure: lipids (CH_2 stretching, 2845 cm⁻¹), water (OH stretching, 3250 cm⁻¹) and proteins (CH_3 stretching, 2950 cm⁻¹). This allowed imaging the water, lipid, and protein distribution of the SC and the viable epidermis (Figure 55.3A and B). The corneocytes and the intercellular spaces clearly appeared, as well as the sebaceous glands in the epidermis, which appeared both in lipid and water images, i.e., when the incident laser frequency was tuned to the lipids (CH_2 stretching) or water (OH stretching) vibrations. Sebaceous glands appeared clear when the frequency was tuned to that of lipid vibration and dark when it was tuned to the water vibration.

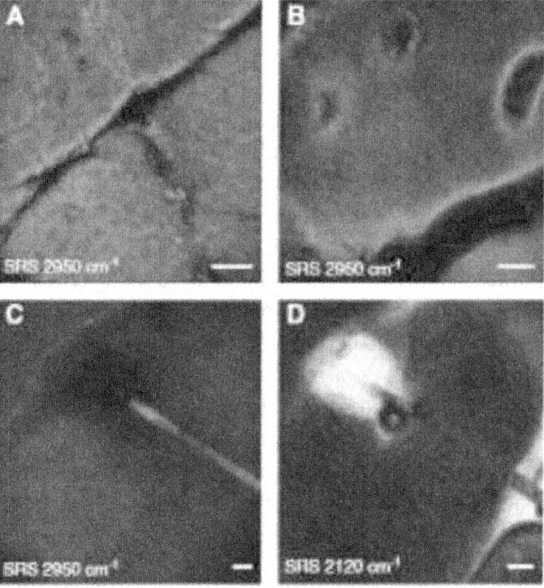

FIGURE 55.3   SRS skin imaging of the forearm of a volunteer; A to C: the frequency was tuned to the CH_3 stretching vibration of proteins at 2950 cm⁻¹: (A): stratum corneum; (B): viable epidermis; (C) hair shaft; (D) SRS skin imaging after applying deuterated DMSO-d_6 (the frequency was tuned to the specific vibration of DMSO-d_6 2120 cm⁻¹) in the same region as shown in (C).

It was possible to detect hairs by SRS imaging the ear of living mice with a frequency tuned to the protein vibration (CH_3 stretching) (Figure 55.3C).

55.4.2.4   Intraindividual and Interindividual Variability Studied by CRM

Assessing intraindividual and interindividual variability in Raman signatures of components of interest is important for establishing the reproducibility of a CRM protocol across a study population, as well as interpreting possible differences in the penetration kinetics of permeants.

Chrit et al. (2005) studied intraindividual and interindividual variations in Raman spectra by analyzing (1) spectral replicates from one area (the fingertip) of one volunteer; (2) spectra from one volunteer across three body sites (fingertip, thenar or palm, and the volar forearm); (3) spectra from the volar forearm of seven volunteers 28 to 60 years of age; and (4) spectra from the fingertip of a volunteer at different depths into the skin. Replicate spectra from the fingertip of a single volunteer revealed differences in the intensities of the amide I band, as well as a band at 855 cm^{-1} attributed to lactate. The authors suggested a difference in sweat content of the skin yielded this difference. Spectra from the fingertip, thenar, and volar forearm of a single volunteer showed intensity differences in the amide I and amide III regions, as well as for the 855, 880, 935, and 1420 cm^{-1} bands. Further analysis of these spectral differences revealed different ratios of α-helix (1652 cm^{-1}), β-sheet (1660 cm^{-1}), and random coil (1666 cm^{-1}) keratin conformation. Differences between the three regions were also found in lipid conformation (*trans* or ordered vs. gauche or disordered) and in the content of pyrrolidone-5-carboxylic acid, a component of NMF. Comparing the spectra of the forearm of seven volunteers, they found a range of differences in lipids, NMF, and amino acid contents. Cluster analysis depicted that these spectral differences could accurately discriminate the volunteers. Depth-dependent analysis (skin surface to a depth of 48 μm in 12 μm increments) showed differences mainly in the 885 cm^{-1} and 1420 cm^{-1} bands. In the forearm, the water bands in the high wavenumber region (3100 to 3600 cm^{-1}) varied the most.

More recent studies on volunteers have shown overall low interindividual and intraindividual variability, with interindividual variability greater than intraindividual variability. Mogilevych et al. (2015) performed their statistical analysis on four integrated areas of the fingerprint region (996 to 1018 cm^{-1}, 1288 to 1314 cm^{-1}, 1388 to 1498 cm^{-1}, and 1558 to 1722 cm^{-1}). Dos Santos et al. (2016) analyzed the fingerprint and high wavenumber spectra in their entirety, while Quatela et al. (2016) focused their analyses on functional aspects of the skin, i.e., the I_{2880}/I_{2850} intensity ratio (lipid conformation order and lateral packing), the $(I_{1130} + I_{1060})/I_{1085}$ ratio (*trans*/gauche packing), the keratin β-sheet/α-helix ratio, the unbound/partially unbound water ratio, and the maximum in the 2930 cm^{-1} band, an indicator of the folding/unfolding process of proteins. Taken together, the results from these studies lead to the conclusions that confocal Raman spectroscopic data are, to a satisfactory extent, reproducible and comparable. In contrast to Chrit et al. (2005), the populations in these studies covered narrower age intervals (22 to 30, 18 to 37, and 20 to 30 years, respectively), and Raman spectra were acquired only from the volunteers' volar forearms, the most commonly used body site for percutaneous penetration studies. Furthermore, Quatela et al. (2016) showed no significant interday variability over five consecutive days of measurements. A spectral variability study performed by Franzen and Windbergs (2014) using excised human skin from three donors similarly found no statistical interindividual and intraindividual differences.

Another matter of variability is that related to different body sites. As an example, Egawa et al. (2007) determined the water content profiles using the method of Caspers et al. described earlier and deduced the SC thickness of 15 volunteers' cheek, upper arm, volar forearm, back of the hand, and the palm. Body site variation was found, particularly in the water content of the upper SC, which was 30% to 40% at all body sites, except in the palm, where it was 20% to 30%. Differences in SC thickness, in particular that of the palm (mean: 173 μm), were in agreement with results from other methodologies.

A recent work illustrates the use of CRM for a less widely studied epithelium, namely lip skin. Using a dental tongue fixation device, Bielfeldt et al. (2019) developed a novel method for investigation of the lip skin barrier by Raman spectroscopy. Total water, ceramide, and NMF–depth profiles were acquired on the lower lip of volunteers. As for skin at other body sites, water content profiles show two distinct slopes, corresponding to the lip SC and the tissue below, and enabling estimation of the lip SC thickness. Overall, average total water content of the lip was a little higher than the average forearm value. SC thickness in the lip skin was similar to volar forearm and leg values; however, lip SC was thicker than cheek skin SC. Ceramide content was also similar to forearm values, whereas NMF content was lower in lip skin than in forearm skin. For each measured parameter, a detailed statistical analysis showing the number of volunteers required to obtain a given error is provided.

55.4.2.5 Effects of Age on Major Skin Components

Water and NMF. A number of studies have formally investigated the effect of age (young vs. elderly volunteers) on the distribution of major skin components using CRM. In general, the SC of elderly volunteers contains less water and is thicker than for younger populations (up to about 30 years of age). It also contains higher amounts of NMF and t-UCA in the forearm skin (Egawa and Tagami 2008; Binder et al. 2017). Egawa and Tagami (2008) did not observe any significant differences in water or NMF in the cheeks of their studied populations. Comparing the age groups 18 to 30, 30 to 40, 40 to 55, and 55 to 70 years of age and estimating SC thickness from water content profiles, Boireau-Adamezyk et al. (2014) showed an increase in facial, volar, and dorsal forearm SC thickness with age. This increase was more pronounced in the forearms than in the facial skin. There was, however, no significant difference between the SC thickness increase in the two forearms, leading the authors to conclude that SC thickness increase is more related to chronological aging rather than photoexposure (extrinsic aging). Interestingly, their data from volunteers aged 50 to 70 years are more widely dispersed than that of their younger subjects. The increased variability in the data of elderly could be due to more pronounced cumulative lifestyle factors (e.g., sun exposure, stress, smoking, cosmetics application).

Nakagawa et al. (2010) compared the water content of forearm dermis (depth of 70 µm in the skin) and showed significantly higher dermal water content in skin of the elderly.

Choe et al. (2018a) used CRM to compare the hydrogen bonding state of water in an older vs. younger population. They tracked the ratio of the DA (single donor–single acceptor, weakly bound) to DDAA (double donor–double acceptor, strongly bound) water molecule types in the high wavenumber region, i.e., the ratio of intensities I_{3450}/I_{3250}, as a function of depth in the SC. Within the top 10% to 30% of the dermis, elderly skin was shown to contain more hydrogen-bound water. This finding may be linked to the dryness of elderly skin compared to younger skin. Furthermore, these authors showed a significantly higher mean NMF amount in elderly skin within the top 20% to 40% of the SC, in agreement with previously mentioned studies.

Nguyen et al. (2013) investigated the hydration of collagen in the dermis of elderly vs. young volunteers and in relation to relative humidity. The Raman spectra were obtained in the reticular dermis at depths of 500 µm from the skin surface. The intensities of the ν(C–C) peak at 938 cm^{-1} and the wavenumber downshift of the amide I maximum from 1672 cm^{-1} to 1665 cm^{-1} were observed with an increase in relative humidity (RH). The ratio of intensities I_{1658}/I_{1668}, a marker of collagen/water interactions, was used to differentiate between the skin samples of the two populations. The authors surmised that these differences could result from differences of compactness of the collagen fiber bundles. The younger skin contains thinner diameters of collagen fiber bundles and consequently a more compact collagen structure.

Fluhr et al. (2012) compared the water content of the volar forearm of full-term newborns (1 to 15 days), babies aged 5 to 6 weeks, babies aged 6 ± 1 months, children aged 1 to 2 years, children aged 4 to 5 years, and adults aged 20 to 35 years. They showed that the SC is less hydrated in the first 2 weeks of postnatal life. There is a decrease in SC water content towards the skin surface for all age groups, but this gradient is lower for the newborns. The mean total amount of NMF in the SC was greater for the newborns than for all other age groups.

Lipid components. Tfayli et al. (2012b) studied the skin of 20 volunteers aged 22 to 64 years old. Overall, a lower total amount of lipids was detected in the skin of the elderly volunteers. In order to specify lipid markers of aging, they analyzed "subtracted" skin spectra, that is, the difference between normal skin spectra and spectra for skin from which the lipid components had been extracted through rubbing of the skin with an alcohol mixture. A principal component analysis on the 2845 to 3020 cm^{-1} region of the subtracted spectra yielded good discrimination between three groups: the younger population, the elderly population, and a "middle-aged" group. Hence, the 2845 to 3020 cm^{-1} region is a significant marker of aging in SC. Additional analysis showed the relative intensity of the 2850 to 2960 cm^{-1} region to be higher for younger SC lipids, indicating small changes in the lateral packing. Within this spectral region, the authors point out the decrease in relative intensity of the 2930 cm^{-1} peak as relating to a decrease in intermolecular and organizational order in the elderly skin. Therefore, this peak could be a marker of the weaker barrier function of elderly skin. Another marker of age is the ratio of intensities I_{2880}/I_{2845}, which was lower in aged skin. This points to a lower amount of *trans* conformers *gauche* conformation in the alkyl chain of the lipids of aged skin.

Corroborating Tfayli et al.'s (2012b) results, Boireau-Adamezyk et al. (2014) observed a significant decrease in the lipid-to-protein ratio in the dorsal and volar forearm of volunteers with increasing age. Differences between the two sides of the forearms were only significant in their oldest subpopulation (55 to 70 years of age). Analyzing the fingerprint region of Raman spectra, they found the ratio *trans/gauche* lipid conformation ($I_{1055-1070} + I_{1120-1140}/I_{1080-1090}$) to decrease significantly with age only on the dorsal (sun-exposed) forearm. Again only the oldest subpopulation presented differences in this ratio between the two sides of the forearm. They showed that SC ceramide content decreases with age only on the forearm site. Cholesterol content decreases with age on face and the dorsal forearm, not the volar forearm. Unlike SC thickness, which is a function of chronological aging, their results indicated that SC lipid content and conformation are functions of extrinsic (e.g., photo-) aging.

In accordance with previous results on lipid content, Binder et al. (2017) showed lower ceramide and cholesterol relative intensities as a function of depth in the skin of volunteers more than 50 years old compared to those less than 25 years old.

Choe et al. (2018a) analyzed the effect of age on SC lipid spectral markers in both the fingerprint and the high wavenumber region. The ratio of intensities indicative of lateral packing order according to C–H vibrations (a modification of the I_{2880}/I_{2845} ratio used by Tfayli et al. (2012b) is greater in elderly skin within the top 20% to 30% of the SC thickness. The ratio $I_{1080}/(I_{1130} + I_{1060})$, indicating the relative amount of *gauche* to *trans* conformation according to the skeleton C-C vibration, was significantly lower in elderly skin at depths corresponding to 30% to 40% of the SC thickness. Thus, elderly SC has prevalence of *trans* conformation and therefore higher-ordered packing at those depths. However, they did not find a significant difference in the ratio ($I_{2850} + I_{2880})/I_{2930}$ representative of the mean amount of lipid normalized to the keratin present in SC.

Protein conformation. Choe et al. (2018a) also focused on the spectral intensities centered around 2390 cm^{-1}, indicative of folding or unfolding properties of keratin filaments. This marker did not reveal a significant difference in the studied populations.

55.4.2.6 Effects of Water/Moisturizer Exposure and Environmental Humidity on Skin Components

Water and NMF. The permeability of skin for hydrophilic molecules increases dramatically with skin hydration. Hydration by occlusion or exposition to high humidity level results in an increase of the SC water content from 13% (standard value) to near 400% of the dry tissue weight (Williams and Barry 2004). Water in SC can be either bound to structural elements (NMF, functional groups) or free. The free water acts as a solvent for hydrophilic molecules in the SC, thus increasing the solubility of drugs in the tissue. Drug partition between the cosmetic product and the SC is then modified, and the increase in solubility leads to higher transdermal fluxes of hydrophilic substances in hydrated skin. It is not clearly established whether water can enhance the skin penetration of lipophilic drugs. It has been proposed that swelling of the polar head group regions of the lipid bilayers by water could disrupt the lipid domains and cause higher permeability for lipophilic permeants such as steroids. However, several researchers have shown that water does not cause modification of the lipid bilayer packing (Bouwstra ct al. 1991, 1996, 2003; Gay et al. 1994). Van Hal et al. (1996) incubated human skin explants with a saline phosphate buffered solution for 24 hours under occlusive or non-occlusive conditions. They proved that water penetrated the corneocytes, inducing their swelling, but also between the cells in the intercellular lipid region, mainly located in separated water pools. The images revealed these water pools and some vesicle-like structures were occasionally found. Nevertheless, the majority of the lipid bilayers exhibited a smooth fracture plane and no change in appearance. The amount of water in these smooth regions was low, and swelling of lamellae or lateral swelling of lipids was not observed.

CRM is well suited to the investigation of the effects of water or moisturizer application onto the skin. Research in this area has a number of applications in biological, pharmaceutical, and cosmetic R&D. Chrit et al. (2006, 2007) demonstrated this by studying the effects of commercially available and novel moisturizers in the skin of volunteers. In the first study, they tracked the effects of water, of a placebo (emollient without a hydrating agent), and of a 3% glycerol-containing cream by following the ratio of the bands OH/CH_3 (water content relative to proteins). Application of the latter yielded a highly significant increase in water content within the SC compared to application of water only (Chrit et al. 2006). In the second study, the authors investigated the effects of a biocompatible moisturizer, poly(2-methacryoyloxyethylphosphorylcholine) (pMPC) (Chrit et al. 2007). In vitro pilot tests on extracted human SC were performed to show a significant increase in the water content of the skin following application of pMPC in microspheres. Extracted SC samples treated with microspheres containing the combination of pMPC and hyaluronic acid was more efficient in reuptake of water by about 85% compared to glycerol 3% used as a reference. In vivo tests on volunteers showed that application of both polymers in microspheres yielded a significantly higher hydration level compared to bare skin.

Crowther et al. (2008) demonstrated the possibility of comparing the effects of three commercially available moisturizers. One of them (product A) yielded significant increases in SC water content and thickness compared to the other two. Further along this line, Tippavajhala et al. (2018) used CRM to compare the efficacy of four commercial moisturizers. They compared the short-term (7 days after treatment) and long-term (30 days after treatment) effects of the products—relative to control—on the total water and NMF contents measured in volunteers' SC. This study interestingly shows diverging effects of the products. One product increased the water content over time while decreasing the NMF content. For other products, the number of days following treatment was crucial, with water content and/or NMF content decreasing 7 days after treatment, but increasing during the following period of study, to day 30 after treatment. One product failed to hydrate the skin, with both water and NMF contents steadily decreasing over time.

Egawa et al. (2007) and Egawa and Tagami (2008) investigated the effects of forced hydration and humidity on the water and NMF composition of skin in vivo. Tracking water content as function of depth following Caspers et al.'s method (Section 55.4.2.1), they showed that a 15-minute application of water could drastically alter the SC water content and depth of penetration of water. Water could reach the stratum granulosum (beyond a depth of 12 μm) and was only gradually released by the skin, even after discontinuation of the forced hydration. Egawa and Tagami (2008) also investigated the effect of season. While no seasonal change in water content of the skin was observed, they did find that NMF content decreased during hot and humid months. Overall they found that the decreases in NMF, sweat, and lipid components of skin correlated to a subjective feeling of dry skin reported by the volunteers.

Dąbrowska et al. (2016) used CRM to compare the effects of changes in environmental RH on skin. They showed that water exposure changed the hydration level of the superficial SC much more significantly than relative humidity at 90%. An increase in RH from 40% to 90% yielded an increase in the hydration level of the superficial SC from ~24% to ~28% after 60 minutes. Within the same time frame, water exposure yielded an increase in superficial SC hydration level from 26% to 60% water. Comparing water content–depth profiles obtained following the method of Caspers et al., they showed that the largest change in hydration level caused by external factors occurred within the first 10 µm. Application of water for different durations yielded changes in the hydration that were more evident in the initially drier outer layers of the skin. As SC thicknesses were derived from the water-content profiles, the forced hydration through water exposure and increased RH modified this parameter in different ways. Water exposure yielded an increase in SC thickness linear with increasing exposure time. The SC thickness increased linearly with water exposure time, from ~18 µm prior to exposure to ~21 µm after 60 minutes of exposure. Changes in SC thickness due to RH changes were smaller, from ~17 µm with 40% RH to ~19 µm with 90% RH for 60-minute exposures.

Vyumvuhore et al. (2013) investigated the effect of RH on the different types of bound water molecules within isolated human SC. They deconvoluted the Raman spectra in the high wavenumber region associated with water (3100 to 1700 cm^{-1}) to assess the effect of humidity change on the presence of totally bound water (3210 cm^{-1}), partially bound water (3280 cm^{-1} and 3345 cm^{-1}), and unbound water (3470 cm^{-1}). Whereas totally bound water was not affected by RH, the total amount of partially bound water increased for RH = 28% to 60%, then decreased for RH > 60%. The total amount of unbound water increased slightly to RH = 44%, then significantly for RH = 66% and 75%. The amount of partially bound water affects the conformational order and compactness of the lipid phase of the SC barrier (see "Lipid components" later). Conversely, Vyumvuhore et al. (2015) studied the impact of drying stress (reduction of RH) and the kinetics of water desorption from hydrated SC samples. With respect to water types, comparison of the ratios of spectral bands of unbound water (3420 to 3620 cm^{-1}) to global water (3100 to 3620 cm^{-1}) and partially bound water (3245 to 3620 cm^{-1}) to global water showed that the fraction of unbound water decreases with drying time in a 7% RH environment, while the fraction of partially bound water increases. A relationship between the change in skin water content and the change in skin biomechanical stress due to drying (at 7% RH over 8 hours) was shown. Highly hydrated SC corresponded to weakly stressed SC. The decrease in water content was accompanied by a linear increase in the stress. Within the last hours of drying time the low water content corresponded to a constant maximum in the mechanical stress. The authors concluded that the loss of unbound water during drying was primarily due to the increase in skin biomechanical stress.

In another interesting study, Kim et al. (2017) focused on the effect of water content in excised porcine skin on the skin's optical properties. They observed that the peak intensity of the Raman spectra varies with the water content of the sample, even though the laser power on the sample surface remained constant. They observed a decrease of the peak intensity with an increase in water content from 40 to 55wt%. Further Kim et al. depicted a twofold increase in the reduced scattering coefficient μ_s' of skin with the same increase in water content. Diffuse reflectance and simulation work indicated that the water content of skin samples could alter the backscattered light over a larger angular range, leading to variation in Raman spectra intensity. The authors conclude that the effect of cutaneous water content on Raman intensities should be taken into account when analyzing different types of skin, e.g., diseased skin.

Lipid components. Egawa and Tagami (2008) showed a reduction in ceramide 3 and cholesterol. Their total amount was reported in Caucasian skin in winter compared with summer, while a decreased tendency in ceramides was reported in most parts of the body in Japanese subjects in summer. Using a mixture of commercially available ceramides that make up the SC lipid barrier function, Tfayli et al. (2013) investigated the effect of RH variation (2.5%, 20%, 50%, 65%, and 88%) on polar interactions, interchain organization, and alkyl chain conformation of these ceramides. The effect of RH on polar interactions, lateral packing, and the conformational order of the ceramides depends on their structure. CER III and 5 showed a more compact and ordered organization with stronger polar interactions at the intermediate RH values, while CER 2 showed opposite tendencies to those observed with CER III and 5. Investigations on the effect of RH on human SC samples showed that the *trans/gauche* conformation [ratio $(I_{1060} + I_{1130})/I_{1080}$] increases with RH = 44% and 60%, then decreased for RH = 75%. The same trend was observed for the conformational state and lateral packing (I_{2882}/I_{2852}) (Vyumvuhore et al. 2013). Hence, a more organized SC lipid barrier is present at intermediate RH. A drying experiment on hydrated SC samples by Vyumvuhore et al. (2015) showed that the compactness of the lipid matrix in the SC increases according to drying time at 7% RH, similarly to the relative amount of partially bound water compared to the global water content.

Protein conformation. Skin protein conformation is linked to skin water content due to the water present in corneocytes. Vyumvuhore et al. (2013) showed that the decrease in bound water content below 60% RH destabilizes protein conformation. This was evidenced by a decrease in the content of exposed tyrosine (830 cm^{-1}) compared to the buried conformation (850 cm^{-1}) and a shift in the protein conformation (2932 cm^{-1} band) towards lower wavenumbers. Additionally, an increase in RH up to 60% yielded an increase in the water sub-band of 1690 cm^{-1} representing conformational turns and random coils. The interpretation is that the increase in RH caused a swelling of keratin filaments, corresponding to unfolding of long α-helixes and β-sheets and yielding turns and a random coil protein secondary structure. Similar results were obtained by Vyumvuhore and coworkers during the drying of SC from 98% to 7% RH (Vyumvuhore et al. 2015). In highly humidified SC, multilayered water molecules fill spaces between keratin fibers, favoring keratin β-sheet conformation. The drying process removes this water, leaving spaces between the fibers and decreasing β-sheet conformation.

55.4.2.7 Probing the Barrier of Diseased Skin

With its sensitivity to lipid and protein conformation and organization in skin, CRM lends itself well to the characterization of dermatological pathologies that result in a weakened skin barrier and, therefore, a propensity towards increased penetration of compounds compared to healthy skin. Atopic and psoriatic skin in particular have been studied via CRM, with a focus on the same Raman bands and intensity ratios.

Wohlrab et al. (2001) used CRM to highlight the decrease in lipid order in non-lesional skin of patients compared to healthy skin through the study of CH$_2$ symmetric stretching mode at 2848 cm^{-1} and its shift towards higher wavenumbers and the lower intensity of the 1128 cm^{-1} band. Osada et al. (2004) and Verzeaux et al. (2018) showed a decrease in the lipid matrix structure of psoriatic and mildly atopic skin using the lipid packing order ratio $v_{asym}CH_2 / v_{sym}CH_2$ (I_{2890}/I_{2850} or I_{2885}/I_{2850}), also used by Tfayli and coworkers investigating the effects of age and relative humidity on the lipidic aspect of the skin barrier (Sections 55.4.2.5 and 55.4.2.6). Verzeaux et al. (2018) further compared the vCC *trans*/vCC *gauche* conformation ratio [$(I_{1060} + I_{1130})/I_{1080}$] in mildly atopic vs. healthy skin, also showing a significant decrease in pathological skin.

With regard to protein in the skin, the consensus revealed through CRM is a shift of the amide I band towards higher wavenumbers in the diseased skin compared to healthy skin, indicating a loss in protein conformational structure (Osada et al. 2004; Bernard et al. 2007). Verzeaux et al. (2018) showed a significant increase in the α-helix and β-sheet structures in atopic skin compared to healthy skin by measuring the ratio between the α-helix (1656 cm^{-1}) and β-sheet (1672 cm^{-1}) conformations to the overall amide I (1600 to 1700 cm^{-1}) band.

Comparing lipid and protein contents, lipid-to-protein ratios are decreased in diseased skin compared to healthy skin (Verzeaux et al. 2018), as well as in non-lesional skin of atopic eczema volunteers compared to their lesional skin (Janssens et al. 2014).

Richters et al. (2017) studied whether indicators of sensitive skin could be reliably detected using CRM. Sensitive skin is defined as "a condition characterized by the perception of skin discomfort following mild stimuli, frequently without objective signs of skin irritation." They compared water, NMF, and ceramide/fatty acid levels in volunteers' sensitive skin to those from non-sensitive skin individuals as well as atopic dermatitis (AD) and allergic rhinoconjunctivitis (AR) volunteers.

Trends observed in NMF levels between the groups were not statistically significant. With respect to ceramides and fatty acids, statistical significance was found only in the higher levels in sensitive skin compared to atopic skin. Overall, the study served to show that sensitive skin was not a subclinical form of atopic dermatitis. The skin barrier of sensitive skin was shown to be unmodified with respect to SC thickness and water, NMF, and lipid content.

55.5 DRUG PENETRATION AND PENETRATION ENHANCEMENT STUDIES

CRM is a useful tool to follow label-free and simultaneously the distribution of an active drug and vehicle components such as penetration enhancers, as well as to record modifications of endogenous skin components arising from the application of a given product. CRM allows studying whether or not an active drug and vehicle components have similar distribution patterns in the skin. Conversely, it allows one to control for possible adverse effects due to the formulation. This is, for instance, of interest in the study of sunscreens, which are supposed to remain on the skin surface. CRM is also helpful for efficacy purposes. Detection of the active agent and quantification of metabolites help to gain insight into the protective potential of novel formulations and to reevaluate existing ones. Moreover, this method is also useful to establish in vitro/in vivo correlations.

The penetration of various drugs spanning a range of chemical structures and physicochemical properties has been studied (Table 55.2 and Table 55.3) insofar as these drugs possess a specific Raman signature allowing their identification within the skin. In general, penetration profiles of compounds as a function of depth inside SC consist of qualitative or semi-quantitative data (Zsikó et al. 2019). The methodology of Caspers et al. involves fitting a reference spectrum of the compound of interest to the spectra of skin onto which the compound has been applied. Since the collected Raman signal weakens with increasing depths into the skin due to scattering in the tissue, the compound signal is normalized by the signal of endogenous keratin, whose concentration in the skin is assumed constant as a function of depth in the skin (Pudney et al. 2007). This assumption of constant keratin concentration as a function of depth, and the general methodology based upon it, have recently been challenged by Darvin et al. (2019).

Recently, Caspers et al. (2019) introduced a new methodology yielding fully quantitative skin penetration–depth profiles from in vivo CRM, that is, in terms of mass of compound penetrated per cm^2 of skin. Their method, illustrated by the tracking of retinol in the skin of volunteers, is reviewed in the next section.

55.5.1 Methodologies to Assess Drug Skin Penetration

Similarly to classical skin penetration experiments, CRM lends itself to the tracking of chemicals from solutions or more complex formulations (with or without penetration enhancers) in ex vivo human and animal skin. Studies on skin explants may be conducted to define methodological parameters in view of performing in vivo CMR studies.

Caffeine has been selected as a model hydrophilic drug in a number of several CRM studies (Franzen et al. 2013, 2014, 2015; Tfaili et al. 2013, 2014; Alonso et al. 2018). Widely used in cosmetics as an active substance, it is also one of the most frequently used compounds in transdermal delivery studies. This hydrophilic molecule is not metabolized in the skin and has interesting physicochemical properties, with a low octanol/water partition coefficient ($\log P = -0.07$) and low molar mass ($M_W = 194$ g·mol^{-1}).

Caffeine penetrates the skin rapidly (Bolzinger et al. 2008). However, it is difficult to track with CRM because it does not accumulate in the upper layers of skin. Tfaili et al. (2013) followed caffeine penetration in human skin samples. Solutions of caffeine at two concentrations, 2.57×10^{-1} mg·mL^{-1} and 5.15×10^{-2} mg·mL^{-1}, were applied on human skin samples. Raman spectra were collected every half-hour from the surface to a depth of 50 μm in a 6-μm increment. The total duration was 4 hours after application. Raman analysis was not possible with the most concentrated solution

TABLE 55.2
Confocal Raman Microspectroscopy in Drug Penetration Studies Utilizing Excised Human and Animal Skin

Compound	Functionality	Excised Skin	References
Caffeine	Pharmaceutical and cosmetic active ingredient	Skin surrogate and Human stratum corneum	Franzen et al. 2013
		Human stratum corneum	Franzen et al. 2014
		Human stratum corneum	Franzen et al. 2015
		Porcine skin	Alonso et al. 2018
		Human skin	Tfaili et al. 2013
Caffeine and resveratrol	Active ingredients	Human skin	Tfaili et al. 2014
Caffeine nanocrystals and propylene glycol	Pharmaceutical and cosmetic active ingredient and excipient	Porcine skin	Ascencio et al. 2016
Dimethyl sulfoxide (DMSO)	Excipient	Human stratum corneum	Anigbogu et al. 1995
		Porcine skin	Zhang et al. 2007c
		Films of SC lipids	Tfayli et al. 2012a
Flufenamic acid, propylene glycol/ ethanol (75/25) versus hydrophobic enhancers (octanol)	Anti-inflammatory drug and excipients	Human skin	Pyatski et al. 2016
Hyaluronic acid	Active cosmetic ingredient	Human skin	Essendoubi et al. 2016
Iminosulfuranes	Penetration enhancers	Hairless mouse skin, human cadaver skin	Song et al. 2005
Lidocaine	Anti-inflammatory drug	Human skin	Bakonyi et al. 2018
Metronidazole	Antibiotic drug	Human skin	Tfayli et al. 2007
Perdeuterated acyl-chain 1,2-dimyristoylphosphatidylcholine (DMPC-d_{54})	Excipients used for the preparation of liposomes	Porcine skin	Xiao et al. 2005a
Perdeuterated acyl-chain 1,2-dipalmitoylphosphatidylcholine (DPPC-d_{62}) and 1-palmitoyl-d_{31},2-oleoylphosphatidylcholine (P-d_{31}OPC)	Excipients used for the preparation of liposomes	Porcine skin	Xiao et al. 2005b
Perdeuterated sodium laureth sulfate	Excipient	Porcine and human skin	Mao et al. 2012
Pro-5-fluorouracil and 5-fluorouracil	Antitumor pro-drug and drug	Porcine skin	Zhang et al. 2007b
Procaine	Local anesthetic	Porcine skin	Lunter and Daniels 2014
Propylene glycol and oleic acid	Excipients	Rat skin	Atef and Altuwaijri et al. 2018
Sulphadiazine sodium	Antibiotic drug	Porcine skin	Binder et al. 2019
Sulfathiazole sodium, sodium laureth sulfate, sodium dodecyl sulfate, DMSO	Antibiotic drug and excipients	Porcine skin	Binder et al. 2018
Trans-cinnamaldehyde and vehicles (ethanol, water, PG and oils)	Perfumes ingredient (skin sensitizer)	Porcine skin	Bonnist et al. 2011
Trans-retinol	Antioxidant	Porcine skin	Förster et al. 2011a,b
β-Carotene	Antioxidant	Human stratum corneum	Ashtikar et al. 2013

due to the crystallization of caffeine on the skin surface; the strong signals from caffeine crystals hid the Raman signal from the skin. Caffeine from a diluted solution, however, could be tracked in the skin using the vibrational bands δ(C=O-N) at 555 cm^{-1} and υ(CN) at 1360 cm^{-1}. The maximum of caffeine signal intensity at 12 μm under the skin surface was recorded after 2 hours and

TABLE 55.3
Confocal Raman Microscopy for In Vivo Skin Penetration and Penetration Enhancement Studies on Volunteers

Compound	Functionality	Body Site of Application	References
2-Butoxyethanol, toluene and pyrene	Occupational toxicants	Volar forearm	Broding et al. 2011
Dimethyl sulfoxide (DMSO)	Excipient	Palm	Caspers et al. 2002
Fruit wax (Rhus vernicula peel cera) Natural oil-based (Cocos nucifera fruit oil and Olea europea oil)	Lip care	Lips	Bielfeldt et al. 2019
Ibuprofen in propylene glycol and mixed propylene glycol/water	Anti-inflammatory drug and excipients	Volar forearm	Mateus et al. 2013
Ibuprofen, ketoprofen	Anti-inflammatory drugs	Mice	Saar et al. 2011
Jojoba, almond, paraffin, and petrolatum oils	Excipient	Volar forearm	Choe et al. 2015
Monoacyl-phosphatidylcholine mixtures	Nanocarrier formulations	Volar forearm	Wolf et al. 2018
Mycosporine-like amino acids (MAAs) and Gadusol (Gad) incorporated in polymer gel	Photoprotection	Forearm	Tosato et al. 2015
Niacinamide	Anti-aging, decrease of photoaging, reduction of sebum production	Volunteers	Mohammed et al. 2014
Paraffin, jojoba, almond	Moisturizers	Forearm	Stamatas et al. 2008
Paraffinum liquidum, petrolatum, paraffin, and tocopheryl acetate	Ingredients of products used for oral or genital mucosa	Volar forearm	Laing et al. 2019
Petrolatum oil	Excipient	Volar forearm	Choe et al., 2014
p-phenylenediamine	Hair dye ingredient	Forearm	Pot et al. 2016
Retinyl acetate and α-tocopheryl acetate	Antiaging, photoprotection, antioxidant	Volar forearm	Dos Santos et al. 2018
Retinyl acetate and vitamin A	Photoaging, acne	Volar forearm	Dos Santos et al. 2016
Salicylic acid	Management of dandruff, seborrheic dermatitis, ichthyosis, psoriasis, acne, wart removal	Volar forearm (and ex vivo porcine skin)	Mateus et al. 2014
Sunscreens	Photoprotection	Volar forearm	Tippavajhala et al. 2018
Trans-retinol	Antioxidant	Volar forearm	Pudney et al. 2007
Trans-retinol	Antioxidant	Volar forearm	Mélot et al. 2009
Trans-retinol	Antioxidant	Mice	Saar et al. 2010
Trans-retinol and propylene glycol	Antioxidant and excipient	Volar forearm	Caspers et al. 2019
Urocanic acid	Sunscreen	Chicken and volar forearm	Egawa and Iwaki 2008
Vitamins A, E and C esters	Skin homeostasis and protection	Volar forearm	Mogilevych et al. 2015

35 minutes. After 4 hours, caffeine was no longer detected in the skin by Raman analysis. Several causes were proposed by the authors: a too low concentration in the skin due to rapid caffeine diffusion, heterogeneous diffusion possibly resulting in too low a concentration of caffeine in the analyzed volume, and a too low depth of analysis (50 μm) enabled by the Raman method.

The same team applied the methodology to investigate skin absorption from low concentrations of caffeine and resveratrol solutions in real time (Tfaili et al. 2014). The study was limited to a small skin region, and all samples originated from one person's human abdominal skin. Kinetic profiles were recorded over approximately 9 hours; data were processed to monitor the spectral modifications induced on skin signal after actives application. Caffeine was detected as described earlier.

Spectral modifications in the vibration bands at 1003 cm^{-1} and in the 1604–1654 cm^{-1} (amide I) and 2800–3000 cm^{-1} spectral regions were observed after application of resveratrol. For both actives, the concentrations were directly related to the intensities of the Raman vibrational bands and were higher at 6 μm of depth compared to deeper skin layers. A marked variability in the caffeine and resveratrol diffusion profiles at different depths was shown. This heterogeneity is most probably related to the microvariability of skin constituents.

Franzen et al. (2013, 2014, 2015) proposed a new approach to obtain Raman intensity depth profiles that account for Raman signal attenuation arising from the inhomogeneous nature of skin. They first obtained spectra of an artificial skin surrogate containing homogeneously distributed caffeine. These spectral data were used to develop a mathematical algorithm describing the Raman signal attenuation within the surrogate. Spectra from excised human skin incubated in a caffeine solution could then be corrected for Raman signal attenuation. Without the correction, caffeine intensity decreases with depth into the skin. Conversely, the corrected intensity is roughly constant with depth, as expected from an incubation (i.e., complete soaking) experiment.

Later on, the same team applied CRM for quantification of caffeine penetration into freeze-dried excised human SC. Freeze-drying the sample slows down diffusion of the penetrating substance during analysis, facilitating depth profiling. A linear dependency of substance amount and Raman signal intensity at the surface of the freeze-dried SC samples was observed. The Raman signal intensity of caffeine was measured at 0, 2.5, 5, 7.5, and 10 μm depth inside the SC. The Raman signal decreased according to depth. Utilization of the Raman peak of the unspecific C-H vibration (1388 to 1497 cm^{-1}) as an internal standard allowed finding a linear correlation of Raman data and substance concentration independent of depth inside the freeze-dried skin (Franzen et al. 2014). Similarly, the authors conducted a systematic validation study of quantitative caffeine intensity–depth profiling in human SC sheets by CRM and HPLC (Franzen et al. 2015). A linear relationship between peak ratio determined by CRM and caffeine concentration per mass of SC determined by HPLC was obtained independently from skin depth. However, the limit of quantification is high because of the intense baseline coming from endogenous skin components.

Alonso et al. (2018) used caffeine to illustrate a new protocol yielding the relative concentration of a permeant from its relative Raman intensity. The caffeine contents in SC and in the viable epidermis of porcine skin were evaluated by CRM and HPLC. The caffeine peak (556 cm^{-1}) of skin samples was correlated to the aromatic amino acids (1004 cm^{-1}) and amide I peaks (1650 cm^{-1}) of skin. Linear correlations were obtained between the Raman peak ratios in the SC and viable epidermis at depths up to 35 μm and the concentration of caffeine determined by HPLC. Semi-quantitative penetration profiles of caffeine into the pig skin were obtained by CRM for each internal skin reference. The results showed a decrease in relative caffeine intensity with increasing depth. Using the amino acid (AA) intensity and the amide I (AI) intensity as references yields qualitatively similar profiles; however, the values are different due to differences in the AA and AI intensities. Quantitative caffeine penetration profiles were obtained by combining the semi-quantitative data and the AA- or AI-based correlations linking caffeine Raman intensity to concentration in solution.

As previously mentioned, to date, CRM can generate semi-quantitative active intensity–depth profiles, where the Raman intensity of the active of interest is expressed relative to the intensity of a reference component of skin. Often, the endogenous keratin signal is taken as a reference (Caspers et al.'s method, see Section 55.4). The methodology developed by Alonso et al. (2018) expresses the concentration of the active relative to skin mass.

Recently Caspers et al. (2019) developed a methodology to track the penetration of topical compounds into skin quantitatively, the goal being to obtain a cumulative amount of active (e.g., cumulative mass/skin diffusion area), or a flux, that can be directly compared to the output of classical skin penetration experiments (Section 55.2). The method is based on the premise that the ratio of Raman intensities of two products in skin is proportional to the ratio of their concentrations in skin. Taking an active of interest and its solvent, the first steps consist in calculating an active mass/solvent mass ratio as a function of their relative Raman intensities, and similarly for the solvent compound to

SC protein. From these an active/protein mass ratio can be calculated and, using the mass of protein in the SC, a concentration of active in the SC. Integrating the active concentration over the SC thickness then yields a mass of active normalized by the skin surface area, in other words, an amount of active expressed as mass/cm². Demonstration of the method was provided using Pudney et al.'s (2007) in vivo Raman data of *trans*-retinol applied in propylene glycol.

55.5.2 TRACKING DRUGS, FORMULATION INGREDIENTS, COMBINATIONS OF BOTH, AND SKIN CARE PRODUCTS

55.5.2.1 The Performance of Penetration Enhancers for Improved Skin Delivery

The major drawback of the skin as a route of administration is its barrier function that extensively limits the absorption of various interesting active substances, depending on their physicochemical properties. Molecules of medium polarity with a log$P$ ranging between 1 and 3 and having a low molar mass (< 500 g·mol⁻¹) generally penetrate through the skin. Very hydrophobic molecules or hydrophilic molecules or molecules of high molar mass do not penetrate to a large extent despite their interesting pharmacologic properties. For example, cosmetic agents showing a useful activity, such as antiaging agents (vitamins, hyaluronic acid), anesthetics, antibiotics, or anti-inflammatory drugs such as ibuprofen are poor penetrants because of limitations stemming from inadequate log$P$ and molar mass values. Penetration enhancers are widely used to promote the penetration of actives by disturbing the skin barrier. Enhancers may fluidize the lipid bilayer (glycols, alcohol), extract lipids (surfactants), induce phase separation of lipids, and alter the polar head groups of SC lipids, as reviewed by Williams and Barry (2012).

CRM is a useful investigation tool to obtain a better understanding of the role of penetration enhancers on intrinsic skin components and to study their mechanisms of action alone or in combination with a drug. For example, the role of dimethyl sulfoxide (DMSO) has been extensively studied by CRM and interesting conclusions could be reached, as discussed next.

55.5.2.1.1 Modification of Skin Components by Enhancers

Several studies aimed to explain the penetration enhancement mechanism of DMSO, one of the most common penetration enhancers. DMSO enhances the penetration of both hydrophilic and lipophilic drugs; its action in the skin is complex and remains largely an open question. Upon interaction with keratin, DMSO changes the keratin conformation from α-helical to a β-sheet structure. DMSO can also interact with the polar headgroups of intercellular lipids, resulting in a perturbation of their packing. Finally, DMSO can alter the drug partition between the formulation and the skin layers due to its good solvent properties for a large number of molecules (Williams and Barry 2004). Caspers et al. (2002) investigated the penetration of DMSO from an 80% v/v mixture of DMSO in 5% aqueous solution of PG into the palm skin of volunteers. The mixture alone presented some characteristic bands: a doublet at 671 and 702 cm⁻¹ assigned to the ν(CSC) modes and a broad band at 1030 to 1048 cm⁻¹ assigned to ν(S=O) stretching. After application to the skin of volunteers, there was a shift of these bands, indicating interaction of DMSO with water and possibly other components of the SC. The SC depth profile was calculated as a function of time from the ratio of DMSO/proteins bands (ν(CSC) 677 cm⁻¹/δ(CH₂) 1450 cm⁻¹). They showed that most of the applied DMSO permeated through SC within 20 minutes and reached the viable epidermis where a small fraction was detected. Data collected for a longer time showed evidence of a progressive penetration of DMSO through the SC. DMSO could still be detected inside skin 72 hours after application. Other conclusions about DMSO–lipids or DMSO–protein interactions could not be drawn during this study. Anigbogu et al. (1995) showed using Raman spectroscopy that DMSO penetrated the SC and altered both the keratin conformation from α-helix to β-sheets and the lipid bilayer from a crystalline phase with alkyl chains of lipid molecules in their all-*trans* conformation (called "gel") to a liquid crystalline phase where the alkyl chains of lipids undergo equilibrium between *gauche* and *trans* conformations. After the immersion of the SC obtained from human abdominal skin into aqueous solutions of DMSO or deuterated DMSO-d_6 for 1 hour, CRM was performed, and the spectra showed an alteration of the keratin conformation: α-helix progressively converted into β-sheets as the concentration of DMSO increased. A plateau was reached at a concentration of DMSO above 60% for which the protein conformation was approximately 50% α-helix and 50% β-sheets. Lipid bilayer organization was only altered at high DMSO concentrations (70% to 100%). This behavior can be related to the penetration enhancement power of DMSO, which is generally significant when used at concentrations above 60% (Williams and Barry 2004). Zhang et al. (2007b) showed a reversible alteration of the keratin secondary structure using CRM when DMSO was applied in a keratinocyte culture. They reported an appearance of β-sheet structures in the cellular keratin after treatment with DMSO; this change was reversible, and the original α-helix structure was recovered upon rehydration. This result was explained by strong complex formation between DMSO and water, which displaced the bound water that stabilizes the secondary structure of keratin.

Saar et al. (2010) explored DMSO penetration on human skin by SRS imaging using a specific vibration of deuterated DMSO-d_6 at 2120 cm⁻¹. As shown in Figure 55.3d, DMSO was found in the area surrounding the hair follicles, confirming the initial rapid penetration of DMSO into those appendages. However, DMSO was not found to penetrate the hair itself.

Tfayli et al. (2012a) studied the modification of the lipids' conformational order, lateral packing, and polar interactions induced by three penetration enhancers. The Raman investigation was carried out on thin films of ceramides, the main lipid class of SC lipids, differing by their hydrocarbon chain length, polar head group, and the presence of a lateral group (ester or hydroxyl groups). The DMSO penetration enhancer mainly affected the polar interactions between lipid chains and their lateral packing, and its effect was dependent on the structure of the ceramides. As an example, adding DMSO to ceramides IIIb resulted in the increase of the band at 1633 cm⁻¹ indicating weak H-bonds at the expense of the amide I band at 1614 cm⁻¹ characteristic of strong H-bonds. DMSO also induced a slight change of the peak height ratio of the bands ν(CH₂ sym) at 2850 cm⁻¹ and ν(CH₂ asym) at 2880 cm⁻¹ that reflected a looser lateral packing of all ceramides. Such decrease of packing density is associated with higher skin permeability.

In another example of SRS use, Wanjiku et al. (2019) evaluated the effect of different concentrations of ethanol on the protein (2934 cm⁻¹)-to-lipid (2850 cm⁻¹) ratio of frozen human and mouse skin, as well as reconstructed human skin (RHS). With ethanol concentrations varying from 12% to 70% and exposure times from 30 to 300 minutes, the lipid signal was consistently more affected than the protein signal. For human skin, the ratio remained low and relatively constant compared to the mouse skin value, indicating faster lipid dissolution in the latter. The ratio for the RHS was almost twice as high. Contrary to human and mouse skin, the RHS ratio decreased slightly with increasing exposure time to ethanol at concentrations of 35% and 70%. This suggested that lipid dissolution in the RHS might be counter balanced by protein structural changes. This interesting result reflects different susceptibilities to ethanol-induced protein and lipid changes between the natural and artificial skins.

A novel group of chemical penetration enhancers, iminosulfuranes, was studied by Song et al. (2005) on mouse and human skin. The objective was to design new penetration enhancers having high efficacy and less toxicity and irritation potency. The iminosulfurane enhancers were easily detected in the skin by their specific Raman peak at 670 cm⁻¹; their intensity was normalized to that of the amide I vibration band (1743 cm⁻¹). The results showed penetration of the enhancer into the SC to a depth of approximately 20 μm, the maximum content being found 5 to 10 μm below the skin surface. This new enhancer did not penetrate into the viable epidermis, which meant that it might bind to the protein and/or the lipids in the SC. Furthermore, its penetration-enhancing activity was proved both for a lipophilic drug (hydrocortisone) and a hydrophilic one (caffeine). The penetration enhancement of caffeine was lower than for hydrocortisone.

Atef and Altuwaijri (2018) studied the permeability enhancement effect of oleic acid and propylene glycol and their mixture on rat skin. Raman spectra indicated that oleic acid disrupted rat skin lipid after 2 hours of treatment by changes in the lipid peak. The lipid disruption of the skin decreased the barrier effect by SC lipid fluidization and increased the permeability. The results also showed that propylene glycol and oleic acid improved their diffusion and created faster, yet reversible changes of the skin peaks.

55.5.2.1.2 Combination of Penetration Enhancers and Active Substances

As previously mentioned, studies using CRM are useful to evaluate the disruption of the skin barrier by penetration enhancers. Choosing the best possible enhancer to improve the skin absorption of a specific active molecule is an important task in drug formulation design. CRM is helpful to track simultaneously enhancers and active drugs in the skin. The best strategy to enhance cutaneous drug delivery is to combine a drug and an enhancer with similar penetration profiles and distribution patterns. If the fluxes or distribution of both molecules is different, the flux of the active molecule may decrease because of its partial recrystallization in the skin. Several examples are reported next.

55.5.2.1.2.1 Lipophilic drugs **Retinol and derivatives.** The penetration of β-carotene, a lipophilic molecule ($\log P = 17.62$, $M_W = 537$ g·mol^{-1}) dissolved in DMSO, using CRM was studied by Ashtikar et al. (2013). Three main bands were used to identify β-carotene in the skin, the C=C bound stretching at 1510 and 1153 cm^{-1} and the C-CH$_3$ bound rocking at 1004 cm^{-1}. Raman analysis showed that β-carotene hardly penetrated the skin; it was essentially found in the first 10 μm of the SC and presented a heterogeneous distribution. This result was quite expected with such a lipophilic molecule that shows poor skin permeability. DMSO may have enhanced the penetration of β-carotene, but this was not proved by the authors.

Trans-retinol is a common antiaging active substance (vitamin A) in cosmetic products. It is frequently used as a hydrophobic model drug in skin absorption experiments (Failloux et al. 2004; Pudney et al. 2007; Mélot et al. 2009). This molecule with a $\log P = 5.68$ mostly remains in the lipid phase of the superficial SC. Raman spectroscopy is an appropriate detection technique, as *trans*-retinol possesses a characteristic peak due to the C=C bond at 1594 cm^{-1} (Mélot et al. 2009) or 1585 cm^{-1} (Förster et al. 2011a), which is well-resolved from other peaks of major skin components (Figure 55.4).

Various types of penetration enhancers for *trans*-retinol were investigated such as glycol, nonionic surfactants, or fatty acids such as oleic acid.

Pudney et al. (2007) compared 0.3% *trans*-retinol applied in a propylene glycol (PG)/ethanol (EtOH) vehicle and in caprylic/capric acid triglyceride (Myritol 318), an oil widely used in skin

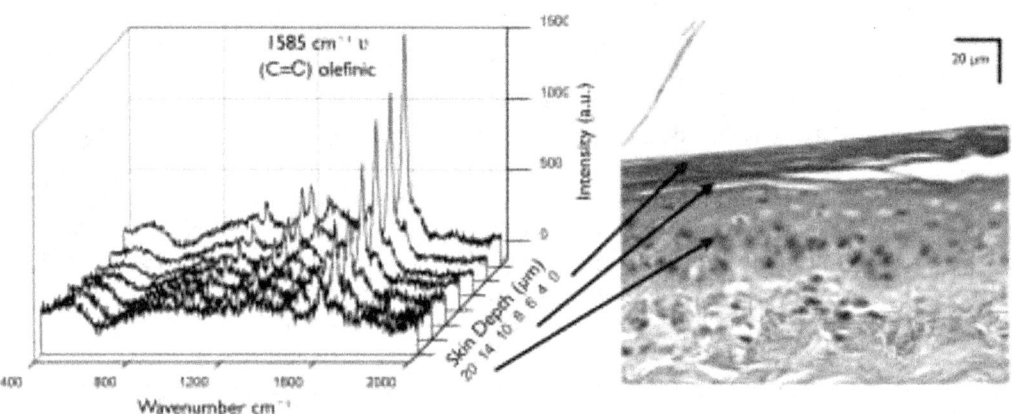

FIGURE 55.4 Raman spectra of pig skin after application of a surfactant solution containing 0.5% *trans*-retinol for 24 hours. The Raman profile was measured at the surface (0 μm) and at 2, 6, 8, 10, 14, and 20 μm skin depth. Arrows indicate skin depths in the image of histological section (magnification of ×40). (From Förster et al. 2011a with permission.)

creams. Retinol intensity–depth profiles revealed significantly greater penetration of *trans*-retinol from the PG/EtOH vehicle through the SC and into the viable epidermis; this penetration profile was correlated with that of PG alone. In contrast, penetration from capric/caprylic triglycerides was low. The correlation between the retinol and PG skin penetration suggested that PG is an efficient enhancer to promote *trans*-retinol penetration into the viable epidermis.

Mélot et al. (2009) monitored the effect of two penetration enhancers on the delivery of *trans*-retinol through human skin. Three formulations for the combination of 0.3% *trans*-retinol and Myritol 318 were tested: the first one (used as a control) contained no enhancer; the second one contained a lipid fluidizer, oleic acid; and the third contained a lipid extractor octoxynol-9 (Triton X100)—both enhancers were introduced at 1%. These were compared to the very efficient PG/EtOH vehicle. From Raman spectra acquired on the volar forearm of two male volunteers, concentration–depth profiles of *trans*-retinol and Myritol were obtained. Improved delivery of *trans*-retinol was observed with addition of the penetration enhancers in the formulation; oleic acid was found to be more efficient than Triton X100. In the absence of a penetration enhancer, the Raman signal of *trans*-retinol was mainly confined in the first 5 μm within the SC. *Trans*-retinol penetrated into deeper layers of the skin in the presence of each penetration enhancer. Oleic acid yielded penetration to the same depth as the PG/EtOH formulation; however, the amount of *trans*-retinol penetrated into the skin was tenfold higher from the PG/EtOH system. Oleic acid caused a phase separation in SC lipids because it is not miscible with the SC lipids.

Saar et al. (2010) used SRS (Section 55.3) to follow *trans*-retinol skin penetration in a living mouse by tuning the excitation wavelength to the vibration of *trans*-retinol, the C=C stretch at 1596 cm^{-1}. Images showed that penetration of *trans*-retinol occurred through the hair shaft. SRS was also used to image human skin in vivo up to a depth of 50 μm showing the localization of *trans*-retinol around the hair and in the top of the sebaceous gland.

Dos Santos et al. (2019) evaluated the penetration of retinyl acetate and alpha-tocopheryl acetate into young and elderly skin using in vivo CRM. Retinyl acetate (vitamin A acetate)– depth profiles did not differ significantly between the two age groups. Alpha-tocopheryl acetate (vitamin E acetate) penetration in the elderly SC was significantly lower than in the younger skin up to a depth of 12 μm, i.e., half of the SC depth probed. The different effect of age on the penetration of these two compounds is related to intrinsic changes in the skin coupled with the physicochemical parameters of the permeants in elderly skin using in vivo CRM. The authors argued that the decrease in lipid levels in elderly skin, which they observed via ceramide 3–depth profiling, hinders the partitioning of the highly lipophilic compound vitamin E ($\log P = 12.20$, $M_W = 431$ g·mol^{-1}) into the SC compared to vitamin A ($\log P = 9.40$, $M_W = 328$ g·mol^{-1}).

Anesthetic drugs. The penetration of procaine chlorhydrate, a local anesthetic, has been studied by CRM. Lunter and Daniels (2014) investigated the influence of the penetration enhancers propylene glycol and polyoxyethylene (POE)-23-lauryl ether on the penetration of procaine ($\log P = 2.14$, $M_W = 236$ g·mol^{-1}) contained in hydroxypropyl methylcellulose (HPMC)–poloxamer gels in cross-sections of porcine skin. The results of the CRM study were compared to those of a conventional skin penetration experiments in Franz cells. The HPMC–poloxamer gels containing a penetration enhancer and procaine were applied to the skin for 14 hours. The spectral range used for visualization of the procaine distribution in the skin covered the "fingerprint region" between 720 and 1820 cm^{-1}. For the calculation of color-coded images, the peak at 1600 to 1625 cm^{-1}, which results from the υ(C=C) (β NH$_2$)-scissoring mode, was used to identify procaine in the skin. For semiquantitative analysis of the procaine content in the skin samples, the procaine peak (1600 to 1625 cm^{-1}) was normalized to the δ (CH$_2$, CH$_3$) mode (1430 to 1490 cm^{-1}). This procedure differs from the frequently used normalization to the signal at 2910–2950 cm^{-1} assigned to the υ(CH$_3$) mode of keratin. No traces of propylene glycol and POE-(23)-lauryl ether were detected in skin. Results indicated that the highest procaine content was found in the SC, corresponding to the highest intensity of the procaine relative peak. Without penetration enhancers, the procaine was detected to a depth of 20 μm. In presence of the propylene glycol, the procaine was also found in the skin up to a depth of 20 μm. With the formulation containing POE-(23)-lauryl ether, Raman imaging showed a higher procaine content in an area of high lipid content at a depth of 40 to 50 μm (dermis) than in adjacent, more hydrated tissue. This behavior was explained by the lipophilic nature of procaine. Raman imaging also showed the presence of the procaine in skin up to a depth of 60 μm. The overall procaine content decreased with increasing depth. The penetration depths achieved with different vehicles increased in the following order: formulation with propylene glycol = formulation without enhancer > formulation with POE-(23)-lauryl ether. The enhancement of penetration by POE-ethers occurred via increases of the solubility and partition coefficient of procaine in the skin. The CRM results showed a good correlation with those of conventional penetration experiments.

Antiinflammatory drugs. The penetration of ketoprofen ($\log P = 3.20$, $M_W = 254$ g·mol^{-1}) and ibuprofen ($\log P = 3.97$, $M_W = 206$ g·mol^{-1}) applied as solutions in propylene glycol on skin samples were followed by SRS (Saar et al. 2011). 3D images of the skin during drug penetration and drug concentration profiles in the skin depth were obtained as a function of time. Ketoprofen presented a specific vibration band at 1599 cm^{-1} corresponding to the aromatic C–H stretching, whereas no specific bands could be detected for ibuprofen and propylene glycol. These two molecules were used in deuterated form to create a specific vibration band around 2120 cm^{-1} corresponding to the CD$_2$ bond stretching. The incident laser wavelength was tuned either to 1599 cm^{-1} to observe ketoprofen penetration or to 2120 cm^{-1} in order to image ibuprofen and propylene glycol in the skin. The results showed that propylene glycol penetrated the skin more rapidly and more efficiently than ketoprofen. Furthermore, the authors observed that the propylene glycol concentration was the same throughout the experiment time (158 minutes) on a hair shaft area, whereas it increased continuously in another area of the SC. This was explained by a rapid penetration of propylene glycol in the hair shaft, which was saturated before the first measurement time. In the case of ibuprofen, formation of crystals at the skin surface was observed before the first measurement, less than 30 minutes after application. This was explained by a rapid penetration of propylene glycol, which increased the ibuprofen concentration at the skin surface above its solubility, leading to its crystallization. This study shows the role of the enhancer as a solubilizing agent that may increase the penetration rate, but it also points out that similar kinetics for drugs and the formulation excipients are desirable.

This point has been demonstrated by Pyatski et al. (2016) with flufenamic acid (FluA), a non-steroidal antiinflammatory drug ($\log P = 5.25$, $M_W = 281$ g·mol^{-1}). They studied the permeation and spatial distribution of FluA in human skin in the presence of a hydrophilic (propylene glycol/ethanol (75/25)) vs. a hydrophobic enhancer (octanol). The authors also assessed the spatial distribution of both enhancers to provide mechanistic information regarding transport pathways. The FluA pathway was tracked by the C=C stretching mode at 1618 cm^{-1}. Deuterated versions of the enhancers allowed spectroscopic discrimination of exogenous chemicals from endogenous SC lipids. The CD$_2$ and CD$_3$ stretching (1941 to 2341 cm^{-1}) was used to track skin penetration of the vehicles. Discrete, small inclusions of both enhancers were observed throughout the SC. Although several features of the enhancer domains were similar, the spatial distribution of the relative concentration of FluA in the skin was significantly different between the two vehicles. In the SC it appeared to be predominantly driven by its solubility in the enhancers used and by the capacity of the vehicle-induced perturbation of the SC barrier. High concentrations of FluA were co-localized with octanol domains, which appeared to provide a pathway to the viable epidermis for the drug. The lipid barrier was significantly perturbed by octanol penetration, where time-dependent lipid extraction was suspected, as endogenous lipids were observed in octanol pockets. In contrast, with the hydrophilic agent, FluA concentrated in the upper SC and endogenous lipids appeared unperturbed in regions outside the enhancer pockets. The evolution and spatial distribution of the propylene glycol domains coincide with the development of the water pockets, whereas the distribution of octanol inclusions is complementary to regions with a relatively high water concentration.

55.5.2.1.2.2 Hydrophilic molecules Tfayli et al. (2007) studied the penetration of metronidazole ($\log P = -0.02$, $M_W = 171$ g.mol^{-1}), a drug used in the treatment of rosacea, on excised human skin samples. The drug was applied on the skin as a solution in diethylene glycol monoethyl ether

(DGME), a penetration enhancer. They first determined specific vibrations of the metronidazole Raman signature, which can be detected in the skin: two vibration bands were selected at 1191 and 1369 cm^{-1}. Metronidazole was applied at the concentration of 18 μg·mL^{-1} in DGME, and Raman spectra were acquired at several depths in the skin after 1- and 2-hour application times. Metronidazole was detected down to 23 to 24 μm in the skin after 1 hour and between 15 and 40 μm after 2 hours. These results were confirmed by Raman images obtained on thin slices of the skin samples used in the penetration experiment. Spectral images were reconstructed by integration of the metronidazole vibration (1191 cm^{-1}) intensity. They showed that metronidazole was present at depths of 40 to 45 μm in hair follicles and 25 μm in the SC. Furthermore, the authors used CRM to study the effect of metronidazole–DGME solution on the skin structure. A decrease in the intensity of the 1084 cm^{-1} peak was observed after applying the solution, corresponding to a decrease of the lipid chain organization. Such fluidization of lipid chains in skin can be related to the drug or DGME penetration.

Propylene glycol appears to be a gold standard among penetration enhancers for hydrophobic molecules. It has, however, a limited effect on the penetration of hydrophilic molecules. Ascencio et al. (2016) investigated the penetration of caffeine nanocrystals and propylene glycol as penetration enhancers, applied topically on porcine ear skin in the form of a gel, using CRM. Nanocrystals have been employed as a new alternative to increase the skin penetration of active components. Spectral ranges of 526 to 600 cm^{-1} for caffeine and 810 to 880 cm^{-1} for propylene glycol were chosen for analysis of penetration into the skin. Data reduction using statistical methods showed that propylene glycol penetrates significantly deeper than caffeine (20.7 to 22.0 μm versus 12.3 to 13.0 μm) without any penetration enhancement effect on caffeine, probably due to its size. Considering the measured SC thickness of 18.1 ± 1.0 μm, it was concluded that caffeine did not deeply penetrate SC and accumulated to saturate the upper 70% to 80%, while propylene glycol easily penetrated the SC and reached the stratum spinosum layer.

CRM was also applied to monitor the skin penetration of hyaluronic acids (HAs) on human skin sections (Essendoubi et al. 2016). HA is a highly hydrophilic polymer used as an active in cosmetics formulations. However, the skin penetration of HA is the matter of controversy because of its molecular size. According to the literature, chemical substances with a molar mass greater than 500 g·mol^{-1} may not penetrate skin. In this study, the penetration of three HA derivatives were investigated: Cristalhyal (1000 to 1400 kDa), Bashyal (100 to 300 kDa), and Renovhyal (20 to 50 kDa). HA solutions were deposited on skin surface for 8 hours at 32°C. Raman spectral analyses were then performed from cryo-sections of skin samples. The major bands of HA were found in two spectral windows: 800 to 1660 and 2700 to 3000 cm^{-1}. The results showed a skin permeability of low-molar-mass HA (20 to 300 kDa) and impermeability of high-molar-mass HA (1000 to 1400 kDa). Renvhyal and Bashyal were present in the skin section at an epidermal depth of about 100 μm for Renovhyal and 50 μm for Bashyal. The penetration depth of Cristalhyal was less than 25 μm. Raman images demonstrated that Renvhyal was present in the deepest layers of the epidermis, whereas Bashyal HA was localized in the superficial layer of the epidermis beneath SC, and Cristalhyal was only found in SC.

55.5.2.2 Metabolism of Active Substances Studied by CRM

The use of Raman may provide simultaneous information on the penetration and metabolism of drugs and pro-drugs. For instance, Zhang et al. (2007c) observed the spatial distribution of a pro-drug (1-ethyloxycarbonyl-5-fluorouracil or pro-5-fluorouracil (pro-5FU)) and a drug (5-fluorouracil, 5FU) inside pig skin using CRM. The pro-drug was applied before the drug because this is known to enhance transdermal delivery of 5FU. The pro-drug is converted to the active molecule, an important systemic antitumor drug, by endogenous enzymes or simple chemical hydrolysis once in the epidermis. Aqueous solutions of pro-5FU were topically applied to the SC (5 μL·cm^{-2}) for 20 hours at two different temperatures (22°C and 34°C). Raman bands at 866 and 637 cm^{-1} were chosen to monitor the relative concentrations of pro-drug and drug, respectively. The presence of several bands arising from 5-FU within the skin confirmed the hydrolysis of the pro-drug into drug. The difference of spectra recorded for treated and untreated skin disclosed the presence of both pro-5FU and 5-FU at depths of 2, 7, and 12 μm below the SC; the permeation into viable epidermis was not detected. Additionally, image planes of the spatial distribution showed that penetration of both species at 22°C was restricted to the SC, whereas both compounds were distributed throughout the SC and viable epidermis at 34°C, suggesting that hydrolysis was taking place in both the SC and in the viable epidermis. The highest relative amounts of drug with respect to pro-drug were observed in the viable epidermis at depths between 40 and 70 μm from the skin surface.

55.5.2.3   Tracking Formulation Excipients and their Influence on Skin Delivery

Mao et al. (2012) studied the distribution of alkyl chain perdeuterated sodium dodecyl sulfate (SDS-d_{25}) in human and porcine skin by CRM and IR. The band intensities of the CD_2 stretching vibrations were used for analysis of the permeation profiles of SDS-d_{25} in skin. The interaction between SDS and skin was evaluated through the CH_2 and CD_2 stretching frequencies and the amide I and II bands. The results indicated that SDS-d_{25} penetrated both porcine and human skin, with slightly deeper penetration through the SC of porcine skin. The chains of SDS are more ordered inside SC than in SDS micelles, giving evidence of an intercellular lipid penetration pathway for SDS in SC.

Binder et al. (2018) studied the penetration of sulfathiazole sodium (STZ) together with three excipients: sodium laureth sulfate (SLES), sodium dodecyl sulfate (SDS) and DMSO, in porcine skin by CRM and other methods. The penetration profiles of all compounds obtained by CRM and ATR-IR spectroscopy combined with tape stripping were comparable, showing good agreement between the methods. Both techniques showed the penetration depth increased in the order DMSO > SDS > SLES > STZ.

More recently, Binder et al. (2019) investigated the effect of viscosity of hydrogels made of hydroxyethyl cellulose (HEC) or hydroxypropyl methylcellulose (HPMC) on skin penetration of sulphadiazine sodium (SDZ) ($\log P = 0.39$, $M_W = 272$ g·mol^{-1}) by CRM and HPLC analysis. The SDZ was detectable at 1120 and 1600 cm^{-1} bands related to the SO_2 symmetric stretching of the sulfonamide group and a ring-stretching mode, respectively. Highly similar SDZ concentrations were observed in case of all gelled formulations, independently of the gelling agent concentration. This suggests that the specific viscosity of the investigated hydrogels had a subordinate effect on the skin penetration of SDZ. Conversely to drug amounts observed in the tape stripping studies, which were similar to CRM results, the penetration depths observed for SDZ showed a different trend. In fact, the gelling agent concentration seemed to have an influence on the total penetration depth of SDZ. In case of tape stripping, penetration depths between 47% and 78% of total SC thickness were observed. In case of CRM, these values ranged between 90% and 113% of SC thickness. For both hydrogels with HEC and HPMC, penetration depths were reduced as the viscosity of the gels increased. The diffusion of the model drug out of the formulation and into the skin might have been hindered by the high viscosity of the systems and thus resulted in a limited total penetration depth. In conclusion, drug distribution within the skin appeared to be affected by the viscosity of the vehicle. A direct comparison of the results obtained with the CRM and HPLC analysis revealed different absolute drug penetration depths. However, similar trends could be observed despite the varied experimental setup. The authors concluded that moderately enhanced hydrogel viscosity is advisable to allow for convenient dermal application while maintaining satisfactory skin penetration.

Bakonyi et al. (2018) investigated and compared the penetration profiles of four different lidocaine-containing formulations in human skin (hydrogel, oleogel, lyotropic liquid crystal [LLC], and nanostructured lipid carrier [NLC]) by Raman microscopic mapping of the drug. Raman spectra of the lidocaine-free blank formulations and lidocaine-containing formulations were detected in the wavenumber range of 300 to 1700 cm^{-1}. The penetration of lidocaine from the LLC and the NLC reached deeper skin layers and a higher amount of the drug penetrated into the skin, compared to the hydrogel and oleogel vehicles. In the case of hydrogel and oleogel, the drug was present in the epidermal and the dermal skin layers. In the case of LLC, the drug was present in the dermal layers of the skin, whereas with NLC the drug was distributed in the epidermal and dermal layers (Figure 55.5).

Förster et al. (2011b) studied the penetration behavior of *trans*-retinol from two kinds of formulations (o/w emulsion and surfactant solution) by using CRM along a diffusion experiment carried out in classical Franz cells. They used two hydrophilic surfactants (polyoxyethylene(20) monolaurate) and polyoxyethylene(20) monooleate), one lipophilic (polyoxyethylene(6) monooleate), and dodecane as the oil phase to prepare three solutions of retinol and three o/w emulsions loaded with retinol. Retinol penetration was higher when applying surfactant solutions than the corresponding o/w emulsions. The retinol penetration enhancement was the largest when using the PEG6C18:1 surfactant.

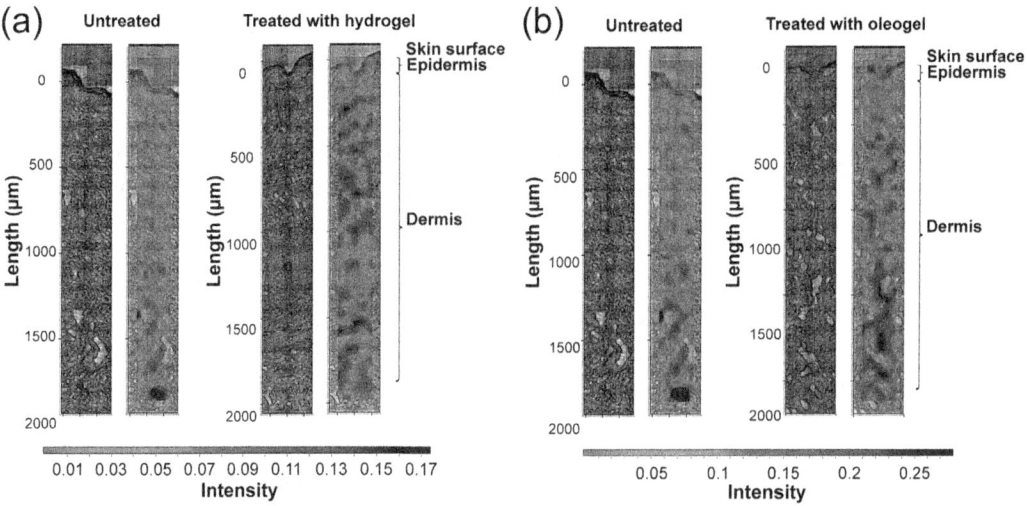

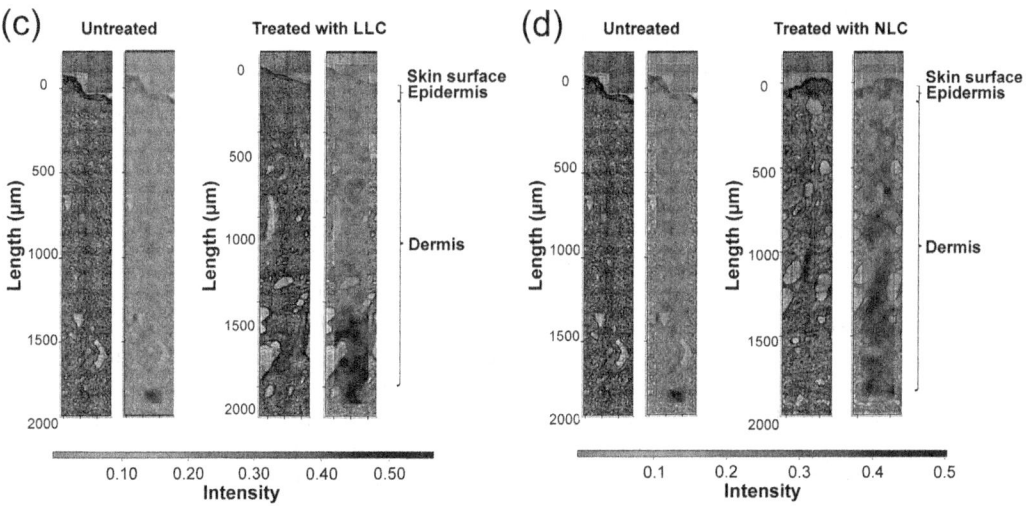

FIGURE 55.5 Video images and qualitative Raman maps of lidocaine distribution in human skin specimens after 6 hours following treatment with: hydrogel (a), oleogel (b), LLC (c) and NLC (d). Untreated skin is also displayed as control in all cases. (From Bakonyi et al. 2018 with permission.)

Indeed the unsaturated alkyl chain and the small polar head are two surfactant parameters known to cause increased penetration of drugs (Cappel and Kreuter 1991). CRM also allowed researchers to study the organization of SC lipids by measuring the intensity ratio I_{2880}/I_{2850} of the Raman bands $v_{asym}(CH_2)$ and $v_{sym}(CH_2)$ reflecting the lateral packing of the lipids. A low I_{2880}/I_{2850} ratio corresponds to a disorganized lipid bilayer, that is, a fluid medium. Fluidization of lipids was observed when applying a surfactant solution, especially PEG6C18:1, in dodecane, as well as pure dodecane, resulting in a significant decrease of the I_{2880}/I_{2850} ratio. The strong decrease of the I_{2880}/I_{2850} ratio by PEG6C18:1 was correlated with the highest penetration of *trans*-retinol into the deeper skin layers (epidermis and dermis). This ratio was not correlated with the total quantity of *trans*-retinol penetrating the skin (including SC). CRM analyses of *trans*-retinol absorption were in agreement with skin penetration experiments performed in Franz diffusion cells.

55.5.2.4 Tracking the Components of Nanocarriers in the Skin

Nanocarriers are useful to modulate and control the skin delivery of drugs. However, it is difficult to track them or their components without any labeling of the components. Labeling may increase the molar mass of the molecule and therefore influence its skin distribution.

Xiao et al. (2005a, b) monitored the penetration of liposomes made from perdeuterated acyl chain 1,2-dimyristoylphosphatidylcholine (DMPC-d_{54}), 1,2-dipalmitoylphosphatidylcholine (DPPC-d_{62}), and 1-palmitoyl-d_{31}, 2-oleoylphosphatidylcholine (P-d_{31}OPC) into excised pig skin using IR imaging and Raman spectroscopy. IR imaging was performed on histological skin sections, while CRM provided spatial information by non-destructive depth profiling. DMPC-d_{54} penetrated at a depth of 25 to 35 μm. The penetration of the gel phase DPPC-d_{62} was limited to 5 to 15 μm, whereas the liquid-crystalline phase P-d_{31}OPC penetrated to substantially greater depths (35 to 100 μm), at times ranging up to 24 hours after application. Further, the results showed that vesicles made of other lipid components did not overcome the skin barrier in their intact structure.

Wolf et al. (2018) tested the effects of two NLCs and a nano-sized emulsion based on monoacylphosphatidylcholine on physiological skin parameters in vivo during daily application over 4 weeks. A number of invasive and non-invasive different tests were performed. Among the latter, water, NMF, and urea profiling of volunteers' skin was studied using CRM. Treatment with the three formulations yielded a decrease in NMF content ranging from 20% to nearly 40% within 2 to 6 μm below the SC surface. Similarly, the treatment decreased the urea content by 18% to nearly 50% and particularly within the top 4 μm of the SC. Taken together with other tests on trans-epidermal water loss, skin pH, and penetration of curcumin followed by tape stripping and UV-vis spectroscopic analysis, CRM provided complementary information showing that these formulations impaired the skin barrier and increased delivery of the active substance.

55.5.3 *In Vitro - In Vivo* Correlations

Mateus et al. (2014) and Mohammed et al. (2014) studied the in vitro and in vivo skin permeation of salicylic acid and niacinamide, respectively. Salicylic acid ($\log P \sim 2$, $M_W = 138$ g·mol^{-1}) is a model drug widely used to manage dandruff, seborrheic dermatitis, ichthyosis, psoriasis, and acne and to remove warts. Niacinamide is a rather hydrophilic molecule ($\log P = -0.4$, $M_W = 122$ g·mol^{-1}), which reinforces the barrier function, decreasing photoaging signs and sebum production. A comparison was performed between in vivo CRM studies and in vitro Franz cell studies for both molecules. Salicylic acid was formulated in gels, while niacinamide was formulated in vehicles containing penetration enhancers (dimethyl isosorbide [DMI], Miglyol 812N [MG], mineral oil [MO], propylene glycol [PG], propylene glycol monolaurate [PGML], and N-methyl 2-pyrrolidone [NMP]). The study with niacinamide demonstrated that the vehicle that most enhanced its penetration (combination of PG:PGML:MG) was the one which itself was most taken up into the skin. In the case of salicylic acid entrapped in a gel, CRM was useful to validate the choice of the vehicle because it allows determining very quickly where the salicylic acid was located in the skin. Both studies showed a linear correlation between in vitro Franz cell results and the in vivo data collected by CRM.

55.5.4 CRM AND EFFICACY OF FORMULATIONS

At variance with the previous studies where tracking of molecules through skin was expected, CRM was also useful to study the deposit of active substances, particularly when they must remain on the skin surface such as sunscreen molecules. As explained earlier, this method is able to detect at the same time some physiological parameters that may assess the quality of the photoprotection.

The UV-protective agent should stay in the upper skin layers to absorb the harmful radiation. The possibility of non-destructive detection of UV absorbers in the skin drew attention to CRM as a tool for in vivo evaluation of sunscreens. Moreover, to evaluate the quality of UV-protective agents in sunscreen formulations, the amount of urocanic acid (UCA) can be measured. UCA is known to isomerize from *trans-* to *cis-*form upon UV exposure. Egawa and Iwaki (2008) tracked the *trans-*UCA content in the SC of 27 volunteers throughout 1 year. The lowest detected amounts in summer on the temporarily UV-exposed forearms indicated the feasibility of confocal Raman microspectroscopy to evaluate UV protection. Therefore, a second group of volunteers was artificially exposed to UV radiation with and without sunscreen. No statistical difference between no-exposure and exposure to sunscreen-treated skin proved the UV-blocking capacity of the applied agent. Furthermore, Egawa et al. (2010) determined the transition rate of *cis-* and *trans-*UCA simultaneously by confocal Raman microscopy. The detected isomerization upon UV exposure was confirmed by HPLC results after tape stripping and extraction of the SC. Further, Caspers et al. (2006) proved by CRM the excellent penetration of a commercially used UV absorber inside the deep part of SC only within few minutes after application.

Since the main region of interest for the evaluation of sunscreen formulations is located in the upper skin regions, the intrusion depth as one of the major limitations of CRM becomes irrelevant. Furthermore, the detection of the active agent and the quantification of metabolites indicating the protective potential make CRM a valuable tool to gain new insights into skin absorption of sunscreens and to reevaluate existing formulations.

Tippavajhala et al. (2008) investigated the penetration of two commercial sunscreen products in the SC of volunteers. Control spectra prior to product application and spectral 15, 60, and 120 minutes after application were acquired. SC containing the products was distinct from control SC in the 1590 to 1626 cm^{-1} region, with the product peak centered at 1606 cm^{-1}, as confirmed by comparison of average spectra and principal component analysis (PCA). PCA further showed discrimination of the spectra acquired in exposed SC at 0 to 8 μm depth from the control SC spectra and the exposed SC spectra acquired below 8 μm. However, application time did not significantly alter the product intensity in the SC.

Laing et al. (2019) employed CRM to show the lack of penetration of oils from a proprietary topical medical device containing paraffinum liquidum, petrolatum, paraffin, and tocopheryl acetate. Using references spectra of the oils of interest fitted to the skin spectra after topical application, they showed low Raman intensities of the oils at the skin surface and at a depth of 5 μm below the surface. No intensity pertaining to the product was detected at 10 μm inside the SC and below. Focusing on the depth interval 10 to 20 μm below the SC surface, the total product detected after 90 minutes of application (i.e., the AUC of the intensity–depth profile) corresponded to the detection limit in Raman obtained with a pure solution. The product intensity in the skin had a 95% confidence interval lower limit equal to the upper limit of the baseline 95% confidence interval. With a detection limit of 0.5 wt%, the authors concluded there was no statistically significant amount of product below 10 μm.

Tosato et al. (2015) used CRM to study in vivo the biochemical changes in human skin following mycosporine-like amino acids (MAAs) and Gadusol exposure incorporated in polymer gels containing Pluronic F127 under UV radiation. Distribution of MAAs and Gadusol was tracked from the 1280 and 920 cm^{-1} Raman bands, respectively. The effect of treatment on urocanic acid (1490 to 1515 cm^{-1} region and 1650 cm^{-1} peak) and histidine (1381 cm^{-1}) levels in SC, as well as lipid conformational changes, were monitored. Tracking the MAA and Gadusol Raman peaks, it was demonstrated that the polymer gel concentrated the actives at a depth of 2 μm in the SC, with no higher amounts at greater depths. CRM data further showed the photoactive properties of the actives, with urocanic acid levels in treated UV-exposed skin closer to those of normal skin than UV-exposed, non-treated skin. Conversely, Raman intensities of histidine decreased in UV-exposed treated skin, as urocanic acid is synthesized by histidine. UV-exposed skin contained a higher amount of *gauche* lipids. Application of the gels yielded an increase in the Raman intensities corresponding to lipids in *trans* conformation (1063 and 1128 cm^{-1}) compared to normal skin and a disappearance in the intensity assigned to *gauche* conformation (1085 cm^{-1}).

55.5.5 Tracking Potential Toxicants

Broding et al. (2011) demonstrated the ability of CRM to monitor the skin penetration of potentially hazardous substances, specifically 2-butoxyethanol, toluene, and pyrene. Intensity of the chemicals in the skin was normalized by the skin protein content and expressed as mmol per gram of keratin. Overall, for each compound, relative concentrations in the skin obtained by CRM were in the range reported in the occupational medicine literature, despite significant variability due to skin, analytical methods, and other assumptions.

CRM was also used to follow the penetration of a potent skin sensitizer, trans-cinnamaldehyde, continuously over 24 hours after topical application in different vehicles. The authors also investigated the delivery all four vehicles (absolute ethanol, 50% aqueous/ethanol, propylene glycol, and acetone:olive oil mixture) into porcine skin. Cinnamaldehyde penetration from the vehicle followed this relative ordering (fastest to slowest): acetone > aqueous ethanol > absolute ethanol > propylene glycol > olive oil (Bonnist et al. 2011).

Pot et al. (2016) demonstrated the use of CRM to obtain cutaneous penetration profiles of *para*-phenylenediamine (PPD), the well-known hair dye component that can cause skin sensitization. The 1% PPD patch test, used to confirm sensitization to PPD, was performed on volunteers. PPD penetration profiles, expressed as PPD mass/mass of keratin as a function of depth, were obtained for patch application times (0.5 to 23 hours) and for different time intervals after removal of the patch following a 3 × 1 hour repeated application scenario. This second experiment serves to track PPD clearance from the SC as a function of time. The first experiment showed substantial amounts of PPD detected after just 0.5 hour of application, namely ~70 mg PPD/g keratin at a depth of 4 μm. The PPD was detectable to a depth of about 20 μm in the skin, where the limit of detection of 13 mg PPD/g keratin was reached. The clearance experiment showed a decreased in PPD intensity with time, particularly from 0 to 10 μm depth. The baseline reading was reached approximately 20 μm below the SC surface. From these curves the half-life of PPD was estimated at 3 hours. Pot et al. also tracked metabolites of PPD known to form in the skin, as well as Bandrowski's base, a trimer that is classified as an extreme sensitizer. None of these compounds were detected, which may be due to concentrations below the limit of detection.

55.5.6 Compound Penetration in Reconstructed Human Skin

Recent changes in European Union directives (2010/63/EU) encourage the replacement of human and animal tests by reconstructed skin models in transdermal delivery experiments. RHE models are an essential tool for studying the penetration and permeation of cosmetic and pharmaceutical ingredients, although the permeability is higher compared to excised human and pig skin. However, the ranking of compounds is similar, and the results are reproducible (Fleischli et al. 2015). Utilization of CRM as a method to analyze skin penetration of topically applied actives into reconstructed human epidermis has been studied by different authors in order to validate artificial skin models for future use in place of clinical studies (Fleischli et al. 2013, 2015; Miloudi et al. 2018). Fleischli et al. (2013) used CRM to follow the penetration of the hydrophilic active glycerol and the lipophilic octyl methoxycinnamate in the RHE models. The distribution maps indicated a higher glycerol concentration in water-rich domains, while octyl methoxycinnamate was accumulated in the lipid-rich area droplets.

The same team compared the penetration in RHE and human skin of other hydrophilic (caffeine, benzoic acid, and salicylic acid) and lipophilic (octyl methoxycinnamate and 4-methylbenzylidene camphor) compounds. The results showed a strong correlation between the concentration of the compound in skin and their lipophilic/hydrophilic character. Moreover, different concentration profiles for RHE models and human skin in vivo were observed. This behavior was explained by the substantial differences in the molecular constitution of RHE models and human skin, mainly for water, lipids, and NMF (Fleischli et al. 2015).

Later, the penetration and distribution profiles of Delipidol (BioEurope Solabia, France), a hydrophobic anticellulite molecule, in RHE were monitored by confocal Raman spectroscopic imaging after different incubation times (1, 2, and 3 hours). Delipidol penetration was increased for longer exposition times. After 1 hour, the Delipidol showed a limited diffusion and its presence was restricted to the SC, whereas higher contribution of the SC was observed after 2 hours and 3 hours, with a deeper diffusion after 3 hours. This profile across the SC is a result of the barrier function of the lipid rich layer to the Delipidol which confers hydrophobicity to the molecule and retards its diffusion into the epidermis during the first hours. After 3 hours exposure, significant concentrations have penetrated the interface with the epidermal layer resulting in an accumulation of the molecule in this region (Miloudi et al. 2018).

Dancik et al. used CRM and skin permeation to show the effect of different storage conditions on the barrier function of RHE (Dancik et al. 2020).

55.6   CONCLUSION

With roughly 30 years' worth of studies in the area of skin research, CRM has established itself as a very efficient tool for fundamental study of the skin barrier function, investigation of skin penetration kinetics, and of mechanisms and effects of penetration enhancers. It is a highly versatile technique applicable, depending on instrumentation, to in vivo analysis with volunteers as well as excised human or animal skin and reconstructed skin models. As such, it can simultaneously complement several classical and invasive methods such as immunohistochemical analysis of biopsies and skin cryo-sections and transepidermal water loss, diffusion cell, and tape stripping protocols. In addition to the significant advantages of being label-free and non-invasive, CRM is a sensitive and reproducible technique. Above and beyond the classical techniques, it gives access to molecular-level information pertaining to the nature, physical state, and amount of cutaneous water, NMF, lipids, proteins, and other fundamental constituents of our skin physical barrier.

Development of CRM tools and methodologies in skin research is ongoing on several fronts. From the viewpoint of instrumentation, there is the development of handheld Raman probes for the in vivo analysis of dermatological pathologies (e.g., St-Arnaud et al. 2018). Such instruments will undoubtedly also find strong interest in pharmaceutical and cosmetic R&D, akin to the handheld TEWL, corneometry, and sebumetry instruments currently on the market. As no single technique can reveal everything there is to observe in skin, current research also pertains to the integration of Raman spectroscopy with multiphoton imaging and/or optical coherence tomography for multimodal approaches yielding morphological and molecular information (Sarri et al. 2019; Andreana et al. 2019). From the viewpoint of spectral data analysis and interpretation, developments are ongoing to provide not only semi-quantitative but also quantitative amount or concentration profiles of a given compound in skin (Caspers et al. 2019). More broadly, research in chemometrics provides advanced statistical methods enabling the extraction of relevant and critical information from complex, multidimensional datasets (Gautam et al. 2015; de Oliveira Mendes et al. 2016).

Despite the many publications utilizing CRM for skin analysis and percutaneous penetration research, what is missing is a set of guidelines outlining best practices for in vivo and ex vivo/in vitro Raman analysis, spectroscopic parameter selection, and data analysis and reporting. With respect to classical in vivo and in vitro skin penetration, the Organisation for Economic and Co-operation Development (OECD 2004a,b) and the Scientific Committee on Consumer Safety (SCCS 2010) published guidelines can enable a certain degree of homogeneity in published methodologies and reported results. It is the authors' opinion that CRM in skin R&D has reached a point where a similar document is necessary for effective cross-comparison of bioavailability and bioequivalence data and establishment of effective in vitro–in vivo correlations.

REFERENCES

Alonso C, Carrer V, Barba C, Coderch L. Caffeine delivery in porcine skin: a confocal Raman study. Arch Dermatol Res. 2018;310:657–664.

Andreana M, Sentosa R, Erkkilä MT, Drexler W, Unterhuber A. Depth resolved label-free multimodal optical imaging platform to study morpho-molecular composition of tissue. Photochem Photobiol Sci. 2019;18(5):997–1008.

Anigbogu ANC, Williams AC, Barry BW, Edwards HGM. Fourier transform Raman spectroscopy of interactions between the penetration enhancer dimethyl sulfoxide and human stratum corneum. Int J Pharm. 1995;125:265–82.

Ascencio SM, Choe C, Meinke MC, Müller RH, Maksimov GV, Wigger-Alberti W, Lademann J, Darvin ME. Confocal Raman microscopy and multivariate statistical analysis for determination of different penetration abilities of caffeine and propylene glycol applied simultaneously in a mixture on porcine skin ex vivo. Eur J Pharm Biopharm. 2016;104:51–58.

Ashtikara M, Matthäus C, Schmitt M, Krafft C, Fahr A, Popp J. Non-invasive depth profile imaging of the stratum corneum using confocal Raman microscopy: First insights into the method. Eur J Pharm Sci. 2013;50:601–608.

Atef E, Altuwaijri N. Using Raman spectroscopy in studying the effect of propylene glycol, oleic acid, and their combination on the rat skin. AAPS PharmSciTech. 2018;19:114–122.

Babita K, Kumar V, Rana V, Jain S, Tiwary AK. Thermotropic and spectroscopic behavior of skin: Relationship with percutaneous permeation enhancement. Curr Drug Deliv. 2006;3:95–113.

Bakonyi M, Gácsi A, Kovács A, Szűcs MB, Berkó S, Csányi E. Following-up skin penetration of lidocaine from different vehicles by Raman spectroscopic mapping. J Pharm Biomed Anal. 2018;154:1–6.

Barry BW, Edwards H, Williams A. Fourier transform Raman and infrared vibrational study of human skin: assignment of spectral bands. J Raman Spectrosc. 1992;23:641–645.

Bernard G, Auger M, Soucy J, Pouliot R. Physical characterization of the stratum corneum of an in vitro psoriatic skin model by ATR-FTIR and Raman spectroscopies. BBA-General Subjects. 2007;1770(9):1317–1323.

Bielfeldt S, Laing S, Sadowski T, Gunt H, Wilhelm KP. Characterization and validation of an in vivo confocal Raman spectroscopy led tri-method approach in the evaluation of the lip barrier. Skin Res Technol. 2020;26:390–397.

Binder L, Kulovitsa EM, Petza R, Ruthofera J, Baurechtb D, Klang V, Valenta C. Penetration monitoring of drugs and additives by ATR-FTIR spectroscopy/tape stripping and confocal Raman spectroscopy – A comparative study. Eur J Pharm Biopharm. 2018;130:214–223.

Binder L, Mazál J, Petz R, Klang V, Valenta C. The role of viscosity on skin penetration from cellulose ether-based hydrogels. Ski Res Technol. 2019;25:725–734.

Binder L, SheikhRezaei S, Baierl A, Gruber L, Wolzt M, Valenta C. Confocal Raman spectroscopy: in vivo measurement of physiological skin parameters–a pilot study. J Dermatol Sci. 2017;88(3):280–288.

Böhling A, Bielfeldt S, Himmelmann A, Keskin M, Wilhelm KP. Comparison of the stratum corneum thickness measured in vivo with confocal Raman spectroscopy and confocal reflectance microscopy. Skin Res Technol. 2014;20(1):50–57.

Boireau-Adamezyk E, Baillet-Guffroy A, Stamatas GN. Mobility of water molecules in the stratum corneum: effects of age and chronic exposure to the environment. J Invest Dermatol. 2014;134(7):2046–2049.

Bolzinger M-A, Briancon S, Pelletier J, Fessi H, Chevalier Y. Percutaneous release of caffeine from microemulsion, emulsion and gel dosage forms, Eur J Pharm Biopharm. 2008;68:446–451.

Boncheva M, Damien F, Normand V. Molecular organization of the lipid matrix in intact stratum corneum using ATR-FTIR spectroscopy. Biochim Biophys Acta. 2008;1778:1344–1355.

Bonnist EYM, Gorce J-P, Mackay C, Pendlington RU, Pudney PDA. Measuring the penetration of a skin sensitizer and its delivery vehicles simultaneously with confocal Raman spectroscopy. Skin Pharmacol Physiol. 2011;24:274–283.

Bouwstra JA, Cheng K, Gooris GS, Weerheim A, Ponec M. Phase behavior of isolated skin lipids. Biochim Biophys Acta. 1996;1300:177–186.

Bouwstra JA, Gooris GS, Ponec M. Skin lipid organization, composition and barrier function. IFSCC Magazine. 2007;10:297–307.

Bouwstra JA, Gooris GS, van der Spek JA, Bras W. Structural investigations of human stratum corneum by small angle X-Ray scattering. J Invest Dermatol. 1991;97:1005–1012.

Bouwstra JA, Honeywell-Nguyen PL, Gooris GS, Ponec M. Structure of the skin barrier and its modulation by vesicular formulations. Prog Lipid Res. 2003;42:1–36.

Bouwstra JA, Ponec M. The skin barrier in healthy and diseased state. Biochim Biophys Acta – Biomembranes. 2006;1758:2080–2095.

Broding H C, van der Pol A, de Sterke J, Monsé C, Fartasch M, Brüning T. In vivo monitoring of epidermal absorption of hazardous substances by confocal Raman micro-spectroscopy. J Dtsch Dermatol Ges. 2011;9(8):618–627.

Bronaugh RL, Maibach HI. Percutaneous absorption. Drugs – Cosmetics – Mechanisms – Methodology. 3rd ed, Marcel Dekker, New York 1999.

Cappel MJ, Kreuter J. Effect of nonionic surfactants on transdermal drug delivery: I. Polysorbates. Int J Pharm. 1991;69:143–153.

Caspers PJ, Lucassen GW, Bruining HA, Puppels GJ. Automated depth-scanning confocal Raman micro-spectrometer for rapid in vivo determination of water concentration profiles in human skin. J Raman Spectrosc. 2000;31:813–818.

Caspers PJ, Lucassen GW, Carter EA, Bruining HA, Puppels GJ. In vivo confocal Raman microspectroscopy of the skin: Noninvasive determination of molecular concentration profiles. J Invest Dermatol. 2001;116:434–442.

Caspers PJ, Lucassen GW, Puppels GJ. Combined in vivo confocal Raman spectroscopy and confocal microscopy of human skin. Biophys J. 2003;85:572–580.

Caspers PJ, Lucassen GW, Wolthuis R, Bruining HA, Puppels GJ. In vitro and in vivo Raman spectroscopy of human skin. Biospectroscopy. 1998; 4(S5):S31–S39.

Caspers PJ, Nico C, Bakker Schut TTC, de Sterke J, Pudney PD, Curto PR, Illand A, Puppels GJ. Method to quantify the in vivo skin penetration of topically applied materials based on confocal Raman spectroscopy. Translational Biophotonics. 2019;e201900004.

Caspers PJ, van der Pol A, de Sterke J. Penetration of sunscreen agents monitored in vivo by confocal Raman spectroscopy. J Invest Dermatol. 2006;126:S3–S73.

Caspers PJ, Williams AC, Carter EA, Edwards HG, Barry BW, Bruining, HA, Puppels GJ. Monitoring the penetration enhancer dimethyl sulfoxide in human stratum corneum in vivo by confocal Raman spectroscopy. Pharm Res. 2002;19(10):1577–1580.

Choe C, Lademann J, Darvin ME. Gaussian-function-based deconvolution method to determine the penetration ability of petrolatum oil into in vivo human skin using confocal Raman microscopy. Laser Phys. 2014;24(10):105601.

Choe C, Lademann J, Darvin ME. Analysis of human and porcine skin in vivo/ex vivo for penetration of selected oils by confocal Raman microscopy. Skin Pharmacol Physiol. 2015;28(6):318–330.

Choe C, Lademann J, Darvin ME. Depth profiles of hydrogen bound water molecule types and their relation to lipid and protein interaction in the human stratum corneum in vivo. Analyst. 2016;141(22):6329–6337.

Choe C, Schleusener J, Lademann J, Darvin ME. Age related depth profiles of human stratum corneum barrier-related molecular parameters by confocal Raman microscopy in vivo. Mech Ageing Dev. 2018a;172:6–12.

Choe C, Schleusener J, Lademann J, Darvin ME. Human skin in vivo has a higher skin barrier function than porcine skin ex vivo—comprehensive Raman microscopic study of the stratum corneum. J Biophotonics. 2018b;11(6), e201700355.

Chrit L, Bastien P, Biatry B, Simonnet JT, Potter A, Minondo AM, Flament F, Bazin R, Sockalingum GD, Leroy F, Manfait M, Hadjur C. In vitro and in vivo confocal Raman study of human skin hydration: assessment of a new moisturizing agent, pMPC. Biopolymers: Original Research on Biomolecules. 2007;85(4):359–369.

Chrit L, Bastien P, Sockalingum GD, Batisse D, Leroy F, Manfait M, Hadjur C. An in vivo randomized study of human skin moisturization by a new confocal Raman fiber-optic microprobe: assessment of a glycerol-based hydration cream. Skin Pharmacol Physiol. 2006;19(4):207–215.

Chrit L, Hadjur C, Morel S, Sockalingum GD, Lebourdon G, Leroy F, Manfait M. In vivo chemical investigation of human skin using a confocal Raman fiber optic microprobe. J Biomed Opt. 2005;10(4):044007.

Crowther JM, Sieg A, Blenkiron P, Marcott C, Matts PJ, Kaczvinsky JR, Rawlings AV. Measuring the effects of topical moisturizers on changes in stratum corneum thickness, water gradients and hydration *in vivo*. Br J Dermatol. 2008;159:567–577.

Dąbrowska AK, Adlhart C, Spano F, Rotaru GM, Derler S, Zhai L, Spencer ND, Rossi RM. In vivo confirmation of hydration-induced changes in human-skin thickness, roughness and interaction with the environment. Biointerphases. 2016;11(3):031015.

Damien F, Boncheva M. The extent of orthorhombic lipid phases in the stratum corneum determines the barrier efficiency of human skin in vivo. J Invest Dermatol. 2010;130:611–614.

Dancik Y, Bigliardi PL, Bigliardi-Qi M. What happens in the skin? Integrating skin permeation kinetics into studies of developmental and reproductive toxicity following topical exposure. Reprod. Toxicol. 2015;58:252–281.

Dancik Y, Kichou H, Eklouh-Molinier C, Souce M, Munnier E, Chourpa I, Bonnier F. Freezing Weakens the Barrier Function of Reconstructed Human Epidermis as Evidenced by Raman Spectroscopy and Percutaneous Permeation. Pharamceutics. 2020;12(11):1041–1060.

Dancik Y, Sriram G, Rout B, Zou Y, Bigliardi-Qi M, Bigliardi PL. Physical and compositional analysis of differently cultured 3D human skin equivalents by confocal Raman spectroscopy. Analyst. 2018;143(5):1065–1076.

Darvin ME, Choe CS, Schleusener J, Lademann J. Non-invasive depth profiling of the stratum corneum in vivo using confocal Raman microscopy considering the non-homogeneous distribution of keratin. Biomed Opt Express. 2019;10(6):3092–3103.

de Oliveira Mendes T, Pereira LP, Dos Santos L, Tippavajhala VK, Soto CT, Martin AA. Statistical strategies to reveal potential vibrational markers for in vivo analysis by confocal Raman spectroscopy. J Biomed Opt. 2016;21(7):075010.

dos Santos L, Rangel JL, Tippavajhala VK, da Silva MGP, Mogilevych B, Martin AA. In vivo intra-and inter-individual variability study of human stratum corneum by confocal Raman spectroscopy. Vib Spectrosc. 2016;87:199–206.

dos Santos L, Tippavajhala VK, Mendes TO, da Silva MGP, Fávero PP, Soto CAT, Martin AA. Evaluation of penetration process into young and elderly skin using confocal Raman spectroscopy. Vib. Spectrosc. 2019;100:123–130.

Downes A, Elfick A. Raman spectroscopy and related techniques in biomedicine. Sensors 2010;10:1871–1889.

Egawa M, Hirao T, Takahashi M. In vivo estimation of stratum corneum thickness from water concentration profiles obtained with Raman spectroscopy. Acta Derm Venereol. 2007;87:4–8.

Egawa M, Iwaki H. In vivo evaluation of the protective capacity of sunscreen by monitoring urocanic acid isomer in the stratum corneum using Raman spectroscopy. Ski Res Technol. 2008;14:410–417.

Egawa M, Nomura J, Iwaki H. The evaluation of the amount of cis- and trans-urocanic acid in the stratum corneum by Raman spectroscopy. Photochem Photobiol. Sci. 2010;9:730–733.

Egawa M, Tagami H. Comparison of the depth profiles of water and water-binding substances in the stratum corneum determined in vivo by Raman spectroscopy between the cheek and volar forearm skin: effects of age, seasonal changes and artificial forced hydration. Br J Dermatol. 2008; 158(2):251–260.

Essendoubi M, Gobinet C, Reynaud R, Angiboust JF, Manfait M, Piot O. Human skin penetration of hyaluronic acid of different molecular weights as probed by Raman spectroscopy. Ski Res Technol. 2016;22:55–62.

Evans CL, Xie XS. Coherent anti-Stokes Raman scattering microscopy: chemical imaging for biology and medicine. Annu Rev Anal Chem. 2008;1:883–909.

Failloux N, Bonnet I, Perrier E, Baron M-H. Effects of light, oxygen and concentration on vitamin A_1. J Raman Spectrosc. 2004;2:140–147.

Fleischli FD, Mathes S, Adlhart C. Label free non-invasive imaging of topically applied actives in reconstructed human epidermis by confocal Raman spectroscopy. Vib Spectrosc. 2013;68:29–33.

Fleischli FD, Morf F, Adlhart C. Skin concentrations of topically applied substances in reconstructed human epidermis (RHE) compared with human skin using in vivo confocal Raman microscopy. Chimia. 2015;69(3):147–151.

Fluhr JW, Darlenski R, Lachmann N, Baudouin C, Msika P, De Belilovsky C, Hachem JP. Infant epidermal skin physiology: adaptation after birth. Br J Dermatol. 2012;166(3):483–490.

Förster M, Bolzinger M-A, Ach D, Montagnac G, Briançon S. Ingredients tracking of cosmetic formulations in the skin: a confocal Raman microscopy investigation. Pharm Res. 2011b;28:858–872.

Förster M, Bolzinger M-A, Montagnac G, Briançon S. Confocal Raman microspectroscopy of the skin. Eur J Dermatol. 2011a;21:851–863.

Francoeur ML, Golden GM, Potts RO. Oleic acid: its effects on stratum corneum in relation to (trans)dermal drug delivery. Pharm Res. 1990;7:621–627.

Franzen L, Anderski J, Planz V, Kostka K.-H, Windbergs M. Combining confocal Raman microscopy and freeze-drying for quantification of substance penetration into human skin. Exp Dermatol.2014;23:942–944.

Franzen L, Anderski J, Windbergs M. Quantitative detection of caffeine in human skin by confocal Raman spectroscopy – A systematic in vitro validation study. Eur. J. Pharm. Biopharm. 2015;95:110–116.

Franzen L, Selzer D, Fluhr JW, Schaefer UF, Windbergs M. Towards drug quantification in human skin with confocal Raman microscopy. Eur J Pharm Biopharm.2013;84:437–444

Franzen L, Windbergs M. Accessing Raman spectral variability in human stratum corneum for quantitative in vitro depth profiling. J Raman Spectrosc. 2014;45(1): 82–88.

Freudiger CW, Min W, Saar BG, Lu S, Holtom GR, He C, Tsai JC, Kang JX, Xie XS. Label-free biomedical imaging with high sensitivity by stimulated Raman scattering microscopy. Science 2008;322:1857–1861.

Fu D, Lu F-K, Zhang X, Freudiger C, Pernik DR, Holtom G, Xie XS. Quantitative chemical imaging with multiplex stimulated Raman scattering microscopy. J Am Chem Soc. 2012;134:3623–3626.

Gautam R, Vanga S, Ariese F, Umapathy S. Review of multidimensional data processing approaches for Raman and infrared spectroscopy. EPJ Tech Instrum. 2015;2(1):1–38.

Gay CL, Guy RH, Golden GM, Mak VHW, Francoeur ML. Characterization of low temperature (i.e., < 65 degrees C) lipid transitions in human stratum corneum. J Invest Dermatol. 1994;103:233–239.

Gniadecka M, Nielsen OF, Christensen DH, Wulf HC. Structure of water, proteins, and lipids in intact human skin, hair, and nail. J Invest Dermatol. 1998;110(4):393–398.

Groen D., Poole DS, Gooris GS, Bouwstra JA. Is an orthorhombic lateral packing and a proper lamellar organization important for the skin barrier function? Biochim Biophys Acta Biomembranes 2011;1808:1529–1537.

Hancewicz TM, Xiao C, Weissman J, Foy V, Zhang S, Misra M. A consensus modeling approach for the determination of stratum corneum thickness using in-vivo confocal Raman spectroscopy. J Cosmet Dermatol Sci Appl. 2012;2:241–251.

Janssens M, van Smeden J, Puppels GJ, Lavrijsen APM, Caspers PJ, Bouwstra JA. Lipid to protein ratio plays an important role in the skin barrier function in patients with atopic eczema. Br J Dermatol. 2014;170(6):1248–1255.

Kim S, Byun KM, Lee SY. Influence of water content on Raman spectroscopy characterization of skin sample. Biomed Opt Express. 2017;8(2): 1130–1138.

Klossek A, Thierbach S, Rancan F, Vogt A, Blume-Peytavi U, Rühl E. Studies for improved understanding of lipid distributions in human skin by combining stimulated and spontaneous Raman microscopy. Eur J Pharm Biopharm. 2017;116:76–84.

Knudsen L, Johansson CK, Philipsen PA, Gniadecka M, Wulf HC. Natural variations and reproducibility of in vivo near-infrared Fourier transform Raman spectroscopy of normal human skin. J Raman Spectrosc. 2002;33(7):574–579.

Laing S, Bielfeldt S, Wilhelm KP, Obst J. Confocal Raman spectroscopy as a tool to measure the prevention of skin penetration by a specifically designed topical medical device. Ski Res Technol.2019;25(4):578–586.

Li L, Wang H, Cheng J-X. Quantitative coherent anti-Stokes Raman scattering imaging of lipid distribution in coexisting domains. Biophys J. 2005;89:3480–3490.

Lu F-K, Ji M, Fu D, Ni X, Freudiger CW, Holtom G, Xie XS. Multicolor stimulated Raman scattering microscopy. Mol Phys. 2012;110:1927–1932.

Lunter D, Daniels R. Confocal Raman microscopic investigation of the effectiveness of penetration enhancers for procaine delivery to the skin. J Biomed Opt. 2014;19:126015.

Mahrhauser DS, Nagelreiter C, Gehrig S, Geye A, Ogris M, Kwizda K, Valenta C. Assessment of Raman spectroscopy as a fast and non-invasive method for total stratum corneum thickness determination of pig skin. Int J Pharm. 2015;495(1):482–484.

Mao G, Flach CR, Mendelsohn R, Walters RM. Imaging the distribution of sodium dodecyl sulfate in skin by confocal Raman and infrared microspectroscopy. Pharm Res. 2012;29:2189–2201.

Mateus R, Abdalghafor H, Oliveira G, Hadgraft J, Lane ME. A new paradigm in dermatopharmacokinetics–confocal Raman spectroscopy. Int J Pharm. 2013;444(1–2):106–108.

Mateus R, Moore DJ, Hadgraft J, Lane ME. Percutaneous absorption of salicylic acid–in vitro and in vivo studies. Int J Pharm. 2014;475(1–2):471–474.

Mélot M, Pudney PDA, Williamson AM, Caspers PJ, Van Der Pol A, Puppels GJ. Studying the effectiveness of penetration enhancers to deliver retinol through the stratum corneum by in vivo confocal Raman spectroscopy. J Control Release 2009;138:32–39.

Miloudi L, Bonnier F, Tfayli A, Yvergnaux F, Byrne HJ, Chourpa I, Munnier E. Confocal Raman spectroscopic imaging for in vitro monitoring of active ingredient penetration and distribution in reconstructed human epidermis model. J Biophotonics. 2018;11(4):e201700221.

Min W, Freudiger CW, Lu S, Xie XS. Coherent nonlinear optical imaging: beyond fluorescence microscopy. Annu Rev Phys Chem. 2011;62:507–530.

Mogilevych B, dos Santos L, Rangel JL, Grancianinov KJ, Sousa MP, Martin AA. Analysis of the in vivo confocal Raman spectral variability in human skin. Biophotonics South America. 2015; 9531:95312.

Mohammed D, Matts PJ, Hadgraft J, Lane ME. In vitro –In vivo Correlation in Skin Permeation. Pharm. Res. 2014;31:394–400.

Naik A, Pechtold LARM, Potts RO, Guy RH. Mechanism of oleic acid-induced skin penetration in vivo in humans. J Control Release 1995;37:299–306.

Naito S, Min YK, Sugata K, Osanai O, Kitahara T, Hiruma H, Hamaguchi HO. In vivo measurement of human dermis by 1064 nm-excited fiber Raman spectroscopy. Skin Res Technol. 2008;14(1):18–25.

Nakagawa N, Matsumoto M, Sakai S. In vivo measurement of the water content in the dermis by confocal Raman spectroscopy. Skin Res Technol. 2010;16(2):137–141.

Nandakumar P, Kovalev A, Volkmer A. Vibrational imaging based on stimulated Raman scattering microscopy. New J Phys. 2009;11:033026.

Nguyen TT, Happillon T, Feru J, Brassart-Passco S, Angiboust JF, Manfait M, Piot O. Raman comparison of skin dermis of different ages: focus on spectral markers of collagen hydration. J Raman Spectrosc. 2013;44(9):1230–1237.

Niehues H, Bouwstra JA, El Ghalbzouri A, Brandner JM, Zeeuwen PL, van den Bogaard EH. 3D skin models for 3R research: The potential of 3D reconstructed skin models to study skin barrier function. Exp Dermatol. 2018;27(5):501–511.

Norlén L. Skin barrier structure and function: The single gel phase model. J Invest Dermatol. 2001;117:830–836.

OECD (2004a), Test No. 428: Skin Absorption: In Vitro Method, OECD Guidelines for the Testing of Chemicals, Section 4, Ed. OECD, Paris.

OECD (2004b), Test No. 427: Skin Absorption: In Vivo Method, OECD Guidelines for the Testing of Chemicals, Section 4, Ed. OCDE, Paris.

Osada M, Gniadecka M, Wulf HC. Near-infrared Fourier transform Raman spectroscopic analysis of proteins, water and lipids in intact normal stratum corneum and psoriasis scales. Exp Dermatol. 2004;13(6):391–395.

Pilgram GSK, Engelsma-van Pelt AM, Bouwstra JA, Koerten HK. Electron diffraction provides new information on human stratum corneum lipid organization studied in relation to depth and temperature. J Invest Dermatol. 1999;113:403–409.

Pot LM, Coenraads PJ, Blömeke B, Puppels GJ, Caspers PJ. Real-time detection of p-phenylenediamine penetration into human skin by in vivo Raman spectroscopy. Contact dermatitis. 2016;74(3):152–158.

Pudney PD, Bonnist EY, Caspers PJ, Gorce JP, Marriot C, Puppels GJ, Singleton S, van der Wolf MJG. A new in vivo Raman probe for enhanced applicability to the body. Appl. Spectrosc. 2012;66(8):882–891.

Pudney PDA, Mélot M, Caspers PJ, van der Pol A, Puppels GJ. An in vivo confocal Raman study of the delivery of trans-retinol to the skin. Appl Spectrosc. 2007;61:804–811.

Pyatski Y, Zhang Q, Mendelsohn R, Flach CR. Effects of permeation enhancers on flufenamic acid delivery in ex vivo human skin by confocal Raman microscopy. Int J Pharm. 2016;505:319–328.

Quatela A, Miloudi L, Tfayli A, Baillet-Guffroy A. In vivo Raman microspectroscopy: intra-and intersubject variability of stratum corneum spectral markers. Skin Pharmacol Physiol. 2016;29(2):102–109.

Richters RJ, Falcone D, Uzunbajakava NE, Varghese B, Caspers PJ, Puppels GJ, van Erp PE, van de Kerkhof PC. Sensitive skin: assessment of the skin barrier using confocal Raman microspectroscopy. Skin Pharmacol Physiol. 2017;30(1):1–12.

Saar BG, Contreras-Rojas LR, Xie XS, Guy RH. Imaging drug delivery to skin with stimulated Raman scattering microscopy. Mol Pharm. 2011;8:969–975.

Saar BG, Freudiger CW, Reichman J, Stanley CM, Holtom GR, Xie XS. Video-rate molecular imaging in vivo with stimulated Raman scattering. Science. 2010;330:1368–1370.

Sarri B, Chen X, Canonge R, Grégoire S, Formanek F, Galey JB, Potter A, Bornschlögl T, Rigneault H. In vivo quantitative molecular absorption of glycerol in human skin using coherent anti-Stokes Raman scattering (CARS) and two-photon auto-fluorescence. J Control Release. 2019;308:190–196.

SCCS. Opinion on Basic Criteria for the In Vitro Assessment of Dermal Absorption of Cosmetic Ingredients, SCCS (Scientific Committee on Consumer Safety). (2010); SCCS/1358/10.

Schallreuter KU, Moore J, Wood JM, Beazley WD, Gaze DC, Tobin DJ, Marshall HS, Panske A, Panzig E, Hibberts NA. In vivo and in vitro evidence for hydrogen peroxide (H_2O_2) accumulation in the epidermis of patients with vitiligo and its successful removal by a UVB-activated pseudocatalase. J Invest Derm Symp Proc. 1999;4(1):91–96.

Sdobnov AY, Darvin ME, Schleusener J, Lademann J, Tuchin VV. Hydrogen bound water profiles in the skin influenced by optical clearing molecular agents—Quantitative analysis using confocal Raman microscopy. J Biophotonics. 2019;12(5):e201800283.

Slipchenko MN, Chen H, Ely DR, Jung Y, Carvajal MT, Cheng J-X. Vibrational imaging of tablets by epi-detected stimulated Raman scattering microscopy. Analyst. 2010;135:2613–2619.

Song Y, Xiao C, Mendelsohn R, Zheng T, Strekowski L, Michniak B. Investigation of iminosulfuranes as novel transdermal penetration enhancers: enhancement activity and cytotoxicity. Pharm Res. 2005;22:1918–1925.

Sriram G, Alberti M, Dancik Y, Wu B, Wu R, Feng Z, Ramasamy S, Bigliardi PL, Bigliardi-Qi M, Wang Z. Full-thickness human skin-on-chip with enhanced epidermal morphogenesis and barrier function. MaterToday. 2018;21(4):326–340.

Stamatas GN, de Sterke J, Hauser M, von Stetten O, van der Pol A. Lipid uptake and skin occlusion following topical application of oils on adult and infant skin. J Dermatol Sci. 2008;50(2):135–142.

St-Arnaud K, Aubertin K, Strupler M, Madore W-J, Grosse AA, Petrecca K, Trudel D, Leblond F. Development and characterization of a handheld hyperspectral Raman imaging probe system for molecular characterization of tissue on mesoscopic scales. Med Phys. 2018;45(1):328–339.

Tfaili S, Gobinet C, Josse G, Angiboust JF, Baillet A, Manfait M, Piot O. Vibrational spectroscopies for the analysis of cutaneous permeation: experimental limiting factors identified in the case of caffeine penetration. Anal Bioanal Chem. 2013;405:1325–1332.

Tfaili S, Gobinet C, Josse G, Angiboust JF, Manfait M, Piot O. Confocal Raman microspectroscopy for skin characterization: a comparative study between human skin and pig skin. Analyst 2012a;137:3673–3682.

Tfaili S, Josse G, Angiboust J.-F, Manfait M, Piot O. Monitoring caffeine and resveratrol cutaneous permeation by confocal Raman microspectroscopy. J. Biophotonics. 2014;7:676–681.

Tfaili S, Josse G, Gobinet C, Angiboust JF, Manfait M, Piot O. Shedding light on the laser wavelength effect in Raman analysis of skin epidermises. Analyst 2012b;137:4241–4246.

Tfayli A, Guillard E, Manfait M, Baillet-Guffroy A. Molecular interactions of penetration enhancers within ceramides organization: a Raman spectroscopy approach. Analyst 2012a;137:5002–5010.

Tfayli A, Guillard E, Manfait M, Baillet-Guffroy A. Raman spectroscopy: feasibility of in vivo survey of stratum corneum lipids, effect of natural aging. Eur J Dermatol. 2012b;22:36–41.

Tfayli A, Guillard E, Manfait M, Baillet-Guffroy A. Thermal dependence of Raman descriptors of ceramides. Part I: effect of double bonds in hydrocarbon chains. Anal Bioanal Chem. 2010;397:1281–1296.

Tfayli A, Jamal D, Vyumvuhore R, Manfait M, Baillet-Guffroy A. Hydration effects on the barrier function of stratum corneum lipids: Raman analysis of ceramides 2, III and 5. Analyst. 2013;138(21):6582–6588.

Tfayli A, Piot O, Pitre F, Manfait M. Follow-up of drug permeation through excised human skin with confocal Raman microspectroscopy. Eur J Biophys. 2007;36:1049–1058.

Tippavajhala VK, Magrini TD, Matsuo DC, Silva MG, Favero PP, De Paula LR, Martin AA. In vivo determination of moisturizers efficacy on human skin hydration by confocal Raman spectroscopy. AAPS PharmSciTech. 2018;19(7):3177–3186.

Tosato MG, Orallo DE, Ali SM, Churio MS, Martin AA, Dicelio L. Confocal Raman spectroscopy: In vivo biochemical changes in the human skin by topical formulations under UV radiation. J Photochem Photobiol B Biol. 2015;153:51–58.

Touitou E, Meidan VM, Horwitz E. Methods for quantitative determination of drug localized in the skin. J Control Release. 1998;56:7–21.

Van Hal DA, Jeremiasse E, Junginger HE, Spies F, Bouwstra JA. Structure of fully hydrated human stratum corneum: a freeze-fracture electron microscopy study. J Invest Dermatol. 1996;106:89–95.

Verzeaux L, Vyumvuhore R, Boudier D, Le Guillou M, Bordes S, Essendoubi M, Manfait M, Closs B. Atopic skin: In vivo Raman identification of global molecular signature, a comparative study with healthy skin. Exp Dermatol. 2018;27(4):403–408.

Vyumvuhore R, Tfayli A, Biniek K, Duplan H, Delalleau A, Manfait M, Dauskardt R, Baillet-Guffroy A. The relationship between water loss, mechanical stress, and molecular structure of human stratum corneum ex vivo. J Biophotonics. 2015;8(3):217–225.

Vyumvuhore R, Tfayli A, Duplan H, Delalleau A, Manfait M, Baillet-Guffroy A. Raman spectroscopy: a tool for biomechanical characterization of stratum corneum. J Raman Spectrosc. 2013;44(8):1077–1083.

Wanjiku B, Yamamoto K, Klossek A, Schumacher F, Pischon H, Mundhenk L, Rancan F, Judd MM, Ahmed M, Zoschke C, Kleuser B, Rühl E, Schäfer-Korting M. Qualifying X-ray and stimulated Raman spectro-microscopy for mapping cutaneous drug penetration. Anal Chem. 2019;91(11):7208–7214.

Williams AC, Barry BW, Edwards HG, Farwell DW. A critical comparison of some Raman spectroscopic techniques for studies of human stratum corneum. Pharm Res. 1993;10(11):1642–1647.

Williams AC, Barry BW. Penetration enhancers. Adv Drug Deliv Rev. 2004;56:603–618.

Williams AC, Barry BW. Penetration enhancers. Adv Drug Deliv Rev. 2012;64(Suppl):128–137.

Wohlrab J, Vollmann A, Wartewig S, Marsch WC, Neubert R. Noninvasive characterization of human stratum corneum of undiseased skin of patients with atopic dermatitis and psoriasis as studied by Fourier transform Raman spectroscopy. Biopolymers: Original Research on Biomolecules. 2001;62(3):141–146.

Wolf M, Klang V, Stojcic T, Fuchs C, Wolzt M, Valenta C. NLC versus nanoemulsions: Effect on physiological skin parameters during regular in vivo application and impact on drug penetration. Int J Pharm. 2018;549(1-2):343–351.

Xiao C, Moore DJ, Flach CR, Mendelsohn R. Permeation of dimyristoylphosphatidylcholine into skin—Structural and spatial information from IR and Raman microscopic imaging. Vib Spectrosc. 2005a;38:151–158.

Xiao C, Moore DJ, Rerek ME, Flach CR, Mendelsohn R. Feasibility of tracking phospholipid permeation into skin using infrared and Raman microscopic imaging. J Invest Dermatol. 2005b;124:622–632.

Zhang G, Flach CR, Mendelsohn R. Tracking the dephosphorylation of resveratrol triphosphate in skin by confocal Raman microscopy. J Control Release. 2007a;123:141–147.

Zhang G, Moore DJ, Flach CR, Mendelsohn R. Vibrational microscopy and imaging of skin: from single cells to intact tissue. Anal Bioanal Chem. 2007b;387:1591–1599.

Zhang G, Moore DJ, Sloan KB, Flach CR, Mendelsohn R. Imaging the prodrug-to-drug transformation of a 5-fluorouracil derivative in skin by confocal Raman microscopy. J Invest Dermatol. 2007c;127:1205–1209.

Zsikó S, Csányi E, Kovács A, Budai-Szűcs M, Gácsi A, Berkó S. Methods to evaluate skin penetration in vitro. Sci Pharm. 2019;87(3):19:1–21.

56 Microscopy Methods for Assessing Percutaneous Drug Penetration

Percutaneous Absorption-Drugs-Cosmetics-Mechanism-Methodology

Miko Yamada, Peter Hoffmann, and Tarl Prow
Future Industries Institute, University of South Australia, Adelaide, Australia

CONTENTS

56.1   INTRODUCTION

Technical advances in microscopy imaging techniques have been applied to assess the fate of drugs for transdermal delivery in ex vivo and in vivo experiments for the last few decades. The skin offers the most accessible and convenient administration route for medications. Scientists continue to develop safe and efficacious means of delivering drugs through the skin [1]. The first challenge when topically applying drugs is to know how the dug penetrates through the skin. First, the drug must penetrate the outmost layer of lipophilic skin, the stratum corneum. The layers beneath the stratum corneum are the epidermis and dermis, which are made of compact and organized cells mainly composed of keratinocytes. These layers make it difficult for any actives to penetrate through. Any topical drug penetration assessment needs to indicate the localization of actives in each skin strata or adnexal structures, e.g., sweat ducts, sebaceous glands. Therefore, visual confirmation of the drug profile using microscopy is crucial.

Many studies have used fluorescent-labeled drugs. Tracing fluorescence, assuming the drug is firmly attached, has been the most common approach for the assessment of transdermal drug delivery [1, 2]. Fluorescence-based microscopes range from affordable fluorescence microscopy to expensive, sophisticated equipment, such as multiphoton or fluorescent-lifetime imaging microscopy (FLIM), has been discussed [3, 4]. Image analysis is often done by fluorescent signal intensity plotted against skin depth. A limitation of fluorescent-based microscopy is autofluorescence of the skin. More advanced microscopy approaches such as multiphoton or FLIM can better differentiate the signal of active molecules from skin autofluorescence by counting photons from each fluorophore lifetime. Another limitation of fluorescence-based microscopy is that dye labeling can change the molecular structure of the drugs and consequently might influence the penetration profiles. In addition, histologically prepared samples or ex vivo samples may show different drug penetration profiles compared to in vivo samples. The penetration process of nonfluorescent substances can be analyzed by Raman spectroscopy and electron microscopy measurements. Using these methods, semiquantitative analysis of actives in different depths of the skin can be detected by moving the laser focus from the skin surface into deeper layers. However, despite the high spatial resolution of these methods, the sensitivity and chemical specificity are limited, which leads to uncertainty regarding the interpretation of the images. The latest advancement in the analysis of drug penetration assessment is matrix-assisted laser desorption/ionization (MALDI) mass spectrometry imaging (MSI). This approach allows imaging of a tissue sample whereby the laser is rastered across the sample [5]. Mass spectra are then collected for each pixel. The distribution of the molecules within the tissue samples can be presented as a 2D image, with pixel intensity related to the abundance of a particular mass peak. MALDI mass spectrometry can also detect specific drug molecules and metabolites by using an accurate mass measurement within biological samples, which gives more accurate quantification of drugs compared to any of the other techniques mentioned so far. This technology would be greatly beneficial in a clinical setting. At present, a reflectance confocal microscope (RCM) is being used in volunteer studies related to percutaneous drug penetration [6]. RCM is increasingly being used as a noninvasive adjunctive tool in dermatology. With RCM, penetration can be viewed in horizontal sections of skin with resolution comparable to histology, observed drug affects in living skin, and monitored treated area longitudinally if the active has the requisite reflectance properties [7, 8]. A summary of advantages and disadvantages of each microscopy technique in topical drug penetration studies is shown in Table 56.1.

A range of microscopic methods have been used to evaluate cutaneous absorption of drugs in the development of novel formulations to be administered through the skin. Table 56.2 gives an overview of actives that have been applied to the skin and the methodologies used to determine penetration that appear in the recent literature. Selecting the right model for each active ingredient is important to assess topical drug penetration. The cost, requirement for training, and availability of equipment are other important factors to consider when selecting an imaging methodology. We will now describe each of the current imaging technologies and give examples of microscopy-based approaches that have been used for cutaneous drug delivery assessments.

56.2 FLUORESCENCE MICROSCOPY

A fluorescence microscope is an optical microscope that reveals fluorescence emission. The term refers to any microscope that uses fluorescence to generate an image, including epifluorescence microscopes or more complicated design such as confocal microscopes, which use optical sectioning to get a better resolution. Topical drugs that are labeled with fluorescence can be traced by a fluorescence microscope. It enables users to directly visualize and quantify fluorescence drugs within the skin. Skin autofluorescence is a major limitation of this technology, which makes straightforward identification of specific drugs challenging.

Lee et al. (2015) used fluorescent images to assess the penetration of rhodamine-labeled human beta-defensins (hBDs), using nude mice skin ex vivo [9]. hBDs are crucial factors of intrinsic

TABLE 56.1

Summary of Advantages and Disadvantages of Current Microscopy for Topical Drug Penetration Assessment

Imaging Modality	Advantages	Disadvantages
Fluorescent microscopy	• Affordable • Widely available • Minimum training	• No optical section • Physical sectioning, which leads to confounding factors • Strong background
Confocal microscopy	• Widely available • Optical section • En face imaging • Limited background	• Some training is required • Imaging depth is limited to 100 μm • Relatively expensive • Semiquantitative
Multiphoton microscopy	• High resolution • 3D visualization • En face imaging	• Expensive • Less available • produces high intensities which can destroy cells • Semiquantitative
FLIM	• High spatial resolution • In vivo imaging • Signal-to-noise ratio is good	• Expensive • Less available • Training is required • Semiquantitative
CARS	• Dye-free imaging • In vivo imaging • Low background	• Expensive • Less available • Training is required • Only specific metabolites can be imaged
Electron microscopy	• Super high resolution	• Expensive • Less available • Hight maintenance • Extremely sensitive to vibration and external magnetic field • Sample preparation including sectioning and sputter coating, which leads to confounding factors • Semiquantitative
OCT	• In vivo imaging • Resolution is up to 10 μm	• Expensive • Less available • Training is required • Signal diminishes in deeper skin • Best for optically transparent tissue • Semiquantitative
Reflectance microscopy	• Affordable • Feasible to use in clinic • Resolution is up to superficial dermis • Large field of view	• Less available • Training is required • Cannot be used on small and curved area • Semiquantitative
MALDI-IMS	• Visualization of spatial distribution of drugs • quantitative	• Expensive • Intensive training is required • High maintenance • Less available • Sample preparations including sectioning and matrix coating, which leads to confounding factors

TABLE 56.2

List of Targets that Have Been Studied by Each Microscopic Methodology

Methodology	Targets	Model	References
Fluorescence microscopy	Human beta-defensins	In vivo (human)	[9]
	Diclofenac	In vivo (human)	[32]
	5-fluorouracil	Ex vivo (human)	[33]
	Hyaluronic acids	Ex vivo (pig)	[10]
Confocal microscopy	Nanoparticles	In vitro (macrophages cell	[34]
	TOLL receptor 7	line)	[35]
	Mitochondrial calcium	In vitro and in vivo	[36]
	Nanoparticles	Ex vivo (mice)	[12]
	Imiquimod	Ex vivo (pig)	[11]
	Liposomal doxorubicin	In vivo (mice)	[37]
	Hyaluronic acid	Ex vivo (human)	[38]
	Farnesol	Ex vivo (pig)	[39]
	Minoxidil	In vitro (Streptococcus	[40]
	Berbermin hydrochloride	mutants)	[41]
	Chitosan nanosphere	Ex vivo (human)	[42]
	Ozonated oil	In vivo (rat)	[43]
	Capsaicin	In vivo (pig)	[44]
Multiphoton microscopy	Glucocorticoid	In vivo (mice)	[45]
	Benzyl alcohol/benzyl benzoate with	In vivo (human)	[46]
	4',6-diamidino-2-phenylindole and eosin	In vivo (human)	[15]
	Doxorubicin	In vivo/in situ (human)	[13]
	Gold nanoparticles	In vivo (human)	[13]
	Fluorescein and Texas Red	In vivo (pig)	[14]
	Retinoids	Ex vivo (human)	[17]
	Zinc oxide nanoparticles	Ex vivo (human)	[47]
FLIM	Calcium	In vivo (mice)	[48]
	Dexamethasone	Ex vivo (human)	[49]
	Genetically encoded fluorescent proteins	Ex vivo (human)	[16]
	Minocycline	Ex vivo (mice)	[50]
	Gold nanorods	In vivo (pig)	[51]
	Hemagglutinin (HA)	In vitro (keratinocytes cells)	[52]
	Extracellular vehicles (EVs)	Ex vivo (human)	[17]
	Zinc oxide nanoparticles	Ex vivo (mice)	[20]
CARS	Ketoprofen	In vivo (human)	[53]
	Plasma	In vivo (pig)	[21]
	Trans-retinol	In vivo (mice)	[19]
	Triglycerides	Ex vivo (human)	[54]
	Nanodiamonds	Ex vivo (human)	[20]
	Ibuprofen	Ex vivo (pig)	[55]
Electron microscopy	Plasmid DNA nanoparticles	Ex vivo (human)	[22]
	Colloidal nanoparticles	In vitro (fibroblast cells)	[23]
	Roflumilast, tofacitinib, ruxolitinib	In vivo (mice)	[28]
	Gold nanoparticles	Ex vivo (human)	[24]
OCT	Gold nanoparticles	Ex vivo (human)	[56]
	Indocyanine green (ICG)-encapsulated biocompatible	Ex vivo (pig)	[57]
	poly(lactic-co-glycolic) acid (PLGA) nanoparticles	Ex vivo (human)	[26]
	Ferumoxytol nanoparticles	Ex vivo (pig)	[27]
	Ingenolmebutate	In vivo (mice)	[6]
RCM	Gold nanoparticle	In vitro (keratinocytes cells)	[28]

(Continued)

TABLE 56.2 (*Continued*)

List of Targets that Have Been Studied by Each Microscopic Methodology

Methodology	Targets	Model	References
	Sodium fluorescein	In vivo (human)	[29]
	Gold nanoparticles	In vivo (human)	[6]
	Garcinia mangostana	In vivo (human)	[58]
MALDI-MSI	Roflumilast, tofacitinib, ruxolitinib	Ex vivo (human)	[29]
	Bleomycin	In vivo (human)	[30]
TOF-SIMS	Ceramide	Ex vivo (human)	[31]
	Liposomal doxorubicin	Ex vivo (pig)	[59]
		Ex vivo (pig)	
		Ex vivo (pig)	

immunity against a variety of invading enveloped viruses, bacteria, and fungi. Three different hBD peptides were synthesized (hBD3-1, hBD3-2, and hBD3-3) and labeled with rhodamine 123 (peak excitation wavelength = 507 nm). The rhodamine-labeled peptides were applied in separate locations on the back of the neck in mice. After three hours of treatment, the skin was collected and embedded for frozen sections. The skin tissues were sectioned and placed onto histological slides for imaging. Fluorescence microscopic images show positive rhodamine (emission = 575 nm, Figure 56.3 [9]). hBD3-3 shows a strong signal throughout the epidermis, whereas hBD3-1 and hBD3-2 show fluorescent staining of the stratum corneum. These results were consistent with the in vitro (macrophages) cell penetration of peptides. The skin autofluorescence creates a strong background in images, which makes it hard to define the true signal from rhodamine. Another problem was that the low resolution of images from each skin sample, which illustrates one of the limits of this approach. This limits the information on the drug penetration profile. There was no quantitative analysis in this study. Overall, the fluorescence microscopy approach used in this study reveals the utility and feasibility of visualizing a situation where there is minimum transdermal peptide delivery in the skin.

Smejkalova' et al. (2017) [10] assessed cosmetically relevant active hyaluronic acid (HA) penetration in pig skin using fluorescence microscopy. HA is one of the most hydrophilic molecules in nature. They made hydrophobic HA using derivatives and formulated these into polymeric micelles loaded with cosmetic active coenzyme Q10 (C). Nile red (excitation = 558 nm) was encapsulated within the core of the micelles for visualization. They tested other emulsion formulations as controls. They applied these formulations on excised pig skin. After 20 hours, they cryomoulded the tissue and sectioned it onto histology slides. Images were taken by fluorescence microscopy (Figure 56.1). Nile red was detected in the skin after 20 hours of treatment. The skin orientation and location were confirmed with the same image under phase contrast. The fluorescent images showed that delivery of the hydrophobic compounds in HAC6 and HAC18 polymeric micelles were enhanced by hydrophobic HA. The conclusion from the imaging data was that the more hydrophobic the drug becomes (HAC18), the deeper the dye can penetrate into the dermis. The sections were later homogenized to extract Nile red for a relative quantification (T = 5 hours and T = 20 hours) (Figure 56.1, bottom graph). The quantitative analysis results supported the visual data from fluorescent imaging data. The imaging data were limited by the lack of quantitative measurements, sample preparation for frozen sectioning could create artifacts, and ice crystal formation may interfere with polymeric micelles structure, as well as its delivery profile into the skin. The staining process (physical washing or PBS for washing solution) may also affect the delivery profile of the polymeric micelles. This study is a relevant example of visual assessment of cutaneous drug penetration using cross-section imaging with fluorescent microscopy.

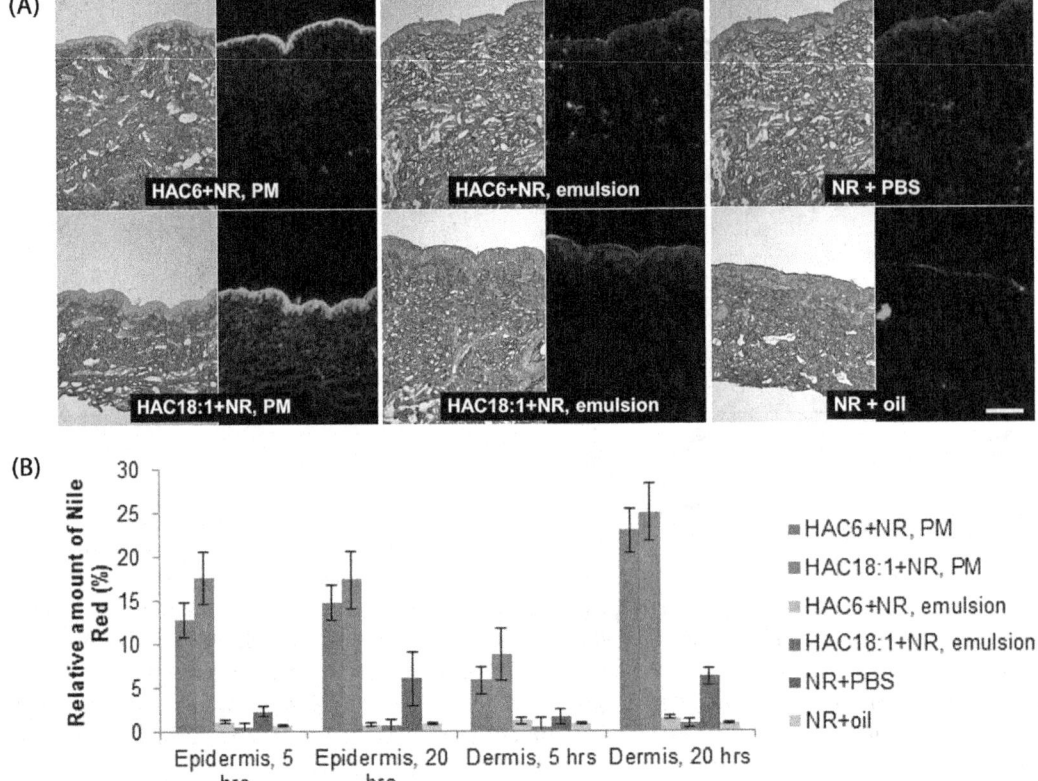

FIGURE 56.1 (a) Cross-sectional images of porcine skin after 20 hours of treatment with Nile red (NR) loaded in two different concentrations of coenzyme Q1O (HAC6 and HAC18 polymeric micelles (PM), Scale bar = 200 μm. (b) Determination of NR amount in epidermis and dermis after its skin extraction ($n = 3$). The porcine skin was treated with NR loaded in HAC6 and HAC18 PM, NR mixed with HAC6 and HAC18 in an emulsion, and NR dissolved in oil and dispersed in PBS (T = 5 hr and T = 20 hr). (Reprinted with permission from Smejkalova'et al. 2017.)

56.3 CONFOCAL MICROSCOPY

The key optical difference between conventional and confocal microscopy is the presence of confocal pinholes in the confocal microscope, allowing light from only the plane of focus to reach the detector. Confocal microscopy offers several advantages over fluorescence microscopy: (1) the depth of the field can be controlled; (2) the background fluorescence can be largely eliminated from the focal plan; and (3) it is possible to collect serial optical sections deep into thick tissue. Images from confocal microscopy give more information about the drug/nanoparticle penetration profile because the depth of the image is known and the background is reduced.

Sun et al. (2018) [11] conducted a clinically relevant topical drug penetration study using confocal microscopy. They applied nanoparticles to imiquimod-induced psoriatic mouse skin to investigate how nanoparticles penetrate diseased skin. They used different-sized FluoSpheres (40, 100, and 500 nm) and confocal laser scanning microscopy to trace fluorescent signals from the FluoSpheres. Psoriatic mouse skin was excised fresh and treated with FluoSpheres for 24 hours at 32° in a Franz cell system. After the treatment, the skin was embedded for cryosectioning. For 40-nm and 100-nm FluoSpheres, the excitation was 552 nm, and for 500-nm FluoSpheres, the excitation was 488 nm. Bright field images were taken to confirm the orientation of the skin. The confocal images of skin exposed to FluoSpheres showed that the fluorescent signal was increased in vertical sections of psoriatic skin samples compared to that in normal skin. All three FluoSpheres sizes seemed to deposit homogeneously into the epidermis of the imiquimod-induced psoriatic model. In normal skin, the dye was found only around the hair follicles. There were no quantitative measurements from these images. Preparation of cryosectioning, including ice crystal formation and the direction of sectioning, may affect the nanoparticle penetration profiles.

Smejkalova et al. used confocal microscopy coupled with spectroscopy to image HA in polymeric micelles (HAC18:1, medium-chain length) with Nile red (excitation = 460 nm) encapsulated (HAC18:1+NR, polymeric micelles) and applied these formulations to ex vivo pig skin [10]. HA delivery into the skin is a major focus for cosmetic products. They also used HAC18:1 + polymeric micelles with no dye inside but covalently labeled with Nile blue (excitation = 500 nm) (HAC18:1+NB), which helps to indicate the fate of HA by tracking the vehicle. The skin was incubated with the formulations for 24 hours, then the skin was embedded for cryosectioning, followed by assessing fluorescence to indicate penetration using confocal microscopy. Nuclei were stained with DAPI. Fluorescence intensity profiles at different deptsh were measured in the treated skin. In addition, they measured HA derivatives using Fourier-transform infrared spectroscopy (FTIR). FTIR is a technique used to obtain an infrared spectrum absorption or emission. Images from confocal microscopy (Figure 56.2) confirmed that both Nile red from polymeric and Nile blue–labeled

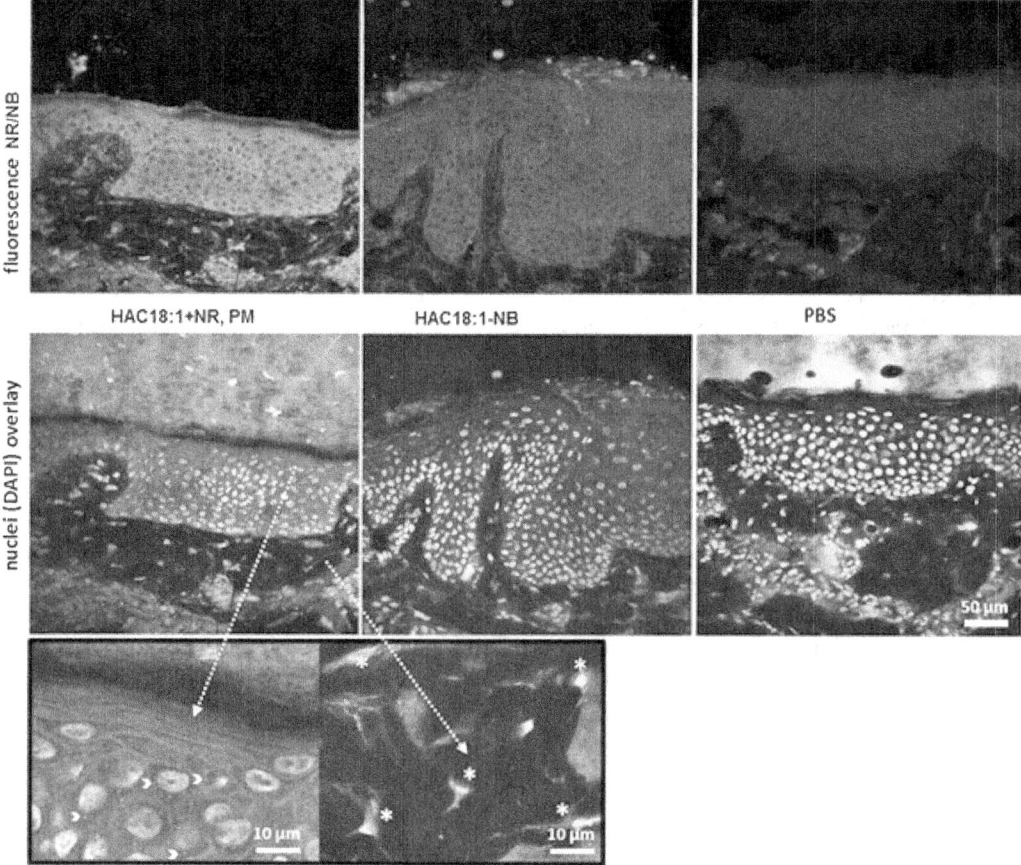

FIGURE 56.2 Confocal images of cross-sections of porcine skin after 20 hours of treatment with (left) HAC18:1 polymeric micelles loaded with NR (HAC18:1 + NR, PM), (middle) HACl8:1 polymeric micelles not loaded with any drug but covalently labeled with Nile blue (HAC18:1-NB), and (right) PBS (= control). (Reprinted with permission from Smejkalova'et al. 2017.)

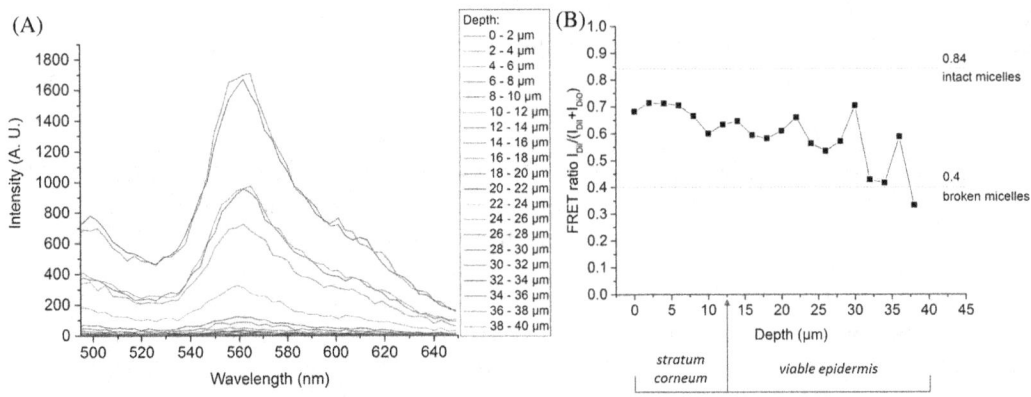

FIGURE 56.3 Emission spectra of HAC 18:1 + FRET polymeric micelles as a function of different skin depth (A) and the corresponding FRET ratio (B). (Reprinted with permission from Smejkalova'et al. 2017.)

polymeric micelles were able to penetrate the stratum corneum. Nile red penetrated the dermis after 20 hours. Together with nuclei staining, the fluorescent signal from both loaded and unloaded polymeric micelles was detected in the cytoplasm surrounding the cell nuclei in the epidermis and dermal strata. Semiquantitative analysis was done by calculating the emission ratio between intact and broken micelles in the individual skin strata (Figure 56.3). The limitation was that autofluorescence from the skin was present, which made it challenging to differentiate between exogenous and endogenous signals. Overall, laser scanning confocal microscopy produced images with improved signal to noise compared to fluorescent microscopy.

The use of nanoparticles as formulation components of topical drug delivery has resulted in questions about the ultimate deposition site or penetration depth of nanoparticles within the skin. Campbell et al. [12] investigated how the different sizes of nanoparticles affect their capacity to penetrate skin when the skin barrier was modestly compromised. The model that they used was ex vivo pig skin. Intact skin was exposed to an aqueous suspension of 20, 100, and 200 nm FluoSpheres or to water alone. The samples were incubated for up to 16 hours. Subsequently, the same experiments were repeated with skin that had been partially compromised by removal of four tape strips. The skin samples were directly imaged by confocal microscopy to observe FluoSphere penetration in each group, and cross-sections of skin images were converted from stacks of serial x-y images. The results show the FluoSpheres (green color) were visible in the top layers of stratum corneum and by 16 hours, FluoSphere (200 nm) in intact skin had penetrated to the dermal-epidermal junction (Figure 56.5a, and b [12]). Tape-stripped skin showed the least FluoSphere penetration. When the signal intensity was calculated against the depth of skin in each group, there was no time-dependent penetration of any of the FluoSpheres examined (Figure 56.7 [12]). Confocal images were used to perform quantitative analysis to visualize the depth of FluoSphere penetration. Although there was no visualization of individual particles, the analysis of fluorescence derived from the particles and penetration of particles into the skin provided safety information on the nanoparticles.

56.4   MULTIPHOTON MICROSCOPY

Multiphoton microscopy (MPM) is based on fluorophore excitation with two or three photons of longer wavelength that interact with the fluorophore at the same time, resulting in fluorophore emission. MPM has become a powerful biomedical research tool that enables noninvasive three-dimensional imaging of tissue with high resolution at greater depth than single photon microscopy. One major advantage is that visualization can be performed without mechanical destruction of the sample through tissue sectioning. MPM can provide information that can be used to assess the bioavailability of drugs and to visualize drug penetration pathways into skin with higher precision and less background than other forms of microscopy.

In 2006, Stracke et al. [13] used MPM to investigate the penetration of nanoparticle-born drugs into ex vivo human skin for over five hours. Polymer particles that were labeled with fluorescein (excitation = 488 nm) and Texas Red (excitation = 543 nm) were used as a drug model. Freshly excised abdominal skin was mounted on a Franz cell system. The tissue was treated with fluores-cent-labeled nanoparticles and incubated at 37° for five hours. After treatment, the skin tissue was taken from the system and imaged directly from the skin surface using multiphoton microscopy (Figure 56.4). Two channels were used to discriminate between particle-bound and release drug model, as well as skin multifluorescence and a white light for visualization of the skin structure. The skin autofluorescence images were also shown. This tracking experiment showed the distribution

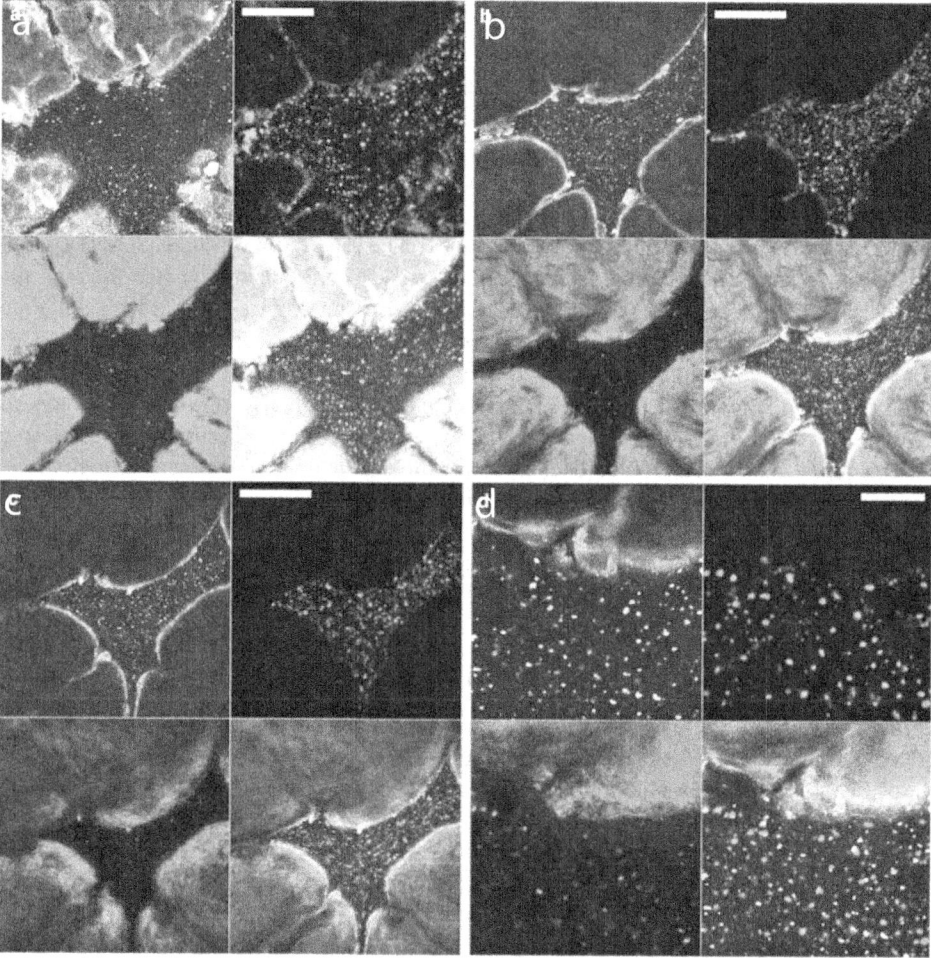

FIGURE 56.4 Multitracking experiments. (a–c) 325 × 325 μm² combined optical sections in –4, –20, and –32 μm depth (bar = 100 μm). (d) A detailed image of particles and skin surface (bar = 25 μm). Each panel consists of a multiphoton excited image (predominantly keratin autofluorescence and fluorescein, grayscale, top-left image), a 488-nm excited image (fluorescein, green scale, top right image), and a 543-nm excited image (Texas Red, orange scale, bottom-left image), as well as an overlay (bottom-right image) (d). The excitation powers for the optical sections in the multitracking study were P_{EX}(800 nm) = 10 mW, P_{EX}(488 nm) = 50 μW, and P_{EX}(543 nm) = 36μW, and the pixel acquisition time was always t_{px} = 3.2 μS. (Reprinted with permission from Strake et al. 2006.)

and penetration of Texas Red, fluorescein, and autofluorescence (Figure 56.4). The skin strata from the surface to viable epidermis was visualized, as well as changing signal intensity as the image was taken deeper into the skin to compensate for light scattering and signal loss. By using multiphoton microscopy, they could collect skin autofluorescence data. In this study, multiphoton microscopy with dual-labeled nanoparticles in human skin was shown to be sufficient to investigate nanoparticle penetration for cutaneous drug delivery.

Tancrède-Bohin et al. published a study where they used multiphoton microscopy to assess the effects of cosmetically relevant active retinoids (retinol and retinoic acid) in volunteer skin [14]. They recruited 20 healthy females, and two products (retinol 0.3%, and retinoic acid 0.025%) were applied to the dorsal of the forearm in separate locations as well as an untreated area. Multiphoton images were taken of the treated areas on days 0, 12, 18, and 32. Quantitative analysis was performed by measuring signal intensity from the retinoids against changing epidermal thickness. The z-stacks from multiphoton microscopy were used to construct a 3D image of the skin. Two-photon excited fluorescence from NAD(P)H, flavins, keratin, melanin, or elastin was collected in addition to second harmonic generation from collagen. MPM, utilizing autofluorescence signals, was used to measure the cutaneous effects of topical retinoids. The findings showed increased epidermal thickening and increased DEJ undulation with decreased melanin content after treating for 12 days. There was no quantification of actives in the skin. This study illustrates the use of MPM to quantify topical drug effects on the skin biology and structure.

Labouta et al. (2011) [15] used multiphoton microscopy to investigate the penetration of gold nanoparticles (AuNP) into skin based on gold luminescence. Their aim was to explore if a combined multiphoton-pixel analysis could be used to semiquantify AuNP penetration into the stratum corneum and deeper skin layers. They used ex vivo human skin. The skin was treated with a thiol-coated AuNP dispersion and incubated in a Franz cell system at 32° for 24 hours. After treatment, the skin was longitudinally cryosectioned and imaged by two-photon microscopy. A light image was taken to visualize the skin orientation. Figure 56.5 shows the representative overlay of multiphoton images with AuNP as a white dot. AuNP penetrated both the epidermis and dermis. Images were taken every 1 μm depth, and pixel data from each positive AuNP signal was used to calculate the weighted number of particles to determine the amount of AuNP penetrating into viable epidermis and dermis. This study extended the application of MPM to quantify nanoparticles in the skin. There are limitations to this study, like light scattering and interparticle distances that affect interpretation, but this study is an important example of where MPM image analysis can be taken beyond signal intensity.

56.5 FLUORESCENCE- LIFETIME IMAGING MICROSCOPY

MPM imaging can be used to generate fluorescence lifetime data when the appropriate hardware is integrated with the MPM. The result is MPM-fluorescence lifetime imaging microscopy, or MPM-FLIM, or FLIM. FLIM is an imaging modality that is based on the differences in the exponential decay rates of photon emission from fluorophores within a sample. FLIM images are produced by visualizing a subset of the lifetime data from the emission decay, rather than its intensity. This information can be used in a number of ways, including fingerprinting specific fluorophores within a sample and inferring fluorophore binding status within living skin.

The Evan group (Jeong et al. 2018) [16] studied the distribution of topical minocycline gel (an antibiotic that is used for acne vulgaris) on human facial skin. Thawed ex vivo human facial skin was treated with gel formulations containing 1%, 2%, and 4% minocycline, as well as placebo and incubated at 32°C for 24 hours. After the treatment, the samples were embedded for frozen sectioning. The frozen tissue was cross-sectioned along the plane perpendicular to the skin surface. The sections were mounted on microscope slides for MPM and FLIM imaging (Figure 56.6). The bright field and FLIM images of epidermis, hair follicle, and sebaceous glands were collected. Then 590-nm to 650-nm emission signals were collected from the active ingredient of gel, minocycline chelated with magnesium ions (MNC-Mg^{2+}). Two-photon excitation microscopy images were confirmed with FLIM images. The MNC-Mg^{2+} fluorescent signal was concentrated at the topmost layers of the epidermis and the deep

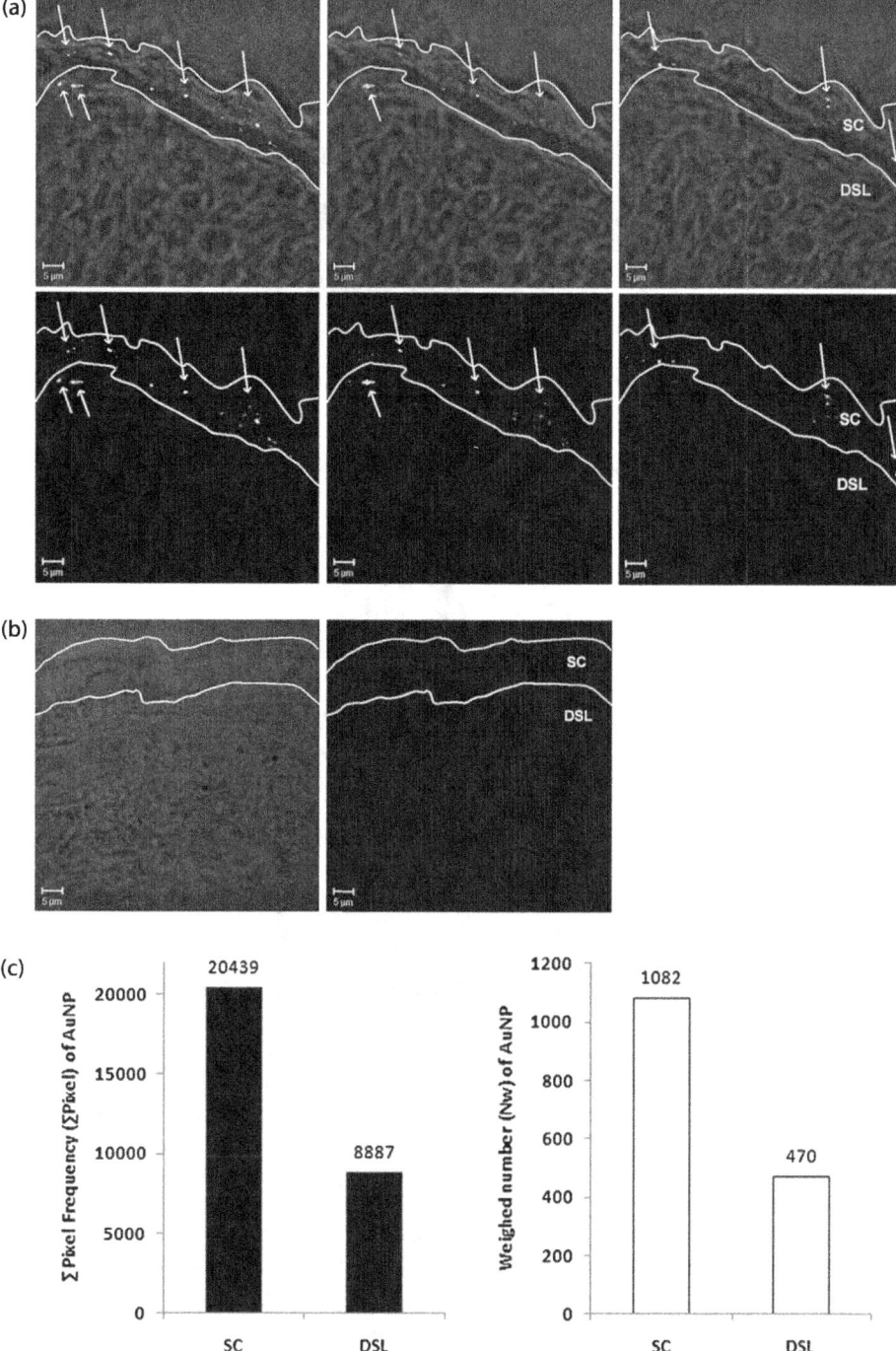

FIGURE 56.5 (a) Representative overlaid multiphoton/transmission images (upper panel) and the corresponding AuNP track (lower panel), each showing AuNP (indicated as white spots) at different optical layers of a z-stack of a longitudinal skin section, in which different amounts of AuNP in the SC and DSL after 24 hours of skin exposure were detected in each layer. A single layer is not descriptive for the overall penetration pattern. This is in comparison to (b), a vehicle-treated-only control skin specimen; the left image is an overlaid multiphoton/transmission image, and the right image is the gold track only. (c) Skin penetration of AuNP into the SC and DSL, expressed as pixel frequency of AuNP (Pixel) in all optical layers of the z-stack, was determined and the respective weighed number of particles (Nw) were then calculated, as shown, revealing the depth profile for AuNP concentrating more in the SC rather than in the DSL. Note that pixel values due to AuNP nanoparticles were recorded following the thresholding of background intensity. Therefore, zero pixels were recorded for control skin specimens (not displayed). (Reprinted with permission from Labouta et al. 2011.)

Bright field   TPEF images   FLIM images
                   (Red)

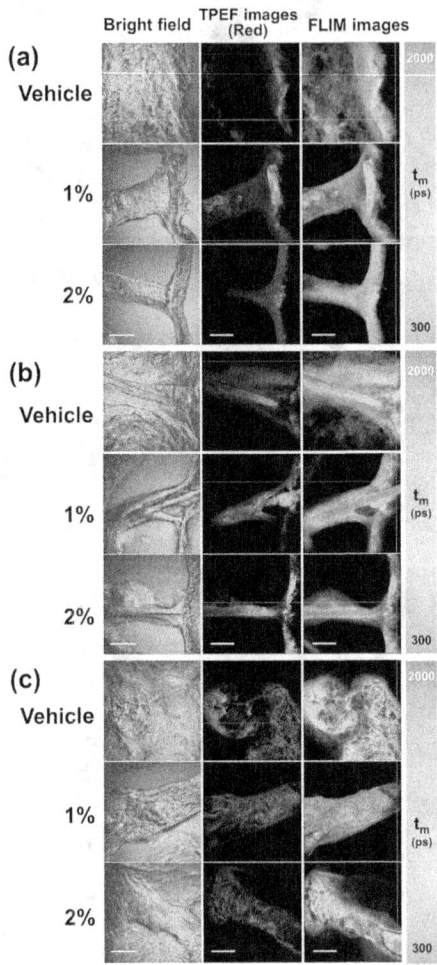

FIGURE 56.6 Uptake of the active pharmaceutical ingredient (MNC-Mg^{2+}) in facial skin, as illustrated by the TPEF and FLIM images of BPX-01–treated facial skin at three anatomical sites: (a) epidermis, (b) hair follicle, and (c) sebaceous gland. The facial skin was treated with 2.5 mg/cm^2 BPX-01 containing 0% (vehicle), 1%, and 2% MNC-Mg^{2+} for 24 hours. The TPEF and FLIM images were acquired from the red fluorescence channel (590 to 650 nm). The scale bar is 50 μm. (Reprinted with permission from Jeong et al. 2018.)

layers of skin strictly along the hair shaft and into the follicle. The limitation in this study was that although the uptake of active ingredient of the drug MNC-Mg^{2+} was successfully visualized using FLIM, it was challenging to accurately discriminate and separate the MNC-Mg^{2+} signal from autofluorescence. This study demonstrated visualization of topical drug penetration using two-photon excitation microscopy and FLIM in a challenging application with a weakly fluorescent active molecule.

Leite-Silva et al. (2013) [17] used FLIM imaging to show how cosmetically relevant nanoparticles in various formulations penetrate volunteer skin. There is controversy about the safety of nanoparticle-based sunscreens. Zinc oxide nanoparticles (ZnO- NP) are one of the most widely studied nanoparticles. Leite-Silva et al. (2013) aimed to assess the extent of ZnO-NP penetration and epidermal metabolic effects using viable epidermal redox state for a number of topical formulations. ZnO-NP was formulated in three ways: gel, emulsion (o/w) (E1), and a water-in-oil emulsion (w/o) (E2). Both E1 and E2 were dispersed in caprylic capric triglyceride. Formulations were applied to volunteers' right and left volar forearms with a light massage of 20 seconds at 2 mg/cm^2. After six hours of treatment, MPM-FLIM images were taken from the treatment sites (Figure 56.7). For each formulation, they took images at

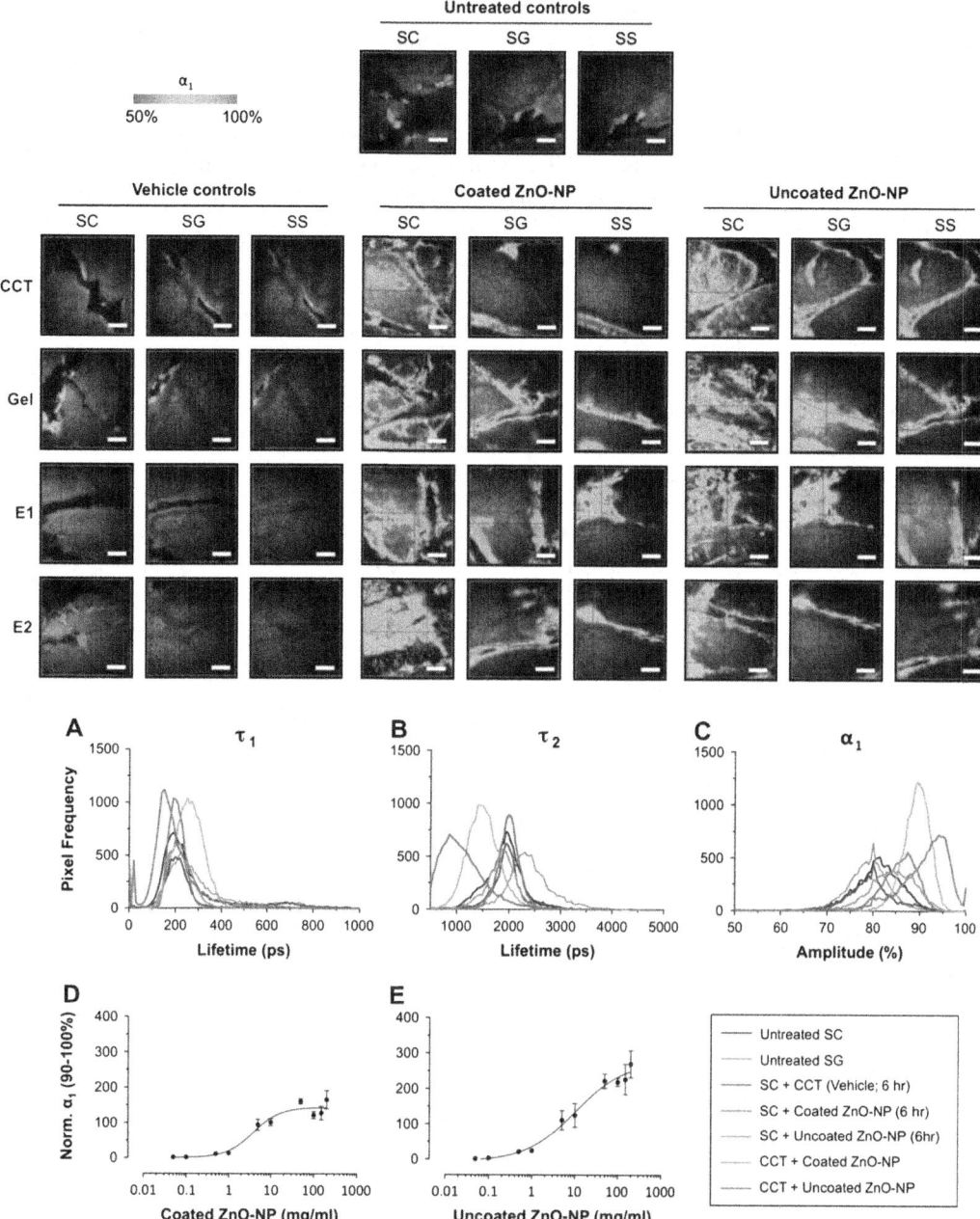

FIGURE 56.7 In vivo pseudo-colored MPT–FLIM images of volunteer skin, at various depths, 6 hours after the topical application of ZnO-NP formulations. Each image is $214 \times 214 \times 1$ µm³. The color scale bar represents α_1 (50% to 100%) from blue to red, with cellular autofluorescence (50% to 90%) associated with blue-green, while ZnO appears yellow-red (90% to 100%). Scale bars (white) indicate a length of 40 µm. Bottom: Fluorescence (τ) lifetime and amplitude (α) coefficient histograms of in vivo human skin and ZnO-NP. (A–C) The τ_1, τ_2, and α_1 % histograms of untreated SC, untreated SG, CCT, and coated/uncoated ZnO-NP treated SC after six hours and coated/uncoated ZnO-NP in CCT. (D–E) In vitro coated and uncoated ZnO-NP in CCT, standard curve of the mean normalized α_1 90% to 100% data. Nonlinear regression was used to obtain a line of best fit and interpolate unknown ZnO-NP signals. Error bars represent the SD. (Reprinted with permission from Leite-Silva et al. 2013.)

three different depths within the epidermis (stratum corneum [SC], stratum granulosum [SG], and stratum spinosum [SS]), which were determined by skin morphology. The results show neither coated nor uncoated ZnO-NP (yellow-red color) was detected in negative or formulation treatment groups. Positive signals from ZnO-NP were detected on the SC surface, and most of them were within the furrows surrounding and between viable epidermis cells in the SG and SS. Fluorescent lifetimes were recorded for each pixel after topical application of ZnO-NP formulations to in vivo human skin (Figure 56.7). Both NAD(P)H skin autofluorescence and ZnO-NP had two lifetimes—one short and one long—that correspond to unbound and protein-bound NAD(P)H. Figure 56.7c shows optical discrimination for the ZnO-NP response from an NAD(P)H epidermal fluorescence lifetime background (amplitude coefficient of ZnO-NP). Figure 56.8 shows the semiquantification of coated/uncoated ZnO-NP in each skin strata calculated from a standard curve. From these results, there was a predominant accumulation of coated and uncoated ZnO-NP within the SC of in vivo human skin. Some coated ZnO-NPs penetrated into the viable epidermis. The quantity of coated/uncoated ZnO-NP progressively decreased deeper within the skin. The topical application of coated and uncoated ZnO-NP did not alter the redox state of viable epidermal cells (data not shown). They were the first group to report lifetime differences between coated and uncoated ZnO-NP. The limitation was that MPM-FLIM could not detect individual nanoparticles, and therefore, it is difficult to accurately quantify ZnO-NP on or in skin. Overall, cosmetically relevant nanoparticle penetration assessment in human skin was possible using the MPM-FLIM approach. This was achieved by using the different fluorescent lifetime between ZnO-NP and skin autofluorescence.

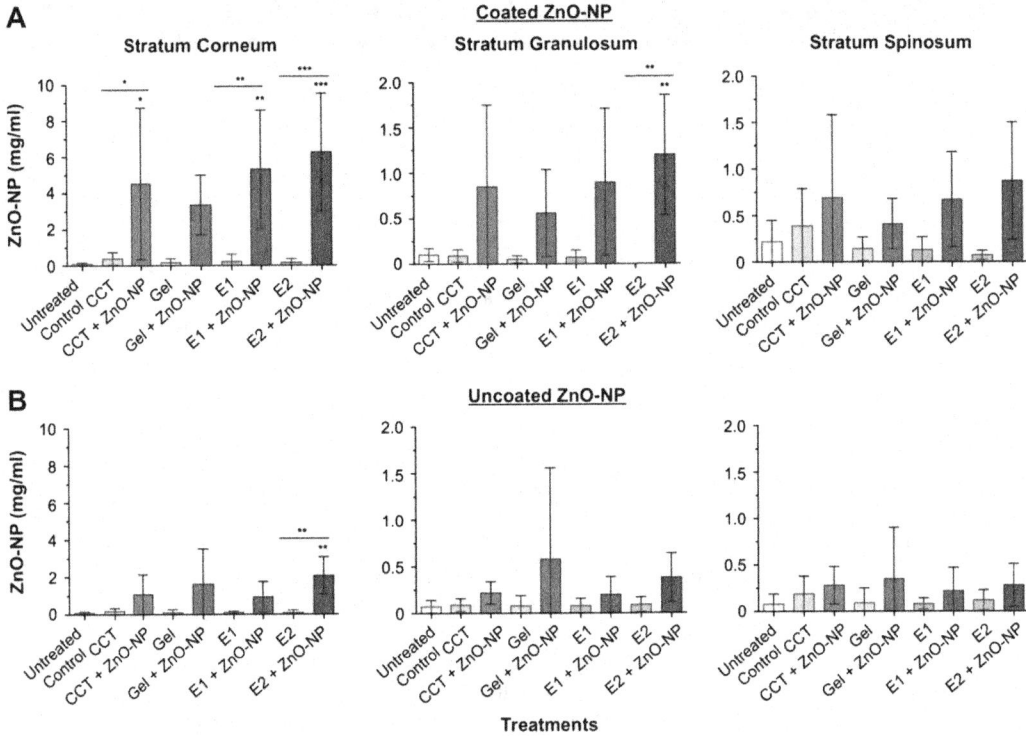

FIGURE 56.8 Quantification of in vivo ZnO-NP signal within the various skin strata in treated and untreated skin. (A-B) The concentration (mg/mL) of coated/uncoated ZnO-NP calculated from the mean normalized mean pixel intensity (photon count/pixel frequency) of the ZnO-NP signal within the SC, SG, and SS regions of interest. The region of interest within the SG and SS corresponded to the VEC (i.e., the furrows were excluded). The skin penetration profiles of ZnO-NP from CCT, gel, El, and E2 formulations ($n = 6$) were compared, along with untreated and vehicle controls ($n = 6$). Error bars represent the SD with significant differences indicated by an asterisk (Student's t-test, $*p < 0.05, **p < 0.01, ***p < 0.001$). (Reprinted with permission from Leite-Silva et al, 2013.)

In 2015, Witting et al. investigated the skin penetration of macromolecules using MPM-FLIM [4]. They hypothesised that HA would enhance the transdermal delivery of bovine serum albumin (BSA). HA was labeled with fluorescent N-methylanthraniloyl (MANT)-guanine nucleotide, and BSA was tagged with rhodamine B (RhB). They used pig skin as a model and tape-stripped 30 times to establish a barrier-deficient model. The tissue was placed in Franz cells. The skin was first treated with HA with different molecular weights (5 kDa, 100 kDa, and 1 MDa) and the penetration profile observed using FLIM. Then they selected the most efficient HA (5 kDa) and applied it together with BSA. All the samples were incubated at 32°C for 24 hours before being prepared for frozen sections. The resulting cross-sections of treated skin were imaged by MPM-FLIM. Bright-field images were also taken to show skin orientation. MPM-FLIM images were analyzed using fluorescence decay curves based on photon counts. MPM-FLIM images show that higher-molecular-weight HA stayed as a cluster on the surface of the skin in normal skin and penetrated to the dermis when the skin barrier was disrupted. The lowest-molecular-weight HA was found in clusters that were mostly on the stratum corneum in both normal and tape-stripped skin, but some signal was detected in the dermis. These observations were confirmed by FLIM photon counts. BSA penetrated to the dermis when it was delivered with 5 kDa HA. This study demonstrated that MPM-FLIM images and analysis were able to show the topical drug delivery enhancement deep into pig skin. The limitation was the overlap between HA emission and RhB absorption, which could result in false-positive signals in the FLIM images.

In 2018, Alex et al. used FLIM in a phase 1 clinical trial to assess topical antiinflammatory treatment in healthy volunteers [18]. Their aims were to investigate the distribution and residency of two topical drugs within the epidermis and dermis in vivo using FLIM. Seven healthy men (Fitzpatrick skin I to IV) were recruited for this study. Each participant received two topical creams (1% concentration of active ingredient) (A and B). Cream A was applied on one volar arm and cream B was applied to the other volar forearm once daily for seven days. FLIM images were taken every day for seven days following treatment. Prior to imaging, double-sided tape was used to place a a glass coverslip on a magnetic coupling ring, which was then attached to the volar forearm imaging site. The articulated arm of the system was attached to the magnetic coupling ring. FLIM images were taken in 5-μm steps from the skin surface down to a depth of 200 μm. Most of the drug signal was detected on the skin surface on treatment days 2 to 7. Accumulation of the topical formulation along skin ridges was also visible in images obtained on days 2, 4, and 9. By day 10, there was no detectable fluorescence from formulation residing in the skin. Semiquantitative analysis from the FLIM images was performed by the readout counts from the drug fluorescence signal against the depth of penetration and residency in one study participant for cream A and B. There was significant variation in the day-to-day observation of drug fluorescence from both formulations shown by FLIM. The signal reached the lower limit of detection after nine days. Accurate quantification of topical drug penetrating was challenging. Overall, this small pilot study of investigational topical drugs described the in vivo distribution and semiquantified measurement of drugs in the skin by using MPM-FLIM.

56.6 COHERENT ANTI-STOKES RAMAN SPECTROSCOPY

Raman scattering microscopy has been developed as a label-free chemical imaging tool that is used to acquired high-resolution images of multiple chemical components of a topical formulation penetrating mammalian skin. Coherent anti-Stokes Raman spectroscopy (CARS) has been used for fast imaging of biological samples, primarily with lipid contrast.

In 2018, we combined two transdermal technologies to investigate the enhancement of topical drug delivery [19]. In Yamada et al. (2018), we coated elongated microparticles with nanoemulsion formulations for topical application on ex vivo human skin. Our initial experiment was to use lipophilic dye, DiI in the core of a nanoemulsion to visualize the delivery under confocal microscopy. We proceeded to use a dye-free imaging system, CARS microscopy, to confirm the location of the lipid components of the nanoemulsion. Medical-grade glycerol (as a surrogate for a hydrophobic drug) was encapsulated into the core of nanoemulsion to enhance CARS imaging.

The microparticles with nanoemulsion were applied with an applicator to freshly excised human skin and incubated at 37° for 30 minutes. The samples were imaged en face by CARS. We captured reflectance images of the skin to confirm skin strata. The scattering signal from the lipid (i.e., glycerol) is shown in red (Figure 56.9). The images from CARS indicated enhanced delivery of the lipid from the nanoemulsion to the dermal and epidermal junction.

Belsey et al. (2014) conducted a feasibility study where they used CARS imaging to investigate the delivery of fluorescent nanoparticles using a porcine abdominal skin model [20]. The excised skin was treated with a poration device prior to mounting the skin in a Franz cell system. Yellow-green fluorescent 0.02 µm and 2 µm diameter carboxy-modified FluoSpheres were applied to the skin, which was then incubated at 37°C for one hour. The skin was imaged en face by two-photon microscopy and CARS. The fluorescent signal from the FluoSphere particles are shown in green, and lipids from the cells were detected with CARS imaging and shown in red. Skin images were taken at 2-µm-depth intervals, and a 3D skin model was reconstructed from z-stack images. The nanoparticles accumulated along the burnt edge of skin and in the "opened surface" by poration of the skin. CARS signal from endogenous lipids was detected from the surface to the deep dermis.

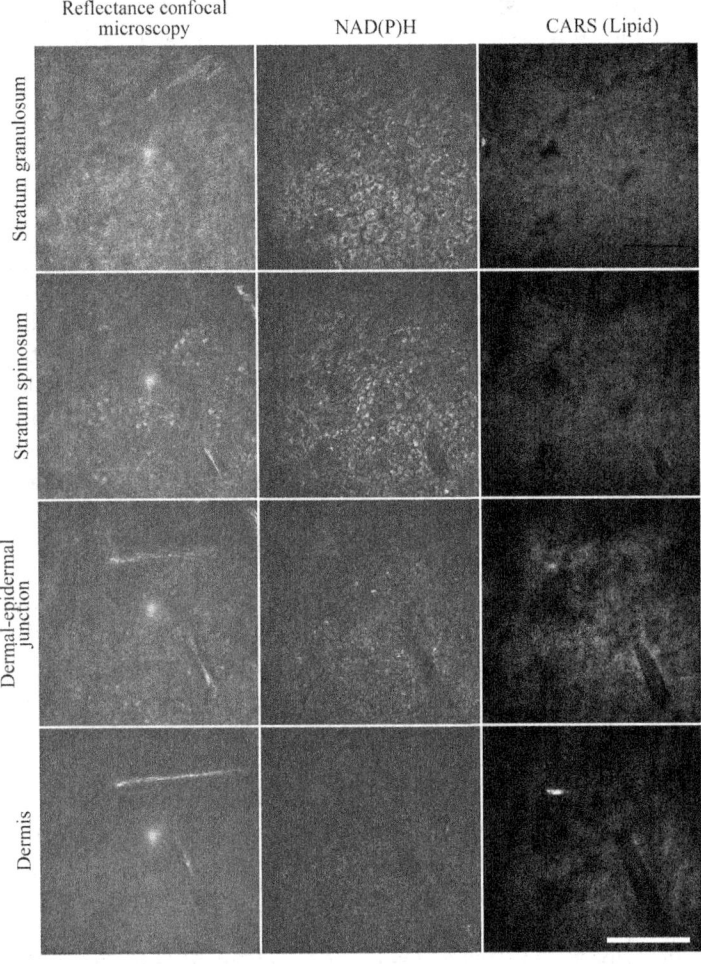

FIGURE 56.9 Depth effects of EMP coated with P20TNE using alginate by reflectance confocal microscopy, NAD(P)H imaging, and CARS imaging for lipid signal. Reflectance confocal microscopy showed the presence of EMP through the skin. The NAD(P)H imaging revealed a dark halo around the EMP, suggesting that there was a gap between the EMP and viable skin. CARS imaging showed the presence of lipid signal hot spots primarily at the surface and dermal-epidermal junction. Bar indicates 50 µm.

This was shown in a graph of the signal intensity versus depth. CARS images were dark where the lipid was absent. One limitation is that the visualization of small particles is difficult to differentiate from skin autofluorescence. This makes it difficult to perform accurate quantification of small particles at lower concentrations. However, both fluorescence and CARS imaging were successfully able to solve this problem and detect the uptake of nanoparticles into thermal ablated skin.

Stimulated Raman scattering (SRS) has overcome some CARS imaging limitations, such as spectral distortion and limited sensitivity, that make quantitative interpretation and applications beyond lipid imaging difficult. SRS microscopy allows highly sensitive optical imaging based on vibrational spectroscopy. By increasing imaging speed (as fast as the video rate), SRS can collect more backscattered signal, which allows the detection of lipid, water, and proteins in *in vivo* settings. One SRS study assessed the penetration of *trans*-retinol in the ear of a living mouse by Saar et al. (2010) [21]. The images demonstrate the penetration of retinol (green color in Figure 56.10) into mouse skin from the stratum corneum to the sebaceous gland. In addition, SRS could capture

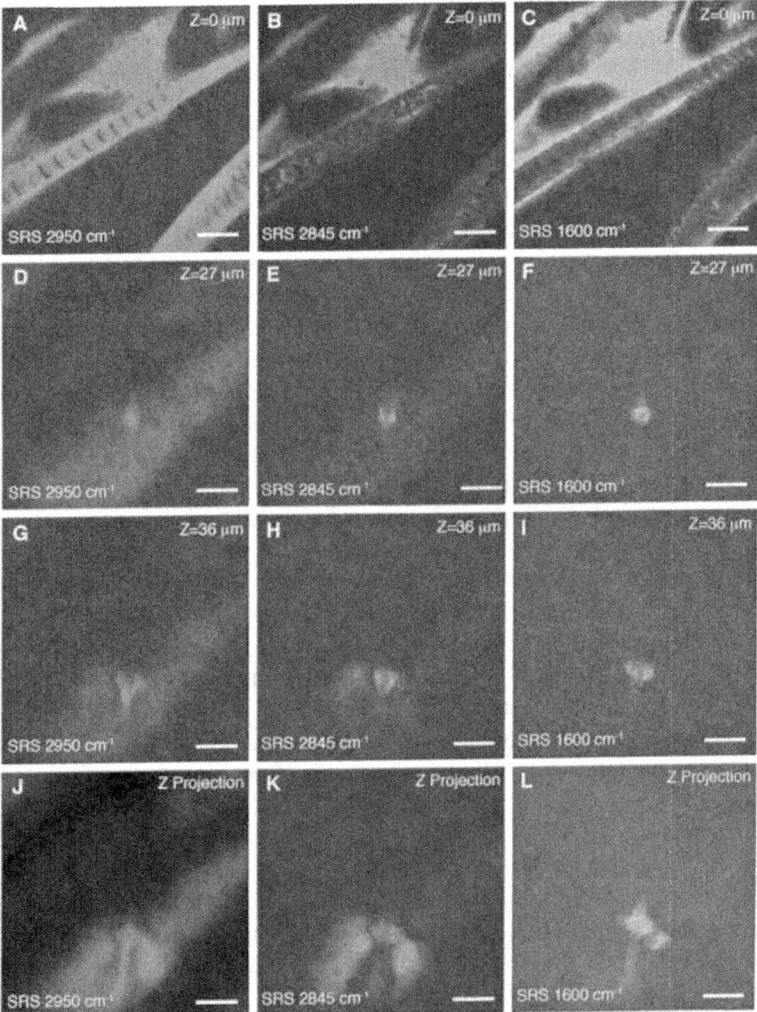

FIGURE 56.10 In vivo imaging of drug penetration of *trans*-retinol. (A-C) SRS images of hair and stratum corneum in the era of a living mouse. (D-F) Images of a hair shaft within the viable epidermis. (G-1) Images of a sebaceous gland within the viable epidermis. (J-L) Depth projection of the three-dimensional image stacks of the viable epidermis. Contrast coming primarily from protein (2950 cm^{-1}) and lipid (2845 cm^{-1}). Scale bar: 25 µm. (Reprinted with permission from Saar et al. 2010.)

the protein (purple) and lipid (red). We see that retinol has penetrated via the hair shaft into the sebaceous gland, which was one of three hypothesized penetration routes into the skin. In addition, they were able to visualize with SRS that drug penetration of the topically applied trans-retinol (Figure 56.10c) occurred along the hair shaft. This study has shown the possibility of using high-speed imaging SRS in in vivo settings. However, there was no quantification from the images in this study. Label-free optical imaging is likely to play an increasingly important role in drug penetration assessment in humans.

56.7   ELECTRON MICROSCOPY

Transmission and scanning electron microscopy can provide ultrastructural evidence on the penetration profile of electron-dense nanoparticles. Transmission electron microscopy (TEM) uses a beam of electrons that is transmitted through a specimen to form an image. The contrast comes from differences in electron density with the sample, e.g., gold is black due to absorbed electrons. The specimen is usually an ultrathin section less than 100 nm thick or a suspension on a grid. The most important difference between a transmission and scanning microscope is that a scanning electron microscopy (SEM) beam is focused to a fine point and scans line by line over the surface of the sample, whereas the TEM images are focused through a thin sample. TEM and SEM approaches in topical drug delivery research are generally focused on tracing electron-dense nanoparticles applied to skin. These technologies can be used to characterize nanoparticles made of gold, silver, iron oxide nanoparticles, and silica-based nanoparticles in skin tissue.

In 2015, a study done by Colombo et al. described the use of SEM to investigate the delivery of Fe_3O_4 nanoparticles in cream formulations to ex vivo human skin [22]. Freshly excised human skin was mounted in a Franz cell, and nanoparticle-containing cream was applied. The skin was collected at three time points (1 to 3 hours, 5 to 7 hours, and 24 hours) and then fixed in formalin solution for paraffin sectioning. The cross-sections of the treated skin were subsequently imaged by SEM (Figure 56.11). The skin architecture was viewed at high resolution. The nanoparticles were distinguished in all skin layers based on the differences between the electron density of the skin, which is relatively low, compared to the relatively high electron density of the nanoparticles. The images showed that a small number of nanoparticles penetrated into viable epidermis, and some of them reached the deeper dermis. There seemed to be no difference in enhancement of penetration between solution or cream formulations. This study shows that the SEM system can detect nanoparticles and trace them in fixed human skin sections. One of the limitations of this type of analysis is the limited field of view of the skin section due to the super high resolution.

The effects of preparation for sectioning on skin morphology have also been the subject of concern in the field. In 2014, a clinically relevant drug penetration study was done by Sjovall et al. revealing substantial cutting artifacts from the sample preparation [23]. Their SEM images and analysis from these images by time-of-flight secondary ion mass spectrometry (TOF-SIMS) showed asymmetric and uneven tissue distribution on either side of the central cartilage and morphological distortions caused by the drying of the tissue (Figure 56.12). SEM images can identify the architecture of the skin strata, and TOF-SIMS can analyze the presence of a variety of lipids in the mouse ear cross-sections, including phospholipids, cholesterol, fatty acids, and triglycerides. The antiinflammatory drug roflumilast was applied topically to mouse ear daily for one week. At the end of the treatment, the ear tissue was collected for frozen sections. The sections were imaged by SEM and analyzed by TOF-SIMS. The spatial distribution of roflumilast in the mouse ear cross-section are shown in SEM images (Figure 56.13) confirmed by TOF-SIMS. Roflumilast was homogenously distributed through the stratum corneum but did not penetrate any farther into the skin. TOF-SIMS could identify lipid and ceramide from the cell membrane and locate them accurately on the skin tissue section. A drug penetration profile can be confounded by the distortion of skin while being prepared for imaging unless the study is done in vivo. In addition, they pointed out that there was a strong signal from TOF-SIMS analysis, indicating there was a contamination possibly due to the

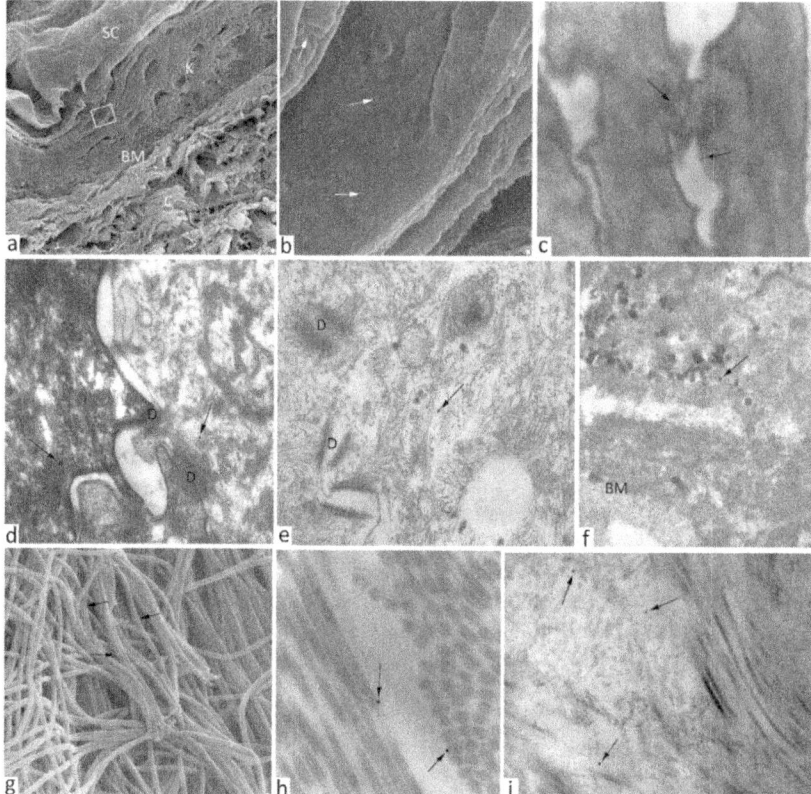

FIGURE 56.11 Images of skin samples treated with PMNP cream or suspension obtained with transmission and scanning electron microscopy. Selected micrographs show (a) SEM image of transversal skin section treated with PMNP solution for 24 hours, SC = stratum corneum, K = keratinocytes, BM = basal membrane, C = collagen. (b) High magnification of (a), PMNP are detected on the surface of the keratinocytes (white arrows). TEM images of PMNP nanoparticles (black arrows) inside the corneocytes of the skin treated with cream (c and d) or suspension (e and f). PMNP nanoparticles in proximity of the basal membrane, D = desmosomes. (g–i) Photomicrographs of PMNP nanoparticles (black arrows) intercalated between the collagen fibers of the dermis (g), SEM image (h), and (i) TEM images. (Reprinted with permission from Colombo et al. 2015.)

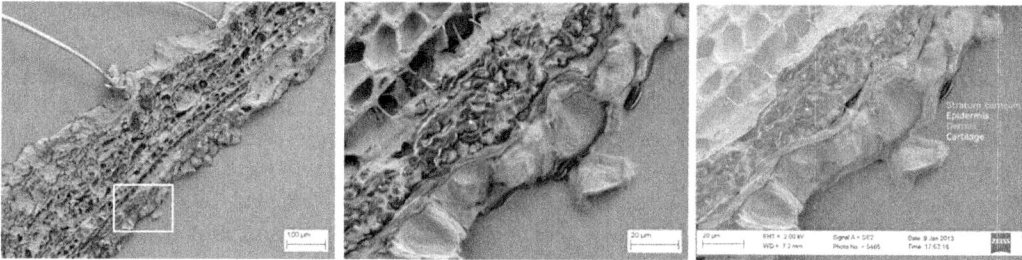

FIGURE 56.12 Scanning electron micrographs of a mouse ear cross-section as analyzed by TOF-SIMS. The area imaged (middle) is indicated by the yellow box in the left panel. Histological features of the cross-section are outlined in the left panel, including the stratum corneum (blue), epidermis (yellow), dermis (green), and cartilage (white). (Reprinted with permission from Siovall et al. 2014.)

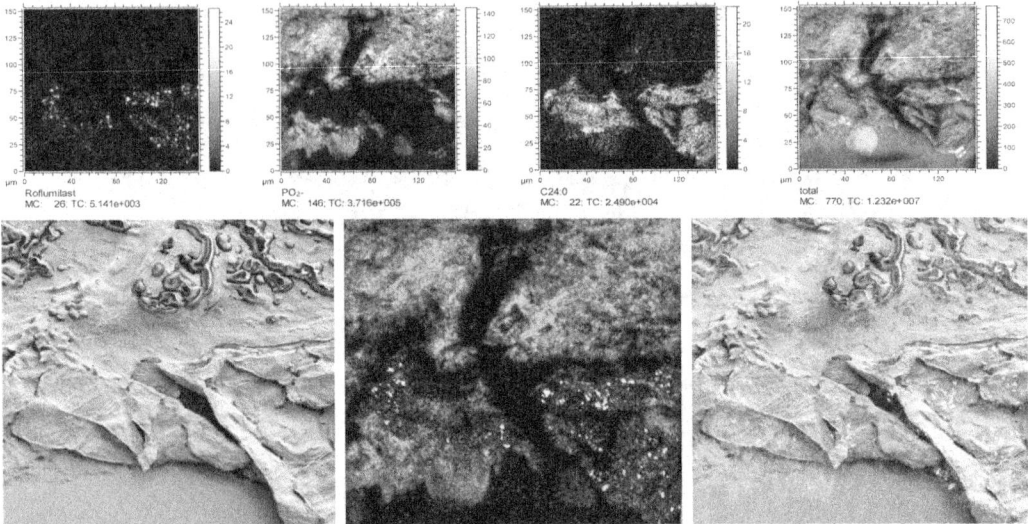

FIGURE 56.13 High-resolution TOF-SIMS images (top panels) and SEM images (bottom panels) showing the distribution of roflumilast in the stratum corneum of a roflumilast-treated mouse ear. Field of view is 150×150 µm^2. In overlay images, roflumilast is shown in green, lipid is red, and cholesterol is blue. (Reprinted with permission from Siovall et al. 2014.)

biopsy of the sample using a blade. The combination of TOF-SIMS and SEM was beneficial to study drug distribution and penetration.

56.8   OPTICAL COHERENT TOMOGRAPY

Optical coherence tomography (OCT) is a noninvasive, label-free optical imaging approach that detects scattered near-infrared (NIR) laser light signals from tissue, which predominantly avoids disruption of the skin tissue. Optical imaging tools such as reflectance microscopy (described later in this chapter) and OCT can provide a real-time "optical biopsy" in clinics. It is useful to detect early stage skin cancer by visualization of target tissue morphology with micrometer resolution in real time. NIR dyes and microparticles and nanoparticles have been explored as OCT contrast agents.

Kim et al. (2009) hypothesized that gold nanoparticles (AuNPs) would be a good candidate for an OCT contrast agent, as well as delivering biological molecules [24]. AuNPs are biocompatible, easy to synthesize, and can be functionalized with additional modalities. The aim of this study was to improve the penetration and distribution of AuNPs using microneedles and ultrasound and therefore enhance contrast in vivo OCT images of oral dysplasia in a hamster model. One side of the cheek pouch of a hamster was treated topically with 0.5% (v/v) 9,10-dimethyl-1,2-benzanthracene (DMBA) three times a week for five months to induce cancer. AuNPs were conjugated with monoclonal antibodies binding to epidermal growth factor, which is overexpressed in oral cancer. The check pouch was attached to a microscope using a custom-built clamp to fasten it to the stage. Microneedles were applied to the pouch and then AuNPs solution was applied to the site for 10 minutes. Ultrasound was then applied to the same spot for one minute to improve nanoparticle delivery. OCT images (Figure 56.14) show AuNPs penetrated deeper into the tissue when microneedles were applied. There was a visible difference between carcinogen-treated and untreated tissue. Ultrasound seems to distribute AuNPs more homogenously on the surface of the skin. When they took an enlarged image of dysplasia (Figure 56.14, bottom) and used scion image analysis software for data processing, considerably greater light scattering in the stratum corneum and upper epithelial layers

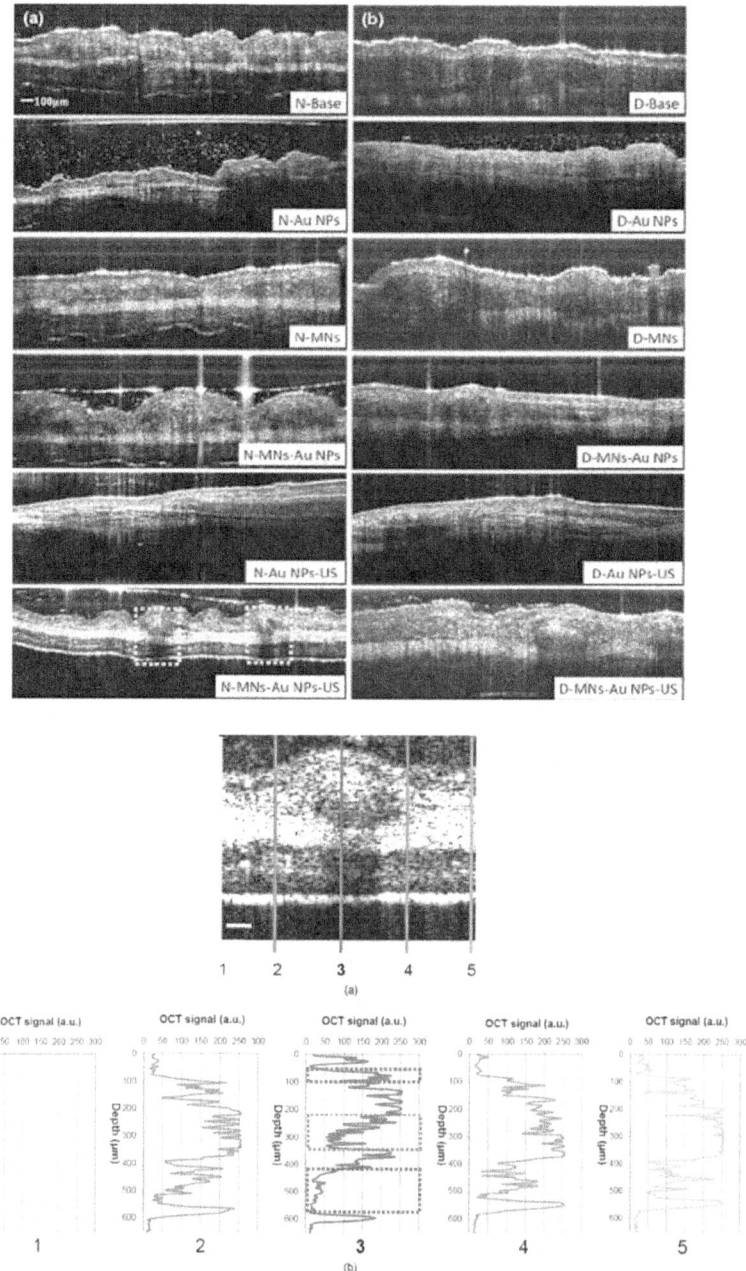

FIGURE 56.14 (A): In vivo OCT images of (a) normal (DMBA-untreated) and (b) DMBA-treated sides of hamster cheek pouches. MN = microneedle treated; AuNPs= gold nanoparticles administrated; US= ultrasound applied. (B): (a) Enlarged OCT image of dysplasia area. (b) Depth-resolved OCT signal profile in dysplastic and normal region. Scale bar: 100 μm. (Reprinted with permission from Kim et al. 2009.)

was observed. However, there was no information about the nanoparticle penetration profile. Lack of skin morphology detail was also a disadvantage of this technology. Overall, AuNPs worked as an OCT contrast agent to show the difference between dysplasia and normal tissue in vivo.

The same group (Kim et al. 2010) published another study in which they delivered AuNPs using dissolvable microneedles and imaged the delivery by OCT [25]. Their hypothesis was that enhanced delivery of AuNPs with dissolvable microneedles in the skin would enhance the OCT image contrast between normal and disease skin. AuNPs (87 nm in diameter) were mixed in sodium carboxymethyl cellulose solution (CMC). CMC is water soluble and mechanically robust in dry form. They developed dysplasia in one cheek pouch by applying 0.45%(w/v) 9,10-dimethy-1,2-benzanthracene in mineral oil topically three times a week for 10 weeks. They applied AuNPs with dissolvable microneedles and dissipated them by ultrasound (US) on the cheek pouch. After the treatment, the cheek pouch tissue was harvested, fixed in 10% formalin buffer, and embedded in paraffin for sectioning. The tissue sections were imaged by spectral domain-OCT (SD-OCT). The OCT images showed morphological differences between dysplasia and normal skin. Quantitative analysis was performed from image data. The data showed alternations in epithelial stratification, one with disruptive and the other one with well-aligned morphologies. Analysis of quantitative depth-dependent distributions of OCT signal intensity indicated that OCT signal intensity was increased in the stratum corneum in dysplastic tissue after treatment. In normal skin, there were significant signal intensity differences before and after the AuNP application. However, little information was obtained in terms of the nanoparticle penetration profile. Overall, their hypothesis was supported by the data that the application of AuNPs could achieve clear quantitative imaging-based differences between dysplastic and normal tissues.

In 2019, Ruini et al. employed OCT to investigate the effect of ingenol mebutate in actinic keratosis (AK) and subclinical AK (sAK) [26]. Twenty patients (Fitzpatrick skin type II-III) with multiple AKs were recruited. Ingenol mebutate 00.015% gel was applied within a 25 cm^2 area on the face or scalp at the time of enrollment and the following two consecutive days. Clinical, dermoscopic, reflectance confocal microscopy, and OCT images were taken at the time of enrollment (T = 0), at day 4 (T1), at day 14 (T2), and at day 56 (T3). OCT images show hyperkeratosis and crusting, irregular layering, and a broadened epidermis. By day 56, thickening of the epidermis was improved by the treatment. For sAK, there was a restoration of the epidermal dermal junction by OCT images after 56 days. These findings were confirmed by images from RCM and dermoscopy. OCT images were analyzed by measuring the mean epidermal thickness. There was a significant reduction in epidermal thickness AK from 0.22 mm to 0.15 mm after 56 days and from 0.2 mm to 0.11 mm in sAK after 56 days. The limitation is that OCT does not provide cellular resolution, but it does allow the visualization of structural patterns. The main histological features of AKs that OCT can provide are hyperkeratosis, thickening, and disruption of the dermal layers. No drug penetration profile was obtained from the OCT images. This study shows the multiple noninvasive in vivo imaging modalities to monitor the pharmacological effects on skin disease over a period of time.

56.9   REFLECTANCE CONFOCAL MICROSCOPY

RCM is a widespread imaging approach technology that is being used clinically to monitor skin morphology with quasi-histological skin images to a depth of 200 to 250 μm, including the entire epidermis and upper dermis. Recently, Haedersdal et al. (2019) published a study that used both RCM and OCT imaging approaches to visualize and quantify gold nanoparticle delivery in the facial skin of acne patients and healthy participants. They also applied laser treatment to the skin to enhance the nanoparticle delivery. RCM images from the initial experiment showed the morphology of channels created by laser application in each skin layer (epidermis, dermoepidermal junction, and papillary dermis). Gold nanoparticles were seen as hyperreflective spots in RCM images that resembled previously reported signatures. Nanoparticle penetration was confirmed by OCT. RCM imaging is useful for this application to 150 to 200 um deep, whereas OCT can image much deeper but has less information in that data. The quantitative measurement of gold nanoparticle delivery in skin strata was calculated by analyzing the signal from the laser channels in the RCM images. This study demonstrated that RCM and OCT can successfully be used to visualize gold nanoparticle delivery into the skin and the effects on skin caused by applications.

In 2018, Banzhaf et al. conducted an explorative experiment to determine whether the combined technologies of RCM and fluorescence confocal microscopy could provide information on drug uptake, distribution, and kinetics in ablative fractional laser-exposed skin [27]. Thawed human skin was used as a model, and sodium fluorescein in a prototypical gel formulation was applied to the skin as a surrogate hydrophilic drug as well as for visualization. Ablative fractional laser was applied to the skin and then the gel was gently massaged into that area. RCM and fluorescence confocal microscopy images were taken at 15 minutes, 60 minutes, and 4 hours. RCM images revealing the morphology of the skin strata (stratum corneum, epidermis, and upper dermis) were recorded at every second micron from the skin surface to a depth of 200 μm (Figure 56.15, left). Fluorescence confocal microscopy images provided a fluorescein signal from the gel. Merged images of RCM and fluorescence confocal microscopy indicated that the ablative fractional laser created channels in the skin, creating a coagulation zone that penetrated to the upper dermis. RCM and fluorescence confocal microscope z-stacks were analyzed with ImageJ to assess the fluorescein delivery according to the skin depth (Figure 56.15, right). RCM has a limitation of decreasing resolution in deeper skin layers; however, this proved for the first time that using both RCM and fluorescence confocal microscopy were useful to investigate uptake, biodistribution, and kinetics of a test drug in ablative fractional laser-treated skin.

Labouta et al. (2011) measured the penetration and metabolic effects of AuNPs in aqueous and toluene solutions on excised human skin [28]. They used both frozen and freshly excised human skin for multiple imaging techniques, including RCM, TEM, MPT, and FLIM. The freshly excised

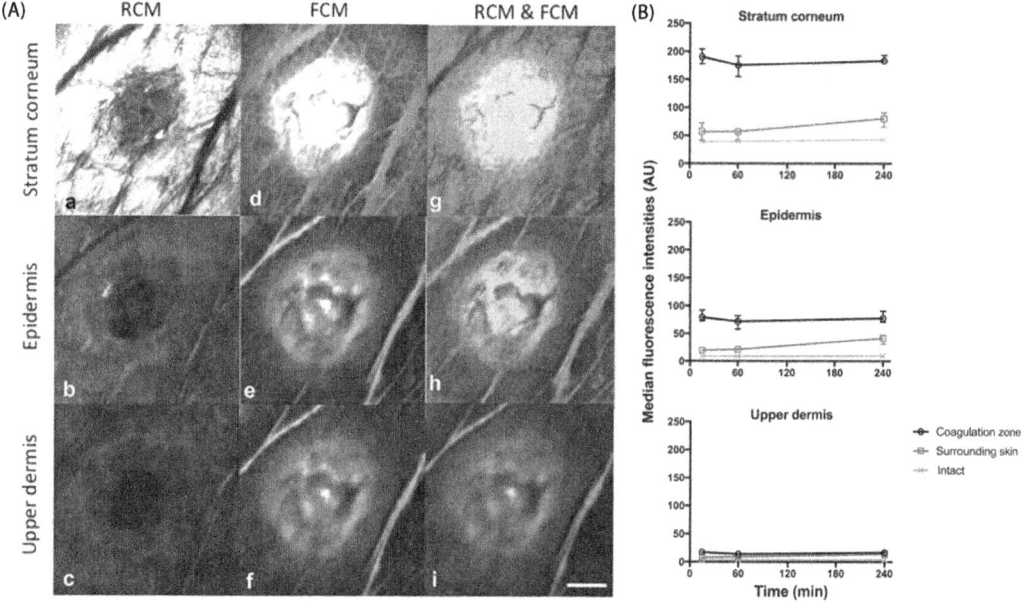

FIGURE 56.15 (A) Laser scanning confocal microscopy images from specific skin compartments after AFXL exposure and sodium fluorescein (NaF) application. (a–c) Representative reflectance confocal microscopy (RCM) images of a laser channel, including coagulation zone (CZ) at the stratum corneum, epidermal, and dermal level and (e and f) corresponding fluorescence confocal microscopy (FCM) images. (g–i) Merged red-green-blue (RGB) channels of RCM and FCM images illustrating the distribution of NaF in CZ and surrounding skin throughout the skin compartments (scale bar 100 μm). (B) Fluorescence intensities (FI) of sodium fluorescein (NaF) in the stratum corneum, epidermis, and upper dermis after 15 minutes, 60 minutes, and 4 hours, respectively. The highest FI occurs in the coagulation zone (CZ) in the stratum corneum and epidermis. FI from surrounding skin at four hours is increased in the epidermis and upper dermis, suggesting enhanced delivery of NaF (P = 0.03). (Reprinted with permission from Banzhaf et al. 2017.)

human skin from abdominoplasty was mounted on a Franz cell system, and two AuNP formulations (aqueous and toluene) were applied to the skin. After 24 hours at 32°C treatment, en face skin was visualized using RCM with dermoscopy. 3D reconstructed images from RCM z-stacks confirmed the aggregates were present within the furrows in the AuNP-aqueous group but were absent in the toluene-containing groups. The limitation of RCM is the resolution of images, especially greater than 100 um deep in the skin. It is challenging to accurately identify small particles in these images. Several imaging techniques were employed in this study to confirm the findings both qualitatively and quantitatively. This study is a good example showing that nanoparticle skin penetration is a multifactorial and multistep process that can be confirmed by complementary imaging techniques that each have strengths and weaknesses.

56.10 MATRIX-ASSISTED LASER DESORPTION/IONIZATION MASS SPECTROMETRY IMAGING

MALDI mass spectrometry imaging technology is an emerging label-free imaging technology that can provide information about drug distribution profiles across the tissue. The quantification of drug molecules on the skin is the unique strength of this technology. The major limitation is the cost of equipment and extensive training needed to apply this powerful technology to topical drug delivery characterization. Equipment access and funding currently limit the uptake of this approach in the field of drug delivery. But most of the large pharmaceutical companies have a mass spectrometry imaging group to look at drug distribution and quantification in tissue.

Bonnel et al. (2018) [29] used MALDI-MSI to conduct a feasibility study to show (1) if this technique could be useful for pharmacokinetics studies; (2) if the results can be reproducible; (3) if this method could be used to compare two different formulations; (4) if the results could be quantified; and (5) if the high spatial resolution data could be varied. Excised human skin from abdominoplasty surgery was mounted in a Franz cell system. The skin was treated topically with three different drugs (ruxolitinib, tofacitinib, and LEO29102 [undisclosed drug]) in two different formulations (transcutol solution and cream) and incubated at 37°C for three hours. An 8-mm punch biopsy was collected for each sample and embedded for frozen sections at the end of the experiment. For each tissue section, three individual sections spaced more than 100 μm apart were analyzed by MALDI-MSI. Histology staining (H&E) was done on the same sections after the MALDI-MSI imaging. Image analysis was done based on molecular distributions in skin and signal intensity per pixel of each drug molecule extracted from the image data set. Figure 56.16 shows drug penetration from the stratum corneum to the fat layers. Tofacitinib in solution remained at the surface of the skin but was not distributed homogenously, whereas in a cream formulation, tofacitinib was distributed evenly on the skin surface and penetrated deeper in some areas. There was a significant contamination signal from punch biopsy (Figure 56.16, red circles), which needed to be subtracted from the total signal. Overall, MALDI-MSI technology can provide pharmacokinetic data on the skin. Biopsy preparation or sample handling contribute to higher variability of the data, which needs to be taken into consideration when the data are analyzed. Images were able to show the different penetration profiles between the two formulations. In skin, there is high spatial variation due to the individual skin layers, hair follicles, and sweat glands. Some limitations of MALDI-MSI are that the sample preparation can introduce artifacts, increasing the resolution decreases sensitivity, and the mass of the active needs to be sufficiently different from the matrix (n.b. OCT, commonly used to embed skin for cryosectioning, is problematic for MALDI-MSI and must be avoided). These need to be taken into consideration when developing experiments to detect drug levels at pharmacologically relevant concentrations.

Hendel et al. (2019) published a study where they quantified fractional laser-assisted delivery of a topical drug, bleomycin, by a liquid chromatography-mass spectrometry (LC-MS), and its skin distribution was visualized by MALDI-MSI [30]. Bleomycin is a hydrophilic molecule, and their hypothesis was that ablative fractional laser-assisted delivery could enhance topical drug delivery of large and hydrophilic molecules in skin. Thawed excised pig skin was treated with a fractional

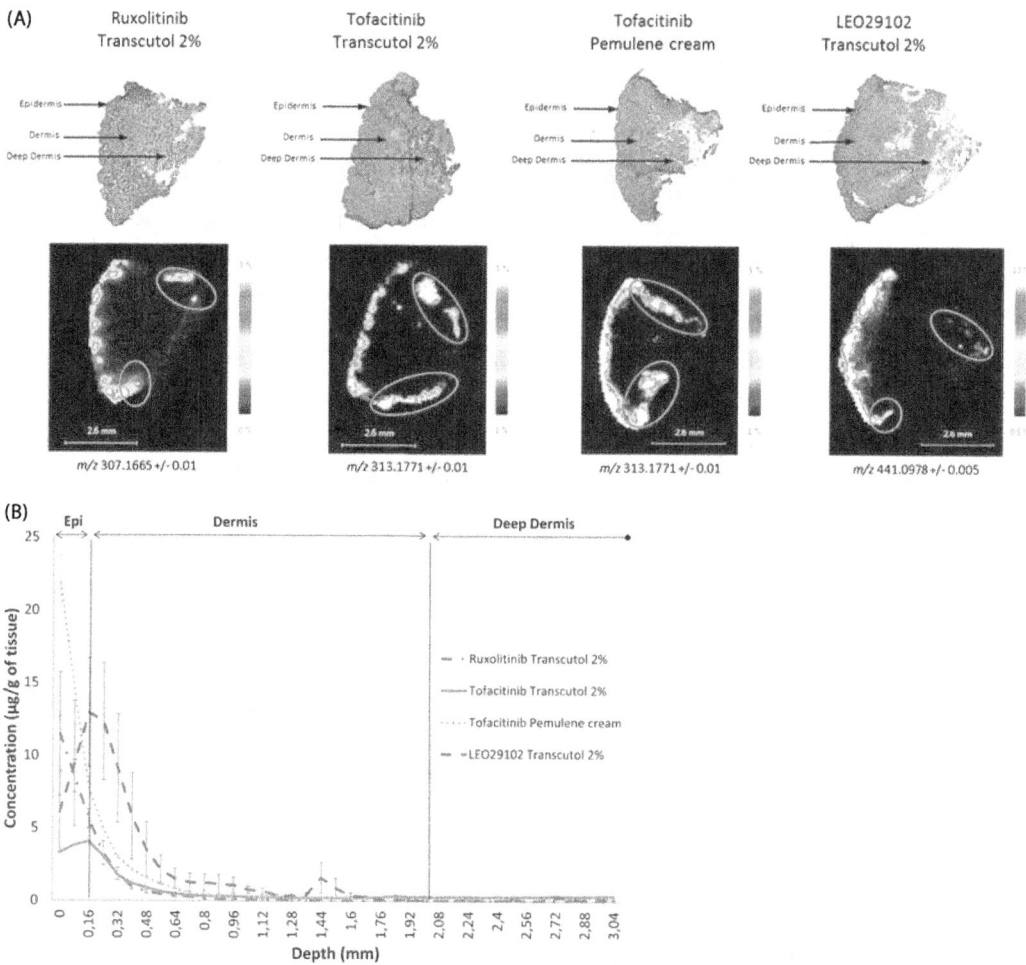

FIGURE 56.16 APIs distribution ([M+H] + ion forms) by 7T MALDI-FTICR imaging at 50 μm of spatial resolution in human expiant sections following a topical application. (A) HE staining pictures were obtained on the analyzed tissue sections after MALDI matrix removal. The signal of each APIs is mainly distributed in the epidermis and in the dermis. A significant contamination signal is observed on the section due to the punch preparation (red circles): APIs are carried on the sides of the biopsies during the punch sampling. (B) Comparison of the APIs penetration profiles through the skin sections generated from the MALDI imaging data sets. Each profile (based on a triplicate of analysis) is generated based on a region of interest defined on the MALDI image without the contamination signal due to the punch biopsy preparation.

CO_2 laser and the skin was mounted on a Franz cell. Bleomycin in solution was applied to the skin and incubated up to 24 hours at 37°C. The skin samples were biopsied using an 8-mm punch biopsy after 0.5, 4, and 24 hours of treatment. A biopsy from each sample was embedded for frozen section (30 μm thickness for LC-MS and 10 μm for MALDI-MSI). The cross-sectional view MALDI-MSI image showed that the laser channels could easily be seen with high concentrations of bleomycin that appeared to spread into the surrounding tissue. Horizontally cut sections taken from samples treated in a time course showed increasing concentrations of bleomycin over time in the superficial dermis. In the deeper dermis, there was no visible bleomycin in the center of the treated area at 0.5 hour, but by 4 and 24 hours the drug had reached the deeper dermis (Figure 56.17). These results were confirmed by quantitative LC-MS analysis. MALDI-MSI showed that bleomycin remained on the surface of the skin when there was no fractional laser applied to the skin, which was also

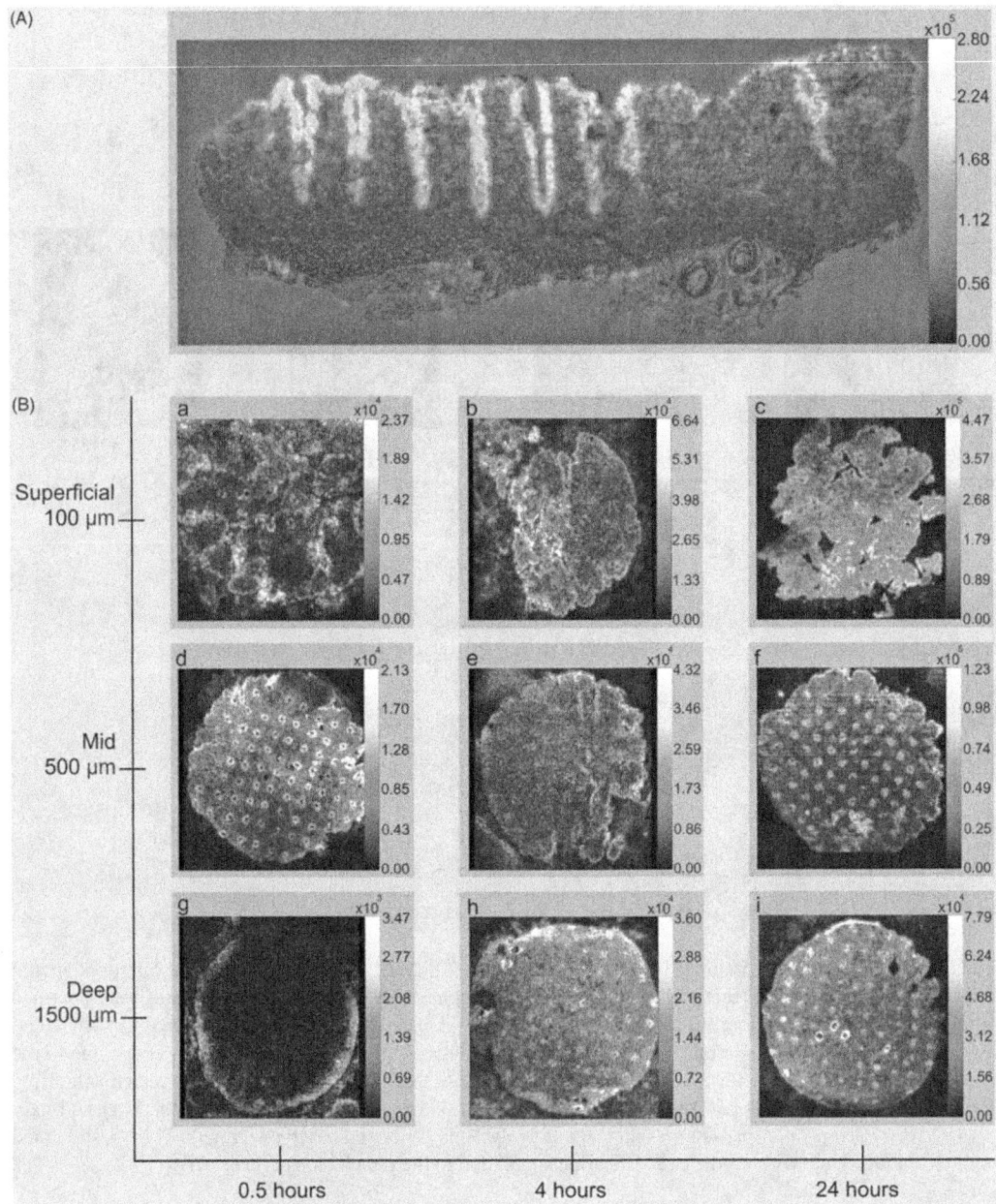

FIGURE 56.17 Mass spectrometry imaging. MALDI-MSI of bleomycin B2 (m/z1425.56323) with MAZ-Deep laser channels. (A) Vertically cut skin cryosection after 24 hours of topical drug exposure. Laser channels are easily seen with high concentration of bleomycin (yellow) in the coagulation zones and drug dissemination into the surrounding tissue. (B) Horizontally cut skin cryosections. A trend towards higher concentrations is seen along the x-axis of time, and lower down the y-axis of skin depth. The depicted intensity values for each image are based on maximum bleomycin detection within the individual skin sample and thus cannot be compared interindividually. MAZ-Deep: Microscopic ablation zone reaching the deep dermis.

confirmed by LC-MS. This study was the first to show the laser assisted large molecule delivery in skin quantified with LC-MS and visualized with MALDI-MSI.

56.11 TIME-OF-FLIGHT SECONDARY ION MASS SPECTROMETRY

TOF-SIMS is a surface-sensitive analytical technology that uses a pulsed ion beam to remove molecules from the very outmost surface of the sample. These molecules are then accelerated into a tube, and their mass is determined by measuring the exact time at which they reach the detector. It can generate high mass resolution and high sensitivity for trace chemicals or compounds. In skin, TOF-SIMS can provide material information, distribution of materials, and depth of the materials.

In 2018, Luengo et al. performed TOF-SIMS to map endogenous lipids in skin cross-sections [31]. The main advantage of using this technology is the spatial resolution, which is in the sub-micrometer range, as compared to 10 to 50 μm for MALDI imaging. Afterwards, they studied the distribution of endogenous lipids in skin treated with carvacrol oil, oregano essential oil, and ceramide. TOF-SIMS was used to investigate the lipid distribution and penetration. Their aim was to differentiate between the exogenous lipid signal from the cosmetic ingredients and the endogenous signal from skin cells using their different molecular weights. Ex vivo human skin was mounted on a Franz cell model. The skin was treated with three different ingredients and incubated at 37°C for 24 hours. The samples were then embedded for frozen sections before imaging.

Their paper shows the cross-sectional TOF-SIMS images after the skin was treated with ceramide. They found that the molecular weight of ceramide in topical formulation is 565 Da and the endogenous ceramide from the stratum corneum was 650 to 750 Da. The TOF-SIMS data revealed a clear localization of the exogenous ceramide in the stratum corneum and epidermis, but minimal ceramide was detected at the deeper epidermal layers. TOF-SIMS can be used to detect the presence of endogenous and exogenous compounds in skin cross-sections. One of the limitations is that this technique cannot be used in vivo. Second, preparation of the cross-section samples is critical and can be problematic, particularly embedding the samples. Embedding processing in a medium can compromise the effect on skin structure, skin lipid distribution, and potentially affect drug distribution. The final limitation is the decreased sensitivity of using cross-section samples compared to direct analysis of the skin via destructive approaches like LC-MS.

56.12 CONCLUSION

Microscopic assessment of topical drug delivery provides valuable information about drugs and nanoparticles via cutaneous delivery in skin. However, it is important to understand the advantages and disadvantages of each technology, as described in Table 56.1. Skin models (ex vivo, in vivo, or fixed samples) and active ingredients need to be considered for each experimental approach. The sample preparations, including skin biopsy, embedding, and frozen sectioning, might have some impact on modifying active molecules or drug penetration profiles. Based on our experiences, we have generated a diagram showing the most applicable methodologies to study topical drug penetration in different skin models. (Table 56.3). Although there have been many innovations in drug delivery systems, the number of effective cutaneous drugs remains small, primarily because of the stratum corneum permeability barrier. Overcoming this barrier safely and reversibly to deliver large hydrophilic drugs topically is still one of the major challenges in the field of dermatologic therapy. Sweat glands or hair follicles might be a new route for delivering actives deep into skin, as they are easily visible and distributed evenly throughout the skin. Noninvasive microscopy is an ideal approach to evaluate the penetration of topical drugs in this context.

The future of microscopy is going to provide higher resolution and faster imaging, which will generate increasing amounts of data. Our study with nanoelmulsions (Yamada et al. 2018) [19] generated a total of over 800 GB. As imaging systems become more accessible, we need to develop automated solutions like artificial intelligence or computer vision to help us get the most out of this exciting technology.

TABLE 56.3

A Flow Chart of Selection of Imaging Modality Based on Skin Models

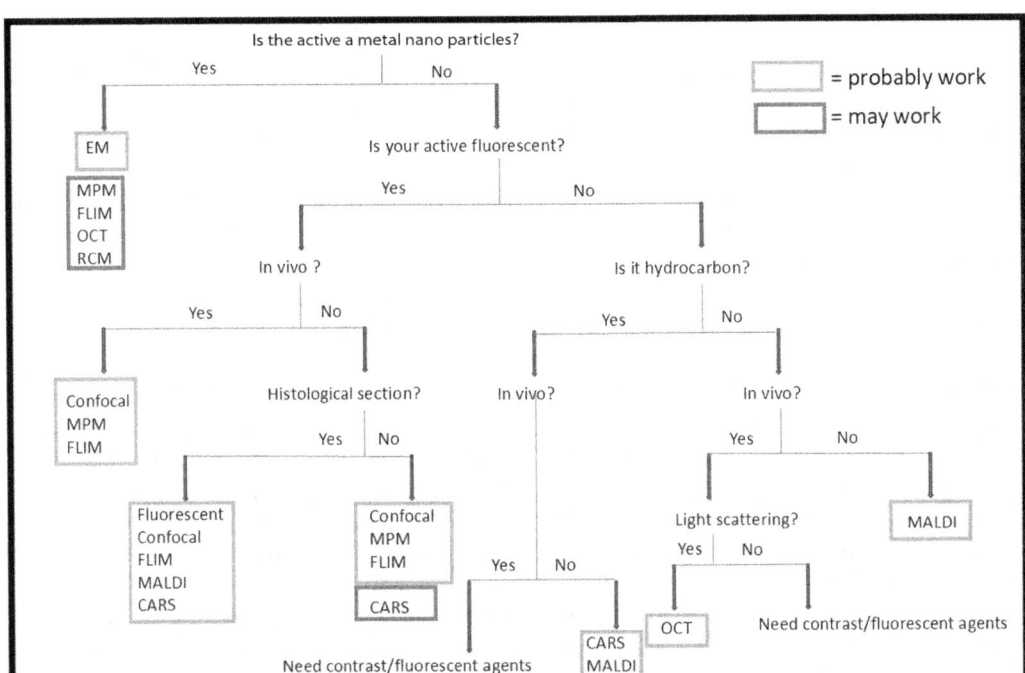

REFERENCES

1. Calienni MN, Temprana CF, Prieto MJ, Paolino D, Fresta M, Tekinay AB, et al. Nano-formulation for topical treatment of precancerous lesions: skin penetration, in vitro, and in vivo toxicological evaluation. Drug Deliv Transl Res. 2018;8(3):496–514. Epub 2017/12/31.
2. Volz P, Schilrreff P, Brodwolf R, Wolff C, Stellmacher J, Balke J, et al. Pitfalls in using fluorescence tagging of nanomaterials: tecto-dendrimers in skin tissue as investigated by Cluster-FLIM. Ann N Y Acad Sci. 2017;1405(1):202–14. Epub 2017/10/07.
3. Romero G, Qiu Y, Murray RA, Moya SE. Study of intracellular delivery of doxorubicin from poly(lactide-co-glycolide) nanoparticles by means of fluorescence lifetime imaging and confocal Raman microscopy. Macromol Biosci. 2013;13(2):234–41. Epub 2013/01/15.
4. Witting M, Boreham A, Brodwolf R, Vavrova K, Alexiev U, Friess W, et al. Interactions of hyaluronic Acid with skin and implications for the dermal delivery of biomacromolecules. Mol Pharm. 2015;12(5):1391–401. Epub 2015/04/15.
5. Russo C, Brickelbank N, Duckett C, Mellor S, Rumbelow S, Clench MR. Quantitative investigation of terbinafine hydrochloride absorption into a living skin equivalent model by MALDI-MSI. Anal Chem. 2018;90(16):10031–8. Epub 2018/07/20.
6. Fuchs CSK, Ortner VK, Mogensen M, Philipsen PA, Haedersdal M. Transfollicular delivery of gold microparticles in healthy skin and acne vulgaris, assessed by in vivo reflectance confocal microscopy and optical coherence tomography. Lasers Surg Med. 2019. Epub 2019/03/06.
7. Banzhaf CA, Ortner VK, Philipsen PA, Haedersdal M. The ablative fractional coagulation zone influences skin fluorescence intensities of topically applied test molecules-An in vitro study with fluorescence microscopy and fluorescence confocal microscopy. Lasers Surg Med. 2019;51(1):68–78. Epub 2018/12/26.
8. Banzhaf CA, Wind BS, Mogensen M, Meesters AA, Paasch U, Wolkerstorfer A, et al. Spatiotemporal closure of fractional laser-ablated channels imaged by optical coherence tomography and reflectance confocal microscopy. Lasers Surg Med. 2016;48(2):157–65. Epub 2015/08/13.

9. Lee JY, Suh JS, Kim JM, Kim JH, Park HJ, Park YJ, et al. Identification of a cell-penetrating peptide domain from human beta-defensin 3 and characterization of its anti-inflammatory activity. Int J Nanomedicine. 2015;10:5423–34. Epub 2015/09/09.

10. Smejkalova D, Muthny T, Nesporova K, Hermannova M, Achbergerova E, Huerta-Angeles G, et al. Hyaluronan polymeric micelles for topical drug delivery. Carbohydr Polym. 2017;156:86–96. Epub 2016/11/16.

11. Sun L, Liu Z, Lin Z, Cun D, Tong HH, Yan R, et al. Comparison of normal versus imiquimod-induced psoriatic skin in mice for penetration of drugs and nanoparticles. Int J Nanomedicine. 2018;13:5625–35. Epub 2018/10/03.

12. Campbell CS, Contreras-Rojas LR, Delgado-Charro MB, Guy RH. Objective assessment of nanoparticle disposition in mammalian skin after topical exposure. J Control Release. 2012;162(1):201–7. Epub 2012/06/27.

13. Stracke F, Weiss B, Lehr CM, Konig K, Schaefer UF, Schneider M. Multiphoton microscopy for the investigation of dermal penetration of nanoparticle-borne drugs. J Invest Dermatol. 2006;126(10):2224–33. Epub 2006/05/20.

14. Tancrede-Bohin E, Baldeweck T, Decenciere E, Brizion S, Victorin S, Parent N, et al. Non-invasive short-term assessment of retinoids effects on human skin in vivo using multiphoton microscopy. J Eur Acad Dermatol Venereol. 2015;29(4):673–81. Epub 2014/09/16.

15. Labouta HI, Kraus T, El-Khordagui LK, Schneider M. Combined multiphoton imaging-pixel analysis for semiquantitation of skin penetration of gold nanoparticles. Int J Pharm. 2011;413(1-2):279–82. Epub 2011/04/26.

16. Jeong S, Hermsmeier M, Osseiran S, Yamamoto A, Nagavarapu U, Chan KF, et al. Visualization of drug distribution of a topical minocycline gel in human facial skin. Biomed Opt Express. 2018;9(7):3434–48. Epub 2018/07/10.

17. Leite-Silva VR, Le Lamer M, Sanchez WY, Liu DC, Sanchez WH, Morrow I, et al. The effect of formulation on the penetration of coated and uncoated zinc oxide nanoparticles into the viable epidermis of human skin in vivo. Eur J Pharm Biopharm. 2013;84(2):297–308. Epub 2013/03/05.

18. Alex A, Frey S, Angelene H, Neitzel CD, Li J, Bower AJ, et al. In situ biodistribution and residency of a topical anti-inflammatory using fluorescence lifetime imaging microscopy. Br J Dermatol. 2018;179(6):1342–50. Epub 2018/07/11.

19. Yamada M, Tayeb H, Wang H, Dang N, Mohammed YH, Osseiran S, et al. Using elongated microparticles to enhance tailorable nanoemulsion delivery in excised human skin and volunteers. J Control Release. 2018;288:264–76. Epub 2018/09/19.

20. Belsey NA, Garrett NL, Contreras-Rojas LR, Pickup-Gerlaugh AJ, Price GJ, Moger J, et al. Evaluation of drug delivery to intact and porated skin by coherent Raman scattering and fluorescence microscopies. J Control Release. 2014;174:37–42. Epub 2013/11/16.

21. Saar BG, Freudiger CW, Reichman J, Stanley CM, Holtom GR, Xie XS. Video-rate molecular imaging in vivo with stimulated Raman scattering. Science. 2010;330(6009):1368–70. Epub 2010/12/04.

22. Santini B, Zanoni I, Marzi R, Cigni C, Bedoni M, Gramatica F, et al. Cream formulation impact on topical administration of engineered colloidal nanoparticles. PLoS One. 2015;10(5):e0126366. Epub 2015/05/12.

23. Sjovall P, Greve TM, Clausen SK, Moller K, Eirefelt S, Johansson B, et al. Imaging of distribution of topically applied drug molecules in mouse skin by combination of time-of-flight secondary ion mass spectrometry and scanning electron microscopy. Anal Chem. 2014;86(7):3443–52. Epub 2014/02/27.

24. Kim CS, Wilder-Smith P, Ahn YC, Liaw LH, Chen Z, Kwon YJ. Enhanced detection of early-stage oral cancer in vivo by optical coherence tomography using multimodal delivery of gold nanoparticles. J Biomed Opt. 2009;14(3):034008. Epub 2009/07/02.

25. Kim CS, Ahn YC, Wilder-Smith P, Oh S, Chen Z, Kwon YJ. Efficient and facile delivery of gold nanoparticles in vivo using dissolvable microneedles for contrast-enhanced optical coherence tomography. Biomed Opt Express. 2010;1(1):106–13. Epub 2011/01/25.

26. Ruini C, Hartmann D, Bastian M, Ruzicka T, French L, Berking C, et al. Non-invasive monitoring of subclinical and clinical actinic keratosis of face and scalp under topical treatment with ingenolmebutate gel 150 mcg/gby means of reflectance confocal microscopy and optical coherence tomography: new perspectives and comparison of diagnostic techniques. J Biophotonics. 2019:e201800391. Epub 2019/01/18.

27. Banzhaf CA, Lin LL, Dang N, Freeman M, Haedersdal M, Prow TW. The fractional laser-induced coagulation zone characterized over time by laser scanning confocal microscopy-A proof of concept study. Lasers Surg Med. 2018;50(1):70–7. Epub 2017/12/02.

28. Labouta HI, Liu DC, Lin LL, Butler MK, Grice JE, Raphael AP, et al. Gold nanoparticle penetration and reduced metabolism in human skin by toluene. Pharm Res. 2011;28(11):2931–44. Epub 2011/08/13.

29. Bonnel D, Legouffe R, Eriksson AH, Mortensen RW, Pamelard F, Stauber J, et al. MALDI imaging facilitates new topical drug development process by determining quantitative skin distribution profiles. Anal Bioanal Chem. 2018;410(11):2815–28. Epub 2018/03/17.

30. Hendel KK, Bagger C, Olesen UH, Janfelt C, Hansen SH, Haedersdal M, et al. Fractional laser-assisted topical delivery of bleomycin quantified by LC-MS and visualized by MALDI mass spectrometry imaging. Drug Deliv. 2019;26(1):244–51. Epub 2019/03/13.

31. Sjovall P, Skedung L, Gregoire S, Biganska O, Clement F, Luengo GS. Imaging the distribution of skin lipids and topically applied compounds in human skin using mass spectrometry. Sci Rep. 2018;8(1):16683. Epub 2018/11/14.

32. See GL, Sagesaka A, Sugasawa S, Todo H, Sugibayashi K. Eyelid skin as a potential site for drug delivery to conjunctiva and ocular tissues. Int J Pharm. 2017;533(1):198–205. Epub 2017/10/03.

33. Sahu P, Kashaw SK, Jain S, Sau S, Iyer AK. Assessment of penetration potential of pH responsive double walled biodegradable nanogels coated with eucalyptus oil for the controlled delivery of 5-fluorouracil: In vitro and ex vivo studies. J Control Release. 2017;253:122–36. Epub 2017/03/23.

34. Etrych T, Lucas H, Janouskova O, Chytil P, Mueller T, Mader K. Fluorescence optical imaging in anti-cancer drug delivery. J Control Release. 2016;226:168–81. Epub 2016/02/20.

35. Darvin ME, Thiede G, Ascencio SM, Schanzer S, Richter H, Vinzon SE, et al. In vivo/ex vivo targeting of Langerhans cells after topical application of the immune response modifier TMX-202: confocal Raman microscopy and histology analysis. J Biomed Opt. 2016;21(5):55004. Epub 2016/05/28.

36. Davidson SM, Duchen MR. Imaging mitochondrial calcium fluxes with fluorescent probes and single- or two-photon confocal microscopy. Methods Mol Biol. 2018;1782:171–86. Epub 2018/06/01.

37. Caracciolo G, Palchetti S, Digiacomo L, Chiozzi RZZ, Capriotti AL, Amenitsch H, et al. Human biomolecular corona of liposomal doxorubicin: The overlooked factor in anticancer drug delivery. ACS Appl Mater Interfaces. 2018;10(27):22951–62. Epub 2018/06/16.

38. Olson E, Levene MJ, Torres R. Multiphoton microscopy with clearing for three dimensional histology of kidney biopsies. Biomed Opt Express. 2016;7(8):3089–96. Epub 2016/08/30.

39. Sims KR, Liu Y, Hwang G, Jung HI, Koo H, Benoit DSW. Enhanced design and formulation of nanoparticles for anti-biofilm drug delivery. Nanoscale. 2018;11(1):219–36. Epub 2018/12/14.

40. Kumar P, Singh SK, Handa V, Kathuria H. Oleic acid nanovesicles of minoxidil for enhanced follicular delivery. Medicines (Basel). 2018;5(3). Epub 2018/09/19.

41. Torky AS, Freag MS, Nasra MMA, Abdallah OY. Novel skin penetrating berberine oleate complex capitalizing on hydrophobic ion pairing approach. Int J Pharm. 2018;549(1-2):76–86. Epub 2018/07/28.

42. Donalisio M, Leone F, Civra A, Spagnolo R, Ozer O, Lembo D, et al. Acyclovir-loaded chitosan nanospheres from nano-emulsion templating for the topical treatment of herpesviruses infections. Pharmaceutics. 2018;10(2). Epub 2018/04/13.

43. Lu J, Chen M, Gao L, Cheng Q, Xiang Y, Huang J, et al. A preliminary study on topical ozonated oil in the therapeutic management of atopic dermatitis in murine. J Dermatolog Treat. 2018;29(7):676–81. Epub 2018/02/23.

44. Ghita MA, Caruntu C, Rosca AE, Caruntu A, Moraru L, Constantin C, et al. Real-time investigation of skin blood flow changes induced by topical capsaicin. Acta Dermatovenerol Croat. 2017;25(3):223–7. Epub 2017/12/19.

45. Ropke MA, Alonso C, Jung S, Norsgaard H, Richter C, Darvin ME, et al. Effects of glucocorticoids on stratum corneum lipids and function in human skin-A detailed lipidomic analysis. J Dermatol Sci. 2017;88(3):330–8. Epub 2017/09/16.

46. Carlson M, Watson AL, Anderson L, Largaespada DA, Provenzano PP. Multiphoton fluorescence lifetime imaging of chemotherapy distribution in solid tumors. J Biomed Opt. 2017;22(11):1–9. Epub 2017/12/01.

47. Behne MJ, Sanchez S, Barry NP, Kirschner N, Meyer W, Mauro TM, et al. Major translocation of calcium upon epidermal barrier insult: imaging and quantification via FLIM/Fourier vector analysis. Arch Dermatol Res. 2011;303(2):103–15. Epub 2011/01/05.

48. Frombach J, Unbehauen M, Kurniasih IN, Schumacher F, Volz P, Hadam S, et al. Core-multishell nanocarriers enhance drug penetration and reach keratinocytes and antigen-presenting cells in intact human skin. J Control Release. 2019;299:138–48. Epub 2019/02/25.

49. Herman P, Holoubek A, Brodska B. Lifetime-based photoconversion of EGFP as a tool for FLIM. Biochim Biophys Acta Gen Subj. 2019;1863(1):266–77. Epub 2018/11/06.

50. Xu Y, He R, Lin D, Ji M, Chen J. Laser beam controlled drug release from Ce6-gold nanorod composites in living cells: a FLIM study. Nanoscale. 2015;7(6):2433–41. Epub 2015/01/08.

51. Thaa B, Herrmann A, Veit M. Intrinsic cytoskeleton-dependent clustering of influenza virus M2 protein with hemagglutinin assessed by FLIM-FRET. J Virol. 2010;84(23):12445–9. Epub 2010/10/01.

52. Saari H, Lisitsyna E, Rautaniemi K, Rojalin T, Niemi L, Nivaro O, et al. FLIM reveals alternative EV-mediated cellular up-take pathways of paclitaxel. J Control Release. 2018;284:133–43. Epub 2018/06/16.

53. Lademann J, Meinke MC, Schanzer S, Richter H, Darvin ME, Haag SF, et al. In vivo methods for the analysis of the penetration of topically applied substances in and through the skin barrier. Int J Cosmet Sci. 2012;34(6):551–9. Epub 2012/09/11.

54. Pope I, Payne L, Zoriniants G, Thomas E, Williams O, Watson P, et al. Coherent anti-Stokes Raman scattering microscopy of single nanodiamonds. Nat Nanotechnol. 2014;9(11):940–6. Epub 2014/10/13.

55. Aissaoui A, Chami M, Hussein M, Miller AD. Efficient topical delivery of plasmid DNA to lung in vivo mediated by putative triggered, PEGylated pDNA nanoparticles. J Control Release. 2011;154(3):275–84.

56. Subhash HM, Xie H, Smith JW, McCarty OJ. Optical detection of indocyanine green encapsulated biocompatible poly (lactic-co-glycolic) acid nanoparticles with photothermal optical coherence tomography. Opt Lett. 2012;37(5):981–3. Epub 2012/03/02.

57. de Schellenberger AA, Poller WC, Stangl V, Landmesser U, Schellenberger E. Macrophage uptake switches on OCT contrast of superparamagnetic nanoparticles for imaging of atherosclerotic plaques. International journal of nanomedicine. 2018;13:7905.

58. Mahendra J, Mahendra L, Svedha P, Cherukuri S, Romanos GE. Clinical and microbiological efficacy of 4% Garcinia mangostana L. pericarp gel as local drug delivery in the treatment of chronic periodontitis: A randomized, controlled clinical trial. J Investig Clin Dent. 2017;8(4). Epub 2017/03/23.

59. Lukowski JK, Weaver EM, Hummon AB. Analyzing liposomal drug delivery systems in three-dimensional cell culture models using MALDI imaging mass spectrometry. Anal Chem. 2017;89(16):8453–8. Epub 2017/07/22.

57 Dermal Sampling Techniques with a Focus on Dermal Open Flow Microperfusion

Thomas Birngruber, Beate Boulgaropoulos, and Frank Sinner
Medical University of Graz, Graz, Austria

CONTENTS

57.1 INTRODUCTION

Assessment of percutaneous drug penetration is highly relevant for the development of dermal topical drug products, as these drug products aim to penetrate the skin, deliver a therapeutically effective drug concentration, and exert a local effect [1]. However, there is a complex relationship between the applied drug dose and the therapeutically effective drug concentration at the site of action. Dose–response assessment, which requires the availability of pharmacokinetics (PK) profiles, is therefore a key step in drug development. Drug development of topical drugs is particularly fraught with risk, because PK data from the site of topical drug action are difficult to access, and systemic PK data derived from blood samples may not be predictive for topical drugs that exert their therapeutic effect in the skin. To establish relevant PK profiles, knowledge of the effective drug concentrations at the site of action is required, which includes consideration of the amount of effective unbound drug in the target tissue.

Dermal PK can be mapped by sampling and analyzing dermal interstitial fluid (ISF). ISF represents the immediate environment of cells and serves as a transport medium for nutrients, signaling molecules, and for waste products among cells, as well as blood and cells [2–4]. ISF defines the physical and biochemical microenvironment of the cells in several tissues, and its relevance has recently been reassessed [5]. The interstitial space is the largest fluidic compartment of the body [6] and it is crucial for drug PK processes. ISF and plasma together contain all extracellular fluids of the body, with ISF being the much larger of these two extracellular compartments. ISF is considered a plasma ultra-filtrate, and one may expect that it contains various dissolved substances in similar concentrations as in plasma. However, ISF contains 50% to 80% less protein than plasma [3, 6, 7], and it contains slightly more anions than plasma, which is attributed to the net-negative charge of plasma proteins that attracts positively charged ions (Donnan effect) [8]. Small, water-soluble molecules circulate relatively freely between the two compartments, and their concentrations are similar in ISF and plasma [9, 10].

Nonetheless, sampling of dermal ISF is challenging, and the limited accessibility of dermal PK data contributes to the underrepresentation of topical drugs on the market.

Data on the dermal PK is also a prerequisite for the development of more cost-effective generic drug products, which requires proof of bioequivalence (BE) of the prospective generic drug relative to the respective reference-listed drug. For topical generic drugs acting in the skin, systemic PK data derived from blood samples are of limited value, because the measured drug concentrations are mostly below the lower limit of quantification of the analytical method used. Clinical endpoint studies are often performed to show BE of the generic and the respective reference-listed drug, because methods to assess effective drug concentrations directly in the skin are very limited. However, such clinical endpoint studies are expensive and have a high risk of failure, as the therapeutic effect of the drug is highly variable [11–13]. The lack of dermal PK data and the urgent need to access PK data of topical drugs directly in the skin promote the development of techniques capable of directly monitoring percutaneous drug penetration.

57.2   OVERVIEW OF DERMAL SAMPLING TECHNIQUES

Techniques to monitor percutaneous drug penetration and to assess dermal PK data by extracting and analyzing dermal ISF samples include a range of models and may be applied ex vivo and in vivo. Ex vivo dermal sampling can be performed with skin explants from humans or animals. In vivo assessment of percutaneous drug penetration can be performed in preclinical (animal studies) or in clinical studies with human participants. Although drug absorption into animal skin can predict the drug absorption kinetics in human skin to a certain degree, human studies are the gold standard against which all methods for measuring percutaneous absorption should be judged [14, 15].

The applied sampling techniques to gain dermal ISF deliver either snapshots of the drug concentration in the targeted skin layers or provide time-resolved data delivering PK profiles of the respective topical drug in the skin. Also, the collected dermal sample fluids differ regarding their composition, i.e. protein content, unbound drug content, contamination with intracellular fluid or with drug from the stratum corneum depot of the skin, etc., depending on the applied technique.

Dermal ISF can be collected using wicks or capsules implanted into tissue [16–18]. Further, access to dermal ISF is provided by tissue centrifugation, skin biopsies, and suction blisters. In addition to these rather invasive sampling techniques, minimally invasive continuous dermal ISF sampling can be performed with microdialysis (MD) [39] and open flow microperfusion (OFM) [43].

Skin biopsies and suction blister are well established in vivo sampling techniques to assess dermal drug concentration. Skin biopsies involve surgical removal of a piece of the skin for analysis and represent a commonly applied diagnostic procedure in dermatology practice [19]. However, the relevance of biopsies as tools in topical PK studies is limited due to several reasons: Their invasiveness prevents repeated sampling and thus excludes monitoring of PK concentration–time profiles. The concentrations derived from biopsy samples may not reflect the concentrations at the drug target site in the skin due to sample contamination with the drug from the stratum corneum depot of the skin or due to metabolic activity. Data reliability is highly dependent on the quality and standardization of the biopsy procedure, and the lack of standardized procedures when taking biopsy samples presents a major hurdle for reliable data collection.

For suction blisters, a partial negative pressure is applied to the skin, which disrupts the epidermal–dermal junction and leads to the formation of a blister filled with ISF and serum [21, 22]. Topical drugs can be quantified in collected blister fluid [23] and penetration properties of topical formulations can be compared. However, the collected samples may contain very low levels of the drug due to potential binding to skin tissue, especially when the compounds of interest are lipophilic [24]. Further, the resulting protein ISF-to-serum ratios are highly variable [7, 25, 26]. Certain commercial devices that allow simultaneous generation of multiple blisters are available [27], but the application is generally restricted by the risk of scar formation.

Tape stripping is a less invasive method that removes non-viable cells from the stratum corneum of the skin [28]. Use of tape stripping to assess PK profiles of topical drugs in the dermis that exert their effects in the underlying viable tissue is limited because reproducible correlations between drug levels in the stratum corneum and those in the underlying viable tissue remain contradictory [29, 30], and use of such correlations is under debate by the respective agencies such as the European Medicines Agency (EMA) or the U.S. Food and Drug Administration (FDA). While the EMA regards tape-stripping data as a potentially suitable surrogate to characterize drug absorption to the underlying tissue for drugs that have their sites of action below the stratum corneum [31], the FDA withdrew their skin-stripping approach [32] in 2002 [33] due to inconsistent study results [34, 35].

Two minimally invasive methods to sample diluted dermal ISF are the probe-based, continuous dermal sampling techniques MD [37, 39] and OFM [43]. Continuous dermal ISF sampling provides time-resolved data and allows assessment of drug concentration–time profiles in the skin. To continuously sample dermal ISF, the probe is implanted into the dermis parallel to the skin surface and it is perfused with a physiological solution (perfusate) which equilibrates with the extracellular fluid of the surrounding tissue.

During MD sampling, passive diffusion of compounds between the probe and the ISF of the surrounding tissue leads to compound exchange across a semi-permeable membrane [36, 37]. Compounds smaller than the molecular weight cutoff value of the MD membrane can enter the probe [38]. In contrast, dermal OFM allows unrestricted exchange of compounds via an open steel mesh which forms the open exchange area of the OFM probe, and the exchange of compounds between the probe and the surrounding fluid occurs non-selectively in either direction driven by convection (Figure 57.1).

Dermal sampling with MD is usually restricted to compounds with a molecular size of up to about 20 kDa (CE-certified), and the membrane cutoff is chosen according to the size of the compound of interest [39]. Exclusion of high-molecular-weight compounds allows assessment of unbound drug concentrations in dermal ISF. Moreover, high-molecular-weight cutoff MD probes are available that enable recovery of molecules with a size of 100 kDa and beyond are available [40, 41]. However, these probes are not CE-certified which hinders their application in clinical trials. Limitations of MD as a dermal sampling technique for the assessment of percutaneous drug

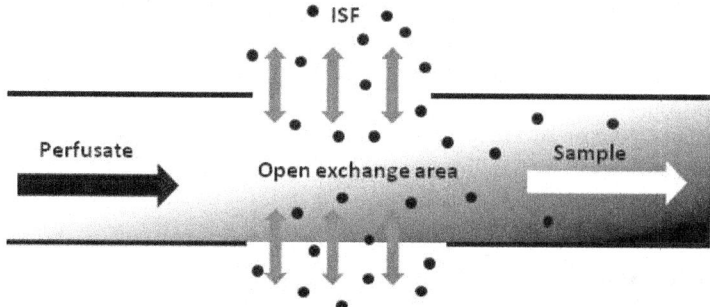

FIGURE 57.1 Nonselective exchange of compounds between perfusate and the surrounding ISF across the open exchange area of the probe with dermal OFM sampling.

penetration are attributed to the size exclusion of compounds. Further, adsorption of especially lipophilic and high-molecular-weight compounds to MD material excludes these substances from entering the probe. Protein clotting to the probe surface and to the membrane leads to membrane fouling, which may result in a change of probe recovery during prolonged sampling and contribute to biased results [42]. When intending to analyze drugs with poor permeation ability, the drug quantities collected during sampling are rather small. Adsorption of compounds to the MD membrane also results in very low drug concentrations present in the MD sample which restricts the routine application, especially for lipophilic compounds in PK studies of topical drugs.

Standardization of procedures needs to be handled rigorously when applying MD or OFM to get reliable data. The use of MD in bioavailability studies is limited by a lack of such standardized procedures.

MD sampling is most successful with target compounds with high skin permeation characteristics, reasonable aqueous solubility, and low protein-binding properties. However, molecules with these properties have limited relevance as dermatological drugs. The MD performance for highly lipophilic molecules can be enhanced by adding e.g., albumin, cyclodextrin, and cosolvents such as ethanol and dimethyl sulfoxide to the perfusate. However, due to drug extraction processes the resulting absolute tissue concentration may be falsified.

57.3 CONTINUOUS SAMPLING WITH DERMAL OPEN FLOW MICROPERFUSION

Dermal OFM is a minimally invasive continuous dermal sampling technique with unrestricted exchange of compounds between the perfusate and the dermal ISF in the open exchange area of the probe [43] (Figure 57.1). Compounds are exchanged nonselectively in either direction between the perfusate and the surrounding ISF, regardless of their molecular size, lipophilicity, or charge [44–46]. Dermal OFM is capable of sampling lipophilic [47, 48] and hydrophilic compounds with low skin permeation ability [49] and compounds with high protein binding properties.

The collected dermal ISF samples contain diluted and unfiltered ISF and contain compounds ranging from small molecules, peptides, and proteins to protein-bound drug molecules and high-molecular-weight antibodies [50], up to entire immune-competent cells. This complex composition of the dermal OFM samples provides large inherent informational content, but it also poses challenges for the subsequent analytical method used. In particular, the presence of proteins and peptides, which may not be compounds of interest, present major challenges, as the analytical methods need to be highly specific, highly sensitive, and often specifically adapted by including sophisticated sample preparation.

Dermal OFM probes are certified for clinical use for up to 48 hours [51], which allows long continuous assessment of dermal PK. Dermal OFM sampling has been successfully performed in a clinical study for 36 hours [49]. Although the ISF sample collection with dermal OFM relies on the same sampling principles as MD, highly standardized procedures enable collection of high-quality data capable of BE assessment. Dermal OFM allows performance of GCP-certified clinical studies, as demonstrated within an FDA grant promoting the development of new approaches for topical generic drug approval.

The same dermal OFM set-up can be applied ex vivo and in vivo in preclinical and clinical studies, which further supports the reliability of results. Thus dermal OFM provides a strong platform to foster translational projects [52, 53].

57.3.1 DERMAL OFM DESIGN

Skin anatomy and physiology pose certain challenges for dermal sampling applications and need to be taken into account when optimizing sampling-related procedures. Skin is a large but very thin organ (about 1.5 mm thick) and also highly flexible and tough, which challenges probe insertion.

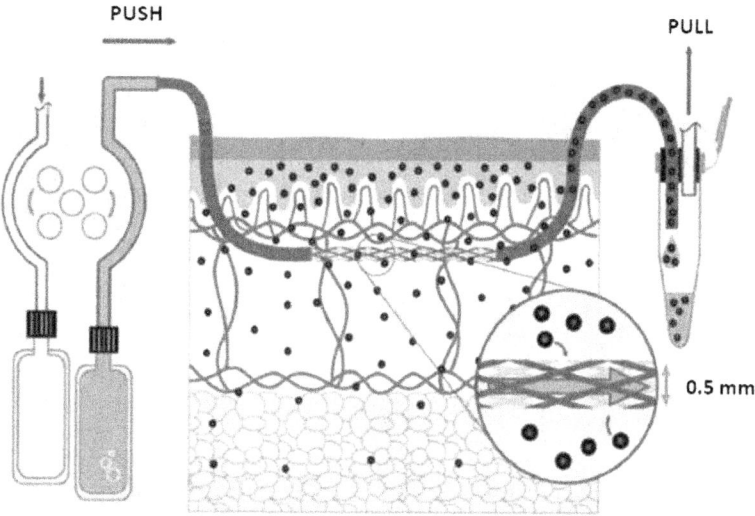

FIGURE 57.2   Dermal OFM setup. After dermal OFM probe insertion, the inlet tube of the probe is connected to a pump for continuous perfusion with sterile perfusate (push) and the outlet tube to a sampling vial that is evacuated by the pump to control the sampling rate from the probe (pull). The open exchange area of the dermal OFM probe (insert) allows free exchange of compounds between the perfusate and the surrounding ISF.

The dermal OFM setup consists of a probe with an open exchange area implanted into the dermis and a push/pull pump for continuous perfusion of the dermal OFM probe with sterile perfusate [54]. The open exchange area is designed to provide sufficient mechanical support. This push-pull pump setup enables volume-controlled ISF sampling from the dermis for subsequent analysis (Figure 57.2).

The dermal OFM probe comprises a braided steel mesh with an exchange area of cylindrical structure (diameter: about 100 µm) with macroscopic openings (size: about 0.2 mm). Adsorption of compounds is minimized by the Teflon coating of the probe's inner lumen except for the exchange area and by ensuring short sampling distance through a direct connection of the probe with a sample vial.

The linear, CE-certified dermal OFM probe is highly flexible and the demarcated exchange area is 15 mm long. Imprinted position markers facilitate accurate positioning of the permeable section of the probe exactly underneath the treated skin. The probe's outer diameter is 0.5 mm, and it is inserted over a length of 30 mm with a hollow insertion needle (outer diameter: 0.9 mm). During sampling, the perfusate is actively pushed into the probe lumen and pulled into a sampling vial using a small, wearable multichannel, push-pull peristaltic pump. The pump can operate several sampling probes and allow the study participants to move freely. The pump provides variable perfusion modes (including push, pull, or both). The generated flow rates range from 0.1 µL/min to 10 µL/min and are independently adjustable for push and pull. Performance of several quantification protocols, such as zero flow, no net flux, OFM recirculation, and OFM suction is feasible [20, 44, 46, 50, 55, 56].

The treatment sites where the dermal OFM probes are implanted are stabilized by self-adhesive plastic rings (diameter: about 60 mm), which prevents the skin from being stretched and fixates the probes in the skin during sampling (Figure 57.3). Precise insertion of dermal OFM probes and application of topical drugs are ensured by predefined insertion patterns and application templates.

The volume-controlled ISF sampling prevents loss of perfusate into the tissue and ensures stable recovery of the compound of interest in the collected samples. Stable sampling performance in a clinical trial over 36 hours has been verified based on glucose concentrations of 240 dermal OFM probes in 20 participants. Linear regression analysis revealed a change of the glucose concentration from a mean of only 0.01% per hour (Bodenlenz, unpublished data). All dermal OFM procedures are highly standardized (GCP, GLP) and allow performance of drug approval studies. Prolonged sampling periods of 36 hours in a clinical setting were well tolerated by the study participants [49].

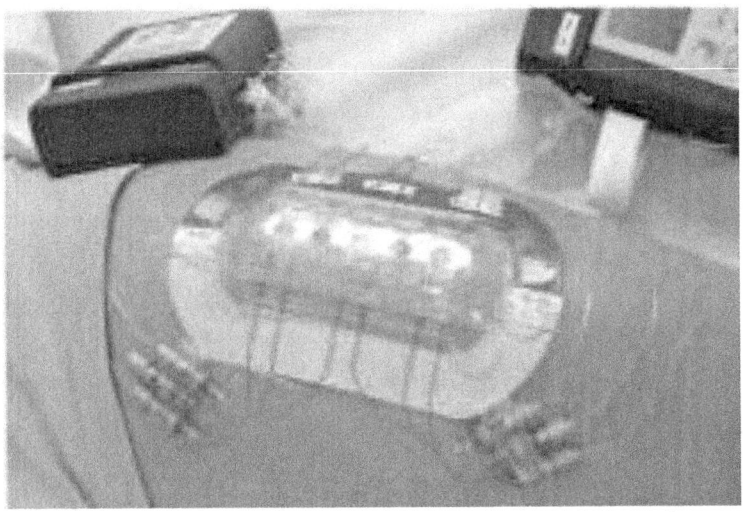

FIGURE 57.3 Picture of three dermal OFM treatment sites (two dermal OFM probes per treatment site) stabilized by a self-adhesive plastic ring. Dermal ISF is sampled continuously using wearable OFM pumps, a push-pull tubing set, and a sampling unit with sampling vials.

Source: Reference [49].

57.3.2 QUANTIFICATION AND ANALYTICAL ASPECTS

The transport of compounds from the surrounding ISF into the dermal OFM probe is unrestricted and occurs nonselectively, but equilibration of compound concentrations between the ISF and perfusate is not achieved with the commonly applied flow rates of above 0.5 µl/min. Therefore, the collected dermal OFM samples contain lower concentrations of compounds than those present in the ISF. Consequently, knowledge of the degree of dilution, i.e., of the relative recovery is required to quantify compounds in the ISF. The degree of dilution of the sampled ISF depends primarily on the perfusion flow rate, the length of the exchange area, and the physicochemical properties of the compound of interest (e.g., lipophilicity, molecular weight, aqueous solubility).

Dermal OFM sampling and subsequent analysis of the samples can be used for either relative or absolute quantification of analytes in tissue. Relative quantification of analytes is most commonly used. When performing relative quantification the change in analyte concentration in the tissue is determined while a constant recovery rate is maintained. For absolute quantification of an analyte in the tissue special methods have to be applied which are described in the following sections.

57.3.2.1 Determination of Absolute Tissue Concentration from Diluted ISF Samples

Quantification of compounds from diluted ISF samples requires application of calibration methods in combination with OFM, such as zero flow rate, no net flux, and ionic reference.

Zero flow rate is based on the assumption that the recovery of an analyte correlates with the perfusion flow rate. The relative recovery is measured for different flow rates, and the equilibrium analyte concentration is assessed by extrapolation to a flow rate of zero, where the recovery should be 100% [57]. Zero flow rate has been successfully used with dermal OFM by Schaupp et al. to quantify potassium, sodium, and glucose in adipose ISF samples [44].

No net flux allows reference-independent analyte quantification in the ISF [46, 58]. To quantify analytes with no net flux, the OFM probe is perfused with perfusates to which different concentrations of the analyte of interest have been added, e.g., two perfusates with concentrations higher and two with concentrations lower than the expected analyte concentration in the ISF. A net flux of substances occurs according to the concentration gradient. Thus, the perfusates with analyte concentrations higher than that in the ISF become diluted, and perfusates with analyte concentrations below that in the ISF become more concentrated. Quantification is done via determination of that concentration, where no net flux occurs. To do so, linear regression analysis of the influent perfusate concentration versus the associated net loss or net gain, as determined from the concentrations in the effluent samples, is performed. The concentration at the x-intercept of the linear regression line represents the mean dermal ISF concentration of the analyte over the sampling period.

No net flux has been successfully applied to quantify several analytes in OFM studies in adipose, muscle, and dermal ISF: The absolute lactate concentrations [60] and the absolute glucose concentrations in adipose ISF [44], the absolute albumin concentration in muscle ISF [45], and the absolute insulin concentration in adipose and muscle ISF have been successfully determined [46]. Dragatin et al. used no net flux in combination with dermal OFM to assess the absolute dermal ISF concentration of a fully human therapeutic antibody [50].

Ionic reference is based on the assumption that ion concentrations in the ISF are constant, known, and very close to those in plasma [44, 55, 61]. Thus, the ionic recovery can be determined as the ratio of ion concentrations in the sample to those of ISF or plasma. Assuming the recovery of ions and analytes to be the same, and performing simultaneous measurements of analyte and ions in the sample, the analyte concentration in the ISF can be assessed as the ratio of analyte concentration in the sample to ionic recovery.

Ionic reference has been used in combination with OFM to assess the absolute glucose concentration [44] and the absolute lactate concentration in adipose ISF [60] using sodium as the ionic reference. Dermal OFM in combination with ionic reference has also been used to quantify the concentrations of human insulin and an insulin analogue in the ISF with inulin as exogenous marker (Bodenlenz, unpublished data).

57.3.2.2 Determination of Absolute Tissue Concentration from Undiluted ISF Samples

Dermal OFM has been further advanced to deliver pure ISF samples that contain unfiltered and undiluted ISF and thus provide direct access to the analyte concentration in the ISF without applying additional calibration techniques. These advancements include OFM-recirculation and OFM-suction [20].

OFM-recirculation is based on the OFM-recirculation method developed by Schaupp et al. [56], where the perfusate has been recirculated in a closed loop. Schaupp et al. quantified ISF analytes from recirculation samples, which had not yet reached complete equilibrium concentrations, by monitoring the analyte concentrations with a sensor and calculating the absolute analyte concentration in the ISF.

OFM-recirculation to collect undiluted ISF samples recirculates the perfusate in a closed loop until equilibrium concentrations are established between the perfusate and ISF. For albumin as an analyte, 20 recirculation cycles were sufficient to reach equilibrium ISF concentrations [20].

OFM-suction is performed by applying a mild vacuum, which pulls ISF from the tissue into the OFM probe. The obtained samples from OFM-recirculation and OFM-suction contain unfiltered and undiluted ISF and enable direct quantification of analytes [20].

57.3.2.3 Analytical Aspects

All compounds present in the dermal ISF are able to enter the OFM probe through the open exchange area, which on the one hand widens the application range of the method, but on the other hands adds challenges to the chemical analysis of the dermal OFM samples. The complex matrix, mainly the presence of proteins, requires special and sophisticated sample preparation processes to be included into the subsequent analytical method, as proteins must be removed without losing the analyte of interest. Further, possible enzymatic degradation of the compound of interest by certain matrix components may bias the results and needs to be taken into account. Small sample volumes and diluted analytes occurring in small quantities in the ISF also have to be dealt with.

57.4   APPLICATIONS OF DERMAL OFM SAMPLING

Dermal OFM allows continuous assessment of several target compounds in dermal ISF [43] for time-resolved quantification of lipophilic [47, 48] and hydrophilic compounds [49], and compounds with low skin permeation capacity [49]. Further, high-molecular-weight compounds, e.g., antibodies [50], molecule clusters, nanoparticles, and entire immune-competent cells can be investigated. A unique feature of the samples collected by dermal OFM is that they contain the same amount of protein-unbound drug as the dermal ISF, unbiased by equilibrium shifts which may occur when one drug fraction is continuously removed from the ISF during sampling. Wearable push-pull pumps and highly standardized procedures (GLP, GCP) allow dermal OFM sampling of up to 48 hours [51], and the resulting data are highly reproducible over 36 hours of sampling [49].

Applications of dermal OFM sampling involve PK/pharmacodynamics (PD) assessment in ex vivo studies with animal skin and human skin explants [62], in preclinical studies, and in clinical studies with healthy participants and patients [49]. The same OFM set-up can be used in these different study designs to assess percutaneous penetration of a topical drug. High data reliability is ensured following this translational research approach.

Dermal OFM has shown its value in vivo in clinical studies through the assessment of the PK/PD profiles of lipophilic compounds [47, 48] and compounds of high molecular weight e.g., antibodies [50], up to entire cells in humans, following highly standardized procedures. Additionally, dermal OFM has shown its value in sampling hydrophilic, slowly permeating compounds [49] and has proven its utility to evaluate topical BE via comparative bioavailability assessment [49].

In the following paragraphs, selected applications for dermal OFM sampling with subsequent analytical analysis of the ISF samples are presented, which deliver time-resolved data that are indispensable for basic research on drug actions in the skin, topical drug development processes, or topical bioavailability/BE studies for development of generic topical drugs.

57.4.1 Ex Vivo Dermal OFM Sampling: Use Case

The benchmark to assess dermal PK data of topical drug products is to perform in vivo permeation studies in human skin. However, dermal drug development processes include several models such as in vitro models, ex vivo models (human or animal skin explants), and animal models (preclinical studies) to assess the PK of the active pharmacological ingredient of the respective topical drug product in the skin. These models require considerations regarding the different metabolic capacity of e.g. in vivo skin compared to explanted skin that is influenced by skin explant pretreatment, the missing clearance in skin explants, or species-related differences of the skin (animal versus human skin) that may add bias to the results.

In an ex vivo study with fresh human skin explants, dermal OFM was used to assess the concentrations of two topical phosphodiesterase (PDE) 4-inhibitors [63]. One is metabolized by skin esterase, while the other spontaneously degrades in dermal ISF. The results were used to investigate the clinical efficacy of these two inhibitors. Both have similar in vitro potencies and have reached similar skin exposures in clinical studies and revealed the same high skin concentrations assessed by punch biopsies. However, dermal cAMP levels that serve as a biomarker for the inhibition of dermal PDE4 activity were increased only for one of the two inhibitors. This finding indicated that high skin concentrations found in the biopsies may not reflect the actual concentrations at the drug target site in the skin. These differences may be due to sample contamination by the inhibitors from the stratum corneum depot of the skin or due to the existing different metabolic activities of punch biopsy samples and skin explants.

Dermal OFM studies were applied to explain the differences in target engagement of the two inhibitors. First, a dermal OFM study was performed to investigate the predictive capacity of fresh and frozen ex vivo pig skin with regard to in vivo pig skin (unpublished data). Dermal OFM was applied in vivo and ex vivo in fresh and in thawed skin explants from the same pig to assess the dermal concentrations of the two PDE4 inhibitors. Dermal OFM was able to assess esterase activity in vivo and ex vivo in fresh pig skin and thus confirmed that fresh pig skin explants retain esterase activity and skin metabolism. These findings led to the conclusion that OFM results derived from fresh ex vivo pig skin can be predictive of human skin.

Results from a subsequent ex vivo dermal OFM study with fresh human skin explants explained the differences in target engagement of the two inhibitors by differences in drug exposure in the ISF [64].

These results illustrate that the application of dermal OFM on fresh human skin explants has the potential to generate data that serve as an integrated model for preclinical assessment of topical drug candidates.

57.4.2   IN VIVO CLINICAL DERMAL OFM STUDY: PK/PD

57.4.2.1   Biomarker: PK/PD Profile Assessment

Dermal OFM has demonstrated its feasibility to assess PK/PD profiles of a lipophilic topical drug and a high-molecular-weight compound in a clinical trial [48]. The target drug was BCT194 (logP = 3.1), which acts by inhibiting the p38 pathway and thus the intradermal release of pro-inflammatory cytokines. The clinical dermal OFM study with psoriasis patients monitored the PK/PD profiles of the lipophilic topical drug and the inflammatory biomarker and high-molecular-weight compound TNF-alpha (molecular weight: 51 kDa as a trimer) in vivo in the skin of psoriasis patients.

Another clinical dermal OFM application with psoriatic patients successfully assessed intradermal PK/PD profiles of the highly lipophilic corticoid clobetasol-17-propionate (CP-17) (logP = 3.49) [47]. CP-17 is a topical drug widely used for the treatment of psoriasis, which activates glucocorticoid receptors and triggers antiinflammatory and immunosuppressive activities. PK and PD data of the drug and vehicle were comparatively assessed in lesional and non lesional skin. Further, time-resolved and probe-depth-dependent kinetic data were collected, which revealed slower penetration kinetics of CP-17 into lesional than into non lesional skin and showed that skin penetration into lesional skin normalized after repeated dosing. Results also showed that CP-17 does not significantly accumulate in the dermis independently of the skin condition.

The reduced penetration rate into hyperkeratosed psoriatic skin supported the assumption that the thickened psoriatic stratum corneum functions as a trap compartment for lipophilic topical drugs. The results of this clinical dermal OFM study further highlight the accuracy, sensitivity, and reproducibility of in vivo dermal OFM to assess dermal PK/PD profiles of lipophilic topical drugs and inflammatory biomarkers.

57.4.2.2   Antibody Assessment

Dermal OFM sampling was used in a clinical study with healthy participants and psoriatic patients to perform absolute quantification of a fully human monoclonal antibody. The concentration profile of the therapeutic antibody secukinumab was determined to assess the ability of a single subcutaneous dose to neutralize IL-17A in the skin [50]. The absolute tissue concentration of secukinumab was determined using dermal OFM in combination with no net flux in the skin of healthy human participants. No net flux was performed with an external reference substance, and the results were validated with results from suction blisters and punch biopsies. Secukinumab levels in the dermal ISF of psoriatic patients were quantitatively assessed one week after drug injection, and the resulting secukinumab levels were sufficiently high to completely neutralize IL-17A in the lesional skin of psoriatic patients.

57.4.2.3   Proteomics

The ISF samples collected during this antibody study [50] underwent proteomic and gene transcription analyses. A total of 170 proteins were further analyzed, including cytokines, chemokines, growth factors, cell adhesion molecules, and soluble receptors [65]. Early proteomic changes that occur in the dermis after secukinumab treatment were complemented with gene expression changes extracted from skin biopsy. Beta-defensin-2 was identified as a biomarker of IL-17A–driven pathology in patients with psoriasis.

57.4.3   IN VIVO CLINICAL DERMAL OFM STUDY: BIOEQUIVALENCE ASSESSMENT

The utility of clinical dermal OFM as a dermal PK approach to assess BE was recently performed as part of an FDA-granted collaborative research effort to evaluate PK-based methods for topical BE assessment [49]. Acyclovir, a hydrophilic, poorly permeating topical drug, was used to assess the rate and extent of percutaneous penetration by continuous sampling with dermal OFM and

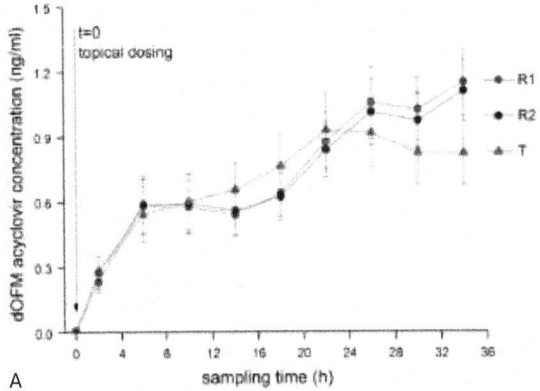
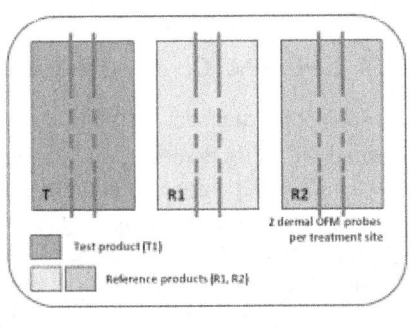

A   sampling time (h)   B

FIGURE 57.4 Dermal OFM acyclovir concentration profiles and scheme of three dermal OFM treatment sites. (a) Dermal OFM acyclovir concentration profiles. T: Acyclovir 1A Pharma cream (5% 1A Pharma Austria), R1, R2: Zovirax cream, 5% (GlaxoSmithKline US) (mean ± standard error, 20 participants). Acyclovir was analyzed from one pre-dose sample. Post-dose samples were taken every 4 hours for 36 hours. The post-dose concentrations were plotted in the mid-point of each time interval. The figure was taken from [49]. (b) Scheme of three dermal OFM treatment sites. Two replicate dermal OFM probes were inserted in each of the three treatment sites. On each thigh T was applied once and R twice. R was compared with itself as a positive control, and T was compared with R as a negative control.

subsequent analysis of the collected ISF samples. In each healthy participant, dermal PK profiles were monitored simultaneously on six treatment sites for 36 hours (Figure 57.4, left side). Products were applied in three dermal OFM treatment sites on each thigh (Figure 57.4, right side).

Dermal OFM showed the necessary accuracy and reproducibility to confirm BE for topically applied acyclovir, and it was sufficiently sensitive to discriminate between two different non-Q1-topical acyclovir cream products, based on conventional PK endpoints [49]. Results from this clinical study show that dermal OFM can support BE evaluations for topical acyclovir creams.

57.4.3.1 Data Variability

BE assessment based on dermal OFM [49] was only possible due to highly standardized dermal OFM sampling procedures that ensure low data variability. However, to further minimize this variability, an explorative statistical analysis of the extensive data set from the dermal OFM BE study was performed to assess and characterize the sources of dermal PK data variability [69]. The data set included data on the dermal PK and on biological-methodological factors (e.g., skin characteristics, OFM probe depths), and it thus enabled investigation of dermal PK data variability after topical drug application. The study also assessed data variability due to different skin characteristics and OFM method-related parameters on topical BE evaluation. Results from statistical analysis of bioavailability data assessed by dermal OFM identified inter-subject variability as a source of variability, but due to the head-to-head design of the experiment, inter-subject variability did not influence BE OFM results.

Investigation of the intra-subject variability and its sources showed that site and site-related methodological factors did not significantly contribute to BE variability. This indicates that a significant ratio of the intra-subject variability is caused by local biological skin factors, e.g., hair follicles, when applying a hydrophilic drug with low permeation capacity such as acyclovir.

57.4.3.2 Impedance Measurements

The combination of results from a drug penetration study using CP-17 in human skin explants with results from skin impedance measurements showed that the measured passive electrical properties of the skin (i.e., low-frequency skin impedance and skin admittance) linearly correlated with the drug concentration–time profiles derived from dermal OFM sampling [62]. Applying this known correlation of skin permeability and skin impedance data and preselect donors based on impedance data of the skin may offer the possibility to select donors with homogeneous permeation skin characteristics. Working with study populations that have homogeneous skin penetration characteristics can greatly improve the statistical outcome of any dermal study.

57.4.3.3 Reference-Scaled Average BE Statistical Approach

Because skin is highly variable, a fairly high number of study participants is still required when performing dermal PK measurements for BE evaluation of topical drug products [66, 67]. Such high participant numbers can be reduced by applying the reference-scaled average BE (SABE) statistical approach instead of the commonly applied average BE (ABE) statistical approach on dermal PK data. SABE scales the BE acceptance limits to the intra-subject variabilities of the reference product [68], and its use is recommended for reference products with an intra-subject standard deviation of more than 0.294.

Results from the clinical dermal OFM study on acyclovir [49] indicated that the variabilities of the dermal PK data for acyclovir can meet these criteria and that application of SABE may be appropriate. We further compared results from SABE and ABE and a power calculation revealed that SABE achieved a statistical power of at least 80% with a sample reduction of about 40% in the clinical study (unpublished data).

We additionally performed an ex vivo study using an identical study design as in [49], and assessed the PK profiles of the same acyclovir products as in the clinical study. This allows for the first time a direct comparison of dermal PK data obtained from a clinical study and an ex vivo study. BE evaluations applying SABE yielded similar results in the ex vivo and in the clinical study (unpublished data). Ex vivo data can thus provide preliminary PK parameters for subsequent clinical studies, and they might serve as test systems for clinical BE studies to compare the penetration behavior of topical drug products. Thus, results indicated that dermal OFM studies in combination with SABE are highly promising tools for BE evaluations of topical drug products.

57.5   OUTLOOK

57.5.1   Basic Research

For future basic research, dermal OFM studies can be used as valuable tools to investigate the skin microenvironment, allow assessment of skin pathology, and promote a mechanistic understanding of dermal drug action in various skin diseases.

57.5.1.1   Immune Cells

The active immune system of patients with commonly occurring chronic inflammatory skin diseases such as psoriasis or atopic dermatitis can be investigated by sampling immune competent cells from lesional skin and from healthy unaffected skin close to the lesions of psoriasis patients. Preliminary results from dermal OFM sampling experiments revealed that the immune cell populations between the different skin regions are notably different. This finding can foster further research efforts and might open doors to pursue novel, innovative approaches in drug target investigations.

57.5.1.2   Biomarker in Skin Cancer

Dermal OFM sampling can also be promising for biomarker research in skin cancer by monitoring interactions between cancer microenvironment in the skin and circulating cancer cells, microvesicles, and other compounds in the blood.

57.5.1.3   Protein Binding

The effect of a drug on numerous aspects of clinical PK/PD in the skin is, among other factors, influenced by the ratio between bound and unbound drug fraction at the site of action, which determines the degree to which a drug is distributed in body tissue rather than plasma (volume of distribution). It is generally believed that only the unbound fraction of a drug is available for interactions with the relevant receptors. Thus, accurate determination of unbound drug concentrations at the site of action is essential during therapeutic drug monitoring [70]. However, since the drug concentration is difficult to assess in the skin, the degree of protein binding of a drug is commonly determined in blood, and the resulting unbound drug concentration from blood is used as a surrogate parameter to estimate the unbound drug concentration at the site of action. Such unbound drug concentrations derived from blood are often biased due to different association strengths of the drug with plasma or tissue proteins, and consequently, the resulting volumes of drug distribution differ. Drugs strongly bound to plasma proteins (e.g., penicillin) are restricted to blood, whereas drugs with weak association to plasma proteins that are therefore present in an unbound state in plasma can also be distributed beyond the vascular system. Further, tissue-binding properties of a drug also affect its volume of distribution. Some drugs although highly bound to plasma proteins (e.g., tricyclic antidepressants) have an even greater affinity to tissue proteins and thus also show a large volume of distribution.

With dermal OFM sampling, the amount of the unbound topical drug fraction can be assessed directly in skin ISF. Results from dermal OFM studies showed that the unbound protein concentration in skin ISF significantly differs from that in blood, which highly influences the therapeutic effect of the respective drug at its site of action (unpublished data).

57.5.2 DEVELOPMENT OF NEW TOPICAL FORMULATIONS

Dermal OFM sampling in combination with other techniques such as skin biopsies or in vitro release testing covers a large part of the topical drug development process and guides the development of topical drugs from early drug formulation development to clinical studies. Development of a new topical formulation involves preclinical drug development and clinical studies.

A major aspect of drug development is compliance with regulations of drug licensing authorities, such as EMA or FDA. New Drug Applications (NDA) and Abbreviated New Drug Applications (ANDA) [32] are the FDA's regulatory pathways for drug approval, where NDA regulates the approval of new drugs and ANDA the approval of generic drug products.

NDA regulations describe a number of in vitro and ex vivo tests to determine the major toxicities of a novel compound prior to first use in human and preclinical animal studies to demonstrate the complex interplay of metabolism and drug exposure. Dermal OFM is a promising tool in several of these required stages of the topical drug approval process.

Besides NDA and ANDA, there is an additional pathway, called 505(b)(2) [71], which can accelerate the approval of a new drug. Following this pathway, a connection between the 505(b)(2)-eligible product, or its active ingredients, and a reference product needs to be established. This can be done, for example, with the use of results from bioanalytical testing, preclinical studies, or even clinical trial results. A dermal OFM clinical study offers an elegant way to bridge the developed drug to the reference product based on dermal PK profiles.

In early drug development, dermal OFM can be used to assess the properties of an active pharmaceutical ingredient (API) in a realistic matrix by sampling pure dermal ISF from skin in vivo. This can be performed, e.g., by sampling pure, undiluted ISF with OFM-recirculation from the skin of anesthetized pigs [20]. Results from stability and degradation assessments of the API are of great value for API design optimization and toxicity assessment.

An ex vivo dermal OFM study can be performed to investigate the stability and metabolism of the API in skin and to predict clinical efficacy. The drug effect of a new chemical entity to be tested may be predicted by assessing skin penetration and dermal metabolism of the API. Such dermal ex vivo OFM studies determine the transport across the skin barrier in a highly sensitive manner due to the absence of blood circulation in the skin explants that would drain compounds from the skin.

Further, dermal OFM proves its value when performing a preclinical proof-of-concept studies which elucidate the mode of action of an API in vivo. Dermal OFM has already been used to investigate the in vivo effect of an in a psoriatic inflammation rat model. The study assessed the dermal PK properties for dose response, the dermal PD effect on cytokine level, and the dermal PD properties at the immune cell level [59].

Also in the clinical study as the last and most relevant step of the topical drug development process, dermal OFM can be used in the same setup as in the previous steps, thus providing a set of consistent data from early ex vivo studies to clinical endpoint studies in healthy volunteers as well as patients with skin diseases. In a clinical setting, dermal OFM also allows assessment of in vivo PK and PD profiles. This highly translational research approach of dermal OFM promotes translation of basic research outcome into positive impacts on human health [72].

57.5.3 GENERIC DRUG PRODUCTS

Generic drug products are very attractive alternatives for consumers because they are equivalent to the brand-name drug products in terms of quality, safety, and efficacy, but are generally available at considerably reduced costs. However, the number of topical generic drug products available on the market is limited, especially in the United States.

One major reason for this restricted market availability of topical generic drug products is that only a limited number of established approaches exist by which the manufacturer can prove that the topical generic drug is comparable in dosage form, strength, route of administration, quality, performance characteristics, and intended use to the reference-listed drug [32]. This comparability must be proved by chemical analysis and BE evaluations.

Apart from the vasoconstrictor assay [73] and certain product-specific guidelines for several topical drugs [74–77], clinical endpoints studies are commonly used to evaluate BE of topically applied and locally acting drugs, although they are among the least sensitive and time and money requiring methods to demonstrate BE [12, 13, 78]. Dermal OFM offers a promising PK-based approach for BE evaluation of locally acting, topical dermatological drug products by comparatively assessing their bioavailability in the dermis [43, 79]. With dermal OFM, the skin bioavailability of the generic drug product and its reference-listed drug can be monitored in one subject from several treatment sites simultaneously and recently, BE has been successfully evaluated by comparative assessment of the PK profiles of acyclovir creams in a clinical study using dermal OFM [49].

REFERENCES

1. Nair A, Jacob S, Al-dhubiab B, Attimarad M, Harsha S. Basic considerations in the dermatokinetics of topical formulations. 2013;49:423–34.
2. Wiig H, Swartz MA. Interstitial fluid and lymph formation and transport: physiological regulation and roles in inflammation and cancer. 2018;8(1):1–8.
3. Wiig H, Tenstad O, Iversen P, Kalluri R, Bjerkvig R. Interstitial fluid: the overlooked component of the tumor microenvironment? Fibrogenesis Tissue Repair. 2010;3(1):12.
4. Skobe M, Detmar M. Structure, function, and molecular control of the skin lymphatic system. J Investig Dermatol Symp Proc. 2000;5(1):14–9.
5. Benias PC, Wells RG, Sackey-Aboagye B, Klavan H, Reidy J, Buonocore D, et al. Structure and Distribution of an Unrecognized Interstitium in Human Tissues. Sci Rep. 2018;8(1):1–8.
6. Fogh-Andersen N, Altura BM, Siggaard-Andersen O. Composition of interstitial fluid. Clin Chem. 1995;41(10):1522–5.
7. Vermeer BJ, Reman FC, Van Gent CM. The determination of lipids and proteins in suction blister fluid. J Invest Dermatol. 1979;73:303–305.
8. Guyton A, JE H. Textbook of medical physiology. Philadelphia: Elsevier Saunders; 2006.
9. Schmook F, Nefzger M, Laber G, Georgopoulos A, Czok R, Schütze E. Composition of fluids from diffusion chambers implanted in the soft tissue and kidneys of rabbits. Infection. 1980;8(4):156–61.
10. Kayashima K, Arai S, Kikuchi T, Nagata M, Ito N, Kuriyama N, et al. Sution effusion fluid from skin and constituent analysis: new candidate for interstitial fluid. Am J Physiol. 1992;263:1623–7.

11. Shah VP. Bioequivalence of topical dermatological dosage forms—methods of evaluation of bioequivalence. Pharm Res. 1998;15:167–171.

12. Raney SG, Franz TJ, Lehman PA, Lionberger R. Pharmacokinetics-Based Approaches for Bioequivalence Evaluation of Topical Dermatological Drug Products. Clin Pharmacokinet. 2015;54(11):1095–106.

13. Miranda M, Sousa J, Veiga F, Cardoso C, Vitorino C. Bioequivalence of topical generic products. Part 1: Where are we now? Eur J Pharm Sci. 2018;123:260–7.

14. Hooijmans CR. Progress in Using Systematic Reviews of Animal Studies to Improve Translational Research. 2013;10(7):1–4.

15. Franz PA, Lehman SG, Raney TJ. Percutaneous Absorption in Man : In vitro-in vivo Correlation. 2011;97086:224–30.

16. Aukland K, Fadnes HO. Protein concentration and colloid osmotic pressure of interstitial fluid collected by the wick technique: analysis and evaluation of the method. Microvasc Res. 1977;14(1):11–25.

17. Heltne JK, Husby P, Koller ME and Lund T. Sampling of interstitial fluid and measurement of colloid osmotic pressure (COPi) in pigs: evaluation of the wick method Lab. Anim. 1998;32 439–45.

18. Guyton A. A concept of negative interstitial pressure based on pressures in implanted perforated capsules. Circ Res. 1963;12:399–414.

19. Elston DM, Stratman EJ, Miller SJ, Carolina S. Skin biopsy issues in specific diseases. J Am Dermatology. 2019;74(1):1–16.

20. Hummer, J., Schwingenschuh, S., Raml, R., Boulgaropoulos, B., Schwagerle, G., Augustin, T., Sinner, F., & Birngruber, T. OFM recirculation and OFM suction: Advanced in-vivo open flow microperfusion methods for direct and absolute quantification of albumin in interstitial fluid. Biomedical Physics & Engineering Express. 2020. https://doi.org/10.1088/2057-1976/abc3a7

21. Kiistala U. Suction blister device for separation of viable epidermis from dermis. J Invest Dermatol. 1968;50(2):129–37.

22. Volden G. Thorsrud, A. K., Bjornson, I., & Jellum, E. Biochemical composition of suction blister fluid determined by high resolution multicomponent analysis (Capillary Gas Chromatography - Mass Spectrometry and Two-Dimensional Electrophoresis). The Journal of Investigative Dermatology. 1980;75:421–424.

23. Makki S, Treffe P, Humbert P, Agache P. High-performance liquid chromatographic determination of citropten and bergapten in suction blister fluid after solar product application in humans. J Chromatogr B Biomed Sci Appl. 1991;563(2):407–13.

24. Surber C, Wilhelm KP, Bermann D MH. In vivo skin penetration of acitretin in volunteers using three sampling techniques. Pharm Res. 1993 Sep;10(9):1291–4.

25. Staberg B, Groth S, Rossing N. Passage of albumin from plasma to suction skin blisters. Clin Physiol. 1983;3(4):375–80.

26. Hommel E, Mathiesen ER, Aukland K, Parving HH. Pathophysiological aspects of edema formation in diabetic nephropathy. Kidney Int. 1990;38(6):1187–92.

27. Herkenne C, Alberti I, Naik A, Kalia YN, Guy RH. Expert review in vivo methods for the assessment of topical drug bioavailability. Pharmaceutical Research. 2008;25(1):87–103. https://doi.org/10.1007/s11095-007-9429-7

28. Denda M, Wood L, Emami S, Calhoun C, Brown B, Elias P, et al. The epidermal hyperplasia associated with repeated barrier disruption by acetone treatment or tape stripping cannot be attributed to increased water loss. Arch Dermatol Res. 1996;288(5–6):230–238.

29. Rougier A, Dupuis D, Lotte C, Roguet R, Schaefer H. In vivo correlation between stratum corneum reservoir function and percutaneous absorption. J Invest Dermatol. 1983;81(3):275–8.

30. Dupuis D, Rougier A, Lotte C RR. An original predictive method for in vivo percutaneous absorption studies. Acta Derm Venereol Suppl. 1987;134:9–21.

31. European Medicines Agency. Draft guideline on quality and equivalence of topical products Draft Guideline on quality and equivalence of topical products. 2018 p. 1–36.

32. U.S. FDA. United States Food and Drug Administration Draft Guidance for Industry: Topical Dermatological Drug Product NDAs and ANDAs - In Vivo Bioavailability, Bioequivalence, In Vitro Release, and Associated Studies. 1998.

33. U.S. FDA. Draft Guidance for Industry on Topical Dermatological Drug Product NDAs and ANDAs-In Vivo Bioavailability, Bioequivalence, In Vitro Release and Associated Studies; Withdrawal. 2002; Federal Reg: 35122–3.

34. Pershing LK, Nelson JL, Corlett JL, Shrivastava SP, Hare DB, Shah VP. Assessment of dermatopharmacokinetic approach in the bioequivalence determination of topical tretinoin gel products. J Am Acad Dermatol. 2003;740–51. https://doi.org/10.1067/mjd.2003.175

35. Franz TJ. Study #1, Avita gel 0.025% vs Retin-A gel 0.025%. Transcribed presentation. In: Advisory Committee for Pharmaceutical Sciences Meeting, Center for Drug Evaluation and Research (CDER), Food and Drug Administration (FDA). 2001.

36. Schnetz E. Microdialysis for the evaluation of penetration through the human skin barrier — a promising tool for future research? European Journal of Pharmaceutical Science. 2001;12:165–74.

37. Kreilgaard M. Assessment of cutaneous drug delivery using microdialysis. Adv Drug Deliv Rev. 2002;54:99–121.

38. Stahle L. On mathematical models of microdialysis: geometry, steady-state models, recovery and probe radius. Advanced Drug Delivery Reviews. 2000;45:149–67.

39. Shippenberg, T. S., & Thompson, A. C. (2001). Overview of microdialysis. Current Protocols in Neuroscience. 7, 1–27. https://doi.org/10.1002/0471142301.ns0701s00

40. Sjögren F, Svensson C, Anderson C. Technical prerequisites for in vivo microdialysis determination of interleukin-6 in human dermis. Br J Dermatol. 2002;146(3):375–82.

41. Clough GF. Microdialysis of large molecules. AAPS J. 2005;7(3):E686–92.

42. Rosenbloom AJ, Sipe DM, Weedn VW. Microdialysis of proteins: performance of the CMA/20 probe. J Neurosci Methods. 2005;148(2):147–53.

43. Bodenlenz M, Aigner B, Dragatin C, Liebenberger L, Zahiragic S, Höfferer C, et al. Clinical applicability of dOFM devices for dermal sampling. Ski Res Technol Technol. 2013;19(4):474–83.

44. Schaupp L, Ellmerer M, Brunner GA, Wutte A, Sendlhofer G, Trajanoski Z, et al. Direct access to interstitial fluid in adipose tissue in humans by use of open-flow microperfusion. Am J Physiol. 1999;276(2):401–8.

45. Ellmerer M, Schaupp L, Brunner GA, Sendlhofer G, Wutte A, Wach P, et al. Measurement of interstitial albumin in human skeletal muscle and adipose tissue by open-flow microperfusion. Am J Physiol - Endocrinol Metab. 2000;278(2):352–6.

46. Bodenlenz M, Schaupp LA, Druml T, Sommer R, Wutte A, Schaller HC, et al. Measurement of interstitial insulin in human adipose and muscle tissue under moderate hyperinsulinemia by means of direct interstitial access. Am J Physiol Endocrinol Metab. 2005;289(2):E296–300.

47. Bodenlenz M, Dragatin C, Liebenberger L, Tschapeller B, Boulgaropoulos B, Augustin T, et al. Kinetics of clobetasol-17-propionate in psoriatic lesional and non-lesional skin assessed by dermal open flow microperfusion with time and space resolution. Pharm Res. 2016;33(9):2229–38.

48. Bodenlenz M, Höfferer C, Magnes C, Schaller-Ammann R, Schaupp L, Feichtner F, et al. Dermal PK/PD of a lipophilic topical drug in psoriatic patients by continuous intradermal membrane-free sampling. Eur J Pharm Biopharm. 2012;81(3):635–41.

49. Bodenlenz M, Tiffner KI, Raml R, Augustin T, Dragatin C, Birngruber T, et al. Open flow microperfusion as a dermal pharmacokinetic approach to evaluate topical bioequivalence. Clin Pharmacokinet. 2017;56(1):91–8.

50. Dragatin C, Polus F, Bodenlenz M, Calonder C, Aigner B, Tiffner KI, et al. Secukinumab distributes into dermal interstitial fluid of psoriasis patients as demonstrated by open flow microperfusion. Exp Dermatol. 2016;25(2):157–9.

51. Joanneum Research Forschungsgesellschaft mbH. EG -Zertifikat, medical device certification GmbH. 2018.

52. Fort DG, Herr TM, Shaw PL, Gutzman KE, Starren JB. Mapping the evolving definitions of translational research. J Clin Transl Sci. 2017;1:60–6.

53. Fudge N, Sadler E, Fisher HR, Maher J, Wolfe CDA, Mckevitt C. Optimising translational research opportunities : A systematic review and narrative synthesis of basic and clinician scientists' perspectives of factors which enable or hinder translational research. PLOSone.2016;11(8):1–23. https://doi.org/10.1371/journal.pone.0160475

54. Bodenlenz M, Hoefferer C, Birngruber T, Schaupp L. Filament-based catheter. Canada; CA 2737634, 2011.

55. Ellmerer M, Schaupp L, Trajanoski Z, Jobst G, Moser I, Urban G, et al. Continuous measurement of subcutaneous lactate concentration during exercise by combining open-flow microperfusion and thin-film lactate sensors. Biosens Bioelectron. 1998;13(9):1007–13.

56. Schaupp L, Feichtner F, Schaller-Ammann R, Mautner S, Ellmerer M, Pieber TR. Recirculation–a novel approach to quantify interstitial analytes in living tissue by combining a sensor with open-flow microperfusion. Anal Bioanal Chem. 2014;406(2):549–54.

57. Jacobson I, Sandberg M HA. Mass transfer in brain dialysis devices–a new method for the estimation of extracellular amino acids concentration. J Neurosci Methods. 1985;15(3):263–8.

58. Löhnroth P, Jansson P, Smith U. A microdialysis method allowing characterization of extracellular water space in humans. Am J Physiol. 1987;253:228–31.

59. Birngruber, T., Eberl, A., Kollmann, D., Bodenlenz, M., Florian, P., Subramaniam, A., Kainz, S., Rauter, G., & Sinnerc, F. (2017). Characterization of the Psoriasis-like Inflammation in the Imiquimod Rat Model using Dermal Open Flow Microperfusion. 47th Annual Meeting of the ESDR, Salzburg, Austria.

60. Ellmerer M, Schaupp L, Sendlhofer G, Wutte A, Brunner GA, Trajanoski Z, et al. Lactate metabolism of subcutaneous adipose tissue studied by open flow microperfusion. J Clin Endocrinol Metab. 1998;83(12):4394–401.

61. Trajanoski Z, Brunner G, Schaupp L, Ellmerer M, P W, Pieber T, et al. Open-flow microperfusion of subcutaneous adipose tissue for on-line continuous ex vivo measurement of glucose concentration. Diabetes Care. 1997;20(7):1114–21.

62. Schwingenschuh S, Scharfetter H, Martinsen OG, Boulgaropoulos B, Augustin T, Tiffner KI, et al. Assessment of skin permeability to topically applied drugs by skin impedance and admittance. Physiol Meas. 2017;38(11):138–50.

63. Felding J, Sørensen MD, Poulsen TD, Larsen J, Andersson C, Refer P, et al. Discovery and early clinical development of 2-{6-[2-(3,5-Dichloro-4- pyridyl)acetyl]-2,3-dimethoxyphenoxy}-N-propylacetamide (LEO 29102), a soft-drug inhibitor of phosphodiesterase 4 for topical treatment of atopic dermatitis. J Med Chem. 2014;57(14):5893–903.

64. Eirefelt, S., Hummer, J., Basse, L. H., Bertelsen, M., Johansson, F., Birngruber, T., Sinner, F., Larsen, J., Nielsen, S. F., & Lambert, M. (2020). Evaluating Dermal Pharmacokinetics and Pharmacodymanic Effect of Soft Topical PDE4 Inhibitors: Open Flow Microperfusion and Skin Biopsies. Pharmaceutical Research, 37(12), 243. https://doi.org/10.1007/s11095-020-02962-1

65. Kolbinger F, Loesche C, Valentin M-A, Jiang X, Cheng Y, Jarvis P, et al. β-Defensin 2 is a responsive biomarker of IL-17A-driven skin pathology in patients with psoriasis. J Allergy Clin Immunol. 2017 Mar 5;139(3):923–32.

66. Akomeah FK, Martin GP, Brown MB. Variability in human skin permeability in vitro: Comparing penetrants with different physicochemical properties. J Pharm Sci. 2007;96(4):824–34.

67. Pinnagoda J, Tupker RA, Smit JA, Coenraads PJ, Nater JP. The intra- and inter-individual variability and reliability of transepidermal water loss measurements. Contact Dermatitis. 1989;21:p. 255–9.

68. Davit BM, Chen M-L, Conner DP, Haidar SH, Kim S, Lee CH, et al. Implementation of a reference-scaled average bioequivalence approach for highly variable generic drug products by the US Food and Drug Administration. AAPS J. 2012;14(4):915–24.

69. Bodenlenz, M., Augustin, T., Birngruber, T., Tiffner, K. I., Boulgaropoulos, B., Schwingenschuh, S., Raney, S. G., Rantou, E., & Sinner, F. (2020). Variability of Skin Pharmacokinetic Data: Insights from a Topical Bioequivalence Study Using Dermal Open Flow Microperfusion. Pharmaceutical Research, 37(10), 204. https://doi.org/10.1007/s11095-020-02920-x

70. Wright J, Boudinot F, Ujhely M. Measurement and Analysis of Unbound Drug Concentrations. Clin Pharmacokinet. 1996;30(6):445–462.

71. U.S. FDA. Guidance for Industry Applications Covered by Section 505(b)(2); 1999.

72. Balas E, Boren B. Managing clinical knowledge for health care improvement. Yearbook of Medical Informatics. Schattauer Verlagsgesellschaft mbH, editor. Stuttgart; 2000: 65–70.

73. U.S. FDA. Guidance for Industry: Topical Dermatologic Corticosteroids: in Vivo Bioequivalence. Guid Ind.. 1995.

74. FDA. US. Draft Product Specific Guidance on Benzyl Alcohol. 2014.

75. U.S. FDA. Draft Product Specific Guidance on Acyclovir Cream. Guid Ind. 2016.

76. U.S. FDA. Draft Product Specific Guidance on Acyclovir Ointment. Guid Ind. 2012.

77. U.S. FDA. Draft Product Specific Guidance on Docosanol. Guid Ind. 2017.

78. Shah VP. Progress in methodologies for evaluating bioequivalence of topical formulations. Am J Clin Dermatol. 2001;2(5):275–80.

79. Pieber TR, Birngruber T, Bodenlenz M, Höfferer C, Mautner S, Tiffner K, et al. open flow microperfusion: an alternative method to microdialysis? In: Müller M, editor. Microdialysis in drug development (AAPS advances in the pharmaceutical sciences series). Springer New York; 2012: 283–302.

58 Dermal-Epidermal Separation Methods
Research Implications

Ying Zou
Shanghai Skin Disease Hospital, Shanghai, P. R. China

Howard I. Maibach
University of California, San Francisco, California

CONTENTS

58.1 INTRODUCTION

Skin contains three primary layers: epidermis, dermis, and hypodermis, and separation into epidermal and dermal components is an important technique in basic investigation of dermatology, pharmacology, toxicology, and biology.

The epidermal-dermal junction (EDJ) attaches the epidermis and dermis [4] and separates these distinct compartments, providing adhesion and a dynamic interface between them, thus governing overall structural integrity. Ultrastructurally, the EDJ is composed of four components: (1) cell membranes of basal keratinocytes, which contain hemidesmosomes; (2) an electron-lucent area, the lamina lucida; (3) an electron-dense area, the lamina densa; and (4) the sub-basal lamina. Each zone contains several components, including laminin and nidogen in the upper regions, type IV collagen and heparan sulphate proteoglycan predominantly in the lamina densa, and type VII collagen within the anchoring fibrils in the sub-basal lamina densa [5].

Therefore, it is important to preserve structure and function as far as possible during epidermal separation. We review here studies on epidermal separation in order to identify those optimal for a given research question.

58.2   MATERIALS AND METHODS

PubMed, Embase, and Web of Science were searched with combinations of the following keywords: skin, cutaneous, epidermis, dermis, isolation and separation.

58.3   RESULTS AND DISCUSSION

58.3.1   CHEMICALS

Collagen works similarly to gelatin in behavior. As a hydrophilic colloid, it swells on either side of the isoelectric point. Either acids or bases will affect the formation of electric double layers on the surfaces of the colloid micelles, resulting in repulsion between similarly ionized particles and then epidermal-dermal separation (Table 58.1).

58.3.1.1   Acid

58.3.1.1.1   Acetic Acid

Separation of epidermis by maceration in dilute acetic acid was first accomplished by Menschel [29]. Acid can swell collagen fibers, which decreases cohesive strength and binding of epidermis to dermis. Felsher [12] investigated the effect of acetic acid and an acid–salt mixture at different concentrations; after immersion in 0.1N acetic acid solution for two hours, the epidermis could be easily removed with forceps. In an acid solution, separation of the epidermis takes place exactly at its junction with the dermis. There is marked swelling of collagen fibrils and no separation of epidermis cells from each other.

TABLE 58.1
Chemical Separation

	Year	Author	Chemical		Concentration	Solution	Duration Time
1	1947	Felsher Z[12]	Acid	Acetic acid	0.1N	/	2 hr (4°C)
2	1942	Baumberger J[1]	Alkali	NH$_4$OH	0.32 mole/L (isosmotic)	H$_2$O	35 min
	1947	Felsher Z[12]	Alkali	NaOH	0.01 N	/	1 hr (20°C)
3	1947	Felsher Z[12]	Neutral salt	Sodium thiocyanate	2N	/	5 min
				Sodium iodide	2N	/	14 min
				Sodium bromide	2N	/	25 min
	1995	Ohata Y [31]	Neutral salt	EDTA	2mM	PBS and 2mM PMSF	48 hr (4°C)

58.3.1.2 Alkali

58.3.1.2.1 Ammonium Hydroxide

Ammonium hydroxide (NH_4OH) has a large concentration of undissociated NH_4OH and NH_3 molecules, which penetrate quickly and elevate pH to about 12. Baumberger [1] found the optimum choice i.e., the use of isomotic NH_4OH applied for 35 minutes.

58.3.1.2.2 Sodium Hydroxide

Felsher [12] verified the effect of sodium hydroxide (NaOH) and alkali salt mixtures, observing that the time required for separation of the epidermis decreases as the pH and swelling effect increased. It was unfeasible to utilize solutions below pH 10; pH 12 was recommended. Bases not only separated epidermis from dermis but caused the separation between epidermal cells.

58.3.1.3 Neutral Salts

Felsher [12] demonstrated that 2N sodium thiocynate, iodide, and bromide caused rapid epidermal swelling and glazing, yielding ease of separation. Diaz et al. [7] extended Felsher's sodium thiocynate separation method. Immunofluorescence and electron microscopy verified that a clean cleavage occurred at the lamina. Separation of epidermis by neutral salts resembles that caused by acids; however, edema between individual collagen fibrils is not as marked as in the acetic acid method. Epidermal separation occurs exactly at the EDJ and the basal cells remain preserved.

58.3.2 ENZYME DIGESTION

Several enzymes separate the epidermis from dermis (Table 58.2). The enzymes produce separation at the EDJ by digesting different structures specifically.

58.3.2.1 Trypsin

Basement membrane elastic fibers play an important part in anchoring the epidermis to the underlying tissue. Medawer [28] observed human skin incubated in trypsin and found that it is possible to disengage the epidermis in the form of an intact sheet. Klein et al. [21] separated mouse epidermis using trypsin and elastase. A shorter incubation period was required for elastase than trypsin. Ease or difficulty of separation was directly related to the total amount and dimensions of skin samples being incubated. Trypsin separation remains widely used, and it is reported to be less damaging to keratinocytes than the other physical and chemical procedures [9]. Separation predominantly occurs between basal and suprabasal cells by disruption of desmosomes, which may cause basal cells to remain loosely attached to the basement membrane [26]. Trypsinization causes loosening of the keratinocytes' intercellular connections. Therefore, vigorous washing of the isolated epidermal sheet to remove contaminating dermal fibroblasts also dissociates keratinocytes. Slight modification of trypsinization conditions also causes separation at the suprabasal layer.

58.3.2.2 Pancreatin

Becker et al. [2] described the pancreatic enzyme method; results resembled those of Medawer [28] obtained with trypsin. Fan [11] showed that crystalline trypsin and purified trypsin separated epidermis using an equal or smaller amount than pancreatin. Purified trypsin freed the epidermis the most efficiently.

58.3.2.3 Pronase

Einbinder et al. [8] compared pronase, a broad-spectrum proteinase, and the relative digestive action with five other proteolytic enzymes, namely trypsin, collagenase, pancreatic elastase, fungal

TABLE 58.2

Enzyme Separation

	Year	Author	Enzyme	Concentration	Ideal Dilution	Duration Time
1	1941	Medwar PB [28]	Trypsin	0.5%	Tyrode's solution	Depends on skin thickness
	1962	Klein M [21]	Trypsin	0.5%	Tyrode's	30 min(back skin), 25 min(ear skin)
	1966	Einbinder JM [8]	Trypsin	0.025%	Tris buffer (0.05M)	90 min~4 hr (37°C)
	1958	Fan J [11]	Purified trypsin; crystaling trypsin	0.5% 0.1%	Isotonic solution (NaCl 0.042%, KCl 0.42%, CaCl₂ 4.2%, NaHCO₃ 0.15%, glucose 0.1%)	45 min (40°C)
	1985	Takahashi H [35]	Trypsin	0.25%	CMF-BSS (Ca⁺⁺ and Mg⁺⁺ free Hank's balanced salt solution)	12~13 hr (4°C)
2	1952	Becker SW [2]	Pancreatin	0.25%~0.5%	Ringer-sodium bicarbonate solution	10~15 min (38°C)
	1958	Fan J [11]	Pancreatin	0.5%	Isotonic solution (NaCl 0.042%, KCl 0.42%, CaCl₂ 4.2%, NaHCO₃ 0.15%, glucose 0.1%)	45 min (40°C)
	1966	Einbinder JM [8]	Pancreatic elastase	0.05%	Tris buffer (0.05M)	90 min~4hr (37°C)
3	1962	Klein M [21]	Elastase	0.012%	Tyrode's	20~25 min(back skin),10~15 min(ear skin)
	1966	Einbinder JM [8]	Fungal elastase	0.1%	Tris buffer (0.05M)	90 min~4 hr (37°C)
4	1966	Einbinder JM [8]	Keratinase	0.1%	Tris buffer (0.05M)	30 min (37°C)
5	1966	Einbinder JM [8]	Collagenase	0.1%	Tris buffer (0.05M)	30 min (37°C)
6	1966	Einbinder JM [8]	Pronase	0.1%	Tris buffer (0.05M)	30 min (37°C)
7	1989	Walzer C [40]	Thermolysin	250 & 500 ug/ml	Mg⁺⁺-free PBS	1 hr (4°C)
8	1983	Kitano Y [20]	Dispase	500 & 1000 U/ml	PBS, Eagle MEM, or Eagle MEM supplemented with 20% fetal bovine serum	24 hr (4°C)
	1985	Takahashi H [35]	Dispase	1000 U/mL	M-199 containing 10% FCS	24 hr (4°C)
	1995	Ohata Y [31]	Dispase	1000 U/mL	Dulbecco's modified Eagle medium	45 min (37°C)

elastase, and keratinase (Table 58.3). The endpoint of digestion was similar. Optimal enzyme concentration, pH, and time varied. Pronase was extremely active, although its proteolytic and elastolytic activity were not significantly different from the others. Separation at the EDJ was followed by acantholysis and subsequently loss of dermal appendages and fibrous elements. Mature keratin structures or basement membrane structures did not appear altered.

58.3.2.4 Dispase

Dispase is a bacterial neutral protease obtained from the *Bacillus polymyxa* culture filtrate, and its cytotoxicity is low. Kitano et al. isolated epidermal sheets *in vivo* without dissociating cells [20]. After 24 hours human skin treatment with 500 and 1000 U/mL dispase, epidermal sheets were easily peeled from the dermis, and its undersurface retained rete ridges. Electron microscopic observation showed the basal surface composed of cells with numerous slender villi and cytoplasmic

TABLE 58.3

Heat Separation

	Year	Author	Temperature (°C)	Duration Time	Ideal Solution	Detail
1	1942	Baumberger J [1]	50	2 min	/	/
2	1947	Felsher Z [12]	56	4-5 min	/	/
			56	1 min	2N sodium chloride	Immersed in salt solution for 4 hr
			56	1.5 min	2N potassium chloride	subsequent to heat treatment
3	1968	Sonderga J [33]	60	10 min	Water bath	/
4	1978	Wadskov S [39]	60	10 min	Water bath	/
5	1982	Kassis V [17]	60	1 min	Water bath	/
6	1995	Ohata Y [31]	56	30 s	PBS	/
7	2012	Lau WM [23]	60	1 min	/	Esterase activity reduced

projections. Although the intercellular spaces of the spinous as well as the basal layers were wide, desmosomes were intact with their accompanying tonofilaments.

Einbinder et al. [8] compared the relative digestive action on skin of six proteolytic enzymes. Optimal enzyme concentration, pH, and time were varied. They ascertained that skin must be incubated in enzyme solutions for consistent separation, as topical application *in vivo* or *in vitro*, as well as intracutaneous injection *in vivo*, did not produce consistent results.

Takahashi et al. [35] compared trypsin with dispase isolation on rat skin. Quantitative estimation was made of yield, viability, and the number of attached epidermal cells. The dispase method was superior to trypsin, especially for cell yield, which was four times higher (1.1 *10^7 vs. 0.24*10^7 cells/10 cm^2 of skin, respectively). Viability and the rate of attachment of the recovered epidermal cells were also higher with dispase than with trypsin.

58.3.2.5 Thermolysin

Thermolysin is isolated from cultured filtrates of *Bacillus thermoproteolyticus*. Walzer et al. [40] reported that human epidermis could easily be separated from dermis following incubation at 4°C for 1 hour in a solution containing 250 to 500 ug/ml thermolysin. Light and electron microscopy revealed that the dermo-epidermal separation occurred at the basement membrane between the sites of bullous pemphigoid antigen and laminin and that the hemidesmosomes were selectively disrupted. They concluded that thermomlysin treatment appears to be a useful alternative to trypsin incubation for epidermal-dermal separation.

Gragnani et al. compared keratinocyte isolation methods using trypsin and thermolysin [15]. In histological evaluation, thermolysin caused detachment in the basal membrane zone, while trypsin made a chaotic segmentation and digestion of keratinocytes. There was no contamination with fibroblasts in the thermolysin group; however, this occurred with trypsin. The number of keratinocyte colonies in the thermolysin group was significantly greater than that with trypsin.

58.3.3 HEAT

Epidermal-dermal separation by heat was introduced in 1942 by Baumberger [1]. As an increase in temperature probably leads to a softening of collagen fibers, temperatures much lower than the boiling point of water may be used to separate epidermis from dermis. After exposure for two minutes on a slide warming table at 50°C, epidermis could be peeled readily and completely with forceps. Incompleteness occurred at 48.2°C, but complete division occurred with ease and completeness at 49.2°C. With temperatures above 51°C, detachment difficulty is encountered.

Felsher [12] detected the influence of salts on the subsequent separation of epidermis by heat. Heat separation is facilitated by ions that promote collagen swelling, and is depressed by ions that shrink it.

In the studies of Sonderga et al. [33] and Wadskov et al. [39], separation of epidermis from the dermis of normal human skin by heat was reported possible after 10 min at 60°C.

Kassis et al. [17] analyzed epidermal and dermal prostaglandins (PG) by heating separation. They kept frozen biopsy specimens in a water bath for various times and found that heating at 60°C for one minute produced a distinct separation of epidermis from dermis. Since no significant change in prostaglandin E1 (PGE1) activity occurred after one minute of heating, the heat-separation method seemed to be a reliable and quick method for PG analysis of skin.

Esterases are important for topical or transdermal delivery of drugs, since the enzymes may catalyze the hydrolysis of pharmaceuticals containing ester bonds. Lau et al. [23] detected esterase activity in fresh and heat-separated porcine ear skin. Esterase activity was diminished significantly in common heat-separated skin than in the fresh one. After heating at 60°C for one minute, neither epidermis nor the stratum corneum exhibited positive staining for esterase activity by histochemical staining. Therefore, heat separation should not be used to study the permeation of ester-containing permeants.

58.3.4 MECHANICAL METHODS

The methods described earlier have the disadvantage of altering to some degree the physical and/ or chemical integrity of one or both layers and may therefore be unsatisfactory for skin studies that require an isolated, but otherwise intact, epidermis or dermis. There is a need for techniques by which the epidermis can be separated from the dermis by purely mechanical forces, avoiding chemical or thermal damage.

58.3.4.1 Mechanical Stretching

Van Scott [38] streched the skin and then removed the epidermis as a continuous sheet by means of a razor blade or scalpel. When skin is stretched, the epidermis slips off easily by the latter procedure and can be rapidly removed. Gilbert et al. [14] and Sputt [34] improved this technique, so the skin only need stretching to a relaxed length. However, these methods require comparatively large surgical necropsy specimens and when scraped off with a scalpel, they may lack a basal cell layer.

58.3.4.2 Suction

As with unidirectinal stretching, dermal-epidermal separation has been achieved by the application of pressure gradients causing multidirectional distension. In 1878 Unna [37] described separation of the epidermis from dermis along the DEJ during dry cupping. Blank et al. [3] separated epidermis from dermis by the use of a vaccum. Bullae formed during an attempt to pull water through the skin when trying to pull water through a piece of skin by vacuum. A histological section of bullae demonstrated EDJ separation. This method therefore became a mechanical method to separate the epidermis. *In vivo* separation of the complete human epidermis by suction was accomplished in 1964.

Kiistala et al. [18] found that suction at a pressure of 20 cm Hg applied to intact human healthy skin within two hours produced blisters, the roof of which consisted solely of the epidermis and included the basal cell layer. They constructed a device that produced standard suction blisters of preselected size and number on human skin without discomfort in about two hours by suction of 150 mmHg [19] and permitted separation of epidermis from cadavers and certain furry animals. The blister roof consisted of viable, full-thickness epidermis; the clear fluid was a noninflammatory transudate, and no resultant scarring occurred. The suction trauma of the dermis was small and of standard nature. Thus the suction epidermis appeared useful for tissue culture and biochemical analyses. Today this suction blister method is widely applied in dermatological research and practice for epidermal grafting [10, 16, 25]; for creating standardized wound healing models [6, 22]; and for studying morphological, physiological, or pharmacological phenomena [24, 32].

58.3.5 COMPARISON

Many techniques relying on different mechanisms of separation have been described. Each method has advantages and disadvantages. Heat is simple, yet tedious. Although the heat process has been used successfully, chemical reagents are effective, but disturb the electrolyte cellular equilibrium. Digestion by enzymes gives complete separation, but it destroys important components. Mechanical division necessitates a relatively large tissue piece, but has the advantage that chemical changes do not occur. Many research studies compared these methods and documented different influences on the structure and function of skin biochemistry.

Baumberger [1], when comparing the separation methods of NH_4OH and heat, found that the epidermal tissues treated were not destroyed, but were only temporarily loosened, and there was a marked decrease in oxygen consumption by the epidermis by both methods. However, the heat technique may be superior because the tissue is not brought into water and there is no loss of material (Table 58.4).

Quantitative determinations of stratum corneum sulfhydryl and disulfide concentration revealed relatively consistent values in certain skin diseases. Epidermal sulfhydryl in different methods of separation showed that sulfhydryl values obtained after ammonium hydroxide separation resembled

TABLE 58.4
Comparison of Separation Methods

	Year	Author	Separation Methods	Results	Conclusion
1	1942	Baumberger J [1]	NH_4OH heat	• Epidermal tissues treated not killed, but temporarily loosened • Oxygen consumption rate by heat: 23% by NH_4OH 14% (compared with method of razor blade)	• Epidermal tissues are not killed by both methods • Marked oxygen consumption by both methods • Heat technique is superior to water free
2	1960	Ogura R [30]	Enzyme heat NH_4OH mechanical	• Sulfhydryl values obtained after NH_4OH method similar to that of mechanical • Heat and enzymes alter the results significantly	• NH_4OH separation technic appeared procedure of choice
3	1983	Woodley D [42]	Trypsin 1M NaCl PBS suction	• Bullous pemphigoid antigen (BPA) remained associated with epidermis of all specimens with a 1:320 or great dilution except warm PBS separation • Antigenicity of basement membrane heparin sulfate proteoglycan lost after trypsin separation • Laminin, type IV and V collagen remained with dermis by all the methods	• Only trypsin effectively degrades the molecule, making the antibody biding site unrecognized.

(Continued)

TABLE 58.4 (*Continued*)
Comparison of Separation Methods

	Year	Author	Separation Methods	Results	Conclusion
4	1991	Willsteed EM [41]	Suction 1M NaCl thermolysin	• 1M NaCl resulted split within lamina lucid, with intact hemidesmosomes and swollen mitochondria. No other degenerative features. • Thermolysin developed intraepidermal separation in four of five specimens. • Suction causes split through the lamina lucina, associated with hemidesmosome disruption and formation of cytoplasmic vacuoles within keratinocytes.	• 1M NaCl was the most reproducible, convenient, and reliable separation method
5	1994	Fort JJ [13]	EDTA trypsin heat mechanical (stretching and scraping)	• Initial rate of soluble protein: EDTA > heat > scraping > trypsin • Initial rate of tissue: EDTA > heat > scraping > trypsin • Microscopic examination confirmed not known to the extent of contamination of dermis after scraping	• Trypsin was unsuitable • Physical scraping had less consideration for hardness to determine cross-contamination of layers occurred • Heat separation slightly inferior to EDTA • EDTA was favorite
6	1995	Ohata Y [31]	EDTA dispase heat	• Antigen molecules (PV, Pf, BP, EBA) can be detected after these methods treating, at either the cell surface or BMZ, except for negative reactivity with BPAG2 in dispase-treated epidermis.	• Heat separation should be the standard substrate for immunoblotting for the shorter preparation time
7	2007	Trost A [36]	Ammonium thiocyanate, dispase heat 1M NaCl	• 58%-69% and 89%-92% less kallikrein 12 mRNA detected after treating with heat and diapase than with ammonium thiocyanate, respectively • No kallikrein detected after 1M NaCl treating	• Separation with 3.8% ammonium thiocyanate was optimal choice for high-quality RNA isolation from human skin
8	2011	Maharlooei MK [27]	NaBr (2N and 4N), NH₄OH typsin	• No significant difference between total cell counts, dead cell counts, and percentage of live cells of four methods: NaBr(4N) method yielded the most cells (total and live); trypsin method produced the most dead cell counts • A significant higher of live cell counts from NaBr(4N) method compared with the others • Immunocytochemical staining of cytokeratin and melanosome antibodies showed no difference between four methods	• NaBr(4N) method yields more live cells and less toxicity.

those obtained following mechanical separation, while heat and enzymes appeared to alter the results significantly and were therefore not satisfactory [30].

Dermal-epidermal separation is an essential technique for immunoblotting studies and for the diagnostic immunofluorescence of autoimmune bullous diseases. To study the localization of basement membrane components after different separation methods, Woodley et al. [42] separated adult human skin using four methods. Only heparan sulfate proteoglycan of the basement membrane was trypsin-sensitive. Willsteed et al. [41] examined the electron microscopic appearance of specimens separated by three methods, concluding that 1M sodium chloride remains the most convenient and reproducible means of inducing dermal-epidermal separation through the lamina lucida. Ohata et al. [31] compared the autoantigens for bullous skin diseases by immunoblotting using different dermal-epidermal separation techniques; the results suggest that ethylene diamine tetra-acetic acid (EDTA)–, dispase-, and heat-separated skin were similar for detecting various autoantigens, but heat separation is preferable because the preparation time is shorter.

To compare effect of epidermal-dermal separation techniques of hairless mouse skin, the most suitable method was determined by kinetic studies in a homogenate medium [13]. Based on the data of effects of separation methods on soluble protein yield and dermal enzymatic activity using dibutyl methotrexate (DBMTX) as a substrate, EDTA treatment appears a favorable method for epidermal separation.

To obtain rapid, high-quality epidermal-specific ribonucleic acid (RNA) from human skin, Trost et al. [36] investigated the effect of dermal-epidermal separation methods, including ammonium thiocyanate, dispase, heat, and 1M NaCl, and concluded that the fast chemical separation method with 3.8% ammonium thiocyanate is the optimal choice for producing high-quality RNA isolation from human skin.

Epidermal separation is also useful in autologous skin transplantation. The first step in isolating epidermal cells is to separate it from the dermis. Recently, several methods for epidermis isolation and epidermal cell suspension were compared to select the optimum one for clinical use. The sodium bromide (NaBr) (4N) method is considered the least toxic and the most viable cells are produced [27]. Figure 58.1 shows action sites of these dermal–epidermal separation methods.

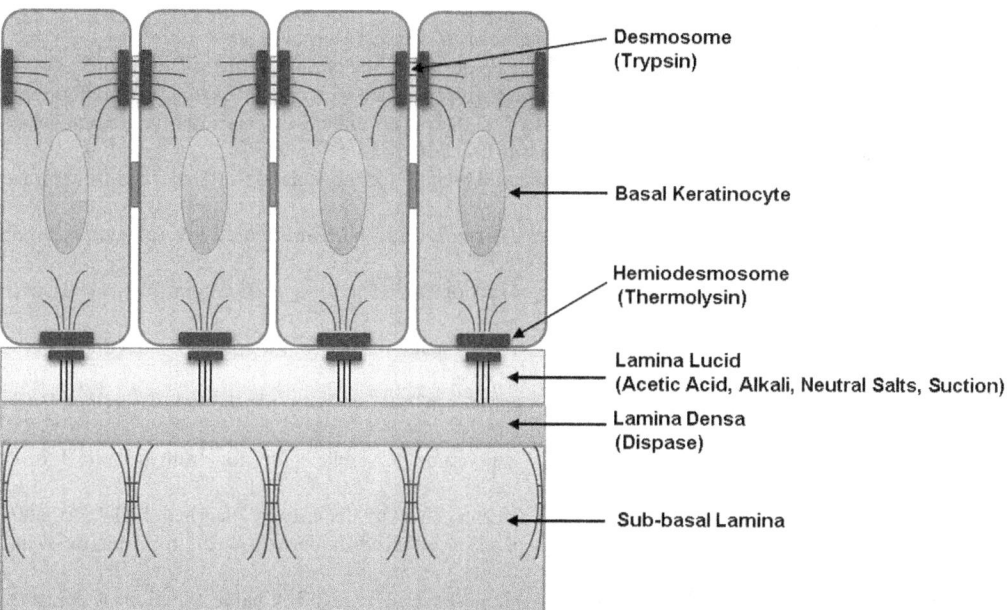

FIGURE 58.1 Diagram of action site of dermal-epidermal separation methods. (Other action sites are not labeled because the exact site has not yet been defined.)

58.4   CONCLUSION

In conclusion, the separation method must be appropriate for the experimental project, and no single method appears to be superior for all purposes. Future comparative investigations should be conducted and will benefit the integrity of research based on this methodology.

ACKNOWLEDGEMENT

The present work was first published in the "reviews" of *Archives of Dermatological Research* as: Ying Zou, Howard I. Maibach. Dermal–epidermal separation methods: research implications. *Arch Dermatol Res* (2018) 310:1–9

REFERENCES

1. Baumberger J (1942) Methods for the separation of epidermis from dermis and some physiologic and chemical properties of isolated epidermis. J Natl Cancer Inst 2: 413–423
2. Becker SW, Fitzpatrick TB, Montgomery H (1952) Human melanogenesis: Cytology and histology of pigment cells (melanodendrocytes). AMA Arch Derm Syphilol 65: 511–523
3. Blank IH, Miller OG (1950) A method for the separation of the epidermis from the dermis. J Invest Dermatol 15: 9–10
4. Briggaman RA, Wheeler CE (1975) Epidermal-dermal junction. J Invest Dermatol 65: 71–84
5. Burgeson RE, Christiano AM (1997) The dermal-epidermal junction. Curr Opin Cell Biol 9: 651–658
6. Czaika V, Alborova A, Richter H, Sterry W, Vergou T, Antoniou C, Lademann J, Koch S (2012) Comparison of transepidermal water loss and laser scanning microscopy measurements to assess their value in the characterization of cutaneous barrier defects. Skin Pharmacol Physiol 25: 39–46
7. Diaz LA, Heaphy MR, Calvanico NJ, Tomasi TB, Jordon RE (1977) Separation of epidermis from dermis with sodium thiocyanate. J Invest Dermatol 68: 36–38
8. Einbinde.JM, Walzer RA, Mandl I (1966) Epidermal-dermal separation with proteolytic enzymes. J Invest Dermatol 46: 492–504
9. Epstein WL (1983) Biochemistry and Physiology of the Skin. Oxford University Press, New York
10. Falabella R (2004) Suction blister device for separation of viable epidermis from dermis. Clin Exp Dermatol 29: 105–106
11. Fan J (1958) Epidermal separation with purified trypsin. J Invest Dermatol 30: 271
12. Felsher Z (1947) Studies on the adherence of the epidermis to the corium. J Invest Dermatol 8: 35–47
13. Fort JJ, Mitra AK (1994) Effects of epidermal/dermal separation methods and ester chain configuration on the bioconversion of a homologous series of methotrexate dialkyl esters in dermal and epidermal homogenates of hairless mouse skin. Int J Pharm 102: 241–247
14. Gilbert D, Mier PD, Jones TE (1963) An improved technic for the isolation of epidermis from human skin. J Invest Dermatol 40: 165–167
15. Gragnani A, Sobral CS, Ferreira LM (2007) Thermolysin in human cultured keratinocyte isolation. Braz J Biol 67: 105–109
16. Gupta S, Shroff S (1999) Modified technique of suction blistering for epidermal grafting in vitiligo. Int J Dermatol 38: 306–309
17. Kassis V, Sondergaard J (1982) Heat-separation of normal human-skin for epidermal and dermal prostaglandin analysis. Arch Dermatol Res 273: 301–306
18. Kiistala U, Mustakallio KK (1964) In-vivo separation of epidermis by production of suction blisters. Lancet 2(7348): 1444–1445
19. Kiistala U (1968) Suction blister device for separation of viable epidermis from dermis. J Invest Dermatol 50: 129–137
20. Kitano Y, Okada N (1983) Separation of the epidermal sheet by dispase. Br J Dermatol 108: 555–560
21. Klein M, Fitzgerald LR (1962) Enzymatic separation of intact epidermal sheets from mouse skin. J Invest Dermatol 39: 111–114
22. Kottner J, Hillmann K, Fimmel S, Seite S, Blume-Peytavi U (2013) Characterisation of epidermal regeneration *in vivo*: a 60-day follow-up study. J Wound Care 22: 395–400
23. Lau WM, Ng KW, Sakenyte K, Heard CM (2012) Distribution of esterase activity in porcine ear skin, and the effects of freezing and heat separation. Int J Pharm 433: 10–15

24. Levy JJ, Vonrosen J, Gassmuller J, Kuhlmann RK, Lange L (1995) Validation of an in-vivo wound-healing model for the quantification of pharmacological effects on epidermal regeneration. Dermatology 190: 136–141

25. Li J, Fu WW, Zheng ZZ, Zhang QQ, Xu Y, Fang L (2011) Suction blister epidermal grafting using a modified suction method in the treatment of stable vitiligo: a retrospective study. Dermatol Surg 37: 999–1006

26. Liu SC, Karasek M (1978) Isolation and growth of adult human epidermal keratinocytes in cell-culture. J Invest Dermatol 71: 157–162

27. Maharlooei MK, Mohammadi AA, Farsi A, Ahrari I, Attar A, Monabati A (2011) A comparison between different existing methods used to separate epidermal cells from skin biopsies for autologous transplantation. Indian J Dermatol 56: 666–669

28. Medawar PB (1941) Sheets of pure epidermal epithelium from human skin. Nature 148: 783

29. Menschel H (1925) Zur kolloidchemie und pharmakologie der keratinzubstanzen und menschlichen haut. Arch Exp Pathol Pharmakol 110: 1–45

30. Ogura R, Knox JM, Griffin AC (1960) Separation of epidermis for the study of epidermal sulfhydryl. J Invest Dermatol 35: 239–243

31. Ohata Y, Hashimoto T, Nishikawa T (1995) Comparative study of autoantigens for various bullous skin diseases by immunoblotting using different dermo-epidermal separation techniques. Clin Exp Dermatol 20: 454–458

32. Panoutsopoulou IG, Wendelschafer-Crabb G, Hodges JS, Kennedy WR (2009) Skin blister and skin biopsy to quantify epidermal nerves A comparative study. Neurology 72: 1205–1210

33. Sonderga J, Zacharia H (1968) Epidermal histamine. Archiv Fur Klinische Und Experimentelle Dermatologie 233: 323–328

34. Sprutt D (1964) An improved technic for the isolation of epidermis from larger specimens of human skin. J Invest Dermatol 42: 285

35. Takahashi H, Sano K, Yoshizato K, Shioya N, Sasaki K (1985) Comparative studies on methods of isolating rat epidermal-cells. Ann Plast Surg 14: 258–266

36. Trost A, Bauer JW, Lanschuetzer C, Laimer M, Emberger M, Hintner H, Oender K (2007) Rapid, high-quality and epidermal-specific isolation of RNA from human skin. Exp Dermatol 16: 185–190

37. Unna P (1878) Zur Anatomie der Blasenbildung an der menschlichenHaut. Vjschr Dermatol Syphil 5: 3

38. Van Scott EJ (1952) Mechanical separation of the epidermis from the corium. J Invest Dermatol 18: 377–379

39. Wadskov S, Sondergaard J (1978) Determination of cyclic-amp in heat-separated human epidermal tissue. Acta Derm Venereol 58: 191–195

40. Walzer C, Benathan M, Frenk E (1989) Thermolysin treatment - a new method for dermo-epidermal separation. J Invest Dermatol 92: 78–81

41. Willsteed EM, Bhogal BS, Das A, Bekir SS, Wojnarowska F, Black MM, McKee PH (1991) An ultra-structural comparison of dermo-epidermal separation techniques. J Cutan Pathol 18: 8–12

42. Woodley D, Sauder D, Talley MJ, Silver M, Grotendorst G, Qwarnstrom E (1983) Localization of basement-membrane components after dermal-epidermal junction separation. J Invest Dermatol 81: 149–153

59 Use of Skin Absorption Data in the Safety Evaluation of Cosmetic Ingredients

Jeffrey J. Yourick and Margaret E.K. Kraeling
Food and Drug Administration, Laurel, Maryland

Disclaimer: This book chapter reflects the views of the authors and should not be construed to represent FDA's views or policies.

CONTENTS

59.1 INTRODUCTION

Exposure of consumers to cosmetic products mainly occurs via the dermal route. Once a chemical contacts skin, absorption begins. Diffusion into and through the stratum corneum typically is the rate-limiting step in percutaneous absorption. However, the rate-limiting barrier to absorption is dependent upon the specific chemical. For a cosmetic chemical that is applied to skin, the accuracy of the exposure assessment and the subsequent safety/risk assessment can be improved by basing potential systemic exposure on an estimate of the dermal exposure that has been corrected with skin absorption data (1). Dermal exposure to a cosmetic ingredient is a function of the concentration of chemical contacting skin, the cosmetic product matrix, and the duration of skin contact. Leave-on cosmetic products would represent product categories resulting in large dermal exposures, while rinse-off product use results in dermal exposures that have skin contact times that are of relatively short duration.

Percutaneous absorption of cosmetic and fragrance ingredients may represent a major route of ingredient uptake and subsequent systemic exposure. Many factors alter the extent of percutaneous absorption of cosmetic ingredients such as physicochemical properties of the ingredient, the hydration state of skin, duration of product contact, vehicle/formulation effects, and area of application, to name a few. To generate data that will be useful for preparing an exposure assessment, the absorption study design should attempt to incorporate testing conditions that approximate realistic consumer product use conditions.

In this chapter, we will focus on how percutaneous absorption data can be used to refine the risk assessment process, especially the exposure estimate, for cosmetic and fragrance ingredients. We will discuss various issues regarding the safety/risk assessment for both noncarcinogenic and carcinogenic cosmetic ingredients.

59.2   HAZARD IDENTIFICATION

The evaluation of cosmetic safety usually begins with the identification of a hazard. Hazard identification may be defined as a determination of whether exposure to a cosmetic ingredient or an impurity in the ingredient can lead to an increased incidence of an adverse health effect and the relative strength of the evidence for biologic causation. Hazard identification can arise from many different sources. Consumer use of products can result in adverse health effects that are reported to physicians, the Food and Drug Administration (FDA), or the company that produced the product. Animal toxicity testing of chemicals can also raise concerns about the safety of chemicals. Toxicology (short-term and subchronic) and carcinogenesis testing, such as that performed at the National Toxicology Program, is one means to identify potential hazardous chemicals. Reports published in the open literature are another source to identify hazardous chemicals. These types of reports may range from human patch testing of cosmetic chemicals for sensitization or irritation to animal toxicity testing.

During the process of hazard identification, it is important to identify toxicity studies that define doses of the chemicals that are toxic and ideally doses at which no toxicity was found. The dosage level at which no observed adverse effects were observed is referred to as the NOAEL. It is rare that a human NOAEL for a cosmetic finished product or cosmetic raw ingredient will be available. For most toxicity testing, a NOAEL is derived from an animal study that administered the chemical by one of several possible routes of exposure such as feed, gavage, drinking water, inhalation, or skin painting. Therefore, some method of extrapolation is needed to estimate human safety from animal toxicity testing. For cosmetics, the extrapolation from animal data to human safety involves using many different uncertainty factors, including the species of animals, body weights, body surface area, quality and length of animal test, and sensitive human populations, just to name a few (2).

59.3   EXPOSURE ESTIMATE

Once a potential hazard has been identified, the next step in the process of safety evaluation is to estimate human exposure. Generally, exposure to a cosmetic ingredient is via the dermal route. Dermal exposure to a cosmetic ingredient is basically the amount of that ingredient that is applied to and in contact with the skin. However, the systemic exposure to that cosmetic ingredient may be much lower given the barrier properties of skin and the rate of absorption. Furthermore, systemic exposure will also be dependent upon the duration of skin contact. For an accurate estimate of systemic exposure for a specific dermally applied chemical, it is important also to know the extent of skin absorption. Once the percentage of applied dermal dose absorbed is experimentally determined, refinement of the systemic exposure estimate can be made from the applied dermal dose. In the absence of any relevant skin absorption data for a chemical, it should be assumed that all (i.e., 100%) of the chemical that is applied to the skin is absorbed ("conservative" exposure approach).

59.3.1   DERMAL EXPOSURE

To estimate dermal exposure to a cosmetic ingredient, it is important to know the use conditions for the specific product(s) containing the ingredient of interest. From the product use instructions, it is possible to determine many factors pertinent to the exposure calculation, such as the approximate frequency of product use, volume/weight of product used, duration of exposure, and other conditions of exposure (e.g., apply heat or cover application area with plastic). An ingredient could be contained in one product intended for leave-on usage (e.g., moisturizing lotion) or in a different product intended as a rinse-off formulation (e.g., hair dye product or shampoo). All use conditions should be defined and considered for a relevant consumer exposure estimate.

A relevant dermal exposure estimate should be based on reliable information regarding the concentration of the ingredient in the finished product. However, this product information is usually proprietary and difficult to obtain. FDA laboratories, Cosmetic Ingredient Review (CIR), and other consumer groups occasionally conduct surveys that directly measure ingredient concentrations in finished cosmetic products. These specific ingredient concentrations can then be used in exposure estimate calculations.

The initial dermal exposure estimate is calculated from as many of the previously mentioned exposure conditions as are deemed pertinent to include. When actual data are unavailable for a specific parameter, an estimate of the parameter must be used. However, any estimates used in the calculation should be clearly noted in the exposure estimate summary. This is important, since uncertainties in the exposure estimate will affect the degree of confidence in the final safety assessment. It is desirable to calculate an exposure in units of ingredient weight/kilogram (kg) body weight/day. This helps to facilitate comparison of dermal exposure to a NOAEL obtained from a dietary or parenteral administration.

59.3.2 Percutaneous Absorption

Ideally percutaneous absorption is measured in fresh, viable human and/or animal skin using in vitro flow-through diffusion cell methodology. However, nonviable skin may be used if metabolic activity is not needed to characterize the absorption profile. These techniques are described in more detail in Chapter 51 of this book. A variety of receptor fluids may be used, the composition of which will depend upon the specific chemical being tested. The application of chemicals to skin should be made in a vehicle that approximates consumer use conditions as closely as possible to generate data providing realistic exposure estimates.

Skin absorption is dependent on many factors, including lipid solubility of the chemical, duration of skin contact, location of skin contact, vehicle for the chemical, environmental conditions, occlusion of the dosing area by clothing, surface area of skin application, and the age of the individual. These factors must be considered when attempting to accurately define the exposure estimate.

Skin absorption studies should be conducted under conditions that approximate specific product use/misuse conditions. A well-designed in vitro absorption study should consider the relevant experimental conditions necessary to replicate consumer use conditions. A typical experimental design should consider the dosing vehicle, the dosing concentration, and the duration of exposure to simulate use conditions (3). To simulate a leave-on product, the dosing solution may be left on the skin for 24 hours, whereas for a rinse-off product, the dosing solution may be removed after one to five minutes (4). The percentage of applied dose absorbed is experimentally determined and is used in estimating systemic exposure to the chemical.

59.4 SAFETY ASSESSMENTS

59.4.1 Noncarcinogenic Cosmetic Ingredient Safety Evaluation: Assume a Threshold for Toxicity

One approach for extrapolating data from animal studies to human hazard/safety is the safety factor approach. The safety factor approach implies that there is a threshold dose for a toxic effect. If the NOAEL is considered the threshold dose, then the NOAEL is divided by a safety factor (usually 100; 10 for interspecies [animal to human] and 10 for intraspecies [human]) variability to determine a safe human dose or an "acceptable daily intake" (ADI) (5).

59.4.1.1   Exposure Estimate: Acute and Chronic Exposure

The systemic exposure estimate for a single exposure to a cosmetic ingredient is a function of the amount applied to skin, the concentration of the ingredient in the product, the duration of skin contact, and the extent of percutaneous absorption. If no data are available for these specific exposure conditions, then these parameters must be estimated. The volume of the product used is the typical amount of product applied to the skin. If the volume of the product applied is not available, then it is possible to use a typical application rate, such as product amount applied per skin surface area (milligrams product applied to skin per cm²), for specific cosmetic product categories (e.g., a lotion is typically applied at 2 mg/cm²). The amount of a cosmetic ingredient systemically absorbed can be estimated as follows:

$$\text{Amount Absorbed / kg body weight} = (\text{Application Rate}) \times (\text{Concentration of Ingredient in Product}) \times (\text{Duration of Exposure}) \times (\text{Surface Area Exposed}) \times (\% \text{ Skin Absorption}) / (\text{Weight of Individual})$$

The estimated daily dose is an exposure estimate based on chronic usage of a specific product. The amount absorbed per kg body weight is multiplied by the estimated frequency of use throughout a lifetime, divided by the total number of days represented by a lifetime of use.

$$\text{Estimated Daily Dose} = (\text{amount absorbed/kg body weight}) \times (\text{estimated frequency of use over a lifetime}) / (\text{total number of days represented by a lifetime of use})$$

59.4.1.2   Safety Assessment

  a. If a NOAEL for the Ingredient Is Available:

$$\text{Acceptable Daily Intake} = \text{NOAEL} / \text{Safety Factor}$$

$$\text{Margin of Safety} = \text{NOAEL} / \text{Estimated Daily Dose}$$

  b. If a NOAEL for the Ingredient is Not Available:

   It is sometimes the case when a toxicology study is completed that all experimental doses caused an adverse effect such that a NOAEL is not determined, but the lowest experimental dose was identified as the lowest observed adverse effect level (LOAEL). It is possible to divide the LOAEL by an additional safety factor to estimate the NOAEL (5). This estimated NOAEL can then be used in the calculation of acceptable daily intake and margin of safety as presented earlier.

59.4.1.3   Assessment

The safety assessment is reviewed, and after a qualitative evaluation of the uncertainties inherent in the exposure estimate, a decision is made by the risk managers as to whether there is a potential safety problem with exposure to a specific cosmetic ingredient or finished product. Furthermore, risk managers will ultimately be responsible for making decisions on any corrective actions that might be necessary to protect public health.

59.4.2   CARCINOGENIC COSMETIC INGREDIENT SAFETY EVALUATION

The safety assessment of a cosmetic ingredient suspected to be carcinogenic (e.g., determined from open literature publications, National Toxicology Program reports, International Agency for Research on Cancer [IARC] reports, unpublished studies) in either animals or humans is currently conducted using a different approach. An initial exposure estimate is completed as outlined in the preceding section to derive an estimated daily dose. Since it may not be appropriate to consider a threshold for carcinogenic potential, quantitative risk assessment calculations are used to determine the relative lifetime cancer risk resulting from the potential exposure. A mathematical model is used to perform the linear regression for the low-dose estimate of cancer risk. The procedure for the cancer risk estimation has been previously outlined (5). Briefly, a direct method (linear-at-low dose approach) for low-dose cancer risk estimation is used. A straight line is drawn from a point on the dose–response curve to the point of origin. The slope of the straight line is used as an index of carcinogenic potency. The upper limit estimate of relative cancer risk (4) is then:

$$\left[\text{risk} = \text{slope} \times \text{dose}\right]$$

59.4.3 RISK MANAGEMENT

Risk management deals with identifying and considering the range of regulatory options and then deciding which approach to use to protect public health. Risk managers review the risk assessment and consider all other legal, economic, social, ethical, and political issues that may arise from a risk management decision (6). A set of decision options is formulated to address the specific risk assessment findings. The risk managers must then decide on the nature of any corrective actions required to protect the public health.

59.5 CONCLUSION

For a cosmetic chemical or contaminant that is applied to skin, the exposure assessment and the subsequent safety/risk assessment can be improved by basing potential systemic exposure on an estimate of the dermal exposure that has been corrected with skin absorption data. In this chapter, we focused on how skin absorption data can be used to refine the exposure estimate and risk assessment for cosmetic ingredients. We discussed various issues regarding the exposure/safety/risk assessment for both noncarcinogenic and carcinogenic cosmetic ingredients and contaminants.

REFERENCES

1. ECETOC: Percutaneous Absorption. Monograph No. 20. Brussels. 1993.
2. Faustman EM, Omenn GS. Risk assessment. In: Klaassen CD, ed. Casarett & Doull's Toxicology: The Basic Science of Poisons, 5th ed. New York: McGraw-Hill, 1996:75–88.
3. Bronaugh RL, Collier SW. Protocol for *in vitro* percutaneous absorption studies. In: Bronaugh RL, Maibach HI, eds. *In Vitro* Percutaneous Absorption: Principles, Fundamentals, and Applications. Boston: CRC Press, 1991:237–241.
4. Kraeling MEK, Yourick JJ, Bronaugh RL. Percutaneous absorption of diethanolamine in human skin in vitro. Food Chem Toxicol 2004; 42(10):1553–1561.
5. Kokoski CJ, Henry SH, Lin CS, Ekelman KB. Methods used in safety evaluation. In: Branen AL, Davidson PM, Salminen S, eds. Food Additives. New York: Marcel Dekker, Inc., 1990:579–615.

60 Bioequivalence, Pharmaceutical Equivalence, and Biowaivers

Topical Dosage Forms for Local Action

Isadore Kanfer
Rhodes University, Grahamstown, South Africa
University of Toronto, Toronto, Canada

CONTENT

60.1 INTRODUCTION

The market approval of a generic product requires demonstration of bioequivalence (BE) against an innovator reference product to ensure safety and efficacy (1). Unlike oral products where well-established methods and regulatory guidelines are available for BE assessment, there are no such procedures or guidelines for the BE of topical dosage forms intended for local action apart from the U.S. Food and Drug Administration's (FDA's) vasoconstrictor assay (VCA) (2), which is restricted to topical corticosteroid products only. Currently, regulatory authorities only accept comparative clinical trials with a clinical endpoint using a randomized, double-blind, parallel, placebo-controlled study design in patients for BE assessment of such products. However, these trials are extremely expensive, time-consuming, and associated with demanding ethical considerations. Furthermore, clinical end-point trials are considered to possess relatively lower sensitivity, are poorly reproducible, and are also the least accurate than the general approaches to demonstrate BE (3). These foregoing issues have resulted in a dearth of generic topical products intended for local action (4). Hence there is an urgent need to develop more economical alternatives for the BE assessment of topical products not intended to be systemically absorbed to ensure speedier market entry of generic products for local action.

BE of oral dosage forms, wherein the active ingredients are intended to be absorbed into the systemic circulation, can be determined using conventional approaches involving the assessment of pharmacokinetic (PK) parameters (1). Since topical dosage forms for local action are not intended for systemic absorption, their BE assessment has proved to be quite complicated, daunting, and extremely challenging. Hence, the PK approach used for the BE assessment of systemically absorbed drugs is deemed inappropriate for BA/BE assessment of topical products intended for local action.

The concentrations of drugs in the systemic circulation following topical administration generally reaches only a fraction of the amount of drug applied to the skin surface, resulting in analytical difficulties. Additionally, systemic drug concentrations following application do not reflect the appropriate concentration in the target organ, the skin. In light of this, the FDA has stated that the BE of products containing active ingredient(s) not intended for systemic absorption may be assessed by (surrogate) measurements intended to reflect the rate and extent to which the active ingredient or moiety becomes available at the site of action (5).

The U.S. Government Accountability Office (GAO) Report in August 2016 provided information for the period from Q1 of 2010 through Q2 of 2015 (6), where they found extraordinary price increases of 57% of the topical drug products on the market during that period. The average price of topical generic drugs was 276% higher at the end of the period analyzed. It is estimated that approximately 80% of topical dermatological drug products have fewer than three generic competitors, and in many cases there are no approved generic products for some certain dermatological indications. This situation has significant economic implications in the quest to provide cost-effective generic drug products in order to save patients and governments many millions of dollars (7). As a result, considerable efforts have been directed towards the development and validation of surrogate models to demonstrate the BE of topical products. This initiative, provided by the Generic Drug User Fee Amendments (GDUFA) (8, 9), makes provision for collaboration within the FDA as well as externally through grants or contracts in the quest to facilitate the availability of such generic products and make these medicines more affordable and more accessible to the wider population.

More recently, the requirements to ensure that topical generic products should be designed to match an approved reference product have been enunciated by regulatory authorities whereby emphasis has been placed on specific quality properties such as qualitative, (Q1), quantitative (Q2), and in particular for semisolid formulations, the similarity in formulation microstructure (9), with the main objective being to ensure pharmaceutical and therapeutic equivalency based on the comparative testing data whereby sameness between test and reference product can be established. Methods involving surrogate assessments to establish pharmaceutical equivalence between test and reference products which can subsequently provide useful information on the clinical performance of a test product must, however, be associated with convincing validation data. Such data should demonstrate that the method has the necessary properties to confirm that it is accurate, sensitive, and most importantly, can discriminate significant differences should such differences exist.

60.2 BIOEQUIVALENCE

The determination of the bioavailability of systemically absorbed products is defined as the rate and extent to which the active ingredient or active moiety is absorbed from the drug product and becomes available at the site of action (10). For such studies, serial blood samples are drawn following the extravascular randomly administered test and appropriate reference dosage forms, such as tablet or capsule, in a cross-over design, and the serum or plasma is harvested and subsequently analyzed to determine the drug concentration in each sample. These data are then processed to provide a profile of drug concentration versus time, where the BE metrics, peak drug concentrations (C_{max}) and area under the curve (AUC) are then used to compute BE.

BE is declared when the relative mean ratios of the test (T) and reference (R) product fall within the prescribed acceptance limits of a confidence interval (CI) of 90% and the relative mean ratios of the test (T) and reference (R) product (using log transformed data) are within 80% and 125%. The assessment of BE is a surrogate approach, which is intended to provide information on the safety and efficacy of products based on the comparative bioavailability between a test and reference product. The latter is usually an innovator's product whose market approval is based on clinical studies in patients. Bioequivalence studies are thus indirect measures of safety and efficacy, justified by the presumption that the concentration of drug in the bloodstream is in equilibrium and reflects the concentration at the site of action, and a relationship between effectiveness and systemic blood concentrations of the

TABLE 60.1

Comparative BE Requirements for Extravascular and Topical Dosage Forms Not Intended to Be Absorbed

Products Intended to be Absorbed into the Systemic Circulation	Topical Products Not Intended to be Absorbed into the Systemic Circulation
Surrogate measures justified by the presumption that concentration of drug in bloodstream is in equilibrium and reflects the concentration at site of action	Surrogate measures cannot be justified on the same basis as for drugs intended to be absorbed into the systemic circulation, since no such relationship is expected
BE methodology well established	Methodology under development
Statistical assessment of data well established	Statistical assessment yet to be defined
Regulatory requirements based upon C_{max} and AUC falling within prescribed limits of CI of 90% and relative means of test to reference being within 80% and 125%	Regulatory requirements? • *Except for topical dermatologic corticosteroids where the FDA Guidance requires that Locke's method, which provides an exact confidence interval from untransformed data, be used* (2)

Since the word "topical" is used both for products intended only for local action (dermatological products) and for products to be absorbed into the systemic circulation (transdermal products), consideration must be given to the meaning of the word, "topical," which is defined as "belonging to a place or spot" and misused interchangeably with the word "local." Clear differences thus exist between the intentions and use of these various topical products and their consequential use and expectations.

drug is implied. However, as previously mentioned, this pharmacokinetic approach, which is used for the BE assessment of systemically absorbed drugs, is not considered appropriate to study the bioavailability (BA) and/or BE of topically applied drugs for local action that are not intended to be absorbed into the systemic circulation, since the use of drug concentrations in the systemic circulation cannot be justified to assess the BE of such drugs where no relationship exists between the effectiveness and blood concentrations of drug.

When considering drug products that contain active ingredient(s) not intended for systemic absorption, the FDA has issued the following statement in the U.S. Federal Register (https://www.govregs.com/regulations/21/314.3): "For drug products that are not intended to be absorbed into the bloodstream, bioequivalence may be assessed by scientifically valid measurements intended to reflect the rate and extent to which the active ingredient or active moiety becomes available at the site of drug action."

Table 60.1 depicts the various issues and challenges associated with assessing the BE of topical drugs for local action where the methodologies and assessment approaches for BE are still being developed and also the statistical assessment is yet to be defined, as are specific regulatory requirements.

Figure 60.1 depicts important distinctions in the types of regions targeted following the local application of topical products. This provides important information relating to specific types of topical products and their ultimate therapeutic target sites and intended activities.

- **Topical** products for cutaneous (dermatologic) use are products where the pharmacologic or other effect is confined to the surface of skin or within the skin and may or may not require percutaneous penetration and deposition.
- **Regional** products for treatment of disease or symptoms in deeper tissue are products where the pharmacological action is effected within musculature, vasculature, joints, and synovial fluid beneath and around the application site, e.g., topical antiinflammatory products. These dosage forms are used where more selective activity is required compared to systemic delivery and requires percutaneous absorption and deposition.
- **Transdermal** products for treatment of systemic diseases are aimed at achieving systemically active drug concentrations and where percutaneous absorption is a prerequisite for activity and ideally, no local drug accumulation should occur.

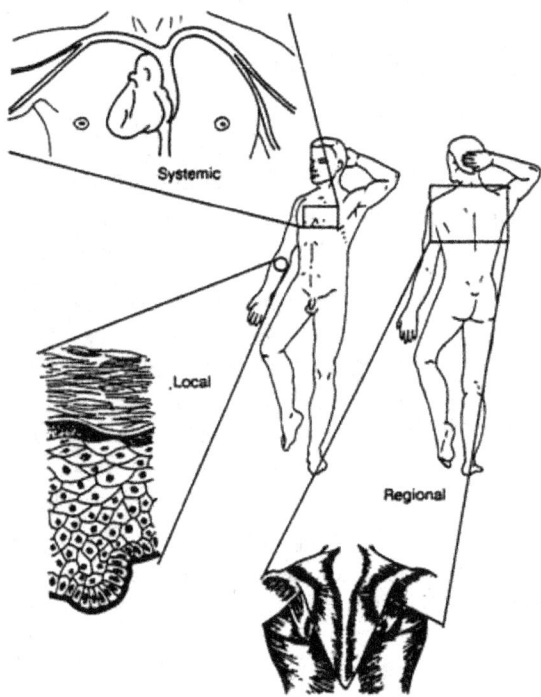

FIGURE 60.1 Specific regions targeted for particular therapy following the local application of various topical products (11).

60.3 PHARMACEUTICAL EQUIVALENCE

According to the FDA, a generic product is required to demonstrate both pharmaceutical equivalence (PE) and BE to be declared therapeutically equivalent to a reference product, the reference listed drug (RLD) (12). A generic product is said to be pharmaceutically equivalent if it contains the same active ingredient in the same amount and same type of dosage form as the RLD. However, it is important to emphasize that pharmaceutical equivalence does not imply bioequivalence per se, as differences in the excipients and/or the manufacturing process can lead to differences in the product performance. According to 21 CFR 314.94 (9) for topical dosage forms, it is necessary for the generic product to have the same excipients and be qualitatively (Q1) and quantitatively (Q2) equivalent to the RLD. Hence, the term *pharmaceutical equivalence* relates to formulation Q1/Q2 sameness where the test and RLD products are qualitatively and quantitatively the same. In addition, as a further requirement, the microstructure, arrangement of matter, and the state of aggregation of the formulation should be established (Q3). Publication of FDA Product-Specific Guidances for Generic Drug Development (13), as well as the recently published draft guideline in 2018 by the EMA (14), address the importance of aspects of the quality (Q1) and equivalence of topical products where the concept of pharmaceutical equivalence is extended to include more comprehensive associated properties such as quantitative (Q2), microstructure aspects (Q3), and product performance. Unfortunately, terms such as "equivalence," "similar," and "sameness," among others, have entered the realm of semantics when describing the development and requirements for market approval of generic semisolid dosage forms intended for local action, thereby creating misunderstandings in the use of methodologies to assess the safety and efficacy of such products to demonstrate BE.

60.4 METHODS TO ASSESS THE BE OF TOPICAL DOSAGE FORMS FOR LOCAL ACTION

When a topical drug product is applied to the skin, the API must be released from the vehicle before it is available for penetration into the stratum corneum and lower layers of the skin (15).

A topical formulation is a complex system, and the kinetics and dynamics of release of the APIs from its vehicle have been the topic of investigation in many research papers (16–20).

BE of topical dosage forms may be demonstrated by comparing the test and reference products using appropriate pharmacokinetic (PK), pharmacodynamic (PD), clinical, or in some instances in vitro tests to obtain a biowaiver (21–33).

Currently, relatively few surrogate approaches to assess the BE of topical dosage forms for local action have been explored apart from the VCA (2) for use to assess the BE of topical corticosteroid products. Most regulatory authorities insist on clinical endpoint studies in patients to confirm BE.

Table 60.2 depicts various options (excluding VCA publications) where descriptions of some methodologies and related data to assess BE have been published:

60.5 BIOWAIVERS

A generic product may be suitable for a biowaiver if its Q1/Q2/Q3 equivalence can be established against the RLD.

In vitro release testing (IVRT) entails measurement of the drug released from the vehicle into a receptor medium, separated by an inert membrane (50) and used to quantify the amount of API released from semisolid dosage forms and to determine its release rate (15). The FDA's SUPAC-SS guidance (51) recognizes IVRT for semisolid dosage forms as a test for product "sameness" following minor formulation, process, and/or manufacturing site related changes to an approved topical dosage form. IVRT has been established as a compendial method by the USP (52) for performance testing of semisolid dosage forms. In addition, IVRT is used to support formulation development, to compare a generic product with innovator formulations, and to determine release data from various formulations used in clinical trials (53). It has been proven to be useful to detect differences in Q1 and Q2 properties between similar products and also the microstructure and arrangement of matter between formulations (Q3) (54). In 2003, the experts from FIP/AAPS pointed out that there was an absence of a standard test protocol that can be applied to all formulations (55). It was suggested that the data obtained from IVRT investigations can be employed as quality indicators and for the screening of the compositions prior to in vivo testing. However, it was noted that in spite of the very fast development of this field, anatomical and physiological factors are not represented in these investigations (56). Until recently, among the numerous publications involving the application of IVRT, comprehensive validation of IVRT systems and methods have been conspicuously absent from the literature. Although various efforts (17, 57, 58) have been made by several researchers to develop a standardized method to measure in vitro drug release from a product using diffusion cells, a comprehensive validation that would be generally applicable to all topical dermatological dosage forms has only recently been published (59).

TABLE 60.2
Options for BE Assessment of Topical Dosage Forms Not Intended to be Absorbed

METHOD	REFERENCES
Dermatopharmacokinetic methods also known as tape stripping (TS)	(34–42)
Dermal microdialysis (DM)	(43–47)
Open-flow microperfusion (dOFM)	(26, 48, 49)
In vitro methods (IVRT) – for "biowaiver" purposes only	See "Biowaivers" section

This is essential to ensure that the developed IVRT method and the associated system have the necessary discriminatory capabilities to determine sameness between products and, more importantly, differences that may affect clinical performance.

Since clinical endpoint studies have been made mandatory by most of the regulatory authorities to establish the safety and efficacy of generic topical products except in the case of topical corticosteroid products wherein a vasoconstrictor or human skin blanching assay is accepted (VCA guidance), an appropriate IVRT method might provide valuable and compelling information to justify waivers of BE studies (biowaivers) for topical semisolid products. In this respect, it is interesting to note that the FDA (13) and the EMA (14) have published guidances recommending the use of IVRT for such purposes.

Over the years, several in vitro methods using excised skin have been developed for the evaluation of drug permeation across the SC, which depends on the interaction between the skin, the drug, and the components in the formulation vehicle (60). The use of vertical diffusion cells (VDC) systems is by far the most commonly used in vitro model for the study of percutaneous absorption. The popularity of this method is due to its simplicity, cost-effectiveness, and easily controllable experimental conditions according to the purpose of investigation.

Historically, in vitro diffusion cells have been employed in the screening of formulations to select promising candidates, in elucidating the effect and mechanism of action of permeation enhancers, and to demonstrate "sameness" after post-approval changes to the product (61).

A simple and reproducible method using VDC system and a synthetic membrane that could be easily adopted for the quality control of semisolid products was first developed and demonstrated by Shah and co-workers in 1989 (62). Since then, IVRT using VDCs has been regarded as one of the most widely accepted and powerful methods for evaluating the release from and stability of semisolid and transdermal dosage forms and for predicting sameness and/or detecting differences (63). It has been acknowledged that sometimes the release of APIs from topical dosage forms during clinical phase trials to establish the therapeutic efficacy could be difficult. A typical example of this is the case of acyclovir ointment where in vitro guidance (64) was published by the FDA in 2012. Subsequently, IVRT has become a promising tool for assessing semisolid dosage forms, including the identification of formulation factors such as Q1/Q2/Q3, which may affect the release of the API (57, 65). More recently, a publication assessing metronidazole topical cream formulations has provided compelling evidence of the value and utility of IVRT to justify a biowaiver for such products (66).

60.6   CONCLUSION

IVRT is acknowledged as a valuable tool in formulation development of topical dosage forms, and a comprehensive review relating to methodology, application, and equipment used in IVRT has been published (67). However, the application of IVRT has many additional benefits such as its use in product development and the provision of some insight of possible in vivo performance and product performance assessment, including batch-to-batch and lot-to-lot uniformity and, importantly, its utility and value to assess the release of API(s) from semisolid dosage forms (67).

A great deal of interest has been shown relating to the use of IVRT data as a surrogate procedure for use as a waiver of BE where the FDA issued the SUPAC guidance issued by the FDA in 1997 (51). Interestingly, whereas in vitro studies have not generally found acceptance by most regulatory agencies to establish bioequivalence, recent FDA draft guidances (13) recommending the use of IVRT provide compelling implications relating to the potential and future applications of IVRT for bioequivalence assessment of topical drug products. Apart from recent publications which have provided important and valuable information and data relating to procedures for validating IVRT methods (59, 67), there are currently no universally acceptable approaches for ensuring the quality, reliability and reproducibility of in vitro release data.

It is important to distinguish differences between the therapeutic intentions and targets of topical dosage forms where such implications are often ignored. A recent editorial entitled "Approaches for Delivery of Drugs Topically" is a clear example that fails to make such an essential distinction in the use of topical drug products (68). Although mention is initially made that "topical dosage forms are being preferred over other dosage forms as they provide local therapeutic effect when applied on the skin or mucous membranes," all further discussion only involves topical dosage forms intended for absorption into the systemic circulation, and no further mention is made of topical dosage forms intended for local action. The main issue involves a consideration whether the active pharmaceutical ingredient (API) is intended for absorption into the systemic circulation, such as application of a transdermal dosage form or whether only local action is required such as in the case of dermatological products. In vitro penetration testing (IVPT) using various types of skin samples as the membranes may be the preferred approach for transdermal products, since topical products intended for the systemic circulation require penetration beyond the stratum corneum and epidermis layers of the skin, whereas topical products used dermatologically for local action are not intended to be absorbed; hence, release only from such dosage forms is the major prerequisite. Since the stratum corneum is the main barrier for percutaneous absorption, the use of human skin as a membrane for topical product diffusion tests is recognized to closely mimic in vivo drug permeation (23). A somewhat incongruous notion is the current regulatory approach which emphasizes the need to apply IVPT to topical products intended for local action (25). The intended use of IVRT is to assess the release of API from the dosage form, whereas application of IVPT is intended to assess permeation into the skin, which is not a prerequisite for topical dosage forms intended for local action.

REFERENCES

1. U.S. FDA, "Guidance for industry: Bioequivalence studies with pharmacokinetic endpoints for drugs submitted under an ANDA," *Guid. Ind.*, no. December, p. 3, 13, 2013.
2. U.S. FDA, "Guidance for industry: Topical dermatologic corticosteroids: In vivo bioequivalence," *Guid. Ind.*, no. June, 1995.
3. United States Food and Drug Administration, Title 21 Code of Federal Regulations (CFR) Part 320, Section 24. http://www.accessdata.fda.gov/scripts/cdrh/cfdocs/cfcfr/CFRSearch.cfm?fr=320.24.
4. Lionberger RA. Innovation for generic drugs: science and research under GDUFA. Clin Pharmacol Ther. 2019; 105(4):878–85.
5. US Code of Federal Regulations, https://www.govregs.com/regulations/21/314.3
6. U.S. Government Accountability Office (U.S. GAO) https://www.gao.gov
7. Gupta R, Shah ND, Ross JS. Generic Drugs in the United States: Policies to Address Pricing and Competition. Clin Pharmacol Ther. 2019; 105(2):329–37.
8. https://www.fda.gov/industry/generic-drug-user-fee-amendments/gdufa-regulatory-science
9. Chang R, Raw A, Lionberger R, Yu L. Generic development of topical dermatologic products: formulation development, process development, and testing of topical dermatologic products. AAPS J. 2013; 15(1):41–52.
10. Generic Drug Product Development: Bioequivalence Issues. Isadore Kanfer and Leon Shargel, Editors, Taylor & Francis, New York, 2007
11. Flynn GL, Weiner ND (1989) Dermal and Transdermal Drug Delivery, Drugs and The Pharmaceutical Sciences, Marcel Dekker, New York, p37.
12. FDA. Orange Book: Approved Drug Products with Therapeutic Equivalence Evaluations 2019. U.S. Food and Drug Administration. https://www.accessdata.fda.gov/scripts/cder/ob/search_product.cfm
13. U.S. FDA. Food and Drug Administration. Office of Generic Drugs. https://www.fda.gov/drugs/guidances-drugs/product-specific-guidances-generic-drugdevelopment.
14. EMA, 2018. Draft guideline on quality and equivalence of topical products. https://www.ema.europa.eu/en/documents/scientific-guideline/draft-guideline-quality-equivalence-topical-products_en.pdf
15. Olejnik A, Goscianska J, Nowak I. Active compounds release from semisolid dosage forms. J Food Drug Anal. 2012; 101(11):4032–45.
16. Shah VP, Elkins JS, Williams RL. Evaluation of the test system used for in vitro release of drugs for topical dermatological drug products. Pharm Dev Technol. 1999; 4(3):377–85.
17. Shah VP, Elkins J, Hanus J, Noorizadeh C, Skelly JP. In vitro release of hydrocortisone from topical preparations and automated procedure. Pharm Res. 1991; 8(1):55–9.
18. Bao Q, Shen J, Jog R, Zhang C, Newman B, Wang Y, et al. In vitro release testing method development for ophthalmic ointments. Int J Pharm. 2017; 526(1–2):145–56.

19. Goebel K, Sato MEO, Souza DF de, Murakami FS, Andreazza IF. In vitro release of diclofenac diethylamine from gels: Evaluation of generic semisolid drug products in Brazil. Brazilian J Pharm Sci. 2013; 49(2):211–9.

20. Rafiee-Tehrani M, Mehramizi A. In vitro release studies of piroxicam from oil-in-water creams and hydroalcoholic gel topical formulations. Drug Dev Ind Pharm. 2000; 26(4):409–14.

21. Shah VP, Flynn G, Yacobi A, Maibach H, Bon C, Fleischer N. Bioequivalence of topical dermatological dosage forms-methods of evaluation of bioequivalence. Skin Pharmacol Appl Skin Physiol. 1998; 11: 117–24.

22. Yacobi A, Shah VP, Bashaw ED, et al. Current challenges in bioequivalence, quality, and novel assessment technologies for topical products. Pharm. Res. 2014;31:837–46.

23. Miranda M, Cardoso C, Vitorino C. Quality and equivalence of topical products: A critical appraisal. Eur J Pharm Sci. 2020;30:148–153.

24. Miranda, M., Sousa, J.J., Veiga, F., Cardoso, C., Vitorino, C., 2018a. Bioequivalence of topical generic products. Part 1: Where are we now? Eur. J. Pharm. Sci. 123, 260–67.

25. Miranda M, Sousa JJ, Veiga F, et al.Bioequivalence of topical generic products. Part 2. Paving the way to a tailored regulatory system. Eur J Pharm Sci. 2018. 122, 264–72.

26. Kanfer I. Methods for the assessment of bioequivalence of topical dosage forms: correlations, optimization strategies, and innovative approaches. In: Topical Drug Bioavailability, Bioequivalence, and Penetration. Springer; 2014. p. 113–51.

27. Syed A R. Approaches for Bioequivalence Assessment of Topical Dermatological Formulations. Advancements Bioequiv Availab.2018; 1(1):5–6. ABB.000503.2018. DOI: 10.31031/ABB.2018.01.000503

28. Lu M, Xing H, Chen X, Xian L, Jiang J, Yang T, et al. Advance in bioequivalence assessment of topical dermatological products. Asian J Pharm Sci. 2016; 11(6):700–7.

29. Narkar Y. Bioequivalence for topical products - an update. Pharm Res. 2010; 27:2590–601.

30. Yacobi A, Shah VP, Bashaw ED, Benfeldt E., Davit B., Ganes D., Ghosh T., Kanfer I., et al. Current Challenges in Bioequivalence, Quality, and Novel Assessment Technologies for Topical Products. Pharm Res.2014; 31:837–46.

31. Borsadia S, Ghanem AH, Seta Y, Higuchi WI, Flynn GL, Behl CR, et al. Factors to be considered in the evaluation of bioavailability and bioequivalence of topical formulations. Skin Pharmacol.1992; 5(3):129–45.

32. Kanfer I, Tettey-Amlalo RNO, Au WL, Hughes-Formella B. Assessment of topical dosage forms intended for local or regional activity. In: Generic Drug Product Development: Specialty Dosage Forms. 2016. p. 54–103.

33. Kanfer I, Strategies for the bioequivalence assessment of topical dosage forms. J Bioequiv Availab 2010; 2: 102–10.

34. Parfitt NR, Skinner M, Bon C, Kanfer I. Bioequivalence of topical clotrimazole formulations: An improved tape stripping method. J Pharm Pharm Sci. 2011; 14(3):347–57.

35. Nallagundla S, Patnala S, Kanfer I. Application of an optimized tape stripping method for the bioequivalence assessment of topical acyclovir creams. AAPS PharmSciTech. 2018; 19(4):1567–73.

36. Au WL, Skinner M, Kanfer I. Comparison of tape stripping with the human skin blanching assay for the bioequivalence assessment of topical clobetasol propionate formulations. J Pharm Pharm Sci.2010; 13(1):11–20.

37. Lademann J, Jacobi U, Surber C, Weigmann HJ, Fluhr JW. The tape stripping procedure -evaluation of some critical parameters. Eur J Pharm Biopharm. 2009; 72(2):317–23.

38. Surber C, Schwarb FP, Smith EW. Tape-stripping technique. J Toxicol—Cut Ocul Toxicol. 2001; 20(4):461–74.

39. Navidi W, Hutchinson A, N'Dri-Stempfer B, Bunge A. Determining bioequivalence of topical dermatological drug products by tape-stripping. J Pharmacokinet Pharmacodyn. 2008; 35(3):337–48.

40. Rath S, Ramanah A, Kanfer I. Dermatopharmacokinetic Assessment of Bio(In)Equivalence of Topical Metronidazole Creams Using Tape Stripping. AAPS Annual Meeting and Exposition, San Antonio, Texas, USA, November 2019

41. Ozdin D, Kanfer, I. Ducharme, MP. Novel Approach for the bioequivalence assessment of topical cream formulations: model-based analysis of tape stripping data correctly concludes BE and BIE. Pharm Res. 2020;37(2), 20–38.

42. Shukla C, Bashaw ED, Stagni G, Benfeldt E. Applications of dermal microdialysis: a review. J Drug Deliv Sci Technol. 2014; 24(3):259–69.

43. Garcia Ortiz P, Hansen SH, Shah VP, Sonne J, Benfeldt E. Are marketed topical metronidazole creams bioequivalent? Evaluation by in vivo microdialysis. Skin Pharmacol Physiol. 2011; 24:44–53.

44. Tettey-Amlalo RNO, Kanfer I, Skinner MF, Benfeldt E, Verbeeck RK. Application of dermal micro-dialysis for the evaluation of bioequivalence of a ketoprofen topical gel. Eur J Pharm Sci. 2009; 36(2–3):219–25.

45. Incecayir T, Agabeyoglu I, Derici U, Sindel S. Assessment of topical bioequivalence using dermal microdialysis and tape stripping methods. Pharm Res. 2011; 28(9):2165–75.

46. Benfeldt E, Hansen SH, Volund A, Menne T, Shah VP. Bioequivalence of topical formulations in humans: evaluation by dermal microdialysis sampling and the dermatopharmacokinetic method. J Invest Dermatol. 2007; 127(1):170–8.

47. Tettey-Amlalo RNO, Kanfer I, Skinner MF, Benfeldt E, Verbeeck RK. Application of dermal micro-dialysis for the evaluation of bioequivalence of a ketoprofen topical gel. Eur J Pharm Sci. 2009; 36(2–3):219–25.

48. Pieber TR, Holmgaard R, Sorensen JA, Nielsen JB, Hofferer C, Sinner F, et al. Comparison of open-flow microperfusion and microdialysis methodologies when sampling topically applied fentanyl and benzoic acid in human dermis ex vivo. Pharm Res. 2012; 29(7):1808–20.

49. Augustin T, Dragatin C, Bodenlenz M, Pieber TR, Kanfer I, Tiffner KI, et al. Open flow microperfusion as a dermal pharmacokinetic approach to evaluate topical bioequivalence. Clin Pharmacokinet. 2017; 56(1):91–8.

50. Shah VP. Progress in methodologies for evaluating bioequivalence of topical formulations. Am J Clin Dermatol. 2001; 2(5):275–80.

51. U.S. Food and Drug Administration. Center for Drug Evaluation and Research. 1997. Guidance for Industry: Nonsterile Semisolid Dosage Forms, Scale-up and Post Approval Changes, Chemistry, Manufacturing, and Control; In vitro Release Testing and In vivo Bioequivalence Documentation (SUPAC-SS). Rockville, USA.

52. USP General Chapter <1724> Semisolid Drug Products — Performance Tests. In: United States Pharmacopeia and National Formulary (USP 41-NF 36). The United States Pharmacopeial Convention. 2018. p. 7944–56.

53. Bashaw ED, Benfeldt E, Davit B, Ganes D, Ghosh T, Kanfer I, et al. Current challenges in bioequivalence, quality, and novel assessment technologies for topical products. Pharm Res. 2014; 31:837–46.

54. Ilić T, Pantelić I, Lunter D, Đorđević S, Marković B, Ranković D, et al. Critical quality attributes, in vitro release and correlated in vitro skin permeation—in vivo tape stripping collective data for demonstrating therapeutic (non)equivalence of topical semisolids: A case study of "ready-to-use" vehicles. Int J Pharm. 2017; 528(1–2):253–67.

55. Aiache J, Aoyagi N, Bashaw D, Brown C, Brown W, Burgess D, et al. FIP/AAPS guidelines to dissolution/in vitro release testing of novel/special dosage forms. AAPS PharmSciTech. 2003; 4(1):1–10.

56. Csoka I, Csanyi E, Zapantis E, Nagy E, Feher-Kiss A, Horvath G, et al. In vitro and in vivo percutaneous absorption of topical dosage forms: case studies. Int J Pharm. 2005; 291:11–9.

57. Klein RR, Bechtel JL, Burchett K, Thakker KD. Technical note: Hydrocortisone as a performance verification test reference standard for in vitro release testing. Dissolution Technol. 2010; 17(4):37–8.

58. Klein RR, Heckart JL, Thakker KD. In vitro release testing methodology and variability with the vertical diffusion cell (VDC). Dissolution Technol. 2018; 25(3):52–61.

59. Tiffner KI, Kanfer I, Augustin T, Raml R, Raney SG, Sinner F. A comprehensive approach to qualify and validate the essential parameters of an in vitro release test (IVRT) method for acyclovir cream, 5%. Int J Pharm. 2018; 535(1–2):217–27.

60. Ng SF, Rouse JJ, Sanderson FD, Eccleston GM. The relevance of polymeric synthetic membranes in topical formulation assessment and drug diffusion study. Arch Pharm Res. 2012; 35(4):579–93.

61. Narkar Y. Bioequivalence for topical products — an update. Pharm Res. 2010; 27:2590–601.

62. Shah VP, Elkins J, Lam S-Y, Skelly JP. Determination of in vitro drug release from hydrocortisone creams. Int J Pharm. 1989; 53(1):53–9.

63. Nallagundla S, Patnala S, Kanfer I. Comparison of in vitro release rates of acyclovir from cream formulations using vertical diffusion cells. AAPS PharmSciTech., 2014; 15(4):994–9.

64. Office of Generic Drugs (OGD), FDA. Draft Guidance on Acyclovir. Recommended Mar 2012.

65. Klein RR, Tao JQ, Wilder S, Burchett K, Bui Q, Thakker KD. Development of an in vitro release test (IVRT) for a vaginal microbicide gel. Dissolution Technol. 2010; 17(4):6–10.

66. Rath SP, Kanfer I. A validated IVRT method to assess topical creams containing metronidazole using a novel approach. Pharmaceutics, Pharmaceutics 2020, 12(2), 119.

67. Kanfer I, Rath S, Purazi P, Mudyahoto NA. In vitro release testing of semi-solid dosage forms. Dissolution Technol. 2017; 24(3):52–60.

68. Murthy, S.N. Approaches for delivery of drugs topically. AAPS PharmSciTech. 2020;21:30.

61 *In Vitro* Human Nail Model to Evaluate Ungual Absorption and Transungual Delivery

Xiaoying Hui and Howard I. Maibach
University of California, San Francisco, California

CONTENTS

61.1 INTRODUCTION

The human nail, equivalent to claws and hooves in other mammals, acts as a protective covering for the delicate tips of the fingers and toes against trauma, enhances the sensation of fine touch, and enables one to retrieve and manipulate objects. The nail is also used for scratching and grooming, as a cosmetic organ, and by some to communicate social status. The appearance of the nail plate is a thin, hard, yet slightly elastic, translucent, convex structure (1).

The human nail anatomy consists of nail plate, nail bed, and nail matrix. The nail plate consists of three layers: the dorsal and intermediate layers derived from the matrix, and the ventral layer from the nail bed (2, 3). The upper (dorsal) layer is only a few cell layers thick and consists of hard keratin. It constitutes the main barrier to drug diffusion into and through the nail plate. The intermediate layer constitutes three quarters of the whole nail thickness, and consists of soft keratin. Below the intermediate layer is the ventral layer of soft keratin—a few cells thick—that connects to the underlying nail bed, in which many pathological changes occur. Thus, in the treatment of nail diseases, achieving an effective drug concentration in the ventral nail plate is of great importance. The nail bed consists of noncornified soft tissue under the nail plate. It is highly vascularized. Beneath the nail bed is the nail matrix, which is a heavily vascularized thick layer of highly proliferative epithelial tissue that forms the nail plate.

The human nail is approximately 100 times thicker than the stratum corneum, and both are rich in keratin. However, they exhibit some physical and chemical differences (4, 5). The nail possesses high sulfur content (cystine) in its hard keratin domain, whereas the stratum corneum does not. The total lipid content of the nail ranges from 0.1% to 1%, as opposed to approximately 10% for the stratum corneum. This suggests that the role of the lipid pathway in the nail plate is probably of much less importance than that in the stratum corneum. The human nail acts like a hydrophilic gel membrane, while the stratum corneum acts like a lipophilic partition membrane.

Under average conditions, the nail contains 7% to 12% water, in comparison to 25% in the stratum corneum. At 100% relative humidity, the maximal water content in the nail is approximately 25%, in sharp contrast to the stratum corneum that can increase its water content to 200% to 300%. The rate of chemical penetration into and through the human nail depends upon its water solubility (4) and its molecular size (5).

Disorders of the nail resulting from a variety of conditions such as infections or physical-chemical damage can result in painful and debilitating states, and often change the appearance of the nail plate. Onychomycosis is the most common nail plate disorder (6). It thickens the nail, makes it white and opaque, and causes pain while wearing shoes. Onychomycosis is a fungal infection of the nail plate—usually caused by the species *Epidermophyton, Microsporum*, and *Trichophyton*— and it affects 14% of the human population. Aging increases the incidence significantly, with the rate estimated to be 48% in persons 70 years of age (7).

To cure the infection, the patient is obliged to take oral systemic medication for an extended period, generally months, or undergo surgical nail removal (8). These treatments have adverse effects such as pain (surgery) and systemic side effects (oral treatment). Thus, topical therapy is the most desirable approach, but has met with limited success to date. Topical therapy is limited by the infection's deep-seated nature and by the ineffective penetration of the deep nail plate by topically applied drugs (9, 10).

Clinical efficacy of a topical anti-onychomycosis drug may be due to keratin-binding affinity, which determines drug permeability into and through the full-thickness nail plate, and free-drug concentrations or anti-dermatophytic activities in the presence of keratin (4). Thus, keratin affinity of topical drugs is an important physicochemical property affecting therapeutic efficacy. To be effective, topical drugs must penetrate the nail bed and retain their antifungal activity within the nail matrix, both of which are adversely affected by keratin binding (5).

Topical therapy for onychomycosis has been largely ineffective, and this failure may be due to poor penetration of drugs into and through the nail plate (9). The nail's unique properties, particularly its thickness and relatively compact construction, make it a formidable barrier to the entry of topically applied agents (10). The concentration of an applied drug across the nail dropped about 1000-fold from the outer surface to the inner surface (11). As a result, the drug concentration presumably had not reached a therapeutically effective level in the inner ventral layer.

The existing clinical evidence suggests that a key to successful treatment of onychomycosis by a topical antifungal product lies in effectively overcoming the nail barrier. Currently available topical treatments have limited effectiveness, possibly because they cannot sufficiently penetrate the nail plate to transport a therapeutically sufficient quantity of antifungal drug to the target sites (12) and eradicate the infection.

To achieve an effective chemical concentration into and through the human nail plate, penetration enhancers that tend to promote diffusion through the skin's horny layer have been studied. However, these studies were conducted on a few limited nail penetration models that may not provide an intimate contact between the receptor compartment and the nail surface, and the nail plate can be easily hydrated beyond normal levels (4, 5, 10, 12, 13). Moreover, nail samples prepared with scalpel or sandpaper are time consuming, and may be not accurate (3, 14).

How can topical drugs be delivered effectively into the nail? And, perhaps as importantly, how can the drug content in the human nail be assessed in order to validate nail drug delivery? Our challenge was to develop a system to assay drug content in the inner nail bed in which the infection resides. During last two decades, we developed a micrometer-controlled drilling instrument that removes and collects from the inner nail bed a powder sample from which—by mass balance recovery—we can determine the amount of penetrated radio-labeled drug. With such an assay procedure, the effectiveness of topical nail drug delivery can be assessed (15, 16). This chapter reviews the results of studies undertaken with the *in vitro* nail incubation device and micrometer controlled drilling-sampling instrument and discusses *in vitro* nail penetration researches conducted with the system.

61.2 *IN VITRO* NAIL STUDY MODEL

61.2.1 NAIL INCUBATION DEVICE

An inline one-chamber diffusion cell (PermeGear, Inc., Hellertown, PA) was selected to hold a human finger (or toe) nail plate (Figure 61.1). The nail plate was placed on a ledge inside the donor chamber with the dorsal surface facing up to the open air. This allows evenly applying 10 ± 5 μl liquid or 15 ± 5 μl ointment formulations on the opened nail surface (1 cm²). The ventral (inner) surface of the nail was placed face down and rested on the wetted cotton pad, as natural cotton fiber has strong absorbent capacity for both hydrophilic and lipophilic chemicals. To approximate physiological conditions, the cotton pad was wetted with approximately 0.3 mL (0.01 M, pH 7.4) and then placed in the receiving chamber to serve as a nail supporting bed that provides moisture for the nail plate. Each cotton pad was removed and replaced at least once daily during the experiment period. If the testing chemical was lipophilic, additional 6% volpo would be mixed with the phosphate buffer solution to increase chemical solubility in the wetted cotton pad (15, 16).

61.2.2 NAIL DRILLING/SAMPLING INSTRUMENT

The human nail plate consists of three layers with different components, thickness, and densities. Therefore, drug penetration rate into and through each layer is also different. To determine drug concentration within each layer of the nail plate, we developed a unique micrometer-controlled nail sampling instrument to sample the inner core of the nail without disturbing the nail surface. The two nail center parts (surface/intermediate and inner core/intermediate) can be collected and assayed separately. The surface contains only residual drug after washing. The drilled out core (from the ventral side) is thus a true drug measurement at the target site where the disease resides (Figure 61.2). Drug penetration into the nail was sampled by this nail sampling instrument that enabled finely controlled drilling into the nail and collection of the powder created by the drilling process. The nail sampling instrument (Figure 61.3) has two parts: a nail sample stage and a drill. The nail sampling stage consists of a copper nail holder, three adjustments, and a nail powder capture. The three adjustments control vertical movement. The first coarse adjustment (on the top) is for changing the copper cell and taking powder samples from the capture. The other two adjustments (lower) are used in sampling. The second coarse adjustment allows movement of 25 mm, while the fine adjustment provides movement of 0.20 mm. The nail powder capture is located between the copper cell and the cutter. The inner shape of the capture is an inverted funnel with the end

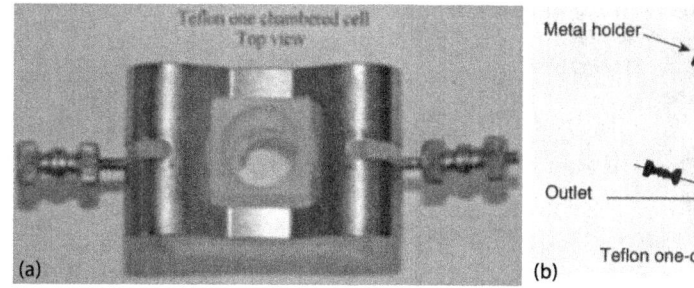
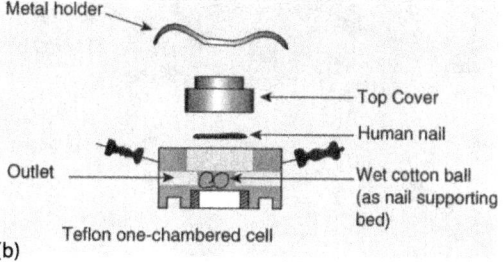

FIGURE 61.1 *In vitro* nail incubation device: (a) one-chamber diffusion cell top view, (b) one-chamber diffusion cell components, and side view. (From reference 17.)

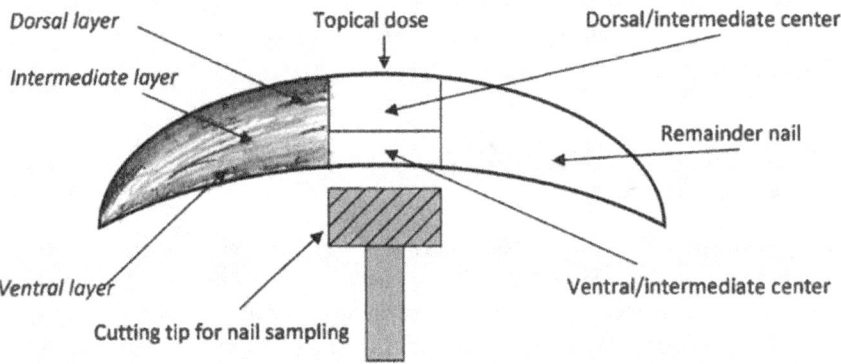

FIGURE 61.2   Schematic of the precise microdrilling technique for assessing depth of penetration.

connected to a vacuum pump. By placing a filter paper inside the funnel, nail powder samples can be captured on the filter paper during sampling. The nail is fastened in a cutting holder below the cutter and surrounded by a funnel containing a filter paper. The funnel is attached to a vacuum pump. During drilling, the vacuum draws the powder debris onto the filter paper so it can be collected and measured.

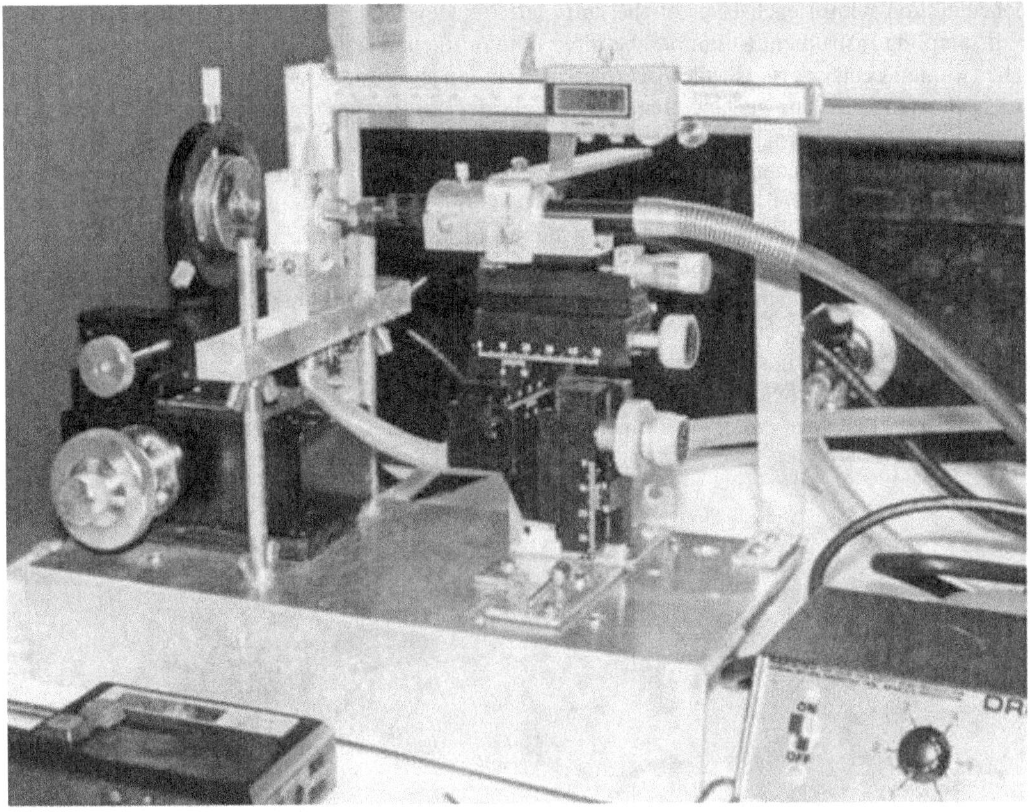

FIGURE 61.3   The micrometer-controlled drilling and nail powder removal instrument. (From reference 17.)

After completion of the dosing, incubation, and surface-washing phases, the nail plate was transferred from the diffusion cell to a clean cutting holder for sampling. The nail plate was secured in position so that the ventral surface faced the cutter and the dorsal-dosed surface faced the holder. The cutting holder was moved to bring the plate surface just barely in contact with the cutter tip. The drill was then turned on and a fine adjustment moved the stage toward the cutter tip, removing a powder sample from the nail. In this way, a hole approximately 0.3 to 0.4 mm in depth and 7.9 mm in diameter was drilled in each nail, enabling the harvest of powder sample from the center of each nail's ventral surface. We will refer to these samples as having been taken from the "ventral/intermediate nail plate."

After the nail had delivered its ventral/intermediate nail plate powder samples, it was removed from the sampling instrument. The nail outside the dosing area was cut and saved separately; we refer to this as the "nondosed surrounding edge." The dorsal layer above the sampling area where the powder samples were taken we referred to as the "dorsal/intermediate nail plate." The ventral/intermediate nail plate powdered samples, the dorsal/intermediate nail plate, and the surrounding edge nail plate were individually collected into a glass scintillation vial and weighed. The nail samples were then dissolved by adding 3 to 5 mL of a Packard Soluene-350 (Packard Instrument Company, Meriden, CT). The total mass of nail collected was measured by the difference in weight of the plate before and after drilling (15, 16).

61.2.3 ADVANTAGES OF THE *IN VITRO* STUDY MODEL

The average of hydration of the wetted cotton pads was 109 ± 6.2 AU (Table 61.1) that resembles the average hydration of the human nail bed, 99.9 ± 8.9 AU measured from fresh human cadavers, where AU is arbitrary units, a digital expression of capacitance. During the experiment, the holding tank for cells had temperature at $25 \pm 2°C$ and relative humidity $44 \pm 8\%$. Thus, there was no statistical difference between hydration conditions for nails treated with either the test formulation or the saline control. The advantage of this incubation device is that it is nonocclusive and hydration controlled, and approximate normal physical condition is reached (17).

The sampling instrument allows well-controlled, accurate, and reproducible sampling of the inside of the nail. Table 61.2 shows that the average depth of nail sampling from the inner center surface was well controlled at 0.33 ± 0.07 mm, which was close to the expected depth of 0.33 mm. The weight of the nail samples collected was consistent for all experiments. The advantage of the micrometer controlled drilling and nail powder removal system is the accuracy of the sampling process.

TABLE 61.1
Hydration of Nail Plate and Nail Bed

Measurement			Hydration (AU)*	
Source	N	Time	Nail Plate	Nail Bed
Human Cadavers	6	24-hr postmortem	7.6 ± 0.9	99.9 ± 8.9
Diffusion Cells	8	Twice/day for 7 days	8.5 ± 2.4	109.9 ± 6.2

Note: During the experiment, the holding device had temperature $25 \pm 2°C$ and relative humidity was $44 \pm 8\%$.

*Hydration of the nail plate and the supporting cotton bed was measured with a Corneometer CM 820 (Courage & Khazaka, Cologne, Germany).

Abbreviations: AU is arbitrary units, a digital expression of capacitance.

Source: From Reference (17).

TABLE 61.2
Nail Core Sampled from the Ventral (Inner) Surface Center of The Human Nail Platt

Test chemicals	Whole Nail Thickness (mm)	Nail Core Sampled from the Ventral (Inner) Surface Center of the Nail Platea		
		Depth of Core (mm)	% Whole Nail Thickness	Powder Sample Collected (mg)
Ciclopirox (8%)[18]	0.65 ± 0.17	0.29 ± 0.10	44.9 ± 11.7	5.3 ± 3.8
Econazole (5%)[19]	0.76 ± 0.17	0.42 ± 0.16	53.8 ± 10.4	9.8 ± 3.9
Efinaconazole (10%)*	0.82 ± 0.19	0.42 ± 0.04	52.8 ± 11.0	5.7 ± 1.3
Ketoconazole (2%)[15]	0.68 ± 0.05	0.28 ± 0.03	41.9 ± 1.2	6.7 ± 2.6
Luliconazole (1%)*	0.85 ± 0.14	0.38 ± 0.11	44.4 ± 11.5	11.2 ± 3.9
Salicylic acid (2%)[19]	0.77 ± 0.07	0.25 ± 0.08	32.6 ± 9.4	6.0 ± 0.5
Tavaborole (10%)[16]	0.68 ± 0.17	0.32 ± 0.11	47.3 ± 10.5	6.9 ± 2.7
Terbinafine (1%)[22]	0.76 ± 0.25	0.31 ± 0.11	42.2 ± 9.1	6.6 ± 3.3

Note: Each number represents mean ± S.D. of five to six samples.

*Unpublished data.

Nail sample area, approximately 0.24 mm in depth and 7.9 mm in diameter, was drilled from the center of the ventral surface of the nail. The amount of nail sample removed was measured by difference in weight and depth of the drilled area before and after sampling.

The mass balance as total applied radioactive recovery of eight [^{14}C]-antifungal agents: ciclopirox (18), econazole (19), efinaconazole, ketoconazole (15), luliconazole, salicylic acid (19), tavaborole (16), and terbinafine (22) following a 14-day nail treatment was summarized in Table 61.3. The overall recovery range of these agents was from 88% to 102%, indicating that essentially the entire doses were accounted for, in which approximately 64% to 98% was removed with the wash method from the dosed surface. The ventral/intermediate nail center (deep nail plate) sample collected beneath the dose area proves the test chemical permeated vertically from the surface. After the deep

TABLE 61.3
Mass Balance of Eight Antifungal Chemicals Following 14-Day Human Nail Incubation *In vitro*

Test Chemicals	Radioactive Recovery as Percentage of Applied Dose (% D)				
	Surface Residue	Nail Plate	Deep Nail Layer	Cotton Pad	Mass Balance
Ciclopirox (8%)[18]	85.2 ± 21.0	3.9 ± 1.6	0.1 ± 0.1	0.05 ± 0.08	89.3 ± 1.6
Econazole (5%)[19]	72.4 ± 4.8	15.5 ± 5.0	1.1 ± 0.8	1.0 ± 0.1	89.0 ± 3.4
Efinaconazole (10%)*	91.5 ± 4.6	1.3 ± 0.5	0.1 ± 0.0	1.3 ± 0.7	94.0 ± 3.2
Ketoconazole (2%)[15]	97.9 ± 27.2	2.6 ± 1.7	0.8 ± 0.3	3.1 ± 2.0	102.8 ± 3.6
Luliconazole (1%)*	65.0 ± 25.4	19.7 ± 7.2	2.2 ± 1.1	16.3 ± 2.6	102.3 ± 10.8
Salicylic acid (2%)[19]	91.2 ± 4.5	8.1 ± 4.7	0.6 ± 0.3	10.7 ± 2.0	86.8 ± 9.6
Tavaborole (10%)[16]	68.4 ± 10.7	26.0 ± 8.2	0.7 ± 0.3	1.4 ± 0.1	95.8 ± 5.9
Terbinafine (1%)[22]	87.4 ± 34.9	7.9 ± 3.1	0.5 ± 0.2	0.3 ± 0.1	95.8 ± 3.3

Note: Each number represents mean ± S.D. of five to six samples.

*Unpublished data.

nail plate, the chemical penetrated further down to the nail supporting bed (cotton pad) samples. These two pieces of data give important information related to the drug's nail absorption/penetration capacities and deep concentrations.

With this *in vitro* nail penetration model, the drug can be measured in the dorsal/intermediate layers, the ventral/intermediate layers, and cotton pad/nail supporting bed samples to determine the distances and levels of the drug penetration. Table 61.4 provides weight normalized concentrations (μg eq./g) of eight antifungal agents: ciclopirox (18), econazole (19), efinaconazole, ketoconazole (15), luliconazole, ME1111 (20,21), tavaborole (16), and terbinafine (22) in the deep nail plate, ventral/intermediate layer and cotton pad, and nail supporting bed samples. These values determined not only the transungual delivery rate and kinetics but also antifungal efficacies with corresponding minimum inhibitory concentration (MIC) values. Antifungal efficacy is calculated by the ratio of an antifungal agent concentration in the deep nail sample (μg/g) to MIC. The MIC is an important laboratory index to determine antifungal potency. The value of an antifungal agent is defined as the lowest antifungal concentration at which no growth is visible in the wells when detected visually (80% to 100% inhibition). The MIC_{90} values, the minimum concentration of eight antifungal agents that inhibited 90% of *T. rubrum* isolates (MIC90), are shown in Table 61.4. The antifungal efficacy of these agents' concentration in the deep nail layer or the nail bed could be a few orders of magnitude greater than the MIC deemed necessary to inhibit the growth of the causative dermatophyte species. However, one has to keep in mind that keratin affinity of each agent should be concluded with related MIC value to assess antifungal efficacy.

Keratin affinity is an important physicochemical property affecting the efficiency of antifungal agents' permeability into and through the nail plate following topical or systemic administration (28). If a high-keratin-affinity drug is administered topically, the drug may cumulate in the nail surface- dorsal layer and has insufficient amount to release and diffusion to the deep part: the ventral layer and the bed. In addition, the drug needs to be an unbound form to exert

---

TABLE 61.4

Analysis of Efficacy Coefficient of Eight Antifungal Agents

Chemicals	MIC_{90} *T. rubrum*	Deep Nail Plate (ventral/intermediate center)		Cotton Pad (nail supporting bed)	
	pH = 7.0 μg/mL	Concentration μg/g	Efficacy	Concentration μg/g	Efficacy
Ciclopirox (8%)[18]	0.25[23]	310 ± 80	1240 ± 320	52 ± 10	206 ± 41
Econazole (5%)[19]	8[24]	8890 ± 3098	1111 ± 387	294 ± 46	37 ± 6
Efinaconazole (10%)*	0.008[23, 27]	67.7 ± 55.6	8459 ± 6950	1.54 ± 0.83	193 ± 104
Ketoconazole (2%)[15]	0.5[25]	810 ± 390	1620 ± 780	180 ± 90	360 ± 180
Luliconazole (1%)*	0.0002[26]	3.49E ± 1.58E (×10⁵)	1.75E ± 0.79E (×10⁹)	1922 ± 309	9.61E ± 1.55E (10⁶)
ME1111 (10%)[20,21]	0.25[20]	2884 ± 924	11536 ± 3696	121 ± 27	484 ± 108
Tavaborole (10%)[16]	81[6]	6000 ± 748	750 ± 94	726 ± 176	91 ± 22
Terbinafine (1%)[22]	0.125[24, 27]	487 ± 132	3896 ± 1056	27 ± 1.2	216 ± 10

Note: Each number represents mean ± S.D. of five to six samples.

*Unpublished data.

The MIC is an important laboratory index to determine of antifungal potency. The value of an antifungal agent is defined as the lowest antifungal concentration at which no growth is visible in the wells when detected visually (80%–100% inhibition). The MIC_{90} values is the minimum concentration of eight antifungal agents that inhibited 90% of *T. rubrum*.

Antifungal efficacy is calculated by the ratio of an antifungal agent concentration in the deep nail sample (μg/g) to MIC isolates (MIC_{90}).

its therapeutic effects. In such a case, high drug concentration in the plate and high calculated antifungal efficacy (nail concentration to MIC_{90}) may not be equivalent to the local treatment efficiency. Additional measurements, such as binding affinity to human nail keratin and keratin effect on antifungal activity, should be considered to estimate the *in vitro* antifungal efficacy coefficients of the antifungal agent (20).

61.3   CASE STUDY OF NAIL ABSORPTION AND PENETRATION WITH THE *IN VITRO* NAIL MODEL

61.3.1   *IN VITRO* HUMAN NAIL PENETRATION AND KINETICS OF PANTHENOL

Panthenol, the alcohol form of pantothenic acid (vitamin B5), is believed to act as a humectant and improve the flexibility and strength of nails. $[^{14}C]$-panthenol (2%) in a polymer gel nail lacquer was dosed daily for 7 days on a human figure nail for 7 days (29). Panthenol concentrations were determined in the dorsal surface, in the interior (by drilling and removal), and in the supporting bed under the human nail (17).

The flux of panthenol through the nail plate reached steady state within 24 hours (Table 61.5). The average flux in the interior nail plate was 10.25 ± 2.75 g equivalent panthenol/cm^2/hr and in the nail supporting cotton bed (completely through the nail) was 1.47 ± 0.79 g/cm^2/hr. The cumulative panthenol concentration in and through the nail layers increased linearly with time (Figure 61.1) and can be mathematically predicted as follows:

Dorsal/intermediate nail layer: Panthenol concentration (mg. eq/g) = $-0.20 + (0.054*hr)$,

$$\text{Slope of the line} = 0.054 \left(R^2 = 0.94, p < 0.001 \right)$$

Ventral/intermediate nail layer: Panthenol concentration. (mg. eq/g) = $-0.29 + (0.021*hr)$,

$$\text{Slope of the line} = 0.021 \left(R^2 = 0.87, p < 0.001 \right)$$

Nail supporting bed cotton ball: Panthenol concentration (mg. eq/g) = $-0.07 + (0.004*hr)$,

$$\text{Slope of the line} = 0.004 \left(R^2 = 0.79, p = 0.003 \right)$$

The main barrier to drug permeation in the human nail plate is attributed to be in the nail surface– dorsal layer that has a very condensed keratin structure and causes low diffusivity of the drug (19). As can be seen in Figure 61.4, the slope of the panthenol concentration vs. time curve of the

---

TABLE 61.5

Flux of Panthenol into and through the Human Nail Plate from the Nail Treatment

	Flux (µg equivalent panthenol/cm^2/hr)							
Incubation time (hours)	24	48	72	96	120	144	168	Average
Ventral/intermediate nail center	12 ± 2.6	8 ± 0.5	7 ± 1.7	8 ± 0.8	13 ± 0.4	13 ± 1.8	14 ± 4.9	10 ± 2.8
Supporting nail bed (cotton pad)	0.5 ± 0.2	2.3 ± 0.9	1.6 ± 0.6	1.4 ± 0.3	1.2 ± 0.2	1.8 ± 0.7	3.0 ± 1.2	1.5 ± 0.8

Note: Each value represents the mean (SD) of three samples. The data gives the daily flux rate of panthenol penetrating into and through the nail plate in the lacquer group. Steady-state fluxes of panthenol were reached within 24 hours and lasted over the dosing period.

Source: The table was modified from reference (29) with permission.

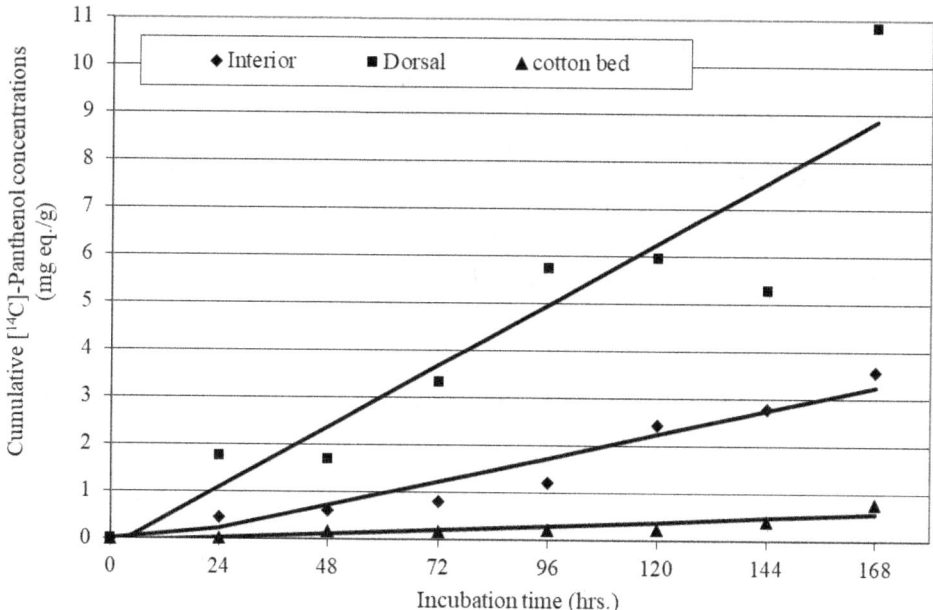

FIGURE 61.4 Each line and symbol represent the mean and standard deviation of three samples This shows that the concentration over time of panthenol was highest at the dorsal layer, suggesting that the affinity of panthenol to the dorsal nail plate was high and therefore, a factor in the relatively low diffusivity compared to that at the deeper layers of the nail plate. (Modified from reference 29 with permission.)

dorsal/intermediate layer (surface) is higher than that of the ventral/intermediate layer (interior), which was higher than that for the supporting bed cotton ball. This shows that the concentration over time of panthenol was highest at the dorsal layer, suggesting that the affinity of panthenol to the dorsal nail plate was high; therefore, it is a factor in the relatively low diffusivity compared to that at the deeper layers of the nail plate.

The variation in the diffusion rates of panthenol as a function of location within the nail plate is similar to the diffusion behavior of 5-fluorouracil, another small water-soluble molecule into the human nail plate, which was explored in an *in vitro* study conducted by Kobayashei et al (30). They concluded that the drug permeation characteristics of the layers of the human nail plate are as follows: the dorsal layer is characterized by low diffusivity to substances; the intermediate layer is characterized by low lipophilicity, and higher diffusion rates of hydrophilic molecules; and the ventral layer is characterized by high lipophilicity and diffusion rates that can be lower than that of the intermediate layer. These researchers found that the diffusion rates of their probe molecules were faster in the interior of the nail plate than the dorsal or ventral layers. Our observed panthenol kinetic data are consistent with their findings (29).

In conclusion, this kinetic study shows the effectiveness of enhancement of transungual panthenol delivery into and through the deep layer of the human nail plate. It thus provide the basis for examining vehicle effects on the delivery of actives into human nail and may stimulate investigation into enhanced activity in nail formulations (29).

61.3.2 ONYCHOPHARMACOKINETICS OF NEW TERBINAFINE HYDROCHLORIDE TOPICAL FORMULATION

Terbinafine HCl is a potent antifungal agent active against a broad spectrum of fungi, including dermatophytes, filamentous and dimorphic organisms, and some yeasts (31). Though terbinafine

HCl is effective after both oral and topical skin administration, it has poor nail penetration. This is because the human nail behaves similarly to a hydrogel rather than a lipophilic membrane such as the stratum corneum. Water solubility and the small molecular size of a drug are the likely characteristics enabling its penetration into the nail plate (32, 33), but not for lipophilic chemicals such as terbinafine HCl. It has relative large molecular weight (327.9), high log P (5.53), and high keratin-binding affinity. This results in the difficulty of its nail absorption and penetration.

To determine the capacity of terbinafine HCl nail penetration, designation of this topical formulation focused on selecting appropriate vehicles and the incorporation of penetration enhancers to alter terbinafine HCl's solubility and allow the chemical to overcome the nail barrier to reach the deeper layers.

The formulation applied in this experiment contained 1% of terbinafine HCl in solid form in a vehicle consisting of ethyl acetate, propylene glycol, urea, polymethylmetacrylate, lactic acid, Tween 80, sodium hydroxide, and EDTA in decreasing order of content. These components can soften the nail plate, increase nail hydration, and enhance nail penetration. Moreover, approximately 90% of the formulation is volatile, and after evaporation, the content of terbinafine HCl retained on the nail surface reaches about 10%. Terbinafine HCl is soluble in the remaining formulation that benefits its nail absorption and penetration. This study determined *in vitro* onychopharmacokinetics of [^{14}C]-terbinafine HCl in this new topical formulation into and through the human finger nail using the *in vitro* finite dose model applied daily for 14 days (22).

To evaluate the effect of a topical antifungal formulation, it is important to know if a sufficient drug concentration is achieved in the treated tissues after topical application. In this *in vitro* nail penetration model, the amount of drug was measured daily in the cotton pad and nail supporting bed samples to determine the penetration rate and kinetics. Figure 61.5 shows the time profile of the terbinafine HCl flux rate (µg/day) in the cotton pad and nail supporting bed samples. After the first dose application, the amount of terbinafine HCl penetrating through the nail plate and

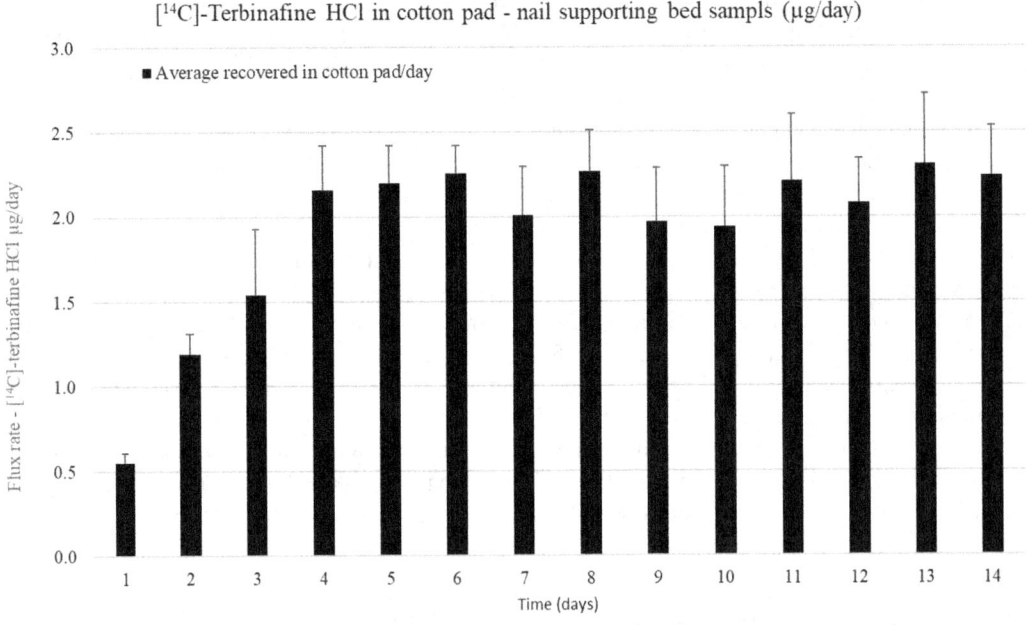

FIGURE 61.5 Time profile of terbinafine HCl flux rate (µg/day) in cotton pad/nail supporting bed samples. After the first dose application, the amount of terbinafine HCl quickly penetrated through the nail plate and the concentration in the cotton pad increased linearly until day 5 and then remained constant. Each bar represents the mean (S.D.) of 10 replicates. (From reference 22.)

the concentration in the cotton pad rapidly increased linearly until day 5 (after 96 hours) and then remained constant. The volume of the receiving chamber of the inline diffusion cell used is approximately 1 mL. Therefore, the amount of terbinafine HCl penetrating through the nail plate daily into the wetted cotton pad sample (as the nail bed model) can be expressed as 1.9 ± 0.6 $\mu g/cm^3$ on average ($\pm$ S.D.), or as the total cumulative amount for 14 days 27 ± 1.2 $\mu g/cm^3$.

Onychomycosis is a disease of the deep nail plate and/or the nail bed. In this *in vitro* nail penetration model, the drug was measured in the dorsal/intermediate layers, ventral/intermediate layers, and cotton pad/nail supporting bed samples to determine the depth and levels of the drug penetration. The percentage of the applied dose retrieved by radioactive recovery from the dorsal/intermediate layers, the ventral/intermediate layers, and the cotton pad/nail supporting bed samples were 0.70 ± 0.05, 2.50 ± 0.47, and $2.03 \pm 0.13\%$, respectively. After weight normalization, the terbinafine HCl mass equivalent was 613 ± 145, the nail weight was 487 ± 132 $\mu g/g$, and the nail bed sample was 27 ± 1.2 $\mu g/nail$ after 14 days of multidose application.

The concentration of terbinafine HCl in the deeper nail plate (ventral/intermediate layers) and the cotton pad and nail bed samples from this study compared with the nail concentration data following oral onychomycosis treatment in the literature show important differences. For example, Faergemann et al. (34) found that 0.39 $\mu g/g$ nail tissue was present in a patient population after 28 days of oral terbinafine treatment. Dykes et al. (35) found 0.6 $\mu g/g$ in the nail after 12 weeks of treatment. Schatz et al. (36) found 0.6 to 1.2 $\mu g/g$ in the nail after 6 and 12 weeks of oral treatment, respectively. The data from this study show that higher amounts of terbinafine HCl were attained in the deep nail plate and/or the nail bed after a 14-day topical treatment with this topical formulation *in vitro*.

In conclusion, this novel terbinafine HCl topical formulation enhanced its penetration into and through human nail and suggested the terbinafine HCl topical formulation has the potential to be an effective topical treatment for onychomycosis. Although a bioequivalent comparison between the oral *in vivo* nail clipping data to our topical onychopharmacokinetic data requires direct comparative studies, the current *in vitro* data appear sufficient to justify controlled clinical trials (22).

61.3.3 COMPARISON NAIL ABSORPTION, DISTRIBUTION, AND PERMEATION RATES OF TWO ANTIFUNGAL AGENTS

The human nail behaves similarly to a hydrogel rather than a lipophilic membrane such as the stratum corneum. To overcome the nail's unique properties such as thickness and compact construction and the infection's deep-seated nature, selecting an appropriate antifungal agent based on its water solubility—more hydrophilicity—and small molecular size is the likely characteristic to enable its penetration into the nail plate (37).

A ciclopirox nail lacquer formulated as Penlac is currently the only topical treatment approved for use against onychomycosis in the United States that has poor clinical efficacy. It is at least partially attributed to its lipophilicity, log P (3.09), and molecular weight (207).

A new class of boron-containing compounds, oxaboroles, recently demonstrated broad-spectrum antifungal activity against yeast, molds, and dermatophytes. Among these compounds 5-fluoro-1,3-dihydro-1-hydroxy-2,1-benzoxaborole (Tavaborole) was the most effective, especially against the dermatophytes *T. rubrum* and *T. mentagrophytes*, fungal pathogens that are the primary cause of onychomycosis (38). Tavaborole has a smaller molecular weight (152) and lower log P (1.24) than ciclopirox. This *in vitro* nail penetration study aimed to compare the *in vitro* nail penetration efficacy of tavaborole in ethanol/propylene glycol (4:1) formulation to the topical onychomycosis drug, ciclopirox, formulated in its commercial nail lacquer in a 14-day experiment (16).

Results provided the concentration of tavaborole or ciclopirox in each section of the nail samples are shown in Table 61.6. After weight normalization, the concentration of tavaborole in the dorsal/intermediate section, ventral/intermediate section, and remainder of the nail samples was

TABLE 61.6

Comparison of Concentrations of Tavaborole and Ciclopirox in Nail Plate and Supporting Bed Samples after 14-Day Treatment

Samples	Time Collected (hours post dose)	Comparison of Two Antifungal Agents		
		Tavaborole	Ciclopirox	p-Value
		(Radioactivity as μg equivalent/mg sample)		
Dorsal/intermediate nail center	360	25.7 ± 8.8	7.4 ± 3.5	0.0008
Ventral/intermediate nail center	360	20.5 ± 4.7	3.1 ± 2.1	0.0001
Remainder nondosed nail edge	360	26.1 ± 12.4	4.4 ± 2.7	0.0022
		(Radioactivity as μg equivalent/sample)		
Cotton pad	72	61 ± 61	1.1 ± 2.0	0.0043
Cotton pad	144	216 ± 187	2.4 ± 4.7	0.0022
Cotton pad	216	605 ± 541	4.2 ± 7.7	0.0022
Cotton pad	288	1283 ± 1175	5.6 ± 9.4	0.0022
Cotton pad	360	2241 ± 1733	8.9 ± 13.1	0.0022

Note: Each number represents the mean ± SD of each group ($n = 6$). Tavaborole has superior penetration compared to ciclopirox and achieves levels within and under the nail plate that suggest it has the potential to be an effective topical treatment for onychomycosis.

significantly higher than that of ciclopirox ($p < 0.002$). The cumulative amounts of tavaborole or ciclopirox found in the cotton ball supporting bed samples were measured every 3 days (72 hours) after the first dose application until the end of the study (Table 61.6). The amount of tavaborole found in the cotton ball samples was significantly higher than that of ciclopirox ($p < 0.05$). By study's end, the amount of tavaborole found in the cotton balls amounted to approximately 250 times that of ciclopirox.

In conclusion, this nail penetration study shows a superior permeation capability of tavaborole into and through the normal human nail plate *in vitro* compared to the commercial treatment, ciclopirox. Concentrations of tavaborole delivered in the deep nail layer and nail bed were significantly higher than the ciclopirox controls. Tavaborole is a good potential to candidate as an antionychomycosis agent due to its hydrophilicity, small molecular weight, and antifungal capacity (16).

61.4 DISCUSSION

A significant difference between the human nail and the stratum corneum is that the lipid content of the nail plate is much less than that of stratum corneum. The absolute rate of water transpiration from the nail therefore is faster than intact skin. A hydrated nail plate could behave like a hydrogel membrane in its barrier properties. This is particularly observed in some *in vitro* human nail studies that use conventional methods to incubate the nail plate in contact with an aqueous solution during the process. As the result, nail plate hydration and swelling were induced and nail porosity increased. This may cause a false-positive result in transungual drug delivery(15, 19)

To mimic physiological conditions for the *in vitro* nail study, we modified one-chamber inline diffusion cells with additional controlled nail hydration and temperature and an environmental humidity device (Figure 61.1). A small piece of saline wetted cotton in the receiving chamber of the cell functions not only as a "nail bed" to moisturize and maintain controlled nail hydration but also as a receiver to deposit drug diffused from above the nail plate. Therefore, the wetted cotton pad can be sampled at successive time points during the incubation to measure permeation kinetics of drug diffusing through the nail layers to reach the bed (16).

Our novel technique was a micrometer-precision nail drilling instrument that was able to take nail samples at different nail layers where fungi reside. It enables finely controlled drilling into the nail core without disturbing its surface and to collect the powder created by the drilling process (16).

The dorsal surface sample contains residual drug, while the core from the ventral to low intermediate sides provides drug measurement at the site of disease. This method permits drug measurement in the intermediate nail plate, which was previously impossible.

The dorsal layer is characterized by low diffusivity to substances. The intermediate layer is characterized by low lipophilicity, and higher diffusion rates of hydrophilic molecules. The ventral layer is characterized by high lipophilicity and diffusion rates that can be lower than those of the intermediate layer (39).

Since the human nail plate has the tendency to hydrate and swell similarly to hydrogel (40). Since the human nail plate has the tendency to hydrate and swell similarly to hydrogel, the penetration into the nail may favor hydrophilic molecules with size smaller than that of the nail pore, in comparison to lipophilic molecules, in particular large ones. The diffusion rates of such small molecules are the likely characteristics enabling their penetrations into the nail plate—faster in the interior (intermediate layer) of the nail plate than the dorsal or ventral layers (39).

Similar observation was reported in our *in vitro* nail penetration studies in which small molecular size and hydrophilic drugs such as tavaborole (MW = 152 and logP =1.2) (16), panthenol (205 and −1.75) (29), and ME1111 (202 and 2.5) (21) were employed. For an example, a 14-day *in vitro* nail study compared the penetration efficacy of tavaborole and ciclopirox (MW = 207 and ClogP = 3.1) and found that the amounts of tavaborole found in the dorsal/intermediate and ventral/intermediate sections and the cotton pad nail supporting bed samples were significantly higher than those of ciclopirox ($p < 0.05$). This superior permeation capability of tavaborole into and through the nail plate *in vitro* is contributed to its hydrophilicity, small molecular weight, and antifungal capacity (16).

The larger-molecular-weight and/or high lipophilic drugs we studied, ciclopirox (MW = 207 and ClogP = 3.1) (18), econazole (382 and 5.4) (19), ketoconazole (531 and 4.3) (15), and terbinafine HCl (328 and 5.5) (22) had poor nail penetrations. Studies found that the mechanism of the human nail permeation process could be affected by hydrophobic and electrical interactions between the drug and the keratin fibers.(41) This suggests drug affinity to keratin, with molecule size and lipophilicity being key factors to determine the nail penetration rate. For example, terbinafine HCl and efinaconazole are similar in molecular size (328 and 348) and lipophilicity (5.5 and 3.5, respectively). Terbinafine HCl is effective after both oral and topical skin administration, but it has a poor nail penetration rate and low antifungal efficiency after topical application (22). Efinaconazole, in contrast, shows high nail permeability and potent antifungal activity *in vitro* (42). The major difference between two drugs is that terbinafine HCl has high affinity to bind keratin but efinaconazole has low affinity.

Keratin affinity is an important physicochemical property affecting the efficiency of antifungal agents' permeability into and through the nail plate following topical or systemic administration. Beneficial or deleterious effects of drug–keratin affinity depend upon the location in the plate and releasing rate of the bound drug (28). If a high-keratin-affinity drug is administered systemically, it diffuses from the capillary in the nail bed to the low part of the plate to the ventral layer and forms a high concentration reservoir that favors local treatment. Nevertheless, if it is applied topically, the drug may cumulate in the nail surface and the dorsal layer and is insufficient to release and diffuse to the deep part, the ventral layer and the bed (20).

Research found, however, that nail permeability could be enhanced by altering the physicochemical properties of a drug and/or formulation characteristics. (39) For example, luliconazole is an imidazole antifungal with an added ketone dithioacetate component. In spite of its large molecular size (354) and high lipophilicity (4.07), a modified molecular structure endows this antifungal with lower keratin affinity and, in turn, potentially improved potency.(26, 43) We previously reported that *in vitro* nail penetration of econazole was increased with additional 2-n-nonyl-1,3-dioxolane as an enhancer to its nail lacquer formulation(19). Total econazole penetration through the nail plate into the nail bed (supporting cotton pad) in the test group was nearly 200-fold greater than that in the control group (without 2-n-nonyl-1,3-dioxolane). 2-n-nonyl-1,3-dioxolane not only causes hydration of the keratin structure and swelling to increase nail plate porosity and effective diffusion but also can soften the lacquer to release more econazole per unit time (19). In the earlier case study, we reported *in vitro* terbinafine HCl nail penetration with a novel permeation enhancing formulation in which high amounts of terbinafine HCl were attained in the deep nail plate and/or the nail bed after a 14-day topical treatment (22). The result agrees with Traynor's conclusion that a novel permeation enhancing system might fundamentally alter the chemical structure of the nail and enhance the efficacy of topical delivery 44).

In conclusion, this *in vitro* nail study device provides reliable experimental conditions similar to normal physiological temperature, hydration, and humidity. The drilling instrument makes it possible to explore drug permeation into the intermediate and ventral nail layers. With weight normalized drug concentration in the deep layers where fungi reside, antifungal efficiency of a drug can be calculated and evaluated in combination with the physicochemical properties of the drug and related vehicle formulation. In addition, the drug needs to be an unbound form to exert its therapeutic effects. In such a case, drug concentration in the plate and antifungal efficacy may not be equivalent to the local treatment efficiency. Additional measurements, such as binding affinity to human nail keratin and keratin effect on antifungal activity, should be considered to estimate *in vitro* antifungal efficacy coefficients of the antifungal agent.

REFERENCES

1 Murdan S: Drug delivery to the nail following topical application. Int J Pharm. 2002;236(1-2): 1–26.
2 Runne U and Orfanos CE: The human nail - structure, growth and pathological changes. Curr Probl Der. 1981;9:102–149.
3 Kobayashi Y, Miyamoto M, Sugibayashi K, and Morimoto Y: Drug permeation through the three layers of the human nail plate. J Pharm Pharmacol. 1999;51:271–278.
4 Martin D and Lippold BC: *In vitro* permeability of the human nail and a keratin membrane from bovine hooves: influence of the partition coefficient octanol/water and the water solubility of drugs on their permeability and maximum flux. J Pharm Pharmacol. 1997;49:30–34.
5 Martin D and Lippold BC: *In vitro* permeability of the human nail and a keratin membrane from bovine hooves: prediction of the penetration rate of antimycotics through the nail plate and their efficacy. J Pharm Pharmacol. 1997;49:866–872.
6 Dorland's Illustrated Medical Dictionary, 27th Edition, Philadelphia: WB Saunders Company (1988).
7 Elewski B, Charif M.A. Prevalence of onychomycosis in patients attending a dermatology clinic in northeastern Ohio for other conditions. Arch Dermatol. 1997;133:1172–1173.
8 Nolting S and Korting HC: Onychmycoses - local antimycotic treatment. Ed. by S. Nolting and H.C. Korting, Sapriner-Verlag, New York (1990).
9 Meisel CW: The treatment of onychomycosis. In: Nolting S and Korting HC (eds). Onychmycoses - local antimycotic treatment. New York: Sapriner-Verlag, 1990;12–28.
10 Walters KA and Flynn GL: Permeability characteristics of the human nail plate. Int J Cosmet Sci. 1983;5:231–246.
11 Stüttgen G and Bauer E: Bioavailability, skin- and nail penetration of topically applied antimycotics. Mykosen 1982;25(2):74–80.
12 Walters KA, Flynn GL, and Marvel JR: Physicochemical characterization of the human nail: solvent effects on the permeation of homologous alcohols J Pharm Pharmacol 1985;37:771–775.
13 Walters KA, Flynn GL, and Marvel JR: Physiocochemical characterization of the human nail: I. Pressure sealed apparatus for measuring nail plate permeabilities. J Invest Dermatol. 1981;76:76–79.
14 Polak A: Kinetic of amorolfine in human nails Mycoses 1993;36:101–103.

15 Hui X, Shainhouse JZ, Tanojo H, Anigbogu A, Markus G, Maibach HI, and Wester RC: Enhanced human nail drug delivery: nail inner drug content assayed by new unique method, J Pharm Sci. 2002;91:189–195.

16 Hui X, Baker SJ, Wester RC, Barbadillo S, Cashmore AK, Sanders V, Hold KM, Akama T, Zhang YK, Plattner JJ, Maibach HI. *In vitro* penetration of a novel oxaborole antifungal (AN2690) into the human nail plate. J Pharm Sci. 2007;96(10):2622–2631.

17 Hui, X., Wester, R.C., Barbadillo, S. and Maibach, H.I. Nail penetration: enhancement of topical delivery of antifungal drugs by chemical modification of the human nail. In: Textbook of Cosmetic Dermatology (Baran, R. and Maibach, H.I., eds), pp.57–64. London and New York: Taylor & Francis (2005).

18 Hafeez F, Hui X, Selner M, Rosenthal B, Maibach H. Ciclopirox delivery into the human nail plate using novel lipid diffusion enhancers. Drug Dev Ind Pharm. 2014;40(6):838–844.

19 Hui X, Barbadillo S, Lee C, Maibach HI, and Wester RC: Enhanced econazole penetration into human nail by 2-N-nonyl-1,3-dioxane, J Pharm Sci. 2003;92:142–148.

20 Kubota-Ishida N, Takei-Masuda N, Kaneda K, Nagira Y, Chikada T, Nomoto M, Tabata Y, Takahata S, Maebashi K, Hui X, Maibach HI. *In vitro* human onychopharmacokinetic and pharmacodynamic analyses of ME1111, a new topical agent for onychomycosis. Antimicrob Agents Chemother. 2017;62(1):1–9.

21 Hui X, Jung EC, Zhu H, Maibach HI. Antifungal ME1111 *in vitro* human onychopharmacokinetics. Drug Dev Ind Pharm. 2017;43(1):22–29.

22 Hui X, Lindahl Å, Lamel S, Maibach HI. Onychopharmacokinetics of terbinafine hydrochloride penetration from a novel topical formulation into the human nail *in vitro*. Drug Dev Ind Pharm. 2013;39(9):1401–1407.

23 Jo Siu WJ, Tatsumi Y, Senda H, Pillai R, Nakamura T, Sone D, Fothergill A. Comparison of *in vitro* antifungal activities of efinaconazole and currently available antifungal agents against a variety of pathogenic fungi associated with onychomycosis. Antimicrob Agents Chemother. 2013;57(4):1610–1616.

24 Zhang J, Chen J, Huang HQ, Xi LY, Lai W, Xue RZ, Zhang XH, Chen RZ. Comparison of a glucose consumption based method with the CLSI M38-A method for testing antifungal susceptibility of Trichophyton rubrum and Trichophyton mentagrophytes. Chin Med J (Engl). 2010;123(14):1909–1914.

25 Yenişehirli G, Tunçoğlu E, Yenişehirli A, Bulut Y. *In vitro* activities of antifungal drugs against dermatophytes isolated in Tokat, Turkey. Int J Dermatol. 2013;52(12):1557–1560.

26 Wiederhold NP, Fothergill AW, McCarthy DI, Tavakkol A. Luliconazole demonstrates potent *in vitro* activity against dermatophytes recovered from patients with onychomycosis. Antimicrob Agents Chemother. 2014;58(6):3553–3555.

27 VK Bhatia, PC Sharma, Determination of minimum inhibitory concentrations of itraconazole, terbinafine and ketoconazole against dermatophyte species by broth microdilution method. Ind J Med Microbiol. 2015;33(4):533–537.

28 Murdan S. The nail: anatomy, physiology, diseases and treatment. In: Murthy SN, Maibach HI, eds. Topical nail products and ungual drug delivery. Boca Raton: CRC Press, Taylor & Francis Group; 2013:1–36.

29 Hui X, Hornby SB, Wester RC, Barbadillo S, Appa Y, Maibach H. *In vitro* human nail penetration and kinetics of panthenol. Int J Cosmet Sci. 2007;29(4):277–282.

30 Kobayashi Y, Miyamoto M, Sugibayashi K, and Morimoto Y, Drug permeation through the three layers of the human nail plate, J. Pharm. Pharmacol. 1999;51:271–278.

31 BalfourJA, Faulds D. Terbinafine: a review of its pharmacodynamic and pharamcokinetic properties, and therapeutic potential in suprefical mycoses. Drugs 1992;43:259–284.

32 Walters KA, Flynn GL, Marvel JR. Physicochemical chemical characterization of the human nail: Permeation pattern for water and the homologous alcohols and difference with respect to the stratum corneum. J Pharm Pharmacol. 1983;35:28–33.

33 Arrese JE, Piérard GE. Treatment failures and relapses in onychomycosis: a stubborn clinical problem. Dermatology (Basel). 2003;207:255–260.

34 Faergemann J, Baran R. Epidemiology, clinical presentation and diagnosis of onychomycosis. Br J Dermatol. 2003;149(S65):1–4.

35 Dykes PJ, Thomas R, and Finlay AY. Determination of terbinafine in nail samples during systemic treatment for onychomycoses. Br J Dermatol. 1990;123(4):481–486.

36 Schatz F, Bräutigam M, Dobrowolski E, Effendy I, Haberl H, Mensing H et al. Nail incorporation kinetics of terbinafine in onychomycosis patients. Clin Exp Dermatol, 1995;20:377–383.

37 Gupchup GV, Zatz JL. Structural characteristics and permeability properties of the human nail: A review. J Cosmet Sci 1999;50:363–385.

38 Baker SJ, Zhang YK, Akama T, Lau A, Zhou H, Hernandez V, Mao W, Alley MRK, Sanders V, Plattner JJ. Discovery of a new boron- containing anti-fungal agent, 5-fluoro-1,3-dihydro-1-hydroxy-,1-benzoxaborole (AN2690), for the potential treatment of onychomycosis. J Med Chem. 2006;49: 4447–4450.

39 Angelo T, Borgheti-Cardoso LN, Gelfuso GM, Taveira SF, Gratieri T. Chemical and physical strategies in onychomycosis topical treatment: A review. Med Mycol. 2017;55(5):461–475

40 Kreutz T, de Matos SP, Koester LS. Recent patents on permeation enhancers for drug delivery through nails. Recent Patents on Drug Delivery & Formulation. 2019;13:203–218.

41 Murdan S. Drug delivery to the nail following topical application. Int J Pharm. 2002;236:1–26.

42 Sugiura K, Sugimoto N, Hosaka S, Katafuchi-Nagashima M, Arakawa Y, Tatsumi Y, Jo Siu W, Pillai R. The low keratin affinity of efinaconazole contributes to its nail penetration and fungicidal activity in topical onychomycosis treatment. Antimicrob Agents Chemother. 2014;58(7):3837–3842.

43 Kawa N, Lee KC, Anderson RR, Garibyan L. Onychomycosis: a review of new and emerging topical and device-based treatments. J Clin Aesthet Dermatol. 2019;12(10): 29–34.

44 Traynor MJ, Turner RB, Evans CRG, Khengar RH, Jones SA, Brown MB. Effect of a novel penetration enhancer on the ungual permeation of two antifungal agents. J Pharm Pharmacol. 2010;62(6):730–797.

62 Drug Permeation through Burn Eschar

Possibilities and Improvements

Hamid R. Moghimi and Seyedeh Maryam Mortazavi
Shahid Beheshti University of Medical Sciences, Tehran, Iran

Howard I. Maibach
University of California, San Francisco, California

CONTENTS

62.1 INTRODUCTION

Burns are one of common injuries of skin or other tissues and are considered a major universal health problem. Burns are caused by different agents such as heat, electricity, and chemicals. The amount of damage and symptoms (erythema, vesication, inflammation, eschar formation, etc.) depend on different factors, including the type and depth of the burn, and thus, the treatment depends on its severity. Survival of burned patients who suffer from extensive and intensive burns depends to a great extent on infection prevention and handling, e.g., by application of antibiotics. Besides these, other molecules are also used in burned tissue, for example, for wound healing. Therefore, drug delivery to burned tissue is an important issue. In severe burns, due to damage to peripheral vessels and the barrier properties of eschar, systemic drug delivery to a burn wound is difficult, and surgical debridement and/or topical drug therapy are the foremost strategies to overcome the problem.

How to treat burned skin remains a challenge in medicine and pharmacy, as the burned skin (especially in severe burns) does not have the same structure as intact skin, and its interactions with drug molecules and its barrier properties are different from those of normal skin. Thus, intact skin permeation data cannot be easily applied to burned skin, and we need to improve our knowledge in barrier properties of such a damaged tissue and develop some methods to overcome this barrier, the subject of the present chapter.

In this chapter, burn wounds, topical drug therapy in burns, drug permeation in burns with an emphasis on burn eschar (a leathery necrotic tissue that is formed in deep second-degree and third-degree burns), permeation enhancement approaches such as chemical and physical methods, factors that affect permeation through damaged tissue including effects of the cause and duration of burning, effects of burning temperature, importance of eschar age and effects of patient age and gender, and finally permeation of nanoparticles through burn eschar are discussed.

62.2   BURN WOUND AND CLASSIFICATION

Burn injuries are created by different physical and chemical agents and are very complicated in nature. The physical category includes thermal, electrical, radiation, and laser burns, and the chemical category includes acid and alkali burns and so on (Hettiaratchy et al. 2004, Tiwari 2012). Based on burn depth, there are four different degrees of the burn wound. First-degree is mildest and the most superficial type and is limited to the epidermis. Second-degree has two levels based on the depth of dermis damage: superficial and deep. The third-degree burn refers to a burn that affects the full skin thickness (Ye et al. 2017) and finally, fourth-degree, the most severe burn, involves deeper tissues.

In first-degree burns, the epidermis remains intact, but erythema is observed. In second-degree burns, the epidermis and dermis are injured and the epidermal integrity is lost. In second-degree superficial burns, vesication and inflammation are seen. The dermis is affected more in deep second-degree burns. In third-degree burns, the epidermis is lost and the whole dermis layer is involved (Dai et al. 2010, Yasti et al. 2015). Eschar, an important barrier against drug delivery, occurs in deep second-degree and third-degree burns, as described next.

62.3   ESCHAR FORMATION AND WOUND HEALING

Eschar is an inelastic dead tissue without any vessels and, in contrast to intact skin, does not have a regular structure so is not considered as having distinct layers. Eschar formation is by nature time-dependent, so that the structure and properties of eschar change with time (Moghimi et al. 2009b). To understand eschar structure and its changes over time, it is necessary to understand its different zones and the wound healing process.

Based on Jackson's description, a severe burn injury has three zones, including coagulation, stasis, and hyperemia (Jackson 1953). The coagulation zone, the area of irreversible injury located in the central part of the wound, is created because of protein denaturation and blood vessel destruction following a burn. As a necrotic tissue, this tissue is irrecoverable. The eschar is formed in 3 to 24 hours postburn (Rowan et al. 2015). The stasis or ischemia zone is located immediately around the coagulation zone. Since this zone is less affected than the coagulation zone, it can be potentially salvaged through therapeutic approaches. Most cells in this area are live at first, but due to the progressive blood circulation impairment that results in the cessation of blood flow and subsequent hypoxia, progressive necrosis is uncontrollable in the absence of intervention. In the case of severe burn injuries, the zone of stasis turns into the eschar (Salibian et al. 2016, Sharif Makhmal Zadeh et al. 2010, Uraloglu et al. 2019). The outermost area of the wound is the zone of hyperemia, where the blood flow increases following inflammatory response to tissue damage. Its outer edge is the border between healthy skin and the burn wound

(Nisanci et al. 2010). The initial eschar tissue (related to the coagulation zone) and the eschar tissue created by conversion of the stasis zone over several days form an avascular structure consisting of coagulated necrotic epidermis and variable degrees of necrotic dermis and hypodermis (Sharif Makhmal Zadeh et al. 2010).

The wound healing process includes consecutive and overlapping phases of hemostasis, inflammation, proliferation, and remodeling. In brief, vasoconstriction, platelet plug formation, and activation of the coagulation system occur in the hemostasis phase to form clots. In the inflammatory phase, the immune response begins by releasing neutrophils and monocytes at the injury site following vasodilation and subsequent extravasation. These two phases frequently take about three days. In the proliferation phase, released cytokines and growth factors activate fibroblasts and keratinocytes that lead to wound closure and revascularization. The extracellular matrix forms a granulation tissue to be replaced by clots. The proliferative phase often takes days to weeks. Finally in the remodeling or maturation phase, replacement of type III collagen (common in the proliferation phase) with type I collagen, rearrangement, and cross-linking of disorganized collagen fibers, as well as the apoptosis of some cells that had been used to heal the wound but that are not needed anymore (like excess amounts of extracellular matrix) occur and take months or years (Arturson 1996, Rowan et al. 2015, Tiwari 2012, Wang et al. 2018). In conclusion, wound healing causes the conversion of eschar (a necrotic tissue) into a scar (a fibrous tissue) in the cases of deep second- and third-degree burns.

62.4 INFECTION, ESCHAR DEBRIDEMENT, AND TOPICAL ANTIMICROBIAL THERAPY

The skin has a defensive function against microorganisms that can lead to infection. This physiological function is affected by burns so that eschar is at high risk of infection due to avascularity and protein coagulation. Eschar loses many qualities of normal skin and turns into a rich growth medium for microorganisms. The distance of third-degree burn eschar surface from the microvasculature of the patient is several millimeters. Thus, antimicrobial agents administered systemically cannot diffuse into the eschar sufficiently to achieve therapeutic levels. On the other hand, the immune system of burned patients does not act efficiently. The combination of these events may cause sepsis, the most common reason for morbidity and mortality (Church et al. 2006, Barret et al. 2003, Greenhalgh 2017, Norbury et al. 2016, Erol et al. 2004, Manafi et al. 2008). To overcome this problem, debridement of eschar remains a good choice, because this procedure makes the wound bed accessible to topical antimicrobials.

Some clinicians believe that debridement is a must, as the coagulated area on the surface of the wound seems almost impermeable and thus, debridement is a necessary step in the management of burned patients (Wang et al. 2009). Other groups like Moghimi et al. describe conditions when debridement is not possible. Efficacy of debridement depends on the time that the procedure is performed and the general condition of the patient. The selection between early excision and conservative treatment associated with delayed excision remains a momentous decision for the medical staff. In many developing countries, burn unit access to resources is insufficient for early excision for all burned patients. Hence, for cases when early excision is not possible, topical therapy should be considered (Barret et al. 2003, Moghimi et al. 2009b, Scott et al. 1997). In such cases, failure of the antimicrobial agents to permeate across the burn eschar could lead to infections.

62.5 PERMEATION THROUGH ESCHAR AND ENHANCING APPROACHES

Drug molecules penetrate intact skin through the transepidermal pathway and/or transappendageal pathway (Barry 2002). Although the transappendageal pathway might be more significant at the early diffusion stages and be more important for nanoparticle permeation, the main route for permeation across the intact skin is the transepidermal pathway for most compounds. Two permeation routes exist in the stratum corneum: intercellular and intracellular pathways. The intercellular route is the main permeation pathway for most hydrophilic and lipophilic compounds (Moghimi et al. 1998). Due to the hydrophobic nature of the intercellular space and its structural properties, lipophilic (logP 1 to 3) and low-molecular-weight compounds (less than 500 Da in the most ideal state) are more susceptible to permeating this barrier (Gorouhi et al. 2009).

Drug delivery to burned skin encounters challenges when eschar is present. Eschar does not have a stratum corneum, which is an important barrier, but this does not result in the loss of its barrier properties. The barrier performance of eschar is sufficient to inhibit permeation of molecules, especially those of a larger size (Moghimi et al. 2009b, Grice et al. 2017). Unfortunately, opposite to intact skin, there is no well-understood pathway for permeation through eschar. Eschar is a melting pot of proteins and lipids; therefore it might be considered a barrier for both hydrophilic and lipophilic permeants (Jelenko et al. 1967, 1968). Following is an attempt to define more about the nature of eschar by reviewing those works that evaluated the permeation of molecules across it.

Is the eschar a permeable tissue at all? Yes, but like normal skin, it has barrier properties, and permeation through it depends certain variables (Rode et al. 1981, Stefanides et al. 1976, Gray et al. 1991). This property was observed in our group with diazepam, nitroglycerin, clindamycin phosphate, chlorhexidine digluconate, and silver sulfadiazine (Ghaffari et al. 2013, Manafi et al. 2008, Moghimi et al. 2009a, Sharif Makhmal Zadeh et al. 2010)

Using the agar diffusion technique and burn clinical isolates, Stefanides et al. evaluated the penetration of topical antimicrobial agents (e.g., gentamicin sulfate, mafenide acetate, nitrofurazone, povidone-iodine, silver nitrate, and silver sulfadiazine) through human eschar. After placing eschar samples or paper discs (as control) on the surface of agar on the inoculated plates, antimicrobial agents were delivered to the center of the eschar or paper disc individually. The plates were then incubated 24 hours and after that the diameter of the inhibition zone (as a measure of antimicrobial agents' permeability across the eschar) was measured and interpreted. Apart from silver nitrate, which did not penetrate even across the paper disc in an effective amount, the remainder of antimicrobial agents penetrated the eschar and showed activity post-penetration (Stefanides et al. 1976).

Although eschar is a permeable tissue, permeation of some antimicrobials through this tissue is insufficient to achieve therapeutic levels (Herruzo-Cabrera et al. 1992, Ward et al. 1995). It has been suggested that chemical penetration enhancers or physical enhancement methods might be used to alter the barrier performance of the burn eschar, as discussed next. These approaches have been applied to increase the permeation of drug molecules across the intact skin.

62.5.1 IMPROVEMENTS BY CHEMICAL PENETRATION ENHANCERS

Different chemicals such as terpenes, sulphoxides, pyrrolidines, fatty acids, fatty alcohols, azones, alcohols and glycols, surfactants, and so on have been used as penetration enhancers to increase permeation of drugs through different biological barriers such as skin over decades (Williams et al. 2004). Such an approach has also been used to increase the permeation of different agents through burn skin and eschar (Table 62.1 and Figure 62.1). These studies are addressed here, and the effects of chemical penetration enhancers on the barrier properties of eschar are discussed.

Moghimi's group (Manafi et al. 2008) investigated the effects of chemical penetration enhancers on the permeation of chlorhexidine gluconate, silver sulfadiazine, and nitroglycerin across human third-degree burn eschar. Antimicrobial studies using plate method and ex vivo permeation studies using diffusion cells were conducted to evaluate the effects of chemical enhancers on the permeation of these drugs through burn eschar. Different classes of enhancers were used in this study, including those expected to mainly influence the membrane hydration (water, NaCl, glycine, and glycerin), those that seemed to mainly affect the lipid domain fluidity (n-hexane, citral, and ethyl acetate), and finally those that affect both hydration and lipid domain (ethanol, urea, and sodium dodecyl sulfate). Chlorhexidine gluconate and silver sulfadiazine were included in the microbial

TABLE 62.1

A Summary of Studies Performed on the Permeation of Compounds through Human Third-Degree Burn Eschar under the Effects of Permeation Enhancers

Permeant	Dosage Form	Permeation Study Type	Chemical Enhancers	ER	Reference
Chlorhexidine digluconate	Aqueous solution 20%	Microbial and diffusion cells studies	Water, saline, glycerin aq*, DMSO** aq, SDS*** aq,	0.7-0.8	(Manafi et al. 2008)
Silver sulfadiazine	Cream 1%		ethanol aq, urea aq, glycine aq, ethyl acetate:ethanol mixture,	1.2–1.8	
Nitroglycerin	Aqueous solution (0.5 mg/mL)		n-hexane:ethanol mixture, and citral solution in PG****	1.8- 2.7	
Silver sulfadiazine	Water: acetonitrile: phosphoric acid (82:16:2) solution (0.6 mg/mL)	Diffusion cells studies	water	9.9-19.8	(Sharif Makhmal Zadeh et al. 2010)
Silver sulfadiazine	Water: acetonitrile: phosphoric acid (82:16:2) solution	Diffusion cells studies	Limonene, eucalyptol, α-pinene oxide, and geraniol	4.3-9.0	(Moghimi et al. 2009a)
Clindamycin phosphate	Saturated phosphate buffer solution	Diffusion cells studies	Trypsin	1.5	(Ghaffari et al. 2013)

* Aqueous solution
** Dimethyl sulfoxide
*** Sodium dodecyl sulfate
**** Propylene glycol

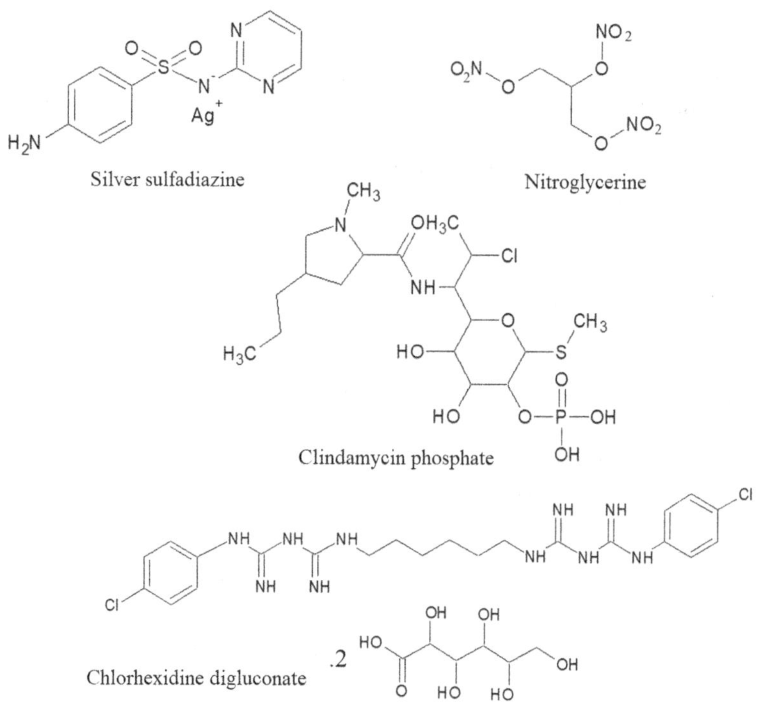

FIGURE 62.1 The chemical structures of permeants used to study permeation through enhancer-treated-burn eschar.

studies, and nitroglycerin was included in the diffusion cell permeation studies. The enhancement ratio (ER) was obtained through dividing the diameter of the inhibition zone of the enhancer-treated eschars by the diameter of the inhibition zone of nontreated eschars (control). To achieve this value in the diffusion cell permeation studies, the permeability coefficients (kp) of nitroglycerin in the presence of permeation enhancers was divided by the kp of nitroglycerin in the absence of enhancers. Results showed that permeation of silver sulfadiazine through eschar was significantly increased by about 1.2 to 1.8 times by glycerin, n-hexane:ethanol, and water as enhancers. Based on the results of the diffusion cell permeation studies, glycine, water, and the n-hexane:ethanol mixture significantly increased the permeation of nitroglycerin across the eschar by 1.8 to 2.7 times. The researchers concluded that the effects of penetration enhancers depended largely on the nature of the permeant, as well as its permeation pathway; for example, water molecules increased the permeation of silver sulfadiazine and nitroglycerin, but not chlorhexidine. This group believed that both groups of enhancers (either those acting on the hydration of the membrane or those acting on the lipid domain) were effective on the permeation of drugs through burn eschar. Thus, it seems that the first group tends to be more effective. Note that the results revealed that some enhancers used for the permeation of chlorhexidine (water, sodium dodecyl sulfate, NaCl, ethanol, and glycerin) not only could not increase permeation through the eschar but also decreased permeability of the compound, a retardation effect (Manafi et al. 2008).

The observed differences should be due to differences in physicochemical properties of drugs. The molecular weight of chlorhexidine gluconate (897.8 Da for salt and 505.4 Da for base) is higher than those of silver sulfadiazine (357.1 Da for salt and 250.3 Da for base) and nitroglycerin (227.1 Da), indicating that chlorhexidine has lower diffusion ability and that its diffusion is very sensitive to any changes in the barrier due to added material. Besides this, the compounds have different Log octanol/water partition coefficients (lipophilicities) and therefore, their tendency to eschar is also different. The calculated logP (clogP) values of chlorhexidine, nitroglycerine, and silver sulfadiazine are 2.8, 1.2, and 0.2, respectively (Tetko et al. 2005, VCCLAB 2005), indicating higher lipophilicity of chlorhexidine, and possibly its lower partitioning into hydrated eschar samples.

Using Franz-type diffusion cells, our group (Sharif Makhmal Zadeh et al. 2010) studied the permeation of silver sulfadiazine across the human third-degree burn eschar at three levels of hydration (fully hydrated, semihydrated, and dry eschars). Permeation studies over 32 hours demonstrated that although the dry eschar seemed to be more permeable than the hydrated during first hours of the study, the hydrated eschars were more effective in the long term, so that the cumulative amounts of permeated silver sulfadiazine through the fully hydrated and semihydrated eschars at the end of study approximated 20 and 1.4 times more than that of dry eschar, respectively. Similar to the study of Manafi et al (2008), the researchers concluded that water acted as a permeation enhancer and decreased the barrier properties of the eschar through interaction with a proteinaceous structure and polar head groups of lipid domains available in the burn eschar structure.

The same group (Ghaffari et al. 2012) observed the importance of water molecules on the permeation of clindamycin phosphate and diazepam through hydrated third-degree burn eschar. Different hydroethanolic solutions containing 10% to 70% (v/v) ethanol were applied. Ethanol had a concentration-dependent effect on the barrier properties of eschar so that the permeability coefficients (kp) of clindamycin phosphate and diazepam were reduced by approximately 1.5 to 5.3 and 2 to 10.7 times, respectively, due to the addition of 20% to 70% ethanol. Using these results and differential scanning calorimetry studies, the authors concluded that ethanol reduced the permeation of these drugs through eschar via dehydration and also affected the internal proteinaceous structure of eschar. These results also confirm water enhancement effects on permeation of drugs through burn eschar.

The effects of terpenes, well-known permeation enhancers, on the permeation of silver sulfadiazine across hydrated third-degree burn eschar have also been evaluated using Franz-type diffusion cells (Moghimi et al. 2009a). Four lipophilic monoterpenes were examined, including three cyclic terpenes of limonene (a hydrocarbon), eucalyptol (an ether), and α-pinene oxide (an epoxide), and one linear terpene (geraniol; an alcohol). These terpenes have molecular weights of 136 to 154 Da and logP values of 2 to 4.6. The obtained enhancement ratio (ER) values showed that all terpenes, irrespective of their types, increased silver sulfadiazine permeation. Limonene showed the most (ER = 9) and α-pinene oxide had the least (ER = 4.3) enhancement effects on silver sulfadiazine permeation through eschar. ER values of geraniol and eucalyptol were 5.5 and 4.7, respectively. There was a good correlation between Log partition coefficients of terpenes and the effects of terpenes on silver sulfadiazine permeation through eschar. The authors concluded that the main mechanism by which terpenes increased the permeation of silver sulfadiazine through eschar was probably improvement of drug partitioning into the eschar; limonene (logP 4.6) showed the highest effect.

Enzymes have also been investigated as eschar permeation enhancers. Permeation of clindamycin phosphate through hydrated third-degree burn eschar pretreated with trypsin solution (1% w/v) has shown that this protease is capable of reducing eschar barrier performance toward this drug in comparison to untreated (control) samples (Ghaffari et al. 2013), possibly by digesting the protein domains available in the eschar structure. This study has also shown that the enhancement effect of trypsin is time-dependent. The clindamycin phosphate enhancement ratio after trypsin pretreatment was shown to be 1.5 and 2.3 for 4 and 24 hours pretreatment times, respectively. Trypsin treatment of eschar for 24 hours caused perforation of some eschar samples. The authors concluded that protein-acting enhancers might be a reasonable approach for improving eschar permeability.

According to these studies, chemical enhancers are able increase the permeation of hydrophilic and hydrophobic drugs, and their effectiveness depends on the structure and physicochemical properties of both permeants and enhancers.

62.5.2 Improvements by Physical Enhancement Methods

Many physical enhancement methods are available to increase the skin permeation of drug molecules such as sonophoresis, iontophoresis, electroporation, and microneedles (Dragicevic et al. 2018). Here, the studies are reviewed in which the effects of physical enhancement methods on permeation of compounds through burn eschar have been studied.

The effects of cathodic and anodic iontophoresis on permeation of clindamycin phosphate through hydrated third-degree burn eschar were investigated using Franz-type diffusion cells by Moghimi's group (Sharif Makhmal Zadeh 2006). Since the charge of this molecule depends on the degree of protonation of the amine and phosphate groups, the researchers applied two drug solutions with pH values of 5.8 and 8 as the donor phase in their permeation studies. Although anodic iontophoresis at a pH of 5.8 was not effective, permeation of clindamycin phosphate was dramatically increased by applying cathodic iontophoresis, especially at pH of 8 (about fiftyfold increase in flux). Given the pKa of this drug, the researchers believed that in the case of cathodic iontophoresis, electromigration force and in the case of anodic iontophoresis, electroosmosis flow were the main causes of increased permeation of clindamycin phosphate through burn eschar.

In another study conducted by Moghimi's group (Ghaffari 2011), the influences of sonophoresis on the permeation of clindamycin phosphate (clogP: 1.0) and diazepam (clogP: 2.6) (Tetko et al. 2005, VCCLAB 2005) through third-degree eschar were studied using Franz-type diffusion cells. Low-frequency, high-intensity (20 kHz, 4 and 13 w/cm²) and high-frequency, low-intensity (1MHz, 2 w/cm²) ultrasound was applied in the permeation studies. Therapeutic ultrasound (high-frequency, low-intensity) failed to increase drug permeation, but low-frequency, high-intensity ultrasound increased the permeation of both drugs through minimal-thickness eschar. Enhancement ratios for clindamycin phosphate and diazepam were 15.4 and 2.76, respectively. Sonophoresis led to perforation in some eschar samples. The authors believed that sonophoresis might be a reasonable approach to increase drug permeation through eschar, especially in thin membranes.

62.6   OTHER EFFECTIVE PARAMETERS ON PERMEATION THROUGH ESCHAR

In addition to formulation-related parameters such as molecular weight, mechanism, and physicochemical properties of drug molecules and chemical enhancers, there are other parameters that affect the drug permeation through eschar, including burning methods (e.g., scalding and branding), temperature and duration of burning, age of eschar, and burn patient age and gender (Behl et al. 1981b, Flynn et al. 1981, Behl et al. 1981a, Flynn et al. 1982, Behl et al. 1980, Daei Hamed 2010).

62.6.1   Effects of the Cause and Duration of Burning

To ascertain the influences of duration of burning as well as burning methods on the permeation through burn eschar, Behl et al. investigated permeation of radiolabeled water, methanol, ethanol, n-butanol, n-hexanol, and n-octanol through burn eschar created in the dorsal side of sacrificed mice by direct contact with 60°C water (wet heat burn) or 60°C branding iron (dry heat burn) (Behl et al. 1981b, Behl et al. 1980). Intact abdominal skin sections of the same mice were used as control. Scalding and branding time ranges of 15 to 480 and 15 to 960 seconds were studied, respectively. Diffusion cell studies showed that both methods of burning increased skin permeability to all mentioned compounds and in terms of enhancement, both methods were similar. In terms of burn duration, both methods for short times produced the same effects at equivalent time periods, so that the eschar permeation of water, methanol, and ethanol increased 1.5- to 2-fold. The permeation of other compounds increased threefold to fourfold. In the case of both scalding and branding methods, for 60°C burning, there was no significant relationship between eschar permeability and duration of burning except at short exposures (less than 30 seconds). Therefore, it was deduced that the relationship between the depth of the burn (changing of second-degree burn eschar into third-degree one occurred at 60 seconds at 60°C) and eschar permeability was not proportional.

62.6.2   Effects of Burning Temperature

To ascertain the effects of scalding and branding iron temperature, Flynn et al. and Behl et al. conducted a similar study, but changed the temperature of the burn instead of the duration (Flynn et al. 1981, Behl et al. 1981a). Sixty-second burns at temperature ranges (60 to 98°C for scalding method and 60 to 200°C for branding method) were applied to mouse skin. In the case of scalding, permeation of all compounds increased with rising temperature. At temperatures between 70°C and 80°C, barrier performance of the skin was extremely affected, so that at temperatures greater than 70°C, scalding coefficient (permeability coefficient of burned skin divided by permeability coefficient of intact skin) increased intensely for all compounds except n-octanol and to some extent n-hexanol. Thus, by increasing the temperature of burning, permeation of polar compounds was more affected than that of hydrophobics. According to the authors, at higher temperatures, some morphological and/or chemical changes occur in the stratum corneum, which decrease its barrier performance. In the case of branding iron, by increasing the temperature up to 70°C, the permeability of skin did not change dramatically, but at higher temperatures, permeation of polar compounds (water, methanol, and ethanol) through eschar increased markedly. Eschar permeability increased moderately for butanol and slightly for hexanol. Permeation of octanol was not significantly affected by rising the temperature. Similar to the scalding method, they believed that with the decrease of the stratum corneum barrier characteristics as a function of temperature increase, penetration of polar compounds increased more than hydrophobics.

62.6.3   Eschar Age Effects

Studies mentioned so far were about the permeation of compounds through eschar immediately postburn. Since properties of burns change gradually with the passage of time, Flynn et al. evaluated effects of eschar age on its permeability in which the permeation of methanol and butanol through burn eschar (created through contact with a metal surface with temperature of 80°C for 15 seconds) was investigated over two weeks postburn. The burning first caused a 50% increase in the methanol permeability and a 300% to 400% increase in the butanol permeability. These changes held over the first four to five days after burning. Then, over time, permeability first gradually and then rapidly increased so that almost on the tenth day it reached a maximum limit (twentyfold increase for permeability of methanol and twelvefold increase for permeability of butanol compared to intact skin). Subsequently, permeability of both compounds began to decrease until end of the investigation (14 days). The dynamic nature of eschar is obvious. In agreement with this study, by investigation of clindamycin phosphate and diazepam permeation through human third-degree eschar in different post-burn ages (3 to 22 days), Moghimi's group (Daei Hamed 2010) also showed that the permeation of drugs altered over time post-burning so that the permeation of clindamycin phosphate and diazepam reached a maximum level on the tenth and sixth day, respectively.

62.6.4 PATIENT AGE AND GENDER EFFECTS

To understand the influences of the age and gender of burn patient on permeation through burn eschar, Moghimi's group (Daei Hamed 2010) investigated the permeation of clindamycin phosphate (clogP: 1.0) and diazepam (clogP: 2.6) through human third-degree burn eschar using Franz-type diffusion cells. Female and male patients (age 16 to 80 years) were included. There was no significant difference between genders in the case of permeation of both permeants through burn eschar. With respect to patient age, the eschars obtained from patients over 60 years were more permeable for clindamycin phosphate, but no differences were observed in diazepam permeation. The authors concluded that age affected the permeation of the drug with lower lipophilicity (clindamycin phosphate) than that of more lipophilic one (diazepam).

62.7 NANOPARTICLES AND ESCHAR PERMEATION

In a study about the deep second-degree burn wound healing process in rats, formulations with and without epidermal growth factor (EGF) were prepared, including EGF-liposome formulation, liposome formulation without EGF, EGF solution, EGF-liposome in chitosan gel formulation, and chitosan gel with EGF (Degim et al. 2011). Formulations containing EGF were generally more effective than the others. Despite the fact that the liposome formulation without EGF was less effective than formulations containing EGF, healing in burns treated by that was also observed; suggesting liposome itself has a healing effect. Perhaps EGF as a macromolecule with molecular weight of 6.2 KDa has difficulty in diffusion through eschar. No permeation data through burn eschar were reported. In another study, this time on basic fibroblast growth factor (bFGF), the effectiveness of liposome containing bFGF formulation on deep second-degree burn eschar was more than that of liposome without FGF (Xiang et al. 2011). Again, there was no report on permeation of this macromolecule through eschar.

Moghimi's group (Ghaffari et al. 2015), determined the permeation of normal and ultra-deformable liposomes containing clindamycin phosphate (clogP: 1.0) through human third-degree burn eschar with Franz-type diffusion cells. Nanoliposomes (either normal or ultra-deformable) containing clindamycin phosphate led to decreased permeation of this drug through eschar. By increasing the concentration of liposomal lipid from 20 to 100 mM, permeation of clindamycin phosphate decreased by almost twice. The authors concluded that the reduction was due either to the entrapment of liposomal clindamycin phosphate in the eschar so that it could not be detected in the receptor phase or due to the increased barrier properties of eschar because of the deposition of liposomal lipids in the microcracks of burn eschar and formation of a lipid barrier.

In agreement with this investigation, by measurement of serum and tissues concentration of drug, as well as assessment of radioactivity in burn dressing, burn tissue, and splanchnic organs,

Price et al. showed that radiolabeled liposomal tobramycin used topically on the rat full-thickness burn eschar had negligible systemic absorption at 24, 48, and 72 hours post-burn, but concentration of drug in the burn tissues was significant at the same times (Price et al. 1992).

At first glance, results of studies mentioned here seem to be controversial. Given the first two studies (Degim et al. 2011, Xiang et al. 2011), liposomes containing drug had an increased effect compared to blank liposomes in terms of wound healing, but according to the third and fourth studies (Ghaffari et al. 2015, Price et al. 1992), compounds failed to permeate through the eschar in liposomal forms. Considering all studies together, it should be said despite the fact that drug molecules in liposomal forms are not capable of permeating through eschar, deposition of liposomes in the eschar increased drug deposition in this tissue, and this is possibly the reason for increased function of drug-loaded liposomal formulations. In contrast to chemical enhancers that lead to increased drug permeation through eschar and possibly provide a deeper treatment, liposomes are effective carriers for delivery of drugs for eschar effect at the site of the burn wound (local effect), e.g., on the microorganisms deposited in the eschar or for healing agents. Further investigations are needed for a better understanding of mechanisms, yet both approaches appear useful for healing such wounds.

62.8 CONCLUSION

Survival of burned patients who suffer from extensive and intensive burns depends to a great extent on infection prevention. Surgical debridement and/or topical drug therapy are the foremost strategies to overcome the problem. Burned skin differs from normal skin and in some injuries (e.g., third-degree burn) a new barrier (eschar) is formed. The first choice of medical teams, especially in developing countries, might be the use of topical antibiotics on intact burn tissue instead of debridement. Besides antibiotics, other molecules are also used in burned tissue for wound healing. Unfortunately, although some drug molecules cannot permeate through burn eschar in therapeutic amounts, the barrier properties of this barrier and overcoming permeation difficulties through this membrane are not well studied. Studies show that drug permeation through this barrier depends on the physicochemical properties of the permeant, burning temperature and type, eschar age, and the vehicle. Current information also shows that there is no difference between men and women and that the effects patient age might occur at ages higher than 60 years. Use of chemical and physical enhancement methods or nanoparticles could improve the drug delivery to the eschar. Many questions remain unanswered on permeation through eschar such as permeation mechanism, molecular weight cutoff, comparison of different burn causes, etc. Therefore, further investigations to fully discover the nature of burn eschar and its permeation properties are needed.

REFERENCES

Arturson, G. 1996. Pathophysiology of the burn wound and pharmacological treatment. The Rudi Hermans Lecture, 1995. Burns. 22 (4):255–74.
Barret, J.P., and Herndon, D.N. 2003. Effects of burn wound excision on bacterial colonization and invasion. Plast Reconstr Surg. 111 (2):744–50.
Barry, B. W. 2002. Drug delivery routes in skin: a novel approach. Adv Drug Deliv Rev. 54 (Suppl 1):S31–40.
Behl, C. R., Flynn, G. L., Barrett, M., et al. 1981a. Permeability of thermally damaged skin IV: influence of branding iron temperature on the mass transfer of water and n-alkanols across hairless mouse skin. Burns. 8 (2):86–98.
Behl, C. R., Flynn, G. L., Barrett, M., et al. 1981b. Permeability of thermally damaged skin II: immediate influences of branding at 60°C on hairless mouse skin permeability. Burns. 7 (6):389–399.
Behl, C. R., Flynn, G. L., Kurihara, T., et al. 1980. Permeability of thermally damaged skin: I. Immediate influences of 60°C scalding on hairless mouse skin. J Invest Dermatol. 75 (4):340–5.
Church, D., Elsayed, S., Reid, O., Winston, B., and Lindsay, R. 2006. Burn wound infections. Clin. Microbiol. Rev. 19 (2):403–434.

Daei Hamed, M. 2010. Evaluation of the effect of third-degree burn eschar age on drug permeability. PharmD Thesis (Supervisor: Moghimi, H.R). School of Pharmacy, Shahid Beheshti University of Medical Sciences, Tehran, Iran.

Dai, T., Huang, Y. Y., Sharma, S. K., et al. 2010. Topical antimicrobials for burn wound infections. Recent Pat Antiinfect Drug Discov. 5 (2):124–151.

Degim, Z., Celebi, N., Alemdaroglu, C., et al. 2011. Evaluation of chitosan gel containing liposome-loaded epidermal growth factor on burn wound healing. Int Wound J. 8 (4):343–354.

Dragicevic, N., and Maibach, H. 2018. Combined use of nanocarriers and physical methods for percutaneous penetration enhancement. Adv Drug Deliv Rev. 127:58–84.

Erol, S., Altoparlak, U., Akcay, M. N., Celebi, F., and Parlak, M. 2004. Changes of microbial flora and wound colonization in burned patients. Burns. 30 (4):357–361.

Flynn, G. L., Behl, C. R., Linn, E., et al. 1982. Permeability of thermally damaged skin V: Permeability over the course of maturation of a deep partial-thickness wound. Burns. 8 (3):196–202.

Flynn, G.L., Behl, C.R., Walters, K.A., et al. 1981. Permeability of thermally damaged skin III: Influence of scalding temperature on mass transfer of water and n-alkanols across hairless mouse skin. Burns. 8 (1):47–58.

Ghaffari, A, Manafi, A, and Moghimi, H. R. 2013. Enhancement effect of trypsin on permeation of clindamycin phosphate through third-degree burn eschar. Iran J Pharm Res. 12 (1):3–8.

Ghaffari, A. 2011. Application of sonophoresis or combination of sonophoresis with iontophoresis, chemical enhancers and liposomes for enhancement of permeation of drugs through third-degree burn eschar. PhD Thesis (Supervisor: Moghimi, H.R). School of Pharmacy, Shahid Beheshti University of Medical Sciences, Tehran, Iran.

Ghaffari, A., Manafi, A., and Moghimi, H. R. 2015. Clindamycin phosphate absorption from nanoliposomal formulations through third-degree burn eschar. World J. Plast. Surg. 4 (2):145–152.

Ghaffari, A., Moghimi, H. R., Manafi, A., and Hosseini, H. 2012. A mechanistic study on the effect of ethanol and importance of water on permeation of drugs through human third-degree burn eschar. Int Wound J. 9 (2):221–229.

Gorouhi, F., and Maibach, H. I. 2009. Role of topical peptides in preventing or treating aged skin. Int J Cosmet Sci. 31 (5):327–345.

Gray, J. H., Henry, D. A., Forbes, M., et al. 1991. Comparison of silver sulphadiazine 1 percent, silver sulphadiazine 1 percent plus chlorhexidine digluconate 0.2 percent and mafenide acetate 8.5 percent for topical antibacterial effect in infected full skin thickness rat burn wounds. Burns. 17 (1):37–40.

Greenhalgh, D. G. 2017. Sepsis in the burn patient: a different problem than sepsis in the general population. Burns Trauma. 5 (23): 1–10.

Grice, J.E, Moghimi, H.R, Ryne, E, et al. 2017. Non-formulation parameters that affect penetrant-skin-vehicle interactions and percutaneous absorption. In *Percutaneous penetration enhancers drug penetration into/through the skin: Methodology and general considerations*, edited by Dragicevic, N and Maibach, H.I, 67–68. Berlin: Springer-Verlag.

Herruzo-Cabrera, R., Garcia-Torres, V., Rey-Calero, J., and Vizcaino-Alcaide, M. J. 1992. Evaluation of the penetration strength, bactericidal efficacy and spectrum of action of several antimicrobial creams against isolated microorganisms in a burn centre. Burns. 18 (1):39–44.

Hettiaratchy, S., and Dziewulski, P. 2004. ABC of burns: pathophysiology and types of burns. Br Med J. 328 (7453):1427–1429.

Jackson, D. M. 1953. The diagnosis of the depth of burning. Br J Surg. 40 (164):588–596.

Jelenko, C., III, Smulyan, W. I., and Wheeler, M. L. 1967. Studies in burns: IV. The relationship of eschar water content to eschar water transmissivity. Ann Surg. 166 (2):278–286.

Jelenko, C. III, Smulyan, W. I., and Wheeler, M. L. 1968. Studies in burns: the role of lipids in the transmissivity of membranes. Ann Surg. 167 (4):521–532.

Manafi, A., Hashemlou, A., Momeni, P., and Moghimi, H. R. 2008. Enhancing drugs absorption through third-degree burn wound eschar. Burns. 34 (5):698–702.

Moghimi, H. R., Makhmalzadeh, B. S., and Manafi, A. 2009a. Enhancement effect of terpenes on silver sulphadiazine permeation through third-degree burn eschar. Burns. 35 (8):1165–1170.

Moghimi, H. R., Williams, A.C, and Barry, B. W. 1998. Enhancement by terpenes of 5-fluorouracil permeation through the stratum corneum: model solvent approach. J. Pharm. Pharmacol. 50 (9):955–964.

Moghimi, Hamid R., and Manafi, Ali. 2009b. The necessity for enhancing of drugs absorption through burn eschar. Burns. 35 (6):902–904.

Nisanci, M., Eski, M., Sahin, I., Ilgan, S., and Isik, S. 2010. Saving the zone of stasis in burns with activated protein C: an experimental study in rats. Burns. 36 (3):397–402.

Norbury, W., Herndon, D. N., Tanksley, J., Jeschke, M. G., and Finnerty, C. C. 2016. Infection in burns. Surg Infect. 17 (2):250–255.

Price, C. I., Horton, J. W., and Baxter, C. R. 1992. Liposome delivery of aminoglycosides in burn wounds. Surg Gynecol Obstet. 174 (5):414–418.

Rode, H., de Wet, P. M., Davies, M. R., and Cywes, S. 1981. An experimental evaluation of the germicidal efficacy of three topical antimicrobial agents in burns. Prog Pediatr Surg. 14:189–208.

Rowan, M. P., Cancio, L. C., Elster, E. A., et al. 2015. Burn wound healing and treatment: review and advancements. Crit Care. 19:243.

Salibian, A. A., Rosario, A. T. D., Severo, L. D. A.M., et al. 2016. Current concepts on burn wound conversion-A review of recent advances in understanding the secondary progressions of burns. Burns. 42 (5):1025–1035.

Scott, J. R., and Watson, S. B. 1997. 7 Surgical management of burns. Baillière's Clinical Anaesthesiology. 11 (3):473–495.

Sharif Makhmal Zadeh, B. 2006. Studying the barrier properties of third-degree burn eschar and improving its permeability by physical and chemical enhancement methods. PhD Thesis (Supervisor: Moghimi, H.R.), School of Pharmacy, Shahid Beheshti University of Medical Sciences, Tehran, Iran.

Sharif Makhmal Zadeh, B., and Moghimi, H.R. 2010. Effect of hydration on barrier performance of third-degree burn eschar. Iran J Pharm Res. 5 (3):155–161.

Stefanides, M. M., Sr., Copeland, C. E., Kominos, S. D., and Yee, R. B. 1976. In vitro penetration of topical antiseptics through eschar of burn patients. Ann. Surg. 183 (4):358–364.

Tetko, I. V., Gasteiger, J., Todeschini, R., et al. 2005. Virtual computational chemistry laboratory - design and description. J. Comput. Aid. Mol. Des. 19:453–463.

Tiwari, V. K. 2012. Burn wound: How it differs from other wounds? Indian J Plast Surg. 45 (2):364–373.

Uraloglu, M., Ural, A., Efe, G., et al. 2019. The Effect of Platelet-Rich Plasma on the Zone of Stasis and Apoptosis in an Experimental Burn Model. Plast Surg (Oakv). 27 (2):173–181.

VCCLAB. 2005. Virtual Computational Chemistry Laboratory, http://www.vcclab.org.

Wang, P.H., Huang, B. S., Horng, H. C., Yeh, C.C., and Chen, Y. J. 2018. Wound healing. J Chin Med Assoc. 81 (2):94–101.

Wang, X. Q., Hayes, M., Kempf, M., et al. 2009. The poor penetration of topical burn agent through burn eschar on a porcine burn model. Burns. 35 (6):901–902.

Ward, R. S., and Saffle, J. R. 1995. Topical agents in burn and wound care. Phys Ther. 75 (6):526–538.

Williams, A. C., and Barry, B. W. 2004. Penetration enhancers. Adv Drug Deliv Rev. 56 (5):603–618.

Xiang, Q., Xiao, J., Zhang, H., et al. 2011. Preparation and characterisation of bFGF-encapsuled liposomes and evaluation of wound-healing activities in the rat. Burns. 37 (5):886–895.

Yasti, A. C., Senel, E., Saydam, M., et al. 2015. Guideline and treatment algorithm for burn injuries. Ulus Travma Acil Cerrahi Derg. 21 (2):79–89.

Ye, H., and De, S. 2017. Thermal injury of skin and subcutaneous tissues: A review of experimental approaches and numerical models. Burns. 43 (5):909–932.

63 Percutaneous Penetration in Humans

Transfer of Chemicals via Skin-to-Skin Contact

Andrew G.D. Ezersky
University of Southern California, Los Angeles, California

Howard I. Maibach
University of California, San Francisco, California

CONTENTS

63.1 INTRODUCTION

Various drugs are applied topically as medications, some of which can produce serious adverse effects. Patients receiving these medications are often aware of these effects based on advice of the prescribing physician and pharmacist. Prior to prescribing the medication, the physician would have weighed the benefits of the medication versus the risk of adverse effects. However, the same is not true for persons who come in skin contact with the patient and their applied medication. It has become increasingly apparent that family, friends, and others in physical contact with the patient could be placed at a similar risk to the patient if proper precautions are not in place to prevent medication transfer.

The basis of the transfer of transdermal medication lies in its initial absorption. Typically, transdermal medication is incompletely absorbed; much medication remains on the skin for hours or even days after application, as shown in studies examining estrogen and testosterone gels [1, 2]. While the average patient may be cognizant of residual medication on the application site immediately post-application, the patient may not be aware that transfer potential does not rapidly cease. Residual medication will largely remain on the skin until absorbed, washed, or rubbed against another object; thus, there is a possibility that the medication can be transferred long past application [1]. Contact between the patient and his or her family members and friends can then pose a risk to their health even when the thought of the medication application is far removed from the patient's mind. Transfer of transdermal medications and the potential for absorption of the transferred medication between the intended users and others pose a public health risk.

63.2   METHODS

We searched PubMed and Google Scholar for articles published between 1970 and 2018 containing data on controlled peer-reviewed studies of the interpersonal and intrapersonal skin-to-skin transfer of chemicals in man. Search terms included "chemical transfer," "interpersonal chemical transfer," "interpersonal skin chemical transfer," "interpersonal skin-to-skin chemical transfer," "skin-to-skin chemical transfer," "skin-to-skin pharmaceutical transfer," "topical gel transfer," "topical skin-to-skin transfer," "occupational chemical exposure," and "paraoccupational skin chemical transfer." Additionally, the reference section of the articles found from databases was used to find more data on studies regarding interpersonal chemical transfer. The UCSF Dermatology textbook library, including those on percutaneous penetration, was reviewed.

63.3   RESULTS

The search provided 12 peer-reviewed controlled studies on interpersonal skin-to-skin chemical transfer. Most studies indicated that it is possible for a transdermal medication to be transferred skin-to-skin and then be significantly absorbed by the recipient (Table 63.1). Of the 12 studies, 9 found that the medication studied was significantly absorbed by the recipient of the transfer [2–7].

Of the three papers not finding significant absorption [1, 8, 9], only one researched the actual transfer of the medication and found that the medication is transferred onto the skin of the recipient but not absorbed [1].

The search provided two peer-reviewed controlled studies on intrapersonal skin-to-skin chemical transfer. One, conducted on tetracycline, concluded that significant medication could be found at the points that had made contact with the application site [10]. Another, conducted on nickel, found that with rubbing, nickel was transferred from the fingers to the cheeks of participants [11]. Consequently, while intrapersonal absorption could not be measured, transfer to different body parts of the same individual was found possible.

Most investigations relating to skin-to-skin transfer of chemicals employed sex hormones as the model for transfer. However, various chemicals have been shown transferable: androgens, estradiol, oxybutynin, tetracycline, and nickel [3–5, 7, 11]. Additionally, certain vehicles used to formulate topical medications are conducive to transfer: patch, gel, emulsion, ointment, and cream [10, 12]. However, other topical formulations like tinctures, lotions, and sprays appear less conducive to skin-to-skin chemical transfer [8, 10].

In a study examining the transfer of testosterone gel from person to person, medication absorption in the recipient when physical contact was made beginning at 2 and 12 hours after application was measured. Time between medication application and contact time did not significantly affect transfer extent [4]. Stahlman et al. [4] also concluded that multiple exposures to the testosterone gel did not significantly increase the testosterone level in the recipient more than a single exposure.

In skin-to-skin transfer of oxybutynin, female recipients absorbed more oxybutynin than their male counterparts, indicating that transfer may be gender related [3]. Stahlman et al. [5] concluded that skin-to-skin contact with the upper arms/shoulders to upper arms/shoulders prompted much more testosterone exposure than abdomen to abdomen. However, even within one individual, the medication does not remain solely at the application point [10]. Thus, it is important to note that transfer can take place at sites other than the application site.

Preventive measures for skin-to-skin transfer were also reviewed, namely washing, and the effect they would have on medication efficacy. Most studies indicated that washing after application has minimal impact on the systemic absorption of sex hormones and other medications [3, 8].

However, the results were not unanimous, as one study found a small but significant effect of washing on estradiol gel absorption [9]. Stahlman et al. [6] found that washing at 2 and 6 hours

TABLE 63.1

Peer-Reviewed Controlled Studies of Skin-to-Skin Chemical Transfer

Drug/Chemical	Concentration	Dose	Vehicle	Dosage per Area	Application Site and Transfer Site	Transfer Method	Method and Compartment of Drug Measurement	Result	Conclusion	Level of Evidence*	Reference
Estradiol	2.5 mg/g	1.74 g per site	Emulsion	n.s.†	Right and left leg from one individual to right and left forearm of another individual respectively	Application and transfer site rubbed for 2 minutes, 2 hours after application	Blood serum concentration (radioimmunoassay)	Systemic average concentration of estradiol increased from 17.0 ± 4.3 to 21.0 ± 4.4 pg/mL.	Estradiol transferred from the donor to the recipient.	IV	[7]
[^{14}C]-estradiol, [4-^{14}C]-NEC-127 estradiol	.6 mg/g	.16 g	Gel	9.6×10^{-4} mg/cm^2	Left ventral forearm of one individual to ventral forearm of another individual	Application and transfer site rubbed for 15 minutes, 1 hour after application	Urinary ^{14}C excretion	10.8 ± 7.9 % of the mean percent dose recovered in the recipient.	Estradiol transferred from the donor to the recipient.	I	[2]
Testosterone	25 mg/g	2.5 or 5 g	Gel	.21 mg/cm^2 or .42 mg/cm^2	Inner side of forearm of one individual to the back of another individual	Application and transfer site rubbed for 10 minutes, 10 minutes after application	Blood serum concentration (reverse-phase high-performance liquid chromatography and UV-detection)	No increase in the testosterone serum levels of the participants.	Testosterone not transferred at a clinically relevant level.	I	[1]

(Continued)

TABLE 63.1 (Continued)

Peer-Reviewed Controlled Studies of Skin-to-Skin Chemical Transfer

Drug/Chemical	Concentration	Dose	Dosage per Area	Vehicle	Application Site and Transfer Site	Transfer Method	Method and Compartment of Drug Measurement	Result	Conclusion	Level of Evidence*	Reference
Testosterone (AndroGel™ 1.62%)	16.2 mg/g	5 g	n.s.	Gel	Abdomen of one individual to abdomen of another individual	Application and transfer site rubbed for 15 minutes, 2 hours after application, once daily for 7 days	Blood serum concentration (validated liquid chromatography/ tandem mass spectroscopy)	Blood collections performed 0, 2, 4, 6, 8, 10, 12, 16, and 24 hours after the day before transfer began (baseline), Day 1, and Day 7. Mean AUC_{0-24} on Day 1 and Day 7 were 105% and 143% higher than baseline, respectively.	Testosterone transferred from the donor to the recipient.	1	[4]
Testosterone (AndroGel 1.62%)	16.2 mg/g	5 g	n.s.	Gel	Abdomen of one individual to abdomen of another individual	Application and transfer site rubbed for 15 minutes, 12 hours after application, once daily for 7 days	Blood serum concentration (validated liquid chromatography/ tandem mass spectroscopy)	Blood collections performed at 0, 2, 4, 6, 8, 10, 12, 16, and 24 hours on the day before transfer began (baseline), Day 1, and Day 7. Mean AUC_{0-24} on Day 1 and Day 7 were 118% and 83% higher than baseline, respectively.	Testosterone transferred from the donor to the recipient.	1	[4]

Drug	Concentration	Dose		Formulation	Application site	Application method	Measurement	Results	Conclusion		Ref
Estradiol (Evamist Estradiol metered-dose spray)	0.042 mg/d	3 90-μL sprays	n.s.	Spray	Inner forearm of one individual to inner forearm of another individual	Application and transfer site held against each other for 5 minutes, 1 hour after application	Blood serum concentration (high performance liquid chromatography/tandem mass spectroscopy)	Blood collections performed 4, 8, 12, 16, and 24 hours on the day before transfer began (baseline) and after transfer. Mean AUC_{0-24} was 2.3% higher than baseline.	Estradiol not significantly transferred from the donor to the recipient.	IV	[8]
Oxybutynin chloride	100 mg/g	1 g	n.s.	Gel	Abdomen of one individual to abdomen of another individual	Application and transfer site vigorously rubbed for 15 minutes, 1 hour after application	Blood serum concentration (high performance liquid chromatography/tandem mass spectroscopy)	The mean C_{max} of oxybutynin in plasma of recipients was 0.94±.75 ng/mL, baseline levels were approximately 0 ng/mL.	Oxybutynin transferred from the donor to the recipient.	I	[3]
Testosterone	16.2 mg/g	2.5 g	n.s.	Gel	Abdomen of one individual to abdomen of another individual	Application and transfer site had contact for 15 minutes, 2 hours after application	Blood serum concentration (validated liquid chromatography/tandem mass spectroscopy)	Mean ratios for the testosterone parameters in the recipients were 24%–27% higher than their baseline.	Testosterone transferred from the donor to the recipient.	I	[5]
Testosterone	16.2 mg/g	5 g	n.s.	Gel	Abdomen of one individual to abdomen of another individual	Application and transfer site had contact for 15 minutes, 2 hours after application	Blood serum concentration (validated liquid chromatography/tandem mass spectroscopy)	Mean ratios for the testosterone parameters in the recipients were 52%–70% higher than their baseline.	Testosterone transferred from the donor to the recipient.	I	[5]
Testosterone	16.2 mg/g	5 g	n.s.	Gel	Shoulders/upper arms of one individual to shoulders/upper arms of another individual	Application and transfer site had contact for 15 minutes, 2 hours after application	Blood serum concentration (validated liquid chromatography/tandem mass spectroscopy)	Mean ratios for the testosterone parameters in the recipients were 266%–280% higher than their baseline.	Testosterone transferred from the donor to the recipient.	I	[5]

(Continued)

TABLE 63.1 (Continued)
Peer-Reviewed Controlled Studies of Skin-to-Skin Chemical Transfer

Drug/Chemical	Concentration	Dose	Dosage per Area	Vehicle	Application Site and Transfer Site	Transfer Method	Method and Compartment of Drug Measurement	Result	Conclusion	Level of Evidence*	Reference
Testosterone	16.2 mg/g	5 g	n.s.	Gel	Abdomen of one individual to abdomen of another individual	Application and transfer site had contact for 15 minutes, 2 hours after application	Blood serum concentration (validated liquid chromatography/tandem mass spectroscopy)	Mean ratios for the testosterone parameters in the recipients were 68%–109% higher than their baseline.	Testosterone transferred from the donor to the recipient.	I	[5]
Estradiol (EstroGel)	0.6 mg/g	1.25 g	n.s.	Gel	An arm of an individual to an arm of another individual	Application and transfer site rubbed for 3 minutes, and then stationary contact for 12 minutes, 1 hour after gel application	Blood serum concentration (validated radioimmunoassay)	Mean AUC_{0-24} for estradiol serum concentration after contact was only 1% higher than the baseline.	Estradiol not significantly transferred from the donor to the recipient.	I	[9]
Tetracycline hydrochloride	16 mg/g	5 g on each site, except for left longitudinal half of body, which was 30 g	n.s.	Ointment and cream	The dominant hand, nondominant hand, preauricular area, dorsal aspect of feet, or left longitudinal half of body to areas in contact during daily activities on same individual	Participants went about their day per usual without bathing for 24 hours	Examination by fluorescence under a Wood's lamp	Areas of fluorescence observed by black light on sites other than where the testosterone was applied.	Tetracycline transferred from the initial application site to other parts of the individual's body. Absorption not measured.	IV	[10]

Tetracycline hydrochloride	16 mg/g	5 g on each site, except for left longitudinal half of body which was 30 g	n.s.	Lotion and tincture	The dominant hand, nondominant hand, preauricular area, dorsal aspect of feet, or left longitudinal half of body to areas in contact during daily activities on same individual	Participants went about their day per usual without bathing for 24 hours	Examination by fluorescence under a Wood's lamp	Extensive areas of fluorescence not observed by blacklight on sites other than where the testosterone was applied	Tetracycline not transferred from the initial application site to other parts of the individual's body. Absorption was not measured.	IV [10]
Nickel	N/A	N/A	N/A	1€ and 2€ coins, which participants rubbed between their fingers for 1 hour	The fingers to the cheeks on the same individual	The participant rubbed their finger on the coin for 30 minutes; every 5 minutes rubbing their cheek with their fingers	Placing adhesive tape on cheeks of individuals (inductively coupled mass spectroscopy)	Concentration of nickel on the cheek on average went from 0.4 ppm to 2.2 ppm.	Nickel transferred from the fingers to the cheek of the individuals. Absorption was not measured.	III [11]

*Based on Cochrane Consumer Network's guidelines on level of evidence.
† Not stated.

after testosterone gel application caused a slight decrease in absorption, but washing 10 hours after application had no impact. The same study indicated that washing decreased the amount of testosterone on the skin by at least 81% [6]. Other studies concurred that washing significantly inhibited interpersonal chemical transfer by removing the chemical from the application site [1, 5, 6].

Hanchenlaksh et al. [13] examined urinary diakylphoshate levels (a biomarker of pesticide exposure) in the spouses of Thai farmers who worked with pesiticides. While the study did not determine that the pesticides were transferred from farmer to spouse via skin-to-skin contact, it concluded that the greatest factor in lowering DAP metabolite levels of the spouses was if the farmer had showered immediately after work [13]. The results indicate that washing is also an effective method of inhibiting transfer of an occupational agent.

63.4   DISCUSSION

While most studies indicate that significant skin-to-skin transfer of chemicals is possible, it is critical to observe the differences in the results of the studies and between groups within the studies. In the oxybutynin study, transfer was greater to females than males. The speculative reason provided was that women have less cornified skin because of better skin care [3]. However, another possible reason is that females are on average smaller than males. The smaller stature means a higher surface area to volume ratio, meaning a similar volume of chemical on a female would, on average, be absorbed more than in a male. Rolf et al. [1] concluded that it is unlikely for transferred testosterone gel to cause side effects in prepubertal males or females or adult female subjects, as has been seen in some case studies. However, unlike in the case studies the paper refers to, Rolf et al. [1] and Schumacher et al. [8] (one of the other studies with negative transfer results), both use only adult male recipients. Even to a further extent than women, children could be subject to adverse effects when exposed to the same dosage that would be insignificant in an adult male due to a relatively high body surface area to volume ratio. Consequently, the testosterone gel in the case studies involving hypergonadism in children may be significant.

Rolf et al. [1] also concluded that the testosterone is transferred, but not absorbed, to a significant extent in the recipient. Rolf et al. [1] reasons from this that in an adult male, this transferred testosterone does not pose a threat via transdermal absorption. However, even the conclusion Rolf et al. [1] drew does not mean that the testosterone remaining on the skin of the recipient is harmless. The transferred testosterone could potentially become bioavailable through other routes such as ingestion. Furthermore, other studies concluded that chemicals could be intrapersonally transferred, so the transferred testosterone could then be transferred to a body part more susceptible to absorption [10, 11].

ZumBrunnen et al. [9] and Wester et al. [2] provide an interesting comparison, as both studies' methods are similar (0.06% estradiol gel transferred arm to arm) but resulted in different conclusions. ZumBrunnen et al. [9] concluded that transferred estradiol was not absorbed to a significant extent in the recipient, while Wester et al. [2] stated the absorption of estradiol was significant. The difference may lie in their diverse methodology. Wester et al. [2] measured the transfer of the ^{14}C in the gel, while ZumBrunnen et al. [9] measured serum concentration of estradiol, estrone, and estrone sulfate individually. The ^{14}C methodology is more sensitive in terms of how much of the gel is absorbed, and unlike in ZumBrunnen et al. [9] where the concentration of each component was compared individually, the entirety of transfer lies in a single parameter [2]. This more inclusive parameter could have meant the difference in terms of significance between the two studies.

We note the likelihood that the factors that control transfer of drugs from one person to another probably holds for exposure to occupational and environmental agents as well. The experimental data, although limited, point to this likelihood. Isnardo et al. [11] concludes that the nickel from a 1€ and 2€ coin can be transferred from the coin to the fingers and then from the fingers to the cheek of the same individual. It is probable that the nickel would also transfer interpersonally, as would other similar agents.

Another aspect of transfer that had an impact was application site. Upper arms/shoulders contact with upper arms/shoulders prompted much more transfer and consequently absorption than abdomen to abdomen [5]. However, no investigation has been conducted on the effect of interpersonal transfer of chemicals from or to the forearms or the back, the transfer sites of many of the previously discussed studies. So, while the difference between shoulders and abdomen makes it apparent that locations of the body have an effect on the level of transfer, the impact the body parts studied had on the outcome of the studies reviewed in this paper remains unclear. The difference in the transfer rates of different body parts may also have implications as to where manufacturers should suggest that their medications be applied. If doing so does not diminish the efficacy of the medication, in order to minimize transfer, more topical medications should likely be applied to areas more inhibitory to transfer such as the abdomen.

Furthermore, as the results conclude that washing has little to no impact on the absorption of medications, washing should be a routine part of the application of the medication, after allowing time for the medication to absorb. However, an exact time when maximal bioavailability is reached is sub judice, and may differ from one medication to another in addition to being dependent on dosage formulation. One study regarding a testosterone gel concluded that washing the application site 2 hours after application reduced the bioavailability of the testosterone from the gel by 10% to 14%, or according to Stahlman et al. [6], not sufficient to be clinically significant in the treatment outcome. Yet another study of an estradiol transdermal spray found that washing after only 1 hour led to no significant differences in estradiol absorption [8]. Consequently, while the application site should be washed post-application, the time at which it should be washed may vary depending on the chemical and vehicle.

Recent overviews of the efficiency in washing chemicals from skin are found in Phuong and Maibach [14]. Food and Drug Administration (FDA)–initiated package label warnings based on adverse reactions of transfer of sex hormones are on the FDA website for each drug [15].

63.5 CONCLUSION

These results strongly suggest the existence of significant transfer and subsequent absorption of transdermal or topical medication. Despite the strong positive results, three studies showed otherwise. While the discrepancy can partially be attributed to demographics of the test subjects and the parameters of the studies, the large differences between the methods of each study implore for a standardized method for measuring the skin-to-skin transfer of chemicals.

The existence of significant skin-to-skin transfer and subsequent absorption by the recipient has many important implications. For example, transfer should be considered during clinical studies that involve a placebo control group, as transfer of the medication by either the researcher or between study participants may confound the true difference between the control group and treatment group, potentially changing a significant difference into insignificance [10].

Additionally, interpersonal chemical transfer has dangerous implications in any industry where workers may inadvertently contact hazardous chemicals. A worker who comes into contact with a dose of a chemical that does not cause visible side effects in himself or herself may be harmful to those that he or she comes into close contact with. Moreover, as shown in this systematic analysis, those using transdermal medications should take precautions, especially when around children, including washing the application site before touching others and ensuring they do not allow areas that have come into contact with the chemicals to touch other parts of their body.

ACKNOWLEDGEMENT

The authors thank Rebecca Law, John H. Cary, and Becky S. Li for their assistance.

REFERENCES

1. Rolf C, Knie U, Lemmnitz G, Nieschlag E: Interpersonal testosterone transfer after topical application of a newly developed testosterone gel preparation. Clin Endocrinol (Oxf) 2002;56:637–641.
2. Wester RC, Hui X, Maibach HI: In vivo human transfer of topical bioactive drug between individuals: estradiol. J Invest Dermatol 2006;126:2190–2193.
3. Dmochowski RR, Newman DK, Sand PK, Rudy DC, Caramelli KE, Thomas H, Hoel G: Pharmacokinetics of oxybutynin chloride topical gel: effects of application site, baths, sunscreen and person-to-person transference. Clin Drug Investig 2011;31:559–571.
4. Stahlman J, Britto M, Fitzpatrick S, McWhirter C, Testino SA, Brennan JJ, Zumbrunnen TL: Serum testosterone levels in non-dosed females after secondary exposure to 1.62% testosterone gel: effects of clothing barrier on testosterone absorption. Curr Med Res Opin 2012;28:291–301.
5. Stahlman J, Britto M, Fitzpatrick S, McWhirter C, Testino SA, Brennan JJ, Zumbrunnen TL: Effect of application site, clothing barrier, and application site washing on testosterone transfer with a 1.62% testosterone gel. Curr Med Res Opin 2012;28:281–290.
6. Stahlman J, Britto M, Fitzpatrick S, McWhirter C, Testino SA, Brennan JJ, Zumbrunnen TL: Effects of skin washing on systemic absorption of testosterone in hypogonadal males after administration of 1.62% testosterone gel. Curr Med Res Opin 2012;28:271–279.
7. Taylor MB, Gutierrez MJ: Absorption, bioavailability, and partner transfer of estradiol from a topical emulsion. Pharmacotherapy 2008;28:712–718.
8. Schumacher RJ, Gattermeir DJ, Peterson CA, Wisdom C, Day WW: The effects of skin-to-skin contact, application site washing, and sunscreen use on the pharmacokinetics of estradiol from a metered-dose transdermal spray. Menopause 2009;16:177–183.
9. Zumbrunnen TL, Meuwsen I, de Vries M, Brennan JJ: The Effect of Washing and the Absence of Interindividual Transfer of Estradiol Gel. Am J Drug Delivery 2006;4:89–95.
10. Johnson R, Nusbaum BP, Horwitz SN, Frost P: Transfer of topically applied tetracycline in various vehicles. Arch Dermatol 1983;119:660–663.
11. Isnardo D, Vidal J, Panyella D, Vilaplana J: Nickel transfer by fingers. Actas Dermosifiliogr 2015;106:e23–26.
12. Busse KL, Maibach HI: Transdermal estradiol and testosterone transfer in man: existence, models, and strategies for prevention. Skin Pharmacol Physiol 2011;24:57–66.
13. Hanchenlaksh C, Povey A, O'Brien S, de Vocht F: Urinary DAP metabolite levels in Thai farmers and their families and exposure to pesticides from agricultural pesticide spraying. Occup Environ Med 2011;68:625–627.
14. Phuong C, Maibach HI: Recent knowledge: Concepts of dermal absorption in relation to skin decontamination. J Appl Toxicol 2016;36:5–9.
15. Administration USFaD: Drugs@FDA: FDA Approved Drug Products. https://www.accessdata.fda.gov/scripts/cder/daf/, U.S. Food and Drug Administration, 2018.

64 Nanoparticles and Their Combination with Physical Methods for Dermal and Transdermal Drug Delivery

Nina Dragićević
Singidunum University, Danijelova 32, Belgrade, Serbia

Howard I. Maibach
University of California, San Francisco, California

CONTENTS

64.1 INTRODUCTION

Dermal and transdermal drug delivery has gained a lot of interest in the past few years, since the skin is readily accessible for drug application. The major problem in both dermal and transdermal drug delivery is low permeability of the most apical layer of the skin, the stratum corneum (SC). Since percutaneous absorption is necessary for the effectiveness of both topical and transdermal systems, significant efforts have been devoted to developing strategies to overcome the impermeability of intact human skin. There are many methods used for overcoming the barrier of the SC. The methods can be drug/vehicle based, such as selection of a correct drug or prodrug, the use of ion-pairs or coacervates, saturated or supersaturated solutions, eutectic systems, nanocarriers, etc. (Dragicevic and Maibach, 2015, 2016a). Besides these, methods based on SC modification are also successfully used, such as enhancing skin hydration, the use of chemical penetration enhancers, the application of methods based on the bypass or removal of the SC (microneedles, ablation, etc.) and electrical methods (ultrasound, iontophoresis, electroporation, magnetophoresis, etc.) (Dragicevic and Maibach, 2016b, 2017).

As to nanocarriers, there are a variety of different nanocarriers which can be, regarding the goal of therapy, used for dermal or transdermal drug delivery (Dragicevic and Maibach, 2016a). They can be lipid-based carriers, such as vesicles (conventional vesicles – liposomes, elastic vesicles – transfersomes, invasomes, ethosomes, etc.), nanoparticles (solid lipid nanoparticles [SLN], nano-structured lipid carriers [NLC]), etc. (Dragicevic-Curic et al., 2008, 2009, 2010; Ascenso et al., 2015; Dragicevic et al., 2016, Müller et al., 2016). Further, polymer-based carriers (Abdel-Mottaleb and Lamprecht, 2016) as well as surfactant-based carriers (Muzzalupo, 2016) are also used. In order to further enhance the penetration enhancing ability of nanocarriers, they are used together with physical penetration enhancement methods such as ultrasound (Oberli et al., 2014; Azagury et al, 2014), electroporation (Engelke et al., 2015; Berkó et al., 2016; Ita, 2016; Mohammad et al., 2016), iontophoresis (Patel et al., 2016; Del Río-Sancho et al., 2017) and microneedles (Arya et al., 2017; Dul et al., 2017; Ripolin et al., 2017).

For a comprehensive review of different nanocarriers used to enhance percutaneous drug penetration, the reader should refer to Dragicevic and Maibach (2016). For a review of physical methods, the reader should refer to Dragicevic and Maibach (2017), and for a detailed review on the combined use of different kinds of nanocarriers with physical methods, the reader should refer to Dragicevic and Maibach (2018).

64.1.1 Nanoparticles – Classification and Their Percutaneous Penetration

For the treatment of skin diseases, it is important to create drug reservoirs in the skin with sustained drug release. Therefore, it is believed that nanoparticles would be a good choice to provide the skin with the drug for a prolonged time, maintaining the required drug concentration in the skin. Further, this would allow dose reduction due to formation of depots with sustained drug release.

As to their composition, nanoparticles can be lipid-based (Pardeike et al., 2009; Mitri et al., 2011; Puglia and Bonina, 2012; Suter et al., 2016; Jain et al., 2017) and polymer-based (Zaric et al., 2013, 2015; Abrego et al., 2016; Parra et al., 2016). First-generation lipid-based nanoparticles are the SLNs produced from solid lipids only, either glycerides or waxes or mixtures of both (Figure 64.1). In order to improve on the drawbacks of the first-generation nanoparticles, second-generation nanoparticles were developed and named as nanostructured lipid nanocarriers (NLC) (Figure 64.1). These new nanoparticles are obtained by blending solid lipids with longer chain fatty acids and oils with shorter chain fatty acids (for details see Müller et al., 2016).

Polymer-based nanoparticles (Zaric et al. 2013, 2015, Abrego et al. 2016, Parra et al. 2016) have also been extensively used for skin delivery of numerous drugs/actives. Depending on the preparation technique, polymeric nanoparticles can be nanospheres (matrix-type nanoparticles) or nanocapsules (reservoir-type nanoparticles) (Figure 64.2). Besides non-biodegradable polymers, various biodegradable polymers (synthetic and natural) have also attracted attention and, hence, are now used for the production of nanoparticles. Polylactides and polyglycolides are commonly used biodegradable polyester polymers. However, other polymers are also used, such as hyaluronic acid, chitosan, etc. (for details see Abdel-Mottaleb and Lamprecht, 2016).

Numerous studies showed that nanoparticles enhanced the drug penetration and drug accumulation in the skin due to the sustained drug release. As to the penetration of the carrier, i.e. the nanoparticles, into the skin, they were not found inside the skin (Alvarez-Roman et al., 2004a, 2004b; Luengo et al., 2006). This was not encouraging as for the treatment of skin diseases, it is crucial to have drug reservoirs inside the skin and not only on the skin surface. Authors reported that nanoparticles are unable to penetrate into the intact skin, thus mostly remaining at the skin surface,

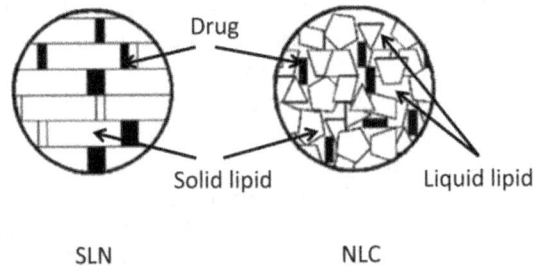

FIGURE 64.1 Schematic representation of lipid-based nanoparticles. Solid lipid nanoparticle (SLN) with an almost perfect solid lipid matrix and nanostructured lipid carrier (NLC) with an imperfect lipid matrix consisting of solid and liquid lipids. (Adapted from Abla et al., 2016.)

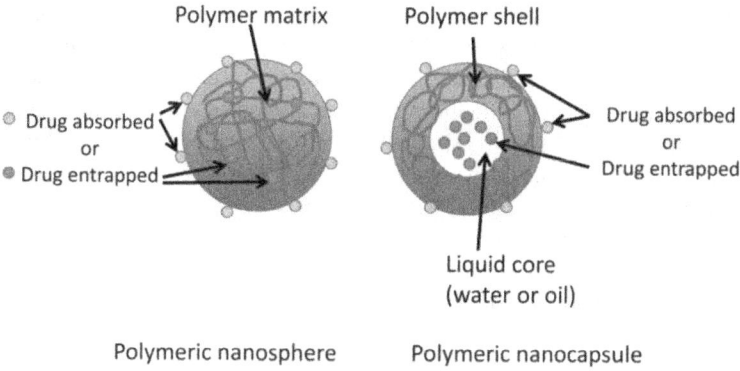

Polymer matrix   Polymer shell

Drug absorbed
or
Drug entrapped

Drug absorbed
or
Drug entrapped

Liquid core
(water or oil)

Polymeric nanosphere   Polymeric nanocapsule

FIGURE 64.2 Schematic representation of polymer-based nanoparticles. Polymeric nanosphere and polymeric nanocapsule. (Modified from Dragicevic and Maibach, 2018).

i.e. at the uppermost SC layer (Lademann et al., 1999; Zhang et al., 2008). Only few nanoparticles permeated the skin passively through the hair follicles (Toll et al., 2004; Lademann et al., 2007; Rancan et al., 2009). Lademann et al. (2007) found a preferential deposition of poly(D,L-lactic-co-glycolic acid) (PLGA) nanoparticles of 320 nm diameter in hair follicles *in vitro* in porcine skin. Rancan et al. (2009) reported deposition of polylactic nanoparticles of 228 and 365 nm diameter in 50% of the available vellus hair follicles. Wang et al. (2008) demonstrated a deposition of PLGA nanoparticles around hair follicles and sebaceous glands *in vitro* in human skin. Further, compared to free drugs (free rhodamine B [Rh B] and fluorescein isothiocyanate [FITC]) showing a negligible skin penetration and localization in hair follicles, the drug-loaded nanoparticles were preferentially deposited in hair follicles (Alvarez-Roman et al., 2004b; Küchler et al., 2009). In conclusion, the consensus is that nanoparticles cannot penetrate the intact skin; however, they can penetrate the follicular pathway, which is insufficient for an effective treatment of skin diseases. In addition, the skin penetration ability of nanoparticles depends on their composition, size, shape and other physicochemical factors.

Hence, to enable sufficient penetration of nanoparticles into the skin, i.e. to overcome the SC barrier, an effective additional penetration enhancement method is needed together with nanoparticles.

64.1.2 Combined Use of Nanoparticles and Microneedles

Microneedle (MN) technology has been used frequently as it facilitates intra/transdermal delivery of drugs in a minimally invasive fashion (Katikaneni, 2015; Arya et al., 2017; Baek et al., 2017; Dul et al., 2017; Kim et al., 2017; Ripolin et al., 2017; Permana et al., 2019; Vora et al., 2020; Courtenay et al., 2020). In brief, the mechanism of action of MNs is based on creating transient microconduits which penetrate through the SC, extend into the viable epidermis and hence facilitate drug permeation, as well as the penetration of drug carriers. It is a powerful enhancement method when used alone, e.g. for intradermal vaccination and gene delivery (Chabri et al., 2004; Prausnitz, 2004; Coulman et al., 2006a, 2006b; Frerichs et al., 2008; Hirschberg et al., 2008; Ali et al., 2016; Puri et al., 2016; Dul et al., 2017; Ita, 2017; Pamornpathomkul et al., 2017b), intradermal lymph targeting of drugs (Permana et al., 2020), intradermal delivery of cosmetic actives (Puri et al., 2016), transdermal delivery of large and small biomolecules(e.g. insulin and other drugs; Martanto et al., 2004; Cormier et al., 2004; Kearney et al., 2016; Modepalli et al., 2016; Kim et al. 2017; Courtenay et al., 2020; Kurnia Anjani et al., 2020), as well as when combined with other physical methods, such as with iontophoresis for the transdermal delivery of methotrexate (Vermulapalli et al., 2008), daniplestim (Katikaneni et al., 2010), and others. It has also been combined with electroporation for the delivery of FITC-dextrans (Yan et al., 2010) or with sonophoresis for the transdermal delivery of calcein and bovine albumin serum (Chen et al., 2010). It has also been shown that the combination of ultrasonic waves and iontophoresis improved the efficiency of hyaluronic acid MNs by shortening the reaction duration, and that this combination strategy could be used for delivery of macromolecules (Bok et al. 2020). In addition to physical methods, MN technology has been used in combination with nanocarriers also, especially nanoparticles for vaccine and gene delivery, as well as delivery of large molecules (Lawson et al., 2007; Combadiere and Mahe, 2008; Manolova et al., 2008; Pamornpathomkul et al. 2017a, Tort et al. 2020).

In an attempt to prove that microconduits created by MNs can act as channels for nanoparticles to penetrate through the SC and epidermis, a lot of studies were performed which will be discussed in following sections. For more details on the mechanism of drug delivery by MNs, MN evaluation in humans and the fabrication of MNs, the reader should refer to the comprehensive references (Kalluri et al. 2017; McAlister et al. 2017, Singh et al. 2017).

The combination of MNs and nanoparticles has been used to date mostly to achieve dermal delivery of low-molecular-weight drugs (Donnelly et al., 2010) and for transcutaneous immunization (Bal et al., 2010; Kumar et al., 2011; Siddhapura et al., 2016; Ali et al., 2017; Pamornpathomkul et al., 2017a).

When using nanoparticles together with MNs, one should differ between the two-step and the one-step delivery strategy. The two-step drug delivery with MNs requires MN puncture followed by drug application. The one-step delivery strategy uses MNs manufactured from biocompatible polymers which contain the drug alone or incorporated in nanoparticles. This strategy combines the advantages of nanoparticles and polymeric MNs showing synergistic effects. Also the nanoparticles are directly deposited across the skin by MN tips which encapsulate nanoparticles.

Donnelly et al. (2010) investigated different possibilities to enhance percutaneous delivery of highly lipophilic photosensitizers used in topical photodynamic therapy (PDT). The authors showed that after insertion of water soluble polymeric MNs containing PLGA nanoparticles (150 nm in diameter) loaded with the hydrophobic model dye, Nile red, into porcine skin, high tissue concentrations of Nile red were observed at 1125 mm depth, but not in the receiver compartment indicating that only intradermal delivery was achieved (without the risk of systemic delivery). As to the application of Nile red-loaded nanoparticles without MNs pretreatment, amounts of Nile red found in the skin were low, i.e. no Nile red was detectable below 1.0 mm. This was expected as it is generally accepted that nanoparticles do not penetrate the intact skin, but accumulate at the skin surface, hair follicles and sweat glands. MNs delivered significantly higher Nile red amounts into the skin (3.59%) compared to the control patch without MNs (0.13%). These results, i.e. high percutaneous drug penetration without delivering the drug into the receiver compartment were very important for topical PDT, indicating that transdermal (systemic) delivery using this system would be very limited, and the prolonged photosensitivity would be overcome. This strategy has also been used in the study by Zaric et al. (2013).

Park et al. (2006) investigated one-step delivery strategy by using biodegradable polymer MNs composed of PLGA, containing drugs. Calcein or bovine serum albumin were directly incorporated into the MN matrix or were first encapsulated into carboxymethylcellulose (CMC) microparticles (mean diameter 9.6 μm) and poly-L-lactide (PLA) microparticles (1–30 μm), which were further incorporated into the PLGA MN matrix. Depending on the encapsulation method, the sustained drug release could be controlled, ranging from hours to months.

This one-step delivery strategy using polymeric MNs with encapsulated nanoparticles has been frequently applied in the past years. Thus, nanoparticles-encapsulated polymeric MNs have nowadays been used for transdermal delivery of various therapeutic cargos, particularly for diabetes therapy, infectious disease therapy, cancer therapy, dermatological disease therapy etc. (Chen et al. 2020).

This strategy has been shown to be effective in the treatment of keloids. 5-fluorouracil (5-FU)-loaded carboxymethyl chitosan (CMC) nanoparticles were prepared and coated on stainless steel solid MNs. 5-FU-loaded CMC nanoparticles showed a significant inhibitory effect on the human keloid fibroblast i.e. up to 16%. The intercellular uptake of the 5-FU-loaded CMC nanoparticles was observed in both controls and keloid fibroblasts (by using a confocal microscope) and nanoparticles showed an inhibition of tumor growth factor-β1 (TGF-β1) by ELISA test. After their application onto the skin, nanoparticles coated onto the MNs were dissolved and diffused at the administration site in the porcine dorsal skin model. Thus, this MN-mediated drug delivery system inhibits the human keloid fibroblasts by delivering drugs effectively into the keloids, and it has the feasibility to self-administer without pain (Park and Kim, 2020).

Electrosprayed micro/nanoparticles loaded with dye or insulin were coated onto MNs (Tort et al. 2020). The authors showed that the optimally coated MNs resulted in higher than 70% transfer rate into porcine skins. Further, insulin-loaded particles coated onto MNs were applied to diabetic rats which resulted in the reduction of blood glucose levels fluctuations as compared to subcutaneous injections. Tort et al. (2020) reported that electrospraying represents an effective method to coat MNs with drug-loaded nanoparticles, which can be effective for the delivery of cosmetics, drugs and proteins.

Generally, in order to achieve its therapeutic effectiveness the drug has to be delivered in its therapeutic dosage to the target in the skin. Hence, the amount of drug-loaded nanoparticles deposited in the skin influence whether the drug amount accumulated in the skin would reach its therapeutic level. This would also decide if this combination of enhancement methods could be an effective approach to achieve a positive therapeutic outcome upon the topical drug application.

64.1.2.1 Influence of Nanoparticles' Properties when Combined with MNs

MNs enhance the intradermal delivery of nanoparticles, and the size of nanoparticles may influence their penetration through microconduits in the skin produced by MNs.

The effect of the nanoparticle size and concentrations of PLGA nanoparticles on the drug penetration in MNs-treated human skin was investigated (Zhang et al., 2010). Confocal laser scanning microscopy (CLSM) showed that nanoparticles were delivered into the microconduits created by MNs. As fluorescence was seen only inside the microconduits and not in other areas, it was clear that SC represented a barrier for the skin penetration of nanoparticles and they could be delivered into the skin only after SC has been broken by MNs. Fluorescence was observed even at the depth of 68.32 µm, indicating that nanoparticles permeated into the viable epidermis and diffused also into the dermis, as human abdominal epidermis is about 60 µm thick. As to the penetration of nanoparticles without using MNs, fluorescence was only seen in hair follicles as nanoparticles could not pass the SC, but could passively permeate into the skin by the follicular pathway. This finding is in accordance with the results of Lademann et al. (2007). Regarding *in vitro* skin permeation studies in full-thickness human skin, MNs significantly enhanced ($P < 0.01$) the permeation of nanoparticles (diameter 205.5 nm) into the skin as compared to the treatment without MNs. Hence, MNs were more effective than the hair follicles for enhancing penetration of nanoparticles into skin. When MNs were used, significantly more ($P < 0.01$) nanoparticles were deposited in the epidermis than in the dermis (as no microconduits were created in the dermis and few nanoparticles diffused from the epidermis to the dermis) (Zhang et al. 2010). Skin penetration of nanoparticles was particle size dependent, i.e. the decrease in the particle size significantly increased ($P < 0.01$) the nanoparticles' accumulation in the skin. Furthermore, permeation increased with increasing the nanoparticle concentration until reaching a threshold value. The efficiency of MNs in enhancing skin penetration of nanoparticles increases as time passes, since after 48 hours the amount of nanoparticles deposited in the skin was significantly higher ($P < 0.01$) than after 3 hours, in contrast to the treatment without MNs where the deposited amount of nanoparticles in the skin did not significantly increase after 48 hours. Obtained results confirmed the enhanced intradermal delivery of nanoparticles by using MNs, which could sustain the drug release in skin, supplying skin with the drug over a prolonged period and maintaining the desired drug concentration in skin. These effects are crucial for an effective dermal drug application (Zhang et al., 2010). The nanoparticles did not reach the receptor solution, despite using MNs, being in accordance with findings of other authors (de Jalon et al., 2001).

In contrast to Zhang et al. (2010) and de Jalon et al. (2001), Coulman et al. (2009) detected polystyrene nanoparticles (100–150 nm diameter) in the receptor solution after their application to human epidermal membrane treated with MNs. The contradictory results may be due to different nanoparticle size, channel size and the physico-chemical properties of the nanoparticle material, as PLGA is lipophilic and accumulates in the skin rather than penetrating the receptor solution. However, Birchall et al. (2006) found *in vitro* that polystyrene nanoparticles could permeate only into the dermis and epidermis, through the microconduits produced by ViaDerm™ confirming an intradermal delivery of nanoparticles by using MNs.

Kohli and Alpar (2004) found, by fluorescence microscopy in porcine skin, that latex nanoparticles of 50 and 500 nm diameter, being negatively charged, were able to permeate through the intact SC into the viable epidermis. In contrast, positively charged and neutral particles of all sizes (50, 100, 200 and 500 nm) and negatively charged 100 and 200 nm particles did not show penetration into the skin. However, Alvarez-Roman et al. (2004b) demonstrated by CLSM in porcine skin that negatively charged polystyrene nanoparticles of 20 and 200 nm diameter could not penetrate through the intact SC. Nanoparticles accumulated in the skin appendages in a time-dependent fashion. They found (Alvarez-Roman et al., 2004c) *in vitro* by CLSM using polystyrene nanoparticles (20–200 nm diameter) that small particles could be delivered into the hair follicles in porcine skin more favorably than big particles, which could be due to their higher specific surface area.

Coulman et al. (2009) investigated permeation of negatively charged polystyrene nanoparticles (size: 100 nm) through untreated, MNs treated and hypodermic needle treated human epidermal membrane. They confirmed previous studies of Alvarez-Roman et al. (2004b) that nanoparticles when applied to intact skin adhered to the skin surface, and identified in dermatoglyphics. After the application of a hypodermic needle (10 punctures) and creating microchannels, 50–100 μm in diameter, 10% of the applied nanoparticle formulation permeated the skin and was found in the receptor phase within 3 hours. The application of MNs to the skin prior the administration of nanoparticles, creating microchannels of comparable size, but greater in number compared to hypodermic needle-induced channels, resulted in more than 20% of the applied nanoparticle formulation permeating the epidermis (found in the receptor phase) within 6 hours of application. The study showed that microchannels are of crucial importance for the permeation of nanoparticles through the epidermis, i.e. without microchannels there is no epidermal permeation of nanoparticles and hence no potential for the therapeutic application of nanoparticles for intradermal drug delivery. Further, Coulman et al. (2009) showed that nanoparticles interacted with the SC and viable epidermis of the MN-treated skin. Nanoparticles were adsorbed at the surface of the skin between disrupted corneocytes and on the interior surface of microchannels and in associated lateral disruptions. This interaction of nanoparticles and MN-treated skin could retard the transdermal delivery of drugs. However, for indications where intradermal delivery is desired, such as gene delivery, vaccination or treatment of skin diseases, this interaction between the formulation and viable skin would be beneficial and thus clinically promising. The retardation in drug delivery was proposed to be a result of two observed phenomena: nanoparticle adherence to the skin surface and the aggregation of nanoparticles due to the instability of colloidal formulation, which occurred when MNs were applied (Coulman et al., 2009). This study also confirmed, by using Isopore® membranes (pore sizes 100 nm, 1.2 μm and 10 μm), the *importance of the surface charge of particles* (due to the electrostatic interaction of the nanoparticles with the membrane or microchannel surface). At pH 7.4, nanoparticles and the membrane surface possess negative zeta potentials and almost 80% of the applied formulation is diffused through 10-μm pores in the receptor phase after 4 hours; while at pH 3 (membrane possess positive surface charge) 50% of the applied formulation is diffused after 2 hours, this being significantly lower. As to the *pore size of microconduits* for nanoparticle permeation, the increase of pore size significantly enhanced the nanoparticle permeation across the skin. At pH 7.4, the diffusion through 1.2-μm pores was significantly reduced compared to the diffusion through 10-μm pores (80% after 4 hours), i.e. only 60% of the applied formulation was found in the receptor phase after 12 hours. At pH 3, the difference was even more significant, i.e. 40% of the applied formulation was found in the receptor phase in case of 10-μm pores and only 0.1% in case of pores of 1.2 μm. As to membranes with 100-nm pores (simulates intact skin), no penetration of nanoparticles into the skin was observed. However, the maximum dimensions of microchannels created in the skin are restricted by the desire for limited invasiveness, pain and safety concerns.

Gomaa et al. (2014) used two dyes, Rh B (hydrophilic model drug) and FITC (hydrophobic model drug), encapsulated in PLGA nanoparticles to gain information on the mechanism of their transdermal drug delivery across MN-treated full-thickness porcine skin. They found that their permeation through MN-treated skin was affected by physicochemical characteristics of nanoparticles and the encapsulated dyes. Dye flux was enhanced by smaller particle size, hydrophilicity, and negative zeta potential of nanoparticles. Reduction in particle size of Rh B nanoparticles from 422.3 to 155.2 nm resulted in significant increase of Rh B permeation, i.e. it led to a fivefold increase in total amount permeated per unit area at 48 hours. The authors explained this finding by faster release of the encapsulated Rh B from smaller nanoparticles with larger surface-to-volume ratio. Further, they suggest deeper and more extensive influx of smaller nanoparticles through MN-created channels leading to enhanced transdermal delivery of Rh B released at the deeper deposition sites of nanoparticles (Gomaa et al., 2014). As for nanoparticle's hydrophilicity, increasing PLGA copolymer hydrophilicity by reducing the lactide-to-glycolide ratio significantly enhanced permeation of Rh B from PLGA 50:50 nanoparticles compared to PLGA 75:25 and 100:0 nanoparticles. This was explained by greater compatibility of the more hydrophilic nanoparticles with the aqueous environment of microchannels, leading to deeper penetration. Regarding the surface charge, negatively charged nanoparticles larger in size (−4.5 mV, 367.0 nm,) allowed significantly greater ($P < 0.05$) permeation of FITC compared to smaller positively charged nanoparticles (122.0 nm, 57 mV), i.e. 2.7-fold and 2.9-fold increases in Q_{48} and flux, respectively, could be observed. The authors suggested that as porcine skin bears a net negative charge at physiological pH, repulsion of negatively charged nanoparticles may reduce adsorption at its surface, inducing influx of nanoparticles deeper into the microchannels and enhancing flux of released FITC.

As to the effect of dye-related variables on skin permeation, drug solubility at physiological pH and potential interaction with skin proteins proved to outweigh molecular weight as determinants of skin permeation. The effect of dye solubility was examined by comparing two encapsulated dyes of different solubility (solubility of 0.99 versus 0.09 g/L for Rh B and FITC, respectively), while other variables were kept constant. Statistically significant 33.2-fold and 35.8-fold differences in Q_{48} and flux values, respectively, were observed for Rh B compared to FITC. CLSM confirmed significantly higher skin permeability of nanoencapsulated Rh B (190 μm) compared to FITC (130 μm). Higher solubility was reported to increase drug flux across MN-treated skin, since the dermis does not represent a distinct barrier to hydrophilic drugs once the SC is bypassed (Gomaa et al., 2014). According to the authors, significantly lower flux of FITC can be ascribed to poor solubility due to the hydrophobic isothiocyanate substituent which probably resulted in slower release from nanoparticles and saturation of the microenvironment, resulting in reduced concentration gradient and molecular diffusion.

As to the effect of the percentage of initial drug loading on skin permeation of nanoencapsulated Rh B and FITC, permeation of Rh B increased significantly ($P < 0.05$) with the increase in dye loading. In contrast, increasing percentage of initial FITC loading led to reduced skin permeation. This was explained by the fact that increasing the initial FITC loading from 5% to 20% w/w was associated with increase in particle size and PDI (higher heterogeinity), and decrease in zeta potential. Gomaa et al. (2014) proposed a mechanism for percutaneous penetration of nanoparticles, particularly of smaller size, deep into MN-created channels, generating reservoirs of the drug. According to the authors, molecular diffusion of the released dye across viable skin layers proceeds at a rate determined by its molecular characteristics. It was confirmed that only the free dye released from nanoparticles permeated skin layers to the receiver compartment.

64.1.2.2 Influence of MN Characteristics and Application Variables on Drug Diffusion

Gomaa et al. (2012) investigated the effect of MN application, MN characteristics and application variables on the transdermal delivery of a hydrophilic small/medium-sized model drug (Rh B) encapsulated in PLGA nanoparticles in full-thickness porcine skin *in vitro*. They reported a 5.4-fold higher ($P < 0.005$) skin permeation of flux of encapsulated Rh B compared to the solution of free Rh B. Nanoparticles were preferentially deposited in the hair follicles (diameter of approximately 200 μm in porcine skin), which has already been found by other groups (Lademann et al., 2007; Wang et al., 2008; Zhang et al., 2010). The authors proposed that Rh B was released from the nanoparticles localized in the follicles and that it laterally diffused into the viable epidermis, which explained the enhanced transdermal drug delivery (as it was found in the receptor solution), while nanoparticles were not detected in the receptor solution. Skin *pretreatment with MNs* enhanced the transdermal flux of free Rh B 3.7-fold compared to free drug without MNs, and significantly more of Rh B loaded in nanoparticles, i.e. 13.76-fold compared to free drug without MNs (2.5-fold higher compared to nanoparticles without MNs), as nanoparticles were preferentially deposited in the microchannels formed by MNs, creating dye reservoirs, releasing Rh B which freely diffused into the skin layers below the SC. This resulted in accelerated drug permeation. However, no particles were detected in the receptor solution, which was in accordance with findings of Zhang et al. (2010). As to the epidermis and deeper skin layers, the highest drug deposition was also obtained by the combined use of nanoparticles and MNs. In conclusion, the combination of Rh B nanoencapsulation and skin treatment with MN produced the greatest apparent dye infiltration into deeper skin layers.

In the same study, use of *different needle lengths* showed that the insertion of 600-μm-long needles yielded a significantly higher permeation enhancement of encapsulated Rh B compared to the insertion of 400-μm-long MNs, as well as compared to the untreated skin. However, the further increase of needle length, i.e. use of 1000-μm-long needles did not lead to further significant permeation increase, which can be explained by the increased frictional resistance characteristic for the longest needles; different threshold needle lengths have been reported by different groups (Gomaa et al., 2012). Kumar et al. (2011) reported that the use of a MN roller with larger MNs (1000 μm long, base diameter 80 μm) allowed more extensive permeation of SLN with conjugated ovalbumin (OVA) than the pretreatment with a roller containing smaller MNs (200 μm long, base diameter 20 μm).

Regarding the *MN density*, the highest density was less effective than the lower densities, i.e. the 361 MNs/array provided a smaller steady-state flux of encapsulated Rh B (5.08 ± 0.34 μg/cm^2/hour, $P = 0.008$) than lower densities, such as the 121 MNs/array (6.19 ± 0.77 μg/cm^2/hour), while the cumulative amount of dye permeated (Q_{48} of 5.44 ± 0.16 mg/cm^2) was almost the same as with lower densities (121 MNs/array, Q_{48} of 5.40 ± 0.39 μg/cm^2)(Gomaa et al., 2012). The authors explained it by the "bed of nails" effect, where the pressure exerted by each needle tip can be decreased to a potentially insufficient level to penetrate as deeply into the skin as an array of lower density when the same force is spread over a very large number of needles (Yan et al., 2010; Gomaa et al., 2012).

As to the *number of array insertions* (one, five or nine insertions), the more insertions were applied the higher was the permeation of encapsulated Rh B, as more microchannels were created in the skin. Values obtained at one and nine insertions differed statistically significantly. The same group (Gomaa et al., 2010) showed in another study that this phenomenon may be due to the finding that when skin poration, i.e. number of pores, is high, pore re-closure may be suppressed to an extent since in that case the skin cannot effectively contract and reduce the pore size. Among different used *durations of MN insertion* (2 second, 3 minutes and 5 minutes), the highest permeation of Rh B was provided by the shortest insertion duration, indicating that the duration of MNs insertion in the skin should be short (Gomaa et al., 2012). This was in accordance with their previous study (Gomaa et al., 2010). The authors explained this by the possibility that accelerated elastic contractions caused by prolonged embedding of MNs in the skin result in partial closing of many microconduits formed by MNs, which inhibits the decrease of the skin barrier function (Gomaa et al. 2012).

64.1.2.3   Transcutaneous Immunization and Other Indications

Transcutaneous immunization (TCI) with needle-free formulations is a noninvasive approach which overcomes the drawbacks of the parenteral vaccination methods. The skin represents an ideal vaccination site as it allows targeted access to professional antigen-presenting cell (APC) populations within the skin, such as Langerhans cells (LCs), various dermal dendritic cells (dDCs), macrophages, etc. In TCI, it is of crucial importance that vaccine components overcome the SC in order to achieve an access to dermal APC populations that induce priming of T cell or B cell responses for protective immunity. Recently, it has been shown that a lot of progress has been made in particle-based systems for TCI, which deliver vaccine antigens together with adjuvants to peri-follicular APCs by diffusion and deposition in hair follicles (Mittal et al., 2013; Pielenhofer et al., 2020). Further, these particle-based carriers (liposomes, transfersomes, ethosomes, nanoparticles, etc.) represent not only noninvasive systems for enhanced percutaneous penetration, but also have other advantages regarding their ability to encapsulate different vaccine antigens, such as DNA, peptides, proteins, attenuated viruses, microorganism fragments, etc., thereby improving their stability and absorption, as well as increasing their antigenicity by mimicking the size of microorganisms. The particle-based systems enable the co-delivery of adjuvants which is important to increase the immunogenicity of the antigen allowing a reduction of the antigen dose. I very attractive for antigen encapsulation (Mittal et al., 2013).

The mechanism of enabling an immune response with TCI is shown in Figure 64.3. Intensive research has been performed in the field of nanoparticle-based transfollicular immunization also as this approach does not compromise the SC barrier (Mittal et al., 2013; Chen et al., 2018). As we are dealing with nanoparticles and physical enhancement methods in this chapter, studies confirming

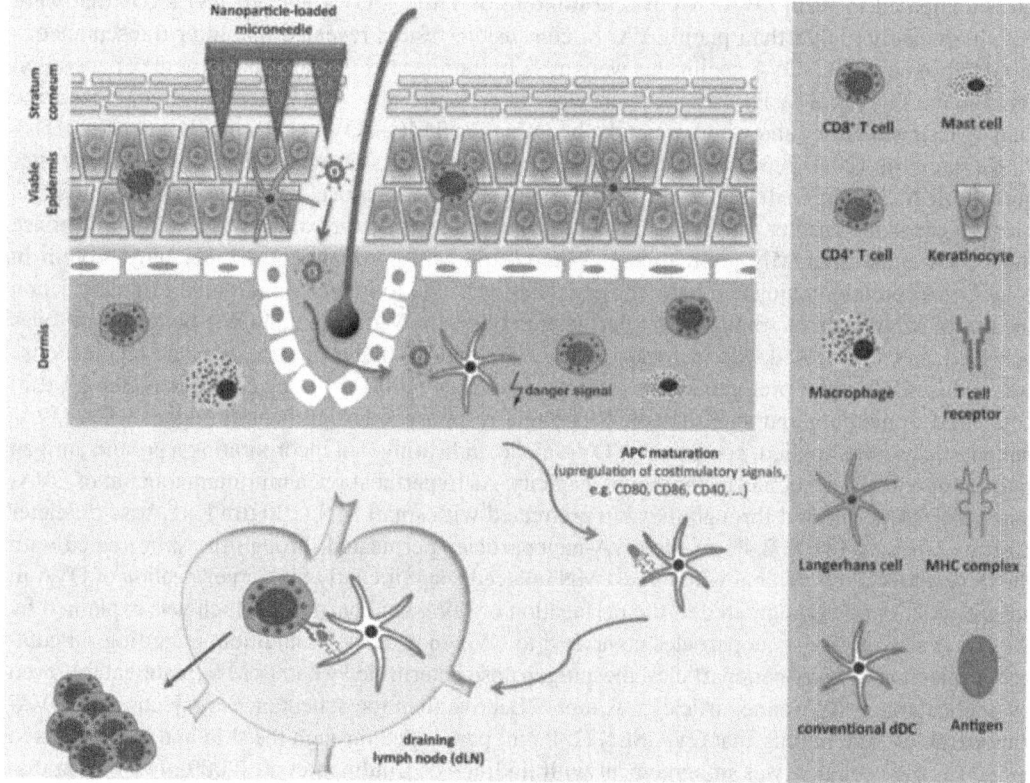

FIGURE 64.3 Particle-based systems for transcutaneous immunization facilitate the targeting of the skin-resident antigen-presenting cells (APCs). Activated APCs incorporate an antigen and migrate to the draining lymph node (dLN) where naive T cells are primed, thereby enabling an antigen-specific cellular immune response. (Pielenhofer et al., 2020.)

the ability of achieving TCI with protein antigens carried by nanoparticles that are applied onto skin pretreated with MNs (without this pretreatment there is no sufficient particle penetration into the skin) will be discussed (Bal et al., 2010, 2011; Kumar et al., 2011, 2012).

As to the choice whether to incorporate the drug inside the nanoparticles or to conjugate it onto the nanoparticle's surface when applying the nanoparticles onto the MNs-treated skin, Bal et al. (2010) reported that incorporation of protein antigens into nanoparticles does not lead to a stronger immune response compared to free antigens. The authors showed that diphtheria toxoid (DT) incorporated into N-trimethyl chitosan (TMC) nanoparticles and applied onto MN-treated skin did not induce a stronger antibody response than DT alone. However, when DT was conjugated with TMC nanoparticles and applied on MN-pretreated skin, it induced a stronger immune response than DT alone, i.e. the immunoglobulin G (IgG) titers after the second boost were eightfold higher compared to application of a solution of DT ($p<0.001$) and comparable to those elicited by subcutaneously applied DT-alum. This result indicated that conjugation of antigen with nanoparticles instead of incorporation of antigens inside nanoparticles was a better solution, which is in agreement with Kumar et al. (2011).

Bal et al. (2011) investigated the effects of formulations of OVA with TMC on the TCI conducted in the skin pretreated with MNs. They prepared three formulations of OVA: TMC + OVA mixtures, TMC–OVA conjugates and TMC/OVA nanoparticles.

After the prime vaccination, TMC–OVA conjugates induced significantly higher IgG titers than the other two formulations. Also after the boost, TMC–OVA conjugates proved to be significantly better than plain OVA, although the TMC/OVA nanoparticles also significantly elevated the IgG titers compared to plain OVA. A physical mixture of TMC + OVA elicited IgG levels that were not significantly higher than plain OVA. In conclusion, results revealed that after transcutaneous administration, TMC–OVA conjugates were most immunogenic, probably because they penetrated through the skin more easily than nanoparticles and consequently were better delivered to dendritic cells (DCs), while they show higher uptake by DCs than TMC + OVA mixtures (Bal et al., 2011).

Kumar et al. (2011) reported that the pretreatment of mice skin with MNs enabled the permeation of SLN, 230 nm in diameter, with OVA conjugated on their surface (not incorporated in SLN) through the skin. Further, this TCI induced a significantly stronger anti-OVA antibody response than OVA alone after MN pretreatment. Without the MN pretreatment, neither only protein in solution nor protein conjugated onto nanoparticles was able to induce an immune response. Upon the use of MNs, even of smallest size, permeation of both OVA alone and OVA-nanoparticles was achieved, and it increased with increasing needle size and the highest permeation and IgG response was induced after the pretreatment with largest needles (1000 μm long, base diameter 80 μm) compared to medium and small needles. The IgG response was significantly higher when OVA-nanoparticles were applied, compared to OVA alone, indicating that incorporating a protein antigen into nanoparticles can enhance its immunogenicity. As to permeation, a minimum amount of OVA-nanoparticles permeated through the skin pretreated with small MN (200 μm long, base diameter 20 μm), whereas 13.6 ± 2.4% of the OVA-nanoparticles permeated through the skin treated with the largest MN. Pretreatment with largest MN induced a significantly higher permeation of OVA in solution (28.3± 6.5%) compared to the permeation of OVA-nanoparticles, which was explained by the larger size of OVA-nanoparticles compared to OVA molecules. In addition, regarding subcutaneous injection of OVA-nanoparticles, the antigen dose determined whether MN treatment followed by application of OVA-nanoparticles was more effective than the subcutaneous injection of OVA-nanoparticles. The finding that OVA-SLN (230 nm) permeated through the skin and were detected in the receiver solution was in agreement with findings of Coulman et al. (2009), but was in disagreement with the reports by Zhang et al. (2010) and Bal et al. (2010) who used PLGA nanoparticles (166, 206, or 288 nm) and DT-N-TMC nanoparticles (211 ± 4 nm), respectively.

Kumar et al. (2012) showed that MN-mediated TCI with plasmid DNA coated on the surface of cationic (PLGA:DOTAP [1,2-dioleoyl-3-trimethylammonium-propane]) nanoparticles induced a stronger immune response than the plasmid DNA alone. Further, the study showed that the surface charge of the DNA-coated nanoparticles influenced their *in vitro* skin permeation and *in vivo* ability to induce immune response. TCI with plasmid-DNA-coated cationic nanoparticles elicited a stronger immune response than the same performed with anionic nanoparticles as well as than the intramuscular injection of the same dose of plasmid DNA alone. Furthermore, TCI by plasmid-DNA-coated cationic nanoparticles applied upon the MN pretreatment or by intramuscular injection induced comparable immune responses (i.e. comparable levels of total IgG) and proliferative reponses, but only TCI induced specific mucosal response, indicating the advantage of TCI. According to the authors (Kumar et al. 2012), the high efficiency of cationic nanoparticles is proposed to be due to their ability to increase the expression of the antigen gene encoded by the plasmid and more effectively stimulate the maturation of APCs.

Zaric et al. (2013) investigated the potential of dissolving MNs loaded with antigen encapsulated in PGLA nanoparticles to increase vaccine immunogenicity by targeting antigen specifically to DC network within the skin. Authors reported that this approach provided complete protection *in vivo* against the development of both tumors and virus. It was found that nanoencapsulation facilitates antigen retention in the skin layers and provides antigen stability in MNs. According to the authors, the use of biodegradable polymeric nanoparticles for selective targeting of antigen to skin DCs through dissolvable MNs is a promising technology for improved vaccination efficacy, compliance and coverage.

Siddhapura et al. (2016) investigated the potential of tetanus toxoid loaded chitosan nanoparticles (TT-Ch) for immunization with and without the use of MNs. The *in vitro* analysis demonstrated higher skin penetration of TT when used in combination with MNs. *In vivo* immunization studies showed that TT-Ch nanoparticles combined with MN treatment induced comparable IgG and IgG1 titer, and higher IgG2a titer than the commercial TT vaccine. The authors showed that MNs, especially hollow MNs applied with TT-Ch nanoparticles could be considered as the best solution for immunization due to induction of more balanced Th1/Th2 biased immune response.

Yang et al. (2017) incorporated ebola DNA vaccine into PLGA-PLL/γPGA nanoparticles and administered them onto the skin using MN patch. The incorporation of ebola DNA vaccine into the nanoparticles increased the vaccine thermostability and immunogenicity compared to the free vaccine. Furthermore, the vaccination by the MN patch produced a stronger immune response than the intramuscular administration of the vaccine.

Seok et al. (2017) developed an intradermal pH1N1 DNA vaccine delivery platform using MNs coated with a polyplex containing poly lactic-co-glycolic acid/polyethyleneimine (PLGA/PEI) nanoparticles. Stainless steel MNs were used, with enhanced hydrophilicity, manufactured by silanization. MNs were further coated with the polyplex encapsulating pDNA vaccine, without severe aggregation of the polyplex in the dry form. After MNs insertion into the porcine skin, the coated polyplex rapidly dissolved (within 5 minutes) and induced a greater humoral immune response compared to the intramuscular polyplex delivery or naked pH1N1 DNA vaccine delivery by a dry-coated MN. The authors showed that intradermal delivery of pDNA vaccines within a cationic polyplex coated on MNs is promising method for TCI (Seok et al., 2017).

Du et al. (2017) developed and compared four types of nanocarriers for vaccine delivery, i.e. PLGA nanoparticles, liposomes, mesoporous silica nanoparticles (MSNs) and gelatin nanoparticles (GNPs), which they loaded with OVA with and without an adjuvant (poly(I:C)). The nanocarrier dispersions were injected precisely into murine skin at a depth of about 120 μm. OVA/poly(I:C)-loaded nanoparticles and OVA/poly(I:C) solution elicited similarly strong total IgG and IgG1 responses, while the co-encapsulation of OVA and poly(I:C) in nanoparticles significantly increased the IgG2a response compared to OVA/poly(I:C) solution. PLGA nanoparticles and liposomes induced stronger IgG2a responses than MSNs and GNPs, correlating with sustained release of the antigen and adjuvant and a smaller nanoparticle size (Du et al., 2017). Regarding cellular responses, OVA/poly(I:C)-loaded liposomes induced the highest $CD8^+$ and $CD4^+$ T cell responses.

Mönkäre et al. (2018) developed hyaluronan (HA)-based dissolving MNs loaded with PLGA nanoparticles (NPs) co-encapsulating OVA and poly(I:C) for intradermal immunization. The authors found that the delivered antigen dose in mice from MNs was 1 μg OVA, in nanoparticles or as free antigen.

The immunogenicity of the nanoparticles after administration of dissolving MNs (NP:HA weight ratio 1:4) was compared with that of hollow MN-delivered nanoparticles in mice. The study revealed that the immunization with free antigen in dissolving MNs resulted in equally strong immune responses compared to the delivery by hollow MNs. However, humoral and cellular immune responses evoked by nanoparticles-loaded dissolving MNs were inferior compared to those elicited by nanoparticles delivered through hollow MNs. However, the authors found that the critical formulation parameters are important for the further development of nanoparticle-loaded dissolving MNs, such as the NP:HA ratio used for the preparation of dissolving MNs, drying conditions during MN preparation, and others, which they can vary to obtain the formulation with desired characteristics (Mönkäre et al., 2018).

Niu et al. (2019) investigated the use of the hollow MNs for the intradermal delivery of polymeric nanoparticles in rats. The model antigen OVA and TLR agonists imiquimod and monophosphoryl lipid A were encapsulated in PLGA nanoparticles. Hollow MNs with encapsulated nanoparticles bearing antigens were used due to their advantages, such as the pharmacokinetic profile, characterized by an early burst transit through the draining lymph nodes and a relatively limited overall systemic exposure compared to subcutaneous or intravenous delivery. OVA-loaded nanoparticles demonstrated faster antibody affinity maturation kinetics compared to soluble OVA-based vaccine. Furthermore, antigen-loaded nanoparticles delivered via a hollow MN array elicited a significantly higher IgG2a antibody response and higher number of interferon (IFN)-γ secreting lymphocytes, both markers of Th1 response, in comparison to antigen-loaded nanoparticles delivered by intramuscular injection and soluble antigen delivered through hollow MN array. The authors confirmed that hollow MN-mediated intradermal delivery of polymeric nanoparticles represents a promising approach to improve the effectiveness of vaccine formulations (Niu et al., 2019).

Nanoparticles combined with MNs besides being used for TCI, are also used to enhance the penetration of various drugs through the skin. Poly (D, L-lactic acid) (PDLLA) nanoparticles loaded with ketoprofen and applied to the skin upon the application of silicon MN arrays enhanced ketoprofen flux and supplied the porcine skin with the drug over a prolonged (24 hour) period of time (Vučen et al. 2013). Nanoparticles provided a 2.4-fold higher amount of drug permeated through MN-treated skin compared to nanoparticles applied to intact skin. The flux of ketoprofen was also more than twofold higher for MN-treated skin compared to intact skin. Thus, the MN- pretreatment of skin significantly enhanced the ketoprofen skin permeation from nanoparticles compared to ketoprofen permeation from nanoparticles through intact skin. MNs were also used with gold nanoparticles and they enhanced the penetration of gold nanoparticles into the skin, leading to a 150% increase in optical coherence tomography (OCT) contrast agent levels, enabling improved early-stage detection of oral cancer *in vivo* (Kim et al. 2009).

64.1.3 Combined Use of Nanoparticles and Iontophoresis

Among electrical physical penetration enhancement methods, iontophoresis has been extensively studied (Takeuchi et al., 2017; Manjunatha et al., 2018; Ronnander et al., 2019). Iontophoresis is a noninvasive method which involves the application of a small electric current to drive ionic and polar drugs exhibiting poor skin permeation into/through the skin. Good candidates for iontophoresis are hydrophilic molecules with high water solubility and little affinity for lipids. Fukuta et al. (2020) investigated the influence of iontophoresis on the skin delivery of biological macromolecular drugs, such as antibodies and fusion protein drugs. The authors confirmed the intradermal delivery of biological macromolecular drugs (FITC-labeled IgG antibody) via iontophoresis as fluorescence was broadly observed in the skin, i.e. it extended from the epidermis to the dermis layer of hairless rats, while passive antibody diffusion was not observed. Antibodies were also delivered via iontophoresis into inflamed skin tissue in a psoriasis model, and upregulation of interleukin-6 mRNA levels (marker for progression of psoriasis) was significantly inhibited by iontophoresis of the anti-tumor necrosis factor-α drug etanercept, which also ameliorated epidermis hyperplasia (symptom of psoriasis). Thus, Fukuta et al. (2020) were the first to demonstrate that iontophoresis can be applied as a noninvasive and efficient percutaneous penetration enhancement method for biological macromolecular drugs. For more details on iontophoresis, its mechanism of action and drugs which were delivered intradermally via iontophoresis, the reader should refer to Chapter 46 in this book and to references (Guy et al. 2000; Grice et al. 2011; Gratieri and Kalia 2017a,b). It can be used to enhance dermal and transdermal drug delivery and noninvasive skin sampling applications, while it has mostly been used for the treatment of palmoplantar hyperhidrosis and the diagnosis of cystic fibrosis (Kalia et al., 2004; Delgado-Charro, 2009, 2011; Del Río-Sancho et al., 2017; Merino et al. 2017). Due to the popularity and high therapeutic effectiveness of nanocarriers, espicially nanoparticles, iontophoresis has also been used in combination with nanoparticles in order to synergistically enhace the drug penetration into/through the skin (Dragicevic and Maibach, 2018; Helmy, 2021).

Huber et al. (2015) investigated the effect of iontophoresis on the skin distribution and antitumor effect of doxorubicin-loaded cationic SLN (DOX-SLN). The encapsulation of DOX increased the distribution of DOX in the SC *in vitro*. The combined use of SLN and iontophoresis increased the *in vitro* skin penetration of DOX and led to the formation of drug reservoirs in the hair follicles. Iontophoresis of cationic DOX-SLN increased the DOX penetration into the viable epidermis by approximately 50-fold, while it increased the skin penetration of DOX from the solution only by approximately fourfold. As to the antitumor effect investigated *in vivo* in squamous cell carcinoma induced in nude BALB/c mice, iontophoresis combined with DOX-SLN was highly effective in inhibiting tumor cell survival and tumor growth, indicating a synergistic effect of iontophoresis and DOX-SLN in the treatment of skin cancer (Huber et al. 2015). These results are in accordance with the results of Taveira et al. (2014), who found that iontophoresis of DOX-SLNs increased DOX delivery to the viable epidermis (56% of DOX), compared to passive DOX-SLN delivery, where most of DOX remained in the SC (43% of DOX) and only a small amount penetrated into the viable epidermis (26% of DOX). Further, DOX-SLNs increased DOX cytotoxicity against melanoma cells by 50%.

Charoenputtakun et al. (2015) investigated iontophoretic delivery of hydrophilic and lipophilic drugs through the skin, when applied as encapsulated lipid nanoparticles. Iontophoresis did not enhance the delivery of the lipophilic all-trans-retinoic acid across human epidermal membrane from SLN and NLC compared to passive delivery. In contrast, iontophoresis significantly enhanced the amounts of the hydrophilic drug salicylate delivered across human epidermal membrane (HEM) from salicylate-loaded lipid nanoparticles and salicylate solution compared to those obtained during passive delivery. In addition, the amounts of salicylate delivered from lipid nanoparticles during iontophoretic delivery were significantly larger than those delivered from the solution (Charoenputtakun et al., 2015). As for the amounts of salicylate extracted from HEM after 5 hours of iontophoretic delivery, they were significantly larger than those achieved after 24 hours of passive delivery, and amounts of salicylate delivered from lipid nanoparticles (SLN and NLC) during iontophoresis into the HEM were significantly larger than those delivered from salicylate solution during iontophoresis. Thus, the combined use of iontophoresis and lipid nanoparticles (SLN and NLC) provided significantly higher permeation of hydrophilic SA into and across HEM than iontophoresis applied with plain salicylate (without lipid nanoparticles). The different effect of iontophoresis on the permeation of salicylate and all-trans-retinoic acid could be explained by the different iontophoresis effect on hydrophilic and lipophilic drugs. Similarly, iontophoresis significantly enhanced the amount of acyclovir permeated from SLN compared to passive acyclovir delivery from SLN and suspension applied with and without iontophoresis. These results suggest that lipid nanoparticles combined with iontophoresis represent a promising penetration enhancement method to improve skin delivery of hydrophilic drugs.

Tomoda et al. (2011, 2012a) applied negatively charged PLGA nanoparticles loaded with indomethacin onto rat skin *in vitro* and *in vivo* with or without iontophoresis. When iontophoresis was applied together with indomethacin-loaded nanoparticles *in vivo* in rats, a significantly higher amount of indomethacin was delivered into the systemic circulation, i.e. plasma concentration increased after 60 minutes and continued to increase in next 5 hours (at 6 hours, approx. 200 ng/ml), compared to indomethacin-loaded nanoparticles and indomethacin solution (at 6 hours less than approx. 20 ng/ml). Thus, the combined use of iontophoresis and nanoparticles can be used for an efficient transdermal/systemic delivery of indomethacin (Tomoda et al. 2012a). Higher indomethacin amounts were delivered through rat skin *in vivo* and *in vitro* when indomethacin was loaded in nanoparticles than when indomethacin was free. Further, the application of iontophoresis enhanced indomethacin permeation from nanoparticles compared to simple diffusion of nanoparticles through the skin. This study showed that the combination of charged PLGA nanoparticles and iontophoresis represents an effective method to enhance transdermal delivery of therapeutic agents (Tomoda et al. 2011, 2012a).

These negatively charged PLGA nanoparticles were also studied for their ability to deliver estradiol through the skin (Tomoda et al. 2012b). Estradiol encapsulation into nanoparticles provided *in vitro* threefold higher permeated amounts of estradiol through rat skin compared to free estradiol, i.e. estradiol in suspension. Iontophoresis further enhanced the permeation of estradiol from nanoparticles, approx. threefold compared to the application of nanoparticles without iontophoresis. Iontophoresis enhanced the permeation of nanoparticles and they were found to penetrate mainly through hair follicles. The effectiveness of the combined use of nanoparticles and iontophoresis for the transdermal delivery of estradiol was confirmed *in vivo* in rats. Namely, significantly enhanced permeation of estradiol by application of nanoparticles and iontophoresis was achieved (measured estradiol concentration in plasma after 9 hours was approx. 8 ng/ml) compared to using nanoparticles or suspension without iontophoresis (approx. 3 ng/ml and 2 ng/ml, respectively). Thus, this approach significantly enhanced accumulation of nanoparticles in follicles where estradiol seemed to be released from the nanoparticles and would migrate to muscle and blood stream and accumulate (Tomoda et al., 2012b).

In another study by Takeuchi et al. (2016) it has also been shown that when iontophoresis was applied with estradiol-PLGA nanoparticles, higher skin permeability of the drug was achieved ex vivo, i.e. 2.6-fold higher plasma concentration and 3.75-fold higher cumulative permeated amounts of drug were obtained than by applying same nanoparticles without iontophoresis (passive delivery). The same trend was seen *in vivo*. The authors showed *in vivo* in ovariectomized female rats that estradiol-loaded PLGA charged nanoparticles combined with iontophoresis were useful to recover bone mineral density of cancellous bone, and that the dosing interval of estradiol could be extended. When the estradiol-loaded PLGA nanoparticles were administrated once a week, at 60 days after the start of treatment bone mineral density (approx. 250 mg/cm^3) was significantly higher than that of the non-treated group (approx. 200 mg/cm^3). In the group where nanoparticles were applied twice a week, the bone mineral density increased significantly at 45 days after the start of treatment (approx. 230 mg/cm^3). Thus, these nanoparticles together with iontophoresis could be used for the treatment of postmenopausal osteoporosis.

Takeuchi et al. (2017) continued their research in the field of PLGA nanoparticles using indomethacin-loaded PLGA nanoparticles. They found that 2 hours after the ex vivo administration of nanoparticles, the amounts of indomethacin permeated through rat skin from 50-nm and 100-nm PLGA nanoparticles applied with iontophoresis were 21.1 ± 4.8 and 14.6 ± 3.7 ng/cm^2, respectively, and that they were significantly higher than those of passively diffused indomethacin from nanoparticles and solution (approx. 2–2.5 ng/cm^2). Thus, without iontophoresis, skin permeability of the drug from 50-nm and 100-nm PLGA nanoparticles was equivalent to the indomethacin solution. Regarding the skin accumulation of the drug, 50 nm PLGA nanoparticles combined with iontophoresis provided a 1.7-fold higher drug amount in rat skin compared to 100-nm PLGA nanoparticles applied with iontophoresis. When nanoparticles passively diffused, skin accumulation of nanoparticles tended to be higher with 50-nm PLGA nanoparticles. The 50-nm nanoparticles applied with iontophoresis delivered the drug more deeply into the SC and hair follicle than the 100-nm nanoparticles. Thus, most efficient transdermal delivery of indomethacin as well as the highest amount in the skin was achieved by the combined use of 50-nm PLGA nanoparticles and iontophoresis. The authors concluded, therefore, that these nanoparticles could be used to treat male and female androgenetic alopecia, for transcutaneous vaccination, topical administrations requiring drug delivery to the hair follicle as well as to treat systemic diseases (Takeuchi et al. 2017).

Shiota et al. (2017) developed redox nanoparticles containing nitroxide radicals as free radical scavengers, which are expected to be useful for the protection against UV-induced melanin production. The authors further applied these nanoparticles together with iontophoresis onto the dorsal skin of hairless mice producing melanin in response to light exposure. It has been shown that iontophoresis provided an accumulation of nanoparticles in the epidermal layer, as well as that this combination decreased UV-induced melanin spots and melanin content in the skin. Thus, Shiota et al. (2017) confirmed that melanin production was prevented by the application of redox nanoparticles in combination with iontophoresis.

Some authors reported that there has been no advantage when a drug, flufenamic acid was encapsulated into PLGA nanoparticles and applied with iontophoresis. The permeation of flufenamic acid through the skin from PLGA nanoparticles was not enhanced compared to free drug formulation, either in passive or iontophoretic delivery regimens (Malinovskaja-Gomez et al., 2016).

In addition, also layer-by-layer polymer coated gold nanoparticles (AuNP) were investigated as carriers for the iontophoretic delivery of drugs. The authors (Labala et al., 2015) showed that AuNP combined with iontophoresis are able to deliver imatinib mesylate into the skin for the treatment of melanoma. Skin penetration studies performed *in vitro* in excised porcine ear skin showed that iontophoresis enhanced the skin penetration of imatinib mesylate from nanoparticles by 6.2-fold compared to passive application. Tape stripping studies revealed that iontophoresis provided a 7.8- and 4.9-fold greater imatinib mesylate amount in the SC and viable skin, respectively, compared to iontophoresis of free imatinib mesylate. Furthermore, AuNP loaded with imatinib mesylate significantly decreased B16F10 cell viability compared to free imatinib mesylate. The obtained results confirmed the potential of AuNPs to be used in combination with iontophoresis for the percutaneous penetration enhancement of drugs. Dohnert et al. (2012) evaluated the therapeutic effects of GNPs and diclofenac diethylammonium used together with iontophoresis on the inflammatory parameters in rats challenged with traumatic tendinitis. The results confirmed the efficacy of drug administration used with nanoparticles and iontophoresis in treating tendinitis in an animal model.

AuNPs applied together with iontophoresis could be used in physiotherapy, i.e. they were investigated for their effects in the skeletal muscle of wistar rats exposed to a traumatic muscle injury. Iontophoresis with AuNPs showed significant differences in inflammation and oxidative stress parameters, preserved morphology in the histopathological evaluation, as well as an improvement in the locomotor response and pain symptoms of treated rats. Thus this approach accelerated the inflammatory response of the injured limb and would be promising method in physiotherapy (da Rocha et al., 2020).

Bernardi et al. (2016) investigated an interesting approach for TCI using OVA as a model antigen, which included a vaccine formulation composed of OVA-loaded liposomes and silver nanoparticles (NPAg). These OVA-liposomes associated with NPAg and applied together with iontophoresis increased OVA penetration *in vitro* into the viable epidermis by 92-fold in comparison to passive delivery. As to *in vivo* studies, TCI with a suitable combination of liposome, nanoparticles and iontophoresis induced indeed the production of antibodies and differentiation of immune-competent, thereby confirming the ability of this approcah to be used for TCI (Bernardi et al., 2016).

64.1.4 COMBINED USE OF NANOPARTICLES AND ELECTROPORATION

Electroporation is a physical technique used to enhance drug penetration into/through the skin. Usually electroporation requires application of high-voltage electric pulses of very short duration (microsecond-millisecond). This protocol is able to reversibly enhance cell or tissue permeability for bioactive molecules such as drugs, dyes, vitamins, peptides, proteins, DNA, RNA etc. (Medi et al. 2017). It holds promise for the percutaneous penetration enhancement of macromolecules, such as peptides and gene-based drugs, enabling their transdermal delivery (Dujardin and Préat 2004; Medi et al. 2017). Electroporation is an efficient penetration enhancing method depending on itself and the properties of drugs, i.e. the cumulative drug permeation increases with increasing drug solubility, decreasing oil–water partition coefficient (logP) and dissociation constant (pKa) (Chen et al., 2020). Nowadays, there are novel electroporation protocols which allow at low voltages sufficient delivery of DNA and siRNA into mouse skin (Huang et al., 2020). For more detail on electroporation, the reader should refer to Chapter 45 of this book and to references (Medi et al., 2017; Angamuthu and Murthy, 2017).

Rastogi et al. (2010) developed insulin-loaded polymeric nanoparticles and investigated *in vitro* and *in vivo* the influence of electroporation on the transdermal delivery of insulin from nanoparticles and solution and compared it with the subcutaneous administration of insulin. Electroporation combined with nanoparticles resulted in fourfold enhancement in insulin deposition in rat skin compared to the solution. *In vivo* studies showed maximum reduction of 77% and 85% in blood glucose levels for the solution and nanoparticles, respectively, while therapeutic levels maintained for 24 and 36 hours. Thus, the authors confirmed that electroporation and polymeric nanoparticles could be an alternative to injectable administration of insulin.

Anirudhan and Nair (2019) investigated electroporation in conjugation with AuNPs, while diclofenac sodium was used as a model drug. The authors developed an electrosensitive patch using skin adhesive matrix, polyvinyl alcohol/poly(dimethyl siloxane)-g-polyacrylate. AuNP/carbon nanotube nanocomposite (AuNP-CNT) was incorporated into the matrix with AuNP and CNT to enhance skin permeability and electrical conductivity, respectively. The diclofenac sodium release study was performed in rat skin at different GNP-CNT contents and variable conditions of applied voltage. Incorporating AuNP-CNT enhanced the diclofenac sodium permeation, while best results were obtained by the device containing 1.5% nanofillers at an applied bias of 10.0 V. Thus, this approach, which has been shown in the viability test to be safe, efficiently enhanced drug permeation by different mechanisms, by affecting/disrupting the intercelullar SC lipids, generation of new aqueous pathway and thermal effect. The authors, thus, reported that this approach represents a promising new method for achieving transdermal drug delivery.

64.2   CONCLUSION

Nanocarriers have been recently intensively studied due to their penetration enhancement ability regarding dermal and transdermal drug delivery, as well as due to their ability to encapsulate hydrophilic and lipophilic drugs, thereby preserving their stability. Among different nanocarriers, lipid-based and polymer-based nanoparticles have gained a lot of interest. However, nanoparticles when applied alone mostly deliver drugs on to the skin, as they accumulate at the skin surface and do not penetrate the intact skin. Therefore, they are mostly used to treat skin diseases. In order to achieve effective systemic drug absorption, nanocarriers are applied together with physical enhancement methods, which are able by different mechanisms to bypass or to disrupt the SC barrier. In this chapter, we described the use of nanoparticles combined with different physical enhancement methods, such as the use of MNs, iontophoresis and electroporation. The described studies revealed that physical methods mostly enhanced the efficiency of nanoparticles and that this combination of different methods was promising, as nanoparticles and physical methods act synergistically in enhancing percutaneous drug penetration, but via different mechanisms of action. Most promising application of this approach is its use in achieving TCI; various studies confirmed that the combined use of nanoparticles and physical methods may be an alternative approach for TCI. In this way with the use of needle-free vaccination, numerous drawbacks of the conventional vaccination (with syringes and needles), such as pain, fear, spread of diseases, would be circumvented. In addition, this approach can be used for the percutaneous penetration enhancement not only of low-molecular-weight drugs, but also of high-molecular-weight drugs, which usually are not able to penetrate the SC (e.g. peptide/protein drugs like antibodies, insulin, genes, etc.).

REFERENCES

Abdel-Mottaleb MMA, Lamprecht A (2016). Polymeric nano (and micro-) particles as carriers for enhanced skin penetration. In: Dragicevic N, Maibach HI, (Eds.), Percutaneous Penetration Enhancers—Chemical Methods in Penetration Enhancement: Nanocarriers, Springer: Heidelberg, 187–199.

Abrego G, Alvarado H, Souto EB, Guevara B, Bellowa LH, Garduño ML, Garcia ML, Calpena AC (2016). Biopharmaceutical profile of hydrogels containing pranoprofen-loaded PLGA nanoparticles for skin administration: *In vitro*, ex vivo and *in vivo* characterization. Int J Pharm 501(1-2):350–361. doi: 10.1016/j.ijpharm.2016.01.071.

Ali AA, McCrudden CM, McCaffrey J, McBride JW, Cole G, Dunne NJ, Robson T, Kissenpfennig A, Donnelly RF, McCarthy HO (2017). DNA vaccination for cervical cancer; a novel technology platform of RALA mediated gene delivery via polymeric microneedles. Nanomedicine 13(3):921–932. doi: 10.1016/j.nano.2016.11.019.

Alvarez-Roman R, Naik A, Kalia YN, Guy RH, Fessi H (2004a). Enhancement of topical delivery from biodegradable nanoparticles. Pharm Res 21:1818–1825.

Alvarez-Roman R, Naik A, Kalia YN, Guy RH, Fessi H (2004b). Skin penetration and distribution of polymeric nanoparticles. J Control Release 99:53–62.

Angamuthu M, Murthy SN (2017). Therapeutic applications of electroporation. In: Dragicevic N, Maibach HI (Eds.), Percutaneous Penetration Enhancers—Physical Methods in Penetration Enhancement, Springer: Heidelberg, 123–137.

Anirudhan TS, Nair SS (2019). Development of voltage gated transdermal drug delivery platform to impose synergistic enhancement in skin permeation using electroporation and gold nanoparticle. Mater Sci Eng C Mater Biol Appl 102:437–446. doi: 10.1016/j.msec.2019.04.044.

Arya J, Henry S, Kalluri H, McAllister DV, Pewin WP, Prausnitz MR (2017). Tolerability, usability and acceptability of dissolving microneedle patch administration in human subjects. Biomaterials 128:1–7. doi: 10.1016/j.biomaterials.2017.02.040

Ascenso A, Raposo S, Batista C, Cardoso P, Mendes T, Praça FG, Bentley MV, Simões S (2015). Development, characterization, and skin delivery studies of related ultradeformable vesicles: transfersomes, ethosomes, and transethosomes. Int J Nanomedicine 10:5837–5851.

Baek SH, Shin JH, Kim YC (2017). Drug-coated microneedles for rapid and painless local anesthesia. Biomed Microdevices 19(1):2. doi: 10.1007/s10544-016-0144-1.

Bal SM, Slütter B, Jiskoot W, Bouwstra JA (2011). Small is beautiful: N-trimethyl chitosan-ovalbumin conjugates for microneedle-based transcutaneous immunisation.Vaccine 29(23):4025–4032.

Bal SM, Ding Z, van Riet E, Jiskoot W, Bouwstra JA (2010). Advances in transcutaneous vaccine delivery: do all ways lead to Rome? J Control Release 148(3):266–282.

Berkó S, Szűcs KF, Balázs B, Csányi E, Varju G, Sztojkov-Ivanov A, Budai-Szűcs M, Bóta J, Gáspár R (2016). Electroporation-delivered transdermal neostigmine in rats: equivalent action to intravenous administration. Drug Des Devel Ther 10:1695–701. doi: 10.2147/DDDT.S102959.

Bernardi DS, Bitencourt C, da Silveira DS, da Cruz EL, Pereira-da-Silva MA, Faccioli LH, Lopez RF (2016). Effective transcutaneous immunization using a combination of iontophoresis and nanoparticles. Nanomedicine 12(8):2439–2448. doi: 10.1016/j.nano.2016.07.001.

Birchall J, Coulman S, Anstey A, Gateley C, Sweetland H, Gershonowitz A, Neville L, Levin G (2006). Cutaneous gene expression of plasmid DNA in excised human skin following delivery via microchannels created by radio frequency ablation. Int J Pharm 312(1-2):15–23.

Bok M, Zhao ZJ, Jeon S, Jeong JH, Lim E (2020). Ultrasonically and iontophoretically enhanced drug-delivery system based on dissolving microneedle patches. Sci Rep 10(1):2027. doi: 10.1038/s41598-020-58822-w.

Chabri F, Bouris K, Jones T, Barrow D, Hann A, Allender C, Brain K, Birchall J (2004). Microfabricated silicon microneedles for nonviral cutaneous gene delivery.Br J Dermatol 150:869–877.

Charoenputtakun P, Li SK, Ngawhirunpat T (2015). Iontophoretic delivery of lipophilic and hydrophilic drugs from lipid nanoparticles across human skin. Int J Pharm 495(1):318–328.

Chen M, Quan G, Sun Y, Yang D, Pan X, Wu C (2020). Nanoparticles-encapsulated polymeric microneedles for transdermal drug delivery. J Control Release 325:163–175. doi: 10.1016/j.jconrel.2020.06.039.

Chen Z, Lv Y, Qi J, Zhu Q, Lu Y, Wu W (2018). Overcoming or circumventing the stratum corneum barrier for efficient transcutaneous immunization. Drug Discov Today 23(1):181–186. doi: 10.1016/j.drudis.2017.09.017.

Chen X, Zhu L, Li R, Pang L, Zhu S, Ma J, Du L, Jin Y (2020). Electroporation-enhanced transdermal drug delivery: Effects of logP, pK_a, solubility and penetration time. Eur J Pharm Sci 151:105410. doi: 10.1016/j.ejps.2020.105410.

Combadiere B, Mahe B (2008). Particle-based vaccines for transcutaneous vaccination. Comp Immunol Microbiol Infect Dis 31:293–315.

Courtenay AJ, McAlister E, McCrudden MTC, Vora L, Steiner L, Levin G, Levy-Nissenbaum E, Shterman N, Kearney MC, McCarthy HO, Donnelly RF (2020). Hydrogel-forming microneedle arrays as a therapeutic option for transdermal esketamine delivery. J Control Release 322:177–186. doi: 10.1016/j.jconrel.2020.03.026.

Cormier M, Johnson B, Ameri M, Nyam K, Libiran L, Zhang DD, Daddona P (2004). Transdermal delivery of desmopressin using a coated microneedle array patch system. J Control Release 97:503–511.

Coulman SA, Allender C, Birchall JC (2006a). Microneedles and other physical methods for overcoming the stratum corneum barrier for cutaneous gene therapy. Crit Rev Ther Drug Carrier Syst 23:205–258.

Coulman SA, Barrow D, Anstey A, Gateley C, Morrissey A, Wilke N, Allender C, Brain K, Birchall JC (2006b). Minimally invasive cutaneous delivery of macromolecules and plasmid DNA via microneedles. Curr Drug Deliv 3:65–75.

Coulman SA, Anstey A, Gateley C, Morrissey A, McLoughlin P, Allender C, Birchall JC (2009). Microneedle mediated delivery of nanoparticles into human skin. Int J Pharm 366:190–200

de Jalon EG, Blanco-Prieto MJ, Ygartua P, Santoyo S (2001). PLGA microparticles: possible vehicles for topical drug delivery. Int J Pharm 226:181–184.

da Rocha FR, Haupenthal DPDS, Zaccaron RP, Corrêa MEAB, Tramontin NDS, Fonseca JP, Nesi RT, Muller AP, Pinho RA, Paula MMDS, Silveira PCL (2020). Therapeutic effects of iontophoresis with gold nanoparticles in the repair of traumatic muscle injury. J Drug Target 28(3):307–319. doi: 10.1080/1061186X.2019.1652617.

Delgado-Charro MB (2009). Recent advances on transdermal iontophoretic drug delivery and noninvasive sampling. J Drug Del Sci Tech 19:75–88.

Delgado-Charro MB (2011). Sampling substrates by skin permeabilization. In: Murthy M (Ed.), Dermatokinetics of Therapeutic Agents, Taylor and Francis Publishers: Boca Raton, 149–174.

Del Río-Sancho S, Serna-Jiménez CE, Sebastián-Morelló M, Calatayud-Pascual MA, Balaguer-Fernández C, Femenía-Font A, Kalia YN, Merino V, López-Castellano A (2017). Transdermal therapeutic systems for memantine delivery. Comparison of passive and iontophoretic transport. Int J Pharm 517(1-2):104–111. doi: 10.1016/j.ijpharm.2016.11.038.

Dohnert MB, Venâncio M, Possato JC, Zeferino RC, Dohnert LH, Zugno AI, De Souza CT, Paula MM, Luciano TF (2012). Gold nanoparticles and diclofenac diethylammonium administered by iontophoresis reduce inflammatory cytokines expression in Achilles tendinitis. Int J Nanomedicine 7:1651–7. doi: 10.2147/IJN.S25164.

Donnelly RF, Morrow DI, Fay F, Scott CJ, Abdelghany S, Singh RR, Garland MJ, Woolfson AD (2010). Microneedle-mediated intradermal nanoparticle delivery: Potential for enhanced local administration of hydrophobic pre-formed photosensitisers. Photodiagnosis Photodynamic Ther 7:222—231.

Dul M, Stefanidou M, Porta P, Serve J, O'Mahony C, Malissen B, Henri S, Levin Y, Kochba E, Wong FS, Dayan C, Coulman SA, Birchall JC (2017). Hydrodynamic gene delivery in human skin using a hollow microneedle device. J Control Release pii: S0168-3659(17)30087-1. doi: 10.1016/j.jconrel.2017.02.028.

Dragicevic-Curic N, Scheglmann D, Albrecht V, Fahr A (2008). Temoporfin-loaded invasomes: development, characterization and in vitro skin penetration studies. J Control Release 127(1):59–69. doi: 10.1016/j.jconrel.2007.12.013.

Dragicevic-Curic N, Scheglmann D, Albrecht V, Fahr A (2009). Development of different temoporfin-loaded invasomes-novel nanocarriers of temoporfin: characterization, stability and in vitro skin penetration studies. Colloids Surf B Biointerfaces 70(2):198–206. doi: 10.1016/j.colsurfb.2008.12.030.

Dragicevic-Curic N, Gräfe S, Gitter B, Fahr A (2010). Efficacy of temoporfin-loaded invasomes in the photodynamic therapy in human epidermoid and colorectal tumour cell lines. J Photochem Photobiol B 101(3):238–50. doi: 10.1016/j.jphotobiol.2010.07.009.

Dragicevic-Curic N, Fahr A (2012). Liposomes in topical photodynamic therapy. Expert Opin Drug Deliv 9(8):1015–32. doi: 10.1517/17425247.2012.697894. Epub 2012 Jun 25. PMID: 22731896.

Dragicevic N, Maibach HI (2015). Percutaneous Penetration Enhancers—Chemical Methods in Penetration Enhancement: Drug Manipulation Strategies and Vehicle Effects, Springer: Berlin.

Dragicevic N, Maibach HI (2016). Percutaneous Penetration Enhancers—Chemical Methods in Penetration Enhancement: Nanocarriers, Springer: Berlin.

Dragicevic N, Maibach HI (2017). Percutaneous Penetration Enhancers—Physical Methods in Penetration Enhancement, Springer: Berlin.

Dragicevic N, Maibach H (2018). Combined use of nanocarriers and physical methods for percutaneous penetration enhancement. Adv Drug Deliv Rev 127:58–84.

Du G, Hathout RM, Nasr M, Nejadnik MR, Tu J, Koning RI, Koster AJ, Slütter B, Kros A, Jiskoot W, Bouwstra JA, Mönkäre J (2017). Intradermal vaccination with hollow microneedles: a comparative study of various protein antigen and adjuvant encapsulated nanoparticles. J Control Release 266:109–118. doi: 10.1016/j.jconrel.2017.09.021.

Dujardin N, Préat V (2004). Delivery of DNA to skin by electroporation. Methods Mol Biol245:215–226. doi: 10.1385/1-59259-649-5:215.

Engelke L, Winter G, Hook S, Engert J (2015). Recent insights into cutaneous immunization: how to vaccinate via the skin. Vaccine 33(37):4663–4674. doi: 10.1016/j.vaccine.2015.05.012.

Escobar-Chávez JJ (2017). Therapeutic application of sonophoresis and sonophoresis devices. In: Dragicevic N, Maibach HI (Eds.), Percutaneous Penetration Enhancers—Physical Methods in Penetration Enhancement, Springer: Heidelberg, 31–58.

Frerichs DM, Ellingsworth LR, Frech, SA, Flyer DC, Villar CP, Yu JM, Glenn GM (2008). Controlled, single-step, stratum corneum disruption as a pretreatment for immunization via a patch. Vaccine 26:2782–2787.

Fukuta T, Oshima Y, Michiue K, Tanaka D, Kogure K (2020). Non-invasive delivery of biological macromolecular drugs into the skin by iontophoresis and its application to psoriasis treatment. J Control Release 323:323–332. doi: 10.1016/j.jconrel.2020.04.044.

Gomaa YA, Morrow DI, Garland MJ, Donnelly RF, El-Khordagui LK, Meidan VM (2010). Effects of microneedle length, density, insertion time and multiple applications on human skin barrier function: assessments by transepidermal water loss. Toxicol In vitro 24(7):1971–1978.

Gomaa YA, El-Khordagui LK, Garland MJ, Donnelly RF, McInnes F, Meidan VM (2012). Effect of microneedle treatment on the skin permeation of a nanoencapsulated dye. J Pharm Pharmacol. 64(11):1592–1602.

Gomaa YA, Garland MJ, McInnes FJ, Donnelly RF, El-Khordagui LK, Wilson CG (2014). Microneedle/nanoencapsulation-mediated transdermal delivery: mechanistic insights. Eur J Pharm Biopharm 86(2):145–155.

Gratieri T, Kalia YN (2017a). Iontophoresis: Basic principles. In: Dragicevic N, Maibach HI (Eds.), Percutaneous Penetration Enhancers—Physical Methods in Penetration Enhancement, Springer: Heidelberg, 61–65.

Gratieri T, Kalia YN (2017b). Iontophoretic transport mechanisms and factors affecting electrically-assisted delivery. In: Dragicevic N, Maibach HI (Eds.), Percutaneous Penetration Enhancers—Physical Methods in Penetration Enhancement, Springer: Heidelberg, 67–76.

Grice JE, Prow TW, Kendall MAF, Roberts MS (2011). Electrical and physical methods of skin penetration enhancement. In: Benson HAE, Watkinson AC (Eds.), Transdermal and Topical Drug Delivery, John Wiley Sons Inc, 43–65.

Guy RH, Kalia YN, Delgado-Charro MB, Merino V, López A, Marro D (2000). Iontophoresis: electrorepulsion and electroosmosis. J Control Release 64:129–132.

Helmy AM (2021). Overview of recent advancements in the iontophoretic drug delivery to various tissues and organs. J Drug Deliv Sci Technol 61:102332. https://doi.org/10.1016/j.jddst.2021.102332.

Huang D, Huang Y, Li Z (2020). Transdermal delivery of nucleic acid mediated by punching and electroporation. Methods Mol Biol 2050:101–112. doi: 10.1007/978-1-4939-9740-4_11.

Huber LA, Pereira TA, Ramos DN, Rezende LC, Emery FS, Sobral LM, Leopoldino AM, Lopez RF (2015). Topical skin cancer therapy using doxorubicin-loaded cationic lipid nanoparticles and iontophoresis. J Biomed Nanotechnol 11(11):1975–1988.

Hirschberg H, De Wijdeven G, Kelder AB, Van Den Dobbelsteen G, Kerstena GFA (2008). Bioneedles (TM) as vaccine carriers. Vaccine 26:2389–2397.

Ita K (2016). Perspectives on transdermal electroporation. Pharmaceutics 8(1). pii: E9. doi: 10.3390/pharmaceutics8010009. Review.

Ita K (2017). Dermal/transdermal delivery of small interfering RNA and antisense oligonucleotides—advances and hurdles. Biomed Pharmacother 87:311–320. doi: 10.1016/j.biopha.2016.12.118. Review.

Kalia YN, Naik A, Garrison J, Guy RH (2004). Iontophoretic drug delivery. Adv Drug Deliv Rev 5:619–658.

Kalluri H, Choi S-O, Guo XD, Lee JW, Norman J, Prausnitz MR (2017). Evaluation of microneedles in human subjects. In: Dragicevic N, Maibach HI (Eds.), Percutaneous Penetration Enhancers—Physical Methods in Penetration Enhancement, Springer: Heidelberg, 325–340.

Katikaneni S (2015). Transdermal delivery of biopharmaceuticals: dream or reality? Ther Deliv 6(9):1109–16. doi: 10.4155/tde.15.60. Epub 2015 Sep 30. Review.

Katikaneni S, Li G, Badkar A, Banga AK (2010). Transdermal delivery of a approximately 13 kDa protein—an in vivo comparison of physical enhancement methods. J Drug Target 18(2):141–7. doi: 10.3109/10611860903287164.

Kearney MC, Caffarel-Salvador E, Fallows SJ, McCarthy HO, Donnelly RF (2016). Microneedle-mediated delivery of donepezil: potential for improved treatment options in Alzheimer's disease. Eur J Pharm Biopharm 103:43–50. doi: 10.1016/j.ejpb.2016.03.026.

Kim CS, Wilder-Smith P, Ahn YC, Liaw LH, Chen Z, Kwon YJ (2009). Enhanced detection of early-stage oral cancer in vivo by optical coherence tomography using multimodal delivery of gold nanoparticles. J Biomed Opt 14:034008.

Kim JY, Han MR, Kim YH, Shin SW, Nam SY, Park JH (2016). Tip-loaded dissolving microneedles for transdermal delivery of donepezil hydrochloride for treatment of Alzheimer's disease. Eur J Pharm Biopharm 105:148–55. doi: 10.1016/j.ejpb.2016.06.006.

Kohli AK, Alpar HO (2004). Potential use of nanoparticles for transcutaneous vaccine delivery: effect of particle size and charge. Int J Pharm 275:13–17.

Küchler S, Radowski MR, Blaschke T, Dathe M, Plendl J, Haag R, Schäfer-Korting M, Kramer KD (2009). Nanoparticles for skin penetration enhancement—a comparison of a dendritic core-multishell-nanotransporter and solid lipid nanoparticles. Eur J Pharm Biopharm 71(2):243–50. doi: 10.1016/j.ejpb.2008.08.019.

Kumar A, Li X, Sandoval MA, Rodriguez BL, Sloat BR, Cui Z (2011). Permeation of antigen protein-conjugated nanoparticles and live bacteria through microneedle-treated mouse skin. Int J Nanomedicine 6:1253–1264.

Kumar A, Wonganan P, Sandoval MA, Li X, Zhu S, Cui Z (2012). Microneedle-mediated transcutaneous immunization with plasmid DNA coated on cationic PLGA nanoparticles. J Control Release 163(2): 230–239. doi: 10.1016/j.jconrel.2012.08.011.

Kurnia Anjani Q, Dian Permana A, Cárcamo-Martínez Á, Domínguez-Robles J, Tekko IA, Larrañeta E, Vora LK, Ramadon D, Donnelly RF (2020). Versatility of hydrogel-forming microneedles in *in vitro* transdermal delivery of tuberculosis drugs. Eur J Pharm Biopharm S0939–6411(20):30361-1. doi: 10.1016/j.ejpb.2020.12.003.

Labala S, Mandapalli PK, Kurumaddali A, Venuganti VV (2015). Layer-by-layer polymer coated gold nanoparticles for topical delivery of imatinib mesylate to treat melanoma. Mol Pharm 12(3):878–888.

Lademann J,Weigmann HJ, Rickmeyer C, Barthelmes H, Schaefer H, Mueller G, Sterry W (1999). Penetration of titanium dioxide microparticles in a sunscreen formulation into the Horny Layer and the follicular orifice. Skin Pharmacol Physiol 12:247–256.

Lademann J, Richter H, Teichmann A, Otberg N, Blume-Peytavi U, LuengoJ,Weiss B, Schaefer U, Lehr CM, Wepf R, Sterry W (2007). Nanoparticles—an efficient carrier for drug delivery into the hair follicles. Eur J Pharm Biopharm 66:159–164.

Lawson LB, Freytag LC, Clements JD (2007). Use of nanocarriers for transdermal vaccine delivery. Clin Pharmacol Ther 82:641–643.

Lee JW, Gadiraju P, Park JH, Allen MG, Prausnitz MR (2011). Microsecond thermal ablation of skin for transdermal drug delivery. J Control Release 25 154(1):58–68. doi: 10.1016/j.jconrel.2011.05.003.

Levin G, Gershonowitz A, Sacks H, Stern M, Sherman A, Rudaev S, Zivin I, Phillip M (2005). Transdermal delivery of human growth hormone through RF-microchannels. Pharm Res 22(4):550–555.

Luengo J, Weiss B, Schneider M, Ehlers A, Stracke F, Konig K, Kostka KH, Lehr CM, Schaefer UF (2006). Influence of nanoencapsulation on human skin transport of flufenamic acid. Skin Pharmacol Physiol 19:190–197.

Malinovskaja-Gomez K, Labouta HI, Schneider M, Hirvonen J, Laaksonen T (2016). Transdermal iontophoresis of flufenamic acid loaded PLGA nanoparticles. Eur J Pharm Sci 89:154–162. doi: 10.1016/j.ejps.2016.04.034.

Manjunatha RG, Sharma S, Narayan RP, Koul V (2018). Effective permeation of 2.5 and 5% lidocaine hydrochloride in human skin using iontophoresis technique. Int J Dermatol 57(11):1335–1343. doi: 10.1111/ijd.14107. Epub 2018 Jul 6. PMID: 29978889.

Manolova V, Flace A, Bauer M, Schwarz K, Saudan P, Bachmann MF (2008). Nanoparticles target distinct dendritic cell populations according to their size. Eur J Immunol 38:1404–1413.

Martanto W, Davis SP, Holiday NR, Wang J, Gill HS, Prausnitz MR (2004). Transdermal delivery of insulin using microneedles *in vivo*. Pharm Res 21:947–952.

McAlister E, Garland MJ, Singh TRR, Donnelly RF (2017). Microporation using microneedle arrays. In: Dragicevic N, Maibach HI (Eds.), Percutaneous Penetration Enhancers—Physical Methods in Penetration Enhancement, Springer: Heidelberg, 273–303.

Medi BM, Layek B, Singh J (2017). Electroporation for dermal and transdermal drug delivery. In: Dragicevic N, Maibach HI (Eds.), Percutaneous Penetration Enhancers—Physical Methods in Penetration Enhancement, Springer: Heidelberg, 105–122.

Merino V, López Castellano A, Delgado-Charro MB (2017). Iontophoresis for therapeutic drug delivery and non-invasive sampling applications. In: Dragicevic N, Maibach HI (Eds.), Percutaneous Penetration Enhancers—Physical Methods in Penetration Enhancement, Springer: Heidelberg, 77–101.

Mittal A, Raber AS, Lehr CM, Hansen S. (2013). Particle based vaccine formulations for transcutaneous immunization. Hum Vaccin Immunother. 9(9): 1950–1955.

Modepalli N, Shivakumar HN, McCrudden MT, Donnelly RF, Banga A, Murthy SN (2016). Transdermal delivery of iron using soluble microneedles: dermal kinetics and safety. J Pharm Sci 105(3):1196–200. doi: 10.1016/j.xphs.2015.12.008.

Mohammad EA, Elshemey WM, Elsayed AA, Abd-Elghany AA (2016). Electroporation parameters for successful transdermal delivery of insulin. Am J Ther 23(6):e1560–e1567.

Mönkäre J, Pontier M, van Kampen EEM, Du G, Leone M, Romeijn S, Nejadnik MR, O'Mahony C, Slütter B, Jiskoot W, Bouwstra JA (2018). Development of PLGA nanoparticle loaded dissolving microneedles and comparison with hollow microneedles in intradermal vaccine delivery. Eur J Pharm Biopharm 129:111–121. doi: 10.1016/j.ejpb.2018.05.031.

Müller RH, Alexiev U, Sinambela P, Keck CM (2016). Nanostructured Lipid Carriers (NLC) – the second generation of solid lipid nanoparticles. In: Dragicevic N, Maibach HI, Percutaneous Penetration Enhancers—Chemical Methods in Penetration Enhancement: Nanocarriers, Springer: Heidelberg, 161–185.

Niu L, Chu LY, Burton SA, Hansen KJ, Panyam J (2019). Intradermal delivery of vaccine nanoparticles using hollow microneedle array generates enhanced and balanced immune response. J Control Release 294:268–278. doi: 10.1016/j.jconrel.2018.12.026.

Oberli MA, Schoellhammer CM, Langer R, Blankschtein D (2014). Ultrasound-enhanced transdermal delivery: recent advances and future challenges. Ther Deliv 5(7): 843–857.

Park JH, Choi SO, Seo S, Choy YB, Prausnitz MR (2010). A microneedle roller for transdermal drug delivery. Eur J Pharm Biopharm 76(2):282–289.

Park J, Kim YC (2020). Topical delivery of 5-fluorouracil-loaded carboxymethyl chitosan nanoparticles using microneedles for keloid treatment. Drug Deliv Transl Res. doi: 10.1007/s13346-020-00781-w.

Patel N, Jain S, Lin S (2016). Transdermal iontophoretic delivery of tacrine hydrochloride: correlation between *in vitro* permeation and *in vivo* performance in rats. Int J Pharm 513(1-2):393–403. doi: 10.1016/j.ijpharm.2016.09.038.

Pamornpathomkul B, Wongkajornsilp A, Laiwattanapaisal W, Rojanarata T, Opanasopit P, Ngawhirunpat T (2017a). A combined approach of hollow microneedles and nanocarriers for skin immunization with plasmid DNA encoding ovalbumin. Int J Nanomedicine 12:885–898. doi: 10.2147/IJN.S125945.

Pamornpathomkul B, Rojanarata T, Opanasopit P, Ngawhirunpat T (2017b). Enhancement of skin permeation and skin immunization of ovalbumin antigen via microneedles. AAPS Pharm Sci Tech doi: 10.1208/s12249-017-0730-4.

Permana AD, Tekko IA, McCrudden MTC, Anjani QK, Ramadon D, McCarthy HO, Donnelly RF (2019). Solid lipid nanoparticle-based dissolving microneedles: a promising intradermal lymph targeting drug delivery system with potential for enhanced treatment of lymphatic filariasis. J Control Release 316:34–52. doi: 10.1016/j.jconrel.2019.10.004.

Pielenhofer J, Sohl J, Windbergs M, Langguth P, Radsak MP (2020). Current progress in particle-based systems for transdermal vaccine delivery. Front Immunol 11:266. doi: 10.3389/fimmu.2020.00266.

Prausnitz MR (2004). Microneedles for transdermal drug delivery. Adv Drug Deliv Rev 56:581–587.

Puri A, Nguyen HX, Banga AK (2016). Microneedle-mediated intradermal delivery of epigallocatechin-3-gallate. Int J Cosmet Sci 38(5):512–23. doi: 10.1111/ics.12320.

Rancan, F, Papakostas, D, Hadam, S et al. (2009). Investigation of polylactic acid (PLA) nanoparticles as drug delivery systems for local dermatotherapy. Pharm Res 26: 2027.

Rastogi R, Anand S, Koul V (2010). Electroporation of polymeric nanoparticles: an alternative technique for transdermal delivery of insulin. Drug Dev Ind Pharm 36(11):1303–1311.

Ripolin A, Quinn J, Larrañeta E, Vicente-Perez EM, Barry J, Donnelly RF (2017). Successful application of large microneedle patches by human volunteers. Int J Pharm 521(1-2):92–101. doi: 10.1016/j.ijpharm.2017.02.011.

Ronnander JP, Simon L, Koch A (2019). Transdermal delivery of sumatriptan succinate using iontophoresis and dissolving microneedles. J Pharm Sci 108(11):3649–3656. doi: 10.1016/j.xphs.2019.07.020. Epub 2019 Jul 30. PMID: 31374318.

Seok H, Noh JY, Lee DY, Kim SJ, Song CS, Kim YC (2017). Effective humoral immune response from a H1N1 DNA vaccine delivered to the skin by microneedles coated with PLGA-based cationic nanoparticles. J Control Release 265:66–74. doi: 10.1016/j.jconrel.2017.04.027.

Shiota K, Hama S, Yoshitomi T, Nagasaki Y, Kogure K (2017). Prevention of UV-induced melanin production by accumulation of redox nanoparticles in the epidermal layer via iontophoresis Biol Pharm Bull 40(6):941–944. doi: 10.1248/bpb.b17-00155.

Siddhapura K, Harde H, Jain S (2016). Immunostimulatory effect of tetanus toxoid loaded chitosan nanoparticles following microneedles assisted immunization. Nanomedicine 12(1):213–22. doi: 10.1016/j.nano.2015.10.009.

Singh TRR, McMillan H, Mooney K, Alkilani AZ, Donnelly RF (2017). Fabrication of microneedles. In: Dragicevic N, Maibach HI (Eds.), Percutaneous Penetration Enhancers—Physical Methods in Penetration Enhancement, Springer: Heidelberg, 305–323.

Sintov AC, Hofmann MA (2016). A novel thermo-mechanical system enhanced transdermal delivery of hydrophilic active agents by fractional ablation. Int J Pharm 511(2):821–30. doi: 10.1016/j.ijpharm.2016.07.070.

Takeuchi I, Fukuda K, Kobayashi S, Makino K (2016). Transdermal delivery of estradiol-loaded PLGA nanoparticles using iontophoresis for treatment of osteoporosis. Biomed Mater Eng 27(5):475–483.

Takeuchi I, Kobayashi S, Hida Y, Makino K (2017). Estradiol-loaded PLGA nanoparticles for improving low bone mineral density of cancellous bone caused by osteoporosis: application of enhanced charged nanoparticles with iontophoresis. Colloids Surf B Biointerfaces 155:35–40. doi: 10.1016/j.colsurfb.2017.03.047.

Takeuchi I, Suzuki T, Makino K (2017). Skin permeability and transdermal delivery route of 50-nm indomethacin-loaded PLGA nanoparticles. Colloids Surf B Biointerfaces 159:312–317. doi: 10.1016/j.colsurfb.2017.08.003. Epub 2017 Aug 4. PMID: 28858661.

Taveira SF, De Santana DC, Araújo LM, Marquele-Oliveira F, Nomizo A, Lopez RF (2014). Effect of iontophoresis on topical delivery of doxorubicin-loaded solid lipid nanoparticles. J Biomed Nanotechnol 10(7):1382–1390.

Toll R, Jacobi U, Richter H, Lademann J, Schaefer H, Blume-Peytavi U (2004). Penetrationprofile of microspheres in follicular targeting of terminal hair follicles. J Invest Dermatol 123:168–176.

Tomoda K, Terashima H, Suzuki K, Inagi T, Terada H, Makino K (2011). Enhanced transdermal delivery of indomethacin-loaded PLGA nanoparticles by iontophoresis. Colloids Surf B Biointerfaces 88(2):706–710.

Tomoda K, Terashima H, Suzuki K, Inagi T, Terada H, Makino K (2012a). Enhanced transdermal delivery of indomethacin using combination of PLGA nanoparticles and iontophoresis in vivo. Colloids Surf B Biointerfaces 92:50–54.

Tomoda K, Watanabe A, Suzuki K, Inagi T, Terada H, Makino K (2012b). Enhanced transdermal permeability of estradiol using combination of PLGA nanoparticles system and iontophoresis. Colloids Surf B Biointerfaces 97:84–89.

Tort S, Mutlu Agardan NB, Han D, Steckl AJ (2020). In vitro and in vivo evaluation of microneedles coated with electrosprayed micro/nanoparticles for medical skin treatments. J Microencapsul 37(7):517–527. doi: 10.1080/02652048.2020.1809725.

Vermulapalli V, Yang Y, Friden PM, Banga AK (2008). Synergistic effect of iontophoresis and soluble microneedles for transdermal delivery of methotrexate. J Pharm Pharmacol 60(1):27–33.

Vora LK, Courtenay AJ, Tekko IA, Larrañeta E, Donnelly RF (2020). Pullulan-based dissolving microneedle arrays for enhanced transdermal delivery of small and large biomolecules. Int J Biol Macromol 146:290–298. doi: 10.1016/j.ijbiomac.2019.12.184.

Vučen SR, Vuleta G, Crean AM, Moore AC, Ignjatović N, Uskoković D (2013). Improved percutaneous delivery of ketoprofen using combined application of nanocarriers and silicon microneedles. J Pharm Pharmacol 65(10):1451–62. doi: 10.1111/jphp.12118.

Wang F, Chen Y, Benson HAE (2008). Formulation of nano and micro PLGA particles of the model peptide insulin: preparation, characterization, stability and deposition in human skin. Open Drug Deliv J 2:1–9.

Yan G, Warner KS, Zhang J, Sharma S, Gale BK (2010). Evaluation needle length and density of microneedle arrays in the pretreatment of skin for transdermal drug delivery. Int J Pharm 391(1-2):7–12.

Yang HW, Ye L, Guo XD, Yang C, Compans RW, Prausnitz MR (2017). Ebola vaccination using a DNA vaccine coated on PLGA-PLL/γPGA nanoparticles administered using a microneedle patch. Adv Healthc Mater 6(1). doi: 10.1002/adhm.201600750.

Zaric M, Lyubomska O, Touzelet O, Poux C, Al-Zahrani S, Fay F, Wallace L, Terhorst D, Malissen B, Henri S, Power UF, Scott CJ, Donnelly RF, Kissenpfennig A (2013). Skin dendritic cell targeting via microneedle arrays laden with antigen-encapsulated poly-D,L-lactide-co-glycolide nanoparticles induces efficient antitumor and antiviral immune responses. ACS Nano 7(3):2042–55. doi: 10.1021/nn304235j.

Zaric M, Lyubomska O, Poux C, Hanna ML, McCrudden MT, Malissen B, Ingram RJ, Power UF, Scott CJ, Donnelly RF, Kissenpfennig A (2015). Dissolving microneedle delivery of nanoparticle-encapsulated antigen elicits efficient cross-priming and Th1 immune responses by murine Langerhans cells. J Invest Dermatol 135(2):425–34. doi: 10.1038/jid.2014.415.

Zhang LW, Yu WW, Colvin VL, Monteiro-Riviere NA (2008). Biological interactionsof quantum dot nanoparticles in skin and in human epidermal keratinocytes. Toxicol Appl Pharmacol 228:200–211.

Zhang W, Gao J, Zhu Q, Zhang M, Ding X, Wang X, Hou X, Fan W, Ding B, Wu X, Wang X, Gao S (2010). Penetration and distribution of PLGA nanoparticles in the human skin treated with microneedles. Int J Pharm 402(1-2):205–212.

Index

Note: *Italicized* page numbers refer to figures, **bold** page numbers refer to tables

A

AAPV (Ala-Ala-Pro-Val) human neutrophil elastase inhibitor, 461–463
Abbreviated new drug application (ANDA), 270
Absorbed materials in skin, 377–380
Accountability (mass balance), 194–195. *See also* Dose response of percutaneous absorption
Acetaminophen, percutaneous absorption of, *227*
Acetic acid, 886
Acetone, 122
Acetyl aspartic acid, 123
Acetylsalicylic acid, 121
    urinary excretion, 177–179
Acid, 886
Acid dissociation constant (pK$_a$), 288
Actinic keratosis, 858
Activated alumina, 332
Activated charcoal, 333
Acyclovir, 674–676, *878*
Adsorbent gloves, 333
Adsorbent powders, 332
Alachlor, **91**, 315–317, *317*, *318*, *320*
Alanine, 674–676
Alginate, 548
Alkali, 887
Allergic contact dermatitis (ACD), 614
Alniditan, **655**, 657
Alopecia, 964
Alpha-tocopheryl acetate, 821
Alumina, 332, 547
Alzheimer disease, 788
4-Amino-2-hydroxytoluene, **399**, 400–405
Ammonium hydroxide, 887
Amylopectin, 548
Analgesics, 490–491
Anesthesia, 581
Anesthetic drugs, 821–822
Antiacne drugs, 494
Antibody assessment, 877
Antigen-presenting cells (APCs), 959, *959*, 961
Antiinflammatory drugs, 490–491, 822
Antioxidants, 494
Antisense oligonucleotides, 473–474
Apocrine sweat glands, 290
Apomorphine, 494
Appendages, 144–145
Arginine, 674–676
Aromatic amines, 393–394
Aromatic hydrocarbon hydroxylase (AHH), 453
Ascorbyl palmitate, 509
Asenapine, 182
Assisted decontamination, 330
Atenolol, **655**
Atopic dermatitis, 779

Atrazine, **454**
Attenuated total reflectance mode (ATR-IR), 801
AuNP/carbon nanotube nanocomposite (AuNP-CNT), 966
Australian Register of Therapeutic Goods (ARTG), 557
Avobenzone, 436–445
Azidothymidine, 626–627
Azone, 237–238, *239*

B

Bacillus thermoproteolyticus, 889
Basic fibroblast growth factor (bFGF), 937
Beauty Mouse, 557
Benzocaine (ethyl aminobenzoate), 276
Benzoic acid
    effect of occlusion on percutaneous absorption, **207**
    penetration of, 107–108, 121
    skin absorption of, 276
    urinary excretion, 177, 179
Benzophenone-3 (oxybenzone), **419**, 422, 423
Benzophenone-4, **420**
Benzyl acetate, **207**, **208**
Benzyl derivatives, **222**
Beta-adrenoceptor antagonists, 452
Beta-carotene, 820
Betamethasone 17-valerate, **454**
Betulin, 719
BHT (butylated hydroxytoluene), 610
Biodegradation, 338
Bioequivalence, 763, 870, 877–879, 904–905, **905**
Biomarker in skin cancer, 879
Biomedica EZ4U cell proliferation kit assay, 718–719
Biowaivers, 907–908
Birch bark (*Betula pendula*), 719
Bis-ethylhexyloxyphenol methoxyphenyl triazine, **419**
Blank, Irvin, 253
Bleomycin, 860–861, *862*
Blood flow measurements, 775–777
    subject selection, 777
    vasoconstrictive test, 776
    vasodilative test, 776–777
Body surface area (BSA), 289
Body weight (BW), 289
Bone volume and total tissue volume (BV/TV), 532
Borosilicate glass, 547
Bovine serum albumin (BSA), 274–275, 375–376
Bovine udder skin (BUS), 704–705. *See also Ex vivo* animal skin models
BrdU assay, 718–719
Brushing/wiping in decontamination, 333
Brushite, 547
Buprenorphine, 182, **655**
Burns, 780, 929–930
    burning temperature, 936
    cause and duration of burning, 936
    classification of, 930

Printed in the United States
by Baker & Taylor Publisher Services